INFERTILITY
Diagnosis, Management and IVF

INFERTILITY
Diagnosis, Management and IVF

Editor

Anil K Dubey PhD HCLD

Professor of Obstetrics and Gynecology
Associate Director of Division Reproductive Endocrinology
Fertility and IVF
Director of IVF Labs
George Washington University
2150 Pennsylvania Ave, NW
Washington, DC, USA

Foreword

Alan H DeCherney

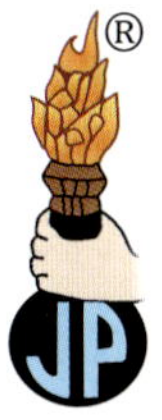

JAYPEE BROTHERS MEDICAL PUBLISHERS (P) LTD

New Delhi • Panama City • London

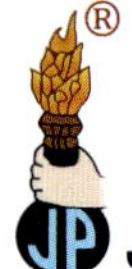

Jaypee Brothers Medical Publishers (P) Ltd.

Headquarter
Jaypee Brothers Medical Publishers (P) Ltd
4838/24, Ansari Road, Daryaganj
New Delhi 110 002, India
Phone: +91-11-43574357
Fax: +91-11-43574314
Email: jaypee@jaypeebrothers.com

Overseas Offices

J.P. Medical Ltd.
83 Victoria Street, London
SW1H 0HW (UK)
Phone: +44-2031708910
Fax: +02-03-0086180
Email: info@jpmedpub.com

Jaypee-Highlights Medical Publishers Inc.
City of Knowledge, Bld. 237, Clayton
Panama City, Panama
Phone: + 507-301-0496
Fax: + 507- 301-0499
Email: cservice@jphmedical.com

Website: www.jaypeebrothers.com
Website: www.jaypeedigital.com

Inquiries for bulk sales may be solicited at: jaypee@jaypeebrothers.com

Infertility: Diagnosis, Management and IVF

First Edition: **2012**

ISBN 978-93-5025-780-7

Printed at : Ajanta Offset & Packagings Ltd., New Delhi

Dedicated to

My Father Prayag N Dubey (1909–2009)
and the Dubey family
with gratitude and love

Contributors

Agarwal Ashok MD
Professor
Lerner College of Medicine
Director, Andrology Laboratory
Director, Center for Reproductive Medicine
Cleveland Clinic
9500 Euclid Avenue
Cleveland, Ohio 44195
United States

Allahbadia N Gautam MD
The Center For Human Reproduction
672, Kalpak Gulistan
Perry Cross Road
Bandra (W), Mumbai
Maharashtra, India

Alper M Michael
Associate Clinical Professor of
Obstetrics and Gynecology
Reproductive Endocrinology and Infertility
Harvard Medical School
Medical Director, Boston IVF
130 Second Avenue
Waltham, MA 02451
United States

Athanasiadis Ioanna MD
Department of Obstetrics and Gynecology
The George Washington University
2150 Pennsylvania Avenue, NW
Washington, DC 20037
United States

Chason J Rebecca
Reproductive Endocrinology and Infertility
Eunice Kennedy Shriver
National Institute of Child Health and
Human Development
National Institutes of Health
10 Center Drive, Bethesda, MD 20892
United States

Cohen Jacques PhD
Senior Editor
Reproductive Biomedicine Online
Tyho-Galileo Research Laboratories
Reprogenetics LLC,
Livingston, New Jersey 07039
United States

Christianson S Mindy MD
Clinical Fellow
Reproductive Endocrinology and
Infertility, Reproductive Surgery
Division of Reproductive Endocrinology
and Infertility
Department of Gynecology and Obstetrics
Johns Hopkins University School of
Medicine
Baltimore, MD 21093
United States

DeCherney H Alan MD
Head
Program in Reproductive and
Adult Endocrinology
Eunice Kennedy Shriver National
Institute of Child Health and
Human Development
National Institutes of Health
10 Center Drive
Bethesda, MD 20892
United States

Domar D Alice PhD
Domar Center for Mind/Body Health
Boston IVF, Waltham, MA
Beth Israel Deaconess Medical Center
Harvard Medical School
Boston, MA
United States

Dube Barbara CMAAC
Boston IVF
Waltham, MA
United States

Dubey K Anil PhD HCLD
Professor of Obstetrics and Gynecology
Associate Director of Division
Reproductive Endocrinology
Fertility and IVF
Director of IVF Labs
George Washington University
2150 Pennsylvania Ave, NW
Washington, DC
United States

Dayal B Molina MD
Associate Professor
Division of Reproductive Endocrinology,
Fertility and IVF
Department of Obstetrics and Gynecology
The George Washington University
2150 Pennsylvania Avenue, NW
Washington, DC 20037
United States

Desai Nina PhD HCLD
Director
IVF Laboratory
Department of Obstetrics and Gynecology
Assistant Professor
Lerner Cleveland Clinic Fertility Center
26900 Cedar Rd.
Beachwood, OH 44122
United States

DiMattina Michael MD
Director
Dominion Fertility
Arlington, VA
United States

Esteves C Sandro MD PhD
Director
ANDROFERT – Andrology and Human
Reproduction Clinic
Av. Dr. Heitor Penteado, 1464
13075, 460 Campinas, São Paulo
Brazil

Fogerty E Annemarie MD
Division of Hematology and Oncology
Massachusetts General Hospital
Harvard University, Boston, MA
United States

Frankfurter David MD
Professor
Department of Obstetrics and Gynecology
Division of Reproductive
Endocrinology and IVF
The George Washington University
2150 Pennsylvania Avenue, NW
Washington, DC 20037
United States

Fru N Karenne
Reproductive Endocrinology and Infertility
Eunice Kennedy Shriver
National Institute of Child Health and Human Development
National Institutes of Health
10 Center Drive
Bethesda, MD 20892
United States

Gandhi Goral PhD
The Center For Human Reproduction
672, Kalpak Gulistan
Perry Cross Road
Bandra (W), Mumbai
Maharashtra, India

Gindoff R Paul MD
Professor and Director
Division of Reproductive Endocrinology
Fertility and IVF
Department of Obstetrics and Gynecology
The George Washington University
2150 Pennsylvania Avenue, NW
Washington, DC 20037
United States

Gordon David John MD
Clinical Professor of Obstetrics and Gynecology
The George Washington University
Co-Director
Dominion Fertility
Arlington, VA
United States

Goyal Deepinder
Department of Endocrinology
Cedars Sinai Medical Center
B-131, 8700 Beverly blvd
Los Angeles 90027, CA
United States

Gupta Sajal MD
Center for Reproductive Medicine
Glickman Urological and Kidney Institute & Obstetrics and Gynecology
Women's Health Institute
9500 Euclid Avenue, A19.1
Cleveland Clinic
Cleveland, Ohio 44195
United States

Hafez Abdel Faten MD
Fertility Center
Department of Obstetrics and Gynecology/ Women's Health Institute, Cleveland Clinic
Beachwood, OH
United States

Hamada Alaa MD
Center for Reproductive Medicine
Cleveland Clinic Cleveland, 44195
Ohio
United States

Harton L Gary BS
Reprogenetics
3 Regent Street
Suite 301
Livingston, NJ 07039
United States

Hawa Nadim MD
Department of Obstetrics and Gynecology
The George Washington University
2150 Pennsylvania Avenue, NW
Washington, DC 20037
United States

Hsu L Albert MD
Department of Obstetrics and Gynecology
Jones Institute for Reproductive Medicine
Eastern Virginia Medical School
Norfolk, VA
United States

Irish Robin RN
Boston IVF
Waltham, MA
United States

Jindal Sangita PhD HCLD
IVF Lab Director & Assistant Professor
Montefiore's Institute for Reproductive Medicine and Health
Albert Einstein College of Medicine
141 South Central Ave
Hartsdale, NY 10530
United States

Kalmbach Keri MS
NYU Langone Medical Center
Department of Obstetrics and Gynecology
550 First Avenue New York, NY 10016
United States

Keefe David MD
Stanley H Kaplan Professor and Chairman of Obstetrics and Gynecology
Chair Departments of Obstetrics and Gynecology (Chair) and Cell Biology (Cell Biology)
NYU Fertility Center
New York, NY 10016
United States

Khaldi Reem
Reproductive Endocrinology
Fertility and IFV
Department of Obstetrics and Gynaecology
George Washington University
2150 Pennsylvania Ave
Washington, DC 20037
United States

Krause KH Walter MD PhD
Department of Dermatology and Allergology
University Hospital
Philipp University
Deutschhausstr. 9
D-35033 Marburg
Germany

Levine A Brian MD MS
Department of Obstetrics and Gynecology
Columbia University, College of Physicians and Surgeons
New York, NY 10032
United States

Liu Lin PhD
NYU Langone Medical Center
Department of Obstetrics and Gynecology
550 First Avenue
New York, NY 10016
United States

Merchant Rubina MD
The Center For Human Reproduction
672, Kalpak Gulistan
Perry Cross Road
Bandra (W), Mumbai
Maharashtra, India

Moawad Gaby MD
Department of Obstetrics and Gynecology
The George Washington University
2150 Pennsylvania Avenue, NW
Washington, DC 20037
United States

Moon S Kimberly
Reproductive Endocrinology and Infertility
Eunice Kennedy Shriver
National Institute of Child Health and Human Development
National Institutes of Health
10 Center Drive
Bethesda, MD 20892
United States

Moragianni A Vasiliki MD MS
Division of Reproductive Endocrinology & Infertility
Department of Obstetrics & Gynecology
Beth Israel Deaconess Medical Center
Harvard Medical School, Boston, MA
United States

Muasher J Suheil MD
Clinical Professor
Division of Reproductive Endocrinology and Infertility
Department of Gynecology and Obstetrics, Johns Hopkins University
School of Medicine, Baltimore
Maryland, United States
The George Washington University
Washington, DC
Virginia Commonwealth University
Richmond, Virginia
Muasher Center for Fertility and IVF
Fairfax, Virginia
United States

Munne Santiago PhD
President
Reprogenetics
3 Regent Street, Suite 301
Livingston, NJ-07039
United States

Naz K Rajesh PhD
Professor of Obstetrics and Gynecology and Vice Chair for Research
Professor of Microbiology, Immunology and Cell Biology
Director, Division of Research
West Virginia University
School of Medicine
2085 Robert C. Byrd Health Sciences Center North Morgantown, WV 26506
United States

Parker Jason DO
4817 Reilly Rd
Fayetteville
NC 28314,
United States

Peak Douglas
Reproductive Endocrinology
Fertility and IVF
Department of Obstetrics and Gynecology
George Washington University
2150 Pennsylvania Ave
Washington, DC 20037
United States

Penzias S Alan MD
Associate Professor of Obstetrics
Gynecology and Reproductive Biology
Director, Fellowship Program in Reproductive Endocrinology and Infertility
Beth Israel Deaconess Medical Center / Boston IVF / Harvard Medical School
Boston, MA, United States

Perfetto O'Hern Candice MD
Reproductive Endocrinology and Infertility
Department of Obstetrics and Gynecology
Stanford University Medical Center
PaloAlto, CA, United States

Petrozza C John MD
Chief, Division of Reproductive Medicine & IVF, Assistant Professor of Massachusetts General Hospital
Obstetrics and Gynecology
Harvard University, Boston, MA
United States

Rebar W Robert MD
Executive Director
American Society for Reproductive Medicine
1209 Montgomery Highway
Birmingham, Alabama 35216-2809
United States

Rooney L Kristin BA
Domar Center for Mind/Body Health
Boston IVF
Beth Israel Deaconess Medical Center
Harvard Medical School
Boston, MA, United States

Sauer V Mark MD
Professor of Obstetrics and Gynecology
Vice-Chairman, Department of Obstetrics and Gynecology
Chief, Division of Reproductive Endocrinology
New York, NY 10019
United States

Segars H James
Head, Reproductive Endocrinology and Infertility
Program in Reproductive and Adult Endocrinology
Eunice Kennedy Shriver National Institute of Child Health and Human Development
National Institutes of Health
10 Center Drive Bethesda, MD 20892
United States

Seifer B David MD
Medical Director
Genesis Fertility and Reproductive Medicine
1355 84th Street
Maimonides Medical Center, Brooklyn
NY 11228
United States

Stadtmauer A Laurel MD
Associate Professor
Department of Obstetrics and Gynecology
Jones Institute for Reproductive Medicine
Eastern Virginia Medical School
Norfolk, VA
United States

Stanic Aleksandar MD PhD
Clinical Fellow, Reproductive Medicine & IVF
Massachusetts General Hospital
Harvard University, Boston, MA
United States

Thornton L Kim
Associate Professor of Obstetrics
Gynecology and Reproductive Biology
Director
Reproductive Endocrinology and Infertility
Beth Israel Deaconess Medical Center/ Boston IVF/Harvard Medical School
Boston, MA
United States

Wasik Monika
Center for Reproductive Medicine
Cleveland Clinic
Cleveland, Ohio 44195
United States

Wolff Foran Erin
Reproductive Endocrinology and Infertility
Eunice Kennedy Shriver
National Institute of Child Health and Human Development
National Institutes of Health
10 Center Drive
Bethesda, MD 20892
United States

Zarek M Shvetha MD
Department of Obstetrics and Gynecology
The George Washington University
2150 Pennsylvania Avenue, NW
Washington, DC 20037
United States

Foreword

Dr Anil K Dubey is a Professor of Obstetrics and Gynecology and the Director of the In Vitro Fertilization Laboratory at the George Washington University School of Medicine, where he has been a faculty member since 1997. Prior to his positions at the George Washington University School of Medicine, Dr Dubey was the Director of the In Vitro Fertilization Program and the Director of the IVF Laboratory at the New England Medical Center, Tufts University School of Medicine in Boston, MA.

Dr Dubey received his education in India, obtaining his Doctorate of Philosophy from the Cancer Research Institute, University of Bombay in 1977 and completed his Post-Doctorate research training at the All India Institute of Medical Sciences, New Delhi and Cambridge University, England. In addition, Dr Dubey spent time at the University of Pittsburgh prior to entering the clinical field.

Dr Dubey has an extensive bibliography of research that he has carried out in the field of Reproductive Physiology, including Preimplantation Genetic Diagnosis and Blastocyst Culture. He has presented a superb book. He has convinced the experts in the field across a broad series of topics to contribute what stands to be the standard textbook in the field of infertility. His exemplary career and reputation has allowed him to construct this prime text.

The chapter focusing on the History of Infertility, including *In Vitro* Fertilization, prepared by Dr Jacques Cohen, is a landmark contribution and contains well-attributed first-hand information. Dr Cohen's chapter is followed by a very comprehensive dissertation on *Male Factor Infertility*, written by Dr Ashok Agarwal, one of the leading investigators in the field. He not only covers diagnosis, but he also mentions medical and surgical management of male factor infertility.

The section on *Female Factor Infertility* is comprehensive and the chapters are written by well-recognized experts in the field. The chapters include: 'Ovarian Reserve Testing' by Dr David B Seifer; 'Female Reproductive Aging' by Dr David Keefe; 'The Molecular and Genetic Basis of Infertility' by Dr James H Segars and 'Evaluation and Diagnosis of Female Infertility' by Dr Alan Penzias. 'Preimplantation Genetic Screening/Diagnosis' by Dr Anil Dubey and Dr Santiago Munne and 'Procedures and Protocols in *In Vitro* Fertilization Laboratory' by Dr Dubey and 'Integrating Quality Management into a Fertility Practice' by Dr Michael M Alper are also comprehensive and well written.

The area of fertility preservation, including: 'Cryopreservation of Human Embryos' and 'Fertility Preservation for Women'. Other interesting portions of this book include chapters like, 'Third Party Reproduction', which explores the current status and future of third party reproduction; 'Sperm Banking: Indications and Regulations' and 'Oocyte Donation Program'. Each chapter is covered well with insight and wisdom.

Finally the book is donated to the future of infertility, including: 'Genetics and Male Infertility in the 22nd century'; 'Assisted Reproductive Technology and Birth Defects'; 'Emotional and Social Aspects of Infertility Treatment' and 'Fertility Testing and Treatment in 2020'.

To conclude, Dr Anil Dubey's book is a superb contribution. It is encyclopedic and will become the standard textbook for infertility management. He is to be congratulated on a fine selection of authors and topics. The text is well organized and will serve both as something that can be read from cover to cover, and as an up-to-date reference. I am proud to be a part of this endeavor.

Alan H DeCherney MD

Head
Program in Reproductive and Adult Endocrinology
Eunice Kennedy Shriver National Institute of
Child Health and Human Development
National Institutes of Health
10 Center Drive, Bldg 10, CRC, Rm 1-3140
Bethesda, MD 20892
United States

Preface

The field of human reproductive endocrinology, infertility and *in vitro* fertilization (IVF) is a dynamic field in modern medicine. Infertility treatment tends to be daunting for most physicians whether they are specialists-in-training, novice reproductive endocrinologists or seasoned practitioners.

Thirty years ago, infertility was a diagnosis with little hope for treatment. However, since the birth of first IVF baby in 1978, infertility diagnosis, management and treatment options have drastically improved. Diagnosis methods have been refined; management and treatment of infertility patients have been vastly improved upon; implementations of vitrification techniques have aided the cryopreservation of embryos, eggs and blastocysts; new technologies for screening embryos for genetic competence have developed. A historic landmark in IVF occurred in 2010, when Professor Robert Edward was recognized with Nobel Prize for contributions in Medicine.

The book *Infertility: Diagnosis, Management and IVF* explores the detailed diagnosis of male and female infertility, treatment of infertility with IVF, and various aspects of the IVF laboratory including protocols, handling of embryo transfers, freezing and biopsy for preimplantation genetic screening. This book also covers the quality management of IVF programs, practice guidelines, ethical and social aspects of infertility and IVF, as well as preservation of future fertility for cancer or delaying childbearing age.

The challenge for both the clinicians and scientists in the 21st century is to vigilantly continue to innovate and advance the science of ART while avoiding their potential abuse. At a minimum, we need to further improve live birth rates and reduce the rate of multiple pregnancy, and remain abreast in this ever-expanding field. Future medical historians will scrutinize how we take these steps, as the choices we make today will have consequences that will last beyond our lifetimes.

I sincerely hope that readers will enjoy reading this new book as much as I enjoyed working on it.

Anil K Dubey

Acknowledgments

The book *Infertility: Diagnosis, Management and IVF* represents a collaborative effort of colleagues and friends with high enthusiasm and dedication to Reproductive Endocrinology and IVF. Each chapter is written by experts who have dedicated their lives to treat infertility patients with the highest moral and ethical standards to diagnose, manage, and treat with IVF. I am ever grateful to all of the authors for their contributions and for sharing their knowledge and time to compose each chapter as a precious gem in this book.

I would like to specifically acknowledge my colleagues Drs Molina Dayal, David Frankfurter, Paul Gindoff, and other faculty members of Obstetrics and Gynecology at Medical Faculty Associates at the George Washington University, without their encouragement and help, this project would not have been completed. I also want to extend my thanks to my IVF lab team, Douglas Peak and Reem Khaldi for their assistance in this project.

My sincere thanks are also due to Dr Alan DeCherney for constant support throughout twenty-five years of my career in this field as well as for this book. Dr Ashok Agarwal and his team from Cleveland Clinic were indispensable contributors to the completion of this book.

I appreciate M/s Jaypee Brothers Medical Publishers (P) Ltd, New Delhi, India particularly Ms Chetna Malhotra Vohra and her team for support and expertise throughout the publication process.

Further, I admire with utmost respect, the patients who have undergone the infertility treatment in the hope of having a child through IVF. It is my absolute privilege to handle their embryos in IVF lab and I remain very humbled for these opportunities and being a part of their quest to have a biological child.

And finally, I lovingly thank my wife, Anita, and my children, Juhi and Neil, for their constructive criticism and support.

Contents

Section 1: Infertility

Section 2: Male Factor Infertility

Section 3: Female Factor Infertility

Section 4: In Vitro Fertilization

Section 7: Regulation of Assisted Reproductive Technology Laboratory

Section 8: Emotional and Social Aspects of Infertility Treatment

1

Infertility

Section Contents

1

A History of Clinical Embryology and Therapeutic IVF: From Pythagoras and Aristotle to Boveri and Edwards

Jacques Cohen

Chapter Contents

"All truths are easy to understand once they are discovered; the point is to discover them."

— Galileo Galilei (1564–1642)

INTRODUCTION

In vitro fertilization (IVF) has become a routine medical intervention over the past three decades, resulting in the birth of millions of children and culminating in the awarding of the 2010 Nobel Prize in physiology or medicine to Robert G Edwards. Yet, just 50 years ago IVF was considered science fiction and not at all an obvious choice for treatment of infertility and subfertility.

As astounding as this relatively quick rise may be, the future of IVF promises to be even more so. Inventor and futurist Ray Kurzweil predicts that our knowledge-base will multiply thousands of times faster during the next few decades compared to the entire history of science, technology and philosophy. *In vitro* fertilization is certain to see major new changes with further integration of genetics, molecular biology and physics. But to anticipate and help shape future possibilities, the past must be understood. Where did we begin and how did we arrive here?

The history of science and technology is defined as a field of history that examines how humanity understands

"This chapter is a reprint from a chapter with the same title by Jacques Cohen to be published in Textbook of Clinical Embryology by Cowan and Wells (Editors) in Cambridge University Press in 2013. Reprinted with permission from Cambridge University Press."

the science and technology that has changed over time. This now-accepted academic discipline also includes the study of cultural, economic, and political impacts of scientific innovation. *In vitro* fertilization is a wonderfully broad discipline that demands both historical reflection and frank discussion of complex and profound issues touching on matters of law, politics, culture and ethics.

The reader is reminded that this text is not written by a science historian. Though intended to be unbiased, the narrative draws not only on written history gleaned from historical documents, but on personal experience, as well as numerous conversations with scientists and physicians in the field.

The history of infertility treatment and IVF in particular, can be told in many different ways. Here the story is told from the perspective of basic science, with emphasis on the final steps that led to the birth of the first IVF baby in the 1970s and tribute made to those responsible for paradigm shifts in philosophy that allowed the new reproductive technologies to take form. Moreover, because no medical intervention is possible without the tools that have been made available in surgery and laboratory practice, this aspect is also covered in some detail, in the hope that future historical reflections on IVF and related technologies will include appropriate reference to this neglected area of science history.

FROM PREFORMATION AND EPIGENESIS TO THE DISCOVERY OF CHROMOSOMES AND MEIOSIS

Antiquity and Procreation

It is evident that humans have long been intrigued by questions surrounding fertilization and procreation. Symbols depicting fertility are at least 35,000 years old, dating from the early Aurignacian period shortly after the earliest representatives of *Homo sapiens* (Cro-Magnon) migrated to Europe (Figures 1A to F). However, it was not until well after the introduction of script that such consideration was recorded in Western thought.

The first written record of deliberations on reproduction starts with those by Greek physicians and philosophers who evidently were quite familiar with the concept of generations and embryology. They held the belief that a new organism could not only arise through sexual and asexual reproduction, but also through the process of spontaneous generation, a now obsolete principle described in detail by Aristotle (384–322 BC) (Figure 2). Earlier, Pythagoras (c570-495 BC) introduced the concept of 'spermism', an erroneous theory asserting that only fathers provide the essential characteristics of offspring while mothers supply only a solid substrate. Two millennia later, the doctrines of spermism and

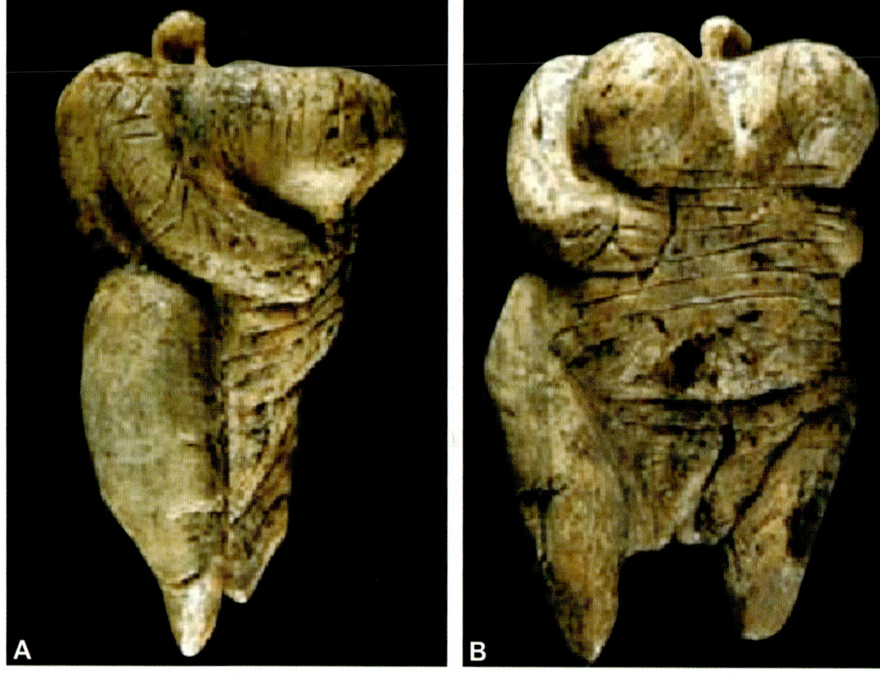

Figures 1A and B

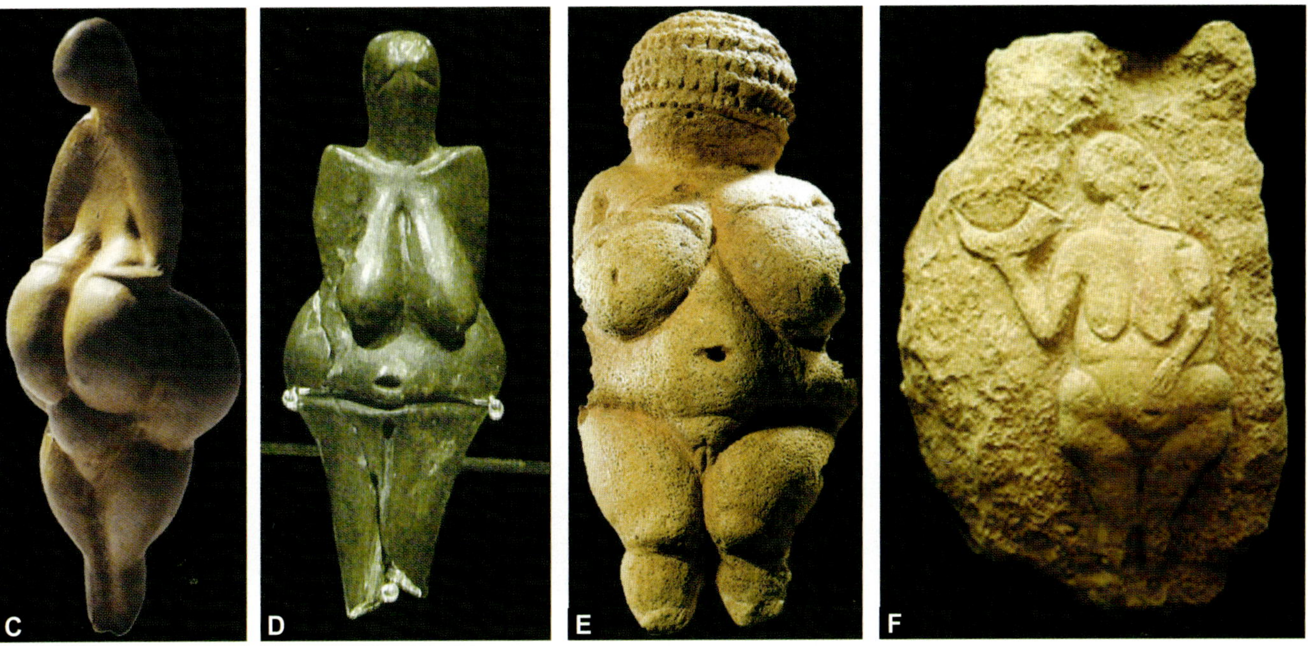

Figures 1C to F

Figures 1A to F Fine examples of so-called small Venus figurines made by European representatives of *Homo sapiens* of the Cro-Magnon culture during the Upper Paleolithic era of prehistory (from 40,000 BCE onwards). These figures either represent an early form of pornography or some form of worship of the female secondary sex characteristics, such as hips, breasts and vulva, possibly reflecting on the need of survival through reproduction. Facial and extremity details are under-represented or absent. Artistic and cultural interpretation may be a reflection of our modern opinion and experience

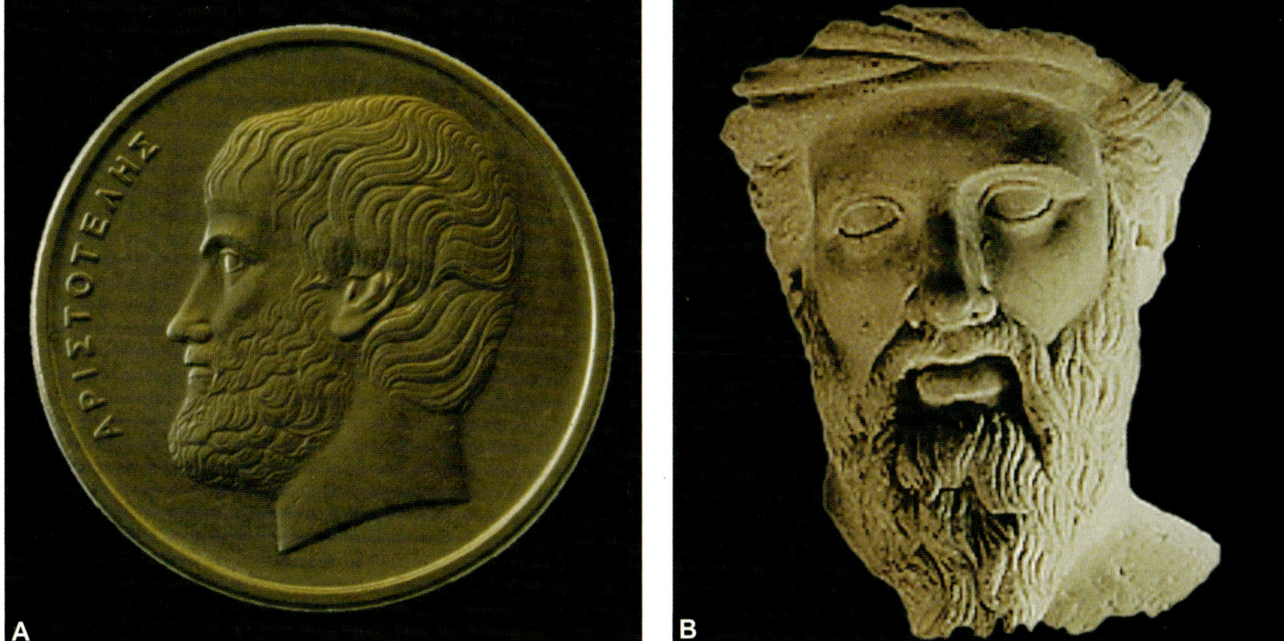

Figures 2A and B

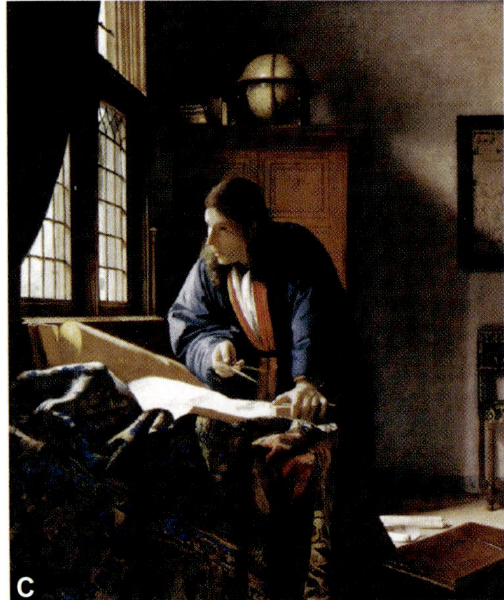

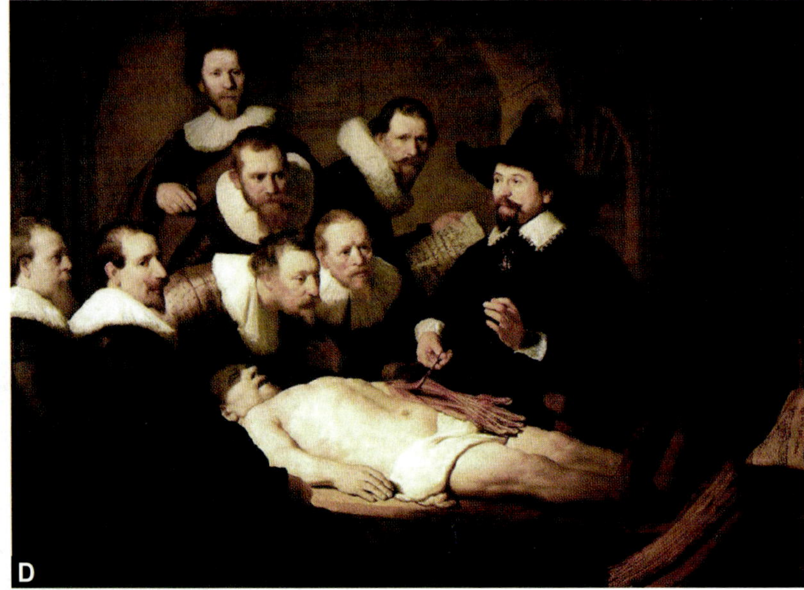

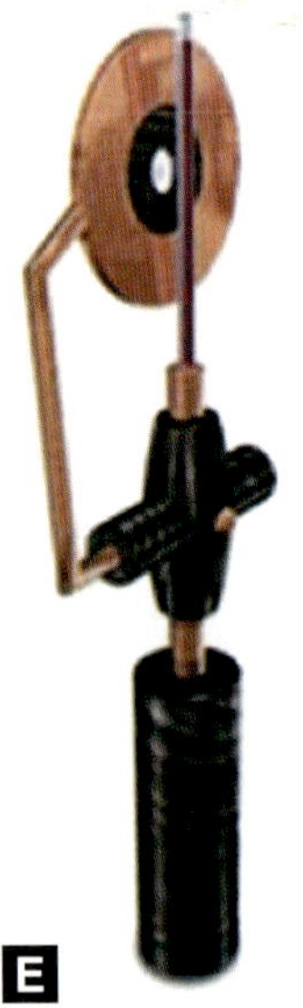

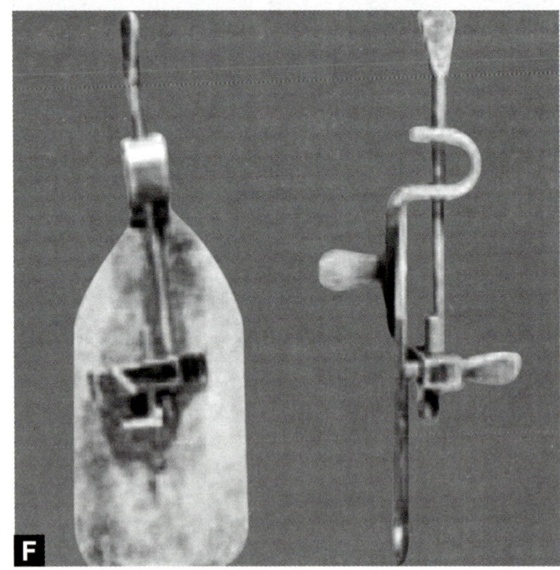

Figures 2C to F

Figures 2A to F (A) A depiction of Aristotle, the great Greek philosopher on a Drachme coin, who first introduced the concept of epigenesis. Reprinted with permission from 123RF. Reprint purchased by author; (B) Rendering of Pythagoras, the Greek mathematician and philosopher, who first formulated spermism; (C) A possible representation of Anton van Leeuwenhoek who first described spermatozoa, in Johannes Vermeer's 'The Geographer'. Vermeer and van Leeuwenhoek knew each other in 17th century Delft, The Netherlands; (D) The figure closest to the pathologist performing the autopsy in Rembrandt's "The Anatomy Lesson" was mistakenly believed to be the great Dutch biologist Jan Swammerdam. No known portraits of Swammerdam exist; (E) Jan Swammerdam's handheld microscope; (F) Anton van Leeuwenhoek's microscope

spontaneous generation were finally proven to be wrong through experiments and observations of Louis Pasteur (1859) who won a contest called by the French Academy of Sciences (Figure 3). However, it must be mentioned that 200 years earlier, the physician and poet Francesco Redi had already raised serious doubts about spontaneous generation by conducting an elegant set of controlled experiments that showed maggots could not arise in a jar of rotting meat covered with gauze. Aristotle's concepts were entirely replaced by germ and cell theories in the 19th century, but it took a great deal of convincing before scientists and philosophers accepted that spontaneous generation was a simply wrong theory.

Aristotle described two historically important models of development based on Pythagoras' doctrine known as the theories of 'preformation' and 'epigenesis'. Preformationism held that an embryo or miniature individual already existed in either the mother's egg or the father's semen and began to grow when stimulated; spermism was the first of these models. Aristotle preferred the theory of epigenesis, which assumed that the embryo began as an undifferentiated mass and that new parts were added during development. Aristotle thought that the female parent contributed only unorganized material to the embryo. The male-centric views of the day helped lead him to the conclusion that semen

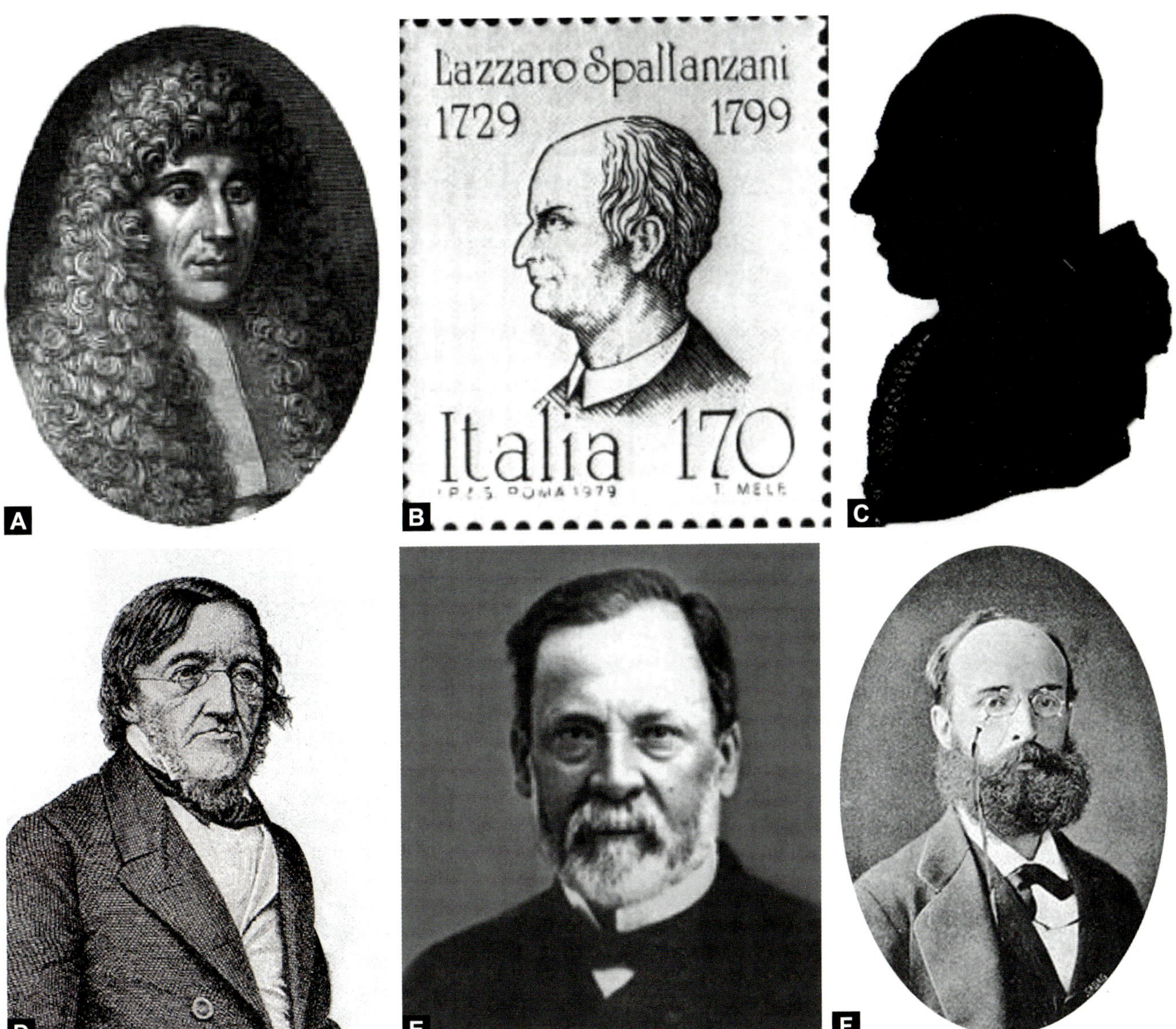

Figures 3A to F (A) Francesco Redi (1629-1697) was a physician, poet and naturalist who in 1668 elegantly showed that maggots did not form from rotting meat through "spontaneous generation"; (B) Lazzaro Spallanzani (1729-1799) was an Italian catholic priest and biologist who discovered that reproduction required semen and an ovum. In frogs and dogs he performed artificial insemination, before John Hunter's experiment in humans; (C) Caspar Friedrich Wolff (1733-1794) was one of the first to reject preformationism. His work opened the doors to germ layer theory and fertilization. He discovered the mesonephros; (D) Hermann Fol (1845-1892) was a Swiss zoologist and one of at least three scientists who observed fertilization microscopically for the first time; (E) Louis Pasteur (1822-1895) was a French chemist and microbiologist, best known for developing the first vaccines against rabies and anthrax and the process of pasteurization. He provided clear evidence that spontaneous generation was not an existent reproductive process; (F) Karl Ernst von Baer (1792-1876) was a multidisciplinary German zoologist born in Estonia. He discovered the ovum in 1826 and the blastocyst later. He also accurately described the germ layer theory of development in the characteristic separation of ectoderm, endoderm and mesoderm

from the male parent provided both the form and the soul. Both Pythagoras and Aristotle were 'spermists'.

PREFORMATION AND THE FOUNDATION OF MODERN EMBRYOLOGY

Aristotle's theory of epigenetic development dominated the science of embryology until the work of English physician William Harvey (1578–1657), although it took another 200 years to be considered archaic by most scientists. Harvey was inspired by the work of his teacher, Girolamo Fabrici (ca1533–1619). Some science historians consider Fabrici the founder of modern embryology, because of the significance of his embryological thesis: *On the Formed Fetus* and *On the Development of the Egg and the Chick.* Harvey's *On the Generation of Animals* was not published until 1651 after he completed his groundbreaking work: *An Anatomical Study of the Motion of the Heart and of the Blood in Animals* which explained how blood was pumped by the heart throughout the body. Although Harvey had hoped to provide experimental confirmation for Aristotle's theory of epigenesis, his observations proved that many aspects of Aristotle's theory were erroneous, yet Harvey held on to certain core beliefs of epigenesis.

Aristotle held the view that the embryo was formed by coagulation in the uterus soon after mating. Harvey's experiments in chick and deer's eggs persuaded him that the generation proceeded by epigenesis, that is, the accumulation of parts over time. Epigenesis or epigenetics is still used in biology, the contemporary sense being aspects of morphogenesis that are not encoded by genes themselves but occur by factors that control the gene activity. Many of Harvey's contemporaries and students rejected Aristotle's epigenesis and turned to the more fundamental theories of preformation.

Naturalists who favored preformationist theories (preformationism) of generation were inspired by the microscope, probably first introduced in primitive form by two Dutch spectacle makers (Hans and Zacharia Janssen around 1590) who used their knowledge of lens manufacturing. Based on this primitive compound microscope, Galileo Galilei (1564–1642) added a focusing control. Later, Anton van Leeuwenhoek (1632–1723) refined the curvature of the lenses and his upgraded device could be used to enlarge objects by as much as 260x (Figure 2). Leeuwenhoek was the first to observe bacteria, yeast and blood cells.

Marcello Malpighi (1628–1694) and Jan Swammerdam (1637–1680), two pioneers of observational microscopy, provided information that seemed to support preformation (Figure 2). Based on Swammerdam's studies of insects and amphibians, naturalists suggested that embryos pre-existed within each other and called the forms homunculi or animalcules. This phenomenon was likened to sets of Russian nesting dolls by the developmental biologist and author Pinto-Correia (1997) in her outstanding book on preformationism.[1] However, the limitation of this theory was that only one parent could be the biological source of the preformed organism. At the time, philosophers were familiar with the eggs of many species, but when the microscope revealed the apparent existence of 'little animals' in male semen, some naturalists argued that the preformed individuals must be present in the sperm (Figure 4).

Respected scientists of the time, such as Charles Bonnet (1720–1793) and Lazzaro Spallanzani (1729–1799) supported preformationism (Figure 3). Bonnet's study of parthenogenesis in Aphids was regarded as an argument in favor of 'ovist' preformationism. Thus, some naturalists argued that the human race was already present in the ovaries of Eve, while others reported seeing homunculi (tiny humans) inside spermatozoa apparently derived in paternal lineage from the theological figure Adam. Clara Pinto-Correia (1997) has argued that the terminology and emphasis on this theory is the result of a more recent historical misrepresentation.[1] The vivid discussions between groups of naturalists and theologians holding these two opposed views would shape the debate on the origins of life for some time to come.

EARLY CELL AND GERM THEORIES

Some 18th century scientists rejected both the ovist and spermist doctrines. One of the most convincing arguments was raised by Casper Friedrich Wolff (1733–1794), who published a groundbreaking article, "Theory of Generation," in 1759. Wolff argued that the organs of the body did not exist at the beginning of gestation, but formed from some originally undifferentiated material through a series of steps. Other naturalists became interested in this attractive model known as natural philosophy. During the 19th century, the basis of cell theory was expanded by the discovery (1827) of the mammalian (dog) ovum in Germany by Karl Ernst von Baer (1792–1876) many years after the finding that semen contained millions of individual moving cells called spermatozoa (Leeuwenhoek, approximately 1677) (described in Anton von Leeuwenhoek and his perception of spermatozoa by Ruestow).[2]

Historians are not always in agreement about who actually witnessed the mammalian fertilization process and sperm-egg interaction first. Was it Schenk in 1978[3]

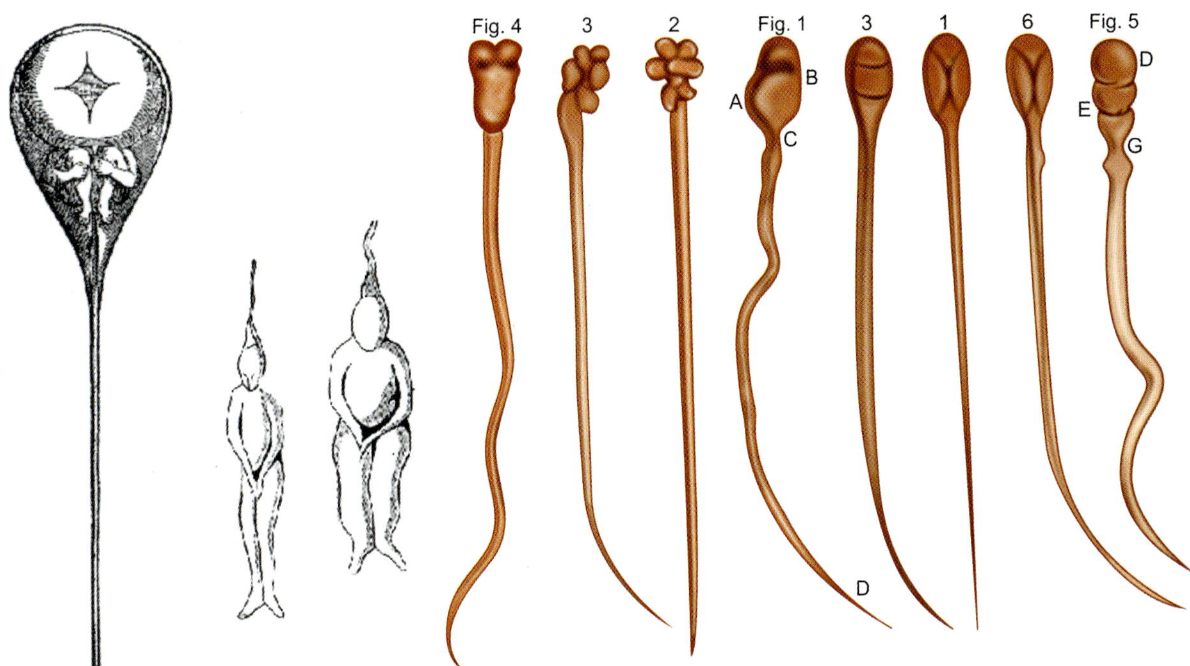

Figure 4 Left panel depicts Nicholaas Hartsoeker's homunculi (1695), the presence of a tiny already complete human in the sperm seen using Hartsoeker's primitive microscope. The right panel shows van Leeuwenhoek's sketches of spermatozoa (1677). The latter showed morphologic disparity as well as detailed head features. The differences between the observations of both microscopists may have been due to subjectivity, visualization and artistic interpretation. Hartsoeker never claimed to have actually seen the homunculi, but suggested the representations to support spermist theory. He apparently was present when Leeuwenhoek noticed spermatozoa in semen for the first time

in Vienna or the Swiss physician and zoologist Hermann Fol[4] a year later (Figure 2)? What is evident is that Schenk was the first to describe the dissolution of cumulus cells in rabbit eggs held in follicular and uterine fluids after exposure to epididymal spermatozoa, thereby clearly establishing the field of experimental embryology. Interestingly, this was reported exactly 100 years before the birth of the first IVF baby in the human (Steptoe and Edwards, 1978) (Figure 5).[5]

Oskar Hertwig, a student of the renowned German biologist and artist Ernst Haeckel, described fertilization in the sea urchin[6] two years before Schenk (in 1876) and it seems that these observations led him to emphasize the important role of sperm and egg nuclei during inheritance and the reduction of chromosomes (meiosis) during the generations. Another German biologist and artist, Theodor Boveri, published some of the most significant principles of preimplantation embryology in the late 1880s and early 1890s (Figure 5)[7]. Oscar Hertwig before this had already proposed that sperm and egg nuclei fuse during fertilization (fusion is typical in invertebrates studied by Hertwig, but does not occur in mammals).

THE BOVERI-SUTTON MODEL AND THE CHROMOSOME THEORY OF INHERITANCE

Boveri studied the maturation of egg cells of *Ascaris megalocephala*, the horse nematode. He observed that as eggs matured, there came a point where chromosome numbers were reduced to half. Boveri was one of the first to see evidence of the process of meiosis. Boveri[7] and Sutton[8] independently advanced the chromosome model of inheritance in 1902 (Figure 5). Boveri performed his studies with sea urchins, in which he found that all the chromosomes had to be present for appropriate embryonic development to occur. Sutton's work with grasshoppers demonstrated that chromosomes are organized in matched pairs of maternal and paternal chromosomes, which detach during meiosis.[8] The Boveri-Sutton chromosome model (the chromosome theory of inheritance) is a fundamental conclusion in genetics. This model identifies chromosomes as the carriers of genetic material. It explains the mechanism essential to the laws of Mendelian inheritance by identifying chromosomes with paired factors as would be

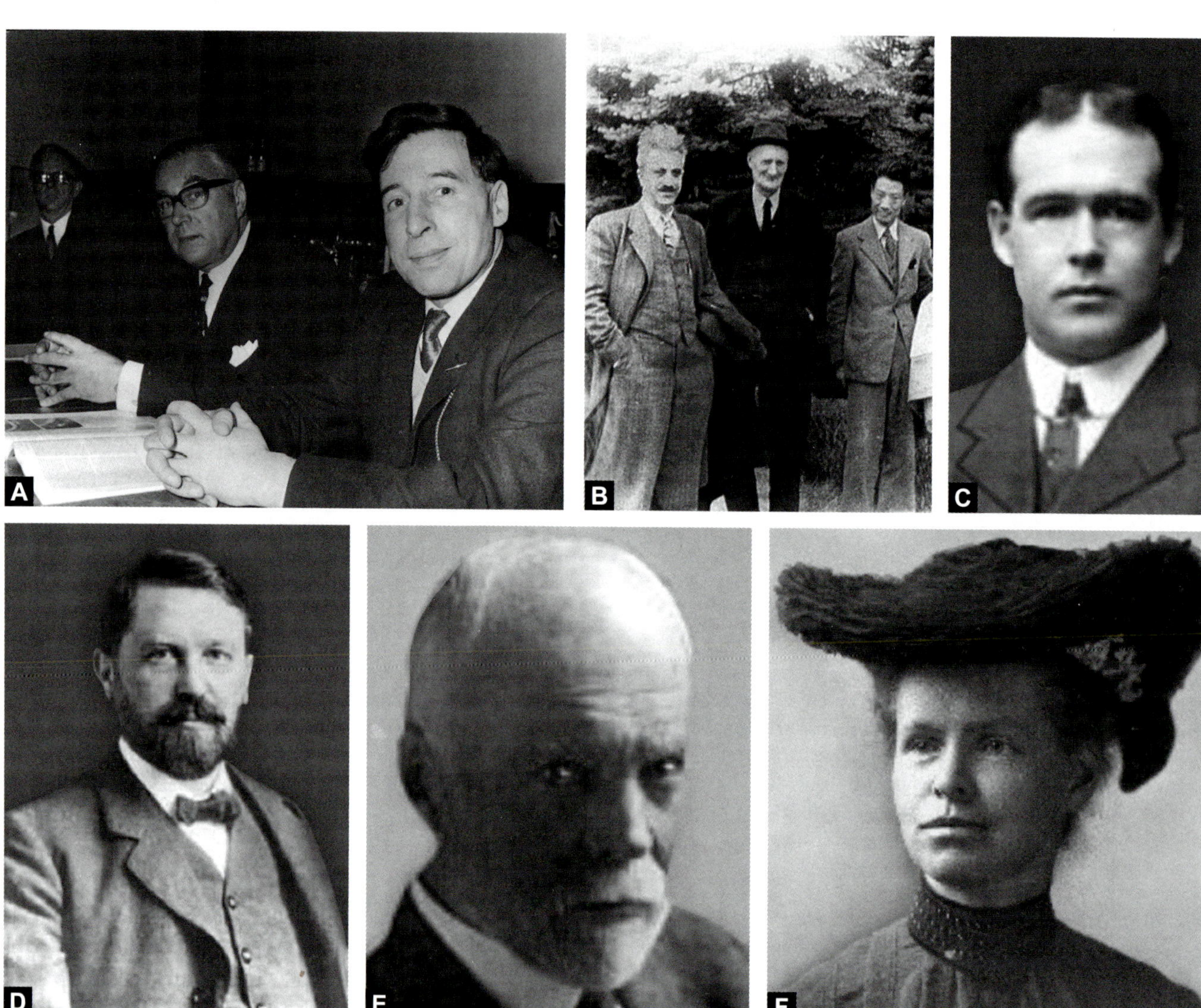

Figures 5A to F (A) Patrick Steptoe and Robert (Bob) Edwards in 1969 tensely answering questions from reporters during their press conference after the announcement of obtaining proof of fertilization using human gametes in the laboratory. Reprinted with permission of Getty Images. Reprint purchased by author; (B) The first wave of IVF pioneers. From left to right: Pincus, Hamilton and Chang; (C) Walter Sutton, one of the co-pioneers of the chromosome theory of inheritance; (D) Theodor Boveri, the other co-pioneer and the most famous of experimental embryologists of his day; (E) EB Wilson who discovered the sex determining chromosomes X and Y, simultaneous with (F) Nettie Stevens

required by Mendel's laws. Boveri-Sutton model also argues that chromosomes must essentially be linear structures with genes located at specific sites along them. The chromosome as an organelle was discovered at least 60 years earlier by Wilhelm Hofmeister in Germany (Campbell, 1925).[9] Just a few years after Boveri-Sutton, E B Wilson[10] and Nettie Stevens[11] (1905) independently discovered the chromosomal XY sex-determination system—that males have XY and females XX sex chromosomes (Figure 5).

Boveri and his partner Marcella Boveri were among the first true experimental embryologists. He was nominated, but never received the Nobel Prize before his sudden death in 1912. He chronicled the development of normal sea urchin eggs, but also when the egg was fertilized by two rather than one sperm cell. Boveri deducted that male sperm and female egg nuclei were similar in the amount of transmissible information. They each had a half set (haploid number) of chromosomes. As long as a set of each was present, defined as the diploid number of chromosomes, there was usually normal sea urchin development. Any more or any less and development would proceed abnormally. Mendel's laws were rediscovered in 1900. Boveri recognized the correlation between Mendel's findings and his own cytological evidence of how chromosomes behaved.

The centriole, which is integral to cell division and flanks the spindle, was also discovered by Boveri earlier in 1888 (Sathananthan et al. 2006).[12] A pair of centrioles, one aligned perpendicular to the other, are found in the centrosome—the microtubule organizing center of animal cells (although some centrosomes, like that of the mouse are acentriolar). Boveri subsequently hypothesized that cancer was caused by errors during cell division. Although scorned at the time, Boveri was later proved to be right. In addition to playing a critical role in mitosis, the centriole apparently also provides structural support. A centriole may have its own unique genetic code, which is distinct from the code of the cell; some scientists now believe that this code allows the centrosome to double and divide with each cell cycle precisely and carry out its various functions in the cell. Boveri correctly argued that only one of the centrioles from the two gametes could survive the fertilization process, the other one being inactivated.

FROM MEIOSIS TO THE CONCEPT OF ECTOGENESIS

Embryo Transfer

Walter Heape (1890) in the UK was the first to successfully transfer a 'segmented ova' (cleaved) embryo from one animal to another.[13] Heape used the characteristics of the Angora rabbit from which the embryos were obtained to describe the offspring after transfer into a Belgian hare. The cohort of siblings was of a mixed nature since the recipient rabbit was mated normally. The embryos were not exposed to laboratory conditions and transfer was done very quickly after washing the embryos from the oviducts. Interestingly, Heape's rabbit experiments were either performed in his laboratory in Cambridge or in Prestwick near Manchester, his family home. Bob Edwards would use a similar venue combination in the 1970s during the first series of human IVF, commuting back and forth between Cambridge and Oldham, a town near Manchester where Steptoe practiced as an NHS consultant. Heape's groundbreaking experiments in rabbits and deer and his suggestion to use the transfer procedures in farm animals in a later book are described in a concise review by Biggers (1991)[14]. Heape's thoughts, to use embryo transfer between two animals, apparently did not translate into the concept of artificial fertilization, at least not explicitly stated as such; however, if his experiments did not lead him to the idea directly, it may have inspired others.

HALDANE, HUXLEY AND ROCK

The idea of achieving extracorporeal fertilization was probably first introduced by the great British Population Geneticist, JBS Haldane,[15] who in a book written for a lay audience and published in 1924 (Daedalus; or, Science and the Future) described how a process he called 'ectogenesis' would soon create individuals outside of the human body (Figure 6). He predicted that the first birth would occur in 1951, only slightly optimistic since the concept would become validated not too long after. Haldane's friend Aldous Huxley, an English writer, popularized reproductive technology mixed with provocative descriptions of sexuality some 600 years into the future in his famous novel, *Brave New World (1932)*[16] (Figure 6). As has unfortunately become commonplace when the future of science is portrayed, *Brave New World* is a dark prophecy. Huxley only admitted to having copied the concept from Haldane's *in vitro* conception theory many years after the publication of his book. Now the Heape-Haldane-Huxley concept of alternative forms of procreation was out of the box and the tantalizing possibility that these could soon be available to anyone was on the horizon.

The second paradigm shift occurred with the idea of applying the ectogenesis model to women with tubal disease. This concept was introduced rather plainly in a short editorial in The New England Journal of Medicine in 1937 by Dr John Rock, who was a highly regarded ObGyn at Harvard University (Figure 6). At the time, the idea was perceived to be so outrageous that even the author avoided claiming it, and the editorial was unsigned.[17] The concept had now matured from being proposed as a futuristic way of general procreation to a specific treatment for women with tubal disease.

DIAGNOSIS AND TREATMENT OF INFERTILITY

Infertility diagnosis and treatment before Louise Brown was more sophisticated than is sometimes believed. Infertility was already an established subspecialty well before World War II. By contrast, andrology is a very new discipline. The success of treatment was sometimes expressed as a function of the duration of infertility. Treatment rarely produced better results than no treatment. There were notable exceptions, for instance tubal disease treatment using surgical intervention was well established and quite successful. Similarly, certain endocrinological and immunological disorders could be treated occasionally. The advent of sperm transfer, artificial insemination using the semen of a donor may have

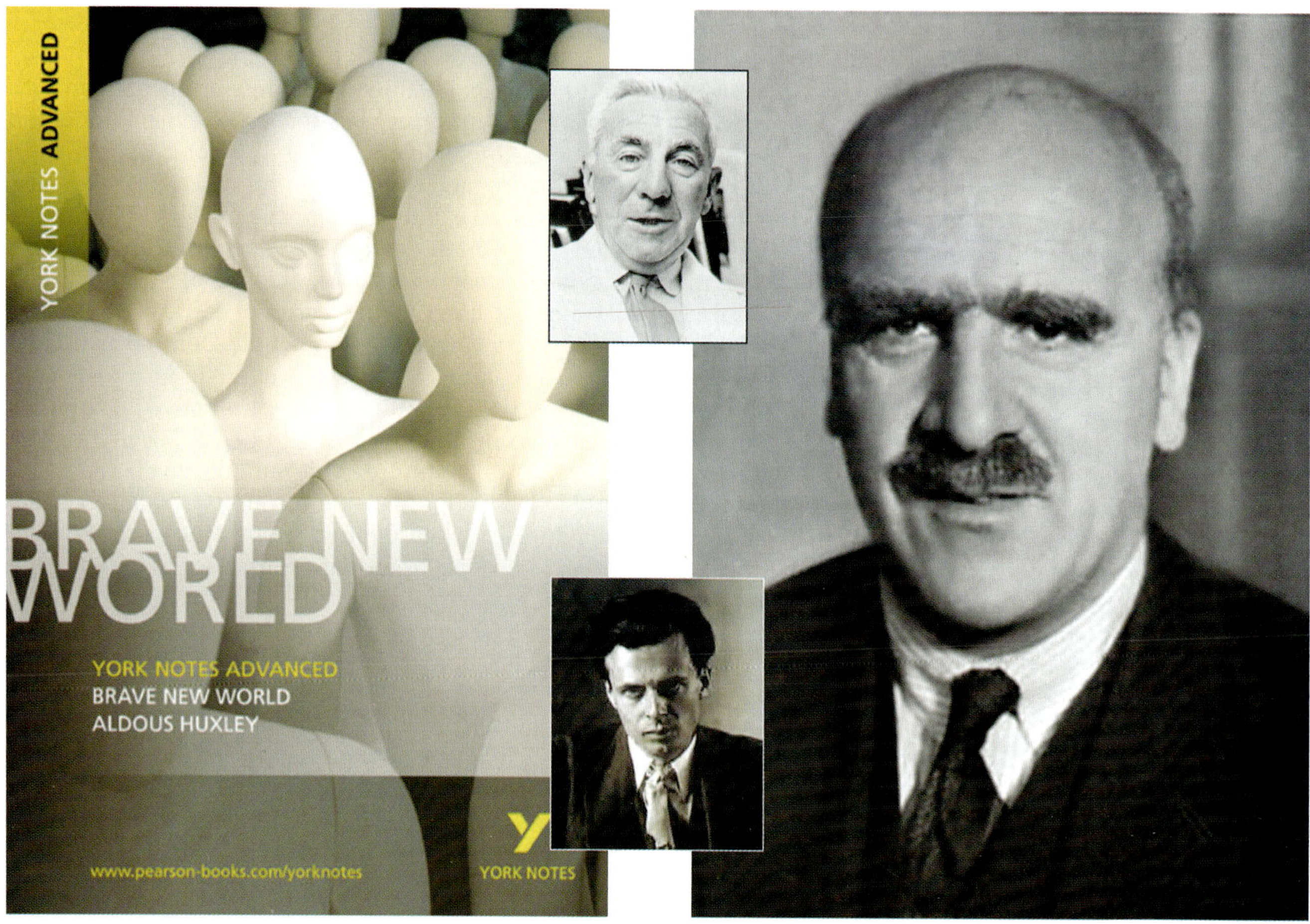

Figure 6 A cover of one of the later editions of 'Brave New World', the novel (1932) by Aldous Huxley (lower panel insert) describing a repressed society where anonymous *in vitro* fertilization and gestation were considered a normal reproductive routine uncoupled from sexual activity. The book was based on JBS Haldane's prophecy of 'ectogenesis' described in 'Daedalus, or, science and the future' (1924). John Rock (upper panel insert), a famous Harvard ObGyn suggested to use ectogenesis for cases of tubal infertility

occurred as early as 1790 in Scotland (Dr John Hunter). In the early part of the 20th century, donor insemination was practiced sporadically until the 1950s when the procedure was first described in medical journals. Chris Polge was the first to deep-freeze spermatozoa from any mammalian species in 1949.[18] Human spermatozoa were first successfully frozen in Iowa (USA) a few years later, by Jerome Sherman, who also established the world's first sperm bank in 1960.[19]

EXPERIMENTAL FERTILIZATION AND PREIMPLANTATION EMBRYOLOGY

Meanwhile scientists would complete the first steps of ectogenesis in the laboratory, planning fertilization experiments *in vitro* in animal models. Although MC Chang's work in 1959[20] is widely regarded as the first proof of IVF in a mammalian model, there were dozens of scientific publications spanning 80 years of research, which paved the way for embryologists (described by Austin in 1961).[21] Of note are the remarkable early experiments by Onanoff in 1893 using eggs flushed from the uterus.[22] Most experimental embryologists later used tubal eggs. Gregory Pincus, the father of the contraception pill, claimed to have fertilized rabbit eggs before World War II, however, the does were inseminated first by a buck and the eggs were flushed quickly from the fallopian tubes after which they were washed vigorously to remove spermatozoa.[23] In the 1950s, when *in vitro* inseminations were more commonplace, it became obvious that spermatozoa could interact with the zona pellucida shortly after insemination and that excess spermatozoa could not be easily removed by washing. Other observations published by Pincus, such as the presence of two polar bodies after activation (disputed by Chang) and a very short interval of only 12 hours between observing the germinal vesicle and the first polar body appearing in the human (disputed by Edwards) were also reasons to perhaps consider the pre-war work in a different light.[5,24]

John Rock and Miriam Menkin at Harvard would collect hundreds of immature ovarian eggs from patients and attempt to fertilize them with modest results during the years after the second world war (Menkin and Rock, 1948).[25] In the 1950s, Thibault in France and MC Chang in the United States carried the field forward by confirming fertilization *in vitro* and obtaining offspring in the rabbit following transfer of the embryos (Thibault et al. 1954; Chang, 1959).[20,26] However, many of the intricate details of the IVF process were still basically unknown. For instance, it was believed that spermatozoa had to mature in the uterus first. By the time Bob Edwards became interested in treating tubal infertility by IVF in 1963, a few others had also attempted to fertilize human eggs *in vitro*, although fertilization was not positively proven in any of those cases.[27] A number of important questions needed to be resolved first: (1) what was a suitable culture fluid or medium? (2) What was the best way of culturing the specimens? (3) How could immature eggs be matured *in vitro*? (4) How could mature rather than immature eggs be obtained routinely? (5) How should spermatozoa be prepared? (6) How could more than one egg be recruited? (7) How could ovulation be timed accurately? (8) At what stage should embryos be returned to the uterus? (9) How and where should embryos be transferred? Although some of these questions were being addressed by experimental embryologists working with animal models, each species had its own specific requirements. The human was very different not only because the women were older and suffered from infertility, but because oocytes were obtained from and embryos were returned to the same individual rather than the egg donor and embryo recipient being two different individuals as is routine in animal work. The concepts of clinical IVF and PGD were accurately described in 11 key points published in Edwards' remarkable 1965 paper in the Lancet.[27] This paper was recently reviewed by one of his first PhD students Martin Johnson.[28]

FERTILIZATION *IN VITRO* AND CULTURING PREIMPLANTATION EMBRYOS

The First Successes in Animal Models

For several years after the success of IVF in the rabbit, as Chang[24] describes, "it was felt that unless living young could be obtained after transplanting such fertilized eggs into recipient rabbits, successful fertilization *in vitro* could not be held to be proven, since such eggs could be abnormally fertilized or may not be fertilized at all". This final confirmation was obtained by Chang in 1959 (Figure 5).[25] He incubated newly ovulated eggs with capacitated sperm for four hours then cultured the eggs in 50% rabbit serum for another 18 hours before transferring the eggs into recipient females. These experiments resulted in the first live births following IVF and embryo transfer in mammals.

It was over a decade after the discovery of *in vivo* capacitation in the rabbit that sperm capacitation *in vitro* was first achieved in the hamster by Yanagimachi and Chang (1963).[29] After another few years, IVF was achieved in the mouse by David Whittingham (1968),[30] opening a tremendous avenue for research into early mammalian development since the period from egg to blastocyst could now be artificially controlled in at least one species. For experimental embryology in mammals to move forward, a reliable embryo culture method was imperative so that the fertilized eggs could be maintained *in vitro* through the cleavage stages. Earlier Hammond (1949) had discovered that mouse embryos collected at the 8-cell stage, but not the 2-cell stage, could be cultured to the blastocyst stage in a physiological saline solution that was supplemented with hen's egg yolk and white.[31] Although the inability to culture 2-cell embryos was and remained for some time a formidable challenge, Hammond's discovery was a significant one and set the stage for abandonment of biological fluids as culture media for embryos. In 1956, Whitten (1956) replaced Hammond's medium with a modification of Krebs-Ringer bicarbonate solution.[32] He supplemented the latter with glucose, antibiotics and bovine serum albumin (BSA) and showed that it could support development of 2-cell and 8-cell mouse embryos to the blastocyst stage. Two years later, McLaren and Biggers (1958) obtained normal young following transfer of blastocysts grown in Whitten's medium, proving that viable blastocysts could be produced *in vitro*.[33]

At this juncture, it was the inability to obtain large numbers of eggs at a time (and in a controlled manner) that hampered research efforts. According to Edwards (1980), the dogma of the time dictated that ovaries of adult females would not respond to gonadotrophic hormones.[34] However, Fowler and Edwards (1957) successfully challenged this theory.[35] They followed the work of Gates in 1954[36] who had artificially induced ovulation in prepubertal mice using a regimen that included injection of pregnant mare serum followed two days later by serum from a pregnant woman. Fowler and Edwards used the same method and induced superovulation and pregnancy in mature mice.[35] Later, it was shown by Gemzell that superovulation could be achieved in the human using pituitary gonadotrophins (1962).[37]

DEVELOPMENT OF A CULTURE SYSTEM

But another hurdle had to be overcome before production, fertilization, culture, and transfer of mammalian eggs would become routine practice. A reliable and efficient embryo culture system had to be devised. In 1963, Brinster introduced culture of eggs and embryos in small drops of culture medium under a layer of paraffin oil.[38] With only minor modifications, this 'micro-drop' method using a 19th century invention called the Petri dish, has become the most widely used and successful system for culture of mammalian embryos *in vitro* today. It would be difficult to think about human embryos growing in the laboratory without contemplating their artificial world and the Petri dish that is temporarily their home. The Petri dish is used in more than 99.9% of ART procedures. By inference, embryologists may have used over 100 million of them to date. In spite of that, the dish has changed little since its inception in the latter part of the 19th century. There have been few secondary changes to adapt the original plain design of the dish to areas of specialized use, such as cell tissue culture (e.g. the square four-well dish) and microbiology. The same can be said about the adaptations made to the Petri dish after its introduction to preclinical embryo research in the 40s and 50s. There have been few such alterations and usually these have been unremarkable, such as place markings for droplets or identification numbers on the bottom. The dish was developed in the latter part of the 19th century, because there was a need in vaccine research to grow micro-organisms on a solid substrate rather than in a broth. This used to be the common way of growing bacteria in culture until the famous German scientist and physician Robert Koch (1843–1910) known as the master of germ theory, suggested replacing the liquid phase. This made a huge difference to the field of germ culture and development of vaccines but the problem was that Dr Koch's assistant had difficulty using glass flasks for this purpose. Koch's assistant was Julius Richard Petri (1852–1921). He decided one day in 1887 to cut off the flask and only use the bottom for pouring the solid media into. The dishes were manufactured in glass and mammalian embryos were cultured experimentally using glass dishes well into the 1970s. In the mid-80s, a sudden increase in the cost of raw material and a better understanding of the injection molding process, allowed most manufacturers to reduce the weight of plastic Petri dishes to the 15–17 grams range. This new thin plastic Petri dish has remained largely unchanged and is now an industry standard.

As mentioned above, one of the most important steps toward contemporary embryo culture was developed by the scientist Ralph Brinster (of sperm stem-cell fame) in 1963, when he successfully cultured mouse eggs to blastocysts. He decided to do away with 'open' culture and protect small amounts of culture medium using a transparent viscous fluid overlaying the media. He used paraffin oil for this purpose. The advantages of this system were huge, although it essentially moved away from Koch's solid substrate approach for which the Petri dish was designed. Oil prevented most microbial infections, allowing fertilization and embryo growth events to take place in less stringent conditions. For example, gametes and embryos could be observed for longer periods since medium evaporation became a problem of the past. The method also allowed the study of minute quantities of metabolites released or absorbed by the cells and later, it facilitated the introduction of micromanipulation methods. Intracytoplasmic sperm injection (ICSI) would have been nearly impossible without the use of oil. The high heat capacity of oil also helped to maintain incubator temperature when the dishes were moved around for observation or manipulation. The problems were oil toxicity and batch-to-batch variation. Paraffin oil has now been largely replaced by other oils, such as mineral oil. This is a variation on light hydrocarbon oils, a distillate of petroleum. Toxicity has been diminished because certain mineral oils are used for human consumption as a lubricant laxative. However, batch-to-batch variation is still a problem. Brinster's technical marvel was for a long time unappreciated by human IVF specialists, as nearly all early practitioners (particularly in the USA) used either organ culture dishes or small test tubes for culture of human gametes and embryos.

TWO DECADES THAT CHANGED HUMAN IVF

The First Test Tube Baby

The basic principles of experimental animal embryology and experience gained in that area, including human oocyte maturation *in vitro* by Edwards in 1965.[27] Bavister, Edwards and Steptoe[39] using a modification of Tyrode's solution devised by Yanagimachi and Chang for hamster IVF,[29] added sperm to nine human eggs and, 11 hours later, recorded the presence of a sperm tail within one egg and the presence of pronuclei in another. This was indisputable evidence of fertilization *in vitro* in the human (Edwards et al. 1969),[40] but it was only the first step since this medium was not able to support further development. It was already known that seminal plasma was not supportive of fertilization and also spermatozoa had to undergo a process called capacitation first, before they could penetrate the oocyte.

The collaboration between Bob Edwards and Patrick Steptoe, one of the most fruitful collaborations ever undertaken between a scientist and clinician, started in 1968 because Steptoe had been able to introduce laparoscopy successfully after others like Palmer (1947)[41] and Fikentscher and Semm (1964) provided the instruments to visualize and manipulate the ovaries.[42]

The first infertile patients were invited to participate in IVF treatment in 1970. Unfortunately for those volunteers, it took over 100 attempts to finally obtain a sustained pregnancy in November 1977. The first pregnancy had been achieved a year earlier in 1976, but it was ectopic and had to be terminated. Wood and Leeton in Australia also reported a biochemical pregnancy in 1975. Other teams in Sweden, Holland, the USA, India and Australia had joined in, but the two pioneers remained the most focused and determined about the work in progress often supported by a third collaborator, nurse Jean Purdy. Purdy played a crucial role in the convergence of experimental embryology and reproductive medicine. She facilitated the transformation of basic research in *in vitro* fertilization to a meticulous clinical discipline with a foundation in quality control. Jean Purdy is without a doubt, the founding mother of QC in clinical embryology.

Louis Joy Brown was born on July 25, 1978 and quickly became the most famous baby. Her name is still well recognized throughout the world. She represents Edwards and Steptoe's quest for knowledge and making human IVF a reality for infertile couples. After the birth of Louise, a short (and remarkably understated) letter was published in the Lancet (Steptoe and Edwards, 1978).[5] Three things stood out in this publication. The first was that the transferred embryo was an 8-cell and not a later stage embryo as was the case during previous transfer attempts. The transfer of blastocysts was based on the assumption that embryos at earlier stages would be received with physiological hostility, since it was believed that the uterus normally accommodates only morulae and blastocysts. We now know that this is only true in animal models and that the human uterus can tolerate any stage of development around the time of ovulation, even prefertilization, if sperm and eggs are injected together as Ian Craft and colleagues demonstrated in 1982.[43]

The second surprising revelation in the Lancet letter was that Lesley Brown's (Louise's mother) diseased fallopian tubes were removed and her ovaries had been relocated into a position of easy accessibility. It escaped no one that this maneuver guaranteed that there would be no doubt about the pregnancy having occurred with the IVF embryos and not per chance from the spontaneous fertilization of a wandering egg.

A third extraordinary aspect of the announcement was that the mature egg had been retrieved from a naturally growing follicle rather than from follicles that had been developing under exogenous hormonal stimulation, as it had been the case in previous patients. The question that was then posed was whether the natural cycle was requisite to success of IVF. It was the team of Alan Trounson that provided the answer a few years later using gonadotropins and clomiphene citrate successfully.[44] Earlier in 1980, another team in Melbourne achieved the first Australian pregnancies.[45]

It should be noted that the initial and subsequent successes of IVF occurred against an extraordinarily unfriendly background, without the support of government agencies, and under a continuous barrage of criticism. Many ethicists, religious leaders, politicians, lawyers, fellow scientists and physicians were appalled by the idea. Edwards confronted them head on and even described scenarios new to them in order to focus the debate. His defense of IVF never wavered and he has written dozens of scholarly articles about the legal, political and ethical issues surrounding reproductive technologies.

ESTABLISHING AND EXPANDING THE CLINICAL ALTERNATIVE: THE 1980s

At the end of 1980, Edwards and Steptoe opened the world's first IVF clinic near Cambridge in an old landhouse called Bourn Hall, which became Bourn Hall Clinic; it had taken the founders some time to establish the facility due to the general lack of interest among financiers. Government funding, both locally and nationally was quite out of the question after the UK Medical Research Council (MRC) and National Health boards again refused to support IVF; an earlier refusal goes back to 1971 when the MRC declined to fund the emerging field of assisted reproduction (for an excellent review on this topic see Johnson et al. 2010).[46] Later in 1983, the MRC would again refuse to grant a broad research application from Edwards and his embryologists. Nevertheless, Bourn Hall Clinic became a legendary place complete with in-patient wards, ethics and visitors committees, endocrinology, embryology, research laboratories, parlors and a dining hall. Other clinics were opened soon: at the Royal Women's Hospital (Alex Lopata) and Monash University (Carl Wood, John Leeton and Alan Trounson) in Melbourne,

Australia with some government support, and in London, UK (Ian Craft) from private funding. At the Eastern Virginia Medical School in Norfolk, Virginia (USA), two famous reproductive gynecologists, Drs Georgianna and Howard Jones, opened the first US-based facility using funds released by the university. Other countries, such as India, Austria, France, Holland, Sweden and Spain followed swiftly and established their own clinics. By 1982, a new discipline was in the making, a field some people were referring to for the first time as ART.

The enthusiasm generated by the success of IVF in Norfolk in 1981, however, did not persuade the US government to lift the moratorium it had placed on all human embryo research a year earlier. In fact, later (in 1995) a law was enacted that prohibits the funding of 'research in which human embryos are destroyed, discarded, or knowingly subjected to risk of injury or death greater than that allowed for research on fetuses *in utero.*' (Dickey-Wicker Amendment, 1995). The US federal government thus does not support clinics or any clinical studies and this sad situation has not changed for over a quarter century.

Although the basis of the technology was now established, many of its aspects were poorly understood. A number of important observations had been made by the first IVF pioneers. They recognized that timing of ovulation and follicular recruitment were complicated processes often limiting a team's ability to plan ahead while many patients became frustrated because of cancellations shortly before egg retrieval. Drugs were needed to recruit follicles at will and control and time ovarian stimulation. The first such family of drugs was the GnRH agonists. These drugs downregulate the secretion of gonadotropins luteinizing hormone (LH) and follicle-stimulating hormone (FSH) resulting in a dramatic decline in estradiol levels. This allowed suppression of endogenous gonadotropin production and the LH surge, and planning for egg retrieval following an injection of human chorionic gonadotropin (hCG) (Fleming et al. 1982).[47]

Another clinical bottleneck during the early days of IVF was the requirement for laparoscopy. Although a magnitude more efficient than laparotomy, laparoscopy had to be performed under general anesthesia in a full operating theater, and required considerable recovery time. Moreover when visualization was hindered, ovaries remained inaccessible and dominant follicles unreachable. The search for a faster and more efficient means of oocyte recovery was on. Ultrasonography, though in its infancy, had already been applied to track growing follicles in the 1970s. [48] The question was whether it could be used during egg retrieval to visualize the follicle and its content. After all, the ovaries were positioned near the vaginal wall. Nevertheless, the first aspiration of a follicle using ultrasound was achieved transabdominally in 1982, a considerably longer route requiring access through the bladder.[49] That same, year abdominal ultrasound was combined with vaginal follicle aspiration.[50] The final and determining step was performed by the Swedish team of Hamberger and Wikland in 1985 using a new narrow vaginal ultrasound probe guiding a needle adjacent to it; this method is still in use now.[51]

In the laboratory meanwhile, experimental embryologists, veterinary researchers and pathology technicians were retrained as clinical embryologists. Their first task was to safely handle and observe gametes and embryos. Laboratory and equipment maintenance, and standardization of methods were other important tasks, as was meticulous record-keeping. These first clinical embryologists were surprised to notice that human embryos varied considerably (Edwards and Purdy, 1982) not just between patients, but also within cohorts.[52] This variability made evaluation of embryos difficult. Even more frustrating was the fact that morphology and rate of development seemed only loosely correlated with outcome. The search for important characteristics that predict implantation has brought under examination many aspects of gamete and embryo development in culture and complicated algorithms have been developed. However, after 30 years, not a single common morphological marker has been identified that can predict the future success of an embryo with certainty. Even algorithms of multiple morphologic criteria do not reveal implanting ability with perfect accuracy. During the past 15 years, researchers have attempted to correlate clinical outcomes with embryo metrics, but only with mixed success. Certainly one of the major challenges remains the identification of accurate (and affordable) embryo selection methods, a crucial step in further reducing multiple pregnancy and facilitating single embryo transfer.[53]

IVF FOR MEN

In vitro fertilization is the first and only general treatment for infertility and subfertility; couples with male infertility can now be treated just as successfully as those with female-related infertility. However, this aspect was not generally accepted in the early 80s. It was feared that spermatozoa from men with male infertility would not be able to penetrate the zona pellucida or that if they did, fetal development could be abnormal. However, when couples with male factor infertility were selected for IVF, many had fertilized eggs although the fertilization rate was only a fraction of that in other groups of infertile couples (Cohen et al. 1984).[54] Moreover, many men with severely reduced sperm counts could not be treated as not enough spermatozoa could be prepared for microdroplet insemination. The notion that micromanipulation could enhance fertilization in male factor cases even further than standard IVF had already been suggested some years back. The first such experiments in some human spare eggs were conducted in Rotterdam in 1979 (Zeilmaker and Cohen, unpublished). The first birth in mice following micromanipulation was achieved by opening the zona pellucida artificially, an approach called zona drilling or dissection.[55] In 1988, human babies were born from a similar mechanical zona dissection, as well as injection of spermatozoa into the perivitelline space.[56,57] Though this improved the prospects for treatment of male factor infertility, fertilization rate were low due to the absence of a quick block to polyspermy on the membrane level. This meant that embryologists could only use very low concentrations of suboptimal spermatozoa after zona dissection or they could only inject one spermatozoon for subzonal insertion. Fertilization rates were improved dramatically with the introduction of ICSI by a team of researchers in Brussels, Belgium.[58] ICSI is now the preferred method of treating those at risk of reduced or failed fertilization.

GAMETE AND EMBRYO PRESERVATION

The most exciting events in science are often marked by the merging of seemingly unrelated disciplines. The field of reproductive science had already experienced this in the 19th century, when the beliefs of both spermists and ovists were shattered by the observation that the spermatozoa penetrate the egg and that this is followed by the formation of two pronuclei in the zygote. Those lucky clinicians and scientists practicing IVF in the 1980s witnessed not one, but two revolutions. The first groundbreaking shift was the enablement of preserving extra embryos for later use. Cryopreservation of the embryo (and later the egg) allowed clinicians to reduce the number of embryos for transfer. In the human, all stages between the zygote and blastocyst were frozen, however, different cryoprotectants and freezing protocols were required.[59-62] Thawing of embryos later allowed transfer in the natural cycle. Some couples did not have to undergo multiple IVF treatments, since the embryos from one cohort could be enough to establish a multisibling family. The effort was well founded in science, since pioneers working with rodents and farm animals had already mastered the technology years earlier.[63-65] The past ten years have seen further refining of egg and embryo cryopreservation, the aims being simplification of methodology and increasing egg and embryo survival rates.

PREIMPLANTATION GENETIC DIAGNOSIS

The other revolution in the 1980s was genetic diagnosis of embryos through blastomere biopsy before transfer, a feat accomplished by a multidisciplinary team in London (UK).[66] Interestingly, the general concept was already introduced 20 years earlier by Bob Edwards and one of his brilliant PhD students at the time, Richard Gardner.[67] They performed trophectoderm biopsy in the rabbit embryo, applied a sexing technique and transferred sexed embryos to the uterus. More than 20 years later and a few years after development of the PCR, this elegant experiment would form the basis for a new field called PGD.

THE EVOLUTION OF REPRODUCTIVE CLINICAL SCIENCE

In vitro fertilization is now considered an industry, a field of its own. More than two thousand clinics specializing in IVF exist worldwide. The largest, in Tokyo, Japan treats more than 15,000 couples a year! A few forward-looking governments support the IVF effort financially. Other governments, such as the ones in Sweden and Belgium, support and guide the practice with smart laws based on clinical data. Many professional organizations have been formed to support the effort and special university-based training programs exist for physicians and embryologists subspecializing in IVF. It is estimated that four million babies have been born through ART; however, the road to this success has not always been easy. In 1934, Dr Gregory Pincus was a young man in his early 30s when he claimed to have achieved *in-vitro* fertilization in rabbits, just a few years after Haldane's prophecies and Huxley's book. While the discovery made international headlines, he was vilified in the press for his research. The New York Times depicted him as Dr Frankenstein, just like others would later describe the work on IVF by Patrick Steptoe and Robert G Edwards as a travesty. It must have been disconcerting for scientific mavericks like Pincus and Edwards to be called names for their sound scientific enquiry. Yet, maybe they found solace in the history of science, since many true innovators, Copernicus, Galileo, Darwin and Boveri among them, were frequently disparaged and often unfairly treated during their lifetime.

ACKNOWLEDGMENTS

I like to thank Dr Mina Alikani for critical review of this chapter and general encouragement and support during the preparations. This chapter is a reprint from a chapter with the same title to be published in Textbook of Clinical Embryology by Cowan and Wells (editors) in Cambridge University Press in 2013. The current chapter was reprinted with permission from Cambridge University Press.

REFERENCES

1. Pinto-Correia C. The ovary of Eve: egg and sperm and preformation. The University of Chicago Press, 1997.
2. Ruestow EG. Images and ideas: Leeuwenhoek's perception of the spermatozoa. J Hist Biol. 1983;16:185.
3. Schenk SL. Das saugetierei kunstlichs befruchtet ausserhalb das muttertieres. Mitth Embryol Instit KK Univ Wien. 1878;1:107.
4. Fol H. Recherches sur la Fécondation et le commencement de L'Hénogénie chez divers animaux.' Mémoires de la Soc. de Physique et d'Histoire Naturelle de Genève. 1879;26.
5. Steptoe PC, Edwards RG. Birth after the reimplantation of a human embryo. Lancet. 1978;12;2(8085):366.
6. Hertwig O. Beitragezurkenntniss der bildung, befruchtung und theilung des thierischen eies. Morph Jb. 1876;1:347.
7. Boveri Th. Über mehrpolige Mitosen als Mittel zur Analyse des Zellkerns. (Regarding multipolar mitosis as a means to analyze the cell nucleus) Verh phys med Ges. 1902;35:67.
8. Sutton WS. On the morphology of the chromosome group in Brachystola magna. Biol Bull. 1902;4:24-39.
9. Campbell, Houghton D. The centenary of Wilhelm Hofmeister. Science. 1925;62 (1597):127.
10. Wilson EB. The chromosomes in relation to the determination of sex in insects. Science. 1905;22(564):500.
11. Stevens NM. Color inheritance and sex inheritance in certain aphids. Science. 1907;6;26(659):216.
12. Sathananthan AH, Ratnasooriya WD, de Silva A, et al. Rediscovering Boveri's centrosome in Ascaris (1888): its impact on human fertility and development. Reprod Biomed Online. 2006;12:254.
13. Heape W. Preliminary note on the transplantation and growth of mammalian ova within a uterine fostermother. Proc R Soc Lond Biol Sci. 1890;48:457-9.
14. Biggers JD. Walter Heape, FRS: a pioneer in reproductive biology. Centenary of his embryo transfer experiments. J Reprod Fertil. 1991;93:173.
15. Haldane JBS. Daedalus; or, Science and the Future (1924), EP Dutton and Company, Inc, a paper read to the Heretics, Cambridge, on February 4, 1923. 2nd edition, London: Kegan Paul, Trench & Co, 1928.
16. Huxley, Aldous. 'Brave New World'. Novel published by Chatto and Windus (London). 1932.
17. Rock J (unsigned editorial). Conception in a Watch Glass. N Engl J Med. 1937;217:678.
18. Polge C, Smith AU, Parkes AS. Revival of spermatozoa after vitrification and dehydration at low temperatures. Nature. 1949;164:666.
19. Sherman JK, Bunge RG. Observations on preservation of human spermatozoa at low temperatures. Proc Soc Exp Biol Med. 1953;82:686.
20. Chang MC. Fertilization of rabbit ova in vitro. Nature. 1959;18:46.
21. Austin CR. Fertilization of mammalian eggs in vitro. Int Rev Cytol. 1961;12:337.
22. Onanoff J. Reserchers de la fecondacion et la gestation des mammifers. Cr Soc Biol. (Paris). 1893;45:719.
23. Pincus G, Enzmann EV. The comparative behavior of mammalian eggs in vivo and in vitro: i. The activation of ovarian eggs. J Exp Med. 1935;62:665.
24. Chang MC. In vitro fertilization of mammalian eggs. J Anim Sci. 1968;1(Suppl 27):15.
25. Menkin MF, Rock J. In vitro fertilization and cleavage of human ovarian eggs. J Obstet Gynecol. 1948;55:440.
26. Thibault C, Dauzier L, Wintenberger S. Cytological study of fecundation in vitro of rabbit ovum. C R Seances Soc Biol Fil. 1954;148:789.
27. Edwards RG. Maturation in vitro of human ovarian oocytes. Lancet. 1965;2(7419):926.
28. Johnson MH. Robert Edwards: the path to IVF. Reprod Biomed Online. 2011;23:245.
29. Yanagimachi R, Chang MC. Fertilization of hamster eggs in vitro. Nature. 1963;200:281.
30. Whittingham DG. Fertilization of mouse eggs in vitro. Nature. 1968;220(5167):592.
31. Hammond J. Recovery and culture of tubal mouse ova. Nature. 1949;163(4131):28.
32. Whitten WK. Culture of tubal mouse ova. Nature. 1956;177(4498):96.
33. McLaren A, Biggers JD. Successful development and birth of mice cultivated in vitro as early as early embryos. Nature. 1958;182(4639):877.
34. Edwards RG, Steptoe PC. A Matter of Life: the story of a medical breakthrough. New York, NY, USA: Morrow; 1980.
35. Fowler RE, Edwards RG. Induction of superovulation and pregnancy in mature mice by gonadotrophins. J Endocrinol. 1957;15:374.
36. Runner MN, Gates A. Conception in prepuberal mice following artificially induced ovulation and mating. Nature. 1954;174(4422):222.
37. Gemzell CA. Induction of ovulation with human pituitary gonadotrophins. Fertil Steril. 1962;13:153.
38. Brinster RL. A method for in vitro cultivation of mouse ova from two-cell to blastocyst. Exp Cell Res. 1963;32:205.
39. Koch R. An address on Bacteriological research. Br Med J. 1890;2(1546):380.
40. Edwards RG, Bavister BD, Steptoe PC. Early stages of fertilization in vitro of human oocytes matured in vitro. Nature. 1969;221(5181):632-5.

41. Palmer R. Instrumentation et technique de la coelioscopie gynecologique. Gynecol Obstet (Paris).1947;46:420-31.
42. Fikentscher R, Semm K. New instruments for insufflation. Int J Fertil. 1964;9:315-20.
43. Craft I, Djahanbakhch O, McLeod F, et al. Human pregnancy following oocyte and sperm transfer to the uterus. Lancet. 1982;1(8280):1031-3.
44. Trounson AO, Leeton JF, Wood C, et al. Pregnancies in humans by fertilization in vitro and embryo transfer in the controlled ovulatory cycle. Science. 1981;212(4495):681-2.
45. Lopata A, Johnston IW, Hoult IJ, et al. Pregnancy following intrauterine implantation of an embryo obtained by in vitro fertilization of a preovulatory egg. Fertil Steril. 1980;33(2):117-20.
46. Johnson MH, Franklin SB, Cottingham M, et al. Why the Medical Research Council refused Robert Edwards and Patrick Steptoe support for research on human conception in 1971. Hum Reprod. 2010;25(9):2157-74.
47. Fleming R, Adam AH, Barlow DH, et al. A new systematic treatment for infertile women with abnormal hormone profiles. Br J Obstet Gynaecol. 1982;89:80-3.
48. Hackeloer BJ. The ultrasonic demonstration of follicular development during the normal menstrual cycle and after hormone stimulation. In: Kurjak A (Ed.). Recent Advances in Ultrasound Diagnosis. Amsterdsm: Excerpta Medica, Amsterdam-Oxford; 1977. pp. 122-8.
49. Lenz S, Lauritsen JG. Ultrasonically guided percutaneous aspiration of human follicles under local anesthesia: a new method of collecting oocytes for in vitro fertilization. Fertil Steril. 1982;38:673-7.
50. Gleicher N, Friberg J, Fullan N, et al. Egg retrieval for in vitro fertilisation by sonographically controlled vaginal culdocentesis. Lancet. 1983;2(8348):508-9.
51. Wikland M, Enk L, Hamberger L. Transvesical and transvaginal approaches for the aspiration of follicles by use of ultrasound. Ann N Y Acad Sci. 1985;442:182-94.
52. Edwards RG, Purdy JM (Eds). Human conception in vitro. London: London, Academic press; 1982.
53. Elder K, Cohen J. Human preimplantation embryo selection. Informa Healthcare, 2008.
54. Cohen J, Fehilly CB, Fishel SB, et al. Male infertility successfully treated by in vitro fertilisation. Lancet. 1984;1(8388):1239-40.
55. Gordon JW, Talansky BE. Assisted fertilization by zona drilling: a mouse model for correction of oligospermia. J Exp Zool. 1986;239(3):347-54.
56. Cohen J, Malter H, Fehilly C, et al. Implantation of embryos after partial opening of oocyte zona pellucida to facilitate sperm penetration. Lancet. 1988;2(8603):162.
57. Ng SC, Bongso A, Ratnam SS, et al. Pregnancy after transfer of sperm under zona. Lancet. 1988;2(8614):790.
58. Palermo G, Joris H, Devroey P, et al. Pregnancies after intracytoplasmic injection of single spermatozoon into an oocyte. Lancet. 1992;340(8810):17-8.
59. Zeilmaker GH, Alberda AT, van Gent I, et al. Two pregnancies following transfer of intact frozen-thawed embryos. Fertil Steril. 1984;42(2):293-6.
60. Trounson A, Mohr L. Human pregnancy following cryopreservation, thawing and transfer of an eight-cell embryo. Nature. 1983;305(5936):707-9.
61. Cohen J, Simons RF, Fehilly CB, et al. Birth after replacement of hatching blastocyst cryopreserved at expanded blastocyst stage. Lancet. 1985;1(8429):647.
62. Lassalle B, Testart J, Renard JP. Human embryo features that influence the success of cryopreservation with the use of 1, 2 propanediol. Fertil Steril. 1985;44(5):645-51.
63. Whittingham DG, Leibo SP, Mazur P. Survival of mouse embryos frozen to -196 degrees and -269 degrees C. Science. 1972;178(59):411-4.
64. Wilmut I. The effect of cooling rate, warming rate, cryoprotective agent and stage of development on survival of mouse embryos during freezing and thawing. Life Sci II. 1972;11(22):1071-9.
65. Willadsen SM. Factors affecting the survival of sheep embryos during-freezing and thawing. Ciba Found Symp. 1977;(52):175-201.
66. Handyside AH, Pattinson JK, Penketh RJ, et al. Biopsy of human preimplantation embryos and sexing by DNA amplification. Lancet. 1989;1(8634):347-9.
67. Gardner RL, Edwards RG. Control of the sex ratio at full term in the rabbit by transferring sexed blastocysts. Nature. 1968;218(5139):346-9.

2

Fertility Testing and Treatment in 2020

Rebecca J Chason, Alan H DeCherney

Chapter Contents

INTRODUCTION

In 2009, 142,241 assisted reproductive technology (ART) cycles were performed in Society for Assisted Reproductive Technology clinics (www.sart.org), of which 64% included intracytoplasmic sperm injection (ICSI) and 4% underwent preimplantation genetic diagnosis (PGD). Comparatively, out of 112, 988 cycles performed in 2003, only 55% utilized ICSI and PGD was not even reported as a national statistic. As we anticipate the continued care of patients with infertility in the coming decade, *in vitro* fertilization (IVF) will continue to be the key to the successful treatment of many men and women. However, the particular ART procedures that will contribute to the success of each cycle, such as ICSI and PGD, may change significantly with the improvement of existing procedures and the advent of novel technologies for diagnostic and prognostic testing.

IMAGING

Anatomic abnormalities of the uterus or fallopian tubes may cause or contribute to infertility, with tubal factor infertility affecting nearly one-third of infertile couples.[1] Uterine abnormalities, such as congenital malformations, leiomyomas and intrauterine adhesions, can either cause infertility or contribute to poor obstetric outcomes once pregnancy is achieved. Currently, the uterus and endometrial cavity are initially evaluated with hysterosalpingography (HSG), transvaginal ultrasound and/or sonohysterography followed by hysteroscopy as indicated, while the fallopian tubes are primarily evaluated with HSG followed by laparoscopy as indicated. In the next decade, anatomic evaluation with radiography will remain routine, with similar imaging modalities offering improvements in resolution and diagnostic certainty.

Technological advances in ultrasound have enabled three-dimensional (3D) imaging, which provides a more accurate morphologic analysis of pelvic structures in the outpatient setting. Furthermore, it offers power Doppler angiography and the potential for more efficiency than conventional two-dimensional scans.[2] While traditional screening with HSG has limitations in the diagnosis of uterine malformations[3] and magnetic resonance imaging requires significantly more time and cost to obtain a definitive analysis of uterine anomalies, 3D ultrasound provides a minimally invasive and accurate means for the diagnosis of congenital uterine anomalies.[4-6] Recent studies have further utilized 3D ultrasound to analyze endometrial and subendometrial vascularity in relation to infertility and treatment outcomes, with promising insights into potential causes and prognostic markers for the infertile population.[7-9] Similar 3D power Doppler imaging indices have also been associated with polycystic ovary syndrome and may help diagnose and explain the pathophysiology of this common syndrome.[10] The clear advantage of 3D ultrasound for identification and classification of congenital uterine anomalies along with the potential exciting uses for in-depth analysis of uterine blood flow and receptivity will secure a role for 3D ultrasound imaging in the routine outpatient evaluation of women with infertility. In addition, advances in Doppler ultrasound have been applied to oocyte retrieval procedures and may improve safety or outcome in the future.[11]

Radiographic testing in 2020 will also include the increased use of more sophisticated imaging techniques to provide comprehensive details regarding pelvic disorders, perhaps even in replacement of the conventional screening modalities such as HSG. While dynamic magnetic resonance-HSG still requires intracervical cannulation and injection of medium, the procedure provides imaging data beyond the endoluminal structures, offers the potential for selective fallopian tube catheterization, and avoids exposure to ionizing radiation.[12,13] Virtual HSG using a mutidetector computed tomography (CT) technique is a minimally invasive test that produces accurate, high-resolution images of both external and internal surfaces of the uterus and fallopian tubes.[14] In addition to evaluation of the female, imaging may also serve a growing role in the noninvasive diagnosis of male infertility, as demonstrated by recent applications of magnetic resonance spectroscopy to identify sites of spermatogenesis in men with non-obstructive azoospermia.[15]

LABORATORY

While follicle-stimulating hormone (FSH) has been the choice biomarker of ovarian reserve, antimüllerian hormone (AMH) will also likely be a routine test in 2020. AMH is produced by the granulosa cells during early follicular development and secreted into serum, where levels are stable until they begin to decrease with the decline in follicular reserve and become undetectable at menopause.[16] AMH is a reliable marker of ovarian reserve and may assist in predicting response to ovarian stimulation, although may not be of additional benefit to the current testing strategies of FSH and/or antral follicle count.[17] However, the future utility of AMH testing may be most profound in its assistance with oocyte selection as it can be measured in follicular fluid to assess oocyte quality.[18]

Recent research has increasingly focused on the endometrium to identify biomarkers of receptivity and causes for implantation failure, a source of significant inefficiency in the current practice of ART. Global gene expression profiles appear to change in conjunction with the phases of the menstrual cycle, although studies to date have found few consensus genes.[19-23] Variation in specific gene expression profiles and polymorphisms also appears to be associated with various aspects of infertility, although which are a cause versus a symptom is yet to be determined.[24-26] Endometrial gene expression and hormonal response may explain one aspect of the subfertility experienced by obese and polycystic ovary syndrome women.[27-29] In addition to the transcriptome, use of new technologies, such as microRNA, to evaluate the multilayered genomic and epigenomic control of endometrial function will further contribute to our understanding of the endometrium's role in implantation over the next decade.[30] The improved understanding of endometrial physiology may introduce additional diagnostic testing, such as endometrial biopsies to evaluate gene expression profiles, and may also maximize current therapies such as embryo transfer.[21]

Infertility testing and treatment will also be affected by advances in the field of metabolomics— the identification and quantification of all metabolites in a biologic sample.[31] Given the recent rapid advances in oocyte vitrification and the increasing success with single embryo transfer, improvements in oocyte selection will be vital to improving the pregnancy rate per embryo transfer and reducing the number of unused embryos in the next decade. The minimally invasive evaluation of follicular fluid with metabolomics may provide the key to oocyte quality and pregnancy potential.[32] Furthermore, investigations into the content of embryo culture medium may also improve embryo selection and IVF success rates.[33]

GENETICS

Genetic testing beyond the conventional karyotype has become a reality with the technical advances that have developed over the past decade. Refinement and implementation of these technologies will enable intimate knowledge of the human genome and provide new mechanisms to study the cause of infertility and to predict the response to subsequent therapy. Microarrays, whole genome sequencing (WGS) and next generation sequencing (NGS) are dominating the current field of genetics and will offer unlimited possibilities to the field of reproductive medicine (Table 1). Microarray experiments use a platform of selected oligonucleotides that represent a genome-wide sample of known sequences (messenger RNA, single-nucleotide

Table 1 Genetic testing technology and terminology

Test	Description
Chromatin Immunoprecipitation	Detection of genomic protein binding site occupancy using immunoprecipitation of a particular protein
Comparative Genomic Hybridization	Comparison of genomic content between samples
Copy Number Variation	Variation in the number of copies of particular regions of the genome ranging in size from one kilobase to several megabases
Gene Expression Profiling	Determination of gene expression levels using mRNA
Microarray	Two-dimensional grid of known DNA fragments arranged on a solid substrate in microscopic spots
Nanotechnology	Functional technologic systems built on a molecular scale, smaller than 100 nanometers
Next Generation Sequencing	Genome-wide sequencing technology in which millions of parallel sequencing reactions produce high coverage of genome in relatively short time period
Single-Nucleotide Polymophism	Variation in the sequence of DNA at a single nucleotide within the genome
Whole Genome Sequencing	Determination of complete DNA sequence including chromosomal and mitochondrial DNA

polymorphisms and copy number variants) that can be used to study the relative amount of genetic material, gene expression level and more. WGS provides the complete DNA sequence of the genome either from de novo or reference-based assembly with NGS significantly improving the time required to obtain the sequencing results. Each sequence can then be evaluated for myriad outputs, from single base-pair alterations to structural alterations to genome-wide profiles. Genome-wide association studies (GWAS) use the data obtained from WGS to compare the variation between individuals and to identify genetic factors that influence the development of disease.[34,35] The data obtained from these genome-wide experiments could be used in reproductive medicine to identify biomarkers for specific reproductive disorders, causes of infertility, likely response to particular therapies (such as stimulation protocol) and viability (in the case of gametes or embryos).

The information supplied by these technologies, however, also presents a variety of technical and ethical challenges that will necessitate the attention of clinicians and scientists during the next decade of infertility testing and treatment. For example, despite its widespread use in the literature, the clinical utility of gene expression profiling is limited by inconsistent results due to the dynamic nature of gene expression, variations in tissue sampling, and differences in microarray platforms, experimental conditions and data analysis techniques.[36] Congruent with its many-fold increase in data output (terabytes of information), WGS presents even further challenges in data storage, management and interpretation.[37] Continued advances in bioinformatics, functional genomics and WGS techniques will certainly improve these issues in 2020.

In addition to technical challenges, WGS will present significant ethical dilemmas. As a means of "presymptomatic" testing, it will give us the capability to identify the carrier status for genetic disorders and genetic risk factors for multifactorial and late-onset diseases. The wisdom of obtaining such information will need to be evaluated carefully in the context of preventability and treatability of each disorder as it pertains to potential parents, gametes and zygotes.

Parental Genetic Testing

Genetic testing certainly has an important role in the current evaluation and treatment of men and women with infertility. Several parental genetic disorders that disrupt large regions of the genome, such as Turner's syndrome and Klinefelter's syndrome, are well-known causes of infertility that are easily diagnosed with a karyotype. While more subtle chromosomal rearrangements and microdeletions (notably, Y chromosome microdeletions) have also been identified in infertile couples, genetic testing in the next decade will utilize more sophisticated methods to improve the detection of submicroscopic genomic abnormalities. Gene expression profiling may provide insight into those couples currently diagnosed with "unexplained" infertility and may guide therapy or provide more accurate prognostic information. An increasing number of gene mutations and polymorphisms have already been implicated in the cause of male factor infertility[38] and could lead to the development of a panel of tests that provide diagnostic and prognostic information beyond the standard semen analysis. WGS may be applied to identify a woman's risk of premature ovarian insufficiency and, thus, influence her family planning timeline or use of oocyte cryopreservation. The possibilities are countless, and clinical applications of such technologies will quickly expand in the coming decade.

Gamete Genetic Testing

Gametogenesis proceeds via unique pathways in sperm and oocytes to produce the mature haploid germ cells necessary for procreation. Germ cells undergo a complex series of mitotic and meiotic divisions[39-41] coupled with extensive epigenetic erasure and establishment[42,43] to obtain competency, thus their reproductive potential is difficult to ascertain yet vital to improving outcomes in ART.

The semen analysis is the current standard for testing male factor fertility and for planning treatment strategies in ART. While the semen parameters are certainly helpful in this regard, the significant overlap between fertile and infertile men suggests additional important parameters that would potentially improve diagnosis and prognostic counseling. A plethora of additional sperm tests have been suggested in the literature for years with variable results, but none substantial enough to secure a position in the routine clinical evaluation. However, both genetic and epigenetic aberrations in the male gamete are likely indicative of reproductive potential and the rapidly advancing technologies may enable more accurate and reliable results in the clinical setting. Recent interest in epigenetic errors as a cause of male factor infertility,[44] in conjunction with technologies better able to assess epigenetic marks, will allow investigation of global sperm DNA structure and function, and perhaps guide counseling or therapy. Microarray studies will also be applied more frequently to sperm testing to evaluate global gene expression patterns,[45] but given the current lack of normative data, the future challenge will be in the interpretation and application of such information.

Embryonic Genetic Testing

The genetic revolution will have its largest impact on ART outcomes through the analysis and selection of embryos for transfer. Moreover, the ethical issues previously discussed will be even more controversial in regards to their management in preimplantation embryos. Currently, PGD is routinely applied to detect single-gene disorders that are lethal or significantly crippling such as Fanconi's anemia and Tay-Sachs disease. Of the monogenic disorders tested, there is a sizable variation in the severity of each disease which is changing as medical advances in other fields impact their treatment. For example, children with spinal muscular atrophy type 1 usually succumb to the disease by age 2 while children with cystic fibrosis now have a median predicted age of survival in the mid-30s. Current notable controversies are the use of PGD for human leukocyte antigen matching and sex selection. However, with the advent of WGS, PGD will assume an even greater capability to provide genetic information about preimplantation embryos, including their risk for polygenic, adult-onset diseases such as Alzheimer's disease and cardiovascular disease. Should such results be provided to prospective parents and should they be used for embryo selection? How will the layperson manage the uncertainty of a disease risk or of variable penetrance? Should parents have the right to decide what is an acceptable medical quality of life for their children in adulthood? What about "favorable" genetic variants—should they be reported and factored into embryo transfer decisions? With such ethical questions, we believe the professional reproductive medicine community should actively anticipate and address the exciting but complicated possibilities that these technologic advances will provide.

MEDICATIONS

While the vast majority of advances in the coming decade will improve infertility testing and prognostics, the development of novel medications and protocols will at least improve the patient experience during controlled ovarian stimulation and may reveal additional benefits with further investigations. In particular, recent use of recombinant technology to modify the beta subunit of FSH has resulted in the production of a long-acting FSH agonist, Corifollitropin alfa, that has a prolonged half-life and slower absorption rate, thus requiring fewer doses to support multifollicular development.[46] Similar pharmaceutical advances may negate the current use of human chorionic gonadotropin as the choice medication for oocyte maturation and release. Instead, use of oral gonadotropin-releasing hormone agonists[47,48] or recombinant luteinizing hormone may more closely simulate the physiologic luteinizing hormone surge with fewer side effects or complications. We anticipate that treatment of infertility in 2020 will continue to enhance the protocols used for IVF and improve the frequency and route of drug administration for patient comfort and safety.

SUMMARY

While the treatment of infertility with IVF and ICSI will likely continue to be the mainstay of therapy in 2020, the most significant advances in the field will be a result of the explosive developments in genetics. Data gleaned from technologies that decipher genetic and epigenetic codes, such as GWAS, will begin to unravel currently unexplained causes of infertility and will hopefully begin to guide an individual's therapy more successfully. However, these developments will require discernment and a keen understanding by the reproductive medicine community to manage and explain the delicate and difficult ethical issues that will arise with the vast knowledge that will be gained. Appropriate applications will maximize ART outcomes and provide optimal care to our patients.

REFERENCES

1. Miller JH, Weinberg RK, Canino NL, et al. The pattern of infertility diagnoses in women of advanced reproductive age. Am J Obstet Gynecol. 1999;181:952-7.
2. Benacerraf BR, Shipp TD, Bromley B. Improving the efficiency of gynecologic sonography with 3-dimensional volumes: a pilot study. J Ultrasound Med. 2006;25:165-71.
3. Braun P, Grau FV, Pons RM, et al. Is hysterosalpingography able to diagnose all uterine malformations correctly? A retrospective study. Eur J Radiol. 2005;53:274-9.
4. Ghi T, Casadio P, Kuleva M, et al. Accuracy of three-dimensional ultrasound in diagnosis and classification of congenital uterine anomalies. Fertil Steril. 2009;92:808-13.
5. Caliskan E, Ozkan S, Cakiroglu Y, et al. Diagnostic accuracy of real-time 3D sonography in the diagnosis of congenital Mullerian anomalies in high-risk patients with respect to the phase of the menstrual cycle. J Clin Ultrasound. 2010;38:123-7.
6. Bermejo C, Martinez Ten P, Cantarero R, et al. Three-dimensional ultrasound in the diagnosis of Mullerian duct anomalies and concordance with magnetic resonance imaging. Ultrasound Obstet Gynecol. 2010;35:593-601.
7. Chen L, Quan S, Li H, et al. A comparison of endometrial and subendometrial vascularity assessed by three-dimensional ultrasonography and power Doppler angiography between healthy fertile women and women with unexplained primary recurrent miscarriage. Fertil Steril. 2011;95:1127-9.
8. Kim A, Han JE, Yoon TK, et al. Relationship between endometrial and subendometrial blood flow measured by three-dimensional power Doppler ultrasound and pregnancy after intrauterine insemination. Fertil Steril. 2010;94:747-52.
9. Ng EH, Chan CC, Tang OS, et al. The role of endometrial blood flow measured by three-dimensional power Doppler ultrasound in the prediction of pregnancy during in vitro fertilization treatment. Eur J Obstet Gynecol Reprod Biol. 2007;135:8-16.
10. Mala YM, Ghosh SB, Tripathi R. Three-dimensional power Doppler imaging in the diagnosis of polycystic ovary syndrome. Int J Gynaecol Obstet. 2009;105:36-8.
11. Risquez F, Confino E. Can Doppler ultrasound-guided oocyte retrieval improve IVF safety? Reprod Biomed Online. 2010;21:444-5.
12. Winter L, Glucker T, Steimann S, et al. Feasibility of dynamic MR-hysterosalpingography for the diagnostic work-up of infertile women. Acta Radiol. 2010;51:693-701.
13. De Geyter C, Steimann S, Frohlich JM, et al. Selective visualization of the Fallopian tube with magnetic resonance imaging. Reprod Biomed Online. 2007;14:593-7.
14. Carrascosa PM, Capunay C, Vallejos J, et al. Virtual hysterosalpingography: a new multidetector CT technique for evaluating the female reproductive system. Radiographics. 2010;30:643-61.
15. Aaronson DS, Iman R, Walsh TJ, et al. A novel application of 1H magnetic resonance spectroscopy: non-invasive identification of spermatogenesis in men with non-obstructive azoospermia. Hum Reprod. 2010;25:847-52.
16. La Marca A, De Leo V, Giulini S, et al. Anti-Mullerian hormone in premenopausal women and after spontaneous or surgically induced menopause. J Soc Gynecol Investig. 2005;12:545-8.
17. La Marca A, Sighinolfi G, Radi D, et al. Anti-Mullerian hormone (AMH) as a predictive marker in assisted reproductive technology (ART). Hum Reprod Update. 2010;16:113-30.
18. Wunder DM, Guibourdenche J, Birkhauser MH, etal. Anti-Mullerian hormone and inhibin B as predictors of pregnancy after treatment by in vitro fertilization/intracytoplasmic sperm injection. Fertil Steril. 2008;90:2203-10.
19. Talbi S, Hamilton AE, Vo KC, et al. Molecular phenotyping of human endometrium distinguishes menstrual cycle phases and underlying biological processes in normo-ovulatory women. Endocrinology. 2006;147:1097-121.

20. Haouzi D, Mahmoud K, Fourar M, et al. Identification of new biomarkers of human endometrial receptivity in the natural cycle. Hum Reprod. 2009;24:198-205.
21. Diaz-Gimeno P, Horcajadas JA, Martinez-Conejero JA, et al. A genomic diagnostic tool for human endometrial receptivity based on the transcriptomic signature. Fertil Steril. 2011;95:50-60, e1-15.
22. Altmae S, Martinez-Conejero JA, Salumets A, et al. Endometrial gene expression analysis at the time of embryo implantation in women with unexplained infertility. Mol Hum Reprod. 2010;16:178-87.
23. Allegra A, Marino A, Coffaro F, et al. Is there a uniform basal endometrial gene expression profile during the implantation window in women who became pregnant in a subsequent ICSI cycle? Hum Reprod. 2009;24:2549-57.
24. Altmae S, Kallak TK, Friden B, et al. Variation in Hyaluronan-Binding Protein 2 (HABP2) Promoter Region is Associated With Unexplained Female Infertility. Reprod Sci. 2011;18:485-92.
25. Fischer CP, Kayisili U, Taylor HS. HOXA10 expression is decreased in endometrium of women with adenomyosis. Fertil Steril. 2011;95:1133-6.
26. Margarit L, Taylor A, Roberts MH, et al. MUC1 as a discriminator between endometrium from fertile and infertile patients with PCOS and endometriosis. J Clin Endocrinol Metab. 2010;95:5320-9.
27. Bellver J, Martinez-Conejero JA, Labarta E, et al. Endometrial gene expression in the window of implantation is altered in obese women especially in association with polycystic ovary syndrome. Fertil Steril. 2011;95(7):2335-41, 2341.e1-8.
28. Savaris RF, Groll JM, Young SL, et al. Progesterone resistance in PCOS endometrium: a microarray analysis in clomiphene citrate-treated and artificial menstrual cycles. J Clin Endocrinol Metab. 2011;96(6):1737-46.
29. Wang A, Ji L, Shang W, et al. Expression of GPR30, ERalpha and ERbeta in endometrium during window of implantation in patients with polycystic ovary syndrome: a pilot study. Gynecol Endocrinol. 2011;27:251-5.
30. Kuokkanen S, Chen B, Ojalvo L, et al. Genomic profiling of microRNAs and messenger RNAs reveals hormonal regulation in microRNA expression in human endometrium. Biol Reprod. 2010;82:791-801.
31. Weckwerth W. Metabolomics: an integral technique in systems biology. Bioanalysis. 2010;2:829-36.
32. Revelli A, Delle Piane L, Casano S, et al. Follicular fluid content and oocyte quality: from single biochemical markers to metabolomics. Reprod Biol Endocrinol. 2009;7:40.
33. Aydiner F, Yetkin CE, Seli E. Perspectives on emerging biomarkers for non-invasive assessment of embryo viability in assisted reproduction. Curr Mol Med. 2010;10:206-15.
34. Ewens KG, Jones MR, Ankener W, et al. FTO and MC4R gene variants are associated with obesity in polycystic ovary syndrome. PLoS One 2011;6(1):e16390.
35. Aston KI, Krausz C, Laface I, et al. Evaluation of 172 candidate polymorphisms for association with oligozoospermia or azoospermia in a large cohort of men of European descent. Hum Reprod. 2010;25:1383-97.
36. Kim K, Zakharkin SO, Allison DB. Expectations, validity, and reality in gene expression profiling. J Clin Epidemiol. 2010;63:950-9.
37. Werner T. Next generation sequencing allows deeper analysis and understanding of genomes and transcriptomes including aspects to fertility. Reprod Fertil Dev. 2011;23:75-80.
38. O'Flynn O'Brien KL, Varghese AC, Agarwal A. The genetic causes of male factor infertility: a review. Fertil Steril. 2010;93:1-12.
39. Sassone-Corsi P. Stem cells of the germline: the specialized facets of their differentiation program. Cell Cycle. 2008;7:3491-2.
40. Yin S, Sun XF, Schatten H, et al. Molecular insights into mechanisms regulating faithful chromosome separation in female meiosis. Cell Cycle. 2008;7:2997-3005.
41. Mehlmann LM. Stops and starts in mammalian oocytes: recent advances in understanding the regulation of meiotic arrest and oocyte maturation. Reproduction. 2005;130:791-9.
42. Boussouar F, Rousseaux S, Khochbin S. A new insight into male genome reprogramming by histone variants and histone code. Cell Cycle. 2008;7:3499-502.
43. Lees-Murdock DJ, Walsh CP. DNA methylation reprogramming in the germ line. Epigenetics. 2008;3:5-13.
44. Oliva R. Protamines and male infertility. Hum Reprod Update. 2006;12:417-35.
45. Ellis PJ, Furlong RA, Conner SJ, et al. Coordinated transcriptional regulation patterns associated with infertility phenotypes in men. J Med Genet. 2007;44:498-508.
46. Loutradis D, Drakakis P, Vlismas A, et al. Corifollitropin alfa, a long-acting follicle-stimulating hormone agonist for the treatment of infertility. Curr Opin Investig Drugs. 2009;10:372-80.
47. Erb TM, Vitek W, Wakim AN. Gonadotropin-releasing hormone agonist or human chorionic gonadotropin for final oocyte maturation in an oocyte donor program. Fertil Steril. 2010;93:374-8.
48. Engmann L, DiLuigi A, Schmidt D, et al. The use of gonadotropin-releasing hormone (GnRH) agonist to induce oocyte maturation after cotreatment with GnRH antagonist in high-risk patients undergoing in vitro fertilization prevents the risk of ovarian hyperstimulation syndrome: a prospective randomized controlled study. Fertil Steril. 2008;89:84-91.

2

Male Factor Infertility

SECTION CONTENTS

3

Evaluation and Diagnosis of Male Infertility

Sandro C Esteves, Alaa Hamada, Ashok Agarwal

Chapter Contents

INTRODUCTION

It is well known that the motivation to have children and the formation of a new family unit are essential components of the individual instinct for existence and well-being. Fertility problems may represent a stressful situation to the individual's life with important negative psychological consequences.[1] The experienced clinician should realize and comprehend the burdensome bearings and frustrated mood of the infertile individual. Most adults are prompted to discuss their sexual issues and behaviors if the interview is conducted in a respectful, confidential, professional and nonjudgmental way.

In the last decades, extraordinary advances have been achieved in the field of male infertility. Significant progress has been made regarding both diagnostic and treatment techniques. Novel tests have been incorporated to the andrological armamentarium. Today, it is possible to correctly classify some cases which were previously believed to be idiopathic. The initial evaluation of common infertility complaint comprises the meticulous history taking, as well as conducting a thorough physical examination along with proper laboratory and imaging studies as needed.

DEFINITION AND EPIDEMIOLOGY OF MALE INFERTILITY

The infertility is defined as failure of the couples to conceive after 12 months of unprotected regular intercourse.[2] Infertility is broadly classified into primary infertility, when the male partner has no previous history of fertility, and secondary infertility, when there was previous man's history of successful impregnation of a woman. Subfertility refers to a reduced but not unattainable potential to achieve pregnancy, while sterility is denoted by permanent inability to induce or achieve pregnancy.[3] Fecundity, on the other hand, indicates the capability of a given male or female to produce live births.

Epidemiology studies indicate that 13–15% of couples face difficulties to conceive.[4] Approximately 8% of men in reproductive age seek medical assistance for fertility-related problems.[5] Isolated male factor infertility, and its combination with female problems accounts for more than 50% of the couples' inability to conceive.[6] The male factor is purely responsible for 20% of infertile couples, while it is contributory in another 30–40% of infertility.[6]

The World Health Organization defines male factor infertility as the presence of abnormalities in the semen analysis, or the presence of sexual or ejaculatory dysfunction.[7] However, modern andrology has revealed that normal semen testing does not guarantee fecundity, and unraveled the predictive power of normal semen to induce natural pregnancy is about 60%.[8] The introduction of novel sperm function testing is revolutionizing the criteria of diagnosis and definitions of male infertility.

Recent reports indicate that sperm counts of men from certain regions of the world have significantly deteriorated. Remarkable differences in sperm production have been detected among men from different countries in Europe and the United States of America. Differences are also seen in individuals of different regions within the same country. Moreover, there is a noticeable epidemiologic increase in the incidence of testicular cancer and urogenital anomalies.[9-12] These observations cause public concerns particularly with regard to the implication of environmental factors and modern life habits.[13-15] Some authors claim that the buildup in the prevalence of infertility among men may be attributed to increased prevalence of obesity.[16-18] Others factors may also be implicated in the apparent rising prevalence of male infertility problems such as exposure to cell phones radiation[19] and certain endocrine disruptors.[20]

PATHOPHYSIOLOGY, ETIOLOGY AND CLASSIFICATION OF MALE INFERTILITY

The male reproductive system consists of the testes, accessory glands and the ductal system for sperm transport. The seminal ducts constitute the pathways for sperm transport; and it includes the efferent ductules and rete testis, epididymis, vas deferens, ejaculatory ducts and urethra. The accessory sex glands include the seminal vesicles, prostate and bulbourethral glands (Figures 1 and 2).

The testes perform two important functions: spermatogenesis and steroidogenesis. Daily sperm production is about 40 million and declines progressively with aging. Recent data suggests that the duration of spermatogenesis is less than 60 days instead of 70 ± 4 days as previously thought for over 40 years.[21] As such, the sperm production of an individual actually represents the result of influencing biological, physical and occupational factors, which acted within the past 2 months from ejaculation. Steroidogenesis and hormone production is another essential testicular function. The hormonal milieu that regulates spermatogenesis depends on complex coordinated interaction between the testes, pituitary gland and hypothalamus that form the hypothalamic-pituitary-gonadal (HPG) axis (Figure 3).

The storage and maturation of spermatozoa occur in the epididymis. However, the maturation process is exclusively completed within the female reproductive tract. Spermatozoa transit throughout the epididymis for

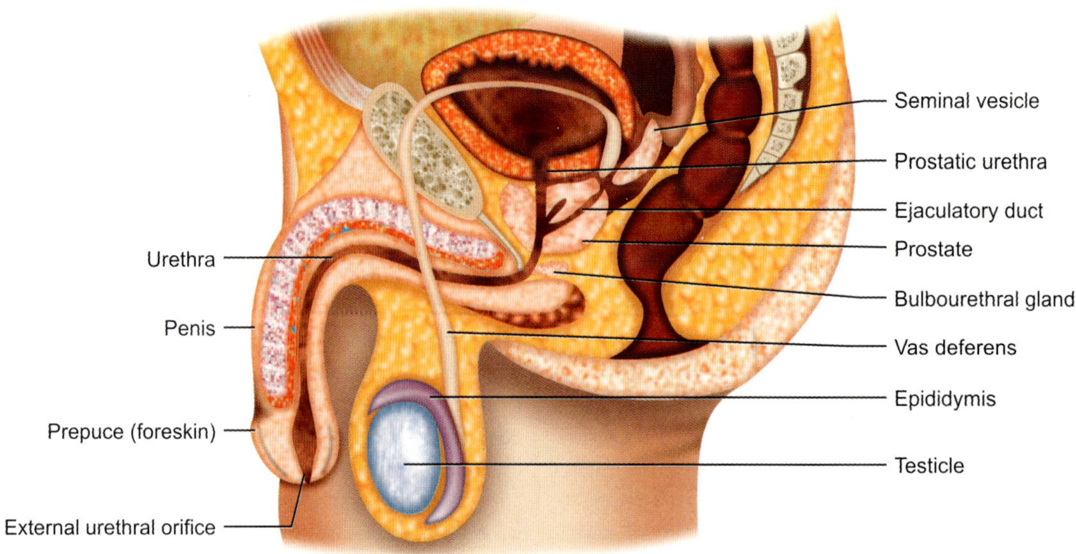

Figure 1 Schematic illustration of the male reproductive organs

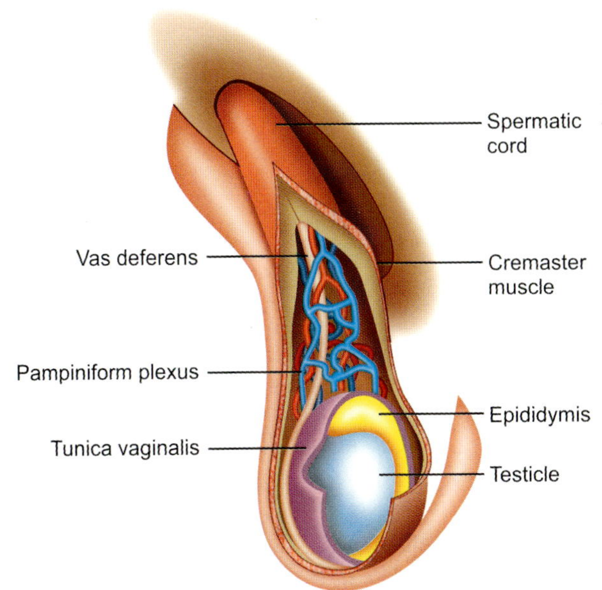

Figure 2 Schematic representation of the testis and its related structures

about 12 days. The epididymides are in continuity with the vasa deferentia, which in turn join the emerging ducts from the seminal vesicles to form the ejaculatory ducts. They enter the prostate, a gland responsible for production of a fluid enriched with zinc, citric acid, acid phosphatase and proteases that contributes to liquefaction and accounts for approximately 0.5 ml of the ejaculate. The seminal vesicles produce an alkaline fluid with prostaglandins and fructose that composes 1.5–2.0 ml of the seminal fluid. Both seminal vesicles and vas deferens have a common embryologic origin. As such, when congenital bilateral absence of vas deferens (CBAVD) is diagnosed, it is often associated with seminal vesicles hypoplasia/agenesis. This is an important aspect in the differential diagnosis of azoospermia. In CBAVD, diminished or no fructose can be found in the seminal fluid and, hence, volume is low (< 1 ml). Under normal conditions, spermatozoa are stored in the epididymides rather than the seminal vesicles. At the time of ejaculation, ductal and epididymal muscle contractions under sympathetic stimulation conduct the spermatozoa towards the prostatic urethra where they join fluids excreted by the prostate, and form the semen. Periurethral muscle contraction is responsible for expelling semen out. Interference in any of these steps may lead to male infertility. Herein, the pathophysiological mechanism involved is dependent on which organ or regulatory system is afflicted.

Male infertility causes may range from simple, reversible and correctable causes to uncorrectable ones. Such conditions may be inherited or acquired. The factors affecting male fertility status can be divided into four major categories: disorders in sperm production, sperm transport and sperm function constitute the essential causes of male infertility. The fourth category is represented by "infertility of unknown origin", a condition in which male infertility has aroused spontaneously, or from an obscure or unknown cause. This category accounts for 37–58% of the cases, and it is divided into two major subtypes: idiopathic and unexplained male infertility.[22-24] Idiopathic male infertility is the cause of about 30% of male infertility, and it is characterized by unexplained reduction in semen quality with no previous history associated with fertility problems, and having normal findings on physical examination and endocrine laboratory testing.[23] The term "unexplained male infertility", on the other hand, is reserved for infertile men with infertility of unknown origin with normal semen profile, and in whom female infertility factors have been ruled out. This category accounts for 6–27% of male infertility, and it strongly depends on how exhaustive evaluation of the patient is done.[22] Table 1 depicts the etiologic classification of male infertility.

The most commonly observed abnormality in infertile men seeking evaluation is varicocele followed by obstruction and cryptorchidism. Table 2 shows the distribution of the causes of male infertility in tertiary care infertility center. It should be noted, however, that the frequency distribution of primary infertility causes is different from secondary infertility causes in which varicocele accounts for 70–80% of the cases, followed by infection of genital tract.[25-27]

PROBABILITIES OF CONCEPTION FOR FERTILE AND INFERTILE COUPLES

Epidemiology studies indicate that the chance of a couple to achieve conception is 80–90% after 1 year of regular well-timed intercourse while the monthly chance for conception is 20–25%.[27] The optimum fertility age for conception in both sexes is 24 years. Henceforth, the fertility potential declines, particularly for female partner after the age of 31 years.[28-30]

On the other hand, the spontaneous pregnancy rate for infertile couples, due to idiopathic reasons, noticeably depends on the result of semen analysis. For non-azoospermic men, the pregnancy rate is 1–3% per month, 23% within 2 years and 10% within another two additional years.[31] However, the cumulative pregnancy rate (PR) for infertile couples whose male partner have normal semen analyses ranges from 50%–80% over a 3-year period as a function of female age, and from 30%–80% as a function of infertility duration.[32] A cumulative PR of 60% may be achieved within 2 years for this category of patient.[33] Infertility periods longer than 3 years are associated with very low PR of 1–3% particularly if the female partner is aged 35 years or older.[34]

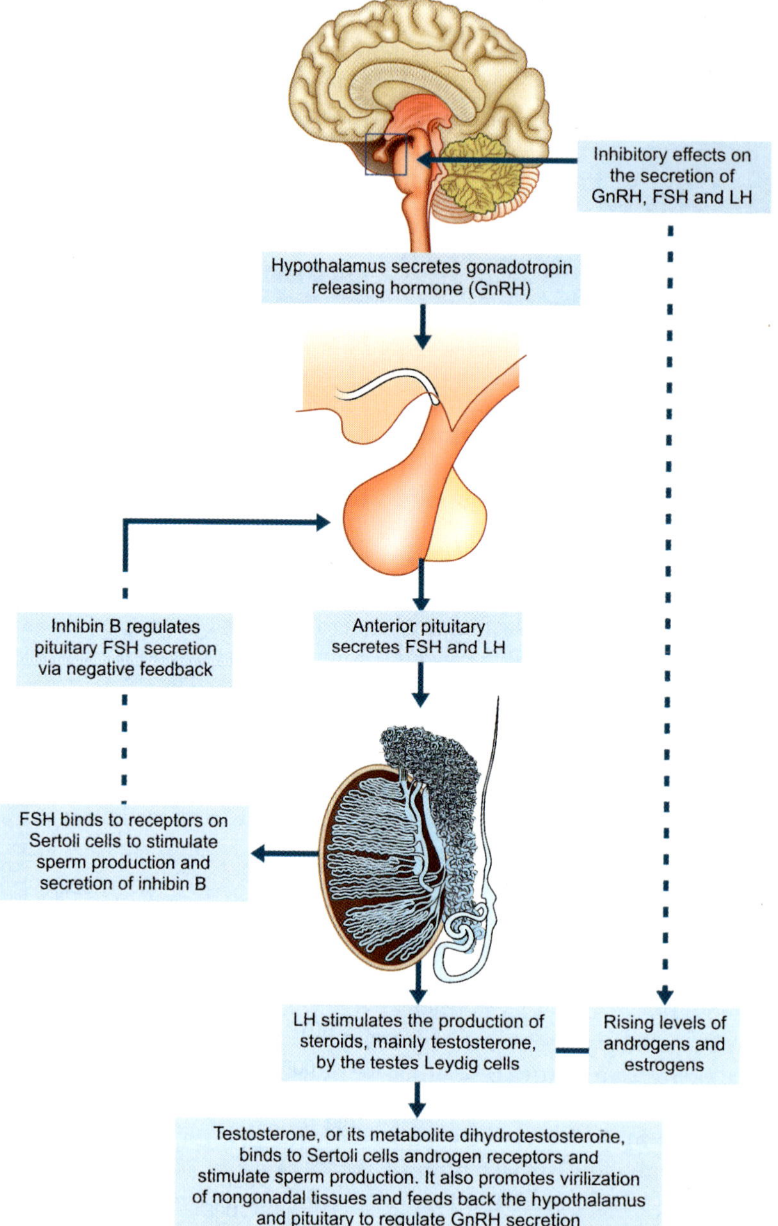

Figure 3 Schematic representation of the components of the hypothalamic-pituitary-testicular axis and the endocrine regulation of spermatogenesis. Luteinizing hormone (LH) and follicle-stimulating hormone (FSH) are secreted by the pituitary gland in response to hypothalamic gonadotropin releasing hormone (GnRH). While FSH acts directly on the germinal epithelium, LH stimulates secretion of testosterone by the Leydig cells. Testosterone stimulates sperm production and also feeds back the hypothalamus and pituitary to regulate GnRH secretion. FSH stimulates Sertoli cells to support spermatogenesis and to secrete inhibin B that negatively feedback FSH secretion

GOALS AND THE PROPER TIMING FOR FERTILITY EVALUATION

Generally, the proper timing for an infertile couple to seek medical advice is after 12 months of regular intercourse. However, immediate attention must be given if any risk factor for infertility is present, such as history of infertility with another partner, cryptorchidism, orchitis and advanced female age either more than or equal to 35 years.[6]

Advanced paternal age is not only associated with a decline in the fecundity potential but also with

Table 1 Etiologic classification of male infertility

1. **Disorders affecting sperm production**
   - i. Hypothalamic and pituitary causes
     - a. Lack of gonadotropin-releasing hormone secretion
       - Kallmann's syndrome
       - Isolated hypogonadotropic hypogonadism
       - Midline facial defects
       - Congenital syndromes such as Prader-Willi syndrome, Laurence-Moon-Biedl syndrome
     - b. Lack of luteinizing hormone (LH) secretion
       - Fertile eunuch syndrome
       - Isolated LH deficiency
     - c. Isolated follicle-stimulating hormone deficiency
     - d. Pituitary disease
       - Tumors
       - Infiltrative disorders
       - Infarction
       - Radiation
       - Hyperprolactinemia
       - Endocrinopathies-induced alterations in pituitary gland responsiveness, such as thyroid dysfunction, glucocorticoid excess, exogenous androgens or estrogens
   - ii. Testicular causes
     - a. Vascular causes: torsion, varicocele
     - b. Infection: mumps, orchitis
     - c. Genetic and congenital causes
       - Congenital causes
         - – Cryptorchidism
         - – Anorchia
         - – Polyorchidism
         - – Microorchidism
       - Genetic causes
         - – Chromosomal aneuploidy and structural defects
         - – Gene defects
         - – Y chromosome microdeletion
     - d. Medications
     - e. Castration, testicular trauma
     - f. Systemic diseases
     - g. Environmental factors
2. **Disorders affecting sperm transport**
   - i. Congenital
     - a. Bilateral absence of vas deferens
     - b. Unilateral absence of the vas
     - c. Prostatic/ejaculatory duct cysts
   - ii. Acquired
     - a. Iatrogenic (surgical procedures)
     - b. Infection
     - c. Trauma

Contd...

Contd...

     - d. Ejaculation
       - Anejaculation
       - Retrograde ejaculation
   - iii. Functional obstruction
   - iv. Coital factors
     - a. Impotence
     - b. Infrequent coitus
     - c. Improper coital techniques
3. **Disorders affecting sperm function**
   - i. Immune infertility
   - ii. Reactive oxygen species and oxidative stress
   - iii. Sperm DNA damage
   - iv. Fertilization defects
     - a. Zona pellucida binding
     - b. Hyperactivation
     - c. Acrosome reaction
     - d. Fusogenic ability
   - v. Immotile cilia syndrome
4. **Infertility of unknown origin**
   - i. Idiopathic
   - ii. Unexplained

Table 2 Distribution of diagnostic categories of couples seeking infertility evaluation in a male infertility clinic

Category	Numbers	Percentage
Varicocele	629	21.9
Infectious	72	2.5
Hormonal	54	1.9
Ejaculatory dysfunction	28	1.0
Systemic diseases	11	0.4
Idiopathic	289	10.0
Normal/Female factor	492	17.1
Immunologic	54	1.9
Obstruction	359	12.5
Cancer	11	0.4
Cryptorchidism	342	11.9
Genetic	189	6.6
Testicular failure	345	11.9
Total	2,875	

Source: ANDROFERT, Campinas, São Paulo, Brazil

increased incidence of miscarriage and inheritance of genetic diseases such as Down's syndrome as well as autism and schizophrenia.[35-40] The yearly decline in sperm parameters has been estimated to be 0.03 ml for volume and 0.7% for motility.[41] The probability of having abnormal sperm counts increases with age. It is 5% at age 30 years, 15% at age 50 years and 50% by age 80 years.[41] As such, the impact of paternal age on male fertility cannot be underestimated. Current recommendations for immediate evaluation include men with advanced paternal age, i.e. more than 45 years, because their fertility potential may be compromised.

The essential goals of male evaluation for infertility encompass the detection of both correctable and uncorrectable causes. The uncorrectable male infertility can be managed by using assisted conception or donor insemination. The identification of genetic and/or chromosomal abnormalities are crucial for proper counseling not only regarding the chances of conception but also for the health of offspring. Evaluation of males complaining of infertility may also identify underlying health-threatening medical pathologies such as endocrinopathies and malignancies.[42]

APPROACHING THE SUBFERTILE MALE

The basic evaluation of men with infertility complaint includes a detailed history, a thorough physical examination and at least two semen analyses. Additional laboratory and imaging testing may be ordered according to the initial findings. The role of the urologist in the management of the subfertile male cannot be under estimated. Whenever possible, he/she is responsible for diagnosing, counseling and treating the existing cause. When no specific treatment is available, the urologist is still responsible for referring the patient to a specialized assisted reproductive technology (ART) center, or for extracting the male gametes from the testicles or epididymides as a member of the ART center's multiprofessional team.

History

The physician's tasks during the medical interview are to address the patient's concerns, and to conduct scientific, courteous and nonjudgmental interview. A comprehensive medical history encompasses all aspects of the male's development from pregnancy to adult life. In Table 3, a comprehensive questionnaire for interviewing a male patient with infertility complaint is provided.

Table 3 Clinical Male Infertility History Outline (Adapted from Esteves SC, Miyaoka R, Agarwal A. An update on the clinical assessment of the infertile male. CLINICS 2011;66(4):691-700, with permission from the Editor)

Infertility History
- Age of partners, time attempting to conceive
- Contraceptive methods/duration
- Previous pregnancy (actual partner/other partner)
- Previous treatments
- Treatments/evaluation of female partner

Sexual History
- Potency, libido, lubricant use
- Ejaculation, timed intercourse, frequency of masturbation

Childhood and Development
- Cryptorchidism, hernia, testicular trauma
- Testicular torsion, infection (e.g. mumps)
- Sexual development, puberty onset

Personal History
- Systemic diseases (diabetes, cirrhosis, hypertension)
- Sexually transmitted diseases, tuberculosis, viral infections

Previous Surgeries
- Orchidopexy, herniorrhaphy, orchiectomy (testicular cancer, torsion)
- Retroperitoneal and pelvic surgery
- Other inguinal, scrotal and perineal surgery
- Bariatric surgery, bladder neck surgery, transurethral resection of the prostate

Gonadotoxic Exposure
- Pesticides, alcohol, cocaine, marijuana abuse
- Medication (chemotherapeutic agents, cimetidine, sulfasalazine, nitrofurantoin, allopurinol, colchicine, thiazide, β-blockers and α-blockers, calcium blockers, finasteride)
- Organic solvents, heavy metals
- Anabolic steroids, tobacco use
- High temperatures, electromagnetic energy
- Radiation (therapeutic, nuclear power plant workers), etc.

Family History
- Cystic fibrosis, endocrine and genetic diseases
- Infertility in the family

Current Health Status
- Respiratory infection, anosmia
- Galactorrhea, visual disturbances
- Obesity

Descriptive Elements

Male age, duration of infertility, primary vs. secondary infertility, as well as age and fertility status of the female partner have prognostic and diagnostic significance. Advanced male or female age and longstanding history of infertility are negative factors for fecundity. The secondary infertility carries a better prognosis than the primary infertility. The secondary male infertility is often associated with correctable causes such as varicocele, infection or ejaculatory problems. A history of early miscarriages, or occurrence of fetal genetic abnormalities may suggest a male factor contribution.[43,44]

The female partner's history of having successful pregnancies and live births renders male infertility more likely. Female age is the most important single variable influencing the outcome in assisted reproduction.[45] Nevertheless, it is now commonplace to see couples delaying family planning due to professional and economic reasons. This delay mainly jeopardizes the female fertilizing potential. There is a 50% reduction in fecundity in woman aged 35 years compared to those aged 25 years.[45]

Sexual and Coital Aspects

Although sexual and coital factors account for only 5% of infertility causes, it is mandatory to analyze these factors, as they may be the sole cause of the problem.[46] It is preferable to discuss these issues with both partners at the same interview, as this will help to disclose the misapprehension undertaken by the partners regarding the physiology of fertilization.

The clinician should address the concept of fertility window, and the importance of frequent and well-timed intercourse. Surprisingly, many couples have infrequent intercourse due to life stressors and irregular working hours, and are unaware of the importance of timed intercourse. The fertility window is defined as the 6-day period within the menstrual cycle when intercourse most likely results in a conception. It is estimated to range from 5 days before ovulation to the day of ovulation for normogonadotropic women.[47-49] The highest probability of a successful pregnancy can be anticipated if intercourse occurs 1 to 2 days prior to ovulation.[48,49] This phenomenon is based on short duration of human ovum longevity and survival that is estimated to be fewer than 16 hours.[50,51] On the other hand, human sperm can survive for up to 6 days in well-estrogenized cervical mucus.[52] This relatively protracted longevity and survival creates an adequate sperm reservoir for fertilization.

Therefore, it is advisable for couples to have intercourse every other day during the 6 days fertile window. Sperm counts are at their maximum after 5 days of ejaculatory abstinence. After that, sperm motility declines. Consequently, it is also advisable to abstain from ejaculation, not longer than 5 days, when attempting to conceive. Woman with regular menstrual cycle can estimate the fertile period by using basal body temperature and calendar calculations. However, these methods are both inaccurate and unreliable. The best methods to prospectively identify the entire fertile window for the purpose to achieve pregnancy would be either the fertility charting of vaginal discharge, or the elevation in urinary estrogen or luteinizing hormone (LH) surge.[51] The former identifies the changes in vaginal discharge that correspond with high ovarian hormones and can roughly estimate the fertile window. The latter method identifies the rises in urinary estradiol 3-glucuronide (E3G) and urine LH surge, and can prospectively predict the 3–6 days fertile window before ovulation and the day of ovulation.[51]

Nonetheless, the best advice for women with unknown fertile window is to have intercourse at a frequency of two to three times a week during the whole menstrual cycle. Unfortunately, some couples find it more stressful and intricate to adhere to frequent schedule of intercourse than to timely assured fruitful intercourse.

A detailed sexual history is also a valuable tool to identify sexual dysfunction problems. A decreased libido may be caused by complex interaction of social, emotional, psychological and hormonal factors. The decreased libido may also be the only sign of hypogonadism, which results in erectile dysfunction (ED) and decrease in the sexual drive. Although erectile dysfunction may be attributed to psychogenic problems, endocrinopathies such as hypogonadism, diabetes, hypothyroidism and hyperprolactinemia may also be involved. The incidence of ED increases with age; it is 52% in men of age between 40–70 years old, and about 2–27% in men less than 40 years old.[53,54]

Though the recommendation to increase the frequency of intercourse in the fertile window is evidence-based, no specific coital technique is praised. Whatever the position is, the ejaculated sperm in the proximal vagina can find the way to the oviduct within five minutes.[55] Consequent to increased coital frequency, vaginal dryness may direct the women to use vaginal lubricants. However, commercially available water-based lubricants are toxic to sperm. These lubricants may either induce poor sperm motility or chromatin damage and, correspondingly, loss of fertilizing potential of sperm.[56] Among the lubricants available in the market, hydroxyethyl cellulose-based lubricant was shown to have the lowest damaging effects on sperm motility and chromatin integrity.[57] Natural lubricants, such as saliva, vegetable oils (canola, vegetable, olive, safflower and peanut), as well as glycerin and petroleum jelly cause mild decrease in sperm motility.[56,58]

Ejaculatory Disorders

Natural fertilization requires successful deposition of semen into the proximal vagina. Therefore, ejaculatory dysfunction can interfere with this process and may render a male infertile. The patient should be asked about volume of the ejaculate during coitus and masturbation. Low semen volume may be attributed to either congenital or acquired obstructive lesion of the genital tract, male hypogonadism or due to retrograde ejaculation. Anejaculation, on the other hand, is a complete absence of antegrade and retrograde ejaculation and is caused by defective seminal emission from seminal vesicles, prostate and the ejaculatory ducts into the posterior urethra. This condition is usually associated with intact orgasm, and its etiology is related to neurogenic or drug induced effect.[59] Anejaculation should be differentiated from anorgasmia, which is a psychological disorder characterized by failure to attain orgasm and is usually associated with anejaculation.[60] The prevalence of premature ejaculation among subfertile males is reported to be around 50%.[61] However, premature ejaculation seems to be related to the stress imposed by the infertility condition rather than to be a primary cause.

Pediatric and Developmental Contribution

The questionnaire about childhood and pubertal development includes prenatal exposure to certain dietary, pharmaceutical and environmental factors that may lead to congenital urogenital anomalies, disordered hormonal milieu and even altered semen parameters. *In utero* exposure to diethylstilbestrol, a medication that has been banned from the market several years ago, leads to appearance of epididymal cyst, cryptorchidism and altered semen quality in the male offspring.[62] History of parental infertility or the mother being subjected to any infertility medical treatment may be associated with a decline in the semen parameters and reproductive potential in the male offspring.[63,64] It has been also assumed that maternal exposure to environmental endocrine disruptors, which are chemicals present in a variety of pesticides, plant constituents and plastic industry, could induce infertility in adult sons. Several compounds have estrogenic activity, as such, they are called xenoestrogens, and they have the ability to impair testicular development and sperm production.[65,66] Maternal cigarette smoking and alcohol consumption have been also linked to altered semen quality in the male progeny.[67-70]

The childhood history of congenital and acquired genitourinary disorders should also be taken into account. Cryptorchidism is the most common genitourinary disorder and affects about 1–3% of term infants. However, its prevalence among infertile men is 9.4%.[71-73] If cryptorchidism is treated by orchidopexy at an early age, there will be higher chance of maintenance spermatogenesis.[74] Though men with unilaterally repaired cryptorchidism have variable semen parameters; their paternity rate seems to be similar to that of general population.[75] However, in those with bilaterally repaired cryptorchidism a 35–53% decrease in the paternity rates (compared to the general population) is observed, with high incidence of disordered semen parameters such as oligozoospermia (31%) and azoospermia (42%).[76] Other rare urogenital anomalies such as microorchidism, polyorchidism, vanishing testis, prune belly syndromes, posterior urethral valve and bladder exstrophy are well known causes of impairment of male fertility potential.

Inquiries should also include questions about accidental and surgical trauma to the testes during childhood as well as about pediatric hernia repair, which is associated with 0.8–2% risk of injury to the inguinal or retroperitoneal vas deferens.[77] Unilateral vas injury may remain unnoticed in the presence of normally functioning contralateral testis and contralateral patent seminal duct. Bilateral pediatric hernia repair, particularly with the use of mesh, forms the highest risk of clinically evident vas injury and male infertility.[78] History of testicular torsion, whether treated by orchidopexy or orchiectomy can lead to abnormal semen analysis in 30–40% of the affected patients.[79]

Now, mumps orchitis during childhood is rare because of the widely conducted vaccination program. Prepubertal mumps orchitis has not been found to affect testicular function.[80,81] However, recent reports have raised concern about an increased incidence of postpubertal mumps orchitis after the age of 15 years.[82] Mumps of postpubertal onset is associated with orchitis in 25% of cases,[83] and in approximately 10–30% of cases, bilateral testicular involvement is documented.[84] Mumps orchitis can lead to subfertility in 13% and 30–87% of patients with unilateral and bilateral testicular involvement, respectively.[84,85]

The age of puberty onset is of paramount importance as it reflects the proper interaction and the integrity of the HPG axis. Most males reach pubertal development at age 11–12 years.[86] Constitutional delay of puberty is the most common cause for such condition and is usually confirmed by positive family history, delayed bone age and low or normal gonadotropins.[86] Nevertheless, this delay may be attributed to primary testicular failure such as Klinefelter syndrome, partial androgen resistance or other acquired causes, or secondary to hypothalamic or pituitary dysfunction. There are many acquired and congenital causes of hypothalamic and pituitary dysfunction such as Kallmann's syndrome, Prader-Willi syndrome, Laurence-Moon-Biedl syndrome, idiopathic hypogonadotropic hypogonadism and pituitary tumors.

Conversely, precocious puberty, which is characterized by appearance of secondary sex features before 9 years of age, is either caused by premature activation of HPG axis (true precocious puberty) or excessive sex steroid production (incomplete precocious puberty). True precocious puberty may cause testicular enlargement and normal spermatogenesis so early that a boy at age of 4 years can father children.[86,87] However, boys with incomplete or pseudoprecocious puberty may have pubic hair and penile enlargement, but no testicular enlargement or production of sperm.[87] Such condition is often caused by adrenogenital syndrome, a form of congenital adrenal hyperplasia, or Leydig cell hyperplasia or tumors. In pseudoprecocious puberty, there is excessive production of androgens, which suppress gonadotropins production. Therefore, there is a lack of stimulatory factor of testicular development and sperm production despite the virilized effects of androgens.

Most men may not memorize the exact timing of their puberty unless there is a marked delay or premature onset. While some of these conditions may respond to hormonal manipulation, others are resistant to hormonal therapy and more aggressive therapies such as sperm retrieval and assisted reproductive techniques may be needed.

Surgical Aspects

Certain surgical procedures in the vicinity of male reproductive organs may inadvertently injure these organs. Surgery in the pelvis, retroperitoneum, scrotum and groin may cause impairment in the male reproductive potential. Ejaculatory and erectile dysfunctions are known complications of retroperitoneal lymph node dissection, deep radical pelvic surgery, bladder neck reconstruction surgery and spinal surgery. Transurethral resection of the prostate and bladder neck incision are often complicated by retrograde ejaculation. Bilateral open or laparoscopic adult inguinal hernia repair, particularly with use of knitted mesh, may result in bilateral vas deferens injury and azoospermia. The prevalence of such condition is estimated to be 0.3%.[88] However, the unilateral injury may go unnoticed if the contralateral testis function and vas deferens are normal. Moreover, inguinal herniorrhaphy may contribute to testicular atrophy in 5% of cases.[89] On the other hand, scrotal surgery for hydrocele and epididymal cyst may injure scrotal vas deferens, epididymal tubules and testicular arteries precipitating vasal and epididymal obstruction as well as testicular atrophy. Considering all these fertility related surgical complications may help to find the cause, direct specific diagnostic investigations and thereby restore fertility potentials.

Medical Aspects

Medical history of urologic and systemic diseases in infertile men may be related to the infertility problem. Recurrent attacks of urinary tract, sexually transmitted infections (STI) and mixed accessory gland infections have all been linked to male infertility. Infected urine is associated with and constitutes a risk factor for genital tract infections. The STI are commonly caused by *Neisseria gonorrhoeae*, *Chlamydia trachomatis*, *Ureaplasma urealyticum*, human immunodeficiency virus (HIV) and other less common microorganisms. Urethral stricture, epididymo-orchitis and postorchitis decline in testicular function are well recognized complications of STI.[90] *Ureaplasma urealyticum* can have deleterious effects on sperm motility and DNA condensation leading to poor fertilization potentials.[91] Moreover, recent reports have shown that *Chlamydia trachomatis* infection is often detected in infertile men. *Chlamydia trachomatis* may attach to the spermatozoa and causes impairment in sperm motility, and DNA integrity as well as acrosome reaction (AR) insufficiency.[92,93] Mixed accessory gland infection (MAGI), which is a syndrome characterized by a chronic inflammatory process that involves the prostate, seminal vesicles or epididymides, is also caused by the same organisms causing STI such as gonococci, *Chlamydia* and gram-negative bacteria. This syndrome is found in about 10% of infertile men, and it is characterized by leukocytospermia, increased reactive oxygen species and high concentrations of inflammatory cytokines.[94,95] Symptoms suggestive of MAGI, such as urethral discharge, pain and/or pus or blood associated with the ejaculate, should be taken in consideration.

Human immunodeficiency virus is one of the STI that impairs male fertility by multiple mechanisms. Orchitis, hypogonadism, enhanced oxidative stress, oligozoospermia and even azoospermia have been described in association with HIV infection.[96,97]

Some men with autosomal dominant polycystic kidney disease may have low semen volume, oligozoospermia, asthenozoospermia and even impaired fertilization potential.[98]

Systemic medical diseases, such as renal insufficiency, liver cirrhosis and endocrinopathies such as thyroid dysfunction, Cushing syndrome and diabetes, are all associated with gonadal dysfunction and disordered spermatogenesis.[99-102] Men with a history of galactorrhea, headache and impaired vision may have prolactinoma. Gastrointestinal diseases, such as celiac disease, inflammatory bowel diseases and other malabsorption syndromes, are associated with delayed puberty, hypogonadism and impaired semen quality.[103,104]

Some respiratory diseases and male infertility may have common genetic origin. More specifically, some syndromes may cause chronic nasal polyps and sinopulmonary infections and sperm transport problems such as Young's syndrome that is associated with obstruction of the epididymides and vasa deferentia due to inspissated secretions; cystic fibrosis which is associated with congenital bilateral absence of the vas deferens; and ciliary dyskinesia syndromes that are characterized by immotile sperm. Other respiratory diseases may affect the fertility potential through centrally induced hypogonadotropic hypogonadism state such as sarcoidosis and obstructive sleep apnea.[105,106] Furthermore, chronic obstructive airway disease may cause pubertal delay and hypogonadism either through hypoxia, or corticosteroid-induced hypogonadotropic hypogonadism.[107] Men with active pulmonary tuberculosis may also have gonadal hormonal dysfunction attributed to central mechanism.[108]

Male infertility is also common in sickle cell anemia, presumably, due to intratesticular ischemia.[109,110] Prolonged fever may cause reversible impairment in semen quality.[111] Malignancy and its treatment, such as radiotherapy and chemotherapy, may also be a risk factor for male infertility due to transient or permanent alterations in sperm production and, less commonly, androgen insufficiency. Testicular cancer, Hodgkin's disease and acute leukemia are the most common malignancies in young adult patients. Men with testicular cancer may be oligozoospermic in 50% and azoospermic in 10–15% of cases before receiving any treatment.[112]

Some specific clinical features have genetic relations with male infertility such as anosmia (Kallmann's syndrome), deafness (deafness-infertility syndrome), early cataract (myotonia dystrophica), bronze discoloration of the skin (hemochromatosis), muscle weakness (myotonia dystrophica, mitochondrial disease) and certain birth marks or scaling skin (X-linked ichthyosis).

Use of Medication

Drugs and medications may undermine male reproductive function in various ways. Personal use of drugs and medications must be thoroughly elucidated. There are four mechanisms explaining their impact on male fertility:

1. By acting as direct gonadotoxins such as chemotherapeutic agents,
2. Through alterations in the hormonal control of testicular function such as exogenous anabolic steroids,
3. Inflicting erectile and ejaculatory dysfunction such as beta-blockers and alpha-blockers, or
4. Mitigating libido such as psychotherapeutic medications and recreational drugs.[113] Table 4 presents a comprehensive list of medications and drugs related to fertility impairment.

Inherited and Familial Aspects

Genetics play essential role in male subfertility. Therefore, exploring the personal history of certain inherited diseases that may affect the reproductive function as well as the family history of involuntary male childlessness are essential components of male fertility evaluation. The retrieved information from such enquiries may shed a light on the genetic etiology of male infertility.

Personal history of cystic fibrosis, Kallmann's syndrome, Klinefelter's syndrome, myotonia dystrophica, Kartagener's syndrome, or adult onset polycystic kidney disease may explain the etiology of childlessness in infertile men. History of recurrent miscarriages may also indicate male chromosomal abnormalities or DNA integrity defects.

The queries about family history must disclose the fertility status of men in the family pedigree of three generations that include first-degree relatives such as father, brothers as well as paternal and maternal uncles. Some studies detected familial clustering of cases of male subfertility due to known genetic, or even due to undiscovered genetic etiology. A single study has shown that 11.8% of 621 couples have involuntary childlessness in at least one first-degree and second-degree relatives on the husband side.[114] Another study demonstrated that men with impaired semen quality, reported higher incidence of subfertility among their brothers than that reported by male relatives of normozoospermic infertile men.[115]

Moreover, the husband's family history of multiple births defects also raises the concern about chromosomal disorders. Husband's parental consanguinity is also considered a risk factor for genetic male infertility.

Environmental Factors and Occupational Exposure

The worldwide rising incidence of male infertility has been recently attributed to environmental toxicants. Exposure to these harmful factors must be assessed such as excessive heat from saunas and hot tubs, use of pesticide and organic solvents, radiation from X-rays or from excessive use of cell phone and heavy metals intoxication such as lead or cadmium.

Certain occupations constitute a hazard for male reproductive health. The foundry and steel workers, specialized welders, and bakers reported to have

Table 4 Effects of medication on male fertility

Medication	Gonadotoxic	Altered HPG axis	Decreased libido	Erectile dysfunction	Fertilization potential
Recreational/illicit drugs					
Alcohol	+	+	+	+	–
Cigarette smoking	+	–	–	–	–
Marijuana	+	–	–	–	–
Opiates	–	+	+	–	–
Cocaine	–	–	–	+	–
Antihypertensive drugs					
Thiazide diuretics	–	–	–	+	–
Spironolactone	–	+	+	+	–
Beta-blockers	–	–	+	+	–
Calcium channel blockers	–	–	–	–	+
Alpha-adrenergic blockers	–	–	–	+	–
Psychotherapeutic drugs					
Antipsychotics	–	+	+	+	–
Tricyclic antidepressant	–	+	+	+	–
MAOIs	–	–	–	+	–
Phenothiazine	–	+	–	–	–
Lithium	–	–	+	+	–
Chemotherapeutic drug					
Alkylating agents	+	–	–	–	–
Antimetabolites	+	–	–	–	–
Vinca alkaloids	+	–	–	–	–
Hormones					
Anabolic steroids	+	+	–	+	–
Testosterone	+	–	–	–	–
Antiandrogens	–	+	+	–	–
Progesterone derivatives	–	–	+	+	–
Estrogens	–	+	+	+	–
Antibiotics					
Nitrofurantoin	+	+	–	–	–
Erythromycin	+	–	–	–	–
Tetracycline	–	–	–	–	+
Gentamicin	+	–	–	–	–
Miscellaneous medications					
Cimetidine	+	+	–	–	–
Allopurinol	–	–	–	–	+

HPG: hypothalamic-pituitary-gonadal axis; MAOIs: monoamine oxidase inhibitors;(+) means that the medication has an effect; (–) means that the medication has no effect

heat-induced decline in semen quality. Sedentary occupations have claimed to increase scrotal temperature and affect the testicular function. Other occupations, including exposure to organic solvents, such as painters, printers, dyes manufacturers are also considered hazardous to male reproductive health.

Cigarette smoking history should be verified, and the patient should be encouraged to quit smoking. As smokers have higher incidence of testicular atrophy, altered semen parameters and sperm function, as well as sperm with oxidative DNA damage and chromosomal aneuploidy.[116] Alcohol, on the other hand, should be taken in moderation because alcohol may suppress testosterone production and consequently impair spermatogenesis.[117]

Lastly, obesity and malnutrition must be considered as both can have detrimental effect on male reproductive function. Such conditions may result in deficiency of vitamins and micronutrients which impairs the highly active biological process of spermatogenesis.

Female Factor Infertility

A comprehensive female evaluation by the gynecologist is an essential step in the integral evaluation of the infertile couple.

Physical Examination

General Aspects

Initially, the physical examination must be performed in a warm room and the patient is asked to undress and stand with his arms outstretched. This position enables the physician to measure the patient's height, weight and arm span as well as to observe abnormal body hair distribution, abnormal body habitus, muscular hypotonic posture, fat distribution and skin pigmentation. Physical signs of hypogonadism depend on age of onset in relation to puberty. Prepubertal hypogonadism onset is characterized by eunuchoidism (arm span exceeds body height by more than 5 cm) due to delayed closure of the epiphyseal plates in long bones with sparse facial, pubic and axillary hair distribution pattern. In contrast, postpubertal hypogonadism (adult onset) may not affect the anthropometric measurements; however, decline in the muscle bulk and bone mass with loss of beard and pubic hair, and thinning of facial skin may be visible. Both conditions affect skin color and texture, due to poor development of androgen-dependent sebaceous gland, resulting in dryness, wrinkling and pallor of the skin. Although testicular and penile size may not be affected to a great extent in adult onset, hypogonadism, preadolescent hypogonadism usually culminates in infantile gonads and penis.

Although rare, particular attention should be paid to the diagnosis of specific inherited syndromes that negatively impact the male reproductive potential. Such conditions include Prader-Willi syndrome, which is characterized by obesity, hypogonadism, short stature, skin hypopigmentation and muscle hypotonia, and Laurence-Moon-Biedl syndrome featured by obesity, mental retardation, and retinitis pigmentosa.

The physical examination of head and neck includes testing for smell, visual field defects, midline craniofacial abnormalities and thyroid enlargement. Anosmia is one of the presenting features of Kallmann's syndrome. Blurred vision and visual field loss are signs of pituitary and intracranial tumors. The combination of galactorrhea, visual field defects and infertility is suggestive of prolactinoma. Thyroid dysfunction is accompanied by relative androgen deficiency and impairment of spermatogenesis.

Chest is examined for the presence of gynecomastia and galactorrhea. The signs of chronic sinopulmonary infections, in association with male infertility, may reveal underlying genetic syndromes such as cystic fibrosis, Young's syndrome and Kartagener's syndrome.

Abdomen is meticulously inspected and palpated to detect signs of chronic liver diseases, such as liver enlargement, and splenomegaly or signs of polycystic kidney diseases.

Genitalia

The genital examination, including digital rectal examination, should be carried out. The inguinal and genital regions must be carefully inspected, in order to identify scars from previous surgical interventions, such as hydrocele correction, inguinal hernia repa irs and surgery for undescended testicle. They may account for damage to the testicle blood supply and to the vas deferens. The genital examination may reveal the presence of a hypospadiac urethral meatus, pathologic curvature of the phallus or active sexually transmitted disease. These factors may ultimately result in misplacement of spermatozoa inside the vaginal vault following ejaculation.

Testis volume can be estimated with the aid of an orchidometer or can be measured by using a pachymeter (Figure 4A). A normal sized adult testicle should have a length of 4 cm and a width of 2.5 cm resulting in a volume around 20 ml. They should present with firm consistency. Eighty-five percent of the testicular parenchyma is involved with spermatogenesis. There is no lower limit for testicular volume to exclude the presence of spermatozoa. As such, testicle size cannot be relied on as a clinical marker to preclude a trial of sperm retrieval.[118]

Bilateral testicular atrophy may be caused by primary or secondary testicular failure. When serum testosterone is low, seminal fluid is often of small volume as well. Endocrine workup helps to distinguish both conditions. High follicle-stimulating hormone (FSH) levels accompanied by normal or low testosterone levels imply primary testicular failure. These patients should be offered genetic evaluation for chromosomal abnormalities and Y chromosome microdeletions. The combined low serum FSH and testosterone levels suggest hypogonadotropic hypogonadism, particularly, if bilateral atrophic testicles are present. In this scenario, serum LH is often low. These men should undergo cranial imaging and serum prolactin measurement to exclude pituitary gland disease as in Kallmann's syndrome.[119]

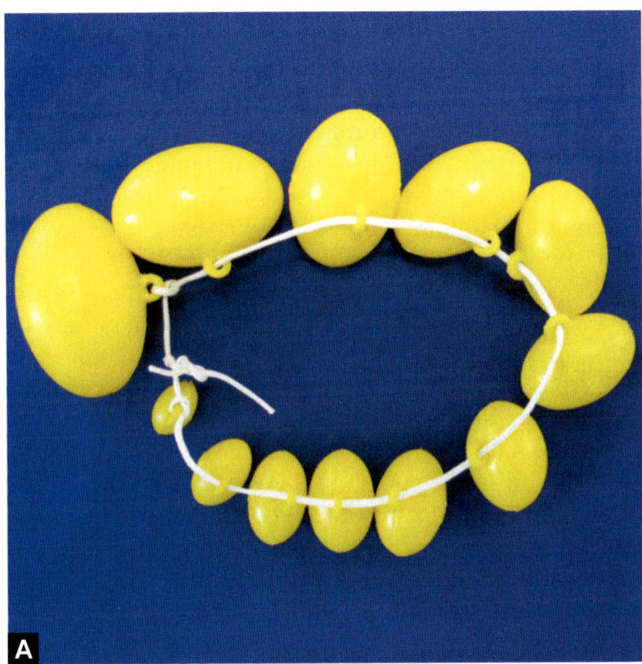

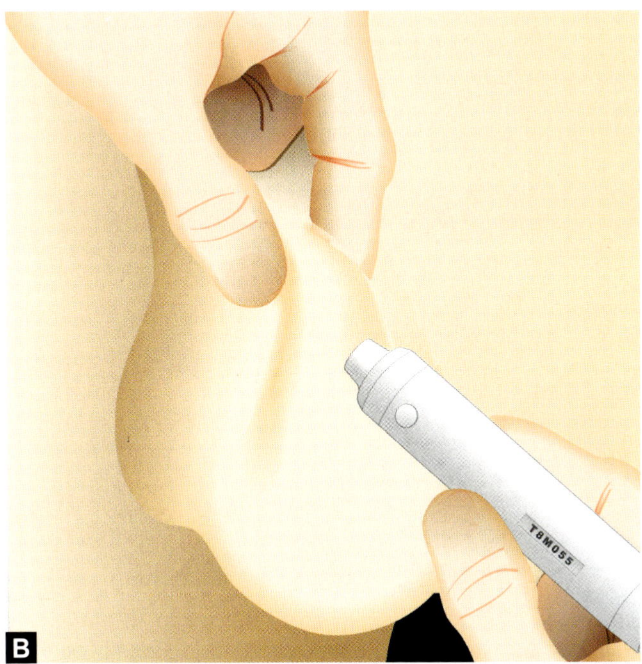

Figures 4A and B Useful tools for the physical examination of the subfertile male. (A) Photograph of the Prader Orchidometer. It is used to measure the volume of the testicles and consists of a chain of 12 numbered beads of increasing size from 1–25 ml. The beads are compared with the testicles of the patient and the volume is read off the bead, which matches most closely in size. Prepubertal sizes are 1–3 ml, pubertal sizes are 4–12 ml and adult sizes are 15–25 ml; (B) Schematic illustration depicting the use of the 9 MHz pencil-probe Doppler stethoscope for varicocele examination. The patient is examined in the upright position and the conducting gel is applied at the upper aspect of scrotum. A venous "rush" may be listened during Valsalva maneuver indicating blood reflux (Reprint with permission from Esteves SC, Miyaoka R, Agarwal A. An update on the clinical assessment of the infertile male. CLINICS 2011;66(4):691-700)

The epididymides have to be evaluated according to their size and consistency as well. The obstructed epididymis is augmented and ingurgitated (soft). A healthy epididymis free of trauma, infection or obstruction should be firm. Partial regression of an epididymis may represent a scenario of CBAVD. The vasa are easily palpable inside the posterior aspect of the spermatic cord as a distinct, firm, round, "spaghetti-like" structure. Unilateral or bilateral congenital absence of the vas results in oligozoospermia or azoospermia, respectively. Narrowing areas of the vasa deferentia may represent an infection or traumatic sequelae.

Absence of the vasa deferentia or vasal agenesis is a clinical diagnosis and does not depend on any complementary imaging study. However, 25% of men with unilateral vasal agenesis and about 10% of those with CBAVD also have unilateral renal agenesis and should undergo an abdominal ultrasound to identify this condition.[120]

Each spermatic cord has to be inspected to assess volume and consistency and to detect existing lipomas or varicocele.

Varicocele may be identified by physical examination with the patient standing in a warm room.[121] A physical examination alone provides a sensitivity and specificity of approximately 70%.[122] Varicoceles diagnosed by this method are termed "clinical" and may be graded according to the size. Valsalva maneuver may reveal differences in blood volume in each cord. Internal spermatic veins and cremasteric veins are filled up, whenever the patient stands. In varicocele patients, a venous dilation exists and may be enhanced during Valsalva maneuver. Large varicoceles (grade III) are varicose veins seen through the scrotal skin (Figure 5). Moderate varicoceles (grade II) and small-sized varicoceles (grade I) are dilated veins palpable without and with the aid of the Valsalva maneuver, respectively.[123] No standardized diagnostic method has been defined for the identification of varicocele.[124]

Lastly, digital rectal examination should assess the pelvic muscle tone in cases of suspected erectile dysfunction and detect any palpable masses including prostatic cysts that may obstruct the ejaculatory ducts.

Investigation

This initial workup consists of semen fluid analysis. Additional testing may be needed depending on the results of semen analysis or the information obtained by history and physical examination.

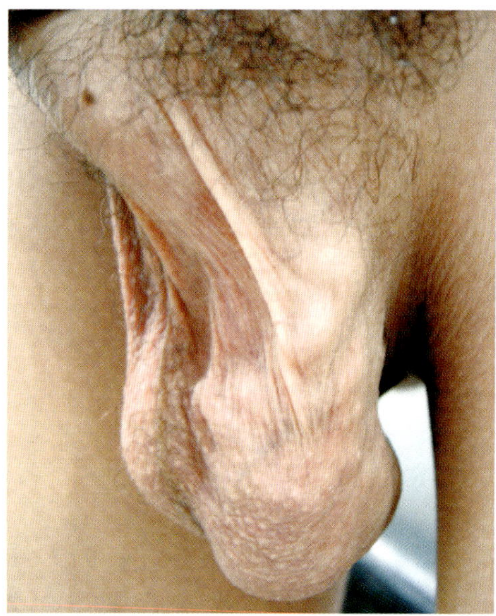

Figure 5 Photograph of a large left grade III varicocele that can be seen through the scrotal skin (Reprinted with permission from Esteves SC, Miyaoka R, Agarwal A. An update on the clinical assessment of the infertile male. CLINICS 2011;66(4):691-700)

Seminal Fluid Analysis

Semen is basically composed of spermatozoa and secretory fluid of the accessory sex glands. The semen analysis is considered as the cornerstone of the laboratory evaluation, although it is not a sperm functional test.[125] It provides information of the functional status of the germ inative cells, epididymides and accessory sexual glands. Semen analysis is of great value on the male initial investigation and its results are often taken as a surrogate measure of male fecundity and pregnancy risk. Reference intervals for values of semen parameters from a fertile population may provide data, on which prognosis of fertility or diagnosis of infertility can be extrapolated. Therefore, it is recommended that evaluation should be undertaken in a specialized andrology laboratory and should be analyzed by well-trained technicians under rigorous quality control standards.[126]

Nonetheless, the prognostic value of semen components such as sperm number, motility and morphology, as surrogate markers of male fertility, is confounded in several ways; the fertility potential of a man is influenced by sexual activity, the function of accessory sex glands and other defined, as well as yet unrecognized conditions. Routine semen analysis itself has its own limitations, and does not account for putative sperm dysfunctions such as immature chromatin or a fragmented DNA. Results from at least two, preferably three separate semen analyses must be obtained before a definitive conclusion can be drawn, as wide biological variability may exist within the same individual. The interval between the semen analyses is arbitrary and is generally recommended to be 1–2 weeks. Ejaculatory abstinence should be a minimum of 2 days to a maximum of 7 days, ideally 2–3 days.[127] Longer abstinence periods lead to higher ejaculatory volume and increased spermatozoa quantity, but motility is usually decreased. The specimen is generally collected by masturbation inside a sterile recipient with a wide opening in order to avoid spillage outside the container that otherwise can be misinterpreted as hypospermia. The collection should be preferentially done in a proper collection room and no lubricant should be used. If collected at home, the specimen should be brought to the laboratory within 30 minutes, and should be kept close to the body in an effort to maintain physiological temperature during transportation. The specimen must be identified and allowed to liquefy for 30–60 minutes before analysis is undertaken. Routine semen analysis should include:

- Physical characteristics of semen, including liquefaction, viscosity, pH, color and odor
- Specimen volume
- Sperm count
- Sperm motility and progression
- Sperm morphology
- Leukocyte quantification
- Fructose detection in cases where no spermatozoa is found especially if the total volume is less than 1 ml.

The criteria used for normality according to the World Health Organization (WHO) have been recently updated,[127] as shown in Table 5. Approximately 2,000 men from eight countries, whose partners had a time-to-pregnancy of either less than or equal to 12 months, were chosen as individuals to provide reference distributions for semen parameters. One-sided lower reference limits (the fifth centile) were generated and have been proposed to be considered the cutoff limits for normality (Table 5). Apart from the total sperm number per ejaculate, the limits of these newly released reference values are lower than the previously presented ones[128-130] but are in agreement with recent observations on the seminal profile of fertile men.[131-133]

The morphometric description of spermatozoa, according to the strict criteria described by Kruger et al.[134] was definitely incorporated in the new WHO guidelines. The low proportions of normal spermatozoa, as defined by those selected in endocervical mucus, inevitably produce very low reference limits for a fertile population. With this method, similar low values of 3–5% normal forms have been found by others to be optimal cutoff values to discriminate fertile from infertile men, whose spermatozoa were used for *in vitro* fertilization,[135] intrauterine insemination[136] and in spontaneous

Table 5 Cutoff values for semen parameters as published in consecutive World Health Organisation (WHO) manuals (Adapted from Esteves SC, Miyaoka R, Agarwal A. An update on the clinical assessment of the infertile male. CLINICS 2011;66(4):691-700, with permission from the Editor)

Semen parameters	WHO, 1992	WHO, 1999	WHO, 2010*
Volume	≥ 2 ml	≥ 2 ml	1.5 ml
Sperm concentration/ml	≥ 20 x 10^6/ml	≥ 20 x 10^6/ml	15 x 10^6/ml
Total sperm concentration	≥ 40 x 10^6	≥ 40 x 10^6	39 x 10^6
Total motility (% motile)	≥ 50%	≥ 50%	40%
Progressive motility†	≥ 25% (grade a)	≥ 25% (grade a)	32% (a + b)
Vitality (% alive)	≥ 75%	≥ 75%	58%
Morphology	≥ 30%‡	14%§	4%"
Leukocyte count	< 1.0 x 10^6/ml	< 1.0 x 10^6/ml	< 1.0 x 10^6/ml

*Lower reference limit obtained from the lower fifth centile value
† Grade a = rapid progressive motility (> 25 μm/s); grade b = slow/sluggish progressive motility (5-25 μm/s); Normal = 50% motility (grades a + b) or 25% progressive motility (grade a) within 60 min of ejaculation
‡ Arbitrary value
§ No actual value given, but multicenter studies refer to > 14% (strict criteria) for *in vitro* fertilization
"Normal shaped spermatozoa according to Tygerberg (Kruger) strict criteria

pregnancies.[137] Interpretation of the reference ranges requires an understanding that they merely provide a description of the semen characteristics of recent fathers. The reference limits should not be overinterpreted to distinguish fertile from infertile men accurately, but they do represent semen characteristics associated with a couple's achieving pregnancy within 12 months of unprotected sexual intercourse; as such, the limits provide only a standardized guide regarding a man's fertility. None of these values were able to solely distinguish fertile and infertile men, although morphology was suggested to be the most important. The coexistence of more than one altered seminal parameter significantly increases the risk for infertility.[131] A man's semen characteristics need to be interpreted in conjunction with his clinical information. The reference limits provided by the WHO manual are from semen samples initiating natural conceptions. As such, they may indicate whether a man would need infertility treatment, but they should not be used to determine the nature of that treatment.

Leukocyte count should also be added to the routine semen analysis. Leukocytospermia (> 1 million leukocytes/ml of semen) incidence in infertile men vary between 3% and 23% and has been correlated with clinical and subclinical genital infections, elevated levels of reactive oxygen species, antisperm antibodies and deficient sperm function.[138] Neutrophils predominate among the inflammatory cells and may be both identified and quantified through different methods and coloring techniques. The Endtz test is one of the most used as it is a simple and low-cost option to detect the presence of peroxidase within neutrophils.[139]

In azoospermic patients, diagnosis must be confirmed by lack of any spermatozoa on centrifuged seminal fluid on two separate occasions at high powered microscopic field evaluation. The WHO recommends centrifugation for 15 minutes at 3000g or greater.[119] Azoospermia with low ejaculate volume (< 1.0 ml) not related to hypogonadism or CBAVD can be caused by ejaculatory dysfunction, although the most common cause is ejaculatory duct obstruction (EDO). When suspected, EDO can be confirmed by assessing seminal pH and fructose as normal seminal vesicle secretions are alkaline and contain fructose.

Endocrine Evaluation

Endocrine evaluation should be performed in the following scenarios:

- Sperm concentration less than 10 million/ml
- Erectile dysfunction
- Hypospermia (semen volume < 1ml)
- Signs and symptoms of endocrinopathies or hypogonadism.

The minimal evaluation includes serum FSH and total testosterone. They reflect germ cells and Leydig cells status respectively. If testosterone level is low, a second analysis will be recommended along with free testosterone, LH, estradiol and prolactin measurements. Isolated FSH elevation is usually indicative of severe germ cell damage. Elevated FSH and LH levels associated with low-normal or below-normal testosterone levels implicate diffuse testicular failure which may have a congenital (e.g. Klinefelter syndrome) or acquired cause. Concomitant low levels of FSH and LH may implicate hypogonadotropic hypogonadism. This may also be congenital, or secondary to pituitary diseases. In these cases, a complete workup of pituitary function is recommended including serum measurement of adrenocorticotropic hormone, thyroid-stimulating hormone, growth hormone and brain magnetic resonance.[140] Gonadotropin values within normal range suggest extraductal obstruction in azoospermic subjects. However, patients with sperm maturation arrest and 10% of those diagnosed with Sertoli-cell-only syndrome may present with nonelevated hormonal measurements. Serum estradiol measurement should be done in obese patients and in those presenting with gynecomastia or hypogonadism. Infertile patients, in whom testosterone to estradiol ratio is less than 10, can harbor significant but reversible seminal alterations.[141] Vaucher et al.[142] suggested that hyperestrogenism secondary to a higher conversion of testosterone into estradiol in Klinefelter syndrome patients inhibits testosterone production via a negative feedback pathway and may indicate overexpression of aromatase CYP19 in the testis at a molecular level. As such, there would be scientific rationale for use of aromatase inhibitors in Klinefelter syndrome patients.[141]

In azoospermic men with normal ejaculate volume, a FSH serum level greater than twice the upper normal limit is reliably diagnostic of dysfunctional spermatogenesis and, when found, diagnostic testicular biopsy is usually unnecessary although no consensus exists in this matter.[119] If FSH level is normal, a unilateral biopsy on the larger testis may be recommended as there is no guarantee of normal spermatogenesis.

Hyperprolactinemia is a rare cause of infertility in healthy men and is more commonly related to erectile dysfunction and pituitary diseases. These men may present micropituitary or macropituitary prolactin-secreting adenomas. Serum prolactin must be determined in infertile men with a complaint of concomitant sexual dysfunction or in those who have clinical or laboratory evidence of pituitary disease. Although hormonal alterations may be present in approximately 10% of men who undergo investigation, clinically significant dysfunctions affect less than 2% (Table 2).[143]

Genetic Evaluation

Genetic factors commonly associated with male infertility include chromosomal aberrations, genetic mutations and Y chromosome microdeletions. Chromosomal aberrations are assessed through peripheral blood lymphocyte culture and Giemsa band staining (G band karyotyping). Genetic mutations and Y chromosome microdeletions assessments are also performed by analysis of peripheral blood sampling. DNA is amplified using polymerase chain reaction technique. Table 6 summarizes the indications and recommended tests for genetic evaluation.

Chromosomal abnormalities can be found in about 6% of infertile men and its prevalence inversely correlates with sperm count. Azoospermic men can present chromosomal alterations in as much as 16% of cases.[144] Sex chromosomal aneuploidy (Klinefelter syndrome; 47,XXY) is the most frequent chromosomal disorder present in infertile men and is generally associated with hypotrophic or atrophic testicles, elevated serum FSH levels and azoospermia, although spermatogenesis can be differently affected in patients with a mosaic karyotype (46,XY/47,XXY).

The mutation of the cystic fibrosis gene located on the long arm of chromosome 7 is the most commonly found genetic mutation. According to the extension of the mutation, cystic fibrosis can be manifested at its full clinical presentation (an autosomal recessive potentially fatal disease) or in a mild form, where congenital bilateral absence of the vasa deferentia exists and affects approximately 1.3% of infertile men. Cystic fibrosis transmembrane conductance regulator (*CFTR*) gene mutations compromise the development of Wolffian ducts derived structures (efferent ducts, epididymides and vasa deferentia) and may even be implicated in seminal vesicles hypoplasia or agenesis, and unilateral renal agenesis. Approximately 80% of men presenting with CBVAD have a CFTR mutation. As the diagnostic methods routinely used are not 100% sensitive, a man with CBAVD should be assumed to harbor a CFTR mutation. Genetic testing should be offered to female partners to exclude the possibility of these being carriers (approximately 4% risk) before using their husband sperm for assisted conception. Genetic counseling should be offered after genetic testing.[119] Recent data suggest that azoospermic men with idiopathic obstruction and those presenting the triad of chronic sinusitis, bronchiectasis and obstructive azoospermia (Young's Syndrome) have an elevated risk for CFTR mutation.[144]

The long and short arms of Y chromosome are respectively related to spermatogenesis and testicle development. The Y chromosome region related to infertility is named azoospermia factor (AZF) locus. The AZF locus can present complete or partial microscopic deletions, isolated or in combination, and in nonoverlapping subregions called AZFa, AZFb, AZFc and AZFd (Figure 6). These subregions contain multiple genes controlling different steps of spermatogenesis.

Table 6 Indications for genetic testing in male infertility (Adapted from Esteves SC, Miyaoka R, Agarwal A. An update on the clinical assessment of the infertile male. CLINICS 2011;66(4):691-700, with permission from the Editor)

Indications	Recommended tests
Men with infertility of unknown etiology and sperm concentration less than 10 million/ml who are candidates for assisted reproductive technology (ART)	Y chromosome microdeletion and G band karyotype
Nonobstructive azoospermia in a male considering testicular sperm retrieval for ART	Y chromosome microdeletion and G band karyotype
Azoospermic or oligozoospermic men with absence of at least one vas deferens at physical examination	CFTR gene mutation
Azoospermic men with signs of normal spermatogenesis (e.g. obstructive azoospermia of unknown origin)	CFTR gene mutation
History of recurrent miscarriage or personal/familiar history of genetic syndromes	G band karyotype

CFTR: cystic fibrosis transmembrane conductance regulator

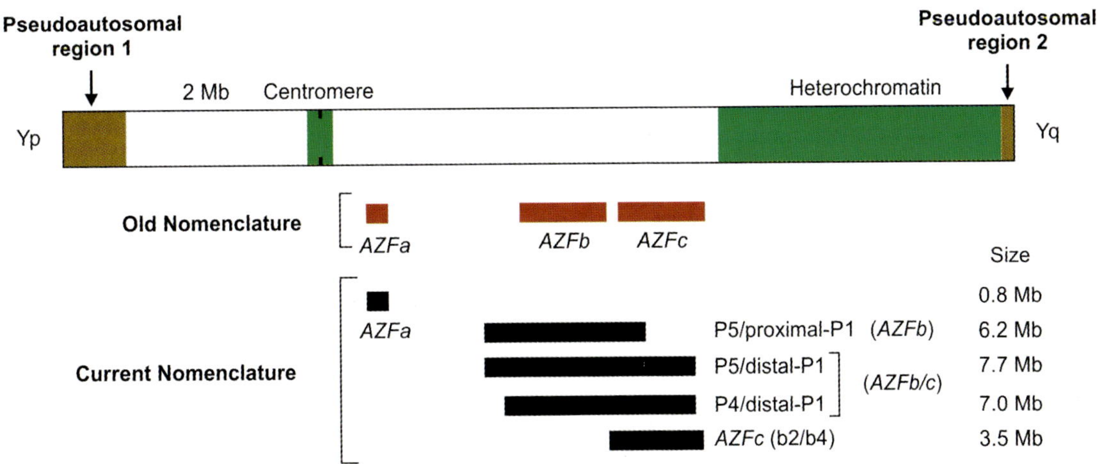

Figure 6 Illustration of the Y chromosome in humans and the regions involved in fertility and infertility. Interstitial or terminal deletions that include AZFa usually produce the severe phenotype of Sertoli-cell-only syndrome. Interstitial or terminal deletions that include AZFb and/or AZFb+c (hereafter, designated AZFb/c) are mediated by recombination between palindromic repeats, either P5/proximal-P1, P5/distal-P1, or P4/distal-P1. These deletions are associated to the maturation arrest phenotype and azoospermia. Interstitial or terminal deletions that include AZFc only are mediated by recombination between the b2/b4 palindromic repeats and result in a variable phenotype, ranging from azoospermia and Sertoli-cell-only syndrome to severe or mild oligozoospermia.

(Adapted from Repping S, Skaletsky H, Lange J, et al. Recombination between palindromes P5 and P1 on the human Y chromosome causes massive deletions and spermatogenic failure. Am J Hum Genet. 2002;71(4):906-22. With permission from Elsevier)

The most common Y chromosome deletion in infertile men is the one affecting the deleted in azoospermia (DAZ) gene located in AZFc region. Severe oligozoospermia or azoospermia can be seen in such cases. Y chromosome microdeletions can be found in 6% of men presenting with severe oligozoospermia (< 1 million/ml) and 15% of those with azoospermia.[144] For sperm counts between 1 million/ml and 5 million/ml, the detection rate drops down to 1.7%.[145] Detection of Y chromosome microdeletions provides predictive information on the success of obtaining spermatozoa from the testicle for intracytoplasmic sperm injection (ICSI). AZFa and AZFb microdeletions present as azoospermia and are associated with germ cell aplasia and maturation arrest, respectively. In such cases, sperm retrieval attempt is not indicated because the chances of finding testicular sperm are unlikely.[146,147] In case of AZFc microdeletion, sperm can be retrieved in approximately 71% of patients.[145] Clinical pregnancy rates after ICSI are virtually the same as for idiopathic nonobstructive azoospermic patients who can have their sperm retrieved as well.

Genetic testing also provides information for genetic counseling, as sons of men with Y chromosome microdeletion will inherit the abnormality and may also be infertile.[148,149]

The prevalence of structural abnormalities in the autosomes, such as inversions and translocations, is also higher in infertile men than in the general population. Gross karyotypic abnormalities are related to an elevated risk for miscarriages and for having children with both chromosomal and congenital defects. As such, men with nonobstructive azoospermia (NOA) or severe oligozoospermia should be karyotyped before their sperm are used for ICSI.[119]

Imaging

Transrectal, scrotal and renal ultrasonography: The indications for transrectal ultrasonography (TRUS) include:

- Low semen volume (< 1.5 ml)
- Abnormal digital rectal examination
- Ejaculatory disorders (anejaculation, hematospermia, painful ejaculation)

It allows for evaluation of the distal extraductal system (seminal vesicles and ejaculatory ducts). Ejaculatory duct obstruction (EDO) EDO may be congenital or acquired, and present either as complete or partial obstruction. The characteristic feature of EDO in TRUS is the enlargement of the seminal vesicles; however visualization of cysts at the level of ejaculatory ducts may coexist.[150] When CBAVD is diagnosed, TRUS can reveal abnormalities at the level of seminal vesicles such as hypoplasia or agenesis. A recent study has suggested that combination of scrotal and TRUS may not only distinguish obstructive from NOA but also determine the etiologic classification of obstructive azoospermia (OA). In this condition, ultrasonographic anatomic abnormalities are more commonly seen than in NOA patients (92.2% vs 2.8%, $p < 0.001$). Sensitivity, specificity and accuracy of combined assessment in discriminating between OA and NOA were 95.3%, 97.2% and 96.0%, respectively.[151] Seminal vesicle aspiration and seminal vesiculography may be performed under TRUS guidance and may help to establish the diagnosis of EDO.[152] In azoospermic men, finding of a large number of sperm in the seminal vesicle aspirate, strongly suggests EDO. Concomitant seminal vesiculography can determine the site of obstruction.

The indication for scrotal ultrasonography is to evaluate palpable nodules or testicular masses. Its use for subclinical varicocele diagnosis is controversial, as several studies demonstrated no clinical benefit from surgical treatment in this situation.[122] When there is doubtful physical examination such as in obese patients or difficulty to assess the contralateral side of a clinically detectable varicocele then ultrasonography is useful, as correction of a subclinical varicocele concomitant to a clinical contralateral one might be justified in this scenario. The commonly accepted color-Doppler ultrasonography criterion for varicocele (maximum vein diameter of 3 mm or greater) has a sensitivity of about 50% and specificity of 90% compared to physical examination.[153] A pencil-probe Doppler (9 MHz) stethoscope is an inexpensive tool that may aid in the diagnosis of the varicocele. The patient is examined in the upright position, and a venous "rush" representing blood reflux is heard with or without the Valsalva maneuver (Figure 4B). Although simple and easily performed in the office, Hirsh et al. demonstrated that more than 50% of men without clinical varicoceles exhibited a Valsalva maneuver Doppler-positive reflux.[154] None of these adjunctive diagnostic methods can differentiate between clinical and subclinical varicoceles. The significance of a positive test result using any of these adjuvant techniques in infertile men remains uncertain.

Urinary tract ultrasonography is indicated to evaluate renal status in patients diagnosed with CBAVD. Renal agenesis may be present in 10% of patients with CBAVD and 25% of those with unilateral absence of vas deferens.[120]

Magnetic resonance imaging: Use of magnetic resonance imaging (MRI) in infertility investigation has gained importance in the recent years. Situations such as varicocele, EDO, seminal vesicle agenesis and undescended testis are male infertility related conditions and can be incidentally seen.[155] Pelvic MRI helps to clarify in detail pictorial changes initially seen at TRUS (Figure 7). Moreover, MRI has traditionally been used to exclude cranial pathologies manifested by hormonal changes including low testosterone levels, low serum LH and FSH values, and high prolactin level.

There is evidence of the optimized usefulness of pituitary MRI in men with hypogonadism when prolactin levels are greater than twice the normal range or when there are worrisome symptoms suggesting intracranial abnormality (headache, visual disturbances, diffuse metabolic derangements and other).[156] In general, pituitary abnormalities can be identified in 25% of hypogonadal men. Of these, however, empty sella and pituitary nonfunctional microadenomas require no specific treatment and make one wonder about the cost-effectiveness of their diagnosis.

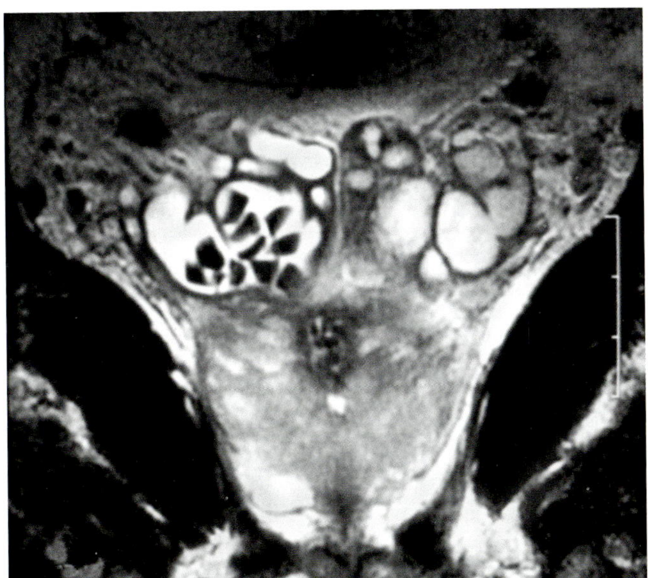

Figure 7 Magnetic resonance imaging showing enlarged seminal vesicles with calculosis (Reprint with permission from Esteves SC, Miyaoka R, Agarwal A. An update on the clinical assessment of the infertile male. CLINICS 2011;66(4):691-700)

Nuclear magnetic resonance spectroscopy has been recently proposed as a possible tool to identify metabolic signatures associated with various histological states in infertile men. Based on *ex vivo* analysis of testicular biopsy specimens, concentrations of 19 tissue metabolites were acquired and then reassessed in men with a diagnosis of NOA. A singular pattern could be determined for two testis histological states: normal and Sertoli-cell-only syndrome. Proliferating germ cells are related to high phospholipid synthesis and with elevated phosphocholine. Normal spermatogenesis spectroscopic pattern presents high peaks of phosphocoline as opposed to Sertoli-cell-only syndrome. Further research in this area may aid in the identification of a distinct metabolic signature for sperm existence sites, regardless of testis histopathology.[157]

Vasography: It is indicated in selected cases of obstructive azoospermia. It can also be performed when there is reason to suspect of unilateral obstruction (e.g. previous surgical intervention) in severe oligozoospermic men with a hypotrophic contralateral testis. Vasography and seminal vesiculography are usually undertaken by scrotal or transrectal routes, but can also be performed transurethrally or perineally. The contrast solution flows through vas deferens, seminal vesicles and ejaculatory duct delineating the anatomy and allowing for identification of obstructive segments. The presence of sperm on microscopic analysis of the fluid recovered from vas deferens and seminal vesicles indicates distal obstruction and rules out testicle or epididymal obstruction. Currently, isolated diagnostic vasography is not recommended, but may be performed concomitantly with surgical approach for obstruction resolution.

Sperm Function Laboratory Testing

In 10–20% of infertile couples who undergo basic investigation, all diagnostic workup will yield normal results and couples will be etiologically classified as having unexplained infertility. Additional tests have been developed in order to identify functional disorders and other sperm abnormalities, which are not addressed in conventional semen analysis. Some of them are only utilized as research tools (computer-assisted semen analysis, acrosome reaction, oxidative stress evaluation using chemiluminescence, hamster egg sperm penetration test, hemizona assay).[158] Others, such as antisperm antibodies and sperm DNA fragmentation have been implemented in clinical practice. The clinical indications of these highly specialized tests are unexplained male infertility or idiopathic male infertility with recurrent failure on multiple *in vitro* fertilization (IVF)/ICSI cycles. A brief overview of sperm function test are provided below.

Antisperm antibodies: Risk factors for antisperm antibodies (ASA) formation include genital infections, testicular trauma or surgical biopsy, cryptorchidism, testicular damage secondary to excessive heat exposure and obstruction of extratesticular ductal system (e.g. vasectomy). Antisperm antibodies can alter sperm motility and sperm-oocyte interaction. The immunobeads test is commonly used for antibodies detection and consists in using human anti-immunoglobulin antibody-coated polyacrylamide beads that are capable to detect IgA and IgG, the two most clinically important immunoglobulin subtypes associated to immunological infertility.[159] It precisely detects antibodies in serum and seminal plasma or bound to sperm surface. The rates of sperm bound to beads above 50% are considered clinically significant and may cause dysfunctional motility, vitality and capability for egg interaction.[127] The detection of antibodies in the serum and seminal plasma are of limited value as antibodies to sperm are the most likely to induce functional alterations.

Sperm DNA fragmentation testing: Sperm DNA fragmentation seems to be one of the most important causes of reduced fertility potential.[160] Advanced paternal age, inadequate dietary intake, drug abuse, pesticide environmental exposure, tobacco use, varicocele, medical disease, scrotal hyperthermia, air pollution, genital inflammation or infectious diseases can be cited as possible causes; some of which are reversible. Fragmentation can be secondary to internal factors such as apoptosis and oxidative stress (a pathophysiological mechanism secondary to a high concentration of free radicals), or external factors such as the presence of leukocytes. Assessment of sperm DNA integrity is indicated in the following situations:

- To investigate infertility in men presenting normal semen analysis as determined by conventional methods
- Cases of recurrent spontaneous abortion
- To aid determining the most appropriate reproductive assisted technology when necessary.

Abnormally fragmented sperm DNA can be found in 5% of infertile men with normal semen analyses and 25% of infertile men with abnormal semen analyses, but is rarely seen in fertile men.[160] Assays to evaluate sperm chromatin/DNA intergrity can be divided in three groups: (a) sperm chromatin structural probes using nuclear dyes (e.g. microscopic acridine orange test (AOT), sperm chromatin structural assay (SCSA), aniline blue test (AB), chromomycin-A3 (CMA3) and toluidine blue (TB), (b) tests for direct assessment of sperm DNA fragmentation (e.g. terminal deoxynucleotidyl transferase mediated dUTP nick end labeling assay (TUNEL) and single-cell gel electrophoresis assay (COMET), and (c) sperm nuclear matrix assays (e.g. sperm chromatin dispersion test). TUNEL technique seems to be one of the most adequate as it offers the possibility to precisely identify all existing endogenous breaks in sperm DNA. It combines both enzymatic and immunohistochemical techniques for direct observation of DNA fragmentation using a fluorescence microscope or flow cytometry. Elevated sperm DNA fragmentation rates significantly diminish the chances for natural or assisted pregnancy.[161]

Reactive oxygen species: It has been shown that 40–88% of nonselected infertile patients have high levels of seminal reactive oxygen species (ROS).[162] Moreover, 11% of normozoospermic infertile men have higher ROS levels and reduced total antioxidant capacity (TAC) levels compared to normospermic fertile counterpart.[163] ROS in low levels have a physiological role for capacitation, hyperactivation and AR.[164,165] ROS also exert their effect on sperm-oocyte interaction. However, the physiological ROS levels are still undetermined.

High ROS levels in semen that often originate from immature spermatozoa and seminal leukocytes can exert pathological impact on sperm.[166] These free radicals have considerable reactivity and the ability to react with and modify the structure of many different kinds of biomolecules including proteins, lipids and nucleic acids.

A natural antioxidant defense system offers protection against ROS. It consists of radical scavengers such as vitamin C and taurine, chain-breaking antioxidants such as alpha-tocopherol and ROS-metabolizing enzymes such as superoxide dismutase and those of the glutathione cycle, but very little catalase. Imbalance between the oxidants load and natural antioxidant defense system is called oxidative stress or oxygen paradox.

The most often used methods for detecting ROS in an andrology setting are divided into two major categories:

1. Direct methods such as chemiluminescence and flow cytometry
2. Indirect methods such as the colorimetric one.

Chemiluminescence uses probes such as luminol to detect ROS.[167,168] Luminol can penetrate the cell and react with intracellular reactive oxygen species; in addition, extracellular ROS exhibit chemiluminescence when mixed with an appropriate oxidizing agent. This property is due to the formation of unstable endoperoxide, which ultimately breaks down with the release of light. The emitted light photons are converted to an electrical signal and measured by luminometer,[169] with ROS generation being measured as counted photons per minute (cpm). The normal range is $< 0.2 \times 10^6$cpm per 20 million spermatozoa.[170] Intracellular ROS can also be measured by flow cytometry using different fluorescent probes such as 2′,7′-dichlorofluorescin-diacetate and hydroethidine that react with ROS to emit a red fluorescence.[171] The colorimetric technique is also widely used for indirectly quantifying ROS. It is based on the principle of spectrophotometry and measures lipid peroxide end products, mainly malondialdehyde, lipid hydroperoxides and isoprostanes.[172]

Sperm-zona pellucida binding: Sperm binding to the zona pellucida (ZP) is attributed to the presence of complimentary binding sites or receptors on the surface of both gametes; Human ZP3 (hZP3) is believed to be the primary ZP receptor for capacitated acrosome-intact sperm binding.[173,174] Sperm binding to ZP3 induces a signal transduction cascade within the spermatozoon, involving multiple proteins that lead to the AR. Defective ZP-binding sperm is present in approximately 15% and 25% of subfertile men with normal and abnormal semen analyzes, respectively.[175-177]

Two tests of sperm binding to the human zona which have been described:

1. The hemizona assay
2. The sperm-zona binding ratio test.

In the former, a single zona is bisected and each zona half is incubated with control and tested sperm suspensions. In the latter, a complete zona is incubated with equal numbers of motile spermatozoa from control and test populations, each labeled with a different fluorescent dye. In each case, the number of spermatozoa from each population bound per whole or half zona is counted and the number of test sperm expressed as a ratio of that of the control.

Acrosome reaction: The AR is defined as the process of fusion of sperm plasma membrane with outer acrosomal membrane leading to release of exocytotic proteolytic enzymes (acrosine and hyaluronidase) in response to sperm-ZP binding. ZP3 is considered the natural stimulus for the AR, which leads to the proteolytic dissolution of the ZP. Artificial stimuli used *in vitro* to challenge the AR are calcium ionophore A23187 and progesterone. Defective AR of clinical significance are: (i) AR prematurity, which is defined as high level of spontaneous AR (> 20% of spermatozoa exhibiting spontaneous AR), and (ii) AR insufficiency, which is defined as poor responsiveness to AR stimulants (when < 15% of spermatozoa responded to the ionophore A23187 challenge).[178] Both conditions are associated with poor fertilization capacity on conventional IVF treatment. Under normal conditions, > 15% AR in response to ionophore treatment is expected.[179] Various techniques are used for visualizing the human sperm acrosome, including lectins, monoclonal antibodies or the triple stain. Replicate (minimum two) slides must be scored for each determination, with at least 100 spermatozoa counted per slide.

The frequency of spermatozoa exhibiting defective ZP induced AR (ZPIAR) is high in subfertile men with idiopathic oligozoospermia (65%) and severe teratozoospermia (62%, strict normal sperm morphology ≤ 5%), but low 25% in normozoospermic subfertile men.[176] Sperm from men with unexplained infertility may be able to bind to the zone but unable to induce the AR, ultimately resulting in reduced sperm-ZP penetration and failure of fertilization. Patients with this condition usually have a long duration of unexplained infertility and normal semen analysis, and have zero or low rates of fertilization with standard IVF.[180] The diagnostic feature is that very low proportions of sperm undergo AR after binding to the ZP. However, those patients achieve high fertilization and pregnancy rates with ICSI.[181]

Although the exact mechanisms of defective AR are unknown, defective ZPIAR is more likely to be related to major structural defects of the sperm head, such as small or abnormal acrosomes, or associated abnormalities in the overlying plasma membrane in severe teratozoospermic subfertile men. In normozoospermic men, it has been shown that the seminal zinc concentration as a decapacitating factor was significantly higher in men with defective ZPIAR.

Sperm penetration testing: The ability of the equatorial region of the acrosome-reacted human sperm to fuse with the vitelline membrane of the oocyte is tested by using the sperm penetration assay (SPA) also known as the zona-free hamster oocyte penetration test. Although this test does not assess sperm-ZP binding it measures the spermatozoon's ability to undergo capacitation, AR, fusion and penetration through the oolemma, and decondensation within the cytoplasm of an oocyte. The ZP is removed from a hamster oocyte, which is then incubated with human spermatozoa. In its original description, sperm penetration ability is scored by calculating the percentage of ova that are penetrated; normal sperm are able to penetrate 10–30% of hamster ova.[182] Recent refinement of this test includes the incubation of sperm in a more potent capacitating media that allow the majority of ova to be penetrated; scores are obtained by calculating the number of subfertile sperm that penetrate each ovum compared to fertile controls. Several studies have evaluated the ability of the SPA to predict success or failure of IVF. Normal SPA results are predictive of fertilization by conventional IVF.[183] Nonetheless, semen samples which fail to fertilize hamster ova usually are unable to fertilize human ova.[182] Although the SPA is considered a research tool, it may be of clinical value for men with unexplained infertility with poor fertilization rate on IVF.

Postejaculatory Urine Examination

Postejaculatory urine (PEU) examination inspects for the presence of sperm to diagnose retrograde ejaculation. It helps to differentiate from other causes of hypospermia (volume < 1.5 ml) such as specimen collection issues, hypogonadism, EDO and congenital bilateral absence of the vas deferens.

Testis Biopsy

Testis biopsy is indicated in selected cases of azoospermia or severe oligozoospermia to distinguish obstructive from nonobstructive cases. Histopathology results may reveal normal spermatogenesis, hypospermatogenesis, germ cell maturation arrest, germ cell aplasia (Sertoli-cell-only syndrome), tubular sclerosis or a combination of these conditions. Biopsy can be performed by percutaneous or open approaches. Intraoperative imprint technique may yield information regarding testicular cytology including the presence of spermatogenesis or Sertoli-cell-only syndrome; however, this method is limited to provide a specific and detailed morphological assessment. In cases biopsies are obtained for diagnostic purposes only, the authors' technical choice is to perform the procedure either percutaneously or using the "window" open technique without testis delivery from the scrotum. Specimens should be placed in an appropriate fixative solution such as Bouin's fixative, Zenker's fixative or glutaraldehyde; formalin should not be used. In cases of NOA, histology results provide important prognostic information on the chances to retrieve spermatozoa to be used in ART.[184] However, as spermatogenesis is often limited and focal in NOA patients who harbor sperm production, it is recommended that biopsy is undertaken preferentially in assisted reproduction specialized centers to allow for immediate fresh sample examination and sperm cryopreservation for future ICSI, and avoiding the need of repeated procedures.

Algorithms for Evaluation and Diagnosis

A detailed medical history, physical examination, semen analyses and complementary tests, as appropriate, are the key to correctly diagnose and to define the better treatment strategies. In Figures 8A and B, we present algorithms summarizing what should be considered when assessing the infertile male.[185]

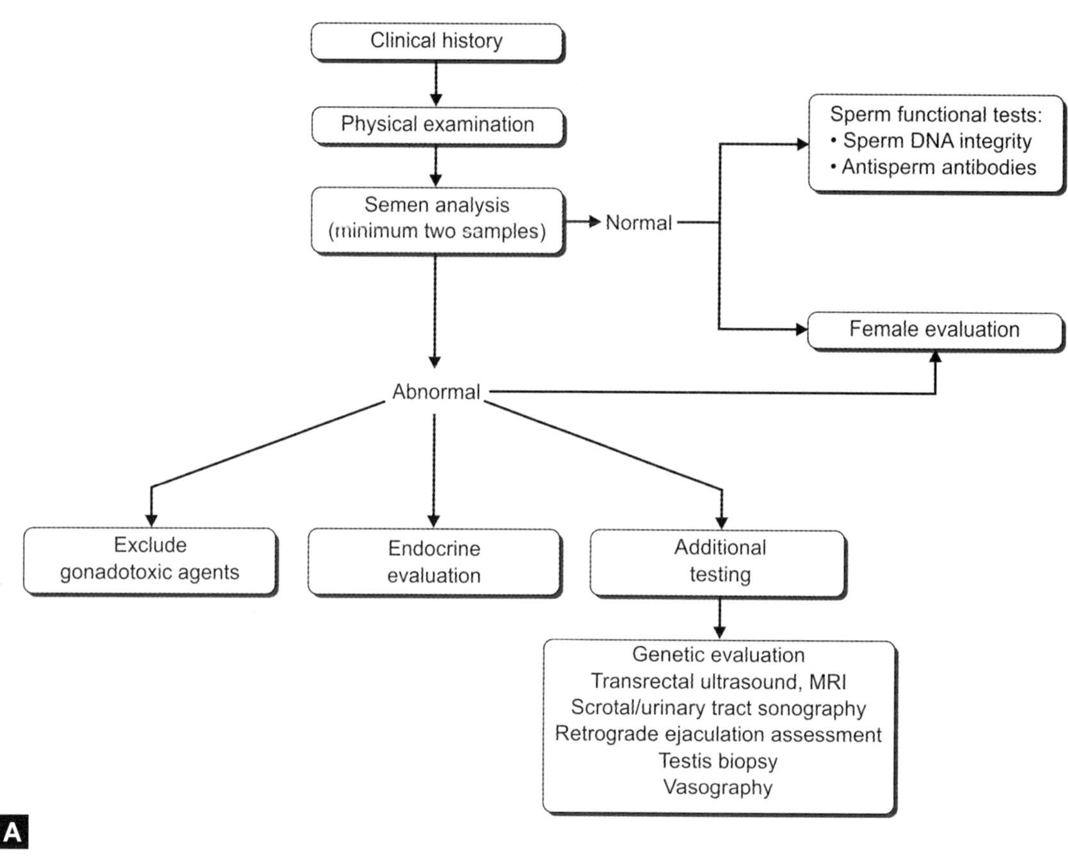

Contd...

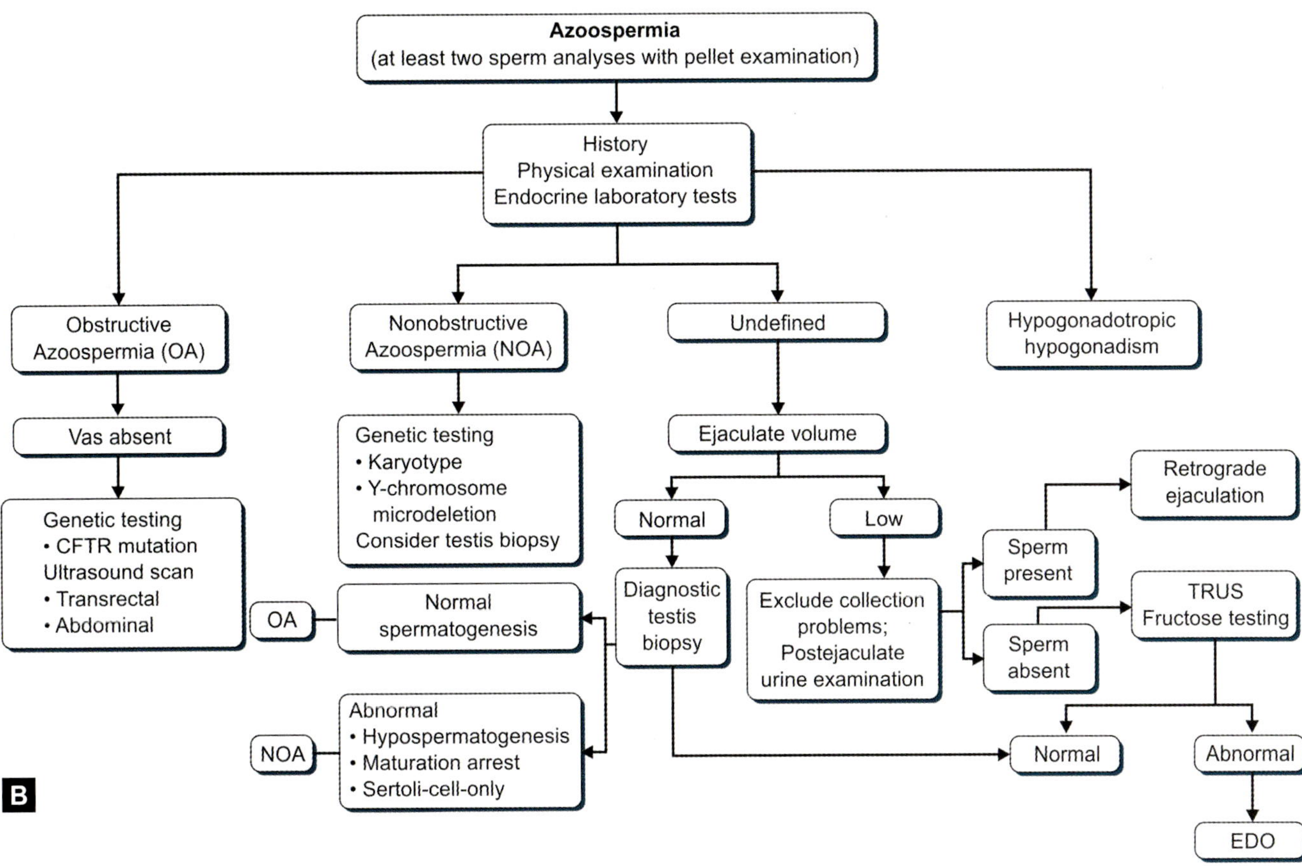

Figures 8A and B Algorithms for the workup of the infertile male. (A) Algorithm to be considered on initial evaluation; (B) Algorithm for the male patient presenting with azoospermia on semen repeated analyzes (Adapted from Esteves SC, Miyaoka R, Agarwal A. An update on the clinical assessment of the infertile male. CLINICS 2011;66(4):691-700, with permission from the Editor)

REFERENCES

1. Kamel RM. Management of the infertile couple: an evidence-based protocol. Reprod Biol Endocrinol. 2010;8 (6): 21-8.
2. Practice committee of the American Society for Reproductive Medicine. Definitions of infertility and recurrent pregnancy loss. Fertil Steril. 2008;90(5 Suppl):S60.
3. Rowe PJ, Comhaire FH, Hargreave TB, et al. WHO manual for the standardized investigation and diagnosis of the infertile couple. Cambridge: Cambridge University Press; 1993. pp. 1-7.
4. World Health Organization. Report of the Meeting on the Prevention of Infertility at the Primary Health Care Level. Geneva: WHO; 1983.
5. Centers for Disease Control and Prevention. (2002). Vital and Health Statistics, series 23, no. 26, CDC, 2002. [online] CDC website. Available from: http://www.cdc.gov/nchs/data/series/sr_23/sr23_026.pdf [Accessed February 2011].
6. Jarow JP, Sharlip ID, Belker AM,et al. Best practice policies for male infertility. J Urol. 2002;167(5):2138-44.
7. Rowe PJ, Comhaire FH, Hargreave TB, et al. WHO Manual for the Standardized Investigation and Diagnosis of the Infertile Male. Cambridge: Cambridge University Press; 2004.
8. Van der Steeg JW, Steures P, Eijkemans MJ, et al. Role of semen analysis in subfertile couples. Fertil Steril. 2011;95(3):1013-9.
9. Auger J, Kunstmann JM, Czyglik F, et al. Decline in semen quality among fertile men in Paris during the past 20 years. N Engl J Med. 1995;332(5):281-5.
10. Irvine S, Cawood E, Richardson D, et al. Evidence of deteriorating semen quality in the United Kingdom: birth cohort study in 577 men in Scotland over 11 years. BMJ. 1996;312(7029):467-71.
11. Swan SH. Semen quality in fertile US men in relation to geographical area and pesticide exposure. Int J Androl. 2006;29(1):62-8.
12. Carlsen E, Giwercman A, Keiding N, et al. Evidence for decreasing quality of semen during past 50 years. BMJ. 1992;305(6854):609-13.
13. Jørgensen N, Andersen AG, Eustache F, et al. Regional differences in semen quality in Europe. Hum Reprod. 2001;16(5):1012-9.

14. Swan SH, Brazil C, Drobnis EZ, et al. Geographic differences in semen quality of fertile US males. Environ Health Perspect. 2003;111(4):414-20.
15. Jørgensen N, Carlsen E, Nermoen I, et al. East-West gradient in semen quality in the Nordic-Baltic area: a study of men from the general population in Denmark, Norway, Estonia and Finland. Hum Reprod. 2002;17(8):2199-208.
16. Magnusdottir EV, Thorsteinsson T, Thorsteinsdottir S, et al. Persistent organochlorines, sedentary occupation, obesity and human male subfertility. Hum Reprod. 2005;20(1):208-15.
17. Nguyen RH, Wilcox AJ, Skjaerven R, et al. Men's body mass index and infertility. Hum Reprod. 2007;22(9):2488-93.
18. Sallmén M, Sandler DP, Hoppin JA, et al. Reduced fertility among overweight and obese men. Epidemiology. 2006;17(5):520-3.
19. Agarwal A, Deepinder F, Sharma RK, et al. Effect of cell phone usage on semen analysis in men attending infertility clinic: an observational study. Fertil Steril. 2008;89(1):124-8.
20. Phillips KP, Tanphaichitr N. Human exposure to endocrine disrupters and semen quality. J Toxicol Environ Health B Crit Rev. 2008;11(3-4):188-220.
21. Misell LM, Holochwost D, Boban D, et al. A stable isotope-mass spectrometric method for measuring human spermatogenesis kinetics in vivo. J Urol. 2006;175(1):242-6.
22. Moghissi KS, Wallach EE. Unexplained infertility. Fertil Steril. 1983;39(1):5-21.
23. Dohle GR, Diemer T, Giwercman A, et al. (2010) Guidelines of male infertility. [online] European Association of Urology. Available from http://www.uroweb.org/gls/pdf/Male%20Infertility%202010.pdf (Accessed February 2011).
24. Rowe PJ, Comhaire FH, Hargreave TG, et al. WHO Manual for the Standardized Investigation and Diagnosis of the Infertile Couple. Cambridge: University Press; 2000.
25. Sigman M, Lipshultz LI, Howard SS. Office evaluation of the subfertile male. In: Lipshultz LI, Howards SS, Niederberger CS (Eds). Infertility in the Male, 4th edition. Cambridge: Cambridge University Press; 2009. pp.153-76.
26. Witt MA, Lipshultz LI. Varicocele: a progressive or static lesion. Urology. 1993;42(5):541-3.
27. Spira A. Epidemiology of human reproduction. Hum Reprod.1986;1(2):111-5.
28. Ford WC, North K, Taylor H, et al. Increasing paternal age is associated with delayed conception in a large population of fertile couples: evidence for declining fecundity in older men. The ALSPAC Study Team (Avon Longitudinal Study of Pregnancy and Childhood). Hum Reprod. 2000;15(8):1703-8.
29. Van Noord-Zaadstra BM, Looman CW, Alsbach H, et al. Delaying childbearing: effect of age on fecundity and outcome of pregnancy. BMJ. 1991;302(6789):1361-5.
30. Schwartz D, Mayaux MJ. Female fecundity as a function of age: results of artificial insemination in 2193 nulliparous women with azoospermic husbands. Federation CECOS. N Engl J Med. 1982;306(7):404-6.
31. Aafjes JH, van der Vijver JC, Schenck PE. The duration of infertility: an important datum for the fertility prognosis of men with semen abnormalities. Fertil Steril. 1978;30(4):423-5.
32. Hull MG, Glazener CM, Kelly NJ, et al. Population study of causes, treatment, and outcome of infertility. Br Med J (Clin Res Ed). 1985;291(6510):1693-7.
33. Brandes M, Hamilton CJ, van der Steen JO, et al. Unexplained infertility: overall ongoing pregnancy rate and mode of conception. Hum Reprod. 2011;26(2):360-8.
34. Collins JA, Rowe TC. Age of the female partner is a prognostic factor in prolonged unexplained infertility: a multicenter study. Fertil Steril. 1989;52(1):15-20.
35. Weiser M, Reichenberg A, Werbeloff N, et al. Advanced parental age at birth is associated with poorer social functioning in adolescent males: shedding light on a core symptom of schizophrenia and autism. Schizophr Bull. 2008;34(6):1042-6.
36. Dalman C, Allebeck P. Paternal age and schizophrenia: further support for an association. Am J Psychiatry. 2002;159(9):1591-2.
37. Durkin MS, Maenner MJ, Newschaffer CJ, et al. Advanced parental age and the risk of autism spectrum disorder. Am J Epidemiol. 2008;168(11):1268-76.
38. Belloc S, Cohen-Bacrie P, Benkhalifa M, et al. Effect of maternal and paternal age on pregnancy and miscarriage rates after intrauterine insemination. Reprod Biomed Online. 2008;17(3):392-7.
39. Fisch H. Older men are having children, but the reality of a male biological clock makes this trend worrisome. Geriatrics. 2009;64(1):14-7.
40. Kidd SA, Eskenazi B, Wyrobek A. Effects of male age on semen quality and fertility: a review of the literature. Fertil Steril. 2001;75(2):237-48.
41. Eskenazi B, Wyrobek AJ, Sloter E, et al. The association of age and semen quality in healthy men. Hum Reprod. 2003;18(2):447-54.
42. Jarrow J, Sigman M, Kolettis PN, et al. (2010). The optimal evaluation of the infertile male. AUA best practice statement. [online] American Urological Association website. Available from http://www.auanet.org/content/media/optimalevaluation2010.pdf. [Accessed March 2011].
43. Kim JW, Lee WS, Yoon TK, et al. Chromosomal abnormalities in spontaneous abortion after assisted reproductive treatment. BMC Medical Genetics. 2010;11:153-8.
44. Puscheck EE, Jeyendran RS. The impact of male factor on recurrent pregnancy loss. Curr Opin Obstet Gynecol. 2007;19(3):222-8.
45. Rowe T. Fertility and a woman's age. J Reprod Med. 2006;51(3):157-63.

46. Center for Male Reproductive Medicine and Microsurgery in Cornell University. (2008) What's new in male infertility treatment at Cornell: the fertility evaluation? [online] Cornell University, Weill Medical College. Cornell Institute for Reproductive Medicine, Center for Male Reproductive Medicine and Microsurgery. Available from http://www.maleinfertility.org/new-evaluation.html. (Accessed March 2011).
47. Wilcox AJ, Weinberg CR, Baird DD. Timing of sexual intercourse in relation to ovulation. Effects on probability of conception, survival of the pregnancy, and sex of baby. N Engl J Med. 1995;333(23):1517-21.
48. Dunson DB, Baird DD, Wilcox AJ, et al. Day-specific probabilities of clinical pregnancy based on two studies with imperfect measures of ovulation. Hum Reprod. 1999;14(7):1835-9.
49. Dunson DB, Weinberg CR, Baird DD, et al. Assessing human fertility using several markers of ovulation. Stat Med. 2001;20(6):965-8.
50. Harrison KL, Wilson LM, Breen TM, et al. Fertilization of human oocytes in relation to varying delay before insemination. Fertil Steril. 1988;50(2):294-7.
51. Stanford JB, White GL, Hatasaka H. Timing intercourse to achieve pregnancy: current evidence. Obstet Gynecol. 2002;100(6):1333-41.
52. Katz DF. Human cervical mucus: research update. Am J Obstet Gynecol. 1991;165(6 Pt 2):1984-6.
53. Laumann EO, West S, Glasser D, et al. Prevalence and correlates of erectile dysfunction by race and ethnicity among men aged 40 or older in the United States: from the male attitudes regarding sexual health survey. J Sex Med. 2007;4(1):57-65.
54. Heruti R, Shochat T, Tekes-Manova D, et al. Prevalence of erectile dysfunction among young adults: results of a large-scale survey. J Sex Med. 2004;1(4):284-91.
55. Settlage DS, Motoshima M, Tredway DR. Sperm transport from the external cervical to the fallopian tubes in women: a time and quantitation study. Fertil Steril. 1973;24(9):655-61.
56. Kutteh WH, Chao CH, Ritter JO, et al. Vaginal lubricants for the infertile couple: effect on sperm activity. Int J Fertil Menopausal Stud. 1996;41(4):400-4.
57. Agarwal A, Deepinder F, Cocuzza M, et al. Effect of vaginal lubricants on sperm motility and chromatin integrity: a prospective comparative study. Fertil Steril. 2008;89(2):375-9.
58. Goldenberg RL, White R. The effect of vaginal lubricants on sperm motility in vitro. Fertil Steril. 1975;26(9):872-3.
59. Wang R, Monga M, Hellstrom WJG. Ejaculatory dysfunction. In: Comhaire FH (Ed). Male Infertility: clinical Investigation. Cause, Evaluation and Treatment. London: Chapman Hall; 1996. pp. 205-21.
60. Pryor JP. Erectile and ejaculatory problems in infertility. In: Hargreave TB (Eds). Male Infertility. Berlin: Springer-Verlag; 1997. pp. 319-36.
61. Shindel AW, Nelson CJ, Naughton CK, et al. Premature ejaculation in infertile couples: prevalence and correlates. J Sex Med. 2008;5(2):485-91.
62. Whitehead ED, Leiter E. Genital abnormalities and abnormal semen analyses in male patients exposed to diethylstilbestrol in utero. J Urol. 1981;125(1):47-50.
63. Jensen TK, Jørgensen N, Asklund C, et al. Fertility treatment and reproductive health of male offspring: a study of 1,925 young men from the general population. Am J Epidemiol. 2007;165(5):583-90.
64. Ramlau-Hansen CH, Thulstrup AM, Bonde JP, et al. Parental infertility and semen quality in male offspring: a follow-up study. Am J Epidemiol. 2007;166(5): 568-70.
65. Sharpe RM, Skakkebaek NE. Are estrogens involved in falling sperm counts and disorders of the male reproductive tract? Lancet.1993;341(8857):1392-5.
66. Sharpe RM. Declining sperm counts in men—is there an endocrine cause? J Endocrinol. 1993;136(3):357-60.
67. Jensen TK, Jørgensen N, Punab M, et al. Association of in utero exposure to maternal smoking with reduced semen quality and testis size in adulthood: a cross-sectional study of 1,770 young men from the general population in five European countries. Am J Epidemiol. 2004;159(1):49-58.
68. Storgaard L, Bonde JP, Ernst E, Spanô M, et al. Does smoking during pregnancy affect sons' sperm counts? Epidemiology. 2003;14(3):278-86.
69. Jensen MS, Mabeck LM, Toft G, et al. Lower sperm counts following prenatal tobacco exposure. Hum Reprod. 2005;20(9):2559-66.
70. Ramlau-Hansen CH, Toft G, Jensen MS, et al. Maternal alcohol consumption during pregnancy and semen quality in the male offspring: two decades of follow-up. Hum Reprod. 2010;25(9):2340-5.
71. Mieusset R, Bujan L, Massat G, et al. Clinical and biological characteristics of infertile men with a history of cryptorchidism. Hum Reprod.1995;(3):613-9.
72. Chilvers C, Pike MC. Epidemiology of undescended testis. In: Oliver RTD, Blandy JP, Hope-Stone HF (Eds). Urological and Genital Cancer. Oxford: Blackwell Scientific; 1989. pp. 306-21.
73. Carizza C, Antiba A, Palazzi J, et al. Testicular maldescent and infertility. Andrologia.1990;22(3):285-8.
74. Coughlin MT, Bellinger MF, Lee PA. Age at unilateral orchiopexy: effect on hormone levels and sperm count in adulthood. J Urol. 1999;162(3 Pt 2):986-8.
75. Miller KD, Coughlin MT, Lee PA. Fertility after unilateral cryptorchidism. Paternity, time to conception, pretreatment testicular location and size, hormone and sperm parameters. Horm Res. 2001;55(5):249-53.
76. Lee PA, Coughlin MT. Fertility after bilateral cryptorchidism. Evaluation by paternity, hormone, and semen data. Horm Res. 2001;55(1):28-32.
77. Lynn HB, Johnson WW. Inguinal herniorrhaphy in children. A critical analysis of 1,000 cases. Arch Surg. 1961;83:573-9.
78. Shin D, Lipshultz LI, Goldstein M, et al. Herniorrhaphy with polypropylene mesh causing inguinal vasal obstruction: a preventable cause of obstructive azoospermia. Ann Surg. 2005;241(4):553-8.

79. Arap MA, Vicentini FC, Cocuzza M, et al. Late hormonal levels, semen parameters and presence of antisperm antibodies in patients treated for testicular torsion. J Androl. 2007;28(4):528-32.
80. Alan L, Manson AL. Mumps orchitis. Urology. 1990;36(4):355-8.
81. Bremner WJ. Endocrinology of the male. In: Becker KL, Bilezikian JP, Bremner WJ, et al. (Eds). Principles and practice of endocrinology and metabolism, part VIII, chapter 115, 3rd edition. Philadelphia: Lippincott Williams & Willkins; 2001. pp. 1125-50.
82. Philip J, Selvan D, Desmond AD. Mumps orchitis in the non-immune postpubertal male: a resurgent threat to male fertility? BJU Int. 2006;97(1):138-41.
83. Barták V. Sperm count, morphology, and motility after unilateral mumps orchitis. J Reprod Fertil. 1973;32(3):491-3.
84. Beard CM, Benson RC Jr, Kelalis PP, et al. The incidence and outcome of mumps orchitis in Rochester, Minnesota, 1935 to 1974. Mayo Clin Proc.1977;52(1):3-7.
85. Casella R, Leibundgut B, Lehmann K, et al. Mumps orchitis: report of a mini-epidemic. J Urol. 1997;158(6):2158-61.
86. Ghai K, Rosenfield RL. Disorders of pubertal development: too early, too much, too late, or too little. Adolesc Med. 1994;5(1):19-36.
87. Root AW. Precocious puberty. Pediatr Rev. 2000;21(1): 10-9.
88. Pollack R, Nyhus LM. Complications of groin hernia repair. Surg Clin North Am. 1983;63(6):1363-71.
89. Reid I, Devlin HB. Testicular atrophy as a consequence of inguinal hernia repair. Br J Surg. 1994;81(1):91-3.
90. Schuppe HC, Pilatz A, Hossain H, et al. (Orchitis and male infertility). Urologe A. 2010;49(5):629-35.
91. Reichart M, Kahane I, Bartoov B. In vivo and in vitro impairment of human and ram sperm nuclear chromatin integrity by sexually transmitted Ureaplasma urealyticum infection. Biol Reprod. 2000;63(4):1041-8.
92. Ouzounova-Raykova V, Ouzounova I, Mitov I. Chlamydia trachomatis infection as a problem among male partners of infertile couples. Andrologia. 2009;41(1):14-9.
93. Hosseinzadeh S, Brewis IA, Eley A, et al. Co-incubation of human spermatozoa with Chlamydia trachomatis serovar E causes premature sperm death. Hum Reprod. 2001;16(2):293-9.
94. Agarwal A, Saleh RA. Role of oxidants in male infertility: rationale, significance, and treatment. Urol Clin North Am. 2002;29(4):817-27.
95. Comhaire FH, Mahmoud AM, Depuydt CE, et al. Mechanisms and effects of male genital tract infection on sperm quality and fertilizing potential: the andrologist's viewpoint. Hum Reprod Update. 1999;5(5):393-8.
96. Krieger JN, Coombs RW, Collier AC, et al. Fertility parameters in men infected with human immunodeficiency virus. J Infect Dis. 1991;164(3):464-9.
97. Shevchuk MM, Pigato JB, Khalife G, et al. Changing testicular histology in AIDS: its implication for sexual transmission of HIV. Urology. 1999;53(1):203-8.
98. Vora N, Perrone R, Bianchi DW. Reproductive issues for adults with autosomal dominant polycystic kidney disease. Am J Kidney Dis. 2008;51(2):307-18.
99. Handelsman DJ, Dong Q. Hypothalamo-pituitary gonadal axis in chronic renal failure. Endocrinol Metab Clin North Am. 1993;22(1):145-61.
100. Spratt DI, Bigos ST, Beitins I, et al. Both hyper- and hypogonadotropic hypogonadism occur transiently in acute illness: bio- and immunoactive gonadotropins. J Clin Endocrinol Metab. 1992;75(6):1562-70.
101. Krassas GE, Poppe K, Glinoer D. Thyroid function and human reproductive health. Endocr Rev. 2010;31(5):702-55.
102. Mulholland J, Mallidis C, Agbaje I, et al. Male diabetes mellitus and assisted reproduction treatment outcome. Reprod Biomed Online. 2011;22(2):215-9.
103. Serghini M, Fekih M, Karoui S, et al. Fertility and inflammatory bowel diseases. Tunis Med. 2010;88(9):623-8.
104. Ozgör B, Selimoğlu MA. Celiac disease and reproductive disorders. Scand J Gastroenterol. 2010;45(4):395-402.
105. Spruit MA, Thomeer MJ, Gosselink R, et al. Hypogonadism in male outpatients with sarcoidosis. Respir Med. 2007;101(12):2502-10.
106. Luboshitzky R, Aviv A, Hefetz A, et al. Decreased pituitary-gonadal secretion in men with obstructive sleep apnea. J Clin Endocrinol Metab. 2002;87(7):3394-8.
107. Kamischke A, Kemper DE, Castel MA, et al. Testosterone levels in men with chronic obstructive pulmonary disease with or without glucocorticoid therapy. Eur Respir J.1998;11(1):41-5.
108. Post FA, Soule SG, Willcox PA,et al. The spectrum of endocrine dysfunction in active pulmonary tuberculosis. Clin Endocrinol. 1994;40(3):367-71.
109. Nahoum CR, Fontes EA, Friere FR. Semen analysis in sickle cell disease. Andrologia. 1980;12(6):542-5.
110. Modebe O, Ezeh UO. Effects of age on testicular function in adult males with sickle cell anemia. Fertil Steril. 1995;63(4):907-12.
111. Carlsen E, Andersson AM, Petersen JH, et al. History of febrile illness and variation in semen quality. Hum Reprod. 2003;18(10):2089-92.
112. Pont J, Albrecht W. Fertility after chemotherapy for testicular germ cell cancer. Fertil Steril. 1997;68(1):1-5.
113. Nudell DM, Monoski MM, Lipshultz LI. Common medications and drugs: how they affect male fertility? Urol Clin N Am. 2002,29(4):965-73.
114. Meschede D, Lemcke B, Behre HM, et al. Clustering of male infertility in the families of couples treated with intracytoplasmic sperm injection. Hum Reprod. 2000;15(7):1604-8.
115. Gianotten J, Westerveld GH, Leschot NJ, et al. Familial clustering of impaired spermatogenesis: no evidence for a common genetic inheritance pattern. Hum Reprod. 2004;19(1):71-6.
116. Künzle R, Mueller MD, Hanggi W, et al. Semen quality of male smokers and nonsmokers in infertile couples. Fertil Steril. 2003;79(2):287-91.
117. Muthusami KR, Chinnaswamy P. Effect of chronic alcoholism on male fertility hormones and semen quality. Fertil Steril. 2005;84(4):919-24.

118. Tsujimura A, Matsumiya K, Miyagawa Y, et al. Prediction of successful outcome of microdissection testicular sperm extraction in men with idiopathic nonobstructive azoospermia. J Urol. 2004;172(5 Pt 1):1944-7.
119. Practice Committee of American Society for Reproductive Medicine in Collaboration with Society for Male Reproduction and Urology. American Society for Reproductive Medicine. Evaluation of the azoospermic male. Fertil Steril. 2008;90(5):S74-7.
120. Schlegel PN, Shin D, Goldstein M. Urogenital anomalies in men with congenital absence of the vas deferens. J Urol. 1996;155(5):1644-8.
121. Dubin R, Amelar RD. Varicocelectomy: twenty-five years of experience. Int J Fertil. 1988;33(4):226-8.
122. Trum JW, Gubler FM, Laan R, et al. The value of palpation, varicoscreen contact thermography and colour Doppler ultrasound in the diagnosis of varicocele. Hum Reprod.1996;11(6):1232-5.
123. Dubin R, Amelar RD. Varicocele size and results of varicocelectomy in selected subfertile men with varicocele. Fertil Steril. 1970;21(8):606-9.
124. Liguori G, Trombetta C, Garaffa G, et al. Color Doppler ultrasound investigation of varicocele. World J Urol. 2004;22(5):378-81.
125. Polansky FF, Lamb EJ. Do the results of semen analysis predict future fertility? A survival analysis study. Fertil Steril.1988;49(6):1059-65.
126. Esteves SC. Espermograma e correlações clínicas. In: Neves PA, Rodrigues Netto Jr N, (Eds). Infertilidade Masculina. São Paulo: Atheneu; 2003. pp. 59-70.
127. World Health Organization. WHO Laboratory Manual for the Examination and Processing of Human Semen, 5th edition. Geneva: World Health Organization, 2010.
128. World Health Organization. WHO Laboratory Manual for the Examination and Processing of Human Semen and Sperm-cervical Mucus Interaction, 2nd edition. Cambridge: Cambridge University Press; 1987.
129. World Health Organization. WHO Laboratory Manual for the Examination of Human Semen and Sperm-cervical Mucus Interaction, 3rd edition. Cambridge: Cambridge University Press; 1992.
130. World Health Organization. WHO Laboratory Manual for the Examination of Human Semen and Sperm-cervical Mucus Interaction, 4th edition. Cambridge: Cambridge University Press; 1999. pp. 128.
131. Guzick DS, Overstreet JW, Factor-Litvak P, et al. Sperm morphology, motility, and concentration in fertile and infertile men. N Engl J Med. 2001;345(19):1388-93.
132. Gunalp S, Onculoglu C, Gurgan T, et al. A study of semen parameters with emphasis on sperm morphology in a fertile population: an attempt to develop clinical thresholds. Hum Reprod. 2001;16(1):110-4.
133. Menkveld R, Wong WY, Lombard CJ, et al. Semen parameters including WHO and strict criteria morphology in a fertile and subfertile population: an effort towards standardization of in vivo thresholds. Hum Reprod. 2001;16(6):1165-71.
134. Kruger TF, Acosta AA, Simmons KF, et al. Predictive value of abnormal sperm morphology in in vitro fertilization. Fertil Steril. 1988;49(1):112-7.
135. Coetzee K, Kruger TF, Lombard CJ. Predictive value of normal sperm morphology: a structured literature review. Hum Reprod Update. 1998;4(1):73-82.
136. Van Waart J, Kruger TF, Lombard CJ, et al. Predictive value of normal sperm morphology in intrauterine insemination (IUI): a structured literature review. Hum Reprod Update. 2001;7(5):495-500.
137. Van der Merwe FH, Kruger TF, Oehninger SC, et al. The use of semen parameters to identify the subfertile male in the general population. Gynecol Obstet Invest. 2005;59(2):86-91.
138. Bar-Chama N, Fisch H. Infection and pyospermia in male infertility. World J Urol. 1993;11(2):76-81.
139. Endtz AW. A rapid staining method for differentiating granulocytes from germinal cells in Papanicolaou-stained semen. Acta Cytol. 1974;18(1):2-7.
140. Sokol RZ, Swerdloff RS. Endocrine evaluation. In: Lipshultz LI and Howards SS, (Eds). Infertility in the male, 3rd. edition. New York: Churchill Livingstone; 1997. pp. 210-8.
141. Raman JD, Schlegel PN. Aromatase inhibitors for male infertility. J Urol. 2002;167(2 Pt 1):624-9.
142. Vaucher L, Carreras E, Mielnik A, et al. Over expression of aromatase CYP 19 in human testis is most likely reason for hypogonadism in men with Klinefelter Syndrome. J Urol. 2009;181(4 Suppl):681.
143. Sigman M, Jarow JP. Endocrine evaluation of infertile men. Urology 1997;50(5):659-64.
144. Foresta C, Moro E, Ferlin A. Y chromosome microdeletions and alterations of spermatogenesis. Endocr Rev. 2001;22(2):226-39.
145. Stahl PJ, Masson P, Mielnik A, et al. A decade of experience emphasizes that testing for Y microdeletions is essential in American men with azoospermia and severe oligozoospermia. Fertil Steril. 2010;94(5):1753-6.
146. Choi JM, Chung P, Veeck L, et al. AZF microdeletions of the Y chromosome and in vitro fertilization outcome. Fertil Steril. 2004;81(2):337-41.
147. Hopps CV, Mielnik A, Goldstein M, et al. Detection of sperm in men with Y chromosome microdeletions of the AZFa, AZFb and AZFc regions. Hum Reprod. 2003;18(8):1660-5.
148. Oates RD, Silber S, Brown LG, et al. Clinical characterization of 42 oligospermic and azoospermic men with microdeletion of AZFc region of the Y chromosome, and of 18 children conceived with ICSI. Hum Reprod. 2002;17(11):2813-24.
149. Kent-First MG, Kol S, Muallem A, et al. The incidence and possible relevance of Y-linked microdeletions in babies born after intracytoplasmic sperm injection and their infertile fathers. Mol Hum Reprod. 1996;2(12):943-50.
150. Netto NR Jr, Esteves SC, Neves PA. Transurethral resection of partially obstructed ejaculatory duct: seminal parameters and pregnancy outcome according to the etiology of obstruction. J Urol. 1998;159(6):2048-53.
151. Du J, Li FH, Guo YF, et al. Differential diagnosis of azoospermia and etiologic classification of obstructive

azoospermia: role of scrotal and transrectal US. Radiology. 2010;256(2):493-503.
152. Jarrow JP. Seminal vesicle aspiration in the management of patients with ejaculatory duct obstruction. J Urol. 1994;152(3):899-901.
153. Chiou RK, Anderson JC, Wobig RK, et al. Color Doppler ultrasound criteria to diagnose varicoceles: correlation of a new scoring system with physical examination. Urology. 1997;50(6):953-6.
154. Hirsh AV, Cameron KM, Tyler JP, et al. The Doppler assessment of varicoceles and internal spermatic vein reflux in infertile men. Br J Urol. 1980;52(1): 50-6.
155. Simpson WL Jr, Rausch DR. Imaging of male infertility: pictorial review. AJR Am J Roentgenol. 2009;192(6):S98-107.
156. Rhoden EL, Estrada C, Levine L, et al. The value of pituitary magnetic resonance imaging in men with hypogonadism. J Urol. 2003;170(3):795-8.
157. Aaronson DS, Iman R, Walsh TJ, et al. A novel application of 1H magnetic resonance spectroscopy: noninvasive identification of spermatogenesis in men with non-obstructive azoospermia. Hum Reprod. 2010;25(4):847-52.
158. Esteves SC, Sharma RK, Thomas A Jr, et al. Evaluation of acrosomal status and sperm viability in fresh and cryopreserved specimens by the use of fluorescent peanut agglutinin lectin in conjunction with hypo-osmotic swelling test. Int Braz J Urol. 2007;33(3):364-76.
159. Esteves SC, Schneider DT, Verza Jr S. Influence of antisperm antibodies in the semen on in vitro fertilization with intracytoplasmic sperm injection (ICSI) outcome. Int Braz J Urol. 2007;33(6):795-802.
160. Shefi S, Turek PJ. Definition and current evaluation of subfertile men. Int Braz J Urol. 2006;32(4):385-97.
161. Collins JA, Barnhart KT, Schlegel PN. Do sperm DNA integrity tests predict pregnancy with in vitro fertilization? Fertil Steril. 2008;89(4):823-31.
162. Lewis SE, Boyle PM, McKinney KA, et al. Total antioxidant capacity of seminal plasma is different in fertile and infertile men. Fertil Steril. 1995;64(4):868-70.
163. Pasqualotto FF, Sharma RK, Kobayashi H, et al. Oxidative stress in normospermic men undergoing infertility evaluation. J Androl. 2001;22(2):316-22.
164. Griveau JF, Le Lannou D. Reactive oxygen species and human spermatozoa: physiology and pathology. Int J Androl. 1997;20(2):61-9.
165. Agarwal A, Nallella KP, Allamaneni SS, et al. Role of antioxidants in treatment of male infertility: an overview of the literature. Reprod Biomed Online. 2004;8(6):616-27.
166. Aitken RJ, Bennetts L. The sperm cell production, maturation, fertilization, regeneration. In: De Jonge C, Barratt C, (Eds). Reactive oxygen species: friend or foe. Cambridge: Cambridge University Press; 2006. pp. 170-93.
167. Aitken RJ, Buckingham DW, West KM. Reactive oxygen species and human spermatozoa: analysis of the cellular mechanisms involved in luminal- and lucigenin-dependent chemiluminescence. J Cell Physiol. 1992;151(3):466-77.
168. Aitken RJ, Baker MA, O'Bryan M. Shedding light on chemiluminescence: the application of chemiluminescence in diagnostic andrology. J Androl. 2004;25(4):455-65.
169. Fraga CG, Motchnik PA, Shigenaga MK, et al. Ascorbic acid protects against endogenous oxidative DNA damage in human sperm. Proc Natl Acad Sci. USA 1991;88(24):11003-6.
170. Agarwal A, Cocuzza M, Abdelrazik H, et al. Oxidative stress measurement in patients with male or female factor infertility. In: Popov I, Lewin G, (Eds). Handbook of Chemiluminescent Methods in Oxidative Stress Assessment. Kerala: Transworld Research Network; 2008. pp. 195-218.
171. Marchetti C, Obert G, Deffosez A, et al. Study of mitochondrial membrane potential, reactive oxygen species, DNA fragmentation and cell viability by flow cytometry in human sperm. Hum Reprod. 2002; 17(5):1257-65.
172. Agarwal A, Makker K, Sharma RK. Clinical relevance of oxidative stress in male factor infertility: an update. Am J Reprod Immunol. 2008;59(1): 2-11.
173. Lefièvre L, Conner SJ, Salpekar A, et al. Four zona pellucida glycoproteins are expressed in the human. Hum Reprod. 2004;19(7):1580-6.
174. Bleil JD, Wassarman PM. Identification of a ZP3-binding protein on acrosome-intact mouse sperm by photoaffinity cross-linking. Proc Natl Acad Sci USA. 1990;87(14):5563-7.
175. Liu DY, Garrett C, Baker HW. Clinical application of sperm-oocyte interaction tests in in vitro fertilization—embryo transfer and intracytoplasmic sperm injection programs. Fertil Steril. 2004;82(5):1251-63.
176. Liu de Y, Liu ML, Garrett C. Comparison of the frequency of defective sperm-zona pellucida (ZP) binding and the ZP-induced AR between subfertile men with normal and abnormal semen. Hum Reprod. 2007;22(7):1878-84.
177. Liu DY, Clarke GN, Lopata A, et al. A sperm-zona pellucida binding test and in vitro fertilization. Fertil Steril. 1989;52(2):281-87.
178. Eisenbach M, Giojalas LC. Sperm guidance in mammals — an unpaved road to the egg. Nat Rev Mol Cell Biol. 2006;7(4):276-85.
179. Garrett C, Liu DY, Clarke GN, et al. Automated semen analysis: 'zona pellucida preferred' sperm morphometry and straight-line velocity are related to pregnancy rate in subfertile couples. Hum Reprod. 2003;18(8):1643-9.
180. Cross NL, Morales P, Overstreet JW, et al. Induction of acrosome reactions by the human zona pellucida. Biol Reprod. 1988;38(1):235-44.
181. Sigman M, Baazeem A, Zini A. Semen analysis and sperm function assays: what do they mean? Semin Reprod Med. 2009;27(2):115-23.
182. Zini A, Sigman M. Evaluation of sperm function. In: Lipshultz LI, Howards SS, Craig S, (Eds). Infertility in the Male. Cambridge: Cambridge University Press; 2009:177-98.
183. Check JH, Nowroozi K, Lee M, et al. Evaluation and treatment of a male factor component to unexplained infertility. Arch Androl. 1990;25(3):199-211.
184. Esteves SC, Verza Jr S, Prudencio C, et al. Sperm retrieval rates (SRR) in non-obstructive azoospermia (NOA) are related to testicular histopathology results but not to the etiology of azoospermia. Fertil Steril. 2010;94(4 Suppl):132.
185. Esteves SC, Miyaoka R, Agarwal A. An update on the clinical assessment of the infertile male. CLINICS 2011;66(4):691-700.

4

Hormonal Management of Male Infertility

Alaa Hamada, Deepinder Goyal, Ashok Agarwal

CHAPTER CONTENTS

INTRODUCTION

Various hormones regulate the male reproductive function through well integrated complex set of interactions in various developmental stages. *In utero* sexual differentiation of the male external genitalia and internal reproductive organs is hormonally mediated through fetal testicular secretion of testosterone. Around 7th to 8th week of gestation, fetal Leydig cells begin *de novo* synthesis and secretion of testosterone. Such secretion is initially maintained by placental human chorionic gonadotropin (hCG) and subsequently by fetal pituitary luteinizing hormone (LH) in the latter half of the gestation. However, neither placental hCG nor fetal pituitary gonadotropins have been proved to be essential for *in utero* differentiation of male reproductive organs.

During puberty, testicular steroidogenesis and spermatogenesis are under the control of hypothalamic pituitary gonadal (HPG) axis. Hypothalamic pituitary gonadal axis mainly consists of three endocrine organs: hypothalamus, anterior pituitary gland and testes, secreting peptide, protein and steroid hormones. The hormonal secretions are under positive and negative feedback control at multiple levels of the HPG axis. Furthermore, contribution of higher brain centers, hypothalamic and pituitary hormonal secretion and other endocrine organs, such as thyroid and adrenal glands, also exerts regulatory role. The scope of this chapter is to present a brief physiological overview about hormone structure, transport in the blood, receptor, metabolism and target organ action. Later, the physiological and the pathological conditions of male reproductive endocrinology will be examined with particular emphasis on the role of endocrine therapy in treatment of male infertility.

PHYSIOLOGICAL OVERVIEW

Hormones are chemical molecules secreted by specialized group of cells to exert specific action or effect on target cells or body system through binding with specific receptors. The secreting cells, scattered or organized in glands, usually release their contents into the extracellular (EC) space. Based upon the mode of hormone delivery and the target cells, three types of hormonal effects are recognized. Paracrine effect is seen when the secreting cells affect other target cells in their vicinity, usually in the same organ or tissue, and the EC fluid is the transporting medium. Autocrine effect is exhibited when the released hormone exerts biological effect on the same cell of origin. Endocrine effect is described when the hormones are transported through the blood stream to bind with their target cell receptors, which are usually in other organs or systems of the body. Lastly, the fourth mechanism, known as intracrine, is demonstrated when the synthesized hormone acts intracellularly in the same cell before release.

Essentially, three classes of hormones are identified based upon the chemical structure: amino acid (usually tyrosine) derivatives, peptides and proteins hormones and steroid hormones. For instance, tyrosine derived hormones encompass thyroxin, epinephrine, norepinephrine (NE) and dopamine (DA). On the other hand, peptide and protein derived hormones constitute the majority of hormones in human body. Specifically, the peptide hormones consists of fewer than 100 amino acids and vary considerably in size, ranging from three amino acids peptide, such as thyrotropin releasing hormone (TRH) to as much as 84 amino acids polypeptide hormone represented by parathyroid hormone. Protein hormone is often composed of more than 100 amino acids and may reach up to 200, such as growth hormone (GH) and prolactin (PRL). Peptide and protein derived hormones are often synthesized in the rough endoplasmic reticulum (RER) as large precursor hormones (preprohormones) that are then cleaved into prohormones and transferred to Golgi apparatus. Inside Golgi apparatus, packaging and storage of prohormones into secretory vesicles occur, where they undergo the final modification and cleavage into active hormones and inactive residues. Certain cellular stimuli, such as increased cytoplasmic calcium or c-AMP trigger fusion of these granules with plasma membranes and release of their contents into interstitial fluid or directly into the blood by the process, known as exocytosis.[1] Peptide hormones are generally water soluble and easily transported to their target organs.

Lastly, steroid hormones, a class of lipids derived from cholesterol, include cortisol, aldosterone, testosterone, progesterone and estrogen. Minor biochemical differences among these hormones result in variable physiological role and function. These hormones are synthesized in the smooth endoplasmic reticulum (SER) and secreted from steroidogenic cells in testes, ovaries, adrenal cortex and placenta. Structurally, these steroid hormones consist of three cyclohexyl rings and one cyclopentyl ring combined into a single structure (Figure 1) and are lipid soluble. There is a limited storage capacity of the steroidogenic cells; however, under effect of specific stimuli large amount of cholesteryl ester can be mobilized from cytoplasmic vacuoles to SER for immediate synthesis and release of steroid hormones.

Hormones are the second key regulator of the human body systems' functions after the nervous system. They are instrumental in maintenance of internal homeostasis, response to stressful condition, water and salt balance, metabolic regulation, energy production, growth and behavior, and human reproduction. The later function is fundamentally based on the integrity of complex set of hormonal interaction, known as HPG axis.

Transport of Hormones in the Blood

Peptide, protein hormones and some amino acid derived hormones, such as catecholamines, are water soluble and therefore freely distribute in the blood stream, reaching their target receptors without the need for carrier proteins. However, steroid and thyroxine hormones are poorly water soluble and circulate in the blood mainly bound to plasma proteins, such as sex hormone binding globulins (SHBGs), corticosteroid binding globulin, thyroxine binding globulins (TBG) respectively and albumins. The biologically inactive protein-bound hormone constitutes the major hormonal fraction, conferring three important physiological properties. Firstly, it acts as a reservoir replacing the biologically active free hormone when they are bound to their target receptors or lost from the circulation and secondly, prevents rapid clearance of small sized molecules in urine or bile and prolongs their half-lives. Thirdly, it ensures ubiquitous hormonal distribution in various body organs. Interestingly, pathological and physiological increase in the carrier proteins may

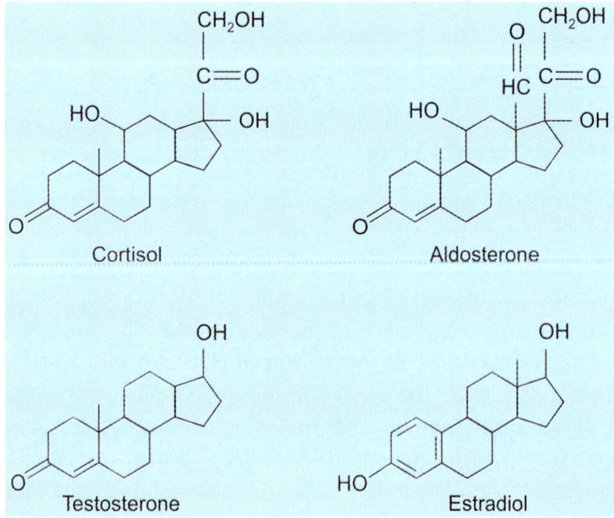

Figure 1 Chemical structure of several steroid hormones

ultimately result in false elevation in total hormone measurement assays. Measurement of the physiologically active component, free hormone fraction, is useful in these situations. However, unreliability of some of these assays necessitates simultaneous determination of total hormone level and hormone binding globulin or preferably calculating the free hormones by equilibrium dialysis method.

Hormone Action at the Target Organ

Covalent binding of a hormone ligand with its specific receptor in the target organ is the first step in the hormonal action, initiating a cascade of events that ultimately result in expression of the response. For a cell to adequately respond there should be at least 2,000–100,000 high affinity receptors, represented by large proteins undergoing dynamic interaction on binding.[1] The receptor sites and number vary based upon the type of hormone and the receptor itself. Protein, peptide and catecholamines usually attach to cell plasma membrane, receptors. The response is relatively fast and depends on signal transduction and activation of a second messenger. Nonetheless, some protein hormones, such as insulin, PRL and gonadotropins can enter the cells as well. Steroid and thyroid hormones, on the other hand, bind to cytoplasmic receptors (and then translocated to the nucleus) and nuclear receptors respectively, resulting in a slower response in the form of hormone-receptor complex induced activation of DNA transcription and translation. For steroid target cells 3,000–10,000 cytoplasmic receptors should be present to illicit a hormonal response.[1]

Two major classes or families of hormone receptors are recognized: cell surface receptors and intracellular receptors[2] (Figure 2). Cell surface receptors are specifically classified according to molecular mechanism of signal transduction into: group A (the receptor is linked to tyrosine kinase activity inducing intracellular phosphorylation) that is further subdivided into subgroup I receptor that has intrinsic tyrosine kinase activity, such as insulin and growth factors' receptors, and subgroup II receptors that recruit tyrosine kinase activity, such as cytokines, GH, PR Land leptin's receptors. On the other hand, group B receptors are coupled with GTP-binding protein (G-protein linked receptor) and there are more than 1,000 known types of G-protein linked receptors. GTP linked receptors have extracellular portion, seven looped transmembrane portion and intracellular cytoplasmic tail. On binding with a ligand, G-protein linked receptors undergo conformational changes replacing GTP for the GDP (already attached to the cytoplasmic tail) and activate either adenylatecyclase with production of cAMP as second messenger or phospholipase C with production of inositol triphosphate (IP3) and diacylglycerol (DAG). Inositol triphosphate increases intracellular calcium as second messenger, while DAG activates protein kinase C with further phosphorylation of intracellular proteins. Examples of G-protein linked receptors that activate adenylatecyclase include LH, follicle-stimulating hormone (FSH), thyroid-stimulating hormone (TSH) and corticotropin-releasing hormone (CRH); whereas, examples of G-protein linked receptors activating phospholipase C encompass LH, FSH, Gonadotropin releasing hormone (GnRH) and thyrotropin-releasing hormone (TRH).

Intracellular receptors are the second major class or family of hormone receptors and include up to 150 members. These receptors are, in fact, hormonally regulated transcription factors which upon binding with specific hormone, bind to specific DNA sequences close to promoter sites controlling the expression of certain genes. This class is further classified into cytosolic receptors, e.g. steroid hormone receptors, and nuclear receptors, e.g. thyroid hormone receptors.

After receptor activation, hormone-receptor complex either dissociates leaving the receptor free or the complex is internalized by endocytosis, degraded inside lysosomes and the receptor is then recycled again. Nevertheless, receptor availability, number and affinity are not static, and instantaneous steady state equilibrium exists between the hormone and its receptors. For instance, increased hormone concentration with consequent increased receptor binding eventually results in decreased availability of the receptors and thus minimizing the target cellular response to the hormone and the process is called 'downregulation,' e.g. continuous administration of GnRH results in decrease in the pituitary gland synthesis and release of FSH and LH. Conversely, some hormones or stimulating substances increase manufacturing of receptors and hence the target cell response to stimulating hormone, e.g. thyroxine increases the receptor response to catecholamines.

Metabolism, Degradation and Clearance of Hormones

Following activation of target receptor tissues, a small fraction of hormones usually undergoes *in situ* enzymatic inactivation and degradation; whereas the remaining large portion is inactivated and excreted through the liver and/or the kidney. Less than 1% of any hormone is excreted unchanged in urine. Metabolic inactivation includes oxidation, hydrolysis, hydroxylation, methylation, decarboxylation, sulfation and glucuronidation. However, some hormones can be enzymatically activated to more potent forms at the target tissues, such as conversion of tetraiodothyronine (T4) to

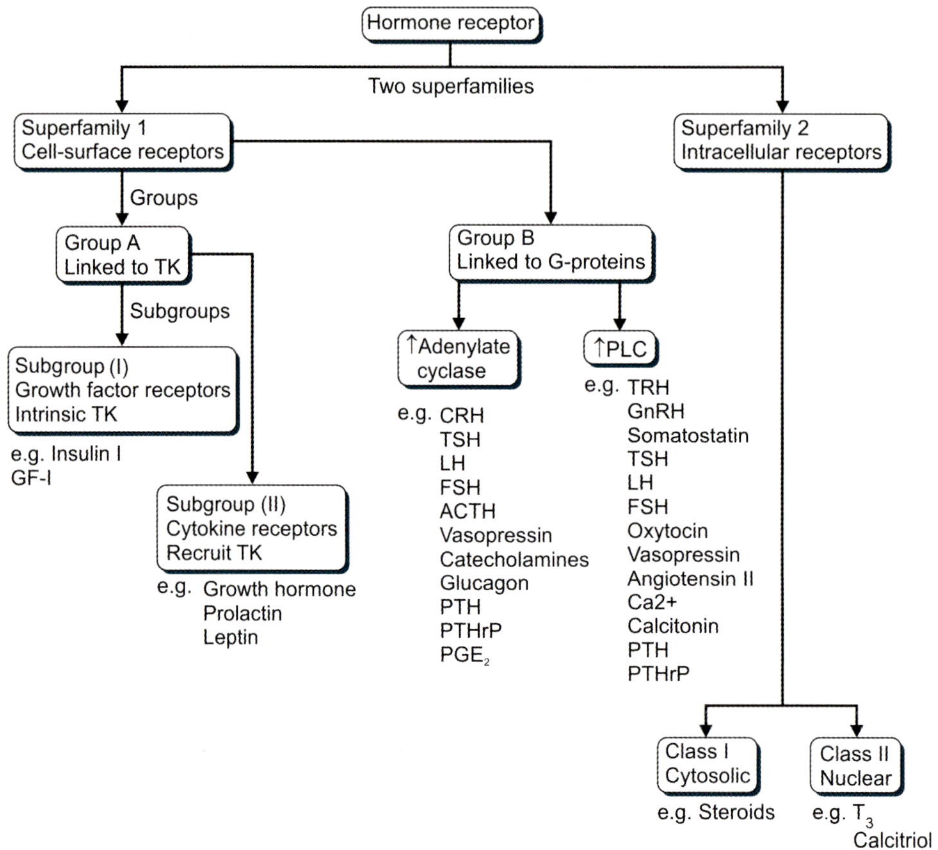

Figure 2 A composite diagram showing the different classes of hormone receptors

Abbreviations: PLC, phospholipase C; TK, tyrosine kinase

Source: Brook CG, Rosalind SB. The application of science to clinical practice. In: Brook CG, Brown RS (Eds). Handbook of Clinical Pediatric Endocrinology, 1st edition. Massachusetts, USA: Blackwell Publishing, Inc; 2008.pp. 1-13

tri-iodothyronine (T3) and conversion of testosterone to dihydrotestosterone (DHT).

HYPOTHALAMIC PITUITARY GONADAL AXIS (HPG)

Hypothalamus

Hypothalamus is a vital neuroendocrine organ, representing an important link between nervous and endocrine systems. Hypothalamus is essentially composed of loose network of neurons defined by arbitrary borders, located below the thalamus and above the brainstem forming the ventral portion of diencephalon. It is a small organ of an almond size (1.5 cm x 1.5 cm x 1.3 cm), weighing about 2.5 gm,[3] bound anteriorly by anterior margin of the optic chiasm and lamina terminalis, posteriorly by the posterior margin of the mammillary bodies, and laterally by a diffuse line extending from the optic tracts, internal capsule, pes pedunculi, globus pallidus and ansa lenticularis[4] (Figure 3). Within this loose network of neurons, several nuclei are discernible. Hypothalamus is mainly divided into two main parts: medial and lateral. In the medial part, three nuclear groups are identified: anterior, middle and posterior. In the anterior group three nuclei are located: suprachiasmatic nuclei (biological clock),[5] paraventricular and supraoptic nuclei. The middle group includes again three nuclei ventromedial, dorsomedial and arcuate nuclei; whereas, in the posterior group of the medial part, two nuclei are seen: posterior nucleus and mammillary body (Figure 3). The lateral portion of the hypothalamus is mainly composed of nerve fibers (lateral forebrain bundle) and loosely arranged nerve cells.

Hypothalamus acts as an integrative unit receiving afferent fibers from limbic structure, brain cortex, taste and olfactory stimuli, gastrointestinal and cardiovascular system. Efferent fibers are widespread and include projections to three main regions: pituitary gland, cerebral cortex and autonomic nervous system. In addition, hypothalamic neurons respond to other stimuli, such

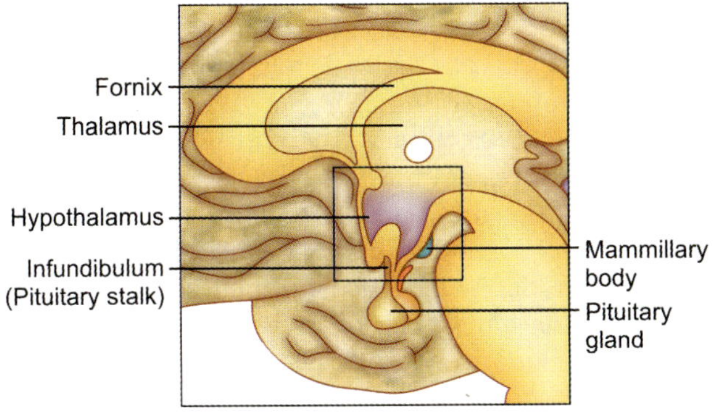

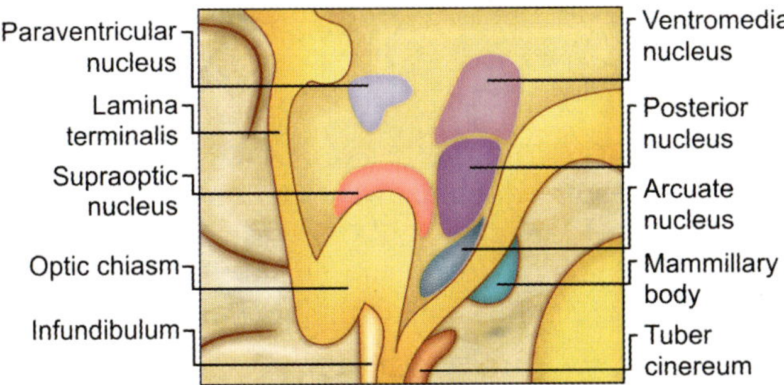

Figure 3 The hypothalamus. Median section through the third ventricle. Some of the major hypothalamic nuclei are shown with colored dots. The size of the dots indicates the relative size of neurons of various nuclei.

Source: Brodal P. The central autonomic system: the hypothalamus. In: Brodal P(Ed).The Central Nervous System Structure and Function, 4th Edition. Oxford: Oxford University Press; 2010.pp. 440-58.

as hormones, changes in blood sodiumconcentration, temperature and volume variations. In response to these stimuli, the hypothalamic neurons activate the regulatory physiological mechanisms achieving homeostasis.

Hypothalamic cells contain specific receptors for hormones, such as sex steroids, thyroid hormones, adrenal steroids, leptin and hormones released from the anterior pituitary. Communication of the hypothalamus and pituitary gland is unique, represented by vascular circuit with the anterior pituitary, and neural circuit with posterior pituitary (Figure 4). Hypothalamic projections from paraventricular and supraoptic nuclei directly release oxytocin and antidiuretic hormone from the nerve terminals endings into the posterior pituitary and thereby, hormones are transferred to the blood stream. Such projections form the neural circuit, hypothalamo-hypophyseal tract. Alternatively, the connection between hypothalamic nuclei and anterior pituitary is mainly through the vascular circuit 'the hypophyseal portal system' and the short neural circuit tuberoinfundibular tract. Axons from the hypothalamic nuclei forming tuberoinfundibular tract secrete releasing and inhibitory factors into the median eminence, whereby vascular networks stemming from superior hypophyseal artery are transporting them through a big vein, hypophyseal portal vein, to another capillary network into the pituitary gland. These releasing and inhibitory factors exert specific effects on a particular group of pituitary cells to elicit a release of a specific hormone.

Specifically, hypothalamic neuropeptides that are mainly concerned with male reproduction are divided into:

Peptides with direct influence on male reproduction. These include GnRH, CRH, and prolactin inhibitory factor (PIF).

Peptides with indirect influence on male reproduction. These include TRH, growth hormone releasing hormone (GHRH) and growth hormone inhibiting hormone (GHIH).

Gonadotropin Releasing Hormone

Gonadotropin releasing hormone is a hypothalamic decapeptide controlling the secretion of gonadotropins, FSH and LH from the anterior pituitary. GnRH is released in a pulsatile pattern from a diffuse network of 1,500 neurons that are mainly concentrated in medial basal hypothalamus, the infundibulum, and periventricular region.[6-8] These neurons act as a single pulse generator for the HPG axis. GnRH pulse release lasts for few minutes at frequency of one pulse every 1–3 hours. The amount of GnRH is determined by the quantity of GnRH secreted at each pulse and the frequency of these cycles (Figure 5). Correspondingly, LH is secreted from the anterior pituitary at pulse frequency exactly coinciding with that of GnRH; whereas, FSH shows nonpulsatile mode of secretion and even when it is pulsatile, there is little concordance with GnRH pulses. Exogenous replacement of GnRH should follow similar physiological regulations to stimulate LH and FSH secretion. Chronic continuous administration of GnRH may result in inhibition of LH and FSH.[9]

Pituitary Gland

Pituitary gland is an essential endocrine organ in the human body. It is composed of three components: anterior lobe (adenohypophysis, predominant part), intermediate lobe (vestigial component) and posterior lobe (neurohypophysis). Pituitary gland is located in the bony sellaturcica at the base of the skull, overlaid by thin diaphragm, through which the pituitary stalk connecting between the pituitary gland and median eminence of hypothalamus is passing through. Its average weight is 400–900 mg and measures about 13 mm in the longest transverse diameter, 6–9 mm vertically, and about 9 mm anteroposteriorly.[10] Adenohypophysis is the major endocrine portion of the

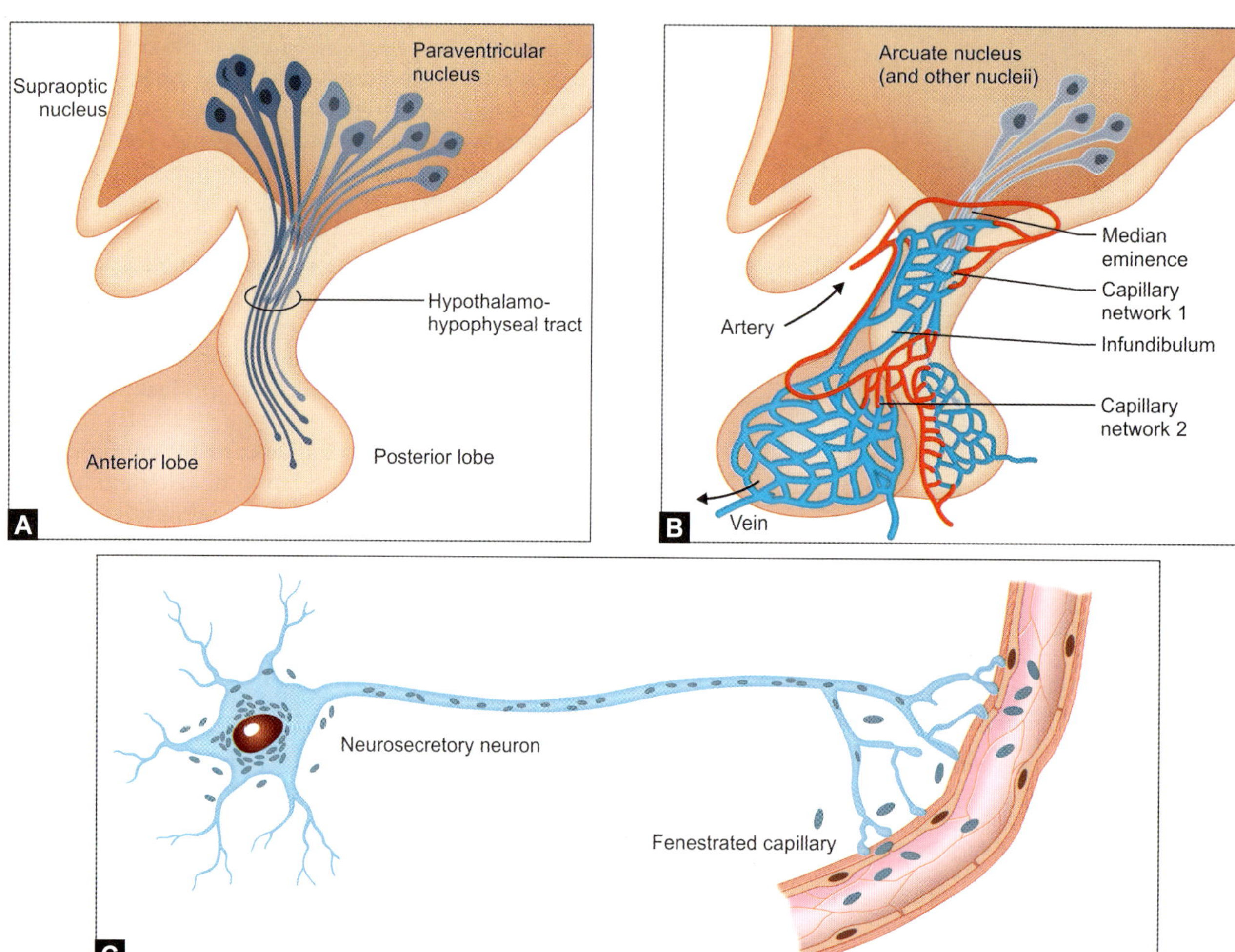

Figures 4A to C Relationship between the hypothalamus and the pituitary gland. (A) Connections from the hypothalamus to the posterior lobe; (B) The portal vessels of the pituitary stalk ensure that releasing hormones (factors) are transported from the median eminence in the upper part of the stalk to the epithelial cells of the anterior lobe; (C) Axonal transport of peptide hormones (neuropeptides) from the hypothalamus to the pituitary

Source: Brodal P. The central autonomic system: the hypothalamus. In: Brodal P(Ed). The Central Nervous System Structure and Function, 4th edition. Oxford: Oxford University Press; 2010.pp. 440-58

pituitary gland, consisting of gonadotrophs (5–10%), somatotrophs, thyrotrophs and corticotrophs.[11] Under the effect of GnRH, gonadotrophs secrete LH and FSH directly into the blood stream to exert their effects on testicular Leydig cells and Sertoli cells, respectively.

Gonadotropins

Luteinizing hormone and FSH belong to a family of glycoprotein hormones that also includes TSH. Each glycoprotein hormone in this family is heterodimeric, i.e. consisting of α-chain and β-chain. The α-chain is a common chain, whereas β-chain confers functional specificity for a particular hormone. These chains are tightly linked by disulfide bonds, yielding specific conformational structure which is necessary for receptor binding and biological activity. Around 60% of gonadotrophs secrete both FSH and LH; whereas, 18% and 22% of cells solely secrete LH and FSH respectively.[10]

Glycosylation of these hormones with various types of oligosaccharides occur before release from the pituitary cells, consisting of various types of sugars, such as sialic acid, mannose, galactose and N-acetylglucosamine. There are two sites of glycosylation in each peptide chain.[12,13] Single branched; di-,tri- and even tetra-branched oligosaccharides are demonstrated in these glycosylation sites that lead to appearance of different isoforms of the gonadotropin. These sugars have effect on hormone assembly, secretion pattern, mode of action and metabolic clearance.[2,12] Sialic acid residues are the most critically important sugar in these oligosaccharides

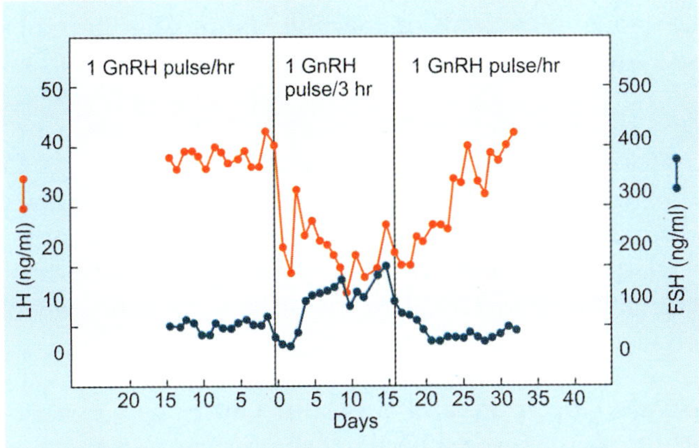

Figure 5 The influence of GnRH pulse frequency on LH and FSH secretion in a female rhesus monkey with an arcuate nucleus lesion ablating endogenous GnRH support of the pituitary. Decreasing GnRH pulse frequency from 1 pulse/hour to 1 pulse/3 hours leads to a decrease in plasma LH concentration but an increase in plasma FSH concentrations. *Source:* Wildt L, Haulser A, Marshall G, et al. Frequency and amplitude of gonadotropin-releasing hormone stimulation and gonadotropin secretion in the rhesus monkey. Endocrinology. 1981;109:376-85.[92]

that leads to appearance of gonadotropin isoforms.[13] Acidic isoforms that have more sialic acid residues in the attached oligosaccharides often have longer half-life and are relatively protected from degradation by the liver, whereas less sialic acid residues render gonadotropins less acidic and more potent.[9] The half-life of LH (< 20 minutes) is relatively shorter than that of FSH (1–4 hours). GnRH and sex steroids play critical role in regulating the process of glycosylation.[9]

Various studies have shown progressive increase in the serum levels of FSH and LH with aging.[14,15] FSH secretion increases in both continuous and pulsatile forms; whereas, LH shows modest but inconsistent elevation in the elderly men.[16] Such rise in gonadotropin level is attributed to impaired testicular feedback regulation of the hypothalamus and pituitary gland.

Testes

Testis is the third component of the HPG axis. Functionally, testis is divided into two compartments: interstitial compartment containing Leydig cells, and seminiferous tubules consisting of Sertoli cells and spermatogenic cells in various stages of development.

Leydig Cell

Leydig cells constitute about 10–20% of interstitial compartment that forms 12–15% of testicular volume.[17] Leydig cells secrete group of hormones collectively known as androgens including testosterone, DHT and androstenedione. Testosterone is the most abundant hormone and 75% of blood testosterone is derived from testes. 200 x 10^6 Leydig cells daily secrete 4–9 gm of testosterone under the effect of LH.[17] Furthermore, insulin-like factor 3 (INSL3) is another protein hormone secreted by Leydig cells, which may be used as an indicator of Leydig cell function. INSL3 has been postulated to play a direct role in regulation of sperm production.[17]

Testosterone: It is the main hormone secreted by the Leydig cells of testes and is the principal androgen in men. It is C19 steroid hormone with OH group at position C17 in the sterol ring. Testosterone is important for regulation and induction of spermatogenesis and development of secondary sexual characteristics. Leydig cells synthesize testosterone, under the effect of LH, from two sources: cholesterol, or synthesized *de novo* or taken directly from the blood. Androstenedione is synthesized by the adrenal glands. LH stimulates mitochondrial uptake of cholesterol by enhanced activity of steroidogenic acute regulatory protein, the first rate-limiting step in testosterone synthesis. Inside the mitochondria, cholesterol undergoes side change cleavage to form pregnenolone that diffuses outside the mitochondria towards SER where it is further processed. Two important pathways are embarked toward formation of testosteroneinside SER: δ5-pathway (pregnenolone, 17OH pregnenolone and dehydroepiandrosterone (DHEA) and androstenediol) and δ4-pathway (pregnenolone, progesterone, 17OH progesterone and androstenedione). δ5-pathway predominates in human testes. Synthesis of testosterone by testis requires the presence of two specific enzymes: 17β-hydroxysteroid dehydrogenase-3 that catalyzes the conversion of DHEA to androstenediol and conversion of androstenedione to testosterone, and 3β-hydroxysteroid dehydrogenase-2 that directly converts androstenediol to testosterone.

As aforementioned, human testis daily produces 4–9 gm of testosterone. In addition, 500 mg of testosteroneis produced either directly from the adrenal glands or from peripheral conversion of androstenedione. DHT is another hormone produced by the testis through enzymatic action of Sertoli cell-derived 5-α-reductase on testosterone. However, only 20% of serum DHT is secreted by the testes and the rest is derived from peripheral conversion at the target tissues. DHT has more than twice the biological activity of testosterone. Alternatively, testosterone and androstenedione can be converted to estradiol and estrone respectively by the action of aromatase enzyme in the gonadal and extragonadal tissues, as will be described below. The major catabolic pathway of testosterone to less active metabolite is mainly through conjugation in the liver and excreted in urine as 17-ketosteroids.

Estrogens: Although small amount (20%) of estrogen in men is directly secreted by the testis, the majority is derived from conversion of testosterone and androstenedione by aromatase enzyme inside gonadal cells, such as Leydig cells and Sertoli cells and extragonadal tissues, such as brain, skin, liver, mammary tissues, and most significantly, the adipose tissue. The plasma level of estradiol is 2–3 ng/dL with production of about 25–40 µg per day. The exact physiological role of estrogen in male reproductive function is under investigation. While estradiol plays an inhibitory role in regulation of HPG axis at the level of hypothalamus and pituitary glands, recent investigations revealed presence of estrogen receptors (ERα) in the efferent ductules, epididymis and Leydig cells. Knockout male mice for ERα suffer alteration of spermatogenesis and infertility. However, exposure to exogenous estrogen can suppress HPG axis and impair spermatogenesis. Further studies on humans may be needed to uncover the complete physiological roles of estrogen. In men, in contrast to women, estradiol level increases with age.

Sertoli Cells

Sertoli cells perform supporting role in orchestrating the process of spermatogenesis and in forming the blood testis barrier. Approximately, 35–40% of the volume of germinal epithelium is represented by Sertoli cells.[18] The intact testis contains 800–1200 × 10^6 Sertoli cells or approximately 25 × 10^6 Sertoli cells per gram testis.[17] Sertoli cells secrete variety of proteins, cytokines, growth factors, opioids, steroids, prostaglandins and modulators of cell division. Specifically, Sertoli cells secrete two structurally related proteins, i.e., inhibin and activin. These proteins are dimers belonging to transforming growth factor-β family. Inhibin consists of an α subunit and a βA or βB subunit, whereas activin is a homodimer (βAβA or βBβB). Inhibin is secreted from Sertoli cells under the effect of FSH and acts to inhibit FSH secretion from the anterior pituitary. Conversely, activin activates secretion of FSH to stimulate spermatogenesis. These hormones are not only secreted by Sertoli cells, but also from other sources, such as Leydig cells, prostate, liver etc.

Regulation of HPG Axis

On each level of HPG axis, three types of regulatory feedback loops are acting to control hormonal output. These regulatory loops are either negative (inhibit hormone secretion) or positive (stimulate hormone secretion). These loops include:

Long feedback loop in which the secretion of testis (the target organ) inhibits or stimulates hypothalamus and anterior pituitary secretion

Short feedback loop in which the anterior pituitary secretions control the hypothalamic hormonal output

Ultrashort feedback loop in which there is intrinsic regulation of hormonal output at each organ or level of HPG axis

In the first loop, testosterone is the major hormone released by testis and regulates GnRH and gonadotropin secretion. Specifically, testosterone or its metabolite DHT reduces the frequency of hypothalamic pulse generator to release GnRH, whereas testosterone or its metabolite estrogen acts on pituitary cells to inhibit GNs release.[17] Higher doses of testosterone can also exert inhibitory effect on GnRH and LH; however, it directly stimulates pituitary FSH secretion through positive feedback loop interaction.[19] Progesterone, on the other hand, acts on dopaminergic arcuate nucleus neurons that inhibit GnRH neurons.[20] Additionally, other testicular factors, such as activin and inhibin, stimulate or inhibit pituitary release of FSH respectively at the level of pituitary gland (Figure 6).

Evidence for pituitary influence on hypothalamic secretion arises from identification of a direct inferior branch of the hypophyseal artery entering the anterior pituitary gland in some mammals and finding that blood flow within the portal system can occur in the reverse (retrograde) direction—from anterior lobe toward hypothalamus. Therefore, the pituitary gland might regulate the hypothalamus by 'short-loop' feedback.[21]

The ultrashort hypothalamic feedback is represented by paracrine and autocrine regulation of GnRH neurons. GnRH neurons can regulate the secretory activity of their own and there is evidence for the presence of receptors for GnRH (GNRHR) in hypothalamic neurons.[21] Neurons from limbic system, brain stem and other hypothalamic areas project to GnRH neurons and influence their secretory activity. Neurons that release glutamate and NE provide stimulatory role to the reproductive axis; whereas, those neurons that release gamma aminobutyric acid(GABA) and endogenous opioid peptides play important inhibitory role.[17]

Within the pituitary gland, nerves and short portal vessels interconnect the pituitary lobes forming potential routes of intrapituitary communication and regulation. Finally, testis is a complex endocrine organ,where various mechanisms of ultrashort regulatory loops exist in the form of paracrine, autocrine and even intracrine systems.

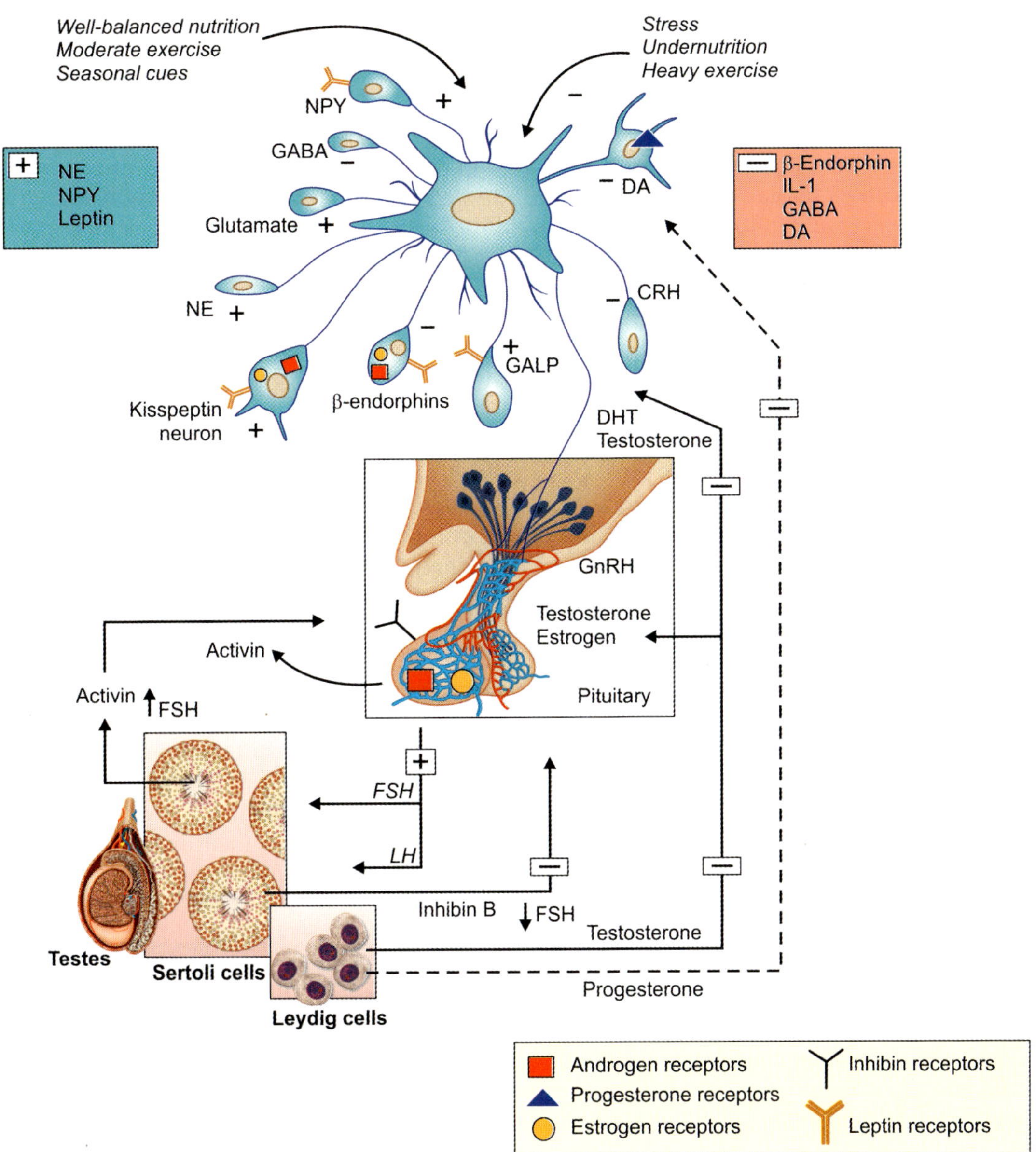

Figure 6 Schematic figure shows the complex regulation of hypothalamic pituitary gonadal axis. Well-balanced nutrition, moderate exercise and seasonal cues have stimulatory effects on the hypothalamus through higher brain centers, whereas excessive exercise, undernutrition may have inhibitory effect on the hypothalamus. Factors stimulating GnRH neurons to release GnRH include norepinephrine (NE), neuropeptide Y (NPY), leptin, galanine like peptide(GALP) and glutamate; whereas, factors inhibiting central GnRH release include beta endorphins, interleukine1, GABA, corticotropin releasing hormone (CRH) and dopamine (DA). The figure also shows negative feedback regulation of gonadotropin synthesis and release. Testosterone, DHT, estrogen, progesterone and inhibin B are factors released from the testes and inhibit gonadotropin release at the level from the hypothalamus and the pituitary gland. Activin is released from many cells in the male reproductive system and locally produced in the pituitary to stimulate FSH release.

Source: Low MJ. Neuroendocrinology. In: KronenberHM, Melmed S, Polonsky KS, Larsen PR(Eds). Kronenberg And Williams Textbook of Endocrinology,11th edition. PhiladelphiaPA: Saunders; 2008. pp. 85-135

CLINICAL ENDOCRINE EVALUATION OF INFERTILE MAN

Initial evaluation of infertile couple should aim at determining whether the problem lies within the male or female partner, or both. If the female partner has regular menstrual cycles; patent fallopian tubes; normal FSH, LH, TSH and PRL levels; male factor infertility is the likely cause.[22] Clinical evaluation of endocrine contribution to male factor infertility should commence with detailed history taking and proper conduction of physical examination. Four important goals of endocrinological evaluation are to assess:

1. Whether male reproductive dysfunction is attributed to male hypogonadism or not.
2. Prepubertal or postpubertal onset of hypogonadism.
3. Whether the problem is localized to the HPG axis or outside this axis.
4. Finally, if the defect has been traced to HPG axis, specific testicular, pituitary or hypothalamic etiology should be sought and then treated.

Certain childhood illnesses, such as unilateral or bilateral empty scrotum, testicular torsion, scrotal trauma, pediatric inguinal hernia repair and mumps orchitis could risk not only the spermatogenesis function, but also Leydig cell function as well. Defective testosterone-synthesis or action in the third trimester could result in male live births born with ambiguous genitalia, cryptorchidism and micropenis. Other risk factors for male hypogonadism include testicular tumors; exposure to certain medications, such as anabolic steroids, cimetidine, ketoconazole, digoxin and spironolactone; cancer chemotherapy or radiotherapy; HIV/AIDS; hemochromatosis; pituitary tumor and surgery and certain systemic inflammatory and infectious conditions, such as sarcoidosis, chronic obstructive airway diseases, chronic liver and kidney diseases, histiocytosis, tuberculosis and fungal infections. Furthermore, substance abuse and recreational drugs, such as marijuana, heavy smoking, cocaine and alcohol have been also implicated in the etiology of male hypogonadism.

Absent or delayed pubertal development is ominous sign of male hypogonadism. In approximately 99.5% of white boys, early signs of secondary sex characteristics may at least become evident by the age of 14 years.[23] Increased testicular volume from 1–2 cc to 3–8 cc accompanied by discernible enlargement of penile size are the first signs of puberty and typically such signs occur at the age of 11.5 years in most US boys.[23] Although the most common cause of pubertal delay is constitutional [idiopathic delay (60%)] and delayed but spontaneous pubertal developmental [functional hypogonadotropic hypogonadism (HH) 20%], permanent endocrine disturbances in the HPG axis (24%) should always be sought.[24]

In adults who have already completed pubertal spurt, features of hypogonadism include loss of energy and decrease in libido. Tables 1 and 2 show signs of male hypogonadism before and after puberty.

Physical examination (general and genital) adds a wealth of information. Tanner staging is essential component of physical assessment. Arms span and its discordance with the body height, excessive skin pallor, sparse pubic and facial hair distribution, female fat distribution, diminished testicular size, and presence of gynecomastia may all pinpoint to potential endocrine deregulation as a cause for infertility. Physical examination could even suggest the possible mechanisms and the exact site of endocrine disturbance. Visual field defects, galactorrhea and impotence may indicate prolactinoma associated hypogonadism. Lack of smell sensation is a diagnostic feature of Kallmann's syndrome. Gynecomastia, bilateral small testes and behavioral problems may indicate Klinefelter's syndrome. Varicocele, bilateral testicular atrophy, testicular mass, signs of chronic liver or kidney diseases, obesity, signs of Cushing's syndrome, acromegaly, thyroid dysfunction all can probably shed a light on the etiology behind hypogonadism.

Semen quality should be determined by analyzing semen samples obtained by masturbation after 2–7 days of abstinence. Semen volume, pH, sperm count,

Table 1 Signs of early onset hypogonadism

- Eunuchoid appearance: arm span > 5 cm than height
- Poor musculinization
- Lack of recession of hair on temporal lobe
- Sparse axillary, pubic, facial and body hair
- High-pitched voice
- Small testes and possibly maldescended
- Infantile external genitalia
- Impaired libido and potency
- Oligospermia to azoospermia

Table 2 Signs of postpubertal onset of androgen deficiency

- Normal body proportions with possibility of osteoporosis
- Atrophy and decreased muscle strength
- Male-pattern baldness
- Sparse facial, pubic, axillary, chest and hair
- Normal pitch of voice
- Small, often soft testes
- No change in the size of external genitalia
- Decreased libido and erectile dysfunction
- Oligospermia to azoospermia

density, motility, morphology and viability are evaluated in accordance with WHO criteria.[25] It is important to obtain multiple semen samples to overcome tremendous variability in sperm parameters.

Indications of Endocrine Testing

In two large retrospective analyses of 1,035 infertile men in two infertility centers, endocrine abnormalities, on repetitive testing, had been detected in only 99 patients (9.6%). FSH elevation was the most frequent abnormality.[26] Furthermore, only 1.75% of these men had clinically relevant endocrinopathy in terms of disease management.[26]

Interestingly, with presence of relatively normal spermatogenesis, detecting low levels of FSH or LH has no clinical significance. The current recommendations of endocrine testing include:

- Sperm concentration less than 10 million/ml
- Erectile dysfunction and decreased libido
- Hypospermia (semen volume < 1 ml)
- Signs and symptoms of endocrinopathies, such as thyroid dysfunction, acromegaly, delayed puberty or hypogonadism
- Presence of gynecomastia
- History suggestive of hyperprolactinemia, such as headache, galactorrhea, impotence, blurred vision
- Testicular mass
- History of exogenous estrogen or androgen exposure
- Significant obesity
- Clinical features of androgen resistance
- Clinical picture consistent with 5-α reductase-deficiency

Clinical fertility centers differ in the extent of hormonal evaluation for infertile men. Current American Urological Association (AUA) guidelines recommend the measurements of at least serum FSH levels and serum testosterone levels in patients suspected of having abnormality in HPG axis.[27] Such measurements are reliable in detecting 99% of endocrine abnormalities.[28] Testosterone is considered the indicator of endocrine balance and normal functioning of Leydig cells, whereas FSH level is thought to be a representative parameter of spermatogenesis.

However, many centers carry out a more extensive laboratory evaluation, which can include measurement of LH, PRL, serum inhibin B, TSH, SHBG, cortisol and estradiol levels, if the clinical findings indicate an endocrine abnormality.

Serum FSH measurement may reflect the state of spermatogenesis in infertile men. As aforementioned, elevated FSH is the most evident endocrine abnormality in infertile men, particularly in cases of nonobstructive azoospermia (NOA) and severe oligozoospermia. High FSH level often indicates significant alteration in spermatogenesis. On the other hand, low FSH in the presence of low testosterone may reflect central disorder in the HPG axis, such as HH. In contrast, normal FSH measurement may not be indicative of normal spermatogenesis and does not exclude severe derangement of spermatogenesis. Specifically, men with spermatogenic arrest at late stages, focal Sertoli cell only syndrome and hypospermatogenesis may all have normal FSH level.[29] Even more specifically, normal FSH is not absolute predictive parameter of sperm retrieval by testicular sperm extraction in men with NOA.[29,30] From the above discussion, it is apparent that the value of serum FSH measurement is particularly limited and determination of other endocrine factors, such as inhibin B, may be required to represent the quality of spermatogenesis.

Inhibin B is a direct product of Sertoli cells and its serum levels have been found to be better correlated to sperm parameters than FSH and thus may serve as a better marker of spermatogenesis.[31] Inhibin B levels can also be useful for monitoring the effects of gonadotropin therapy. However, inhibin B or FSH alone as well as the combination of both hormones cannot predict the finding of spermatozoa by testicular biopsy in patients with azoospermia who are candidates for intracytoplasmic sperm injection(ICSI) treatment.[32]

Testosterone level is, more or less, a good indicator of the integrity of HPG axis and Leydig cell function. Total testosterone level consists of protein (SHBG and albumin) bound fraction (98%) and free fraction (2%), and its measurement correlates well with available testosterone. However, measurement of free testosterone should be considered when alterations in SHBG are expected (Table 3). In order to determine free testosterone reliably, equilibrium dialysis or ultrafiltration-techniques are required. These methods are complicated and not routinely recommended at present. However, a simple and reliable method for clinical practice is the estimation of free testosterone from the levels of total testosterone, and SHBG by using a standard equation and special nomograms (Fig. 7).[33] Calculated free testosterone correlates well with free testosterone estimated by equilibrium dialysis.[34] The serum total testosterone concentration is not diagnostic of hypogonadism in obese patients or those with nephrotic syndrome, hyper- or hypothyroidism, chronic liver disease, or on therapy with anticonvulsants or steroids.[34]

The generally approved reference range for total testosterone in adultmen is wide, from 260 ng/dl to 1,000 ng/dl(9–34.7 nmol/l). Furthermore, testosterone levels have circadian fluctuations, particularly marked in younger men, where there is a striking difference in testosterone levels measured in early morning versus those taken later in the day. The mean maximum level of 720 ng/dl (25 nmol/l) is reached at approximately 8 AM, and declines to a mean minimum of 432 ng/dl (15 nmol/l) at approximately 10 PM. However, such degree of change between morning and evening testosterone levels is less striking in older men. Nevertheless, it is best in all cases to measure the concentration in the morning

Table 3 Factors that affect circulating sex hormone-binding globulin levels

Increase	*Decrease*
Aging	Prepubertal development
Growth hormone deficiency	Obesity
Estrogens	Hyperinsulinemia
Androgen deficiency	Glucocorticoids
Hyperthyroidism	Androgens
Hepatitis	Progestins
	Hypothyroidism
Growth hormone excess	
	Familial

so that peak results can be compared with the usual standards. In general, because of this circadian variations in secretion, serum samples for total testosterone determination should be obtained between 7:00 AM and 9.00 AM.[34] Moreover, because of diurnal variation in testosterone and pulsatile pattern of secretion of LH and FSH, an alternative is to perform hormone assays on three pooled blood samples taken at 10 minutes intervals.[35]

In men who are found to have azoospermia but normal testosterone, LH, and FSH levels and normal testes volume, obstructive disorders should be ruled out by measuring seminal levels of fructose and neutral α-glucosidase. The latter originates in the epididymis.[25] In case of azoospermia or severe oligospermia, normal testosterone and LH levels, but elevated FSH, primary spermatogenic failure should be considered. These patients should get testicular volume assessment, karyotyping and Yq micro deletion screening.

Primary testicular failure (spermatogenesis and steroidogenesis) often presents with low testosterone, and elevated FSH and LH serum levels; whereas, patients

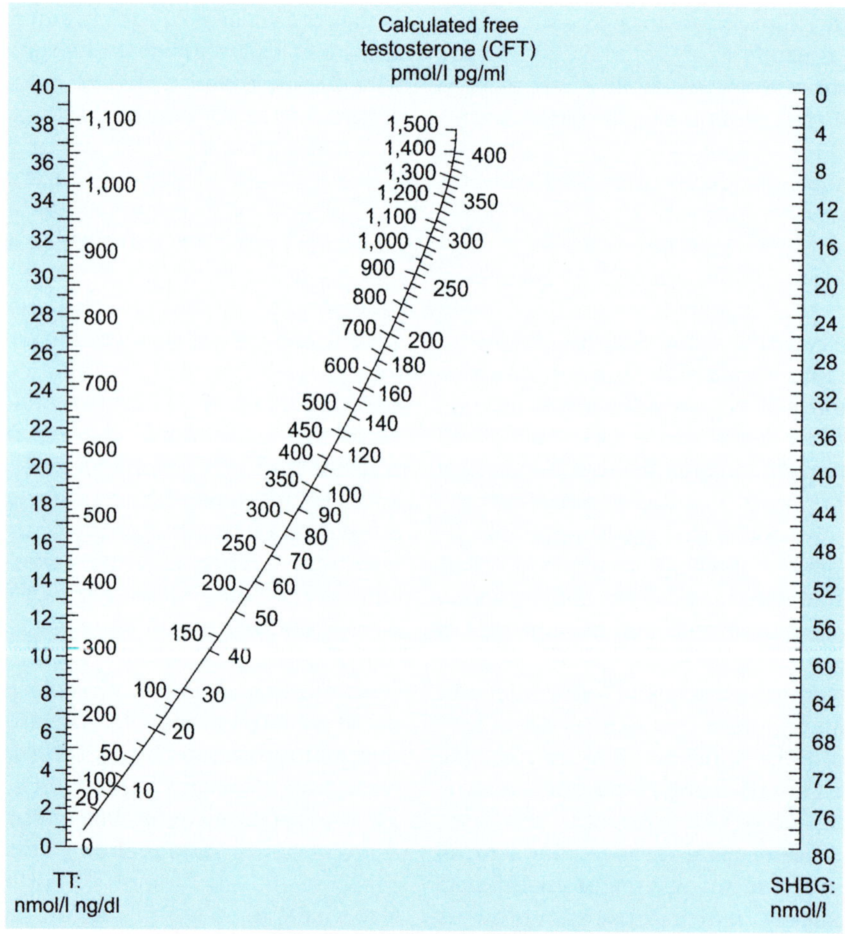

Figure 7 Nomogram for calculating free testosterone (CFT) from total testosterone (TT) and (SHBG)
Source: Carruthers M. Androgen deficiency in the adult male: causes, diagnosis and treatment. London: Taylor & Francis; 2004[93]

with selective spermatogenic failure have normal testosterone and LH, and only elevated FSH. In cases with low testosterone and low or inappropriately normal LH and FSH, it is important to determine PRL, cortisol, serum ferritin, TSH and free thyroxine levels. These patients may need magnetic brain resonance imaging to determine the cause of HH. Normal MRI, PRL level and other measurements in these men point out to the possibility of hypothalamic disorders, such as anosmicHH (Kallmann's syndrome), nonanosmic isolated hypogonadotropic hyp-ogonadism (IHH) and adult onset HH. Direct measurement of GnRH is not feasible in humans due to pulsatile mode of secretion, short half-life, very low concentration and dilution of this hypothalamic hormone by the pituitary portal circulation and then by systemic circulation. In unresolved cases when there is low or normal LH and FSH, GnRH stimulation test can be conducted. Subcutaneous injection of intravenous 100 µg of GnRH should normally cause a three fold rise in LH and 1.5 times in FSH after 30–45 minutes of injection. The rise in LH/FSH helps confirm the diagnosis of anosmic and normosmic HH.[32] In contrast, negative response is usually attributed to failure of pituitary gland to respond to the injected GnRH. Such unresponsiveness may occur due to lack of previous exposure to GnRH (Priming effect) or due to mutated gene coding for GnRH receptor (GNRHR). To discriminate between the two conditions, subcutaneous portable GnRH pump releasing 5 µg of GnRH every (90–120) is undertaken for 36 hours a day for 7 days. Then GnRH stimulation test is repeated. Positive rise confirm the HH diagnosis and exclude the possibility of pituitary unresponsiveness.[32]

Normal PRL level in men is usually less than 18 ng/dl (550 mIU/l). However, due to high assay variability, testing should be repeated, if levels are elevated. If hyperprolactinemia is discovered and secondary causes are ruled out or PRL levels are above 150 ng/dl, a gadolinium enhanced MRI with special attention to the region of hypothalamus and pituitary is indicated for revealing a prolactinoma or another space occupying process.

Both in complete and partial forms of androgen insensitivity, serum testosterone and LH levels are usually elevated, but FSH may be normal or elevated. Estradiol is higher than in normal males. Failure of SHBG to decrease after testosterone administration confirms the androgen insensitivity. An hCG stimulating test demonstrating normal testosterone and DHT production can be used to distinguish partial androgen insensitivity syndrome from defects in testosterone biosynthesis and 5-α reductase activity.[36,37] Karyotyping reveals 46 XY and is indicated especially in cases with ambiguous genitalia and bilateral inguinal hernias. Androgen receptor studies are helpful in cases with incomplete insensitivity.

Serum estradiol determination may be considered in select group of patients, such as ones with Klinefelter's syndrome and in cases with gynecomastia, a testicular mass, a history consistent with exogenous estrogen exposure, or evidence of androgen resistance.[38]

DISEASES OF THE HPG AXIS

Hypothalamic and Pituitary Disorders

Hypogonadotropic hypogonadism results from failure of the hypothalamus or pituitary to stimulate and maintain normal gonadal function.[39] Pituitary functions may be affected in events of pituitary tumors, infarction, inflammatory and granulomatous diseases, surgery and radiation. However, gonadotropin deficiency may also occur in the presence of otherwise normal pituitary function when the secretion or action of GnRH is altered: IHH

Isolated Hypogonadotropic Hypogonadism

Isolated hypogonadotropic hypogonadism is clinically defined as absent or incomplete puberty by the age of 18 years because of low gonadotropin secretion. The GnRH deficiency can be due to impaired migration of the GnRH neurons to the hypothalamus during embryonic development, abnormal maturation or decreased survival of GnRH neurons, or resistance to the action of GnRH at the level of pituitary. IHH can be either sporadic or familial. It may be inherited in an X-linked recessive, autosomal dominant or autosomal recessive mode. However, the genetics are not strictly Mendelian. IHH may be due to mutations in more than one gene, as well as interaction between genes, or between genes and environmental factors.[40] In males, the prevalence is around 1 in 10,000. There are two forms of IHH depending on the presence or absence of the normal sense of smell: normosmic IHH and Kallmann's syndrome.

Kallmann's Syndrome

It is a form of IHH associated with olfactory disturbances (hypo- or anosmia) due to the absence or hypoplasia of the olfactory bulbs and tract. The incidence is estimated to be about 3.7% of all IHH male patients. The male preponderance of cases remains still unexplained. The olfactory and reproductive deficits are combined with various defects, including cryptorchidism, bimanual synkinesis (mirror movements), unilateral renal agenesis, craniofacial or dental abnormalities, syndactyly, sensorineural deafness.[41]

Hyperprolactinemia

It is another endocrine cause of secondary hypogonadism commonly seen in clinical practice. PRL is an anterior pituitary hormone whose excessive concentrations suppress the secretion of FSH and LH and/or impede their action on the gonads. Hyperprolactinemia can be caused by prolactinomas, pituitary tumors secreting both PRL and GH, processes causing pituitary stalk compression or section, empty sella syndrome, medications, primary hypothyroidism, chronic renal failure among other causes or may be idiopathic. Symptoms include depressed libido, erectile dysfunction, and infertility. Galactorrhea is rare in men.

Isolated FSH and LH Deficiency

Rare disorders include isolated FSH deficiency, which may present with oligo- or azoospermia, though such patients have normal virilization and normal testosterone and LH levels.[42] Isolated LH deficiency (Pasqualini syndrome, fertile eunuch syndrome) on the other hand leads to eunuchoid habitus, low testosterone levels, but normal maturation of germinal epithelium with Leydig cell atrophy on testicular biopsy. Serum levels of LH are low, but of FSH are normal.[32]

Other Complex Congenital Syndrome

This syndrome associated with HH includes Prader-Willi syndrome where lack of GnRH secretion leads to LH and FSH deficiency. The hypogonadism in the very rare genetic disorders, Laurence-Moon syndrome and Bardet-Biedl syndrome, is not obligate.[32]

Testicular Diseases

Hypergonadotropic Hypogonadism

This group includes different congenital and acquired disorders primarily affecting the gonads (Table 3). The result in testicular failure and infertility, but some of them can cause only fertility disturbances without obvious signs of hypogonadism. Defects in androgen production, as well as conversion of testosterone to DHT due to the deficiency of enzyme 5-α reductase, affect the phenotype and reproduction. A number of genetic disorders, such as Klinefelter's syndrome and Y chromosome microdeletions, have been implicated in spermatogenic failure. Table 4 demonstrates causes of HH.

Table 4 Disorders causing primary or hypergonadotropic hypogonadism

- Klinefelter's syndrome (47,XXY)
- XX male syndrome
- 47,XYY men
- Gonadal dysgenesis
- Noonan's syndrome
- Defects in androgen biosynthesis
- Bilateral anorchia (vanishing testes syndrome)
- Acquired anorchy
- Orchitis
- Varicocele
- Adult seminiferous tubule failure

Disorders of Androgen Actions

Androgen insensitivity causes undermasculinization of various degrees in 46 XY individuals. The androgen receptor gene is located on the X chromosome between Xq11 and Xq13. Androgen insensitivity syndromes result from defects in androgen receptor number or function. Androgen insensitivity may be complete or partial (incomplete). Complete androgen insensitivity syndrome (testicular feminization syndrome) is characterized by complete feminization of genetic males. Partial androgen insensitivity presents with great variations from normal male phenotype with infertility to individuals with genital ambiguity and gynecomastia.[36,37]

DISEASES OF THE ADRENAL GLANDS

Glucocorticoid excess (hypercortisolism) in Cushing's syndrome of either endogenous or exogenous etiology may also suppress LH secretion and testosterone biosynthesis resulting in testosterone deficiency and hypospermatogenesis.

Androgen excess can induce a hypogonadal state by inhibiting gonadotropin production through negative feedback. The source of androgen excess could be either endogenous production from adrenals or testes, or exogenous anabolic steroids. Deficiency of enzyme 21-hydroxylase is the commonest cause of congenital adrenal hyperplasia. The excess of adrenal androgens in this condition may lead to precocious pseudo-puberty and infertility. It can be diagnosed by high basal and ACTH stimulated plasma 17-α hydroxyprogesterone levels. Men with partial enzyme deficiency may remain undiagnosed until late in adulthood, though they are usually fertile. 'Adrenal or testicular Leydig cell tumors' can also produce excess serum androgens and require radiological imaging for diagnosis.

THYROID DISORDERS

Both hyper- and hypothyroidism may have an adverse impact on male fertility. Hyperthyroidism is known to cause elevation of SHBG and decline in semen quality especially in semen motility.[43] In literature, hyperthyroid men has shown relative primary gonadal insufficiency that might be due to exaggerated SHBG levels and increased gonadotropin levels with co-pulsatility between LH and FSH, which was more pronounced than in healthy men.[44] Evidence is weak though about the possible deleterious effects of hypothyroidism on male reproductive system.[45]

EXCESS ESTROGEN

Estrogen excess can also produce secondary testicular failure by inhibiting pituitary gonadotropins. It can be derived from either estrogen secreting adrenal or testicular tumors or excess peripheral conversion of androgens to estrogens by aromatase enzyme in patients suffering from chronic liver diseases or obesity. Men with high estrogen levels may present with gynecomastia, erectile dysfunction and testicular atrophy.

DIABETES MELLITUS AND METABOLIC SYNDROME

Diabetes mellitus affects the reproductive function mainly through microangiopathy and neuropathy, which in turn leads to erectile dysfunction and ejaculate disturbances. Obesity as well as diabetes mellitus type 2 (DM 2) may cause hypogonadism and infertility. Both low and high body mass index (BMI) are associated with disturbances in spermatogenesis. In obesity, increased peripheral conversion of androgens to estrogens in excess peripheral adipose tissue suppresses the gonadotropin secretion. Another unfavorable effect of obesity may be the oxidative stress leading to impaired spermatogenesis.[46] Dyslipidemia also increases oxidative stress. Metabolic syndrome is not a separate disease by itself but a cluster of abnormalities, including visceral type obesity, dyslipidemia, hypertension and impaired glucose metabolism or DM 2 with insulin resistance as the hypothesized underlying pathogenic mechanism. An association of metabolic syndrome with low testosterone and low SHBG serum levels is widely accepted, but the cause and effect relationship is still unclear. Men with low testosterone and low SHBG levels are more likely to develop insulin resistance and DM 2. On the other hand, insulin is known to inhibit SHBG synthesis, therefore in insulin-resistant individuals SHBG, and consequently total testosterone is decreased. A negative correlation of total testosterone with insulin levels, insulin resistance and BMI in young males with metabolic syndrome was reported.[47]

HORMONAL INTERVENTION IN MALE INFERTILITY

Hormonal therapy was utilized in the field of male infertility many years ago; however, the fertility outcomes confront a great deal of disappointment and frustration. Alternatively, the successful conception rates achieved through assisted reproductive technology has led to infrequent and unenthusiastic demand on hormonal intervention. Nevertheless, appropriately prescribed hormonal treatment is cost-effective and attractive mode of therapy. Currently, therapeutic and fertility preservation roles are the two main sorts of hormonal manipulation.

Therapeutic intervention aiming at restoring the fertility potential is used for specific replacement of a particularly deficient hormone, or used in nonspecific manner in idiopathic male infertility with no identifiable endocrine abnormalities.

Adequate replacement therapy either with GnRH or LH and FSH can induce spermatogenesis in patients with HH. Maturation of the human sperm takes approximately 72 days,[48] so the treatment should last at least 3 months for the sperm to appear in the ejaculate. Usually a much longer period (up to 2 years or even more) is required, especially in congenital HH.

Gonadotropin Releasing Hormone

Rationale: GnRH stimulates anterior pituitary to secrete LH and FSH which in turn regulates T cells production and spermatogenesis. It can thus be used in pulsatile fashion in men with HH caused by hypothalamic dysfunction, but not in those having loss of pituitary function. It can also be used for induction of puberty.

Method of administration: GnRH is administered using portable pump in doses of 4–20 µg per pulse administered subcutaneously every 2 hours as pulsatile therapy. Doses are adjusted until serum testosterone reaches mid-normal levels. GnRH as nasal spray is used for treatment of cryptorchidism.

Indications: GnRH has been demonstrated to be quite effective in inducing androgenization and spermatogenesis in men with IHH.[49-51] It did not differ in efficacy in terms of spermatogenesis and pregnancy rates as compared to the gonadotropin therapy. In preliminary investigations involving infertile men who had cryptorchidism, GnRH analogues have been shown to improve spermatogenesis when used as an adjunct to orchidopexy.[52,53] On the basis of successful treatment of one single case Iwamoto et al. concluded[54] that nasal therapy with GnRH analogue buserelin in low doses avoids pituitary down-regulation exerting stimulatory effect on it and therefore may be an effective and well-tolerated therapeutic option for patients with HH of hypothalamic origin.[54]

Side effects and disadvantages: Wearing of the portable pump is cumbersome and hence discouraging for patients. Formation of anti-GnRH antibodies in certain cases has also raised some concern.[55] Furthermore, at present consensus exists that GnRH has no role as empiric therapy in idiopathic infertility.

Gonadotropins

Various urinary, purified, and recombinant forms of gonadotropins have been used including hCG with LH activity, human menopausal gonadotropin [(hMG) FSH analogue], recombinant FSH and LH.

Mixed Gonadotropin Therapy

Rationale: In all forms of hypogonadism testosteroneal one is sufficient for maturation and maintenance of secondary sex characteristics, libido and erectile function. In HH; however, the anterior pituitary hormones LH and FSH are required together to initiate and maintain spermatogenesis. A combined gonadotropin therapy can thus be used to treat hypogonadotropic infertility arising at the level of pituitary or hypothalamus including IHH, when treatment with GnRH is not desired or indicated. hCG is used as the source of LH activity to stimulate testosterone secretion by Leydig cells, whereas hMG acts as FSH.[56] In recent years, recombinant gonadotropins have been introduced in clinical practice.

Method of administration: The therapy is started with hCG 1,000–2,500 IU two times/week subcutaneously or intramuscularly; adjusting the dose to target mid-normal testosterone levels. Testosterone levels are measured 48 hours after the hCG injection. Alternatively, recombinant LH can be used. After a period of 8–12 weeks of hCG or recombinant human LH therapy, a highly purified hMG or recombinant human FSH is added at the doses of 150–225 IU three times/week subcutaneously.[22] The treatment continues until sperm appear in the ejaculate or pregnancy occurs respectively, but in some cases therapy may be required for 1–2 or more years.

As soon as in men with HH spermatogenesis is induced with combined gonadotropin treatment or with GnRH, it can be maintained qualitatively by hCG alone for long time, but the decreasing sperm counts indicate that FSH is necessary for maintenance of quantitatively normal spermatogenesis.[56]

Indications: Several studies although not placebo controlled have shown induction of spermatogenesis and ability to induce pregnancy with use of mixed gonadotropin therapy[51,57,58] and it is presently the most widely used therapy for hypogonadotropic infertility. Testicular volumes of 8 ml or more and post-pubertal onset of gonadotropin deficiency are more likely to respond than those with testicular volumes of less than 4 ml and pre-pubertal onset.[50] Nevertheless, this treatment is also indicated in cases with cryptorchidism or with small testicular volume.[49] According to a recent study men with BMI less than 30 kg/m^2 have a greater chance of achieving spermatogenesis than men with a BMI equal to or greater than 30 kg/m^2.[39] Low BMI and advanced sexual maturity, especially large baseline mean testicular volume are predictors of a good response to combined therapy with recombinant human FSH and hCG.[39] Recent observations has demonstrated useful effect of hCG therapy in improvement of sperm retrieval rates in men with Klinefelter's syndrome as will be described later.

Side effects and disadvantages: Although spermatogenesis is induced in the majority of cases, some patients may not respond. For quantitatively, normal spermatogenesis both gonadotropins are required. The treatments with gonadotropins and GnRH are expensive, therefore, they should be introduced only when a desire for children is present or once to stimulate testicular function until induction of spermatogenesis is achieved before switching to a long lasting substitution therapy with testosterone.[59]

FSH Monotherapy

Rationale: FSH has an established role in promoting spermatogenesis. It enhances the production of androgen-binding protein by Sertoli cells which are required to maintain high local concentration of testosterone in the seminiferous tubules thus supporting spermatogenesis.[60] However, the role of FSH in the maintenance of spermatogenesis remains controversial.[56]

Method of administration: Purified or recombinant human FSH is given at doses ranging from 50 IUto 300 IU administered subcutaneously threetimes weekly for over 3 months.

Indications: Several randomized controlled trials have evaluated the efficacy of FSH in men with idiopathic infertility with mixed results.[61,62] In these studies, the gonadotrophic status of the patients was not well characterized. Although pregnancy outcomes were not reported in most of these studies, improvement in sperm parameters was noted in some when FSH was used at higher doses.[48,63] When used 50 days before ICSI, FSH has been shown to improve fertilization, implantation and pregnancy rates in men with severe oligozoospermia.[64]

Side effects and disadvantages: Evidence is weak and the consensus is that FSH therapy alone has at the best little efficacy in treating idiopathic male infertility.

Androgen Therapy

Testosterone Therapy

Rationale: Although testosterone has contraceptive properties in men due to its negative feedback on hypothalamic-pituitary axis and thus inhibition of LH and FSH, and spermatogenesis respectively. It has been tried to treat subfertile men with testosterone based on two rationales. Raising serum testosterone would improve epididymal maturation of spermatozoa; gonadotropins and sperm concentration respectively increase transiently upon sudden stopping of testosterone, the so-called 'rebound effect'.

Method of administration: Male infertility is treated using testosterone undecanoate or mesterolone in doses of 120–240 mg/day and 75–150 mg/day respectively.

Indication: Various meta-analyses have demonstrated no improvement in pregnancy outcomes with androgen therapy in idiopathic male infertility.[65,66]

Side effects and disadvantages: Published literature strongly discourages any role of testosterone monotherapy for men with idiopathic infertility.

Anti-estrogen Therapy

Anti-estrogen Monotherapy

*Rationale:*Anti-estrogens indirectly stimulate the secretion of GnRH, FSH and LH by binding to ERα in the hypothalamus and pituitary, thereby blocking estrogen feedback inhibition. The resultant increase of gonadotropin concentration is believed to improve the gametogenic function of the testes.

Method of administration: The two most commonly used nonsteroidal anti-estrogens are clomiphene citrate and tamoxifen. Clomiphene citrate is usually prescribed in doses of 12.5–50 mg/day either continuously or on a 25-day cycle with a 5-day rest period, each month for 3-6 months. Tamoxifen is administered at a dosage of 10–20 mg daily over a period of 3–6 months.

Indication: Cochrane meta-analysis of 10 randomized controlled trials with idiopathic infertility found no improvement in pregnancy rates with anti-estrogen therapy.[67] Similarly, another meta-analysis reported no significant change in pregnancy outcomes with clomiphene citrate or tamoxifen therapy of idiopathic infertile men (OR, 1.54; 95% CI: 0.99-2.40).[65] However, some studies demonstrated improvement in sperm count and sperm motility.[68] Hence, empiric therapy for at least 3 months may have a beneficial effect on fertility status in subfertile men by improving semen parameters which may allow a down-staging of the required ART procedure, i.e. utilizing intrauterine insemination instead of ICSI. Recent reports have shown specific indication and beneficial effect of clomiphene citrate and its isomer enclomiphene in treatment of men with HH and restoration of physiological level of testosterone. Clomiphene citrate can also restore testosterone/estrogen ratio in hypogonadal men.[69,70-72] Lastly, men with Klinefelter's syndrome who have been prescribed clomiphene citrate show an improvement in sperm retrieval rates by testicular extraction as demonstrated below.

Side effects and disadvantages: Literature support remains inconclusive awaiting large randomized prospective trials of empiric therapy in idiopathic male infertility. Unfortunately, deterioration in semen parameters of some men with idiopathic male infertility has been reported after using clomiphene citrate. For replacement of testosterone in men with HH, two regimens have been described either low dose daily regimen of 25 mg[69]or 50 mg given three times a week.[71]

Tamoxifen and Testosterone Combination Therapy

Rationale: Tamoxifen has been shown to primarily increase sperm density without much improvement in other parameters, such as sperm motility and morphology. One of the main reasons could be inferior androgenic environment in the reproductive tract of oligozoospermic men. This in turn may compromise epididymal maturation of the spermatozoa which can be theoretically overcome by supplementing tamoxifen treatment with testosterone.

Method of administration: Tamoxifen and testosterone undecanoate are administered as 20 mg and 120 mg respectively in daily divided doses for 6 months.

Indication: Treatment with tamoxifen and testosterone undecanoate improved sperm variables and led to a higher incidence of pregnancy in couples with subfertility related to idiopathic oligozoospermia.[73]

Side effects and disadvantages: Literature is scarce and primarily restricted to single group of investigators.

Tamoxifen and Kallikrein Combination Therapy

Rationale: While tamoxifen improves sperm count, kallikrein has been shown to improve sperm motility; hence a combination can hypothetically be useful in men with idiopathic oligoasthenozoospermia.

Method of administration: Tamoxifen is administered as 20 mg/day along with 600 IU of kallikrein daily for 3 months.

Indication: Improvement in both sperm count and motility with such a therapy has been demonstrated in few trials when used in idiopathic normogonadotropic men with oligoasthenospermia.[74]

Side effects and disadvantages: Pregnancy outcomes have not yet been studied and further studies are warranted to draw any inferences.

Therapy with Aromatase Inhibitors

Rationale: Aromatase is a P450 cytochrome enzyme that converts androgens to estrogens. Aromatase inhibitors block its activity thereby reducing serum estradiol concentration and its negative feedback on the hypothalamus and pituitary, resulting in elevated serum FSH levels, which in turn, might improve spermatogenesis.[75] On the other hand, aromatase inhibitors lead to increase in testosterone which also might contribute to achievement of fertility.

Method of administration: Two types of aromatase inhibitors are available, steroidal (e.g. testolactone) and nonsteroidal (letrozole and anastrozole). The latter is more effective in increasing testosterone to estrogen ratio and is less likely to cause interruption of the adrenal axis beyond aromatase inhibition. Testolactone is given in doses of 100–200 mg/day, whereas anastrozole is used as 1 mg/day dosage and letrozole 2.5 mg daily orally for 4–6 months.

Indication: Hyperestrogenemia associated with male infertility constitutes the main indication for the use of aromatase inhibitors therapy. Elevated estrogen level or elevated estrogen to testosterone ratio is obviously observed in men with significant obesity associated with idiopathic HH and Klinefelter's syndrome.

In idiopathic oligozoospermic men studied in double blind randomized controlled fashion, testolactone therapy failed to show any improvement in semen parameters.[76] Normal spermatogenesis proven by testis biopsy was achieved with letrozole in one case with azoospermia and normal FSH serum levels.[75] Controlled studies evaluating the efficacy of aromatase inhibitors on pregnancy outcomes are still lacking. Furthermore, Ramasamy et al. (2009) indicated that medications leading to physiological endogenous testosterone secretion, such as aromatase inhibitors, clomiphene or hCG result in a better chance of sperm retrieval in men with Klinefelter's syndrome with either normal or low baseline testosterone than those Klinefelter's men who used exogenous testosterone to induce secondary sexual characteristics [(77% vs. 55%)[77] Level C evidence]. Such observation may be attributed to exogenous testosterone induced suppression of release of pituitary FSH and LH and henceforth suppression of spermatogenesis.

Side effects and disadvantages: Further investigation is needed before drawing any conclusions on the use of aromatase inhibitors in male infertility. Elevation of hepatic enzymes has been reported with both these drugs and hence caution is advised in those who have underlying liver disease.

Growth Hormone Therapy

Rationale: GH acts on gonads directly or through hepatic secreted insulin-like growth factor-1 and plays a significant role in sexual growth and differentiation, gonadal steroidogenesis and gametogenesis.[78]

Method of administration: Recombinant GH is given for 12 weeks.

Indication: GH therapy has shown mixed results in terms of improvement in sperm parameters and pregnancy rate when used in oligo- and asthenozoospermic men.[79,80] When used as an adjunct therapy in a small study of seven men with HH who failed gonadotropin therapy, GH has been demonstrated to help induce spermatogenesis.[81]

Side effects and disadvantages: Available literature is limited and further studies trying combination therapy of GH and gonadotropins for male infertility are awaited.

Oxytocin Therapy

Rationale: Oxytocin has been shown to promote sperm progression through the reproductive tract by improving epididymal contractility. It can thus be used to increase sperm retrieval in men with oligozoospermia.

Method of administration: Oxytocin is given as intravenous injections or intranasal just before ejaculation.

Indication: Oxytocin therapy has failed to improve sperm output in severely oligozoospermic men.[82]

Side effects and disadvantages: This form of therapy lacks evidence in supporting any role in male infertility.

Endocrine Therapy for Hyperprolactinemia

Dopamine agonists are the primary therapy for both micro- and macroadenomas associated hyperprolactinemias, as well as for non-tumor related hyperprolactinemia. Historically, bromocriptine (2.5–10.0 mg, maximal 30 mg a day) was the first effective medical therapy. Cabergoline, a non-ergot DA agonist, is administered at a dosage of 0.25–1.0 mg twice per week. Both normalize PRL levels, decrease tumor size and restore reproductive function. Cabergoline is better tolerated than bromocriptine. However, there are some recent concerns of heart valvular defects with higher doses of cabergoline.[83]

Summary: Therapy for subfertile men generally falls under two categories: specific and empiric, depending upon the etiology. Endocrine evaluation of men presenting with infertility should aim at identifying candidates for specific therapy. For men who have HH, both gonadotropin therapy and pulsatile GnRH are equally effective. However, idiopathic infertility which is a much more frequently encountered clinical problem responds poorly to empiric endocrine treatment. Recently, several hormonal intervention studies have shown promise in management of idiopathic male infertility. Further trials with adequate sample size and study design are warranted before it can be put into routine clinical practice.

CYTOPROTECTIVE HORMONAL EFFECTS ON SPERM IN CANCER PATIENTS

Hormonal manipulation inducing a state of quiescence may protect the testicular germ cells from being heavily damaged by exposure to gonadotoxins, such as cancer chemotherapy, or radiotherapy. This theory stems from the observation of relative resistance of prepubertal testes to cancer chemotherapy and animal studies in which GnRH agonists or antagonists were given to suppress spermatogenesis.

In United States 17,000 men in reproductive ages between 15 years and 45 years are diagnosed with cancer, such as Hodgkin's lymphoma, leukemia, testicular cancer and soft tissue sarcoma each year.[84,85] Of these, more than 3,000 patients receive treatment, such as alkylating agents, platinum based chemotherapy or radiation which may render men azoospermic or severe oligozoospermic.[84,85] Cytotoxic chemotherapy may also be used in the treatment of autoimmune diseases. The mechanisms of deranged spermatogenesis include direct stem cell aplasia or failure of differentiation of surviving stem cells into mature sperm. Restoration of male fertility is very slow and may take upto 6 years. Endocrine alterations, described in these men, particularly with germ cell aplasia, may include a decreased level of serum inhibin and consequently elevated serum FSH level. Chemotherapy or radiotherapy induced testicular ischemia contributes to decline in the systemic distribution of testosterone, elevated LH level and increased intratesticular testosterone.[86,87] Ultimately, successful resumption of spermatogenesis depends on survival of stem cells and their ability to differentiate into sperm.

Various hormonal regimens have been used for protection of testicular tissues during chemo- or radiotherapy. In animals, GnRH, FSH and steroids were administered, whereas in humans GnRH agonists alone or in combination with testosterone or antiandrogen, testosterone and medroxyprogesterone have been used with mixed results. Animal studies have shown protective effect of GnRH given for several weeks (upto 6 weeks) before cytotoxic chemotherapy and continued thereafter or through administration of GnRH after irradiation or chemotherapy to stimulate spermatogenesis.[86,88] Only single small study out of seven trials in humans has shown such promising improvement by the use of testosterone, concomitantly with cyclophosphamide for the treatment of autoimmune nephritis.[89] Nevertheless, further studies are actually required and prolonged pretreatment with hormonal therapy for extended period of time for several weeks should be utilized to show a protective effect.

Other options for fertility preservation encompass sperm or testicular tissue cryopreservation. The transplantation of cryopreserved spermatogonia is being studied and preliminary animal studies have shown beneficial effects of GnRH analogues in maintenance of the survival of transplanted spermatogonia.[90,91]

REFERENCES

1. Guyton AC, Hall JA. Endocrinology and Reproduction. In: Guyton AC, Hall JA (Eds). Text book of Medical Physiology, 11th edition. Philadelphia, Pennsylvania: Elsevier Saunders; 2006. pp.905-17.
2. Brook CG, Rosalind SB. The application of science to clinical practice. In: Brook CG, Brown RS (Eds).

Handbook of Clinical Pediatric Endocrinology, 1st edition. Massachusetts, USA: Blackwell Publishing, Inc; 2008. pp. 1-13.
3. Daniel PM, Treip CS. The pathology of the hypothalamus. J Clin Endocrinol Metab. 1977; 6:3-19.
4. Daniel PM, Prichard MML. Studies of the hypothalamus and the pituitary gland. Acta Endocrinologica. 1975 80:1-216.
5. Brodal P. The central autonomic system: the hypothalamus. In: Brodal P(Ed). The Central Nervous System Structure and Function, 4th edition. Oxford: Oxford University Press; 2010. pp. 440-58.
6. Knobil E. The GnRH pulse generator. Am J Obstet Gynecol. 1990; 163:1721-7.
7. Martinez de la, Escalera G, Choi ALH, et al. Generation and synchronization of gonadotropin releasing hormone (GnRH) pulses: intrinsic properties of the gt1-1 gonadotropin releasing hormone (GnRH) neuronal cell line. Proc Natl Acad Sci USA. 1992;89:1852-5.
8. Styne DM, Grumbach MM. Puberty: ontogeny, neuroendocrinology, physiology, and disorders. In: Kronenberg HM, Melmed S, PolonskyKS, LarsenPR(Eds). Williams Textbook of Endocrinology, 11th edition. Philadelphia USA: Elsevier Inc.; 2008.pp.969-1166.
9. Low MJ. Neuroendocrinology. In: Kronenber HM, Melmed S, Polonsky KS, Larsen PR (Eds). Kronenberg And Williams Textbook of Endocrinology, 11th edition. Philadelphia PA: Saunders; 2008. pp.85-135.
10. Melmed S, Kleinberg D. Anterior pituitary. In: Kronenberg HM, Melmed S, Polonsky KS(Eds). Williams Textbook of Endocrinology, 11th edition. Pennsylvania: Saunders Elsevier; 2008. pp. 240-42.
11. Horvath E, Kovacs K. Fine structural cytology of the adenohypophysis in rat and man. J Electron Microsc Tech. 1988; 8:401-32.
12. Andersen CY, Westergaard LG, van Wely M. FSH isoform composition of commercial gonadotrophin preparations: a neglected aspect? Reprod Biomed Online. 2004; 9(2):231-6.
13. Fares F. The role of O-linked and N-linked oligosaccharides on the structure-function of glycoprotein hormones: development of agonists and antagonists. Biochim Biophys Acta. 2006; 1760:560-7.
14. Vermeulen A. Androgens in aging male. J Clin Endocrinol Metab. 1991; 73:221-4.
15. Bremner W, Vitiello V, Prinz P. Loss of circadian rhythmicity in blood testosterone levels with aging in normal men. J Clin Endocrinol Metab. 1983; 56:1278-81.
16. Handelsman DJ. Ageing in the hypothalamic–pituitary–testicular axis. In: Neil JD (Ed). Knobil and Neill's Physiology. 2008; 2697-2759.
17. Weinbauer GF, Luetjens CM, Simoni M, et al. Physiology of testicular function. In: Nieschlag E, Behre HM, Nieschlag S (Eds). Andrology, Male Reproductive Health and Dysfunction, 3rd edition. Berlin Heidelberg: Springer-Verlag; 2010. pp. 11-59.
18. Raleigh D, O'Donnell L, Southwick GJ, et al. Stereological analysis of the human testis after vasectomy indicates impairment of spermatogenic efficiency with increasing obstructive interval. Fertil Steril. 2004;81:1595-03.
19. Bhasin S, Fielder TJ, Swerdloff RS. Testosterone selectively increases serum follicle-stimulating hormone (FSH) but not luteinizing hormone (LH) in gonadotropin-releasing hormone antagonist-treated male rats. Evidence for differential regulation of LH and FSH secretion. BiolReprod. 1987; 37(1):55-9.
20. Dufourny L, Caraty A, Clarke IJ, et al. Progesterone-receptive dopaminergic and neuropeptides Y neurons project from the arcuate nucleus to gonadotropin-releasing hormone-rich regions of the ovine preoptric area. Neuroendocrinology. 2005; 82:21–31.
21. Krsmanovic LZ, Hu L, Leung PK, et al. The hypothalamic GnRH pulse generator: multiple regulatory mechanisms. Trends Endocrinol Metab.2009; 20:402-8.
22. Bhasin S. Approach to the infertile man. J Clin Endocrinol Metab. 2007; 92(6):1995-2004.
23. Dunkel L. Normal and Delayed Puberty. In: Winters SJ (Ed). Male Hypogonadism, basic, clinical and therapeutic principles. New Jersey USA: Humana Press Inc.;2004. pp.3-79.
24. Sedlmeyer IL; Palmert MR. Delayed puberty: analysis of a large case series from an academic center. J ClinEndocrinolMetab. 2002;87(4):1613-20.
25. WHO laboratory manual for the examination and processing of human semen, 5th edition. WHO, Geneva. 2010.
26. Sigman M, Lipshultz LI, Howards SS. Evaluation of the subfertile male. In: Lipshultz LI, Howards SS(Eds). Infertility in the Male, 3rd edition. St. Louis: Mosby; 1997.
27. American Urological Association. The optimal evaluation of the infertile male [online]. Available from http://www.auanet.org/content/media/optimal evaluation[Accsessed 2010].
28. Turek P. Male infertility. In: TanaghoS, McAninchJW (Eds). Smith's General Urology, 17th edition. 2008. pp. 684-716.
29. Bergmann M, Behre HM, Nieschlag E. Serum FSH and testicular morphology in male infertility. Clin Endocrinol (Oxf). 1994;40:133-6.
30. Vernaeve V, Tournaye H, Schiettecatte J, et al. Serum inhibin B cannot predict testicular sperm retrieval in patients with non-obstructive azoospermia. Hum Reprod. 2002;17(4):971-6.
31. Kumanov P, Nandipati K, Tomova A, et al. Inhibin B is a better marker of spermatogenesis than other hormones in the evaluation of male factor infertility. Fertil Steril. 2006;86(2):332-8.
32. Simoni M, Nieschlag E Nieschlag. Endocrine laboratory diagnosis. In: E, Behre HM, Nieschlag S (Eds). Andrology, 3rd edition. Heidelberg: Springer; 2009. pp. 109-18.
33. Vermeulen A, Verdonck L, Kaufman JM. A critical evaluation of simple methods for the estimation of free testosterone in serum. J Clin Endocrinol Metab. 1999;84:3666-72.
34. Wang C, Nieschlag E, Swerdloff R, et al. Investigation, treatment, and monitoring of late-onset hypogonadism

in males: ISA, ISSAM, EAU, EAA, and ASA recommendations. European Urology. 2009;55:121-30.
35. Bain J, Langevin R, D'Costa M, et al. Serum pituitary and steroid hormone levels in the adult male: one value is as good as the mean of three. FertilSteril. 1988;49:123-6.
36. Balducci R, Ghirri P, Brown TR, et al. A clinician looks at androgen resistance. Steroids. 1996;61(4):205-11.
37. Yong EL, Loy CJ, Sim KS. Androgen receptor gene and male infertility. Hum Reprod Update. 2003;9(1):1-7.
38. Sokol RZ. Endocrinology of male infertility: evaluation and treatment. Semin Reprod Med. 2009;27(2):149-58.
39. Warne DW, Decosterd G, Okada H. A combined analysis of data to identify predictive factors for spermatogenesis in men with hypogonadotropic hypogonadism treated with recombinant human follicle-stimulating hormone and human chorionic gonadotropin. Fertil Steril. 2009;92(2):594-604.
40. Pitteloud N, Durrani S, Raivio T. Complex genetics in idiopathic hypogonadotropic hypogonadism. In: Quinton R (Ed). Front Horm Res. 2010;39:142-53.
41. MacColl GS, Quinton R, Bülow HE. Biology of KAL 1 and its orthologs: implication for X-linked Kallmann syndrome and the search for novel candidate genes. In: Quinton R (Eds): Kallmann Syndrome and hypogonadotropichypogonadism. Front Horm Res. 2010;39:62-77.
42. Al-Ansari AA, Khalil TH, Kelani Y, et al.Isolated follicle-stimulating hormone deficiency in men: successful long-term gonadotropin therapy. Fertil Steril. 1984;42(4):618-26.
43. Krassas GE, Pontikides N, Deligianni V, et al. A prospective controlled study of the impact of hypert hyroidism on reproductive function in males. J Clin Endocrinol Metab. 2002;87(8):3667-71.
44. Zähringer S, Tomova A, von Werder K, et al. The influence of hyperthyroidism on the hypothalamic-pituitary-gonadal axis. Exp Clin Endocrinol Diabetes. 2000;108:282-9.
45. Velázquez EM, BellabarbaArata G. Effects of thyroid status on pituitary gonadotropin and testicular reserve in men. Arch Androl. 1997;38(1):85-92.
46. Kasturi SS, Tannir J, Brannigan RE. The metabolic syndrome and male infertility. J Androl. 2008;29:251-9.
47. Robeva R, Kirilov G, Tomova A, et al. Low testosterone levels and unimpaired melatonin secretion in young males with metabolic syndrome. Andrologia. 2006;38:216-20.
48. Paradisi R, Busacchi P, Seracchioli R, et al. Effects of high doses of recombinant human follicle-stimulating hormone in the treatment of male factor infertility: results of a pilot study. Fertil Steril. 2006;86(3):728-31.
49. Büchter D, Behre HM, Kliesch S, et al. Pulsatile GnRH or human chorionic gonadotropin/human menopausal gonadotropin as effective treatment for men with hypogonadotropic hypogonadism: a review of 42 cases. Eur J Endocrinol. 1998;139(3):298-303.
50. Liu L, Banks SM, Barnes KM, et al. Two-year comparison of testicular responses to pulsatile gonadotropin-releasing hormone and exogenous gonadotropins from the inception of therapy in men with isolated hypogonadotropic hypogonadism. J Clin Endocrinol Metab. 1988;67(6):1140-5.
51. KlieschS, Behre HM, Nieschlag E. High efficacy of gonadotropin or pulsatile gonadotropin releasing hormone treatment in hypogonadotropic hypogonadalmen. Eur J Endocrinol. 1994;131(4):347-54.
52. Hadziselimović F, Herzog B. Treatment with a luteinizing hormone-releasing hormone analogue after successful orchiopexy markedly improves the chance of fertility later in life. J Urol. 1997;158(3 Pt 2):1193-5.
53. Huff DS, Snyder HM, Rusnack SL, et al. Hormonal therapy for the subfertility of cryptorchidism. Horm Res. 2001;55(1):38-40.
54. Iwamoto H, Yoshida A, Suzuki H, et al. A man with hypogonadotropichypogonadism successfully treated with nasal administration of the low-dose gonadotropin-relasing hormone analog buserelin. Fertil Steril. 2009;92(3):1169.e1-3.
55. Lindner J, McNeil LW, Marney S, et al. Characterization of human anti-luteinizing hormone-releasing hormone (LRH) antibodies in the serum of a patient with isolated gonadotropin deficiency treated with synthetic LRH. J Clin Endocrinol Metab. 1981;52(2):267-70.
56. Depenbusch M, von Eckardstein S, Simoni M, et al. Maintenance of spermatogenesis in hypogonadotropichypogonadal men with human chorionic gonadotropin alone. Eur J Endocrinol. 2002;147:617-24.
57. Burgués S, Calderón MD. Subcutaneous self-administration of highly purified follicle stimulating hormone and human chorionic gonadotrophin for the treatment of male hypogonadotrophic hypogonadism. Spanish Collaborative Group on Male Hypogonadotropic Hypogonadism. Hum Reprod. 1997;12(5):980-6.
58. Kung AW, Zhong YY, Lam KS, et al. Induction of spermatogenesis with gonadotrophins in Chinese men with hypogonadotrophic hypogonadism. Int J Androl. 1994;17(5):241-7.
59. Nieschlag E, Behre HM. Testosterone therapy. In: Nieschlag E, Behre HM, Nieschlag S (Eds). Andrology, 3rd edition. Heidelberg: Springer; 2009. pp. 437-56.
60. Dohle GR, van Roijen JH, Pierik FH, et al. Subtotal obstruction of the male reproductive tract. Urol Res. 2003;31(1):22-4.
61. Matorras R, Pérez C, Corcóstegui B, et al. Treatment of the male with follicle-stimulating hormone in intrauterine insemination with husband's spermatozoa: a randomized study. Hum Reprod. 1997;12(1):24-8.
62. Kamischke A, Behre HM, Bergmann M, et al. Recombinant human follicle-stimulating hormone for treatment of male idiopathic infertility: a randomized, double-blind, placebo-controlled, clinical trial. Hum Reprod. 1998;13(3):596-03.
63. Foresta C, Bettella A, Merico M, et al. Use of recombinant human follicle-stimulating hormone in the treatment of male factor infertility. Fertil Steril. 2002;77(2):238-44.
64. Ashkenazi J, Bar-Hava I, Farhi J, et al. The role of purified follicle stimulating hormone therapy in the male partner before intracytoplasmic sperm injection. Fertil Steril. 1999;72(4):670-3.

65. Liu PY, Handelsman DJ. The present and future state of hormonal treatment for male infertility. Hum Reprod Update. 2003;9(1):9-23.
66. Kamischke A, Nieschlag E. Analysis of medical treatment of male infertility. Hum Reprod. 1999;14 (Suppl 1):1-23.
67. Vandekerckhove P, Lilford R, Vail A, et al. Clomiphene or tamoxifen for idiopathic oligo/as the nospermia. Cochrane Database Syst Rev. 2000;(2):CD000151.
68. Kadioglu TC, Köksal IT, Tung M, et al. Treatment of idiopathic and post varicocelectomy oligozoospermia with oral tamoxifen citrate. BJU Int. 1999;83(6):646-8.
69. Shabsigh A, Kang Y, Shabsign R, et al. Clomiphene citrate effects on testosterone/estrogen ratio in male hypogonadism. J Sex Med. 2005;2(5):716-21.
70. Hill S, Arutchelvam V, Quinton R. Enclomiphene, an estrogen receptor antagonist for the treatment of testosterone deficiency in men. I Drugs. 2009;12:109-19.
71. Whitten SJ, Nangia AK, Kolettis PN. Select patients with hypogonadotropic hypogonadism may respond to treatment with clomiphene citrate. Fertil Steril. 2006;86:1664-68.
72. Kaminetsky J, Hemani ML. Clomiphene citrate and enclomiphene for the treatment of hypogonadal androgen deficiency. Expert OpinInvestig Drugs. 2009;18(12): 1947-55.
73. Adamopoulos DA, Pappa A, Billa E, et al. Effectiveness of combined tamoxifen citrate and testosterone undecanoate treatment in men with idiopathic oligozoospermia. Fertil Steril. 2003;80(4):914-20.
74. Maier U, Hienert G. Tamoxifen and kallikrein in therapy of oligoasthenozoospermia: results of a randomized study. Eur Urol. 1990;17(3):223-5.
75. Patry G, Jarvi K, Grober ED, et al. Use of the aromatase inhibitor letrozole to treat male infertility. Fertil Steril. 2009;92(2):829.e1-2
76. Ramasamy R, Ricci JA, Palermo GD, et al. Successful fertility treatment for Klinefelter's syndrome. J Urol. 2009;182:1108-13
77. Clark R, Sherins RJ. Treatment of men with idiopathic oligozoospermic infertility using the aromatase inhibitor testolactone. Results of a double-blinded, randomized, placebo-controlled trial with crossover. J Androl. 1989;10(3):240-7.
78. Hull KL, Harvey S. Growth hormone: roles in male reproduction. Endocrine. 2000;13(3):243-50.
79. Lee KO, Ng SC, Lee PS, et al. Effect of growth hormone therapy in men with severe idiopathic oligozoospermia. Eur J Endocrinol. 1995;132(2):159-62.
80. Radicioni A, Paris E, Dondero F, et al. Recombinant-growth hormone (rec-hGH) therapy in infertile men with idiopathic oligozoospermia. Acta Eur Fertil. 1994;25(5):311-7.
81. Shoham Z, Conway GS, Ostergaard H, et al. Cotreatment with growth hormone for induction of spermatogenesis in patients with hypogonadotropic hypogonadism. Fertil Steril. 1992;57(5):1044-51.
82. Byrne MM, Rolf C, Depenbusch M, et al. Lack of effect of a single i.v. dose of oxytocin on sperm output in severely oligozoospermic men. Hum Reprod. 2003;18(10):2098-02.
83. Klibanski A. Clinical practice. Prolactinomas. N Engl J Med. 2010;362(13):1219-26.
84. Ries LAG, Eisner MP, Kosary CL, et al. SEER Cancer Statistics [Online] Available from www.seer.cancer.gov/csr/1975_2000/. [Accessed July 30, 2007].
85. Shetty G, Meistrich ML. Hormonal approaches to preservation and restoration of male fertility after cancer treatment. J Natl Cancer Inst Monogr. 2005;(34):36-9.
86. Meistrich ML, Wilson G, Huhtaniemi I. Hormonal treatment after cytotoxic therapy stimulates recovery of spermatogenesis. Cancer Res. 1999;59(15):3557-60.
87. Shuttlesworth GA, de Rooij DG, Huhtaniemi I, et al. Enhancement of a spermatogonial proliferation and differentiation in irradiated rats by gonadotropin-releasing hormone antagonist administration. Endocrinology. 2000;141(1):37-49.
88. Meistrich ML, Kangasniemi M. Hormone treatment after irradiation stimulates recovery of ratspermatogenesis from surviving spermatogonia. J Androl. 1997;18(1):80-7.
89. Masala A, Faedda R, Alagna S, et al. Use of testosteroneto prevent cyclophosphamide-inducedazoospermia. Ann Intern Med. 1997;126(4):292-5.
90. Ogawa T, Dobrinski I, Avarbock MR, et al. Leuprolide, a gonadotropin-releasing hormone agonist, enhances colonization after spermatogonial transplantation into mouse testes. Tissue Cell. 1998;30(5):583-8.
91. Dobrinski I, Ogawa T, Avarbock MR, et al. Effect of the GnRH-agonist leuprolide on colonization of recipient-testes by donor spermatogonial stem cells after transplantation in mice. Tissue Cell. 2001;33(2):200-7.
92. Wildt L, Haulser A, Marshall G, et al. Frequency and amplitude of gonadotropin-releasing hormone stimulation and gonadotropin secretion in the rhesus monkey. Endocrinology. 1981;109:376-85.
93. Carruthers M. Androgen deficiency in the adult male: causes, diagnosis and treatment. London: Taylor & Francis; 2004.

5

Immunology of Male Infertility

Walter KH Krause, Rajesh K Naz

Chapter Contents

INTRODUCTION

Definition and Prevalence

Immune infertility is defined as a consequence of immune reaction (antibodies, cytokines, T lymphocytes) that inhibits fertility by interfering with fertilization of the oocyte and/or preimplantation embryonic development. Among these, antisperm antibodies (ASA) directed against the antigens of sperm proteome are the most frequent causative factors. The induction of fertility-relevant ASA requires an immune reaction against the sperm antigens, which are relevant to the fertilization process. Only antigens that are present on the sperm membrane or those externalized after capacitation/acrosome reaction are accessible to antibody binding, thus, are relevant to immune infertility.

ASA are found in 9–12.8% of infertile couples. The presence of ASA indicates a relative decrease of fertility. However, ASA are also present in approximately 1–2.5% of fertile men[1,2] and in 4% of fertile women. The presence of ASA in the fertile population suggests that not all ASA cause infertility.[3-5] These antibodies should not be called 'antisperm' antibodies in a true sense, rather they should be called 'sperm-reactive' immunoglobulins. ASA are usually sperm specific; thus, the presence of ASA does not exert, in most cases any harmful effect on patients, except for their infertility.

SPERM PROTEOME

The spermatozoon is a highly polarized cell with a minimal cytosol.[6,7] The sperm head carries the nucleus that houses the male haploid genome, which is highly condensed by protamines and a large secretory granule called the acrosome, which is oriented over the anterior area of the sperm nucleus. The spermatozoa lack a number of organelles that are found in somatic cells such as endoplasmic reticulum, Golgi body, lysosomes, peroxisomes and ribosomes. As a consequence, they have lost the potential for gene expression; both transcription as well as translation processes are completely silenced.[8] However, there are some residual RNA still present in the mature sperm that are left after spermiogenesis.

The sperm surface is heterogeneous and different regions are responsible for separate functions in the fertilization process. The sperm surface proteome undergoes several modifications during transit from testis to other parts of the genital tract. In the epididymis, a remodeling of the surface membranes takes place by modifying/coating with other antigens. After deposition in the female genital tract, several proteins adsorbed on the sperm surface are removed during capacitation and several enzymes are released during acrosome reaction.

The sperm antigens, against which ASA are directed to, are proteins/glycoproteins that develop during later stages of spermatogenesis and/or adsorbed during the sperm transit in the genital tract. A blood-testis barrier effectively protects the developing germ cells from the immune system. However, the blood-testis barrier is not the only mechanism, which inhibits antibody induction. The testicular macrophages and dendritic cells are also involved in the immune protection of the sperm proteome.[9]

The aim of studying the sperm surface proteome is not only for identifying the localization of proteins in different parts of the sperm, but also for characterizing their role in the fertilization process. The sperm head is involved in zona binding/acrosome reaction/fertilization of the oocyte and the equatorial segment is involved in the fusion with oocyte plasma membrane. These subcellular parts are thus the most interesting for ASA that are relevant to immune infertility.

The standard procedure of proteome analysis includes separation and purification of the sperm heads and their membranes. Different proteins are isolated by two-dimensional gel electrophoresis, followed by protein microsequencing using matrix-assisted laser desorption/ionization time-of-flight mass spectrometry and liquid chromatography mass spectrometry. All steps of the identification procedures have subjected to thorough quality control to ensure that only proteins specific to a defined subcellular area are present in the analytic process.[8] To examine which of these peptides are relevant to immune infertility, the separated peptides are transferred to nitrocellulose membrane and incubated with the serum/seminal plasma/genital tract secretion. The reacted proteins are identified using the Western blot procedure.[10]

The peptide sequences can be used to deduce and synthesize a set of gene-specific oligonucleotides. These can be used to polymerase chain reaction amplify and sequence corresponding cDNA, leading to identification of genes/proteins of unknown sperm components, particularly those associated with acrosome/plasma membrane and are relevant to fertilization.[11] Several sperm antigens have been identified using hybridoma technology and proteomics, genomics, and subtractive hybridization approaches. Of these, fertilization antigen-1 (FA-1), HSP60, HSP70, LDH-C_4, CD52, SP10, TSA-1 and YLP_{12} have drawn considerable attention.

FORMATION OF ANTISPERM ANTIBODIES

Although mature sperm have more potential antigenic components than testicular spermatids, the site of antibody formation in the genital tract is unclear. However, some indications can be drawn from the findings on the risk factors involved in ASA induction (Table 1). Although antibodies can be induced by active immunization with sperm voluntarily, they are also induced involuntarily in infertile couples. The sperm cell has both autoantigen and isoantigen that can form antibodies in both men and women. Some of the antibodies that are present involuntarily are sperm-immobilizing antibodies,[12] antibodies to the proacrosin/acrosin system,[13] antibodies to FA-1 and YLP_{12},[14] and prepubertal antibodies in some cryptorchid young boys.[15-17] ASA can be directed to the peptide moiety or carbohydrate epitopes of the sperm glycoproteins.[18] The sperm immunization antibodies are primarily detected in the serum of infertile women. The antigenic component is within the carbohydrate moieties of CD52, a GPI anchor glycoprotein, expressed in lymphocytes and various

Table 1 Risk factors for antisperm antibodies formation in the male

Pathology	Induction of antisperm antibodies	Site of induction
Chronic obstruction of the genital tract	High frequency	Epididymis/vas deferens/other parts possible
Varicocele	Unlikely	Testis
Cryptorchidism	Unlikely	Testis
Testis trauma/surgery	No probability	–
Testicular torsion	No probability	–
Testis tumor	Unlikely	Testis
Intrarectal sperm deposition	Unlikely	Rectal mucosa

components of the male genital tract including sperm and seminal plasma.[12]

ASA can be present circulating in the blood of male and female patients, and/or locally in the genital tract secretions such as semen, cervical mucus, vaginal secretion and fallopian fluid. The immunoglobulin G (IgG) antibodies in semen and other genital tract secretions are mainly transudate of the serum IgG. The immunoglobulin A (IgA) antibodies, however, can originate locally and/or transudate from serum.[19] The occurrence of ASA in cervical mucus is generally rare. Stern et al. compared retrospectively the concentration of ASA in serum and mucus in patients undergoing infertility evaluation.[20] They found ASA levels in serum not to be correlated with the ASA levels in mucus. Eggert-Kruse et al. examined 192 infertile patients and found that only 2% of them have antibodies in the cervical mucus.[21] In another study, of 48 patients examined, only two cervical mucus samples (4.6%) were positive for ASA.[22] Kamieniczna et al. examined 155 infertile women and found ASA only in 3.2% of cervical mucus samples.[23]

RISK FACTORS OF ANTISPERM ANTIBODIES FORMATION

The obstruction/infection/inflammation of the epididymis and vas deferens frequently induces high titers of ASA.[24-27] Between 50–100% of men that undergo vasectomy subsequently, develop ASA in serum and semen.[28] Following vasectomy, an epididymal distention results due to increased intraluminal pressure. The distensed site frequently develops sperm granuloma. The sperm granuloma is a dynamic structure where active phagocytosis occurs by macrophages. T cells have also been observed in the sperm granuloma. It is plausible that the immune process inducing ASA production initiates here.

ASA can penetrate from circulation into the male genital tract via rete testis, epididymes, vas deferens and accessory glands. They can attach to sperm at any of these regions after transudation. In spermatozoa retrieved directly from the distal end of the vas deferens in patients undergoing vasectomy reversal (vasovasostomy), IgG and IgA, ASA were present in 78.6% and 32.1% of the patients respectively.[29]

The infections and/or inflammation of the male genital tract can cause ASA formation, but the data is inconsistent. Jarow and co-workers described a positive association between prostatitis and ASA using the gel agglutination assay in serum.[30] In a series of 365 patients with documented inflammation/infection of the male genital tract, suffering from—in accordance to the American Urological Association definition—chronic bacterial prostatitis, inflammatory chronic prostatitis/chronic pelvic pain syndrome, noninflammatory chronic pelvic pain syndrome, chronic urethritis, and chronic epididymitis, no association between ASA formation and the intensity of these diseases was demonstrable.[31]

Immunological cross-reactivity between antigens of the sperm membrane and *Chlamydia trachomatis* may occur and explain some cases of an association between infections and ASA formation.[31] Epitopes of chlamydial HSP60 protein cross-react with those of human HSP60. However, clinical data fail to detect an association between chlamydial infections and the presence of ASA in seminal plasma.[31,32]

It is unclear whether varicocele, testicular trauma, surgery or testicular torsion can induce ASA formation. Also, the association between cryptorchidism and ASA remains controversial (Table 2).[28]

Usually, women do not induce an immune reaction after intercourse on coming into contact with spermatozoa. The exact mechanisms that suppress the immune response to sperm antigens are unclear, but there are some hypotheses.[42] Witkin reported that antibody-coated sperms, but not antibody-free sperm, stimulate interferon gamma (IFN-γ) synthesis by lymphocytes from female donors *in vitro*.[43] IFN-γ induces macrophages to express Ia antigen (MHC class II marker). The resulting juxtaposition of sperm antigens and Ia on the macrophage cell surface would facilitate the recruitment of T-helper cells and subsequent initiation of ASA production by B lymphocytes. Another possible hypothesis is that female ASA are anti-idiotype antibodies. It is well known that anti-idiotype antibodies, if produced in sufficient quantities, are able to inhibit production of the related idiotype.[44]

Although suggested by epidemiologic studies, the direct proof of ASA as a cause of infertility is difficult to obtain, since prospective studies comparing pregnancies in patients with and without ASA are limited, and an occurrence of ASA is uncommon.[2,45-47]

In retrospective studies, the degree of sperm-autoimmunization showed a significant inverse correlation with the incidence of spontaneous pregnancies. In the first report by Rumke et al., during a 10-year follow-up of 254 infertile men with serum sperm-agglutinating activity, the ASA titers were inversely correlated with the occurrence of spontaneous pregnancies.[48] If only normozoospermic men were included, no pregnancy was observed with very high ASA titers. In a cohort of 108 infertile couples,[1] the pregnancy rates were significantly higher when males had low antibody titers than in those with high titers. Similar observations were published by Abshagen et al., in 157 infertile couples.[49] The cumulative

Table 2 Randomized studies measuring the effect of corticosteroids on immune infertility

Authors	Patient number	Treatment	Effect on antisperm antibodies	Effect on fertility	Adverse effect
De Almeida et al.[33]	10	T: Prednisolone 1 mg/kg/d, 9 d C: Placebo	None	No difference in CR	No data
Haas et al.[34]	43	T: Methylprednisolone, 96 mg/d, 9 d C: Placebo	None	No difference in CR	No data
Hendry et al.[35]	43	T: Prednisolone 20 mg/d, cyclic C: Placebo	No data	9 conceptions 1 conception	Mild (60%)
Bals-Pratsch et al.[36]	20	T: Prednisolone 40 mg, cyclic + TI C: Placebo	Significant reduction	0 conception 0 conception	Mild (40%)
Robinson et al.[37]	30	T: Corticosteroids + IUI C: Corticosteroids + TI	Significant reduction	11 pregnancies 2 pregnancies	No data
Lahteenmaki et al.[38]	46	T: Prednisolone 20 mg/d + IUI C: Prednisolone 20 mg/d + TI	None	9 pregnancies 1 pregnancy	No data
Räsänen et al.[39]	?	T: Prednisolone 20 mg/d C: Placebo	Significant reduction	No data	No data
Gregoriou et al.[40]	36	T: Corticosteroids + IUI C: IUI only	No data	16.1% CR 21.2% CR	No data
Lahteenmaki et al.[41]	53	T: Prednisolone 20 mg/d, 2 weeks prior to IVF C: No treatment	None	29% CR 32% CR	No data
Omu et al.[4]	77	T: Prednisolon 5 mg/d C: No treatment	No data	20% CR 5% CR	None

C: control group; CR: conception rate; IUI: intrauterine insemination; IVF: *in vitro* fertilization; T: treatment group; TI: timed intercourse

spontaneous pregnancy rates over 6 years were higher (~ 50%) when the immunobead test (IBT) was less than 50%; lower (~ 30%) when test results were 50–90%; and very low (~ 15%) when the test showed more than 90% ASA. Meinertz et al., observed a significant inverse correlation between the degree of sperm autoimmunization and pregnancy rate in a follow-up study of 216 men after vasovasostomy.[50] However, Matson et al., could not confirm this observation.[51]

TESTS FOR SPERM ANTIBODIES

The sperm agglutination (gelatin agglutination test, tube slide agglutination test) and sperm immobilization (sperm immobilization test) are obsolete due to low sensitivity and specificity.[52] The tests, which are used these days, are described below.

Enzyme-Linked Immunosorbent Assay

The visualization of antigen-antibody binding by chromogens amplified by an enzyme is an elegant method to demonstrate the presence of specific compounds and allows the determination of an antibody titer. It is particularly meaningful if either the antigen or the antibody is fixed to a solid phase. However, to obtain informative results, the specificity of antibodies and antigens is required. This prerequisite is not fulfilled in the determination of ASA, since all the antigens specific to the ASA have not been defined. The tests that are marketed, measure the binding of antibodies to sperm extracts containing several antigens. Thus, they are of limited application for the diagnosis of ASA-associated infertility. This is also true for radiolabelled antibody assays, which in addition require the use of radioactive materials.

Flow Cytometry

It is used to detect sperm-bound antibodies and to quantitate the sperm antibody load.[39] However, flow cytometry requires expensive laboratory instruments, and reveals limited results without providing specificity of ASA for fertility-related antigens.

Mixed Antiglobulin Reaction Test

The mixed antiglobulin reaction (MAR) test is based on the Coombs test (antiglobulin test), which detects antibodies bound to erythrocytes, e.g. in the Rh-induced hemolysis in the newborn. The technique of the MAR test is simple. A semen sample is mixed with a suspension of particles, which are covered with immunoglobulins and a second antibody against immunoglobulins. If ASA bound to spermatozoa are present, the particles get attached to the spermatozoa, which is easily visible in the microscope. As a test result, the percentage of motile sperm bearing the particles is counted. An MAR test is considered positive when more than 10% of sperm are attached to a particle and is of clinical significance when more than 80% binding is present.

The MAR test is easy to perform, reproducible and the results are apparent within a few minutes. Different IgG classes can be detected using this test. The test has some limitations: it is difficult to perform when the sperm are less in number and immotile, such as in oligozoospermia and asthenozoospermia, and it requires fresh semen samples (Jager et al., 1978). Commercially available SpermMar kits are based on an antiserum against human IgG to induce mixed agglutination between antibody-coated and latex beads conjugated with human immunoglobulin.[53]

The MAR test can also be used to detect ASA bound in biological fluids such as blood serum and seminal plasma. In these cases, an indirect MAR test is performed. In the first step, donor sperm are mixed with the fluid and then the sperm undergo the MAR test as described above. The reproducibility of the indirect MAR test using different donor sperm is poor.[54]

Quality control of an MAR test comprises inter-assay and intra-assay variation. It was shown that the intra-assay variation is good if different tests are performed using the same spermatozoa. However, an inter-assay comparison of tests using spermatozoa from different donors reveals poor congruence.

Immunobead Test

Immunobead test is similar to the MAR test and is easy to perform. The IBT allows determination of the antibody class attached to spermatozoa, the subcellular localization where the antibodies are attached on the spermatozoa and the percent of antibody-coated sperm. Sperm concentration is usually adjusted to 10–25 x 10^6 motile sperm/ml to optimize the microscopic evaluation. Like the MAR test, the IBT can also be performed indirectly using biological fluids. It was shown that the indirect IBT has a low intra-assay and a high inter-assay variability.[55]

Both the MAR test and IBT are recommended by the World Health Organization (WHO) manual.[56] The MAR test does not require washing the spermatozoa free of seminal plasma, which makes it easier and faster than the IBT. It requires less semen volume and could be applied to samples with a lower sperm concentration compared to the IBT.[39,57] Comparison of IBT and the MAR test have shown a high degree of agreement.[53,58] The sensitivity and specificity also are comparable between these two tests.[59]

The existing consensus indicates that a semen sample having more than 50% of spermatozoa showing binding in the MAR test or the IBT, is suggestive of ASA-mediated immune infertility.[56] There is no correlation between the test positivity and the sperm concentration, motility, and morphology and leukocyte concentration in the semen.

However, ASA levels are usually higher in men with abnormal sperm parameters than in those with normozoospermia. MAR test results were found positive in 48 (10%) of 484 men with normal sperm counts, 18 (23%) of 78 of men with low sperm motility and 19 (15%) of 128 of men with low counts. The presence of antibodies in about 10% of men may provide additional information besides the semen parameters in some cases of unexplained infertility.[60]

TREATMENT OF IMMUNE INFERTILITY

Immunosuppressive Therapy with Glucocorticosteroids

The immunosuppressive treatment using steroids has potential adverse effects. To minimize the side effects, it is usually restricted to the first 7–10 days of the female cycle, irrespective of whether the steroids are given to a male or female partner of an infertile couple. Steroid therapy to suppress ASA was first recommended by Hendry et al.[35] They reported an increasing conception rate in the steroid treated group as compared to the placebo group. Later on, several studies were published, in which corticosteroids did not show an effect on ASA titers, sperm parameters or the conception rate (Table 2). For this reason, the therapy is no longer used for treatment of immune infertility.

In Vitro Techniques

The *in vitro* techniques generally target: (1) prevention of binding of ASA to sperm, (2) elution of bound ASA from sperm surface and/or (3) separation of ASA-free sperm from ASA-coated sperm.

Prevention of Antisperm Antibodies Binding to Sperm

It was erroneously thought that ASA bind to sperm during and/or just after ejaculation, and the antibodies are mostly present in the secretions of prostate and seminal vesicles. It was hypothesized that the antibodies and sperm are ejaculated in different fractions of the semen. To avoid binding of antibodies to sperm, splitting the semen into various fractions during ejaculation was attempted in various laboratories. However, it has been proven ineffective in decreasing ASA binding to sperm.[61] It was examined if the collection of semen into insemination medium containing high concentration of fetal cord/maternal serum would decrease the antibody binding to sperm. Two studies (Bronson et al., 1987 and De Almeida et al., 1987) observed that semen collection into serum supplemented medium results in increased fertilization rates in *in vitro* fertilization (IVF) procedure, and one of these studies also showed an increase in pregnancy rates.[62] A study was conducted to investigate at which site of the male genital tract the antibodies percolate from serum to bind to sperm.[63] I^{125} labeled antibodies to a sperm-specific antigen, the FA-1 antigen, were injected intravenously into male mice and various parts of the genital tract were examined for the antibody penetration. The results indicate that the antibodies preferentially transude into epididymis (especially corpus or caudal regions) and vas deferens, and not into testes to bind to sperm cells. These findings indicate that in men, ASA bind to sperm before ejaculation via transudation through epididymis, vas deferens and probably rete testis.

Immunomagnetic Separation Technique

This technique has been tried to separate the antibodies bound on the sperm surface.[64] The sperm with antibodies are tagged with anti-immunoglobulin antibodies coupled to magnetic microspheres, and then the magnetic field is applied. However, limited success in isolating a sufficient number of ASA-free sperm having good motility makes this procedure theoretically interesting but clinically an unacceptable procedure.

Removing Sperm Surface Antisperm Antibodies

The protease treatment can be used to degrade antibodies on the sperm surface (Bronson, et al., 1987). IgA1 protease treatment was effective in reducing IgA on sperm (Kutteh et al., 1994). In another study, incubation of sperm with chymotrypsin before intrauterine insemination (IUI) resulted in a 25% cycle fecundity versus 3% in controls.[65] However, this needs to be examined whether or not the treatment with proteolytic enzymes affect proteins, especially the oocyte binding receptors, present on the sperm surface.

The use of immunobeads has been suggested as a treatment to remove the sperm bound antibodies. It has been reported that simple incubation of ASA-positive sperm from immunoinfertile men with immunobeads results in a time-dependent decrease in antibody concentration on sperm surface,[64] and even enhanced pregnancies.[66] The explanation that the antibodies are removed from the sperm surface after incubation with immunobeads is not widely accepted, and it is generally believed that the immunobeads just select ASA-positive sperm, leaving ASA-free sperm. Theoretically, there is not a strong rationale why or how incubation with immunobeads should elute antibodies from the sperm surface.

Immunoelution of Bound Antisperm Antibodies Using Sperm Antigens

FA-1 antigen is a well-defined novel sperm-specific surface molecule that is evolutionarily conserved on sperm of various mammalian species, including humans.[63] Antibodies to an FA-1 antigen inhibit human sperm-zona interaction, and also block human sperm capacitation/ acrosome reaction by inhibiting tyrosine phosphorylation.[67] The cDNA encoding for mouse FA-1 and human FA-1 have been cloned and sequenced[68] and vaccination of female mice with recombinant FA-1 antigen causes a long-term reversible contraception by raising sperm-specific immune response.[69]

Fertilization antigen-1 antigen is involved in human immunoinfertility in both men and women. The antibodies are found in sera as circulating antibodies and also locally in genital tract secretions, such as seminal plasma of men, and cervical mucus and vaginal secretions of women.[70] The lymphocytes from immunoinfertile, but not fertile, men and women are sensitized against FA-1 antigen and proliferate on incubation with the antigen *in vitro*.[71] The presence of these antibodies inhibits fertilization in IVF procedure. The involvement of FA-1 antigen in human involuntary immunoinfertility has been confirmed in several laboratories by leading investigators working in the field of ASA. Based upon these findings, a clinical trial was conducted at the University of Michigan Medical School to determine whether immunoadsorption with FA-1 antigen would remove autoantibodies from sperm surface of immunoinfertile men.[72] Adsorption with FA-1 antigen increased immunobead-free swimming sperm on an average of 50% and 76% for IgA ASA and IgG ASA respectively. The acrosome reaction rates increased significantly and showed improvement in 78% of the sperm samples after FA-1 adsorption. The IUI of FA-1 treated antibody-free sperm resulted in normal pregnancies and healthy babies, indicating that the antigen treatment does not have a deleterious effect on implantation or embryonic and fetal development. This study needs to be extended to a larger number of ASA-positive infertile men and constitutes an exciting therapeutic modality using well-defined sperm antigens.

Assisted Reproductive Techniques

Intrauterine Insemination Procedure

Intrauterine insemination has been found to be useful for treatment of ASA-positive infertile men and women. Theoretically, it should circumvent problems related to sperm transport in the female genital tract, especially sperm passage through the cervical canal/mucus. However, in women having ASA in the cervical mucus, pregnancy rates after IUI were identical to women who did not have ASA, if the male partner did not have ASA or male factor infertility.[73] In two other studies of female sperm immunity, IUI treatment did not increase the pregnancy rates per couple or per cycle.[40,74,75] However, the pregnancy outcome significantly improved after including the ovarian hyperstimulation treatment along with IUI.

IUI also has been found to enhance pregnancy rates in some cases of ASA-positive infertile men. A 56% pregnancy rate has been reported after IUI procedure in ASA-positive infertile men who had a poor postcoital test compared with an 83% pregnancy rate in ASA-negative infertile men who also had a poor postcoital test.[76] In another study, after IUI the pregnancy outcome in 19 couples having male immune infertility were compared with 86 couples having other etiologies. No pregnancy was seen in 110 IUIs in the ASA-positive group (0%) versus a 26% pregnancy rate per couple and 5.6% cycle fecundity in the control group.[77] From the Cleveland Clinic Foundation, Agarwal compared 42 ASA-positive couples with 117 ASA-negative infertile couples who were treated with sperm washing and IUI over a 2-year period.[65] There were 15 pregnancies in the ASA-positive group compared with 37 for the entire group.

It is not clear how IUI can circumvent male immune infertility. Washing the sperm in the incubation medium should not elute the antibodies bound to the sperm surface proteins, unless: (1) these antibodies are directed against the adsorbed seminal plasma proteins that are shed off during capacitation/acrosome reaction, (2) the antibodies are of low binding affinity, which does not seem to be the case in immunoinfertility, and/or (3) the swim-up sperm used for IUI are not coated with antibodies like non-swim up sperm, which also seems highly unlikely.

There are mixed reports on simple sperm washing on ASA elution from various laboratories. Adeghe found that washing decreased IgG bound on the sperm surface.[78] Another group did not find the similar positive effects, nor did Haas et al., even after subjecting the sperm to multiple washings.[79,80] Antibodies were also not reduced by passing sperm through percoll gradient.[81]

Gamete Intrafallopian Transfer Procedure

In gamete intrafallopian transfer (GIFT) procedure, sperm and eggs are mixed *in vitro* and then transferred to the fallopian tubes for fertilization. There is not a strong rationale to how it will help either the ASA-positive infertile men or women. Nevertheless, in one study, GIFT was performed in 16 immune infertile couples. This group achieved pregnancy rates of 43% per couple and 24% per cycle.[82] This study did not include any control group, and the pregnancy rates are comparable to those that are reported after GIFT in patients having other etiologies.

In Vitro Fertilization Procedure

Several studies have shown decreased rates of oocyte fertilization in IVF in immune infertile patients.[83] An inverse relationship between ASA titers and fertilization rates has been reported.[64] In a study, 33 ASA-positive infertile couples were subjected to 47 IVF cycles.[84] The couples with high ASA titers had lower fertilization rates than those with lower ASA titers. In contrast, there are also studies that found fertilization to be identical in ASA-positive and ASA-negative population.[62] Interestingly, there are also studies reporting increased rates of IVF outcome, including implantation and pregnancy rates in ASA-positive infertile women compared to women with tubal factor infertility.[85] In IVF procedure, generally albumin instead of female partner's serum is used as a protein source in the insemination medium that circumvents the serum antibodies. Thus, theoretically speaking, IVF can take care of female, but not male immune infertility. Indeed, fertilization and pregnancies have been achieved using oocytes from ASA-positive infertile women where the men had normal semen analysis and were free of ASA.[86,87] In ASA-positive infertile men, both the class/subclass specificity and subcellular localization of the antibodies on sperm have been correlated with various degrees of fertilization failure rates in IVF.[88] ASA that bind to the sperm head may decrease fertilization more than ASA bound to mid-piece or tail regions of the sperm cell. In the IVF procedures involving 21 immunoinfertile couples, it was found that the couples that had ASA bound to the head region of the sperm cell showed more fertilization failure than those having ASA bound to the tail region.[87] Yeh et al. reported that IgA significantly reduces fertilization rates in IVF procedure only when it was associated with immunoglobulin M and was present on the sperm head.[89] Equality of embryo obtained after IVF using sperm from ASA-positive men is generally poor compared to sperm from ASA-negative men.

Intracytoplasmic Sperm Injection Procedure

In vitro fertilization with intracytoplasmic sperm injection (ICSI) have become a routine and widely acceptable procedure in clinics. In ICSI procedure, a single sperm is injected into the cytoplasm of the oocyte. ICSI has been tried using sperm of ASA-positive infertile men. The procedure is successful in the presence of ASA in the male as well as in the female (Nagy, 1999).[90-94] The ICSI procedure leads to pregnancy rates as high as in patients without ASA.

Two of these studies are worth mentioning. One study subjected 29 infertile ASA-positive couples to ICSI, 22 of them were tested before in IVF procedure and had a poor fertilization rate (6%).[84,95] After ICSI, the fertilization (79%) and cleavage (89%) rates in the ASA-positive group were similar to those (68% and 93%, respectively) in the ASA-negative group. Surprisingly, 46% of the pregnancies in the ASA-positive group ended in spontaneous pregnancy loss, compared with none in the ASA-negative group. In contrast, another study did not demonstrate any difference in pregnancy rates (30%) between the ASA-positive and ASA-negative group undergoing ICSI procedure.[96]

Some ASA can have deleterious postfertilization effects on developing preimplantation embryos.[81,97-99] ASA can affect early embryonic development if: (1) an oocyte is fertilized with a sperm cell, which carries these specific antibodies into the ooplasm, and/or (2) these antibodies are cross-reactive with the antigens present on the developing embryos. Some of these antigens and antibodies have been characterized, and the cDNA encoding for a few of these antigens has also been cloned and sequenced.[100] Using the ICSI procedure in immunoinfertile men, one can achieve higher fertilization rates than using the IVF procedure. However, the fertilized zygotes show higher degeneration and mortality, and decreased embryonic development.

Induction of Antisperm Antibodies in the Female by Assisted Reproductive Techniques

Only few studies are available which examined a possible induction of ASA in the female by assisted reproductive techniques. Goldberg et al. looked for ASA in the cervical mucus and blood serum prior to and after repeated IUI.[101] They found only temporary low titers. Prior to a tubal perfusion with sperm suspensions, 11 (8.5%) of the patients had positive IBT results and after 4 cycles of treatment, 6 (4.7%) of the patients developed a positive IBT.[102] However, there was no difference in the pregnancy rates between patients with and without ASA.

REFERENCES

1. Ayvaliotis B, Bronson RA, Rosenfeld D, et al. Conception rates in couples where autoimmunity to sperm is detected. Fertil Steril. 1985;43(5):739-42.
2. Collins JA, Burrows EA, Yeo J, et al. Frequency and predictive value of antisperm antibodies among infertile couples. Hum Reprod. 1993;8(4):592-8.
3. Heidenreich A, Bonfig R, Wilbert DM, et al. Risk factors for antisperm antibodies in infertile men. Am J Reprod Immunol. 1994;31(2-3):69-76.
4. Omu AE, al-Qattan F, Abdul Hamada B. Effect of low dose continuous corticosteroid therapy in men with antisperm antibodies on spermatozoal quality and conception rate. Eur J Obstet Gynecol Reprod Biol. 1996;69(2):129-34.
5. Sinisi AA, Di Finizio B, Pasquali D, et al. Prevalence of antisperm antibodies by SpermMARtest in subjects undergoing a routine sperm analysis for infertility. Int J Androl. 1993;16(5):311-4.
6. Eddy EM and O'Brien DA. The spermatozoon. In: Knobil E, Neild JD (Eds). The Physiology of Reproduction. New York: Raven Press; 1994. pp. 29-78.
7. Yanagimachi R. Mammalian fertilization. In: Knobil E, Neil JD (Eds). The Physiology of Reproduction. New York: Raven Press; 1994. pp. 189-317.
8. Gadella BM. Sperm surface proteomics. In: Krause WKH, Naz RK (Eds). Immune Infertility, Berlin: Springer Verlag; 2009. pp. 33-48.
9. Fijak M, Bhushan S, Meinhardt A. The immune privilege of the testis. In: Krause WKH, Naz RK (Eds). Immune Infertility, Berlin: Springer Verlag; 2009. pp. 69-78.
10. Bhande S, Naz RK. Molecular identities of human sperm proteins reactive with antibodies in sera of immunoinfertile women. Mol Reprod Dev. 2007;74(3):332-40.
11. Shetty J, Herr JC. Methods of analysis of sperm antigens related to fertility. In: Krause WKH, Naz RK (Eds)., Immune Infertility. Berlin: Springer Verlag; 2009. pp. 13-32.
12. Hasegawa A, Koyama K. Sperm-immobilizing antibody and its target antigen (CD52). In: Krause WKH, Naz RK (Eds). Immune Infertility. Berlin: Springer Verlag; 2009. pp. 131-42.
13. Breitbart H. Role and regulation of intracellular calcium in acrosomal exocytosis. J Reprod Immunol. 2002;53(1-2):151-9.
14. Samuel AS, Naz RK. Isolation of human single chain variable fragment antibodies against specific sperm antigens for immunocontraceptive development. Hum Reprod. 2008;23(6):1324-37.
15. Hakimi H, Geary I, Pacey A, et al. Spermicidal activity of bacterial lipopolysaccharide is only partly due to lipid A. J Androl. 2006;27(6):774-9.
16. Cheng GY, Shi JL, Wang M, et al. Inhibition of mouse acrosome reaction and sperm-zona pellucida binding by anti-human sperm membrane protein 1 antibody. Asian J Androl. 2007;9(1):23-9.
17. Jagadish N, Rana R, Mishra D, et al. Immunogenicity and contraceptive potential of recombinant human sperm associated antigen (SPAG9). J Reprod Immunol. 2005;67(1-2):69-76.

18. Kurpisz M, Kamieniczna M. Immune chemistry of ASA. In: Krause WKH, Naz RK (Eds). Immune Infertility. Berlin: Springer Verlag; 2009. pp. 79-90.
19. Yin X, Ouyang S, Xu W, et al. YWK-II protein as a novel G(o)-coupled receptor for Müllerian inhibiting substance in cell survival. J Cell Sci. 2007;120(Pt 9):1521-8.
20. Stern JE, Dixon PM, Manganiello PD, et al. Antisperm antibodies in women: variability in antibody levels in serum, mucus, and peritoneal fluid. Fertil Steril. 1992;58(5):950-8.
21. Eggert-Kruse W, Böckem-Hellwig S, Doll A, et al. Antisperm antibodies in cervical mucus in an unselected subfertile population. Hum Reprod. 1993;8(7):1025-31.
22. Domagala A, Kasprzak M, Kurpisz M. Immunological characteristics of cervical mucus in infertile women. Zentralbl Gynakol. 1997;119(12):616-20.
23. Kamieniczna M, Domagała A, Kurpisz M. The frequency of antisperm antibodies in infertile couples—a Polish pilot study. Med Sci Monit. 2003;9(4):142-9.
24. Gubin DA, Dmochowski R, Kutteh WH. Multivariant analysis of men from infertile couples with and without antisperm antibodies. Am J Reprod Immunol. 1998;39(2):157-60.
25. Jarow JP, Sanzone JJ. Risk factors for male partners antisperm antibodies. J Urol. 1992;148(6):1805-7.
26. Lee R, Goldstein M, Ullery B, et al. Value of serum antisperm antibodies in diagnosing obstructive azoospermia. J Urol. 2009;181(1):264-9.
27. Marconi M, Nowotny A, Pantke P, et al. Antisperm antibodies detected by mixed agglutination reaction and Immunobead Test are not associated with inflammation and infection of the seminal tract. Andrologia. 2008;40(4):227-34.
28. Marconi M, Weidner W. Site and risk factors of antisperm antibodies production in the male population. In: Krause WKH, Naz RK (Eds). Immune Infertility. Berlin: Springer Verlag; 2009. pp. 97-110.
29. Wen RQ, Li SQ, Wang CX, et al. Analysis of spermatozoa from the proximal vas deferens of vasectomized men. Int J Androl. 1994:17(4):181-5.
30. Jarow JP, Kirkland JA, Assimos D G. Association of antisperm antibodies with chronic non bacterial prostatitis. Urology. 1990;36(2):154-6.
31. Marconi M, Pilatz A, Wagenlehner F, et al. Are really antisperm antibodies associated with inflammatory/ infectious diseases of the male reproductive tract. Eur Urol. 2009;56(4):708-15.
32. Eggert-Kruse W, Rohr G, Demirakca T, et al. Chlamydial serology in 1303 asymptomatic subfertile couples. Hum Reprod. 1997;12(7):1464-75.
33. De Almeida M, Feneux D, Rigaud C, et al. Steroid therapy for male infertility associated with antisperm antibodies. Results of a small randomized clinical trial. Int J Androl. 1985;8(2):111-7.
34. Haas GG Jr, Manganiello P. A double-blind, placebo-controlled study of the use of methylprednisolone in infertile men with sperm-associated immunoglobulins. Fertil Steril. 1987;47(2):295-301.
35. Hendry WF, Hughes L, Scammell G, et al. Comparison of prednisolone and placebo in subfertile men with antibodies to spermatozoa. Lancet. 1990;335(8681):85-8.
36. Bals-Pratsch M, Doren M, Karbowski B, et al. Cyclic corticosteroid immunosuppression is unsuccessful in the treatment of sperm antibody-related male infertility: a controlled study. Hum Reprod. 1992;7(1):99-104.
37. Robinson JN, Forman RG, Nicholson SC, et al. A comparison of intrauterine insemination in superovulated cycles to intercourse in couples where the male is receiving steroids for the treatment of autoimmune infertility. Fertil Steril. 1995;63(6):1260-6.
38. Lahteenmaki A, Veilahti J, Hovatta O. Intra-uterine insemination versus cyclic, low-dose prednisolone in couples with male antisperm antibodies. Hum Reprod. 1995;10:142-7.
39. Räsänen M, Lahteenmaki A, Saarikoski S, et al. Comparison of flow cytometric measurement of seminal antisperm antibodies with the mixed antiglobulin reaction and the serum tray agglutination test. Fertil Steril. 1994;61(1):143-50.
40. Gregoriou O, Vitoratos N, Papdias C, et al. Intrauterine insemination as a treatment of infertility in women with antisperm antibodies. Int J Gynecol Obstet. 1991;35(2):151-6.
41. Lahteenmaki A, Rasanen M, Hovatta O. Low-dose prednisolone does not improve the outcome of in-vitro fertilization in male immunological infertility. Hum Reprod. 1995;10(12):3124-9.
42. Clarke G. ASA in the female. In: Krause WKH, Naz RK (Eds). Immune Infertility. Berlin: Springer Verlag; 2009. pp. 121-30.
43. Witkin SS. Production of interferon gamma by lymphocytes exposed to antibody-coated spermatozoa: a mechanism for sperm antibody production in females. Fertil Steril. 1988;50(3):498-502.
44. Naz RK, Ahmad K, Menge AC. Antiidiotypic antibodies to sperm in sera of fertile women that neutralize antisperm antibodies. J Clin Invest. 1993;92(5):2331-8.
45. Witkin SS, David SS. Effect of sperm antibodies on pregnancy outcome in a subfertile population. Am J Obstet Gynecol. 1988;158(1):59-62.
46. Eggert-Kruse W, Christmann WM, Gerhard I. Circulating antisperm antibodies and fertility prognosis: a prospective study. Hum Reprod. 1989;4(5):513-20.
47. Francavilla F, Baronetti A. Male autoimmune infertility. In: Krause WKH, Naz RK (Eds). Immune Infertility. Berlin: Springer Verlag; 2009. pp. 145-54.
48. Rumke PH, Van Amstel N, Messer EN, et al. Prognosis of fertility of men with sperm agglutinins in the serum. Fertil Steril. 1974;25(5):393-8.
49. Abshagen K, Behre HM, Cooper TG, et al. Influence of sperm surface antibodies on spontaneous pregnancy rates. Fertil Steril. 1998;70(2):355-6.
50. Meinertz H, Linnet L, Fogh-Andersen P, et al. Antisperm antibodies and fertility after vasovasostomy: a follow-up study of 216 men. Fertil Steril. 1990;54(2):315-21.

51. Matson PL, Junk SM, Masters JR, et al. The incidence and influence upon fertility of antisperm antibodies in seminal fluid following vasectomy reversal. Int J Androl. 1989;12(2):98-103.
52. Agarwal A, Said TM. Tests for sperm antibodies. In: Krause WKH, Naz RK (Eds). Immune Infertility. Berlin: Springer Verlag; 2009. pp. 155-64.
53. Kay DJ, Boettcher B. Comparison of the SpermMar test with currently accepted procedures for detecting human sperm antibodies. Reprod Fertil Dev. 1992;4(2):175-81.
54. Bohring C, Krause W. The intra- and inter-assay variation of the indirect mixed agglutination reaction test: is a quality control suitable? Hum Reprod. 1999;14(7):1802-5.
55. Franco JG Jr, Schimberni M, Rojas FJ, et al. Reproducibility of the indirect immunobead assay for detecting sperm antibodies in serum. J Reprod Med. 1989;34(4):259-63.
56. World Health Organization. WHO laboratory manual for the examination of human semen and sperm-cervical mucus interaction. Cambridge: Cambridge University Press; 2004.
57. Ackerman S, McGuire G, Fulgham DL, et al. An evaluation of a commercially available assay for the detection of antisperm antibodies. Fertil Steril. 1988;49(4):732-4.
58 Mahmoud A, Comhaire F. Antisperm antibodies: use of the mixed agglutination reaction (MAR) test using latex beads. Hum Reprod. 2000;15(2):231-3.
59. Haas GG Jr, D'Cruz OJ, DeBault LE. Comparison of the indirect immunobead, radiolabeled, and immunofluorescence assays for immunoglobulin G serum antibodies to human sperm. Fertil Steril. 1991;55(2):377-88.
60. Fichorova RN, Boulanov ID. Anti-seminal plasma antibodies associated with infertility: I. Serum antibodies against normozoospermic seminal plasma in patients with unexplained infertility. Am J Reprod Immunol. 1996;36(4):198-203.
61. Lenzi A, Gandini L, Claroni F, et al. Immunological usefulness of semen manipulation for artificial insemination homologous (AIH) in subjects with antisperm antibodies bound to sperm surface. Andrologia. 1988;20(4):314-21.
62. De Almeida M, Herry M, Testart J, et al. In-vitro fertilization results from thirteen women with anti-sperm antibodies. Hum Reprod. 1987;2(7):599-602.
63. Naz RK. Modalities for treatment of antisperm antibody mediated infertility: novel perspectives. Am J Reprod Immunol. 2004;51(5):390-7.
64. Ford WCL, Williams KM, McLaughlin EA, et al. The indirect immunobead test for seminal antisperm antibodies and fertilization rates at in-vitro fertilization. Hum Reprod. 1996;11(7):1418-22.
65. Agarwal A. Treatment of immunological infertility by sperm washing and intrauterine insemination. Arch Androl. 1992;29(3):207-13.
66. Foresta C, Varotto A, Caretto A. Immunomagnetic method to select human sperm without sperm surface-bound autoantibodies in male autoimmune infertility. Arch Androl. 1990;24(2):221-5.
67. Naz RK, Bhargava KK. Antibodies to sperm surface fertilization antigen (FA-1): their specificities and site of interaction with sperm in male genital tract. Mol Reprod Dev. 1990;26(2):175-83.
68. Naz RK, Zhu X. Molecular cloning and sequencing of cDNA encoding for human FA-1 antigen. Mol Reprod Dev. 2002;63(2):256-68.
69. Zhu X, Naz RK. Cloning and sequencing of cDNA encoding for a human sperm antigen involved in fertilization. Mol Reprod Dev. 1998;51(2):176-83.
70. Naz RK, Menge AC. Antisperm antibodies: origin, regulation, and sperm reactivity in human infertility. Fertil Steril. 1994;61(6):1001-13.
71. Naz RK, Chaudhry A, Witkin SS. Lymphocyte proliferative response to fertilization antigen in patients with antisperm antibodies. Am J Obstet Gynecol. 1990;163(2):610-3.
72. Menge AC, Christman GM, Ohl DA, et al. Fertilization antigen-1 removes antisperm autoantibodies from spermatozoa of infertile men and results in increased rates of acrosome reaction. Fertil Steril. 1999;71(2):256-60.
73. Check JH, Bollendorf A, Katsoff D, et al. The frequency of antisperm antibodies in the cervical mucus of women with poor postcoital tests and their effect on pregnancy rates. Am J Reprod Immunol. 1994;32(1):38-42.
74. Margalloth EJ, Sauter E, Bronson RA, et al. Intrauterine insemination as treatment for antisperm antibodies in the female. Fertil Steril. 1988;50(3):441-6.
75. Ombelet W, Vandeput H, Janssen M, et al. Treatment of male infertility due to sperm surface antibodies: IUI or IVF? Hum Reprod. 1997;12(6):1165-70.
76. Check JH, Bollendorf A. Effect of antisperm antibodies on postcoital results and effect of intrauterine insemination on pregnancy outcome. Arch Androl. 1992;28(1):25-31.
77. Francavilla F, Romano R, Santucci R, et al. Failure of intrauterine insemination in male immunolocial infertility in cases in which all spermatozoa are antibody-coated. Fertil Steril. 1992;58(3):587-92.
78. Adeghe AL. Effect of washing on sperm surface autoantibodies. Br J Urol. 1987;60(4):360-3.
79. Windt ML, Menkveld R, Kruger TF, et al. Effect of sperm washing and swim-up on antibodies bound to sperm membrane: use of immunobead/sperm cervical mucus contact tests. Arch Androl. 1989;22(1):55-9.
80. Haas GG, D'Cruz OJ, Denum BM. Effect of repeated washing on sperm-bound immunoglobulin G. J Androl. 1988;9(3):190-6.
81. Almagor M, Margalioth EJ, Yaffe H. Density differences between spermatozoa with antisperm autoantibodies and spermatozoa covered with antisperm antibodies from serum. Hum Reprod. 1992;7(7):959-61.
82. Van der Merwe JP, Kruger TF, Windt ML, et al. Treatment of male sperm autoimmunity by using the gamete intrafallopian transfer procedure with washed spermatozoa. Fertil Steril. 1990;53(4):682-7.
83. Junk SM, Matson PL, Yovich JM, et al. The fertilization of human oocytes by spermatozoa from men with antispermatozoal antibodies in semen. J In Vitro Fertil Embryo Transf. 1986;3(6):350-2.

84. Lahteenmaki A. In-vitro fertilization in the presence of antisperm antibodies detected by the mixed antiglobulin reaction (MAR) and the tray agglutination test (TAT). Hum Reprod. 1993;8(1):84-8.
85. Daitoh T, Kamada M, Yamano S, et al. High implantation rate and consequently high pregnancy rate by in vitro fertilization-embryo transfer treatment in infertile women with antisperm antibody. Fertil Steril. 1995;63(1):87-91.
86. Acosta AA, Van Der Merwe JP, Doncel G, et al. Fertilization efficiency of morphologically abnormal spermatozoa in assisted reproduction is further impaired by antisperm antibodies on the male partner's sperm. Fertil Steril. 1994;62:826-33.
87. Zouari R, De Almeida M, Rodrigues D, et al. Localization of antibodies on spermatozoa and sperm movement characteristics are good predictors of in vitro fertilization success in cases of male autoimmune infertility. Fertil Steril. 1993;59(3):606-12.
88. Ohl D, Naz RK. Infertility due to antisperm antibodies. J Urol. 1995;46(4):591-602.
89. Yeh WR, Acosta AA, Seltman HJ, et al. Impact of immunoglobulin isotype and sperm surface location of antisperm antibodies on fertilization in vitro in the human. Fertil Steril. 1995;63(6):1287-92.
90. Jun JH, Lim CK, Park YS, et al. Efficacy of intracytoplasmic sperm injection (ICSI) treatment in the immunological infertile patients. Am J Reprod Immunol. 1997;37(4):310-4.
91. Mercan R, Oehninger S, Muasher SJ, et al. Impact of fertilization history and semen parameters on ICSI outcome. J Assist Reprod Genet. 1998;15(1):39-45.
92. Check ML, Check JH, Katsoff D, et al. ICSI as an effective therapy for male factor with antisperm antibodies. Arch Androl. 2000;45(3):125-30.
93. Bhattacharya S, Hamilton MP, Shaaban M, et al. Conventional in-vitro fertilisation versus intracytoplasmic sperm injection for the treatment of non-male-factor infertility: a randomised controlled trial. Lancet. 2001;357(9274):2075-9.
94. Lombardo F, Gandini L, Dondero F, et al. Antisperm immunity in natural and assisted reproduction. Hum Reprod Update. 2001;7(5):450-6.
95. Lahteenmaki A, Reima I, Hovatta O. Treatment of severe male immunological infertility by intracytoplasmic sperm injection. Hum Reprod. 1995;10(11):2824-8.
96. Nagy ZP, Verheyen G, Liu J, et al. Results of 55 intracytoplasmic sperm injection cycles in the treatment of male-immunological infertility. Hum Reprod. 1995;10(7):1775-80.
97. Ahmad K, Naz RK. Antibodies to sperm surface antigens and the c-myc proto-oncogene product inhibit early embryonic development in mice. Biol Reprod. 1991;45(6):841-50.
98. Ahmad K, Naz RK. Effects of human antisperm antibodies on development of preimplantation embryos. Arch Androl. 1992;29(1):9-20.
99. Naz RK. Effects of antisperm antibodies on early cleavage of fertilized ova. Biol Reprod. 1992;46(1):130-9.
100. Javed AA, Naz RK. Human cleavage signal-1 protein: cDNA cloning, transcription and immunological analysis. Gene. 1992;112(2):205-11.
101. Goldberg JM, Haering PL, Friedman CI, et al. Antisperm antibodies in women undergoing intrauterine insemination. Am J Obstet Gynecol. 1990;163(1 Pt 1):65-8.
102. Kahn JA, Sunde A, von During V, et al. Formation of antisperm antibodies in women treated with fallopian tube sperm perfusion. Hum Reprod. 1993;8(9):1414-9.

6

Surgical Management of Male Infertility

Sandro C Esteves, Alaa Hamada, Ashok Agarwal

CHAPTER CONTENTS

INTRODUCTION

Infertility is a common problem in the urologic practice. Approximately, 8% of men in reproductive age may ask for medical consultation for fertility problems. Of these, 1–10% carries conditions that compromise the reproductive potential.[1] The essential roles of the urologist in this context are to diagnose, to counsel, to provide medical or surgical treatment whenever possible or to correctly refer the male patient for assisted conception. The urologist can also be part of the multiprofessional reproductive team in the assisted reproduction unit, being responsible for the above-cited tasks as well as for surgical sperm retrieval.

Surgical management can be offered to more than 50% of our patient population in daily practice. In a group of 2,875 infertile couples attending one of the authors (Sandro C Esteves) tertiary center for male reproduction, potentially surgical correctable conditions were identified in 34.4% of the male partners. Azoospermia is identified in about one-third of the individuals. Despite the feasibility of reconstructive surgery in only about 30% of the azoospermic subgroup, most of the remaining would be candidates for sperm retrieval techniques, if enrolled in assisted reproduction programs. These figures are clearly shown in Table 1.

Two major advances have recently occurred in the surgical management of male infertility. The first was the implementation of microsurgery which increased success rates for reconstruction of the reproductive tract. The second was the development of intracytoplasmic sperm injection (ICSI) and the demonstration that spermatozoa retrieved from either the epididymis or the testis were capable of fertilization and pregnancy.[2,3] Thereafter, several sperm retrieval methods have been developed to collect epididymal and testicular sperm for ICSI in azoospermic men. Microsurgery was incorporated to this armamentarium, either for collection of sperm from the epididymis in men with obstructive azoospermia or from the testicle in those with nonobstructive azoospermia (NOA).[2,4]

Surgeries for male infertility can be classified into three major categories:

1. Surgeries to improve sperm production
2. Reconstructive surgeries to correct the sperm transport pathways
3. Surgeries to retrieve spermatozoa from the gonads to be used in assisted conception.

Table 1 Distribution of diagnostic categories of couples seeking infertility evaluation in a male infertility clinic

Category	N	%
Varicocele	629	21.9
Infectious	72	2.5
Hormonal	54	1.9
Ejaculatory dysfunction	28	1.0
Systemic diseases	11	0.4
Idiopathic	289	10.0
Normal/Female factor	492	17.1
Immunologic	54	1.9
Obstruction	359	12.5
Cancer	11	0.4
Cryptorchidism	342	11.9
Genetic	189	6.6
Testicular failure	345	11.9
Total	2,875	

Source: ANDROFERT, Campinas, São Paulo, Brazil

This chapter describes the most common surgical options in the management of male infertility. It includes not only the reconstructive interventions for the male reproductive system but also the sperm retrieval techniques to be used in cases of obstructive azoospermia (OA) and NOA.

SURGICAL TREATMENT TO IMPROVE SPERM PRODUCTION

Varicocele Repair

Varicocele is believed to be the cause or a contributing factor of male infertility/subfertility in up to 35% of the cases.[1] Several hypotheses try to explain the mechanisms underlying the negative impact of varicocele on male fertility. Proposed mechanisms include hypoxia and stasis, testicular venous hypertension, elevated testicular temperature, increase in spermatic vein catecholamine leading to testicular underperfusion and increased oxidative stress. Nevertheless, none of them fully elucidates the unpredictable effect of varicocele on human spermatogenesis and male fertility.[5-8] The association between varicocele and infertility is still a matter of debate. However, there is an unquestionable increased incidence of this condition among infertile men.[9] Moreover, an association of varicocele with reduced semen parameters and testicular size exists,[10] and improvement in semen quality and pregnancy rates after varicocelectomy constitute strong evidence for a cause-effect relationship.[11,12] Despite these facts, it is still unclear why most men with varicocele retain fertility and why fertility status is not always improved after treatment.[13]

Preoperative Planning

Assessment and Patient Selection

The aim of varicocelectomy in infertile men is to restore or improve testicular function. Current recommendations suggest that treatment should be offered for couples with documented infertility whose male partner has a clinically palpable varicocele and abnormal semen analysis. The diagnosis of such condition is mainly clinical. Therefore, a detailed medical history must be taken and prognostic factors identified. Physical examination, with the patient standing in a warm room, is the preferred diagnostic method. Varicoceles diagnosed by physical examination are termed 'clinical' and may be graded according to the size. Large varicoceles (grade III) are varicose veins seen through the scrotal skin. Moderate (grade II) and small-sized varicoceles (grade I) are dilated veins palpable without and with the aid of the Valsalva maneuver, respectively.[14] In the presence of bilateral palpable varicocele, it is recommended to perform surgery on both sides at the same operative time.[15]

However, physical examination may be inconclusive or equivocal in cases of low grade varicocele and, in men with a history of previous scrotal surgery, concomitant hydrocele or obesity. Therefore, imaging studies may be recommended when assessing infertile men for varicocele when physical examination is inconclusive. When a varicocele is not palpable but a retrograde blood flow is detected by other diagnostic methods, such as venography, Doppler examination, ultrasonography, scintigraphy or thermography, the varicocele is termed subclinical.[16,17] The role of subclinical varicocele as a cause of male infertility remains debatable, and current evidence does not recommend surgical intervention for treating infertile men with subclinical varicocele.[18,19] It is our routine, however, to examine the contralateral cord with a pencil-probe Doppler (9 MHz) stethoscope to determine if a subclinical varicocele exists when a clinically palpable varicocele is only identified at one side. In such cases, the subclinical varicocele is treated at the same time as the coexistent clinical varicocele. This is based on the observation that altered blood flow after varicocelectomy may unmask an underlying venous anomaly and results in clinical varicocele formation.[20,21]

Preoperative workup should include hormone profile testing particularly, follicle-stimulating hormone (FSH) and testosterone level. Testicular volume should be assessed using a measurement instrument such as the

Prader orchidometer or a pachymeter. At least two semen analyses must be obtained and evaluated according to the World Health Organization guidelines.[22]

Infertile men either with higher preoperative semen parameters or undergoing varicocele repair for large varicoceles are more likely to show postoperative semen parameters improvement.[23] On the other hand, reduced preoperative testicular volume, elevated serum FSH levels, diminished testosterone concentrations and subclinical varicocele are negative predictors for fertility improvement after surgery.[18,24-29]

Men with clinical varicoceles presenting with azoospermia may be candidates for surgical repair. In such cases, genetic evaluation including Giemsa karyotyping and polymerase chain Yq microdeletion screening for AZFa, AZFb and AZFc regions are recommended. A testis biopsy (open or percutaneous) may be obtained to assess testicular histology, which has been shown to be the only valid prognostic factor for restoration of spermatogenesis.[30,31] The benefit of varicocelectomy in azoospermic men with genetic abnormalities is doubtful and should be carefully balanced. The same caution is valid for patients with atrophic testes and/or history of cryptorchidism, testicular trauma, orchitis, systemic or hormonal dysfunction due to the fact that varicocele in such cases may not be the cause of infertility but merely coincidental.[32]

As for all restorative surgical procedures in male infertility, the evaluation of the female partner's reproductive potential is recommended before an intervention is indicated, and the alternatives to varicocele repair discussed.

Operative Procedure

Overview

The aim of surgical treatment of varicocele in infertile men is to achieve the highest improvement in the male fertility status with lower complication rates. Increase in the likelihood of spontaneous pregnancy after treatment is difficult to ascertain due to a variety of factors that includes the lack of a uniform post-treatment follow-up interval and the female factor parameters such as age and reproductive health. The ultimate treatment goal is to improve the male fertility status regardless of the method to be used for conception (unassisted or assisted). The ideal surgical technique should aim for ligation of all internal and external spermatic and cremasteric veins, with preservation of spermatic arteries and lymphatics.

Anesthesia

Anesthesia for varicocelectomy may be carried out using local, regional or general type, according solely with the surgeon and patient's preferences. The authors routinely perform microsurgical subinguinal varicocele repair using short-acting propofol intravenous anesthesia associated with the blockage of the spermatic cord using 10 ml of a 2% lidocaine hydrochloride in an outpatient basis.[30]

Techniques

Varicoceles are surgically treated either by open (with or without magnification) or laparoscopic approaches. The principle of the surgery is the occlusion of the dilated veins of the pampiniform plexus. The high retroperitoneal and laparoscopic approaches are performed for internal spermatic vein ligation, while the inguinal and subinguinal approaches allow the ligation of the internal and external spermatic and cremasteric veins that may contribute to the varicocele.

Retroperitoneal techniques: High open retroperitoneal varicocele ligation involves incision medial to the anterior superior iliac spine at the level of the internal inguinal ring (Figure 1). The external oblique muscle is split, the internal oblique muscle is retracted and the peritoneum is teased away. Exposure of the internal spermatic artery and vein is carried out retroperitoneally near the ureter. At this level, only one or two internal spermatic veins are present, but the internal spermatic artery may not be easy to identify. The veins are ligated near to the point of drainage into the left renal vein. Neither the parallel inguinal and retroperitoneal collateral veins that may exit the testis and bypass the retroperitoneal area of ligation nor the cremasteric veins can be identified in the retroperitoneal approach. It is believed that these collaterals cause the high recurrence rate seen in high retroperitoneal varicocelectomy. The surgical approach on the right side may be more difficult because the right gonadic vein drains in the inferior vena cava. Laparoscopic varicocelectomy is a retroperitoneal approach using high magnification. The spermatic artery and the lymphatics are easily identified and spared; collateral veins can also be clipped or coagulated. However, external spermatic veins, the second cause of varicocele recurrence, cannot be treated, leading to a recurrence rate of approximately 5%.[33] Laparoscopy varicocele repair is more invasive, costly and associated with higher complication rates than open procedures.[33-35]

Inguinal and subinguinal techniques: The classic approach to the inguinal varicocelectomy involves a 5–10 cm incision over the inguinal canal, opening of the external oblique aponeurosis and isolation of the spermatic cord (Figure 1). The internal spermatic veins are dissected and ligated. An attempt is made to positively identify and

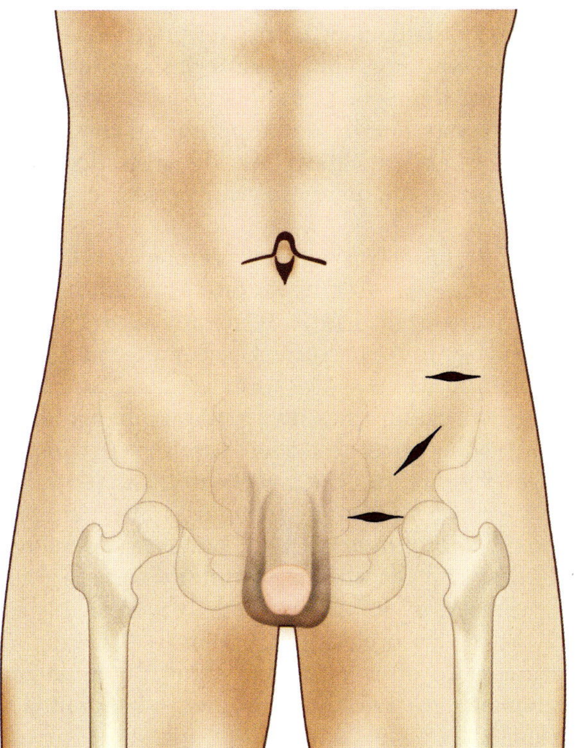

Figure 1 Schematic illustration of the incision sites commonly used for retroperitoneal, inguinal and subinguinal varicocele repair (from top to bottom)

spare the testicular artery and the lymphatics. External spermatic veins running parallel to the spermatic cord or perforating the floor of the inguinal canal can be identified and ligated. Although internal and external spermatic veins can be identified macroscopically, the use of magnification facilitates identification and preservation of internal spermatic artery and lymphatics, which may prevent testicular atrophy and hydrocele formation respectively.[36]

The urologist who opts to treat varicocele using microsurgery should obtain appropriate training. It is also important to have adequate microsurgical instruments and a binocular operating microscope with foot-control zoom magnification. Loupe magnification is insufficient for identification of testicular arteries and lymphatics. Microsurgical varicocelectomy, either using inguinal or subinguinal approaches, requires more skill as compared to other surgical modalities because a higher number of internal spermatic vein channels and smaller diameter artery are seen at the level of the inguinal canal. However, the routine use of microsurgery during varicocele repair may help the urologist to master his/her microsurgical skills, which will be of great benefit when performing more demanding reconstructive procedures.

Microsurgical varicocelectomy can be performed via an inguinal or subinguinal approach. The main advantage of the subinguinal over the inguinal approach is that the former obviates the need to open the aponeurosis of the external oblique, which usually results in more postoperative pain and a longer time before the patient can return to work. The authors treat varicocele with a testicular artery and lymphatic-sparing subinguinal microsurgical repair[12,30] (Figures 2A to D). Briefly, a 2.5 cm skin incision is made over the external inguinal ring. The subcutaneous tissue is separated until the spermatic cord is exposed. The cord is elevated with a Babcock clamp and the posterior cremasteric veins are ligated and transected. A Penrose drain is placed behind the cord without tension. The cremasteric fascia is then opened to expose the cord structures and the dissection proceeds using the operating microscope with magnification ranging from 6X to 16X. Dilated cremasteric veins within the fascia are ligated and transected. Lymphatics and arteries are visually identified and preserved. Whenever needed, the cord structures are sprayed with papaverine hydrochloride to increase the arterial beat. All dilated veins of the spermatic cord are identified, tagged with vessel loops, then ligated using nonabsorbable sutures and transected. Vasal veins are ligated only if they exceed 2 mm in diameter. Sclerosis of small veins is not used.

Postoperative Follow-up and Results

Postoperative care includes local dressing and scrotal supporter for 48–72 hours and 1 week respectively. Scrotal ice packing is always recommended to control local edema for the first 48 hours postoperatively. Patients are counseled to restrain from physical activity and sexual intercourse for 2–3 weeks. Oral analgesics usually suffice to control postoperative pain. Postoperative follow-up aims to evaluate improvement in semen parameters, complications and spontaneous or assisted conception. Semen analysis should be performed every 3 months until the semen parameters stabilize or pregnancy occurs.

In a recent systematic review comparing different surgical modalities to treat varicocele for male infertility,[33] it was concluded that open microsurgical inguinal or subinguinal varicocelectomy techniques resulted in higher spontaneous pregnancy rates and fewer recurrences, and postoperative complications than laparoscopic, radiologic embolization and macroscopic inguinal or retroperitoneal varicocelectomy techniques. Postoperative complications vary with surgical techniques. Hydrocele formation is the most common complication of varicocelectomy, with the incidence ranging from 0% to 10% (Table 2). The lowest and highest reported hydrocele formation rates are seen in the microsurgical and in the high retroperitoneal series

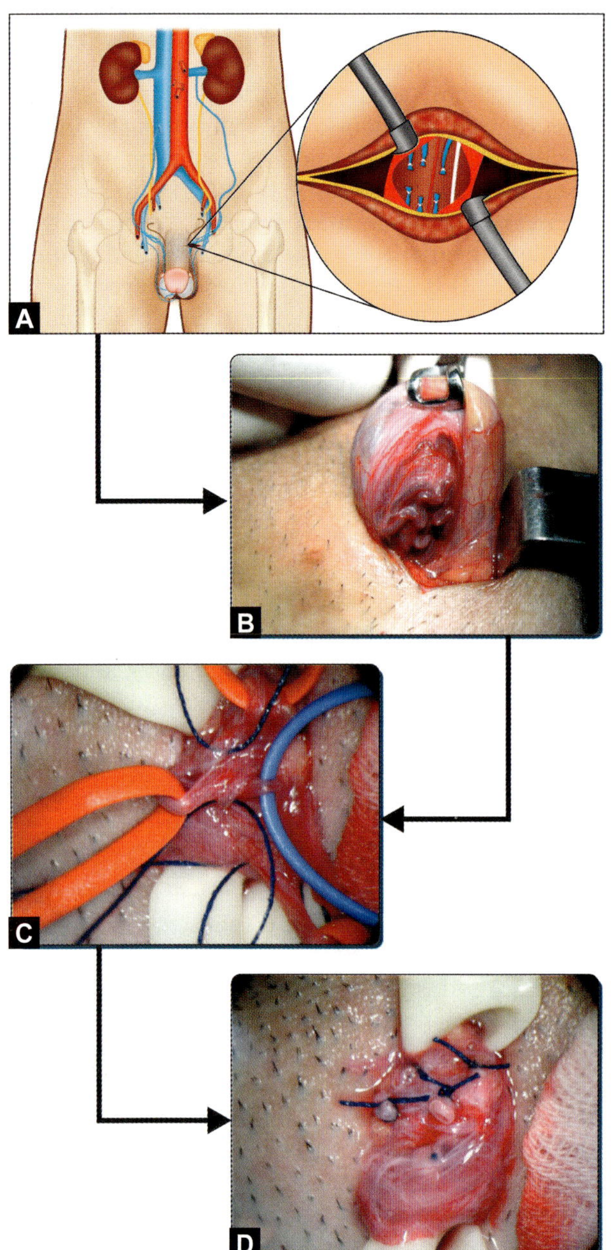

Figures 2A to D Microsurgical subinguinal varicocele repair. (A) A transverse incision is made just below the level of the external inguinal ring. Intraoperative photographs of the spermatic cord are shown in Figures B to D; (B) Dilated cremasteric veins are identified by elevating the spermatic cord with a Babcock clamp; (C) Testicular artery (blue vessel loop), lymphatics (blue cotton suture) and dilated varicose veins (red vessel loops) are demonstrated; (D) Final surgical aspect of varicose veins transected and ligated with nonabsorbable sutures

respectively. Recurrences are reported in the range of 0–35%, varying with varicocelectomy techniques. Overall recurrence rates are low for microsurgical varicocelectomy and high for retroperitoneal and macrosurgical inguinal approaches.[33] Accidental testicular artery ligation during microsurgical varicocelectomy has been reported to be about 1%, and it may cause testicular atrophy. It has been recently demonstrated that the concomitant use of intraoperative vascular Doppler during microsurgical varicocelectomy allows more arterial branches to be preserved, and more internal spermatic veins are likely to be ligated.[37]

Varicocelectomy studies report significant improvements in one or more semen parameters in approximately 65% of men.[38] The meantime for semen improvement and spontaneous pregnancy after surgery is approximately 5 months and 7 months respectively.[39] Overall, sperm concentration, motility and morphology are increased by 9.7 million/ml, 10% and 3% respectively after varicocelectomy.[40] Sperm DNA integrity is also increased after varicocele repair.[41-43] Spontaneous pregnancy rates are higher in men with treated varicoceles (33–36%) as compared to untreated varicoceles (15–20%).[11,44] Our group has recently demonstrated that treatment of clinical varicoceles may improve the outcomes of ICSI in couples with varicocele-related infertility.[12] In our study, the chances of live birth were significantly increased by 1.9-fold while the chance of miscarriage were reduced by 2.3-fold, if the varicocele had been treated before assisted conception.

However, it is still unknown why fertility potential is not always improved after varicocelectomy. Studies evaluating predictors for successful varicocele repair indicate that infertile men either with higher preoperative semen parameters or undergoing varicocele repair for large varicoceles are more likely to show postoperative semen parameters improvement.[38,45] It was also shown that men who achieved a postoperative total motile sperm count greater than 20 millions and decreased sperm DNA fragmentation after surgical varicocelectomy were more likely to initiate a pregnancy either spontaneously or via assisted conception.[41,46] The individual response after varicocele repair may be related to the different profile of antioxidant enzymes genes genotype in infertile men with varicocele. It has been suggested that genetic polymorphisms in the glutathione S-transferase T1 gene may affect individual response to varicocelectomy.[47] Conversely, reduced preoperative testicular volume, elevated serum FSH levels, diminished testosterone concentrations, subclinical varicocele, as well as the presence of Y

Table 2 Treatment results for varicocele repair in infertile men. Postoperative recurrence, hydrocele formation and spontaneous pregnancy rates among different techniques

Technique	Recurrence rate	Hydrocele formation rate	Spontaneous pregnancy rate
Retroperitoneal high-ligation	7-35%	6-10%	25-55%
Laparoscopic	2-7%	0-9%	14-42%
Macroscopic inguinal	0-37%	7%	34-39%
Microscopic inguinal or subinguinal	0-0.3%	0-1.6%	33-56%

Note: Values are expressed as range

chromosome microdeletions seem to be negative predictors for fertility improvement after surgery.[27,48]

The proper management of infertile men with concomitant clinical and subclinical varicoceles at opposing sides is still unresolved. Zheng et al. found that bilateral varicocelectomy had no benefit over the left clinical varicocelectomy;[49] however, the authors used a retroperitoneal approach for vein ligation which is associated with high recurrence rate. Elbendary et al., in a prospective trial, observed that the magnitude of change in sperm count and motility and the spontaneous pregnancy rates were significantly higher in the group of men who had bilateral varicocele repair.[50] Also, it is still debatable whether varicoceles can cause or contribute to azoospermia. A recent meta-analysis reported appearance of sperm in ejaculates of 39% of azoospermic individuals whose varicoceles had been treated.[31] Testicular histopathology results were predictive of success. Postoperatively, appearance of sperm in the ejaculates was increased 9.4-fold in patients with biopsy-proven hypospermatogenesis or maturation arrest than in Sertoli-cell-only (SCO) syndrome. Although motile ejaculated sperm is preferred for ICSI, persistent azoospermia after varicocele repair is still a potential problem and sperm extraction before ICSI will be inevitable for many individuals. In these circumstances, successful sperm retrieval rates of 60% have been reported using testicular microdissection [microsurgical testicular sperm extraction (micro-TESE)] sperm extraction.[51] It has been suggested that varicocele repair may maximize the chances of retrieving sperm for ICSI in men with persistent azoospermia after varicocelectomy.[52]

RECONSTRUCTIVE SURGERIES OF DUCTAL SYSTEM

Vas Deferens and Epididymis

Both microsurgical reconstruction and sperm retrieval combined with *in vitro* fertilization (IVF) coupled with ICSI can be effective treatments for infertility due to OA. A choice between the two must be based not only on the needs and preferences of the individual couple but also on the couple's clinical profile taking into account the cause of azoospermia and any coexisting factors in the female partner. Consequently, both partners should be evaluated thoroughly before making a specific treatment recommendation. Cost issues also play a role in the decision-making process since assisted reproductive technology (ART) is seldom reimbursed by health insurance companies in most countries. Most importantly, infertility clinics and doctors should not limit couple's options for treatment based on their own technical limitations, but always provide all treatment options available for that particular case scenario.

Vasovasostomy and vasoepididymostomy are surgical procedures designed to bypass an obstruction in the male genital tract. While the vast majority of vasovasostomy and vasoepididymostomy procedures are to reverse intentional obstructions, other indications include correction of epididymal or vasal obstructions due to genital infections, iatrogenic injuries related to inguinal or scrotal surgery, especially during the early childhood years, and postvasectomy pain syndrome.[53] Currently, several programs offer microsurgical training for urology residents. Short-term microsurgery courses are of limited value; however, they can help urologists acquire the initial skills needed to use microsurgery in a routine basis. It is important to emphasize that microsurgical procedures for male infertility may be very demanding; therefore, one should only embark on performing either vasovasostomies or vasoepididymostomies after mastering microsurgical skills in the microsurgery laboratory using animals or synthetic models. Among several predictors for a successful microsurgical reconstruction of the male reproductive system, surgeon's skills are the most relevant for treatment outcomes. Surgeon's skills are crucial when vasoepididymostomies are needed, which frequently cannot be anticipated. Therefore, mastering both vasovasostomy and vasoepididymostomy techniques allows for real-time decision making without compromising clinical results.

Preoperative Planning

Patient Assessment

Some historical and prognostic factors must be taken in consideration in preoperative workup. Obstruction intervals from vasectomy to reversal are believed to play a major role in determining surgery outcomes.[54,55] Obstruction intervals longer than 15 years are associated with lower patency and pregnancy rates. Long-interval obstructions are associated with higher incidence of epididymal obstruction and as a result, vasoepididymostomy is likely to be required. A computer model based on obstructive interval and patient age was created to determine the need for vasoepididymostomy. The model was designed to be 100% sensitive in detecting patients requiring vasoepididymostomy. In the test group, the model was 100% sensitive in predicting vasoepididymostomy with a specificity of 58.8%.[56]

A history of a previous vasectomy reversal attempt does not preclude a new one. Satisfactory results are reported for repeated reversals,[57] and the history of conception with the current partner seems to be the only significant predictor for a successful pregnancy. History of genital/inguinal surgery should raise the concern about the possibility of iatrogenic inadvertent surgical obstruction. Repair of obstruction in the inguinal canal or retroperitoneum can be technically challenging.

There are important physical signs that can also predict the success of vasovasostomy. Small and soft testes may indicate impaired spermatogenesis. Indurate, irregular epididymis and the presence of hydrocele are often associated with epididymal obstruction and may suggest the need for vasoepididymostomy. Palpation of a granuloma in the vas deferens should be interpreted as a favorable prognostic sign. Its presence means that sperm has leaked at the vasectomy site preventing from overpressure within the epididymis tubules and rupture.[54,55] If a vasal gap is detected, the patient should be advised that a larger incision into the inguinal region may be needed in order to allow a tension-free anastomosis to be performed. Specific laboratory tests are not necessary before reconstructive surgeries. Serum FSH testing is indicated as a marker of testicular reserve only if testicular damage is suspected on physical examination. The usefulness of antibody testing remains controversial and evidence suggests that late failures following reversals are likely to be technical rather than immunological.[58,59] Besides, overall conception rates are acceptably high and the presence of antisperm antibodies does not correlate closely with postsurgical fecundability.[60]

The female partner fertility has to be carefully assessed before indicating reconstruction procedures and alternatives to vasectomy reversal should be discussed. It has been shown that reversal outcomes in men with the same partners are significantly better than those with new partners. The proven fecundity as a couple, shorter obstructive interval and stronger emotional dedication to achieving conception may act as possible factors for the higher success rate.[54,61] Female age greater than 40 years is a negative predictor for pregnancy achievement.[62,63]

Operative Procedure

Overview

There are several techniques described to perform restoration of the vas integrity. The standard method involves suturing of the vasal segments or the vas to the epididymis tubule. The operating microscope and adequate microsurgical instruments are crucial to facilitate reconstruction. It is not advisable to perform varicocele repair at the same time of vasectomy reversal. In vasectomized men, vasal veins are often compromised which would jeopardize venous return after ligation of internal and external spermatic veins. If necessary, varicocelectomy may be performed 6 months later, when new venous and arterial channels are formed around the anastomosis. Although reconstructive surgery can be performed after percutaneous epididymal sperm aspiration (PESA), the likelihoods for sperm appearance in the semen and pregnancy are decreased.

Anesthesia

Vasovasostomy and vasoepididymostomy may be safely performed using local, regional or general anesthesia. The authors carry out procedures in an outpatient basis. Continuous propofol intravenous anesthesia coupled with the blockage of the spermatic cord using 10–20 ml of a 1% lidocaine hydrochloride solution is our preferred anesthetic method.

Incision

Two centimeters longitudinal scrotal incisions are placed in the anterior aspect of the scrotum on each side. The incision is made onto the palpable granuloma or onto the identified vasal gap. Only the vas ends are delivered through the skin incision. The incision may be extended to the inguinal region when the vasectomy was performed high in the scrotum or a large segment was removed or in repeat reconstructions with difficult vasal mobilization. The testis is delivered only if a vasoepididymostomy or a robotic-assisted anastomosis is to be performed.

Approaching the Vas

Microsurgical dissection is carried out onto the region of the prior vasectomy site to free the vas and its vascular pedicle from surrounding scar tissue. Hemostasis is obtained with great care using either bipolar or hand-held thermal cautery units. After the vas has been mobilized and its scarred ends excised, patency of the abdominal vas end is confirmed with the introduction of a 24-gauge blunt tipped angiocatheter into the lumen and the injection of 20 ml sterile saline through the catheter. The ends of the vas must be adequately mobilized in order to allow a complete tension-free anastomosis. Either a microsurgical clamp or holding sutures can be used according to the surgeon's preference.

Vasal Fluid Examination

Intraoperative factors affecting the success rates of reconstructive procedures include the gross appearance of vas fluid, the presence and quality of sperm in the fluid, the length of the remaining segment adjacent to the epididymis. Fluid emanating from the testicular vas end is examined both macroscopically and under the optical microscope for the presence of sperm. The presence of copious, clear, watery or cloudy fluid and motile sperm is associated with excellent patency rates of 94%, opposed to only 60% when no sperm is found in the vasal fluid.[54] Thick toothpaste-like vasal fluid is suggestive of epididymal obstruction.[54,64] The quality of sperm found in the intravasal fluid and the surgeon's microsurgical skills are the most important factors to determine the type of reconstructive technique. Typically, the presence of sperm or sperm parts, and even a 'dry' vas, are associated with adequate patency rates of about 70–80% following vasovasostomies.[65,66]

Vasovasostomy Techniques

In general, there are four fundamental surgical principles of vasal restorative surgery. These include the accurate mucosa-to-mucosa approximation, a water-tight tension-free anastomosis, preservation of the vasal blood supply and healthy tissue (mucosa and muscularis) and an adequate microscopic atraumatic technique.

Modified One-Layer Technique

The modified one-layer technique was originally described by Sharlip.[67] The anastomosis is completed by placing a total of 12 sutures. Of these, six are through the full thickness of the vas wall at 60° intervals and six are placed in the muscularis only, between the full thickness sutures. The operation is performed entirely with the surgeon located on the patient's right side. One of the authors (Sandro C Esteves) has made some modifications to the modified one-layer technique as described above (Figure 3A). Briefly, the first suture is placed in the medial surface of the right vas (0° position). This suture is placed through the full thickness of the vas wall on the testicular side first taking a generous bite of adventitia and muscularis and a tiny portion of the mucosa. The suture is then passed into the corresponding 0° position of the abdominal side again taking a bite at the edge of the mucosa and a large portion of the muscularis/adventitia layer. This suture is tied and cut long so it is easily identified as the procedure continues. The second suture is placed 180° opposite to the first, again taking the full aspect of the vas wall, firstly on the testicular side and then on the abdominal one. This suture is also tied and cut long. A third full thickness suture is placed at the 60° position, one-third of the distance from the first to the second sutures. Before it is tied, a fourth suture is placed at the 120° position, two-thirds of the distance from the first to the second sutures. Third and fourth sutures are then tied after careful inspection of their proper placement. A fifth suture is placed between these two at the 90° position, but only superficially through the muscularis. This completes the anastomosis of the anterior portion of the vas. At this point, four full thickness stitches and one muscular suture have been placed and half of the total circumference of the vas wall is closed. The vas clamp is then rotated 180° and verification of accidental back-walling and proper position of full thickness sutures is checked. After rotation of the vas, two full thickness sutures are then placed at 240° and 300° positions. These sutures are inserted and inspected before being tied. A final suture is placed in the muscularis at 270° position. These complete the anastomosis, summing-up eight sutures in total instead of twelve as first described by Sharlip. Upon anastomosis completion, the surrounding loose fibrous tissue is sutured over the anastomotic site alleviating tension. Scrotal incision is closed in the routine usual manner.

Two-Layer Technique

This technique, described by Belker, involves placing five to eight interrupted 10-0 nylon sutures in the inner mucosal layer and eight to ten 9-0 nylon sutures in the outer muscular and adventitial layer.[68] The use of an approximating clamp and a holding suture are recommended to stabilize vas ends for the anastomosis. Before the suturing begins, the surgeon looks straight down into the lumen of each end of the vas situated parallel to each other. As suturing proceeds, the transected ends of the vas bend toward each other, bringing the suture together without tension. Firstly, three posterior muscular layer sutures are placed in a row so that the knots are outside. Only 90° of the circumference are approximated, leaving full access to the mucosa.

Then, after three posterior mucosal sutures have been placed and tied, the far-corner and near-corner sutures are placed and tied alternately until space remains for only two or three sutures in the anterior aspect of the anastomosis. These remaining stitches are then placed and left long and untied until back-walling can be safely ruled out. The sutures are finally tied and the closing muscular layer is sutured with caution to visualize the underlying mucosal layer sutures to prevent penetration of the lumen by the outer-layer ones. Placement of these sutures is easier to perform from the assistant side toward the surgeon's side. Closure of scrotal incision is performed in the usual manner.

Multilayer Microdot Technique

This method, originally described by Goldstein, is adequate to treat markedly discrepant diameters in straight or convoluted vas.[69] Vasal ends are prepared with a 90° right angle cut and methylene blue stain can be used to better visualize the mucosal rings. Planned needle exit points can be marked with microtip marking (Figure 3B). Polypropylene monofilament 10-0 double-armed sutures with 70 µm diameter taper-pointed needles are used for the anastomosis. Sutures are placed in an inside-out fashion eliminating the possibility for accidental back-walling. The mucosa and about one-third thickness of the muscularis should be included in each bite, symmetrically on each side of vas ends. Four initial sutures are placed in the anterior aspect of the vas and tied up (Figure 3B). Three 9-0 sutures are then placed exactly in between the previously placed mucosal sutures, just above but not through the mucosa, sealing the gap between the mucosal sutures. The vas is then rotated 180° and four additional 10-0 sutures are placed completing the mucosal part of the anastomosis. Just prior to tying the last mucosal knot, vas lumen is irrigated with heparinized saline solution to prevent formation of clots. After completion of mucosal layer, 9-0 sutures are placed in between each mucosal suture again, avoiding penetrating the mucosa itself (Figure 3B). Sutures are placed but not tied until two or three more have been placed. Superficial additional adventitia 9-0 sutures should be placed only when necessary. Procedure is complete approximating vas sheath with four to six 6-0 sutures.

Robotic-Assisted Technique

Recent reports have shown the possibility to perform the classic above described techniques using robotic assistance. The robot can offer the benefits of enhanced imaging (up to 100X magnification) and control of physiologic tremor.[70,71]

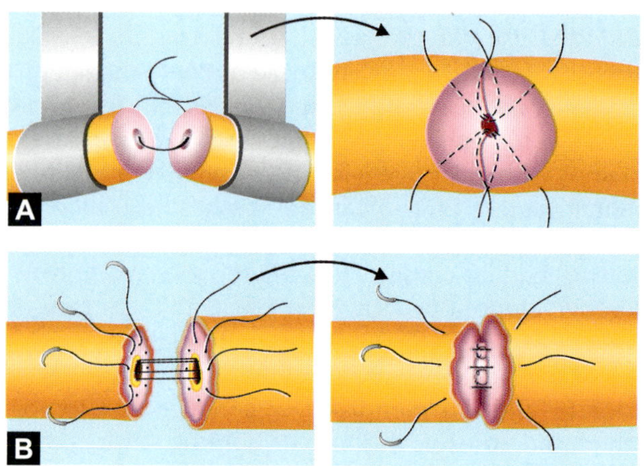

Figures 3A and B Microsurgical vasovasostomy techniques. Schematic illustration of (A) The modified one-layer and (B) The multilayer microdot technique

Vasoepididymostomy Techniques

Vasoepididymostomy is a challenging surgical procedure that should only be attempted by experienced microsurgeons. Meticulous microsurgical technique and high magnification are required for a precise anastomosis of the vas (luminal diameter of 300–400 µm) to the epididymal tubule (150–250 µm).

The procedure starts with the placement of a longitudinal incision in the upper scrotum. The testis is delivered through the incision and the testis and epididymis are thoroughly inspected. The site of obstruction can be often grossly visible as an area where the epididymis transitions from a firm, wide caliber to a smaller, softer structure. The distal end of the vas deferens is mobilized in a similar fashion as that described for the vasovasostomy but often a longer length is required to perform an epididymal anastomosis. At this point, the microscope is brought into the operating field to perform the anastomosis. Currently, three variations of the technique have been used for precise approximation of the vas deferens lumen to a single epididymal tubule: end-to-end, end-to-side, and end-to-side intussusception techniques. Prior to the anastomosis, a dilated epididymal tubule must be identified immediately above the level of obstruction. The tubule must be opened and the fluid inspected for the presence of motile sperm. If no sperm is identified, a more proximal site of the epididymis will be required for the anastomosis. Intraoperative sperm harvesting and cryopreservation can be offered during vasoepididymostomy.[72]

End-to-End Technique

First described by Silber, the end-to-end vasoepididymostomy is the most difficult anastomosis to perform.[73] It involves dissection of a single epididymal tubule, complete transection and anastomosis to the vas lumen. The epididymis is dissected off the testis for 3–5 cm to provide an adequate length to achieve a tension-free anastomosis. Initially, two 9-0 nylon sutures are placed at the 5 O'clock and 7 O'clock positions of the seromuscular surface of the vas, to secure the cut end of the distal vas to the epididymal tunica. Next, four double-armed 10-0 nylon sutures mounted in double-armed 70 µm fishhook-shape taper-pointed needle are placed in a quadrant fashion between the vas mucosa and the epididymal tubule (Figure 4A). These sutures are not tied until all have been positioned. The anastomosis is completed by placing several interrupted 9-0 nylon sutures to approximate the seromuscular layer of the vas to the epididymal tunic layer.

End-to-Side Technique

The end-to-side vasoepididymostomy, popularized by Thomas, is performed by creating a small window in a loop of the epididymal tubule proximal to the obstruction and by suturing the end of the vas lumen to the open window.[74] The advantages over the end-to-end anastomosis include less dissection and bleeding during the anastomosis because hemostasis can be secured before opening the tubule. Moreover, only one tubule is opened making the identification of the patent tubule more precise and easy. With the tubule opened and sperm presence confirmed, three or four double-armed 10-0 nylon sutures are placed in a quadrant fashion through the edge of the epididymal tubule (Figure 4B). The sutures are placed in the corresponding quadrant of the vasal mucosa and tied. The anastomosis is completed with additional 9-0 nylon sutures between the epididymal tunic and the seromuscular layer of the vas deferens. Finally, several 9-0 nylon sutures are used to anchor the vas deferens to the parietal layer of the tunica vaginalis. These final sutures are designed to prevent tension on the anastomosis and are placed well away from the vasoepididymostomy site.

Triangulation End-to-Side Vasoepididymostomy

This technique was introduced by Berger[75] with subsequent modifications by others.[76,77] It is the simplest and fastest among the three techniques described in this chapter. The intention is to combine the precision of the conventional end-to-side anastomosis with a simplified microsuture placement. Rather than a direct approximation of the epididymal tubule to the vas, this method involves pulling the epididymal tubule into the vas lumen. An opening window is made in the epididymal tunic corresponding to the vas diameter. Two 9-0 sutures are used to secure the muscular layer of the vas to the epididymal tunic to avoid tension on the anastomosis site. Three double-armed 10-0 nylon sutures are placed equidistantly in a triangular configuration in the desired epididymal tubule (Figure 4C). Then, the epididymal tubule is carefully opened with microscissors or microknife between the positioned sutures. Once sperm is confirmed in the epididymal fluid, the needles are passed through the lumen of the vas in an inside-out fashion. The sutures are then tied, creating an invagination of the epididymal tubule into the vasal lumen (Figure 4C). Finally, additional 9-0 nylon sutures are placed to approximate the seromuscular layer of the vas to the epididymal tunic.

Recently, a modification of the triangulation end-to-side vasoepididymostomy was described by Marmar.[76] In this technique, a single epididymal tubule is exposed and two 10-0 nylon sutures mounted on double-armed 70 µm bicurve needles are placed on the field. A needle from each suture is mounted on a styrofoam block and positioned parallel to the other with sufficient room for passage of the tip of a microblade between them. A microneedle holder is used to grasp both needles simultaneously and move them from the block to the field while maintaining the parallel arrangement. The tips of both needles are passed through a selected tubule at once. The two sutures are retracted laterally and a tubulotomy is cut between them with a microknife. Then, all four needles from the epididymal sutures are individually placed into the mucosal lumen of the vas and out through the muscularis on the cut end. Needles

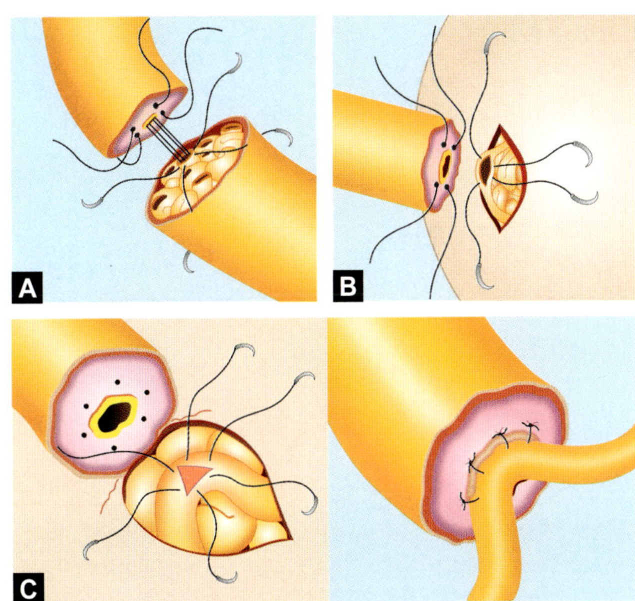

Figures 4A to C Microsurgical vasoepididymostomy techniques. Schematic illustration of (A) The end-to-end, (B) End-to-side and (C) Triangulation end-to-side anastomoses

are placed at the 8 O'clock and 10 O'clock positions on the left side and at the 2 O'clock and 4 O'clock positions on the right side. Sutures are tied allowing the epididymal tubule to invaginate into the vas lumen. The anastomosis is completed with three to four additional 9-0 nylon sutures through the muscularis of the vas and epididymal tunic.

Postoperative Follow-up and Results

Postoperative care involves local dressing and scrotal supporter that are kept for 48–72 hours and 2 weeks respectively. Scrotal ice-packing is always recommended to control local edema for the first 72 hours postoperatively. Patients are counseled to restrain from physical activity and sexual intercourse for 1 or 2 months in cases of vasovasostomy and vasoepididymostomy respectively. Oral analgesics usually suffice to control postoperative pain. Postoperative follow-up is aimed to evaluate improvement in semen parameters, complications and spontaneous or assisted conception. Semen analysis should be performed every 2 months after surgery until the semen parameters stabilize or pregnancy occurs.

Over the past two decades, treatment options for couples with reconstructible OA had a marked improvement. Despite the advances in ART, specifically sperm retrieval techniques for ICSI, microsurgical reconstruction of the vas remains a cost-effective, reliable and effective means of restoring fertility in most individuals with OA[78-82] Nevertheless, a comprehensive understanding of the factors that can affect outcomes, overall cost and the morbidity associated with each treatment modality, respective of the institution providing the treatment, is recommended.

Overall, patency/pregnancy rates following microsurgical vasovasostomy and vasoepididymostomy are 92%/55% and 78%/40% respectively[54,55,61,64,66,73-76,83] (Table 3). Microsurgical techniques are clearly superior compared to macrosurgical or loupe-assisted anastomoses.[54,84] Most pregnancies occur within 24 months after surgery. Pregnancy rates are related to the time elapsed from vasectomy to reversal and female age. Although female partner's age does not affect patency rates after vasectomy reversal (86–90% in female partners aged < 40 years old vs 83% in those older than 40 years), it does affect pregnancy rates (14% in women aged > 40 years vs 56% in those aged < 39 years).[63] Pregnancy rates are also lower after longer duration of vasal obstruction. Approximately 30–40% of couples

Table 3 Treatment results for vasovasostomy and vasoepididymostomy. Type of anastomosis, patency and spontaneous pregnancy rates using different techniques.

Author	Patients (N)	Technique	Patency rate (%)	Pregnancy rate (%)
Vasovasostomy				
Belker et al.[54]	1,247	Modified One-layer	89	57
		Two-layer	86	51
Boorjian and Lipkin[55]	159	Two-layer	95	83
Chan and Goldstein[61]	1,048	Two-layer	99	54
Kolettis et al.[66]	34	Both	76	35
Vasoepididymostomy				
Silber[73]	139	End-to-end	78	56
Thomas[74]	137	End-to-side	79	50
Berger[75]	12	Triangulation intussusception	92	NR
Marmar[76]	9	Modified intussusception	78	22
Chan et al.[83]	68	Triangulation intussusception	84	40
Schiff et al.[64]	153	End-to-end	73	NR
		End-to-side	74	
		3-suture intussusception	84	
		2-suture intussusception	80	

NR: not reported

achieve pregnancy following surgical reconstructions performed in obstruction intervals greater than 15 years as compared to > 50% in shorter intervals.[64,85] Vasectomy reversal has been shown to be feasible in patients, who failed PESA. Marmar et al. showed that PESA procedures cause limited trauma to the epididymis and up to 50% pregnancy rates may be obtained in vasectomy reversal after PESA; however, success is higher for couples whose female partners are 37 years old or less.[86]

As patency and pregnancy rates yielded by the existing surgical procedures do not reach 100% and are technically demanding, efforts continue to be made in order to widen the options for reconstructive repair. Several modifications have been suggested and include intussusception vasoepididymostomy anastomotic techniques, the use of novel biomaterials/sealants, absorbable and nonabsorbable stents, and the use of robotics.[64,71,83,87-90] In a prospective study, Chan et al. reported overall patency and pregnancy rates of 84% and 40% using the vasoepididymostomy intussusception technique.[83] These findings were confirmed by Schiff et al., who reported patency and pregnancy rates of approximately 82% and 45% respectively, using simplified intussusception techniques.[64] It is suggested that anastomoses are more water-tight by using intussusception techniques; therefore, granuloma formation is decreased. The rationale of using sealants around the anastomotic site is to decrease operative time and to simplify the procedure without compromising success rates. Fibrin sealant can stimulate the coagulation cascade producing a fibrin seal around the anastomosis. When mixed with thrombin and calcium, fibrinogen is converted to fibrin monomer which in turn is converted to a stable cross-linked fibrin polymer.[88] Ho et al. achieved 85% patency rates and 23% pregnancy rates using three transmural 9-0 sutures and fibrin glue in a mean follow-up of 6.2 months.[88] There are concerns, however, about the potential contact of the glue with the vas lumen, which may result in possible obstruction, and also about transmission of viral disease because fibrin glue is derived from pooled plasma.[87] The use of nonabsorbable polymeric stent has been reported only in animal model. Preliminary results showed 100% patency rates in a follow-up of 39–47 weeks, and the total sperm count was significantly higher in the stented group.[89] The use of robotics for microsurgical procedures is also a novel concept. The rationale to add this technology to the already existing armamentarium relies on the possibility of physiologic static tremor correction, visual magnification (up to 100X when using a digital microscopic camera) and ergonomics.[90] Animal studies suggest that robotic assisted vasectomy reversal are easier to perform and yields better pregnancy rates than microsurgical reversal.[91] In a preliminary experience in humans, Parekattil et al. reported shorter operative time and higher postoperative sperm count for robot-assisted vasectomy reversal as compared to the microsurgical technique.[90] However, the advantages of the robot over an experienced microsurgeon are yet to be proven in larger series. A robotic system costs more than one million dollars and its annual maintenance surpasses one hundred thousand dollars. These cost issues will certainly represent a barrier to the widely adoption of robotics into microsurgical urologic practice.

EJACULATORY DUCT

Congenital obstructions may be caused either by utricular, Müllerian and Wolffian duct cysts or atresia/stenosis of the ejaculatory ducts. Acquired obstructions may be secondary to trauma or infectious/inflammatory etiologies. Traumatic damage to the ejaculatory ducts may occur after removal of seminal vesicle cysts, pull-through operations for imperforate anus and even prolonged catheterization or instrumentation. Genital or urinary infection and prostatic abscess may cause stenosis or complete obstruction of the ducts.[92] Prostatic infection may also result in calculous formation and secondary obstruction, while tuberculosis produces genital devastation.

Ejaculatory duct obstruction (EDO) is a potential surgically correctable cause of male infertility.

Preoperative Planning

Patient Evaluation

Diagnostic criteria typically included history, physical examination, semen analyses and transrectal ultrasound evaluation. The clinical presentation may be highly variable and, in addition to a history of infertility. Complaints may include painful ejaculation, hemospermia, perineal and/or testicular pain, but patients may be completely asymptomatic. Typically, physical examination is normal. Occasionally, the seminal vesicles or a mass are palpable on rectal examination. Prostatic tenderness and/or epididymal enlargement may exist. Hormone profiles are usually normal.

Semen analyses may reveal oligozoospermia or azoospermia, decreased motility and decreased ejaculate volume. The presence of a low volume (< 1.5 ml) acidic (pH < 7.0) azoospermic ejaculate with absent fructose, palpable vas and epididymal thickening is virtually pathognomonic. However, the typical clinical picture may be complicated whether obstruction is unilateral, partial or functional.[92] Postejaculate urinalyses are often performed to exclude retrograde ejaculation in patients with low-volume ejaculates.

High-resolution transrectal ultrasound evaluation (TRUS) using a 5–7 MHz biplanar transducer is recommended in all cases of suspected EDO. The exact definition of obstruction on TRUS, however, is still a matter of debate due to marked variability in the size and shape of the vas deferens, seminal vesicles, and ejaculatory ducts in fertile and infertile men. Common ultrasound findings include dilation of the seminal vesicles (defined as a cross-sectional width of greater than 1.5 cm) or ejaculatory ducts (defined as an internal duct diameter of greater than 2.0 mm), calcifications or calculi in the region of the ejaculatory duct or verumontanum and midline or eccentrically located prostatic cysts.[93-95] It has been suggested that adjunctive procedures, such as magnetic resonance imaging, chromotubation, seminal vesicle aspiration, seminal vesicle scintigraphy and ejaculatory duct manometry are more sensitive for diagnosis.[96-100] Ultrasound-guided transrectal seminal vesiculography has been shown to provide excellent radiographic visualization of the ejaculatory ducts.[96] TRUS-guided seminal vesicle aspiration and the presence of motile sperm in the aspirates seem to be a useful diagnostic tool, since the seminal vesicles are not sperm reservoirs.[97] The proper management of azoospermic men with EDO involves the confirmation of sperm production. The presence of normal spermatogenesis can be determined by testicular biopsy or 'wet prep'. The presence of motile sperm is highly indicative of ductal obstruction.

Operative Aspects

The standard treatment of EDO is the transurethral resection of the ejaculatory duct (TURED). Resection of the ejaculatory ducts is a technically demanding and critical procedure. The typical patient with EDO is young and has a small prostate. Therefore, TURED is carried out very close to the bladder neck, rectum and sphincter.

Anesthesia

Transurethral resection of the ejaculatory ducts is performed using regional or general anesthesia.

Technique

Our choice is to perform TURED, as originally described by Farley and Barnes,[101] with minor modifications.[92]. First, the obstruction is documented using intraoperative vasotomy and vasography. The vas is delivered using a small scrotal incision and dissected free of the associated perivasal vessels. A mixture of injectable saline and radiographic contrast material in a 1:1 ratio is injected into the abdominal end of the vas, together with methylene blue dye, by direct vas puncture with a 30-gauge lymphangiogram needle. Vasography confirms obstruction, whereas dye injection confirms patency by visualization of the effluxing dye mixture during TURED. A 9-0 nylon suture is placed at the muscular layer of the vas to close the vasotomy site. TURED is performed with the patient in the dorsal lithotomy position. A resectoscope with 24-French loop is used to remove a strip of tissue on the floor of the prostate just proximal to and including a portion of the verumontanum (Figures 5A and B). The ducts are considered adequately opened by visualizing its dilated portion and the dye efflux. If a midline cyst is present, resection is performed to completely unroof the cyst. Resection is performed with pure cutting to avoid thermal injury to the proximal ejaculatory duct. The authors feel more comfortable placing a finger in the patient's rectum to prevent rectal injury during resection and having methylene blue injected through the vasotomy site. Resection is completed by positive identification of free dye efflux into the urethra. An 18-French Foley catheter is left in place for 24 hours and the patient is discharged the next day.

Postoperative Follow-up and Results

An indwelling catheter is kept in place for 24–48 hours and patients are discharged the following day. Oral quinolone antibiotics and anti-inflammatory medication is prescribed for 5 days. Scrotal supporter is recommended for 1 week to avoid scrotal edema due to vasotomy. Frequent ejaculation is recommended 3–4 weeks postoperatively and patients are monitored with monthly semen analyses.

TURED results vary according to the etiology of obstruction being congenital or acquired.[92] Semen quality improvement (ejaculate volume, sperm count and motility) and unassisted conception is observed in approximately 85% and 60% of individuals with congenital obstructions. Conversely, seminal improvement occurs in only about 30% of the individuals with infectious/inflammatory etiologies. Complications occur in approximately one-third of men treated by TURED and

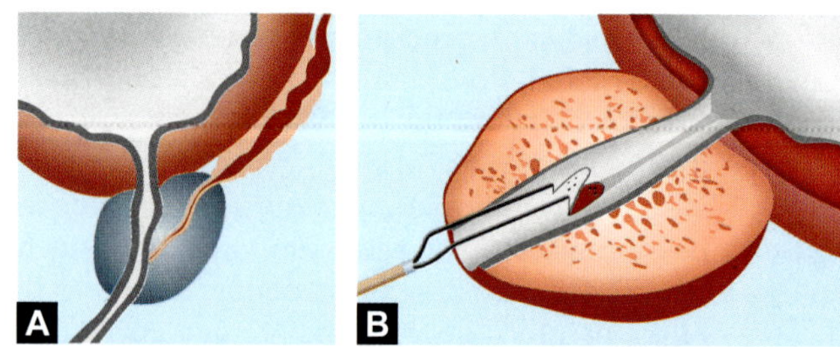

Figures 5A and B Transurethral resection of the ejaculatory duct. (A) Schematic representation of the ejaculatory duct entering into the prostatic urethra; (B) Resectoscope loop is used to remove a strip of tissue on the floor of the prostate just proximal to and including a portion of the verumontanum

mainly include reflux of urine to the unroofed cyst cavity with consequent impairment of the semen parameters, retrograde ejaculation and epididymitis with obstruction.[92] Rectal injury or incontinence is rarely reported.

Modern and less invasive approaches using balloon dilation coupled or not with transurethral incision of the ejaculatory ducts have been proposed to treat EDO. Preliminary data show that such alternatives have similar results and fewer complications than TURED.[102,103]

SPERM RETRIEVAL TECHNIQUES

Azoospermia, defined as the absence of spermatozoa in the ejaculate after centrifugation, is found in 1–3% of the male population and approximately 10% of infertile males.[97] In this scenario, two different clinical situations exist, i.e. obstructive (OA) and nonobstructive azoospermia (NOA). In OA, spermatogenesis is normal but a mechanical blockage exists in the genital tract, somewhere between the epididymis and the ejaculatory duct, or the epididymis and vas deferens are totally or partially absent. Acquired OA may be due to vasectomy, failure of vasectomy reversal, postinfectious diseases, surgical procedures in the scrotal, inguinal, pelvic or abdominal regions and trauma. Congenital causes of OA include cystic fibrosis, congenital absence of the vas deferens (CAVD), ejaculatory duct or prostatic cysts and Young's syndrome.[97] NOA comprises of a spectrum of testicular histopathology resulting from various causes that include environmental toxins, medications, cryptorchidism, genetic and congenital abnormalities, varicocele, trauma, viral orchitis, endocrine disorders and idiopathic. In both OA and NOA, pregnancy may be achieved through IVF associated to ICSI.[2,3]

The goals of surgical sperm retrieval are threefold: (i) to retrieve an adequate number of sperm for both immediate use and for cryopreservation; (ii) to obtain the best quality sperm possible and (iii) to minimize damage to the reproductive tract so as not to jeopardize future attempts of sperm retrieval or testicular function. Several surgical methods have been developed to retrieve epididymal and testicular sperm from azoospermic men. Either percutaneous epididymal sperm aspiration (PESA)[104] or microsurgical epididymal sperm aspiration (MESA)[2] can be successfully used to retrieve sperm from the epididymis in men with OA. Testicular sperm aspiration (TESA) can be used to retrieve sperm from the testes either in men with OA, who fail PESA, or in those with NOA.[105] Testicular sperm extraction (TESE) using single or multiple open biopsies[106,107] and, more recently, TESE using microsurgery (micro-TESE) are indicated for men with NOA.[4,106-109] Sperm can be easily obtained from infertile men with OA whereas individuals exhibiting NOA have historically been the most difficult to treat.

PREOPERATIVE PLANNING

Patient Assessment

It is important to distinguish whether the lack of sperm in the ejaculate is from an obstructive or nonobstructive process since the choice of the retrieval method is based on the type of azoospermia. History, physical examination and hormonal analysis (FSH, testosterone) are undertaken to define the type of azoospermia. Together, these factors provide a 90% prediction of its type (OA and NOA).[110] Men with OA usually have normal testes and hormone profile. Occasionally, the epididymis or the seminal vesicles may be enlarged or a cyst can be palpable on rectal examination. The presence of a low volume (< 1.5 ml) acidic (pH < 7.0) azoospermic ejaculate with absent or low fructose and epididymal thickening is pathognomonic of OA due to either congenital bilateral absence of the vas deferens (CBAVD) or EDO; the differential diagnosis would be the presence of the vas in the latter. Approximately two-thirds of men with CAVD have mutations of the cystic fibrosis transmembrane conductance regulator (CFTR) gene. Failure to identify a CFTR abnormality in a man with CBAVD does not rule out the presence of a mutation, since some are undetectable by routine testing methods. In couples whose male partners have CBAVD, the female partner should be offered cystic fibrosis (CF) testing before proceeding with treatments that utilize their sperm because of the high risk of the male being a CF carrier. If a CFTR gene mutation is identified (approximately 4% of female partners are carriers), testing should be offered to the male as well, and counseling is recommended before proceeding with sperm retrieval and ICSI due to the risk of the transmission of CF to the offspring.[110,111] Azoospermic men with idiopathic obstruction and men with a clinical triad of chronic sinusitis, bronchiectasis and OA (Young's syndrome) may be at higher risk for CF gene mutations as well.

The serum FSH is a critical factor in determining whether a diagnostic testicular biopsy is needed to differentiate the type of azoospermia in men with normal semen volume. Elevated FSH and small testis are indicative of testicular failure (NOA); therefore, a testicular biopsy is not necessary for diagnostic purposes.[111] However, if sperm retrieval with ICSI is being considered, a biopsy may be performed for prognostic purposes, to determine whether spermatozoa are likely to be retrievable by future testicular sperm aspiration or extraction. The absence of sperm in a biopsy specimen taken from a man with NOA, however, does not absolutely predict whether sperm are present elsewhere within the testicle.[4,112] Conversely, men with normal levels of FSH and semen volume may have either NOA or OA.[113] In such cases, there is no non-invasive method to differentiate OA from NOA and a testicular biopsy is usually required to provide a definitive diagnosis. Testicular biopsy can be performed by a standard open incision technique or by percutaneous methods. Histology evaluation of testicular specimens may indicate the presence of normal spermatogenesis in cases of OA while hypospermatogenesis or maturation arrest or SCO syndrome are seen in NOA ones.

All men with primary testicular failure of unknown origin should be offered karyotyping and Y-chromosome microdeletion testing. The frequency of karyotypic abnormalities is reported to be 10–15% in men with NOA, and Klinefelter's syndrome accounts for approximately two-thirds of cases.[114] Genetic testing may provide prognostic information for sperm retrieval.[75] In contrast to partial and complete AZFc deletion patients, in whom sperm can be found within the testis, the chance of finding sperm in men with complete AZFa or AZFb deletions is unlikely.[115,116] Genetic counseling should be offered whenever a genetic abnormality is detected in the male prior to performing ICSI with his sperm.

OPERATIVE PROCEDURE

Surgical sperm retrievals using open or percutaneous methods can be carried out in outpatient basis.

Anesthesia

Sperm retrieval techniques are safely performed using local, regional or general anesthesia. The authors perform percutaneous sperm retrievals under local anesthesia only or in association with intravenous bolus infusion of a short-acting hypnotic agent (propofol). In both cases, a 10–15 ml solution of 2% lidocaine hydrochloride is injected around the spermatic cord near the external inguinal ring. In cases where intravenous anesthesia is used, local injection of the anesthetic is performed after patient unconsciousness is achieved. The authors carry out microsurgical sperm retrievals under local anesthesia, as described above, in association with continuous infusion of propofol using a syringe-drive automated-pump device.

Techniques

Sperm retrieval from the epididymis is indicated in obstructive cases only. Testicular sperm retrieval can be performed either in OA and NOA cases. In OA, testicular retrievals are carried out after failed epididymal retrieval or as a primary retrieval procedure in cases of absent epididymis or intense epididymal fibrosis. In NOA, testicular sperm retrievals are the only viable option to collect sperm.

Percutaneous Sperm Retrieval

Typically, percutaneous sperm retrieval is performed using a needle attached to a syringe. The standard procedure is described below. Minor modifications to the methods have been added, but the main goals remain the same which are to aspirate either epididymal fluid or testicular parenchyma for diagnostic or therapeutic purposes. Loupe magnification may be used to avoid injuring small vessels seen through the scrotal skin.

Percutaneous epididymal sperm aspiration: The epididymis is stabilized between the index finger, thumb and forefinger while the testis is held with the palm of the hand. A 13-gauge needle attached to a 1 ml tuberculin syringe is inserted into the epididymis through the scrotal skin (Figure 6A). Negative pressure is created and the tip of the needle is gently moved in and out within the epididymis until fluid enters the syringe. The amount of epididymal fluid obtained during aspiration is often minimal (~0.1 ml), except in cases of CAVD in which 0.3–1.0 ml may be aspirated. The needle is withdrawn from the epididymis and the aspirate is flushed into a 0.5–1.0 ml 37°C sperm medium. The tube containing the epididymal aspirate is transferred to the laboratory for microscopic examination. PESA is repeated at a different site of the same epididymis (from cauda up to the caput) and/or at the contralateral one until adequate number of motile sperm is retrieved. If PESA fails to retrieve motile sperm for ICSI, TESA is performed at the same operative time.

The adoption of strict criteria to diagnose OA is crucial for obtaining high success retrieval rate using percutaneous techniques. Using PESA, our approach is to perform the first aspiration at the corpus epididymis then proceed up to the caput if necessary, since aspirates from the cauda are usually rich in poor quality senescent spermatozoa, debris and macrophages. Most cases of PESA failures are not necessarily technical failures because immotile spermatozoa are found. However, in certain cases of epididymal fibrosis due to multiple PESA attempts or postinfection, PESA may be ineffective to retrieve sperm.

Testicular sperm aspiration: The epididymis is stabilized between the index finger, thumb and forefinger while the anterior scrotal skin is stretched. A 23-gauge needle attached to a 20 ml syringe is connected to a syringe holder and is inserted through the stretched scrotal skin into the anteromedial or anterolateral portion of the superior testicular pole in an oblique angle towards the medium and lower poles (Figure 6B). Negative pressure is created by pulling the syringe holder while the tip of the needle is moved in and out within the testis in an oblique plane to disrupt the seminiferous tubules and sample different areas. When a small piece of testicular tissue is aspirated, the needle is gently withdrawn from the testis while the negative pressure is maintained. A pair of microsurgery forceps is used to grab the seminiferous tubules that exteriorize from the scrotal skin, thus aiding in the removal of the specimen. The specimen is flushed into a tube containing 0.5–1.0 ml warm sperm medium and is transferred to the laboratory for microscopic examination. TESA or TESE may be performed at the contralateral testis if insufficient or no sperm are obtained.

Microsurgical Sperm Retrieval

The microsurgical approach allows direct visualization of epididymal and seminiferous tubules with high magnification. These techniques have been associated with retrieval of higher sperm numbers and of better quality in OA and higher retrieval success rates in NOA.
Microsurgical epididymal sperm aspiration: A transverse 2 cm incision is made through the anesthetized layers, and the testis is exteriorized. The epididymis is examined and its tunica incised. An enlarged tubule is dissected and opened with sharp microsurgical scissors. Fluid exuding from the tubule is aspirated with a silicone tube or blunted needle attached to a 1 ml tuberculin syringe (Figure 7). The aspirate is flushed into a 0.5–1.0 ml 37°C sperm medium. The tube containing the epididymal aspirate is transferred to the laboratory for microscopic examination. MESA is repeated at a different site of the same epididymis (from cauda up to the caput) and/or at the contralateral one until adequate number of motile sperm is retrieved. If MESA fails to retrieve motile sperm, testicular sperm retrieval may be performed at the same operative time.

Microsurgical testicular sperm extraction: First, the testis is delivered out of the scrotum. Then, a single, large, mid-portion incision is made in an avascular area of the tunica albuginea under 6–8X magnification, and the testicular parenchyma is widely exposed (Figure 7A). Dissection of the testicular parenchyma is carried out at 16–25X magnification searching for enlarged seminiferous tubules. The superficial and deep testicular regions may be examined, if needed, and microsurgical-guided testicular biopsies are performed by removing enlarged tubules which are more likely to harbor active spermatogenesis (Figures 7B to D). If enlarged tubules are not seen, then any tubule different than the remaining ones in size is excised. If all tubules are identical in appearance, random microbiopsies (at least three at each testicular pole) are performed. Testicular tissue specimens

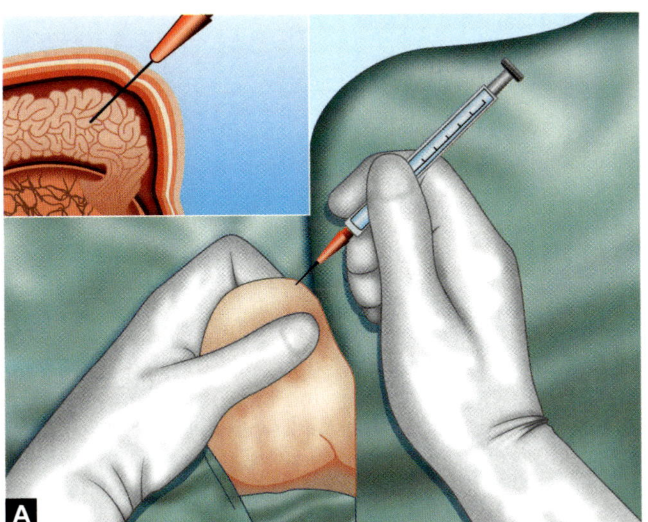

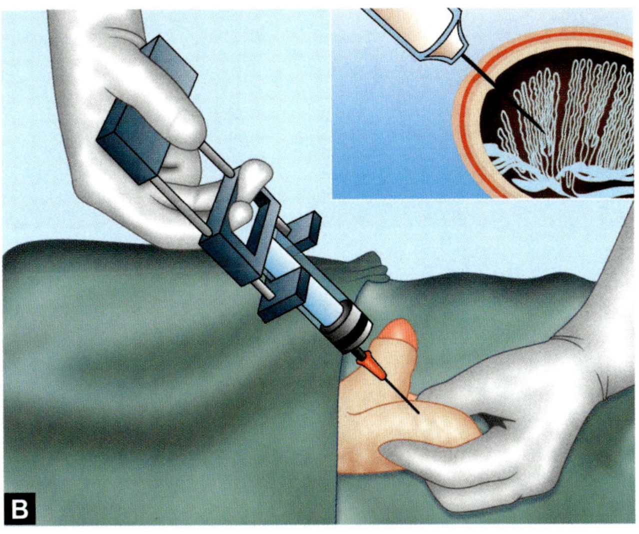

Figures 6A and B Percutaneous sperm retrieval techniques. (A) Percutaneous epididymal sperm aspiration (PESA). Epididymis is stabilized between the index finger, thumb and forefinger. A needle attached to a tuberculin syringe is inserted into the epididymis through the scrotal skin, and fluid is aspirated; (B) Testicular sperm aspiration (TESA). A 20 ml needled-syringe connected to a holder is percutaneous inserted into the testis. Negative pressure is created and the tip of the needle is moved within the testis to disrupt the seminiferous tubules and sample different areas

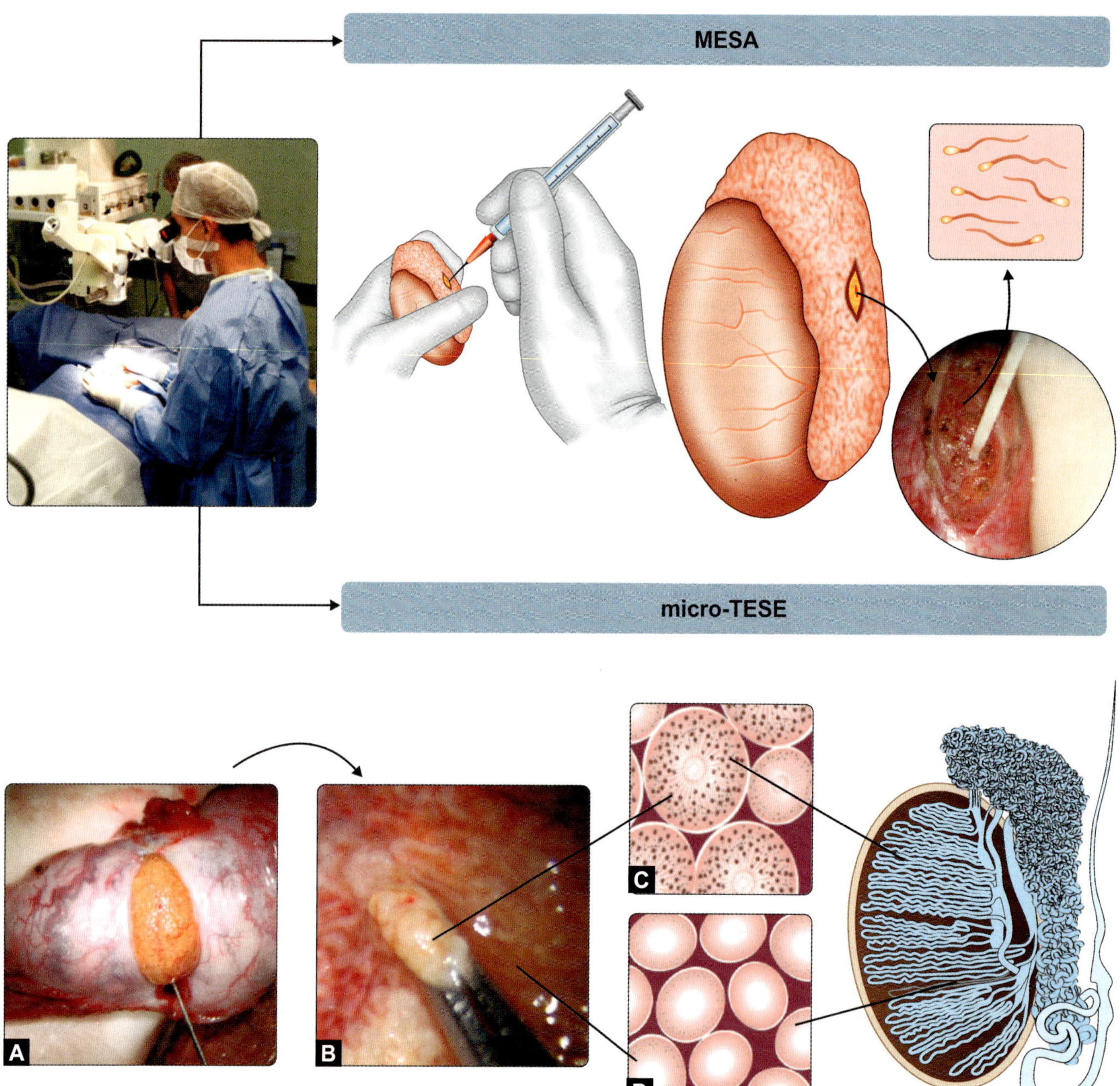

Figures 7A to D Microsurgical sperm retrieval techniques. Operating microscope and microsurgical technique are used throughout the procedures. *On top*: Microsurgical epididymal sperm aspiration (MESA). After exposure of epididymis, a dilated epididymal tubule is dissected and opened. Fluid is aspirated, diluted with sperm medium and sent to the laboratory for examination. *On bottom:* Microsurgical testicular sperm extraction (micro-TESE). (A) After the testicle is exteriorized, a single and large incision is made in an avascular area of the albuginea to expose the seminiferous tubules. (B) Dilated tubules are identified and removed with microforceps (intraoperative photograph at 40X magnification). (C) Illustration of the histopathology cross-section of a dilated seminiferous tubule with active spermatogenesis. (D) Illustration of the histopathology cross-section of a thin tubule with Sertoli-cell-only syndrome

are placed at an outer-well dish containing sperm media. Specimens are washed grossly to remove blood clots and are sent to the laboratory for processing and search for sperm. The albuginea and scrotal layers are closed using nonabsorbable and absorbable sutures respectively.

Conventional Testicular Open-Biopsy Sperm Extraction

Single or multiple open testicular biopsies may be taken to obtain sperm both in OA and NOA, but mainly in cases of NOA. TESE can be also used as a diagnostic tool to obtain testicular parenchyma for histology analysis and search of sperm previous to the ICSI cycle. A transverse 2 cm incision is made through the anesthetized skin, cremaster and parietal tunica vaginalis. Conventional TESE is carried out without magnification. A small self-retaining eyelid retractor is placed to improve exposure of the tunica albuginea, since the testis is not exteriorized. The tunica albuginea is incised for approximately 0.5–1 cm. Gentle pressure is made onto the testis to extrude testicular parenchyma out of the small incision. A fragment of approximately 5x5x5 mm is excised with sharp scissors and placed promptly in sperm culture media (Figure 8). The specimen is sent to the laboratory for processing and microscopic examination. The albuginea is closed using nonabsorbable sutures. TESE can be repeated in a different testicular pole, if the multiple biopsies approach is selected.

POSTOPERATIVE CARE AND RESULTS

Patients are discharged in the same day and can return to normal activities 1 day and 3 days after percutaneous and open techniques respectively. Scrotal ice packing and supporter is recommended to control edema and alleviate pain. Patients should restrain from ejaculation and strenuous physical activity for approximately 7–10 days. Oral analgesics are prescribed, but pain complaint is often minimal.

The best technique for sperm retrieval in men with OA and NOA is yet to be determined. To date, no randomized controlled trial has compared the efficiency of these strategies and thus current recommendations are based on cumulative evidence provided by descriptive, observational and controlled studies.[117] PESA can be performed without surgical scrotal exploration, repeatedly, easily, at low cost, without an operating microscope or expertise in microsurgery, under local anesthesia and it is associated with minimal postoperative discomfort. Microsurgical aspiration has the advantage of retrieving larger number of sperm, which facilitates cryopreservation, and it is associated with a reduced risk of hematoma.[113] Meta-analysis results demonstrated no significant difference in any outcome measure between the use of epididymal or testicular sperm in men with OA.[118] The etiology of the obstruction and the use of fresh or frozen-thawed epididymal/testicular sperm do not seem to affect ICSI outcomes in terms of fertilization, pregnancy or miscarriage rates.[113,119,120] In cases of NOA, the efficiency of TESA for retrieving spermatozoa is lower than TESE[121-123] except in the favorable cases of men with previous successful TESA or testicular histopathology showing hypospermatogenesis. In these circumstances, sperm retrieval rates (SRR) may be as high as 100%.[112] In a recent systematic review, the mean reported SRR for TESE was 49.5%.[122] TESE with multiple biopsies resulted in higher SRR than fine-needle aspiration, a variation of TESA, especially in cases of SCO syndrome and maturation arrest.[112,122] In NOA, current evidence suggests that micro-TESE performs better than conventional TESE or TESA in cases of SCO syndrome, where tubules containing active focus of spermatogenesis can be positively identified using microsurgery. Sperm retrieval rates ranging from 35% to 77% have been reported with micro-TESE.[4,109,112,122-126] To allow for adequate healing and the resumption of spermatogenesis, the minimum recommended interval between sperm retrieval procedures in NOA is 3–6 months.[123-125]

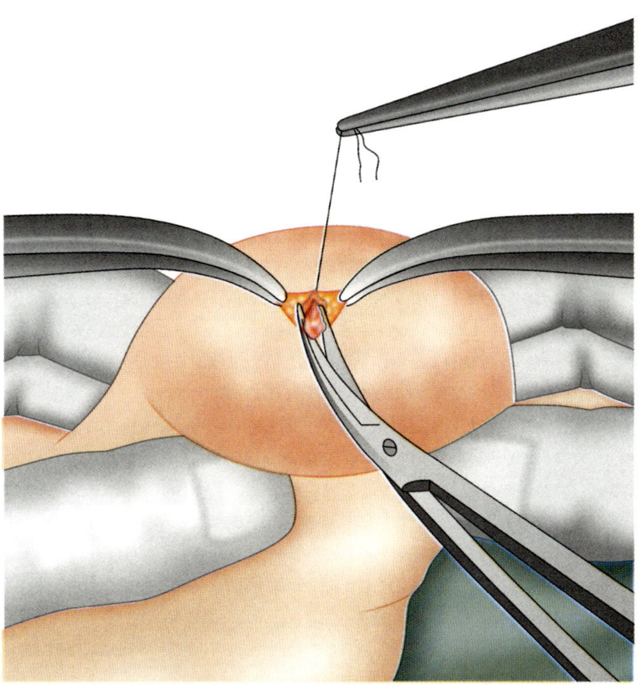

Figure 8 Conventional testicular open-biopsy sperm extraction. Schematic illustration of the extraction of a single fragment of testicular parenchyma using the open biopsy 'window' technique

Postoperative complications of sperm retrieval techniques include persistent pain, swelling, infection, hydrocele and hematoma.[121-127] The development of intratesticular hematoma has been observed in most patients undergoing TESE with single or multiple biopsies based on ultrasounds results performed after surgery, but they often resolve spontaneously without compromising testicular function.[126] In the larger-volume standard testicular biopsy, the risk of transient or even permanent testicular damage (such as complete devascularization) can result in decreased serum testosterone levels.[123,125] Less invasive techniques, such as TESA and micro-TESE, aim to reduce the incidence of complications and long-term consequences of these surgical approaches. Several studies have documented a lower incidence of complications following micro-TESE compared with the conventional technique.[122,123,-125,127] Using micro-TESE, proper identification of testicular vessels under the tunica albuginea is made prior to the placement of an incision into the testis. The use of optical magnification and microsurgery technique allows the preservation of intratesticular blood supply, as well as the identification of tubules more likely to harbor sperm production.[125] Therefore, efficacy of sperm retrieval is improved while the risks of large tissue removal are minimized. The small amount of tissue extracted also facilitates sperm processing.[124] In certain groups of patients, however, such as those with Klinefelter's disease who already have diminished androgen production, a significant decrease on serum testosterone has been documented following micro-TESE.[124] However, testosterone levels return to the presurgical values in most Klinefelter men in a 12-month follow-up period. It is recommended that sperm retrieval should be performed by surgeons who have training in the procedures, because of the potential serious postoperative complications.[123]

The clinical outcomes of ICSI using testicular sperm extracted by TESA or micro-TESE in NOA are significantly lower than those obtained with either ejaculated or epididymal/testicular sperm from men with OA.[118,128,129] Testicular spermatozoa of men with severely impaired spermatogenesis have decreased fertility potential and may have a higher tendency to carry deficiencies, such as the ones related to the centrioles and genetic material, which ultimately affect the capability of the male gamete to activate the egg and trigger the formation and development of a normal zygote and a viable embryo.[130] From the limited data available, it is suggested that the sperm retrieval technique itself has no impact on ICSI success rates.[122] However, frozen-thawed surgically-retrieved sperm from NOA men have significantly impaired reproductive potential than fresh ones.[118,131] Meta-analysis results showed that fertilization rates by ICSI remained similar, but implantation was significantly higher (by 73%) with the use of fresh testicular sperm compared to frozen-thawed testicular sperm.[118]

The question of whether or not ICSI using sperm retrieved from men with either OA or NOA might be associated with increased risk for birth defects is still unresolved. IVF, in general, is associated with multiple gestation and an increased risk of congenital abnormalities (including hypospadias).[132] ICSI in particular, carries an increased risk of endocrine abnormalities, as well as epigenetic imprinting effects.[132] Although the absolute risk of any of these conditions remains low,[132-135] current data is limited and study populations are heterogenic. It is, therefore, recommended that well-defined groups of ICSI with ejaculated sperm, ICSI with epididymal sperm and ICSI with testicular sperm, and a control group of naturally conceived children are closely followed up.

REFERENCES

1. Centers for Disease Control and Prevention. Vital and Health Statistics, series 23, no. 26. [Online] CDC website. Available at http://www.cdc.gov. [Acessed December 2009].
2. Silber S, Nagy ZP, Liu J, et al. Conventional in-vitro fertilization versus intracytoplasmic sperm injection for patients requiring microsurgical sperm aspiration. Hum Reprod. 1994;9:1705-9.
3. Devroey P, Liu J, Nagy ZP, et al. Pregnancies after testicular sperm extraction and intracytoplasmic sperm injection in non-obstructive azoospermia. Hum Reprod. 1995;10:1457-60.
4. Schlegel PN. Testicular sperm extraction: microdissection improves sperm yield with minimal tissue excision. Hum Reprod. 1999;14:131-5.
5. Goldstein M, Eid JF. Elevation of intratesticular and scrotal skin surface temperature in men with varicocele. J Urol. 1989;142:743-5.
6. Chehval MJ, Purcell MH. Varicocelectomy: incidence of external vein involvement in the clinical varicocele. Urology. 1992;39:573-5.
7. Nistal M, Gonzalez-Peramato P, Serrano A, et al. Physiopathology of the infertile testicle. Etiopathogenesis of varicocele. Arch Esp Urol. 2004;57:883-904.
8. Agarwal A, Prabakaran S, Allamaneni SS. Relationship between oxidative stress, varicocele and infertility: a meta-analysis. Reprod Biomed Online. 2006;12:630-3.
9. World Health Organization. The influence of varicocele on parameters of fertility in a large group of men presenting to infertility clinics. Fertil Steril. 1992;57:1289-93.
10. Jarow JP. Effects of varicocele on male fertility. Hum Reprod Update. 2001;7:59-64.
11. Marmar JL, Agarwal A, Prabaskan S, et al. Reassessing the value of varicocelectomy as a treatment for male

subfertility with a new meta-analysis. Fertil Steril. 2007;88:639-48.
12. Esteves SC, Oliveira FV, Bertolla RP. Clinical outcomes of intracytoplasmic sperm injection in infertile men with treated and untreated clinical varicocele. J Urol. 2010;184:1442-6.
13. Redmon JB, Carey P, Pryor JL. Varicocele--the most common cause of male factor infertility? Hum Reprod Update. 2002;8:53-8.
14. Esteves S. Infertilidade masculina. In: Rhoden EL, (Ed). Urologia No Consultório, 1st edition. Porto Alegre: Artmed Editora; 2009. pp. 470-500.
15. Libman J, Jarvi K, Lo K, et al. Beneficial effect of microsurgical varicocelectomy is superior for men with bilateral versus unilateral repair. J Urol. 2006;176:2602-5.
16. Gat Y, Bachar GN, Zukerman Z, et al. Physical examination may miss the diagnosis of bilateral varicocele: a comparative study of 4 diagnostic modalities. J Urol. 2004;172:1414-7.
17. Geatti O, Gasparini D, Shapiro B. A comparison of scintigraphy, thermography, ultrasound and phlebography in grading of clinical varicocele. J Nucl Med. 1991;32:2092-7.
18. Yamamoto M, Hibi H, Hirata Y, et al. Effect of varicocelectomy on sperm parameters and pregnancy rate in patients with subclinical varicocele: a randomized prospective controlled study. J Urol. 1996;155:1636-8.
19. Kantartzi PD, Goulis ChD, Goulis GD, et al. Male infertility and varicocele: myths and reality. Hippokratia. 2007;11:99-104.
20. Nagler HM, Luntz RK, Martinis FG. Varicocele. In: Lipshultz LI, Howards SS (Eds). Infertility in the Male, 3rd edition. St Louis: Mosby Year Book; 1997. pp. 336-59.
21. Dhabuwala CB, Hamid S, Moghissi KS. Clinical versus subclinical varicocele: improvement in fertility after varicocelectomy. Fertil Steril. 1992;57:854-7.
22. World Health Organization. WHO Laboratory Manual for the Examination and Processing of Human Semen, 5th edition. Geneva: WHO Press; 2010. p. 287.
23. Steckel J, Dicker AP, Goldstein M. Relationship between varicocele size and response to varicocelectomy. J Urol. 1993;149:769-71.
24. Marmar JL. The pathophysiology of varicoceles in the light of current molecular and genetic information. Hum Reprod Update. 2001;7:461-72.
25. Marks JL, McMahon R, Lipshultz LI. Predictive parameters of successful varicocele repair. J Urol. 1986;136:609-12.
26. Yoshida K, Kitahara S, Chiba K, et al. Predictive indicators of successful varicocele repair in men with infertility. Int J Fertil. 2000;45:279-84.
27. Cayan S, Lee D, Black LD, et al. Response to varicocelectomy in oligospermic men with and without defined genetic infertility. Urology. 2001;57:530-5.
28. Pryor JL, Kent-First M, Muallem A, et al. Microdeletions in the Y chromosome of infertile men. N Engl J Med. 1997;336:534-9.
29. Kondo Y, Ishikawa T, Yamaguchi K, et al. Predictors of improved seminal characteristics by varicocele repair. Andrologia. 2009;41:20-3.
30. Esteves SC, Glina S. Recovery of spermatogenesis after microsurgical subinguinal varicocele repair in azoospermic men based on testicular histology. Int Braz J Urol. 2005;31:541-8.
31. Weedin JW, Khera M, Lipshultz LI. Varicocele repair in patients with nonobstructive azoospermia: a meta-analysis. J Urol. 2010;183:2309-15.
32. Esteves SC. Editorial comment. J Urol. 2010;183:2315.
33. Cayan S, Shavakhabov S, Kadioglu A. Treatment of palpable varicocele review in infertile men: a meta-analysis to define the best technique. J Androl. 2009;30:33-40.
34. Sautter T, Sulser T, Suter S, et al. Treatment of varicocele: a prospective randomized comparison of laparoscopy versus antegrade sclerotherapy. Eur Urol. 2002;41:398-400.
35. Al-Kandari AM, Shabaan H, Ibrahim HM, et al. Comparison of outcomes of different varicocelectomy techniques: open inguinal, laparoscopic, and subinguinal microscopic varicocelectomy: a randomized clinical trial. Urology. 2007;69:417-20.
36. Hopps CV, Lemer ML, Schlegel PN, et al. Intraoperative varicocele anatomy: a microscopic study of the inguinal versus subinguinal approach. J Urol. 2003;170:2366-70.
37. Cocuzza M, Pagani R, Coelho R, et al. The systematic use of intraoperative vascular Doppler ultrasound during microsurgical subinguinal varicocelectomy improves precise identification and preservation of testicular blood supply. Fertil Steril. 2010;93:2396-9.
38. Schlesinger MH, Wilets IF, Nagler HM. Treatment outcome after varicocelectomy. A critical analysis. Urol Clin North Am. 1994;21:517-29.
39. Colpi GM, Carmignani L, Nerva F, et al. Surgical treatment of varicocele by a subinguinal approach combined with antegrade intraoperative sclerotherapy of venous vessels. BJU Int. 2006;97:142-5.
40. Agarwal A, Deepinder F, Cocuzza M, et al. Efficacy of Varicocelectomy in improving semen parameters: new meta-analytical approach. Urology. 2007;70:532-8.
41. Smit M, Romijn JC, Wildhagen MF, et al. Decreased sperm DNA fragmentation after surgical varicocelectomy is associated with increased pregnancy rate. J Urol. 2010;183:270-4.
42. Zini A, Blumenfeld A, Libman J, et al. Beneficial effect of microsurgical varicocelectomy on human sperm DNA integrity. Hum Reprod. 2005;20:1018-21.
43. Moskovtsev SI, Lecker I, Mullen JB, et al. Cause-specific treatment in patients with high sperm DNA damage resulted in significant DNA improvement. Syst Biol Reprod Med. 2009;55:109-15.
44. Ficarra V, Cerruto MA, Liguori G, et al. Treatment of varicocele in subfertile men: The Cochrane Review—a contrary opinion. Eur Urol. 2006;49:258-63.
45. Shindel AW, Yan Y, Naughton CK. Does the number and size of veins ligated at left-sided microsurgical

subinguinal varicocelectomy affect semen analysis outcomes? Urology. 2007;69:1176-80.
46. Matkov TG, Zenni M, Sandlow J, et al. Preoperative semen analysis as a predictor of seminal improvement following varicocelectomy. Fertil Steril. 2001;75:63-8.
47. Jeng SY, Wu SM, Lee JD. Cadmium accumulation and metallothionein over expression in internal spermatic vein of patients with varicocele. Urology. 2009;73:1231-5.
48. Cocuzza M, Cocuzza MA, Bragais FM, et al. The role of varicocele repair in the new era of assisted reproductive technology. Clinics (Sao Paulo). 2008;63:395-404.
49. Zheng YQ, Gao X, Li ZJ, et al. Efficacy of bilateral and left varicocelectomy in infertile men with left clinical and right subclinical varicoceles: a comparative study. Urology. 2009;73:1236-40.
50. Elbendary MA, Elbadry AM. Right subclinical varicocele: how to manage in infertile patients with clinical left varicocele? Fertil Steril. 2009;92:2050-3.
51. Schlegel PN, Kaufmann J. Role of varicocelectomy in men with nonobstructive azoospermia. Fertil Steril. 2004;81:1585-8.
52. Inci K, Hascicek M, Kara O, et al. Sperm retrieval and intracytoplasmic sperm injection in men with nonobstructive azoospermia, and treated and untreated varicocele. J Urol. 2009;182:1500-5.
53. Lipshultz LI, Rumohr JA, Bennet RC. Techniques for vasectomy reversal. Urol Clin North Am. 2009;36:375-82.
54. Belker AM, Thomas AJ Jr, Fuchs EF, et al. Results of 1,469 microsurgical vasectomy reversals by the Vasovasostomy Study Group. J Urol. 1991;145:505-11.
55. Boorjian S, Lipkin M, Goldstein M. The impact of obstructive interval and sperm granuloma on outcome of vasectomy reversal. J Urol. 2004;171:304-6.
56. Parekattil SJ, Kuang W, Agarwal A, et al. Model to predict if a vasoepididymostomy will be required for vasectomy reversal. J Urol. 2005;173:1681-4.
57. Hernandez J, Sabanegh ES. Repeat vasectomy reversal after initial failure: overall results and predictors for success. J Urol. 1999;161:1153-6.
58. Carbone DJ Jr, Shah A, Thomas AJ Jr, et al. Partial obstruction, not antisperm antibodies, causing infertility after vasovasostomy. J Urol. 1998;159:827-30.
59. Chawla A, O'Brien J, Lisi M, et al. Should all urologists performing vasectomy reversal be able to perform vasoepididymostomies if required? J Urol. 2004;172:829-30.
60. Eggert-Kruse W, Christmann M, Gerhard I, et al. Circulating antisperm antibodies and fertility prognosis: a prospective study. Hum Reprod. 1989;4:513-20.
61. Chan PT, Goldstein M. Superior outcomes of microsurgical vasectomy reversal in men with the same female partners. Fertil Steril. 2004;81:1371-4.
62. Hinz S, Rais-Bahrami S, Kempkensteffen C, et al. Fertility rates following vasectomy reversal: importance of age of the female partner. Urol Int. 2008;81:416-20.
63. Gerrard ER Jr, Sandlow JI, Oster RA, et al. Effect of female partner age on pregnancy rates after vasectomy reversal. Fertil Steril. 2007;87:1340-4.
64. Schiff J, Chan P, Li PS, et al. Outcome and late failures compared in 4 techniques of microsurgical vasoepididymostomy in 153 consecutive men. J Urol. 2005;174:651-5.
65. Sharlip I. Absence of fluid during vasectomy reversal has no prognostic significance. J Urol. 1996;155:365-9.
66. Kolletis PN, Burns JR, Nangia AK, et al. Outcomes for vasovasostomy performed when only sperm parts are present in the vasal fluid. J Androl. 2006;27:565-7.
67. Sharlip ID. Microsurgical vasovasostomy: modified one-layer technique. In: Goldstein M (Ed). Surgery of Male Infertility, 1st edition. New York: WB Saunders Co.; 1995. pp. 67-76.
68. Belker AM. Microsurgical vasovasostomy: two-layer technique. In: Goldstein M (Ed). Surgery of Male Infertility, 1st edition. New York: WB Saunders Co.; 1995. pp. 61-76.
69. Goldstein M. Vasovasostomy: surgical approach, decision making, and multilayer microdot technique. In: Goldestein M (Ed). Surgery of Male Infertility, 1st edition. New York: WB Saunders Co.; 1995. pp. 46-60.
70. Fleming C. Robot-assisted vasovasostomy. Urol Clin North Am. 2004;31:769-72.
71. Parekattil SJ, Cohen MS. Robotic surgery in male infertility and chronic orchialgia. Curr Opin Urol. 2010;20:75-9.
72. Boyle KE, Thomas AJ Jr, Marmar JL, et al. Sperm harvesting and cryopreservation during vasectomy reversal is not cost effective. Fertil Steril. 2006;85:961-4.
73. Silber S. Microscopic vasoepididymostomy: specific microanastomosis to the epididymal tubule. Fertil Steril. 1978 30: 565-71.
74. Thomas AJ Jr. Vasoepididymostomy. Urol Clin North Am.1987;14:527-38.
75. Berger RE. Triangulation end-to-side vasoepididymostomy. J Urol. 1998;159:1951-3.
76. Marmar JL. Modified vasoepididymostomy with simultaneous double needle placement, tubulotomy and tubular invagination. J Urol. 2000;163:483-6.
77. Chan PT, Li PS, Goldstein M. Microsurgical vasoepididymostomy: a prospective randomized study of 3 intussusception techniques in rats. J Urol. 2003;169:1924-9.
78. Lee R, Li PS, Goldstein M, et al. A decision analysis of treatments for obstructive azoospermia. Hum Reprod. 2008;23:2043-9.
79. Robb P, Sandlow JI. Cost-effectiveness of vasectomy reversal. Urol Clin North Am. 2009;36:391-6.
80. Practice Committee of the American Society for reproductive Medicine in collaboration with the Society for Male Reproduction and Urology. The management of infertility due to obstructive azoospermia. Fertil Steril. 2008;90(Suppl 3):S121-4.
81. Malizia BA, Hacker MR, Penzias AS. Cumulative livebirth rates after in vitro fertilization. N Engl J Med. 2009;360:236-43.
82. Hsieh MH, Meng MV, Turek PJ. Markov modeling of vasectomy reversal and ART for infertility: how do obstructive interval and female partner age influence cost effectiveness? Fertil Steril. 2007:88:840-6.

83. Chan PT, Brandell RA, Goldstein M. Prospective analysis of outcomes after microsurgical intussusceptions vasoepididymostomy. BJU Int. 2005;96:598-601.
84. Jee SH, Hong YK. One-layer vasovasostomy: microsurgical versus loupe-assisted. Fertil Steril. 2010;94:2308-11.
85. Bolduc S, Fischer MA, Deceunik G, et al. Factors predicting overall success: a review of 747 microsurgical vasovasostomies. Can Urol Assoc J. 2007;1:388-91.
86. Marmar JL, Sharlip I, Goldstein M. Results of vasovasostomy or vasoepididymostomy after failed percutaneous epididymal sperm aspirations. J Urol. 2008;179:1506-9.
87. Kolettis PN. Restructuring reconstructive techniques -- advances in reconstructive techniques. Urol Clin North Am. 2008;35:229-34.
88. Ho KL, Witte MN, Bird ET, et al. Fibrin glue assisted 3-suture vasovasostomy. J Urol. 2005;174:1360-3.
89. Vrijhof EJ, De Bruine A, Zwinderman AH, et al. The use of newly designed nonabsorbable polymeric stent in reconstructing the vas deferens: a feasibility study in New Zealand white rabbits. BJU Int. 2005;95:1081-5.
90. Parekattil SJ, Atalah HN, Cohen MS. Video technique for human robot-assisted microsurgical vasovasostomy. J Endourol. 2010;24:511-4.
91. Schiff J, Li PS, Goldstein M. Robotic microsurgical vasovasostomy and vasoepididymostomy in rats. Int J Med Robot. 2005;1:122-6.
92. Netto NR Jr, Esteves SC, Neves PA. Transurethral resection of partially obstructed ejaculatory ducts: seminal parameters and pregnancy outcomes according to the etiology of obstruction. J Urol. 1998;159:2048-53.
93. Meacham RB, Hellerstein DK, Lipshultz LI. Evaluation and treatment of ejaculatory duct obstruction in the infertile male. Fertil Steril. 1993;59 393-7.
94. Carter SS, Shinohara K, Lipshultz LI. Transrectal ultrasonography in disorders of the seminal vesicles and ejaculatory ducts. Urol Clin North Am. 1989;16:773-90.
95. Hellerstein DK, Meacham RB, Lipshultz LI. Transrectal ultrasound and partial ejaculatory duct obstruction in male infertility. Urology. 1992;39:449-52.
96. Jones TR, Zagoria RJ, Jarow JP. Transrectal US-guided seminal vesiculography. Radiology. 1997;205:276-8.
97. Jarow JP, Espeland MA, Lipshultz LI. Evaluation of the azoospermic patient. J Urol. 1989;142:62-5.
98. Eisenberg ML, Walsh TJ, Garcia MM, et al. Ejaculatory duct manometry in normal men and in patients with ejaculatory duct obstruction. J Urol. 2008;180:255-60.
99. Orhan I, Duksal I, Onur R, et al. Technetium Tc 99m sulphur colloid seminal vesicle scintigraphy: a novel approach for the diagnosis of the ejaculatory duct obstruction. Urology. 2008;71:672-6.
100. Onur MR, Orhan I, Firdolas F, et al. Clinical and radiological evaluation of ejaculatory duct obstruction. Arch Androl. 2007;53:179-86.
101. Farley S, Barnes R. Stenosis of ejaculatory ducts treated by endoscopic resection. J Urol. 1973;109:664-6.
102. Lawler LP, Cosin O, Jarow JP, et al. Transrectal US-guided seminal vesiculography and ejaculatory duct recanalization and balloon dilation for treatment of chronic pelvic pain. J Vasc Interv Radiol. 2006;17:169-73.
103. Manohar T, Ganpule A, Desai M. Transrectal ultrasound- and fluoroscopic-assisted transurethral incision of ejaculatory ducts: a problem-solving approach to nonmalignant hematospermia due to ejaculatory duct obstruction. J Endourol. 2008;22:1531-5.
104. Craft I, Tsirigotis M, Bennett V, et al. Percutaneous epididymal sperm aspiration and intracytoplasmic sperm injection in the management of infertility due to obstructive azoospermia. Fertil Steril. 1995;63:1038-42.
105. Craft I, Tsirigotis M. Simplified recovery, preparation and cryopreservation of testicular spermatozoa. Hum Reprod. 1995;10:1623-6.
106. Okada H, Dobashi M, Yamazaki T, et al. Conventional versus microdissection testicular sperm extraction for nonobstructive azoospermia. J Urol. 2002;168:1063-7.
107. Tsujimura A, Matsumiya K, Miyagawa Y, et al. Conventional multiple or microdissection testicular sperm extraction: a comparative study. Hum Reprod. 2002;17:2924-9.
108. Ramasamy R, Lin K, Gosden LV, et al. High serum FSH levels in men with nonobstructive azoospermia does not affect success of microdissection testicular sperm extraction. Fertil Steril. 2009;92:590-3.
109. Esteves SC, Verza S Jr, Gomes AP. Successful retrieval of testicular spermatozoa by microdissection (micro-TESE) in nonobstructive azoospermia is related to testicular histology. Fertil Steril. 2006;**86:S**354.
110. Schlegel PN. Causes of azoospermia and their management. Reprod Fertil Dev. 2004;16:561-72.
111. Sharlip ID, Jarow J, Belker AM, et al. Report on Evaluation of the Azoospermic Male. AUA Best Practice Policy and ASRM Practice Committee Report. American Urological Association. 2001.
112. Esteves SC, Verza S Jr, Prudencio C, et al. Sperm retrieval rates (SRR) in nonobstructive azoospermia (NOA) are related to testicular histopathology results but not to the etiology of azoospermia. Fertil Steril. 2010;94:S132.
113. Male Infertility Best Practice Policy Committee of the American Urological Association; Practice Committee of the American Society for Reproductive Medicine. Report on evaluation of the azoospermic male. Fertil Steril. 2006;86(Suppl 1):S210-5.
114. De Braekeleer M, Dao TN. Cytogenetic studies in male infertility: a review. Hum Reprod. 1991;6:245-50.
115. Brandell RA, Mielnik A, Liotta D, et al. AZFb deletions predict the absence of spermatozoa with testicular sperm extraction: preliminary report of a prognostic genetic test. Hum Reprod. 1998;13:2812-5.
116. Hopps CV, Mielnik A, Goldstein M, et al. Detection of sperm in men with Y chromosome microdeletions of the AZFa, AZFb and AZFc regions. Hum Reprod. 2003;18:1660-5.
117. Van Peperstraten A, Proctor ML, Johnson NP, et al. Techniques for surgical retrieval of sperm prior to ICSI for azoospermia. Cochrane Database Syst Rev. 2006;3:CD002807.

118. Nicopoullos JD, Gilling-Smith C, Almeida PA, et al. Use of surgical sperm retrieval in azoospermic men: a meta-analysis. Fertil Steril. 2004;82:691-701.
119. Esteves SC, Verza S Jr, Prudencio C, et al. Success of percutaneous sperm retrieval and intracytoplasmic sperm injection (ICSI) in obstructive azoospermic (OA) men according to the cause of obstruction. Fertil Steril. 2010;94(Suppl):S233.
120. Kamal A, Fahmy I, Mansour R, et al. Does the outcome of ICSI in cases of obstructive azoospermia depend on the origin of the retrieved spermatozoa or the cause of obstruction? A comparative analysis. Fertil Steril. 2010;94:2135-40.
121. Hauser R, Yogev L, Paz G, et al. Comparison of efficacy of two techniques for testicular sperm retrieval in nonobstructive azoospermia: multifocal testicular sperm extraction versus multifocal testicular sperm aspiration. J Androl. 2006;27:28-33.
122. Donoso P, Tournaye H, Devroey P. Which is the best sperm retrieval technique for non-obstructive azoospermia? A systematic review. Hum Reprod Update. 2007;13:539-49.
123. Carpi A, Sabanegh E, Mechanick J. Controversies in the management of nonobstructive azoospermia. Fertil Steril. 2009;91:963-70.
124. Schiff JD, Palermo GD, Veeck LL, et al. Success of testicular sperm injection [corrected] and intracytoplasmic sperm injection in men with Klinefelter syndrome. J Clin Endocrinol Metab. 2005;90:6263-7.
125. Ramasamy R, Yagan N, Schlegel PN. Structural and functional changes to the testis after conventional versus microdissection testicular sperm extraction. Urology. 2005;65:1190-4.
126. Carpi A, Menchini Fabris F, Palego F, et al. Fine-needle and large needle percutaneous aspiration biopsy of the testicle in men with nonobstructive azoospermia: safety and diagnostic performance. Fertil Steril. 2005;83:1029-33.
127. Turunc T, Gul U, Haydardedeoglu B, et al. Conventional testicular sperm extraction combined with the microdissection technique in nonobstructive azoospermic patients: a prospective comparative study. Fertil Steril. 2010;94:2157-60.
128. Verza S Jr, Esteves SC. Sperm defect severity rather than sperm source is associated with lower fertilization rates after intracytoplasmic sperm injection. Int Braz J Urol. 2008;34:49-56.
129. Prudencio C, Seol B, Esteves SC. Reproductive potential of azoospermic men undergoing intracytoplasmic sperm injection is dependent on the type of azoospermia. Fertil Steril. 2010;94(Suppl):S232-3.
130. Tesarik J. Paternal effects on cell division in the human preimplantation embryo. Reprod Biomed Online. 2005;10:370-5.
131. Schlegel PN, Liotta D, Hariprashad J, et al. Fresh testicular sperm from men with nonobstructive azoospermia works best for ICSI. Urology. 2004;64:1069-71.
132. Alukal JP, Lamb DJ. Intracytoplasmic sperm injection (ICSI)--what are the risks? Urol Clin North Am. 2008;35:277-88.
133. Knoester M, Helmerhorst FM, Vandenbroucke JP, et al. Artificial reproductive techniques follow-up project. Cognitive development of singletons born after intracytoplasmic sperm injection compared with in vitro fertilization and natural conception. Fertil Steril. 2008;90:289-96.
134. Belva F, Henriet S, Liebaers I, et al. Medical outcome of 8-year-old singleton ICSI children and a spontaneously conceived comparison group. Hum Reprod. 2007;22:506-15.
135. Woldringh GH, Besselink DE, Tillema AH, et al. Karyotyping, congenital anomalies and follow-up of children after intracytoplasmic sperm injection with non-ejaculated sperm: a systematic review. Hum Reprod Update. 2010;16:12-9.

7

Genetics and Male Infertility

Alaa Hamada, Sandro C Esteves, Ashok Agarwal

CHAPTER CONTENTS

INTRODUCTION

Genes master all aspects of sperm physiology and control not only the hypothalamic pituitary gonadal (HPG) axis necessary for providing the suitable hormonal milieu for spermatogenesis but also the molecular events of sperm production. Additionally, genes bring about the formation of ductal system essential for sperm transport and orchestrate the sperm functions during fertilization events. However, the role of genetics in male infertility is not completely understood and a large number of studies are currently ongoing to elucidate its complex relationship.

Currently, genetic diseases contribute to 15–30% of causes of male infertility.[1] Nevertheless, male factor infertility is responsible for more than 50% of cases of infertility[2] and more than 50% of these cases are of unknown origin.[3–5] Genetics may partly or entirely conduce to the problem of infertility in such men. Exploring the exact hereditary background of male infertility may lead to development of the therapeutic intervention which can modify the genetic error and prevent transmission of such error to the offspring.

With the advent of assisted reproductive techniques and particularly intracytoplasmic sperm injection (ICSI) as a therapeutic option in severe male factor infertility, even sperm with genetic insufficiencies can successfully bypass the genetic barriers that select the healthiest sperm and fertilize the egg. Eventually, embryogenesis and successful pregnancy outcome will depend on the integrity of the genetic information. Genetic abnormalities may explain the 50–60% failure rate of ART in the best centers. Notwithstanding, the final outcome will not end at this part since the male progeny may harbor the same genetic defect that rendered their fathers infertile and that will ultimately lead the sons to be infertile as well.

GENETIC CONCEPTS

Human genome is composed of 23 pairs of nuclear chromosomes, 22 pairs are autosomes and one pair of sex chromosome (XX in female and XY in male). Body's cells are of two types: somatic cells and germ cells (gametes). While somatic cells (nonreproductive cells) are diploid (46 chromosome) and forms the basic units in organ tissues, germ cells (eggs and sperm) are haploid (23 chromosomes and only present in the ovaries and testes respectively. In addition, human genome includes mitochondrial chromosomes where each mitochondrion contains multiple copies of a small chromosome. Mitochondrial chromosomes are of maternal origin because they are entirely inherited from the cytoplasm of the fertilized ovum.

Chromosomes are composed of chromatin which is a complex of unbroken long, double stranded and tightly wound DNA which carries the genes, and proteins which help in packing chromosomes in the nucleus. DNA wrapped around histones forms a nucleosome, which is the basic subunit of chromatin. Single DNA strand is composed of simple units called nucleotides which are essentially formed of nitrogenous bases (adenine, guanine, cytosine and thymine; abbreviated A, G, C and T), sugar (deoxyribose) and phosphate. The two DNA strands are interconnected through specific hydrogen bonds between specific nitrogenous bases forming base pairs. The human genome is formed of approximately 3.1 billion base pairs. Chromosomes are composed of variable lengths of these polynucleotide chains ranging from 50 million base pairs in chromosomes 21 to 250 million base pairs in chromosome 1. Figure 1 shows the basic organization of chromosome, chromatin and DNA.

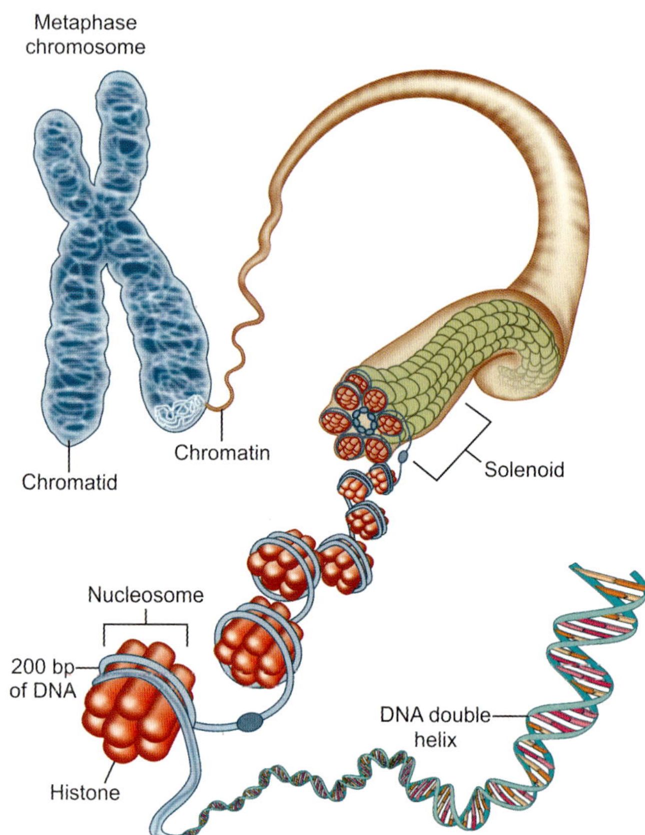

Figure 1 Basic organization of chromosome, chromatin and DNA

Genes are stretches of DNA sequence that encode specific functions such as synthesis of protein through mRNA transcription or synthesis of functional RNA. Human genome contains about 40 million genes. Structurally, genes usually consist of coding regions called exons interrupted by at least one or several noncoding segments called introns. Then by process of splicing, introns are removed from the specifically synthesized RNA and exons are joined together to form mRNA coding for synthesis of specific protein (Figure 2). Gene length is variable and ranges from few kilobases (1 kilobase equal to 1000 base pairs) to millions of base pairs. Interestingly, introns rather than exons constitute greater part of gene length. The exact site or position of a particular gene on a chromosome is called locus while a variant form of a gene is called allele. A gene is usually represented by two alleles. If both alleles are similar the individual is homozygous for this gene. On the other hand, presence of two different alleles of a gene renders an individual heterozygous for such gene.

Genotype is the actual genetic code that controls physical and performance traits. The genotype of an individual cannot be changed by environmental factors. Phenotype is the discernible characteristic or trait of an individual such as specific external feature, biochemical or physiological properties or behavior. Phenotype is the result of the expression of the genotype. However, environmental factors may play a role in alteration of genotype-phenotype correlation.

In general, there are four types of variations in DNA nucleotide sequence. Firstly, single nucleotide polymorphism (SNP), pronounced as "snip", is a single nucleotide (A, T, C or G) alteration along the DNA sequence, occurring at a rate of 1 in every 1,250 bases along the 3 billion base pairs human genome. It has been estimated that up to 20 million SNPs are present in human genome; however, they are not evenly distributed. For instance, SNP may alter the DNA nucleotide sequence from (AAGGTAA) to ATGGTAA. Such variation is reported in at least 1% of the human population and occurs in both coding region of the gene (exon) and noncoding region (introns). The majority of these SNPs are harmless and very few are coding for new amino acids or act as stop codon. Recently, many disease states

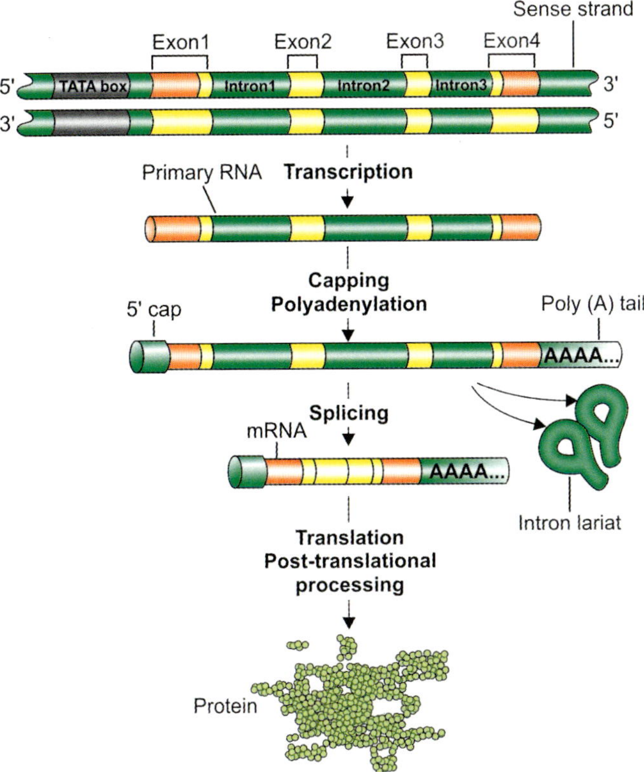

Figure 2 Gene organization and splicing process

such as infertility or certain susceptibility traits have been linked to certain SNPs; however, further studies are needed to thoroughly elucidate their significance.

Secondly, mutations that are the other variation of DNA nucleotide sequence alterations. Some authors consider mutations as a type of SNPs, however, their frequency is less than 1% in the general population and most of them implicate harmful events. Mutations are defined as alterations in DNA sequence contributing to diseases or adverse effects on the host or offspring. Two types of mutations are known: germinal and somatic mutations. Germinal mutations often occur during gametogenesis (sperm or egg formation) and usually are transmitted to the offspring or render the patient infertile. The transmitted mutations may cause various effects in the progeny ranging from minor physiologic modifications to serious disease states, infertility and even death. Somatic mutations usually affect the genetic materials after conception and recently identified to have an essential role in pathogenesis of human diseases such as cancer.

Thirdly, short tandem repeats (STR) are sequences of two to four base pairs such as CG and CAG that repeat in tandems, are flanked by nonrepetitive sequences and occur in the exons, introns and 5′ genomic sequences. Expansion of such repeats has been reportedly associated with certain diseases such as neurodegenerative disorders and fragile X syndrome.

Lastly, the fourth type of structural genetic sequence change is copy number variation (CNV). It is the most common type and accounts for 8–12% of human genome. CNV is defined when long segment of DNA spanning at least 1000 bases or more that has been added, deleted or inserted, deviating from the normal diploidy doctrine. CNV usually affects one gene or complete set of genes and an increase in CNV of a gene results in an increase in the frequency of its expression and the amount of the produced protein. Although CNV is usually harmless, recent association with diseases such as cancer and increased susceptibility to systemic lupus erythematous have been demonstrated.

Genetic diseases are classified into four major types, i.e. chromosomal disorders, single gene mutation related disorders, multifactorial disorders and mitochondrial genetic disorders. Chromosomal disorders include abnormalities in chromosomal number (aneuploidy) or structure. Single gene disorders may follow Mendelian inheritance laws or may be sex-linked. Multifactorial disorders involve alterations in the expression of multiple genes with a postulated role of the environment to affect such expression. Mitochondrial genetic disorders are of maternal origin and contribute to certain debilitating human diseases.

EVIDENCE OF GENETIC CONTRIBUTION FOR MALE INFERTILITY

Infertility is denoted by failure of a couple to conceive after 12 months of unprotected regular intercourse. In the United States, 10–15% of couples face difficulties to conceive and more than 50% of cases are attributed to male factor either as the sole reason or contributory problem.[2] However, 36–58% of male factor infertility is of unknown origin and research is embarked in looking at this dilemma from various views.[3–5] Genetics certainly has a significant role in these unidentified causes and an increasing bulk of evidence are being added to shed light on novel genes or proteins, essential for sperm production and/or function.

Phenotypic characteristics of infertile men are immense including impaired spermatogenesis, reduction of testicular size, hypogonadism and sperm dysfunction. However, as aforementioned, the currently known genetic diseases contribute to less than 15–30% of male infertility and not all these phenotypic abnormalities have been unraveled. Nevertheless, ample evidence of more elaborate genetic implication comes from epidemiological and molecular cytogenetic human and animal studies.

Specifically, in case control studies involving families of infertile men from couples undergoing ICSI, definite genetic etiology was identified in 6.4% in husbands and their first degree relatives while 11.8% of men reported involuntary childlessness in first and second degree male relatives.[6] Another study reported 10% of husbands' brothers having subfertility as compared to 2% among husbands' brothers in control group.[7] Along the same lines, Golde et al. showed statistically significant prevalence of subfertility among brothers and maternal uncles of subfertile men than among brothers and maternal uncles of controls.[8] Moreover, it has been recently demonstrated that high rates of both consanguinity (50%) and family clustering (41%) are seen in men with azoospermia and severe oligozoospermia, respectively.[9] Specific morphological abnormalities have been linked to consanguinity such as tail agenesis, chromatin subcondensation, residual cytoplasmic droplets, rounded head sperm and specific fibrous sheath abnormality.[10]

In animal studies involving the mice, up to 300 null mutations and 50 conditional targeted deletions have produced models of male infertility.[11] Knockout and knockin transgenic mouse models are studied to recognize specific gene loci regulating early and late steps of spermatogenesis as well as genes controlling spermiogenesis. Correspondingly, translational application of such sophisticated genetic studies on human may reveal hereditary basis for infertility problem. However, human genetic research is still far from complete and further studies are certainly needed, including utilization of DNA sequencing as a part of fertility investigations.

SPERM GENOME: DEFINITIONS AND CONCEPTS

Genetic factors control the sperm production process that consists of three phases: mitotic proliferation of spermatogonial series, meiosis of spermatocytes which results in genetic diversity and halves number of chromosomes and lastly, spermiogenesis of the haploid spermatids. Such process eventually results in formation of four haploid spermatozoa from single diploid spermatocytes. The regulating genetic hierarchy has been only recently envisaged from extensive research on animal models and human studies. It has been estimated that 2,000 genes are essential for spermatogenesis, from which only 30 genes are present in Y chromosome and most of the remaining genes are in the autosomes.[12] These autosomal genes regulate not only the metabolism and proliferation of sperm but also control the metabolism in somatic cells. Therefore, autosomal gene mutations may result, in addition to impaired spermatogenesis, in functional alteration of other organ system.

Spermatogenesis usually commences at time of puberty when prospermatogonial germ cells of immature testis give rise to A spermatogonial stem cells (a small population of self-renewal stem cells). Four types of A spermatogonia (A0, A1, A2 and A3) are recognized and appearance of A1 marks the beginning of spermatogenesis. A1 usually undergoes number of mitotic divisions at 42 hour intervals to produce a clone of cells.[13] The number of such divisions is different among various species and determines the number of the produced clone. Interestingly, the produced cells will have different morphological characteristics from the mother cells enabling recognition of first series of A spermatogonia during the first three successive mitoses, type intermediate after the fourth one and type B after the subsequent fifth division. Ultimately, type B will form primary spermatocytes which will then enter into the second phase meiosis.

The characteristics of mitotic phase are the presence of cytoplasmic bridges between the cells originating from a single spermatogonium and this syncytial arrangement persists throughout meiosis. Apoptosis significantly reduces and regulates the total number of proliferating spermatogonial population. Therefore, a fine balance does exist between genes regulating spermatogonial proliferation such as (*Kit*, *Csf*, *Bmp8b*, antiapoptotic genes) and pro-apoptotic genes.[14,15] Disturbance of such balance contributes to hypo- or absent spermatogenesis. Hormonal signals together with other autocrine and paracrine growth factors act to stimulate and maintain spermatogenesis in an orchestrating manner with genetic composition synthesizing proteins necessary for sperm production. Figure 3 presents a list of genes regulating the spermatogonial mitotic proliferation in mouse models.

Meiosis entails two reduction divisions in which the preleptotene primary spermatocytes (diploid) produce four haploid spermatids. Specifically, such process occurs in the adluminal testicular compartment by transiently disrupting the zonular tight junctions between adjacent Sertoli cells. TNFα and TGFB3 are mediators for this transient disruption of blood testis barrier.[17,18] Both genetic diversity and reduction of chromosome number are characteristic features of meiosis. Genetic diversity occurs at the prophase of the first meiotic division in which sister chromatids of paired homologous chromosomes form areas of synaptonemal contacts during pachytene stage. Such contacts enable chromatids to break and to exchange segments of genetic materials between homologous chromosomes with rejoining of the newly exchanged material resulting in formation of new chromosomes. At this stage, primary spermatocyte is very sensitive to exogenous and endogenous gonadotoxins reflecting the fragile properties of genetic material at this stage. Then, separation of the homologous chromosomal pairs is followed by the second round of meiotic division that forms haploid spermatids. Genes regulating sperm meiosis encompass genes controlling chromosomal pairing and synapsis, genes controlling recombination and genes responsible for DNA integrity and synthesis. Mice models reveal that male infertility may result from lack of chromosomal recombination genes and DNA/mismatch repair genes such as *SPO11, DMC1,* ataxia telangiectasia, *MSH4, MLH1* and *MSH5*[19–30] (Figure 3).

The third phase of spermatogenesis is spermiogenesis in which round spermatids undergo cytodifferentiation

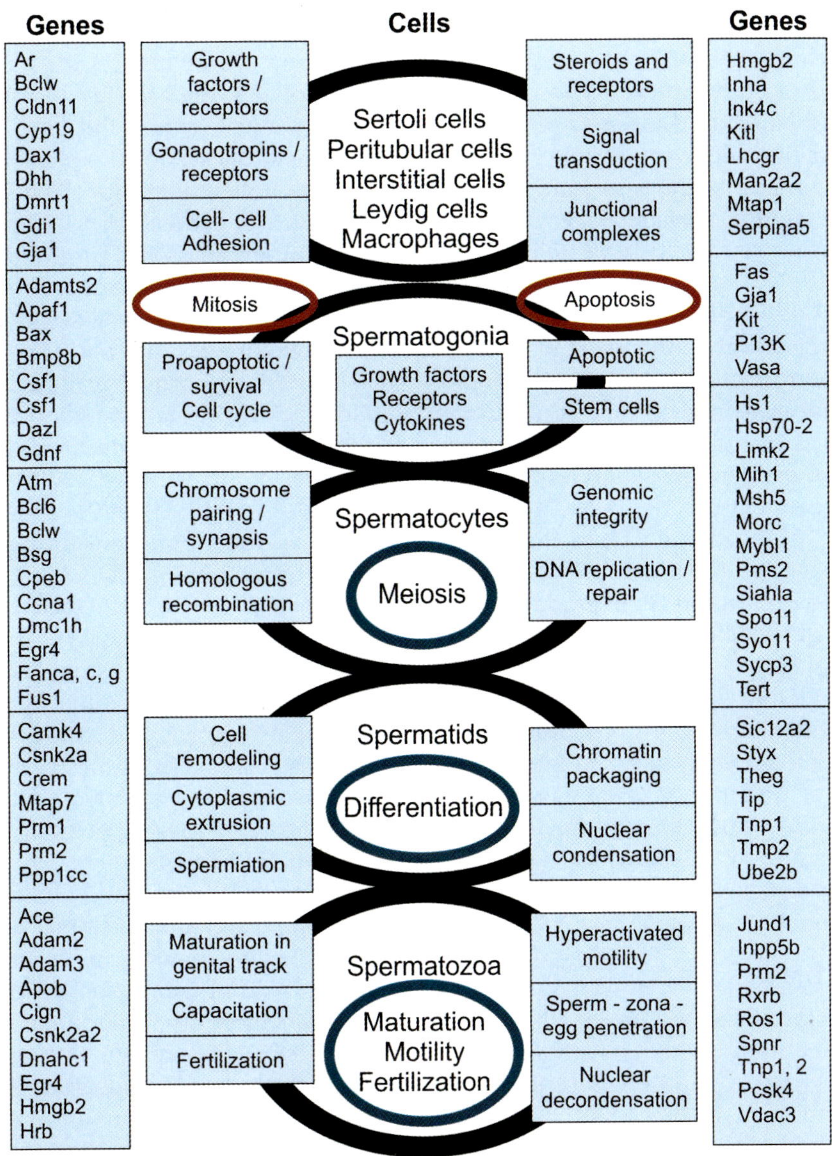

Figure 3 Genes involved in the regulation of male reproduction in the mouse. Spermatogenesis requires a complex interaction of the various cellular compartments of the testis (seminiferous epithelium containing spermatogenic cells, Sertoli cells and peritubular myoid cells, the interstitial cell compartment containing the steroidogenic Leydig cells, macrophages, and other interstitial cells, and the vasculature)

Source: Adapted with permission from: Matzuk MM, Lamb DJ. Genetic dissection of mammalian fertility pathways. Nat Cell Biol. 2002;4(Suppl):s41-9[30]

to form elongated spermatozoon. Three essential steps occur during spermiogenesis as follows:

1. Nuclear chromatin remodeling and condensation to about tenth of its volume
2. Acrosomal cap formation
3. Mid-piece and flagellar structure development.

From animal studies, known genes that regulate cellular differentiation and chromatin remodeling are *Tnp1, Tnp2, Prm1, Prm2, Theg* and *Hsp60*.[16] Lack of such genes has been implicated in defective formation of morphologically normal sperm and male infertility.

It has been shown that RNAs synthesis and protein formation continue throughout mitosis and meiosis (except for those originating from Y chromosome that cease production in meiosis onwards). During spermiogenesis, testis specific genetic transcriptional burst occurs at a faster rate than in any other somatic cells controlling the steps of transitions to spermatozoon formation.[31]

Sperm Chromatin Packaging

Human spermatozoon is a highly organized unit which attains its structural and functional integrity through a very unique packaging system. The coiling of human sperm DNA material is mediated by specific proteins which provide control over condensation and decompression in a time dependent manner. The DNA must be decompressed to expose reading frames for protein synthesis at certain stages of embryo development, yet must be compressed to protect it from degradation and damage.[32] This balance is synchronized by the structural organization of the DNA.

Mammalian sperm DNA is vastly different structurally from that of somatic cell DNA. The majority of sperm DNA is coiled into highly condensed toroids due to the incorporation of protamines, a smaller percent is bound to histones in a much looser form, and the remaining DNA is attached to the sperm nuclear matrix at matrix attachment regions (MARs) at intervals of roughly 50 kb throughout the genome.[33]

Protamine Bound DNA

The most compressed form of spermatozoa DNA exists in toroids. During maturation, the majority of the histone proteins associated with DNA is replaced by protamines. DNA associated to protamine allows for tighter condensation and makes the DNA resistant to nuclease digestion. Protamines contain large bands of positively charged arginine residues that neutralize the negative phosphodiester backbone of the DNA. Such interaction minimizes the repulsion within the DNA backbone, allowing it to double back and fold up onto itself and thus creating the highly compact and tightly wound toroids.[33] These toroids are lined up side by side to provide maximum surface area allocation (Figure 4).

Protamines provide not only substantial compaction to DNA structure but also protection against damage. Mammalian protamines are rich in cysteine residues forming intermolecular disulfide crosslinks that render the sperm chromatin resistant to greater mechanical disruption than somatic cells.[34]

DNA compaction is considered a gene expression control mechanism. Specifically, compaction blocks the reading frame access and thereby causes silencing of gene expression during spermatogenesis.[35] Once the spermatozoon fuses with the oocyte, protamines are completely replaced by histone proteins provided by the oocyte within the first 4 hours. Protamine replacement allows for the paternal chromatin to have increased accessibility for protein generation.[36] This reconstruction process also indicates that the function of protamine toroids is to protect the sperm during their journey in the male and female reproductive tract till the time of fertilization as they do not play a role in embryonic development. This has been demonstrated by the development of normal fertile mice when round spermatids lacking protamine condensation were directly injected into mouse oocytes.[37]

Histone-associated DNA

The second most prevalent form of sperm DNA structure is histone-bound DNA. Approximately 4% of the mature spermatozoa DNA is bound to histones, although between 2% and 15% of the total sperm chromatin can be bound to histones in various mammalian species.[10] Histones are primarily found in association with gene promoter site. Entire gene families, which are vital for spermiogenesis and early fertilization events, are preferentially associated with histones in human spermatozoa.[38–40] More specifically, human histones are associated with miRNA clusters, *HOX* gene clusters, and the promoters of stand-alone developmental transcription and signaling factors.[38]

While DNA binding to histones allows for more accessible reading frame, such accessibility renders DNA more vulnerable to degradation by nuclease activity. Most sperm DNA accessible sites are at the linker regions between protamine toroids in each chromatin fiber, due to the fact that these regions are extremely nuclease sensitive and contain a large amount of histone-bound DNA.[38]

Furthermore, sperm DNA histones are not replaced by those found in the oocyte post-fertilization. This suggests that an inflicted damage to histone-bound sperm DNA will be transmitted to the embryo without detection and possible modification. This may particularly be detrimental due to the fact that most of the DNA

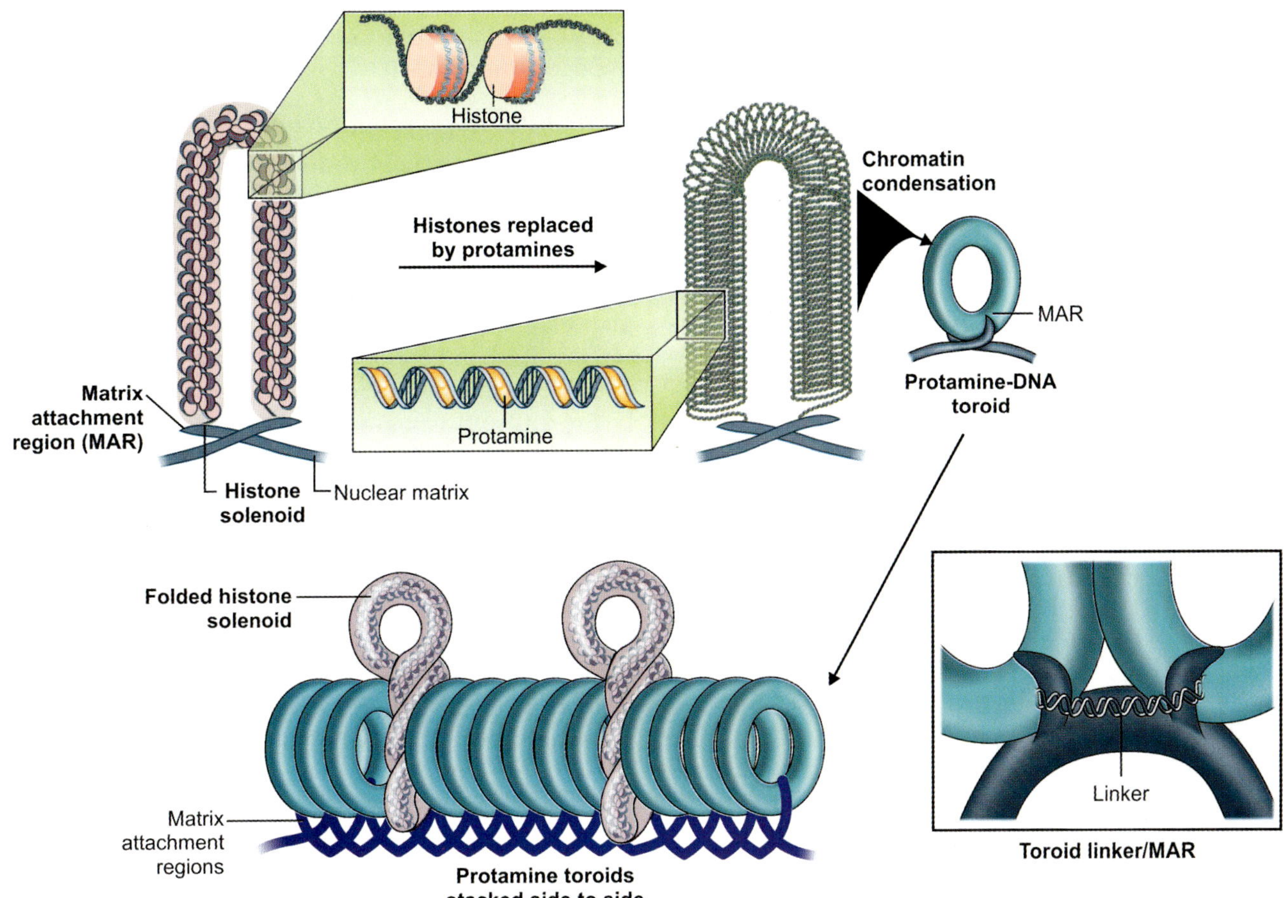

Figure 4 Sperm DNA organization
Source: Adapted with permission from: Ward WS. Function of sperm chromatin structural elements in fertilization and development. Mol Hum Reprod. 2010;16:30-6[33]

bound to histones is significantly rich in gene clusters responsible for early development.[36,38,41]

Matrix Attachment Regions

The third and final form of spermatozoa DNA organization is the nuclear MAR. The MARs are segments of DNA attaching the loop domains of the chromatin to the proteinaceous nuclear matrix. MARs are no larger than 1000 base pairs and are located between each protamine toroid anchoring the toroids into place. As such, they are often called toroid linkers (Figure 3).[42] These toroid linkers contain histone and are thereby extremely sensitive to nuclease activity. In addition to providing association between the DNA and the nuclear matrix, MARs also function as a checkpoint for sperm DNA integrity after fertilization. MAR, along with other histone-bound DNA, are directly derived from the paternal genetic material, inherent to the embryo and vital for proper development.[33] Thus, artificial reproductive techniques (ART) should focus on minimizing damage and maintain genetic integrity of these regions to ensure proper embryo maturation.

GENETIC DISORDERS CAUSING MALE INFERTILITY

Genetic disorders causing male infertility are generally divided into two types according to the genotype integrity of the individual.

Genetic Diseases in Individuals with Abnormal Genotypes in Somatic Cells

Chromosomal abnormalities, monogenic disorders, multifactorial genetic diseases, epigenetic disorders and mitochondrial genetic disorders may contribute to genetic basis of male reproductive failure at various levels as follows:

- Genetic pretesticular disorders
- Genetic testicular disorders
- Genetic post-testicular disorders
- Genetic sperm functional disorders

Chromosomal abnormalities account for approximately 5% of infertility in males, and the prevalence increases to 15% in the population of azoospermic males.[1,43] Abnormalities in number of chromosomes, known as aneuploidy and abnormalities in structure are the two varieties of chromosomal disorders involving both autosomes and sex chromosomes.

Monogenic disorders, on the other hand, include specific gene mutation or polymorphism. Polygenetic disorders usually involve multiple genes and their expression is related to environmental interaction. Epigenetic disorders can modify the gene expression without actual alteration of DNA nucleotide sequence and lastly mitochondrial genetic diseases include mutations in the mitochondrial *DNA* genes.

Genetic Pretesticular Disorders

Pretesticular diseases encompass abnormalities of HPG axis.

Hypothalamic Disorders

Genetic hypothalamic disorder is essentially represented by hypothalamic hypogonadotropic hypogonadism (HH) which is a wide spectrum disease with various genotypes. Deficiency of gonadotropin releasing hormone (GnRH) or its receptor is the fundamental endocrine abnormality detected in this disease. GnRH is a decapeptide that is synthesized by a loose network of neurons located in the medial basal hypothalamus (MBH) and the arcuate nucleus of the hypothalamus.[44] Some GnRH neurons are found outside the hypothalamus in the olfactory organ reflecting the common embryological origin.[45] Developmentally, GnRH neurons originate from olfactory placode/vomeronasal organ of the olfactory system and migrate along vomeronasal nerves to the hypothalamus, where they extend processes to the median eminence and pituitary gland.[46] GnRH is synthesized as a precursor hormone 92 amino acid and then is cleaved to a 69 amino acids prohormone that is further cleaved in the nerve terminals to form the active decapeptide form.[46] Receptors for GnRH are plasma membrane associated receptors which result in increased intracellular calcium as a second messenger on binding to GnRH.[46]

The essential function of GnRH is to stimulate the secretion of luteinizing hormone (LH) and follicle stimulating hormone (FSH) from anterior pituitary gland at time of puberty.[47] The hypothalamic pulse gene triggers pulsatile release of GnRH and considered as a regulatory mechanism of its action. In addition, there is brief postnatal surge during the infantile period lasting for few months allowing proper diagnosis of suspected deficiency at an earlier age.[48]

Genetic HH is mainly divided into two main categories based upon the age of onset: congenital and adult onset HH. Congenital HH is divided into two main subdivisions depending on the presence of intact smell sensation: anosmic HH [Kallmann's syndrome (KS)] and congenital normosmic isolated hypogonadotropic hypogonadism (IHH).

Congenital Hypogonadotropic Hypogonadism

This disease is mainly characterized by early onset of hypogonadism due to dysfunctional release or action of GnRH resulting in delayed or absent pubertal development with low sex steroids in the setting of low or normal gonadotropins level. Normal hypothalamic pituitary gland anatomy on MRI and absence of other causes of HH such as hemochromatosis are prerequisites for diagnosis.[49] Congenital HH incidence is 1–10:100,000 live births with approximately 2/3rds are due to Kallmann's syndrome and 1/3rd is due to normosmic HH.[50]

Kallmann's syndrome: This syndrome is denoted by the presence of complete or partial anosmia in association with congenital HH. Failure of migration of GnRH neurons from olfactory placode to their destination in the hypothalamus and olfactory lobe is the basic embryological defect in this syndrome. It accounts for 60% of congenital HH;[50] however, its molecular genetic bases have not been fully illuminated. Sporadic (2/3) and familial (1/3) varieties have been described.[51] Hereditary studies reveal that familial KS is heterogenetic diseases with variable mode of inheritance (autosomal dominant, autosomal recessive, X-linked) with X-linked being the most common mode. Not only the genotypic characteristics are variable but also the phenotypic features are showing diverse spectrum of physical manifestations. Male is affected five times more than female and its incidence in males is about (1:8,000).[52] Unfortunately, genetic origin of only 50% of familial cases and 10% of sporadic cases has been clarified.[53].

Six known genes account for only 25–35% of all cases of Kallmann's syndrome.[51] These genes are as follows: *KAL-1*; fibroblast growth factor receptor1 (*FGFR-1*); prokineticin 2 (*PROK-2*); *PROKR-2*; *CHD-7* and fibroblast growth factor-8 (*FGF-8*). However, other genetic abnormalities have been described such as chromosomal translocation 46 XY, t (10, 12)[54] and alterations in CNVs.[55] These CNVs account for less than 12% of human genome and are defined as large segments of DNA on a particular chromosome that have been deleted or duplicated.[56,57] Five distinctive chromosomal regions have been implicated and most of these CNV involve the intronic regions of a particular gene reflecting a possible disturbance in the splicing mechanism. These regions are: 1p21.1; 2q32.2; 8q21.13; 14q21.2 and Xp22.31.[55]

KAL-1 gene: It the first discovered gene in Kallmann's syndrome patients. Such gene has been mapped to X chromosome Xp22.32 and consists of 14 exons.[50,58] It encodes for 840 amino acids protein called anosmin 1, an extracellular adhesion protein, which plays a possible role in orchestrating GnRH neurons adhesion and axonal migration.[50,58] Most of the mutations in *KAL-1* gene encompass either nucleotide insertion or deletion resulting in frame shift mutation or premature stop codon.[50] However, in less than 20% of cases such nucleotide insertion or deletion may give rise to amino acid substitution disrupting the tertiary structure of anosmin-1 and attenuating its function.[59] Rarely, contiguous gene syndrome which includes deletion of terminal regions of short arm of X chromosome (Xp22) may contribute to KS. [60,61] Such deletion may cause in addition to KS, short stature, chondrodysplasia punctata, mental retardation and steroid sulfatase deficiency.[60,61] *KAL-1* gene is responsible for X-linked recessive mode of inheritance in familial KS and 10–20% of all cases of KS.[62–64] Specifically, *KAL-1* gene accounts for 30–60% of familial cases and 10–15% of sporadic cases of KS.[64–68] Nevertheless, such gene has not been found in female KS or in isolated normosmic HH.[69] Interestingly, several phenotypic characteristics have been associated with *KAL-1* gene mutations such as midfacial cleft, unilateral renal agenesis in 30%, specific neurological abnormalities such as synkinesis (mirror movement) in 80% of cases, cerebellar dysfunction, deafness, eye abnormality and mental retardation.[51]

Fibroblast growth factor receptor1: *FGFR-1* gene is the second most common genetic mutation in KS. It is also called *KAL-2* gene and is mapped to 8p11.2–p11.1.[70,71] Such gene encodes for tyrosine kinase linked membrane glycoprotein receptor that binds to extracellular acidic and basic fibroblast growth factors.[72] The potential function of fibroblast growth factor is to facilitate GnRH neurons migration, differentiation and survival.[73,74] Dysfunction of FGF receptor results in improper migration and settlement on GnRH neurons which may explain contribution of this gene mutation to normosmic HH as well. *FGFR-1* gene mutation is found in 10% of KS patients.[71,75] This gene is detected in 11% of sporadic cases and 8% of familial cases.[76] More importantly, the observed mode of inheritance in familial type is autosomal dominant form with variable expressivity and incomplete penetrance with equal male to female ratio.[77] Variably expressed *FGFR-1* gene is reflected by occurrence of anosmia alone, hypogonadism alone or both in family members of the proband (affected individual). Moreover, mutated *FGFR-1* gene does not always result in KS (incomplete penetrance) and this phenomenon may highlight another essential factor for loss of function mutation. More than 70% of mutations in *FGFR-1* are nonsense mutations (point mutation) resulting in amino acid substitution in the immunoglobulin-like domain or tyrosine kinase domain and other mutations are either nonsense, frame shift or splice mutation.[52] KS caused by *FGFR-1* gene mutation is characterized by variable severity of hypogonadism from mild to complete form and certain morphogenic abnormalities such as midfacial cleft, synkinesis in 20% and missing teeth.[50,51]

Fibroblast growth factor-8: FGF-8 is considered one of the ligands for *FGFR-1* and is hypothesized to facilitate migration and differentiation of GnRH neurons to hypothalamus as has been described above. Mutation in the gene encoding for such protein is one of the genetic abnormalities of KS and normosmic HH.[78,79] Such gene has been mapped to chromosome10q24 and is responsible for less than 2% of all cases of KS.[51] Autosomal dominant mode of inheritance is also demonstrated in familial cases with variable penetrance.

Prokineticin 2 and Prokineticin Receptor 2: Prokineticin 2 is 81 amino acid proteins encoded by *PROK2* gene, mapped to chromosome 3p13, and is having putative role in chemoattraction of GnRH neurons to migrate to and differentiate in the hypothalamus.[50] This protein act through binding to specific G protein linked receptor which is encoded by prokineticin receptor 2 (*PROKR2*), mapped to 20p12.3.[50,52,53] Frame shift mutation in *PROK2* and missense mutation in *PROKR2* account for 5–10% of KS.[50,52] Both mutations exhibit homozygous (autosomal recessive), heterozygous (autosomal dominant) and compound heterozygous mode of inheritance.[80] Furthermore, both mutations are associated with variable phenotypic manifestations such as fibrous dysplasia, severe obesity, sleep problems and synkinesis. Similarly, these mutations have been described in normosmic HH.[81]

Chromodomain helicase DNA binding protein 7: Chromodomain helicase DNA binding protein 7 (CHD7) is a member of family of proteins whose function is to organize chromatin remodeling (packaging) to regulate gene expression.[82,83] Tightly arranged chromatin is featured by lower gene expression than the loosely arranged chromatin. Such protein is ubiquitous in fetal tissues, brain, eyes, inner ear, olfactory neural tissue and GnRH neurons. The gene encoded for this protein is located in chromosome 8q12.2.[53] Mutations in this gene have been linked to several diseases such KS, normosmic HH and charge syndrome [eye coloboma, heart defect, atresia of nasal choana, retarded growth, genitourinary abnormalities in addition to anosmia and hypogonadism (KS)].[82–84] CHD7 protein is postulated to be an essential factor for migration and differentiation of GnRH neurons. Seven mutations have been described for this gene in sporadic, familial KS and normosmic HH.[50,85] CHD7 accounts for 6% of all cases of KS and 6% of sporadic KS. Moreover, familial KS due to CHD7 exhibits autosomal dominant mode of inheritance.[85]

Normosmic HH: Normosmic HH, also called isolated HH or idiopathic HH, is defined as the lack of GnRH secretion or function resulting in low level of sex steroids in the setting of normal or low pituitary gonadotropins with no anatomical or functional abnormalities detected by MRI and necessary lab testing and presence of a normal smell. Such disease is frequently overlapped with Kallmann's syndrome in the clinical presentation and even in the involved genes.

This disease contributes for 40% of hypothalamic HH and 2/3rds of the disease have sporadic occurrence and 1/3rd of patients has family history of the disease.[51] Familial cases exhibit X-linked, autosomal dominant and recessive mode of inheritance. The pathogenetic mechanism responsible for the disease is attributed to failure of differentiation or development of normally migrated GNRH neurons into the hypothalamus resulting in lack of GnRH secretion or apulsatile secretion.[50,86]

Wide array of gene mutations are identified by nucleotide sequence studies. Nevertheless, the genetic etiology has not been demonstrated in more than 50% of patients. Previously described mutated genes in Kallmann's syndrome have been also implicated in the pathogenesis such as FGFR1, FGF8, PROK2, PROKR2 and CHD7. The other implicated genetic mutations include GNRH, GNRHR, KISS1R, tachykinin 3 (TAC3), tachykinin 3 receptor (TACR3) and DAX1.[50,51,69] However, chromosomal abnormalities have been also demonstrated in 3% of normosmic HH and particularly in the sporadic variety such as 46, XY/46, X, inv(Y) (p11.2q11.2) and mos46, XY, t(3;12)(p13;p13)/46,XY(69,89).

GNRH and GNRHR: Mutations in *GnRH* gene have been recently elucidated as a rare cause of normosmic HH in two human studies on familial HH.[87,88] The gene is mapped to chromosome 8q21–p11.2 and encodes for large precursor (92 amino acid protein). Autosomal recessive mode of inheritance for such trait has been described and homozygous frame shift mutations are detected in the probands.[87,88] On the other hand, mutations in the gene encoding for G-protein coupled receptor for GnRH (GNRHR1) is considered the most common genetic abnormality detected and accounts for 5–40% of normosmic HH (3.5–16% of sporadic cases and up to 40% of familial cases).[89] Such gene is mapped to chromosome 4q13.2–3 and spans over 18.9 Kb and encodes for a 328-amino acid protein.[90] Autosomal recessive with homozygous or compound heterozygous mutations have been shown in familial cases.[91–97] Most of GNRHR1 mutations are missense mutations with single amino acid substitution which result in variable effects on the function of the receptor ranging from mildly impaired to completely inactive receptor.[98] Reversal of hypogonadism has been also reported in this gene mutation.[99]

Other genes: Recent studies have identified other ligand proteins and their receptors whose function is to regulate the differentiation of GnRH neurons and initiate their function at time of puberty such as Kisspeptin (*KSS1*) and neurokinin B. *KISS1* gene has been mapped to chromosome 1q32 and its missense mutation as a cause of normosmic HH are inherited in autosomal recessive pattern.[53,100] Moreover, Kisspeptin receptor (*KISSR1*) gene mutation at chromosome 19p13.3 also exhibit autosomal recessive pattern of inheritance and both *KISS1* and *KISSR1* contribute to less than 5% of normosmic HH.[101] Neurokinin B gene mutation TAC3 at chromosome 12q13–q21 and its receptor (TACR3) gene mutation at chromosome 4q25 have been also implicated in the pathogenesis of normosmic HH with autosomal recessive pattern of inheritance.[102–104] Convertase 1 is endopeptidase encoded by *PCKS1* gene and is involved with post-translational modification of precursor GnRH and release of the mature active form.[50] Mutation in the gene encoding for such protein has been linked to anosmic HH, diabetes and obesity.[105] Lastly, X-linked mode of inheritance of normosmic HH has been linked to *DAX1* gene mutation which causes X-linked adrenal hypoplasia congenital.[106] Table 1 demonstrates the mutated genes in Kallmann's syndrome and isolated normosmic HH.

Clinical features: Both Kallmann's syndrome and normosmic HH share similar clinical presentation with the exception of intact smell sensation in the latter. Various physical signs are detected at different developmental stages such as infancy, adolescence and adulthood period. Infants with HH may have micropenis (stretched penile length is less than 1.9 cm), or unilateral or bilateral cryptorchidism.[51] Interestingly, brief postnatal surge of GnRH for few months provide a window for diagnosis of HH at this period.[48] Adolescents may exhibit delayed sexual maturation with incomplete or absent pubertal development. In adults, testicular volume is characteristically similar to prepubertal size (< 4 ml) with obvious signs of prepubertal hypogonadism such as eunuchoid habitus, lack of axillary or pubic hair, softening of voice, female fat distribution pattern, and decreased muscle and bone mass.[53] Semen analyses of these men usually demonstrate aspermia, azoospermia or oligospermia with hypogonadal erectile dysfunction. However, some genetic mutations cause partial loss of function and some men may have several physical signs indicating some degree of pubertal development. The extreme form of such spectrum is called fertile eunuch variant, in which nocturnal pulsatile secretion of GnRH, mimicking early pubertal development, stimulates testicular spermatogenesis.[99,107] Men with this variant may become fertile with little or no treatment; nevertheless, they still manifest clinical

Table 1 Genes that might be mutated in patients with Kallmann's syndrome or isolated hypogonadotropic hypogonadism

Acronym	Gene Name	Location	Gene ID	MIM	
KAL1	Kallmann's syndrome 1 sequence (anosmin 1)	Xp22.32	3730	308700	Possible function in neural cell adhesion and axonal migration
FGFR1	Fibroblast growth factor receptor 1	8p11.2-p11.1	2260	136350	Binds both acidic and basic fibroblast growth factors
FGF8	Fibroblast growth factor 8	10q24	2253	600483	Member of the fibroblast growth factor family involved in organogenesis
PROK2	Prokineticin 2	3p13	60675	607002	Chemoattractant for neuronal precursor cells in the olfactory bulb
PROKR2	Prokineticin receptor 2	20p12.3	128674	607123	G protein-coupled receptor for prokineticins
CHD7	Chromodomain helicase DNA binding protein 7	8q12.2	55636	608765, 608892	Expressed in undifferentiated neuroepithelium and in mesenchyme of neural crest origin
KISS1	KiSS-1 metastasis-suppressor (METASTIN)	1q32	3814	603286	Ligand of GPR54: stimulation of GnRH secretion
GPR54	G protein-coupled receptor 54	19p13.3	84634	604161	Receptor for Kiss-1: stimulation of GnRH secretion
TAC3	Tachykinin 3 (neurokinin B)	12q13-q21	6866	162330	Influences GnRH secretion
TACR3	Tachykinin 3 (neurokinin B) receptor	4q25	6870	162332	Receptor for tachykinin 3
GNRH1	Gonadotropin-releasing hormone 1	8q21-p11.2	2796	152760	Ligand of GnRH receptor
GNRHR	Gonadotropin-releasing hormone receptor	4q21.2	2798	138850	Receptor for the gonadotropin-releasing hormone

Source: Adapted with permission from: Behre HM, Nieshelag E, Partsch CJ, et al. Diseases of the hypothalamus and the pituitary gland. In: Nieschlag E, Behre HM, Nieschlag S. Andrology Male Reproductive Health and Dysfunction, 3rd edition. Berlin Heidelberg Germany: Springer Verlag; 2010. pp. 169-92.[53]

evidence of hypogonadism and normal or near normal testicular volume with low testosterone level.[99,107,108] In addition, men with Kallmann's syndrome may not be aware of olfactory problem and formal testing of the affected individual and his family members should be contemplated. Reversal phenomenon of hypogonadism has been described in 10% of men with both types of hypothalamic HH particularly after brief stimulation of HPG axis.[109,110] Such phenomenon is attributed to delayed maturation and differentiation of GnRH neurons. About 5–10% of patients with hypothalamic HH show nonreproductive congenital manifestations associated with specific gene mutations which have been already described above.

Treatment: Therapy of hypothalamic HH depends on men's desire for future fertility. For those men planning to impregnate their wives, GnRH or gonadotropin therapy are the best options. Studies showed that successful pregnancy outcome have been achieved even when semen analyses of men remain subnormal.[111] For those men who already have children or have no desire to induce pregnancy testosterone therapy is used to reverse symptoms and signs of hypogonadism.

Genetic Related Adult Onset Hypothalamic Hypogonadotropic Hypogonadism

This category has been described in the last few years, and this term is restricted for men who successfully completed their pubertal development and may already have children and then the disruption of HPG axis occurs. Testicular size in such patients is normal but serum testosterone and gonadotropins levels are low and their LH shows apulsatile pattern of secretion. Single study on 10 men with adult onset HH revealed heterozygous *PROKR2* mutation in one patient.[112] However, good prognosis is expected in these men when medically treated with respect to their future fertility potentials and androgenization status.

Other Genetic Causes of Hypothalamic Hypogonadism

Prader Willi syndrome: Prader Willi is a complex genetic disorder with various systemic involvements. Lack of expression of paternally derived imprinted genes on chromosome 15q11–q13 due to either deletion, maternal uniparental disomy of chromosome 15 or disruption of paternally inherited chromosome 15.[113] Genomic imprinting refers to a phenomenon by which certain genes are expressed in a parent of origin specific manner. Such demeanor is described in less than 1% of genes in which imprinted genes from either parent are silenced to allow expression of nonimprinted genes from the other parent. Obesity, hyperphagia, growth retardation, mild-to-moderate mental retardation, dysmorphic facial features and sleep abnormality are the characteristic features of Prader Willi Syndrome. Hypothalamic HH is a consistent feature of all men with this syndrome.[113] During infancy, 80–90% of affected children have cryptorchidism with poorly developed scrotum and micropenis. Most adolescents will have delayed or incomplete puberty; however, precocious puberty has been described in 4% of patients.[114,115]

Genetic Pituitary Gland Disorders Associated with Male Hypogonadism

Male hypogonadism attributed to genetic pituitary diseases are rare and are divided into two major categories:

1. Generalized or combined anterior pituitary hormone deficiency (CPHD)
2. Selective gonadotropins deficiency.

Generalized anterior pituitary hormone deficiency: Several mutations have been observed in men with CPHD and most of these mutations involve genes expressing signal molecules and transcription factors. Transcription factors are DNA binding proteins that facilitate process of transcription of mRNA from DNA. The affected hormones include growth hormone, prolactin, thyroid stimulating hormone and gonadotropins (LH and FSH). ACTH may or may not be involved. Such mutations may interfere with early or late complex embryonic development of pituitary gland from Rathke's pouch and some of them may give rise to various syndromes such as septo-optical hypoplasia and craniofacial abnormalities.[116,117] In addition to phenotypic variability, MRI appearance of pituitary gland in CPHD is also variable and ranges from enlarged size in *PROP1* gene mutation[116,117] to normal or hypoplastic in *SOX2* gene mutation.[116] Specifically, the implicated mutated transcription factor genes causing hypogonadism are: *PROP1* (most common); *LHX* and *SOX2*. Familial and sporadic cases have been demonstrated with autosomal recessive patterns of inheritance which are the most common mode.[116] To accurately differentiate between hypothalamic and pituitary HH GnRH stimulation test is performed, which results in significant rise in gonadotropin levels in hypothalamic disorder; whereas, no response is observed in pituitary hypogonadism.

Selective gonadotropin deficiency: Follicle stimulating hormone and LH are glycoproteins secreted by anterior pituitary gonadotropes to stimulate testicular spermatogenesis and testosterone production respectively. Each glycoprotein molecule is composed of alpha (α) and beta (β) chain with α chain represents a common chain for LH, FSH, human chorionic gonadotropin (HCG) and TSH whereas the different B chains of these hormones confer immunological and biological hormone specificity. This category includes mutations in the genes coding for synthesis of gonadotropins FSH and LH and their receptors. Specifically, mutations affecting hormone synthesis usually involve B chains genes because mutation in α chain gene (CGA), mapped to chromosome 6q12-21, is usually lethal to embryos due to lack of placental HCG synthesis.[118,119]

Isolated follicle stimulating hormone deficiency: Follicle stimulating hormone exerts its action through receptors in Sertoli cells in stimulating their proliferation in the immature testis as well as stimulating and maintaining spermatogenesis. Mature FSH is composed of α chain composed of 92 amino acids, noncovalently bound to B chain composed of 111 amino acids. Rare B subunit gene mutation (mapped to chromosome 11p13) will result in selective lack of FSH hormone, delayed or normal puberty, and small or normal sized testes with severe oligozoospermia or azoospermia.[120,121,122,123] B subunit gene is composed of three exons and two introns and so far, two missense and three stop codone mutations in such gene with autosomal recessive mode of inheritance have been detected.[121,124–127] In contrast, FSH beta knockout mice did not result in infertility and this indicates different regulation mechanism in humans from mice.[128,129] Furthermore, the rare mutations in the FSH receptor (*FSHR*) genes in Sertoli cells have variable effects on spermatogenesis. In a study on five men, homozygous for FSHR mutation, none had normal semen parameters. Specifically, three had severe and one had moderate oligozoospermia. The fifth patient had low semen volume and teratozoospermia despite normal sperm count.[130] *FSHR* gene has been mapped to chromosome 2p21–16 and consists of 10 exons and 9 introns.[131,132] Such gene codes for the mature form of G-protein linked glycoprotein receptor composed of 678 amino acids that is exclusively expressed in Sertoli cells.[131] Single missense inactivating mutations substituting valine for alanine at position 189 (A189V) with autosomal recessive mode of inheritance have been so far reported. Preliminary studies by Simoni et al.[133] and Ahda et al.[134] have both found differences in the FSHR polymorphisms between fertile and infertile men. Obviously, further research is needed to clarify the genetic background of *FSHR* gene mutation.

Isolated luteinizing hormone deficiency: Luteinizing Hormone initiates male pubertal development through its effect on LH receptors on Leydig cells stimulating release of testosterone. Although reported in only five men, recessively inherited missense mutations in the B subunit (121 amino acids) of *LH* gene, mapped to chromosome 19q13.3, result in delayed or absent pubertal development and oligozoospermia or azoospermia.[135–137] Hormonal profile of such patients reveals normal FSH, high immune reactive LH and low testosterone.[135–137] The detected LH is without biological activity. A variety of autosomal recessive mutations (missense, insertion, deletion and nonsense) have been demonstrated in the gene for G-protein linked LH receptor resulting in variable phenotypic traits and infertility. Interestingly, LH glycoprotein receptors (674 amino acids) respond not only to LH but also to HCG and sometimes called luteinizing hormone/choriogonadotropin receptor gene and present not only in Leydig cells but also in sperm, seminal vesicles, skin thyroid and other organs with unidentified physiological significance. The gene for such receptor has been mapped to chromosome 2p 21(11 exons, 10 introns),[138] close to *FSHR* gene and mutations in this gene result in leydig sell hypoplasia (LCH) or agenesis.[118,139] LCH has a wide spectrum of manifestation which ranges from male pseudohermaphroditism with 46,XY (female external genitalia, undescended abdominal testes, absent breast development) to selective milder undervirilization defect such as micropenis, hypospadias or cryptorchidism.[118]

Genetic Testicular Disorders

Hereditary testicular disorders that cause male infertility can be divided into three categories according to the specific altered function:

1. Genetic testicular disorders primarily affect spermatogenesis and androgen production
2. Genetic testicular disorders primarily affect spermatogenesis
3. Genetic testicular disorders linked to androgen synthesis or action.

Genetic Testicular Disorders Primarily Affecting Spermatogenesis and Androgen Production

Klinefelter syndrome: Klinefelter syndrome, the most common chromosomal abnormality caused by aneuploidy, has a prevalence of 5% in men with severe oligozoospermia and 10% in azoospermic men.[140] The syndrome usually causes the arrest of spermatogenesis at the primary spermatocyte stage, but occasionally later stages of sperm development are observed.[141] There are two forms of Klinefelter syndrome: nonmosaic, 47,XXY; and mosaic, 47,XXY/46,XY. Although previously believed to be sterile, it has been estimated that 25% of nonmosaic Klinefelter syndrome patients have sperm in their ejaculate.[1] Men with both mosaic and nonmosaic form of the disease may have residual spermatogenesis in their seminiferous tubules. Foresta et al. (2005) found that 74% of KS men were azoospermic.[140] Premature degeneration of primordial germ cells before the puberty is essential mechanism for infertility. Besides small firm testes (1–3 ml), gynecomastia (40%) and features of male hypogonadism such as sparse facial and pubic hair growth, loss of libido and erectile dysfunction are also present. Low testosterone is found up to 80% of men and it is attributed to small testicular growth despite presence of Leydig cell hyperplasia. Klinefelter syndrome patients may try to achieve pregnancy using ICSI, but they are at risk of producing offspring with chromosomal abnormalities.[142] This fear was substantiated by several studies that observed that Klinefelter syndrome patients have large numbers of aneuploid gametes.[141] Interestingly, in Klinefelter's men, successful fathering of 60 children has been achieved by testicular sperm extraction (TESE) and ICSI. Karyotypic studies, performed in approximately 50 children, revealed no chromosomal abnormality.[143,144] These genetic findings have been further clarified in a study by Sciurano et al. (2009), detecting foci of spermatogenesis in testicular biopsies of 6/11 nonmosaic Klinefelter's men.[145] While the majority of seminiferous tubules are devoid of germ cells (Sertoli-cell-only syndrome), only 8–24% of them contain germs cells. Sciurano et al. (2009) examined the chromosomal complements in 92 meiotic spermatocytes by fluorescent insitu hybridization (FISH), showing euploidy (normal chromosomal constituents) and the ability of these euploid spermatocytes to form haploid gametes.[145] These new findings may obviously explain the high rate of normal children born after TESE plus ICSI when applied to KS. Nonetheless, even with this high of normal born children, the risk is still there and therefore, it is advised that preimplantation genetic diagnosis (PGD) be performed before ART to ensure that the offspring is not aneuploid.[141]

XX male: This genetic disorder is very rare and heterogeneous with estimated prevalence (1:10,000–1: 20,000).[146] The basic genetic event is translocation of genetic material including testis determining region [sex determining region Y (SRY)] (*SOX A* gene) from Y chromosome to X chromosome during paternal meiosis. *SOX A* gene selectively codes for a transcription factor of about 204 amino acids.[147] Such event results in successful differentiation of indeterminate gonads into testes; however, lack of other genes initiating spermatogenesis renders the male infertile. Furthermore, SRY negative variant has been also described with severe undervirilization defects such as undescended testes, hypospadias and bifid scrotum.[148,149] Phenotypically, these men are very similar to Klinefelter syndrome patients except for their shorter stature than Klinefelter male counterparts.[149,150]

Mutations in X-linked USP 26: *USP26* gene is a single exon gene, mapped to chromosome Xq 26.2, specifically coding for *USP26* protein protease (913 amino acids) which belongs to deubiquitinating enzyme (DUB).[150–152] Ubiquitination and deubiquitination of macromolecules is essential step for regulation of cell cycle, chromosomal structure and gene silencing.[151] Removal of histones and the regulation of protein turnover during meiosis are important functions of this protein. More than 20 alterations in such gene have been reported resulting in severe impairment of spermatogenesis and several of these mutations result in hypogonadism.[153] Studies have found a relationship between this gene and azoospermic men.[154,155] Also, three SNPs have been identified that were thought to be related to spermatogenic failure. However, this finding was challenged by the discovery of the group in a man with normal spermatogenesis.[156] The effects of the SNPs also seem to be influenced by ethnicity; they are relatively common in some groups of African and Asian men.[157]

X-linked SOX3 gene mutation: *SOX* genes are essential developmental genes that control the embryonic ontogenesis of human testes, neural tissue, cartilage and neural crest cell development. Such genes are present only in animal vertebrates and give rise to *SOX* proteins that have a role not only in developing gonads but also in adult gonads. These proteins have a common 79 amino acid DNA binding domains (DBDs), a characteristic of a large protein superfamily called high mobility group because of their high migration rate in electrophoresis polyacrylamide gel.[158] *SOX* proteins, specifically, bind to DNA minor groove and regulate gene expression by acting either as transcriptional activators or repressors.[158] The name SOX is derived from the firstly discovered Y-linked *SOX* gene "SRY" and is called SRY determining box genes (*SOX*). *SOX* genes are divided into groups from A to H with A is the Y linked SRY.[158] X-linked *SOX3* genes, mapped to Xq26.3, belong to SOX B1 group and are specifically expressed in developing testicular and neural tissues producing SOX 3 transcriptional activators proteins.[159,160] Solmon et al. and Woods et al. correlated genetic mutations in *SOX3* gene to hypopituitarism and mental retardation.[161–163] Recessively inherited polymorphic mutations in *SOX3* genes have been demonstrated in men with idiopathic oligozoospermia and in mice with severely impaired sperm production and hypogonadism.[164,165]

Bilateral anorchia: It is a rare congenital disease with estimated prevalence of 1/20,000 males characterized by absence of testicular tissue in 46XY individual.[166] As born male infant has normal genital differentiation, such absence is most likely attributed to testicular regression occurring in the second half of gestation. Micropenis is seen in half of the cases.[166] The exact etiology is unknown; however, a subset of cases shows familial clustering pointing to genetic etiology. Philibert et al. recently pointed out the role of mutated gene (*NR5A1*) for steroidogenic factor-1, member of nuclear receptor regulating transcription of other genes controlling the development of adrenal and gonadal tissues.[167] Such gene has been mapped to chromosome 9q33 and has been correlated with other human diseases such as male infertility, hypospadias, ovarian insufficiency and others.[167]

Noonan syndrome: Noonan syndrome is a relatively common heterogeneous genetic disorder with wide array of clinical manifestations and genotypic abnormalities. Its incidence ranges from 1:1,000 to 1:2,500 live births and is inherited in autosomal dominant fashion.[158,168] So far, nine genes have been implicated in such syndrome or Noonan associated syndromes (*PTPN11, SOS1, KRAS, NRAS, RAF1, BRAF, SHOC2, MEK1* and *CBL*).[169] The basic cellular abnormality caused by these genes is defective signal transduction pathways particularly, GTP linked RAS and the mitogen activated protein kinase signaling cascade.[169] The typical phenotypic features include short stature, webbed neck, facial dysmorphism, congenital pulmonic stenosis and other manifestations. Unilateral and bilateral cryptorchidism is frequent in this syndrome and accounts for up to 77% in Noonan syndrome.[170] Moreover, delayed or absent pubertal development in males with this syndrome attributed to hypergonadotropic hypogonadism due to gonadal failure has been also illustrated.[171] Therefore, altered spermatogenesis with oligozoospermia and azoospermia is multifactorial due to the basic genetic defect itself, associated cryptorchidism or hormonal factor.

45X/46,XY mosaicism (mixed gonadal dysgenesis): In 90% of males with 45X/46,XY mosaicism, normal male external genitalia are observed. Abnormal, ambiguous and female type found in the other 10%. Mixed gonadal dysgenesis (a streak gonad on one side and testis on the other) is found in 10–30% of such mosaicism.[172–174] Abnormal gonadal development results in azoospermia, infertility and low testosterone level.[173]

Genetic Testicular Disorders Primarily Affecting Spermatogenesis

Y chromosome: The Y chromosome is an obvious area of interest in the study of male factor infertility because it contains many of the genes that are critical for spermatogenesis and the development of male gonads. The variation present on the Y chromosome and the occurrence of deletions of large segments of the chromosome involving multiple genes make it difficult to determine the exact cause of certain infertile phenotypes.[175] Furthermore, the same phenotype may be produced by several different deletions or mutations. This fact complicates efforts to distinctively correlate mutations with infertile phenotypes. Y chromosome microdeletions (YCMDs) are a frequent cause of infertility in males. A microdeletion is defined as a chromosomal deletion that spans several genes but is not large enough to be detected using conventional cytogenetic methods.[176] Studies have revealed that microdeletions are more prevalent in men who are azoospermic and severely oligozoospermic.[177] The prevalence of microdeletions in azoospermic men was found to range from 10% to 15%.[178,179] In oligozoospermic men, the prevalence of microdeletions was 5–10%.[178] It is essential to consider these deletions when discussing ART because microdeletions are always passed on to the male offspring[180,181] and fertilization and pregnancy rates are not affected by microdeletions on the AZFc region when using ICSI.[181]

Microdeletions most frequently occur on the long arm of the Y chromosome, Yq, and deletions in this region are specifically related to failure of spermatogenesis.[182,183] A particular area of interest on Yq is the azoospermia factor region (AZF region), which contains genes involved in the growth and development of sperm. The AZF region contains three subregions: AZFa; AZFb and AZFc.[184] The most common aberrations that occur in the AZF region are multiple gene deletions in the AZFb and AZFc areas,[185] which can produce a wide range of infertile phenotypes. Microdeletions in the AZF region are most often found in azoospermic and oligozoospermic men with normal karyotypes.[184] Researchers are attempting to characterize deletions in the AZF region so that they can be used to determine treatment for infertile males.[184] Figure 5 displays the different AZF regions of the Y chromosome and the locations of genes discussed in the following paragraphs.

AZFa: The two main genes located in the AZFa region are USP9Y and DBY (also called DDX3Y).[2] Deletions in the AZFa region that remove both genes cause Sertoli cell-only syndrome, a condition characterized by the

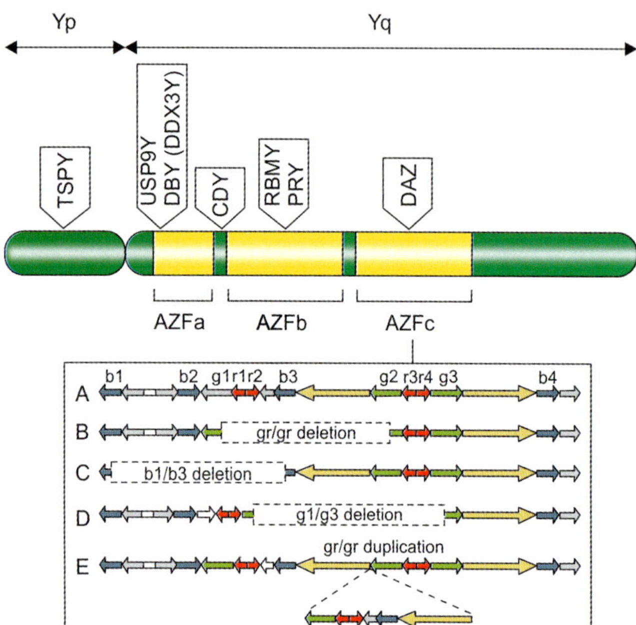

Figure 5 Image of Y chromosome displaying AZF regions and associated genes

Source: Adapted with permission from: O'Flynn O'Brien KL, Varghese AC, Agarwal A. The genetic causes of male factor infertility: a review. Fertil Steril. 2010;93(1):1-12.[397]

presence of complete Sertoli cells in the testes but a lack of spermatozoa in the ejaculate.[184,186] DBY, the major gene located in the AZFa region, has a probable role in infertility because it is localized in the testis and is involved in the development of premeiotic germ cells.[184] Lardone et al., studying the transcriptional activity of several AZF region genes, found that men with Sertoli-cell-only syndrome had reduced levels of DBY transcripts but that the other genes examined were transcribed normally. This finding suggests that DBY may play an important role in spermatogenesis, but further studies must be performed to replicate this result.[187] The *USP9Y* gene is also involved in spermatogenesis.[188] Shortening or deletion of the *USP9Y* gene causes azoospermia,[188] oligozoospermia,[189] or oligoasthenozoospermia.[190] However, it seems that this gene may only be involved in the efficiency of spermatogenesis because it can be passed on to offspring. Furthermore, other animals, such as bonobos and chimpanzees, do not have active forms of the gene.[188] These findings suggest that the *DBY* gene has a more critical role in spermatogenesis than the *USP9Y* gene. Further research studies must be performed to determine the exact roles of each of these genes in fertility to develop more targeted Y chromosome screening practices for infertile males.[190]

AZFb: Deletions of the AZFb region cause arrest of spermatogenesis at the primary spermatocyte stage,[184] indicating that the region is essential for fertility.[186] The main gene in the AZFb region is *RBMY*, and there are six copies of the gene located on the Y chromosome.[183] *RBMY1* codes for an RNA binding protein,[191] which is a testis-specific splicing factor expressed in the nuclei of spermatogonia, spermatocytes and round spermatids.[184] Lavery et al. reported that *RBMY1* expression was reduced in azoospermic men.[192] A family of *PRY* genes is also found in the AZFb region of the Y chromosome. The *PRY* genes are involved in the regulation of apoptosis, an essential process that removes abnormal sperm from the population of spermatozoa.[184] In cases in which all the genes in the AZFb region except *RBMY* and *PRY* are deleted, patients present with hypospermatogenesis.[193] However, if both the *RBMY* and *PRY* genes are removed, spermatogenesis is arrested completely,[194] indicating that *RBMY* and *PRY* are the major genes involved in fertility in the AZFb region.

AZFc: Deletions in the AZFc region produce a wide range of phenotypes, many of which are associated with low sperm concentration due to reduced spermatogenesis.[184] AZFc deletions cause approximately 12% of nonobstructive azoospermia and 6% of severe oligozoospermia.[195] In many cases, men can still achieve fertilization with the assistance of ART.[184] Studies demonstrate that AZFa and AZFb regions are needed to initiate spermatogenesis but spermatogenesis will not be completely normal without the AZFc region.[141] Complete deletions of the AZFc region may occur in two different ways either as a result of a previous deletion within the AZFc or spontaneously from a normal AZFc region. Zhang et al. found that there were more complete deletions of the AZFc region in groups with existing partial deletions in that area of the Y chromosome.[196] This result was replicated in a study of Italian men with a high frequency of partial deletions in the AZFc region.[197] A deletion of the AZFc region may also predispose men to Y chromosome loss, leading to sexual reversal. Several studies have found this deletion to be a premutation for 45,X0[198,199] and for the mosaic phenotype 45,X/46,XY.[200] The AZFc region is prone to many smaller subdeletions that are thought to be caused by intrachromosomal recombinations.[1] These partial deletions produce a wide array of phenotypes, ranging from normospermic to azoospermic, due to many factors, including the interaction of the environment and the genetic background. Genetic studies of ethnic groups produce diverse results because of the variations in their genomes that have evolved over generations to cope with environmental pressures specific to their region.[201] Therefore, studies of the partial deletions of the AZFc region have produced conflicting results that relate to the genetic makeup of the haplogroups studied. The complex interaction of genes and environment makes it difficult to replicate the results of studies and definitively associate subdeletions with infertile phenotypes.[1] The three most frequent subdeletions on the AZFc region of the Y chromosome are gr/gr, b1/b3, and g1/g3 (b2/b3).[202] The gr/gr subdeletion, which removes half of the content in the AZFc region, illustrates the complicating effects of ethnic background on gene function. Several studies have identified the deletion as a risk factor for spermatogenesis loss of, while others failed to find a correlation.[196] Furthermore, a study of the Han Chinese population discovered that duplication of the gr/gr region was detrimental to fertility, contributing to further uncertainty about the role that this region plays in determining a man's fertility status.[203] This finding has not yet been replicated by others. Table 2 summarizes these studies according to geographic region to illustrate the complex effects of environment and genetics on fertility. The AZFc region also contains genes involved in spermatogenesis. The *DAZ* gene has four copies on the Y chromosome.[204] *DAZ* genes are thought to serve a variety of roles throughout the spermatogenic process because they are expressed in all stages of germ cell development.[175] They regulate translation, code for germ cell-specific RNA binding proteins,[205] and are involved in the control of meiosis and maintenance of the primordial germ cell population.[175] Deletions of the *DAZ* genes can cause a spectrum of phenotypes ranging from oligozoospermia to azoospermia.[206] Additionally, *DAZ* gene expression was reduced in azoospermic patients,[193] and partial deletions of *DAZ* genes seem to be related to oligozoospermia.[207] It is critical that azoospermic and severely oligozoospermic men be tested for microdeletions both for accurate diagnosis and genetic counseling before performing ART.[208,209] However, the lack of association between testicular phenotype and genotype in affected men forces clinicians to employ inefficient and costly methods, such as polymerase chain reaction (PCR), to determine diagnosis. The Y chromosome contains 300 sequence tagged sites (STS) which correspond to the AZF regions and could be exploited for easier characterization of microdeletions.[178] Mitra et al. demonstrated the utility of this strategy by developing a targeted multiplex PCR using STS specific to the Indian population. This type of procedure could be used as an initial screen for YCMDs before employing more expensive and technically challenging testing methods.[210] However, to be effective, specific STS would need to be defined for different ethnic populations.

Other Genes on the Y chromosome: Another gene involved in spermatogenesis and located on Yq is *CDY*, the chromodomain protein Y-linked gene. It is expressed exclusively in the testis and is involved in facilitating the replacement of histones in spermatogenesis. It also grants the proteins that regulate transcription easier access to the postmeiotic sperm DNA through the acetylation of histones.[184] The *CDY* gene seems to have diverged functionally from its autosomal homologue

Table 2 Ethnic variation of gr/gr mutation

Variation	Effect	Ethnicity	Study
Deletion	Failure of spermatogenesis	Dutch	Repping et al. 2003[212]
Deletion	Failure of spermatogenesis	Spanish	de Llanos et al. 2005[213]
Deletion	Failure of spermatogenesis	Italian	Giachini et al. 2005;[214] Ferlin et al. 2005[186]
Deletion	Failure of spermatogenesis	Australian	Lynch et al. 2005[215]
Deletion	No correlation	French	Machev et al. 2004[216]
Deletion	No correlation	German	Hucklenbroich et al. 2005[217]
Deletion	No correlation	Brazilian	Carvalho et al. 2006[218]
Deletion	No correlation	Japanese	de Carvalho et al. 2006[219]
Deletion	No correlation	Chinese	Zhang et al. 2006[220]
Deletion	No correlation	Sri Lankan	Fernando et al. 2006[221]
Duplication	Risk for impaired spermatogenesis	Han Chinese	Lin et al. 2007[204]

Source: Adapted with permission from: O'Flynn O'Brien KL, Varghese AC, Agarwal A. The genetic causes of male factor infertility: a review. Fertil Steril. 2010;93(1):1-12.[397]

(CDYL, located on chromosome 6) during evolution and then subsequently migrated to the Y chromosome. This fact makes it an interesting gene to study and demonstrates that there may be a tendency for genes with spermatogenic function to consolidate on the Y chromosome.[184] The *TSPY* gene is located on the short arm of the Y chromosome, Yp, and it also has copies on the long arm of the chromosome.[187] The gene is expressed in the testis, and its protein has been identified in spermatogonia.[211] The *TSPY* gene may regulate the timing of spermatogenesis by signaling spermatogonia to enter meiosis.[186] A study of CNV of the *TSPY* gene found that more copies were found in infertile patients.[212] This finding warrants further investigation of *TSPY* to characterize its role in infertility. Table 3 is a visual representation of the information presented above to serve as an easy reference for the reader.

X-linked TAF7L: The *TAF7L* gene, mapped to chromosome Xq22.1, has also been studied as a possible contributor to infertility in men. It is expressed in the testis and is related to the autosomal *TAF7* gene which is a transcription factor.[186] Transcription factor regulators play integral roles in spermatogenesis because they control the spatial and temporal aspects essential for accurate execution of the process.[213,214] Falender et al. found that TAF genes were involved in spermatogenesis in the mouse,[215] prompting the examination of the role of *TAF7L* in human spermatogenesis by Akinloye et al.[216] The study discovered that an SNP at exon 13 may be a risk factor for an infertile phenotype if combined with additional polymorphisms or mutations.[216] This finding warrants additional research to elucidate the role of this gene in the genetic basis of male factor infertility.[216,217]

Chromosomal Translocations

X; autosome translocations: In general structural abnormalities of X chromosome such as deletion, duplication and translocations correlate with more severe phenotypic manifestations in men than in women. This phenomenon is in part attributed to preferential inactivation of abnormal X chromosome in females.[218] X; autosome translocations are very rare (1–3:10,000) and are of two types—balanced and unbalanced:

Balanced X; autosome translocations: Males with balanced X; autosome translocation are often phenotypically normal; however, they are almost always infertile with azoospermia or severe oligozoospermia.[219] Meiotic errors have been speculated as the underlying causes of defective spermatogenesis in these men. Moreover, there are reports of genital anomalies in men with X; 6 balanced translocation.[220]

Unbalanced X; autosome translocations: Such translocation is usually lethal for males during *in utero* life and if they survive, they may sustain multiple congenital anomalies and mental retardation.[221]

Autosome; autosome translocation: Translocations can cause the loss of genetic material at the break points of genes, which can corrupt the genetic message.[222]

Table 3 Genes on Y chromosome

Gene	Location	Reasons for Investigation
USP9 Y	AZFa	Involved in efficiency of spermatogenesis; deletion or shortening may cause azoospermia, oligozoospermia or oligoasthenozoospermia
DBY	AZFa	Involved in premeiotic germ cell development
PBMY	AZFb	RNA binding protein/testis-specific splicing factor; reduced expression in azoospermic men
PRY	AZFb	Regulation of apoptosis
DAZ	AZFc	Regulation of translation, meiosis and germ cell population; codes for RNA binding proteins; reduced expression in azoospermic men; partial deletions related to oligozoospermia
CDY	Yq	Involved in histone replacement
TSPY	Yp	Regulates timing of spermatogenesis; greater copy number in infertile patients

Adapted with permission from: O'Flynn O'Brien KL, Varghese AC, Agarwal A. The genetic causes of male factor infertility: a review. Fertil Steril. 2010;93(1):1-12.[397]

Autosomal translocations were found to be 4–10 times more likely in infertile males in comparison with normal males.[223,224] Robertsonian translocations, which occur when two acrocentric chromosomes fuse, are the most frequent structural chromosomal abnormalities in humans, and they affect fertility in one out of 1000 men.[1,225] Although the prevalence of Robertsonian translocations is only 0.8% in infertile males, this figure is 9 times higher than in the general population.[226] The translocations can result in a variety of sperm production phenotypes from normal spermatogenesis to an inability to produce spermatogonia.[141] Robertsonian translocations are more common in oligozoospermic and azoospermic men, with rates of 1.6% and 0.09%, respectively.[227,228] Carriers of Robertsonian translocations may exhibit a normal phenotype but could be infertile because of a lack of gamete production.[1] Because of the risk of passing on the translocation to offspring, fluorescent *in situ* hybridization (FISH), with additional probes added for common translocations, is recommended to determine the chromosomal composition of the sperm.[141]

DAZL gene: The autosomal homologue of the *DAZ* gene, *DAZL*, is another gene that is still being studied owing to inconclusive results. The gene is located on chromosome 3 and codes for the RNA binding proteins involved in the regulation of protein expression and meiosis.[229,230] Two different SNPs, one each at exon 2 and exon 3, have been discovered. The SNP at exon 3 is only associated with infertility in populations of Chinese men,[231] but this finding has not been replicated.[186] Tung et al. identified four new mutations in the *DAZL* gene, but further studies are necessary to determine their effects.[232] In the aforementioned study, haplotypes in the *DAZL* gene related to sperm count were also identified.[233] Moreover, Teng et al. discovered haplotypes associated with failure of the spermatogenic process.[234] The findings of these uncoordinated studies suggest that further investigation of the *DAZL* gene must be performed to elucidate the role that the gene plays in infertility.

MTHFR gene: Methylenetetrahydrofolate reductase (MTHFR) gene is located on the short arm of chromosome 1,[229] codes for an enzyme involved in folate metabolism, a critical factor in DNA methylation and the spermatogenetic process.[186] The polymorphism 677C/T causes the substitution of an alanine for a valine, which decreases the activity of the enzyme.[235] The reduced activity of MTHFR can lead to the dysregulation of folic acid metabolism, causing errors in the methylation of genomic DNA and subsequent implications in spermatogenesis.[186] The polymorphism is related to infertility in African, South East Asian, and Indian men,[236,237] but these results were not replicated in the European populations that were studied.[1] Further studies must be performed to confirm the role of this gene in fertility, although it seems likely that the *MTHFR* gene is involved due to its influence on spermatogenesis.[230]

Cryptorchidism: Cryptorchidism is another infertile phenotype that seems to be influenced by genetic factors. Mutations in the *INSL3* gene (insulin-like 3 on chromosome 19) and its receptor LGR8 (relaxin/insulin-like family peptide receptor 2 on chromosome 13)[1,229] have been linked to cryptorchidism.[239] These mutations occur in approximately 5% of men with cryptorchidism.[250] Additionally, the first phase of normal testicular descent is controlled by *INSL3*.[240,241] The *INSL3* gene may also have a role in testicular dysgenesis syndrome (TDS),[242] which consists of a variety of disorders like cryptorchidism, hypospadias, testicular cancer and infertility. It is thought that TDS results from the combination of genetic, environmental and lifestyle factors.[238]

Genetic Testicular Disorders Linked to Androgen Synthesis or Action

Genetic diseases interfering with testosterone action or synthesis that may contribute to male infertility are as follows:

Defective testosterone action: Certain genetic disorders have been linked to defective androgen action.

Sex hormone-binding globulin gene: The sex hormone-binding globulin (*SHBG*) gene, located on chromosome 17, has also been studied for a possible role in spermatogenesis. The gene is involved in both delivering sex hormones to target tissues and controlling the concentration of androgens in the testis.[243] Androgens play important roles in sexual differentiation and the process of spermatogenesis; if androgen levels are disrupted, fertility could decrease. A study that examined the effects of the SHBG (TAAAA)n polymorphism on male factor fertility concluded that shorter SHBG alleles were associated with increased levels of spermatogenesis and higher sperm concentration. Shorter SHBG alleles were related to elevated levels of circulating SHBG, resulting in higher levels of free androgens to stimulate the spermatogenetic process.[243] This study by Lazaros et al. employed a small sample size; consequently, a larger population of subjects should be examined to confirm the relevance of their findings to the field of infertility.

Estrogen receptor 1 and Estrogen receptor 2 genes: Other autosomal genes that have been investigated for a possible involvement in fertility are the estrogen receptor (ESR) genes *ESR1* and *ESR2*.[186] Studies have found an association between abnormal spermatogenesis and estrogen insufficiency, prompting the investigation of the *ESR* genes.[186] *ESR1*, found on chromosome 6, has several different polymorphisms that have been studied for their role in male factor infertility, especially in relation to severe oligozoospermia, and the results have been varied.[229] This variation is most likely due to the interactions of the genes and the environment because the variations are mostly between different ethnic groups. The promoter region of *ESR1* also has a variable number of tandem repeats, (TA)n.[224] The (TA)n polymorphism is related to sperm output, a higher number of repeats on both alleles is correlated with lower levels of spermatogenesis. Sperm production might be negatively affected by the elevated numbers of repeats because it is thought that they result in lower levels of estrogens and increased estrogen activity.[186] The effect of this polymorphism was found to be similar in both fertile and infertile Italian men, although the result was not statistically significant in the fertile population.[224] The correlation with sperm output presents the (TA) polymorphism as a candidate for further studies. The *ESR1* also contains the AGATA haplotype, which is caused by five SNPs located within the gene.[186] A recent study in the Japanese population identified this haplotype as a risk factor for cryptorchidism,[245] but this finding was not replicated in Italian and Spanish populations.[246] In the *ESR2* gene located on chromosome 14, the Rsal polymorphism has been examined, but studies have produced conflicting evidence.[229,230] Nuti and Krausz, and Tuttelmann et al. suggested that the ESR genes be examined further to replicate the results of previous uncoordinated studies to clarify the significance of these mutations on male factor fertility.[186,230]

Androgen receptor gene: The androgen receptor (AR) gene is located on the long arm of the X chromosome[186] (Figure 6). It plays a role in meiosis and the conversion of spermatocytes to round spermatids during spermatogenesis.[247] In normal males, androgens [testosterone (T)/dihydrotestosterone (DHT)] bind to the *AR*, forming a complex that activates the transcription of genes necessary for secondary sexual growth and spermatogenesis. Unlike other autosomal genes, *AR* gene is a single copy gene located on the X chromosome (Xq11-q12) containing eight exons. Exon 1 is the transactivation domain that activates the transcription, exon 2-3 is the DBD, exon 5-8 is the ligand binding domain (LBD) whereas exon 4 is the hinge region that connects DBD and LBD (Figure 6). *AR* gene mutations can severely impair the amount, structure and function of the *AR*, thus causing androgen insensitivity syndrome (AIS) in which various phenotypes may be seen such as ambiguous genitalia, partial labialscrotal fusion, hypospadias, bifid scrotum and gynecomastia.[248] Testosterone hormone level and LH show consistent biochemical elevations in various AIS phenotypes. Mutations range from point mutations, insertions or deletions, or altered CAG repeats of *AR* gene.

A recent study of infertile men determined that approximately 2% had mutations in their *AR* gene while the control population had none.[249] Another possible result of mutations in the *AR* gene is Kennedy syndrome, a neurodegenerative disorder characterized by abnormalities in spermatogenesis.[250] The *AR* gene also has two polymorphisms that have been studied for their role in male factor infertility. The CAG and GGC polymorphisms, both located on exon 1, code for polyglutamine and polyglycine stretches, respectively.[1] Examinations of the role of the GGC polymorphism have produced limited findings. Although it seems to have an inverse relationship with the transactivation activity of the receptor,[251] no significant difference in the lengths of the GGC polymorphisms has been determined between infertile men and the general population.[251,252] The CAG polymorphism has been studied more intensively than the GGC polymorphism. Longer lengths of the CAG polymorphism are associated with decreased transcriptional activity of the *AR* gene in infertile men, suggesting that longer polyglutamine tracts are related to male factor infertility.[1] Some researchers also observed that shorter CAG polymorphisms were related to higher quality sperm and increased levels of spermatogenesis.[243] Conversely, Lazaros et al. discovered a correlation between short CAG repeat length and sperm motility, but there was no observed effect on sperm concentration.[243] This study also identified a

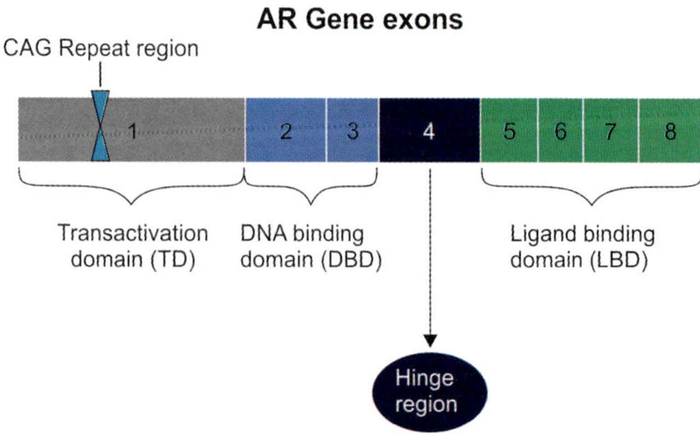

Figure 6 Schematic representation of Androgen receptor gene exons and its functional domains

synergistic effect of the *SHBG* gene and the *AR* gene that influences sperm motility.[243] These polymorphisms may be affected by ethnic influences as well because studies performed in Europe failed to find a correlation between the CAG polymorphism and infertility,[253] while studies in men from Asia,[251] Singapore,[254] and Australia[255] found a relationship. These results warrant further exploration of the role of the CAG polymorphism. There are no specific regions (except CAG repeats) or base changes which are particularly responsible for AIS. It is therefore recommended to screen the entire *AR* gene (8 exons) for mutations/deletions using bidirectional sequencing in a male with normal 46,XY karyotype (46,XY).[256] The direct sequencing of human *AR* gene (*AR*) has allowed researchers to examine the effect of *AR* mutations on the development of the normal male phenotype including spermatogenesis.[257] Most of the mutations are described in the carboxy-terminal domain of *AR*, which includes exons 4 to 8, which can lead to a defect in androgen binding and the loss of receptor function.[254] Screening for the CAG repeats in the *AR* gene is widely performed as they are the most often ones detected in patients with AIS.[254,258,259]

The overall fertility status of affected individuals with AIS depends not only on the AR sequence alteration but also on the emergent phenotype resulting from a dynamic interaction between the genome and proteome. Nevertheless, detailed characterization of the molecular mechanisms of AR dysfunction in AIS, together with a thorough phenotype profiling, may lead to effective therapy and useful genetic counseling for affected individuals and families. In view of the success of testicular sperm aspiration and the prospects of successful conception following ICSI in azoospermic men,[260] screening for AR mutations and appropriate preconception counseling should be offered to subfertile men at risk of having AR mutations. The detailed up to date completion of over 400 mutations of *AR* gene can be found at http://androgendb.mcgill.ca.

Defective androgen synthesis: Androgens play a vital and indispensable role in man's life since fetal and embryonic period till death. Androgens selectively control the differentiation of Wolffian ducts to form the internal genitalia and also regulate the differentiation of external genitalia. During puberty, androgens induce the development of secondary sex characteristics, and stimulate and maintain spermatogenesis. Androgens act as endocrine, paracrine and autocrine hormone. The major secreted androgen is testosterone and the major site of production is Leydig cells that account for 75% of its synthesis. Steroidogenic acute regulatory protein (StAR) which facilitates transfer of cholesterol from outer to inner mitochondrial membranes is the rate limiting step in testosterone synthesis.[261] Then cholesterol is converted by cholesterol side chain lyase to pregnenolone. Upon which, four enzymes subsequently act to synthesize testosterone. Furthermore, testosterone is converted to DHT through the action of 5α reductase A 2 (Figure 7), whom genetic deficiency results in failure of external genitalia development, inability to copulate and subsequently male infertility.

Congenital lipoid hyperplasia: This rare disease is attributed to frameshift, missense and nonsense mutations demonstrated in the gene coding for StAR. The gene spans **8** kb and consists of seven exons interrupted by six introns and mapped to 8p11.2.[262,263] Since StAR is the first essential step in synthesis of all steroid hormones in all steroid synthesizing cells, its classic deficiency results in lack of corticosteroids, mineralocorticoids and testosterones. Males with classic form are born with feminized external genitalia and because the condition is life threatening, delayed institution of proper hormonal replacement may lead to fatal outcomes shortly after birth. However, nonclassic form has been also described due to partial retaining of the protein activity. In such form, males may be born with external genitalia; nonetheless, they may have compromised fertility potentials and azoospermia.[264,265]

3BHSD type 2 deficiency: 3BHSD type 2 is one of the intracellular adrenal and gonadal enzymes necessary for synthesis of all steroids. Mutation in the gene coding for

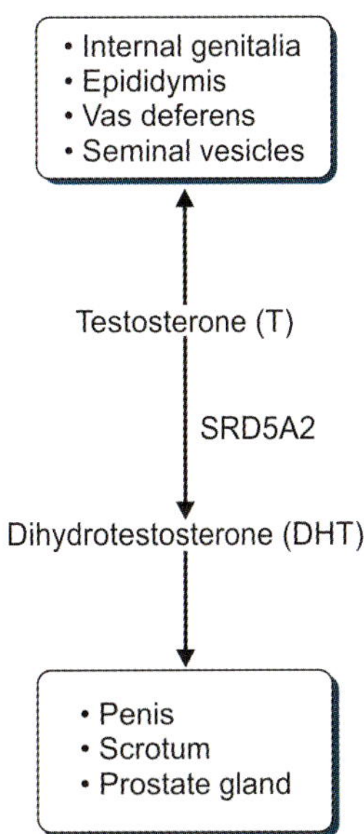

Figure 7 Shows the role of androgens (T and DHT) in development of internal and external genitalia SRD5A2: (steroid-5α reductase type A2)

its synthesis, mapped to 1p11-13, results in salt losing or nonsalting losing varieties with female like genitalia at birth in the 46,XY males. These males may develop secondary sexual characteristics at time of puberty.[265]

Cholesterol 20, 21 desmolase deficiency: Such condition also results in male pseudohermaphroditism.

Other forms of congenital adrenal hyperplasia: More than 90% of congenital adrenal hyperplasia (CAH) is attributed to 21 hydroxylase deficiency (*CYP21A2* gene mutation) and most men with such condition are fertile despite their low sperm count. However, some men with adult onset CAH have reported infertility problems and such problems were attributed to testicular masses (adrenal rest tumors) accompanied by inadequate spermatogenesis.[266]

SRD5A2: SRD5A2 is the gene, mapped to 2p23, coding for 5-α reductase type 2 present in the external genitalia and prostate. Autosomal recessive homozygous mutations in such gene result in feminized external genitalia in males 46,XY. At time of puberty, signs of musculinization develop due to the activity of 5-α reductase type 1 (SRD5A1), in the skin and liver. However, other features such as prostatic hypoplasia, less body hair and female frontal hair line remain. These men are often infertile due to prostatic underdevelopment. Nevertheless, fertility has been reported in some men because of partial enzymatic activity based upon different degrees of mutations. Epidemiologically, this disease has been reported more frequently in isolated area in the Dominican Republic.[267,268]

Genetic Post-Testicular Disorders

This group incorporates the genetic seminal ducts diseases obstructing the normal semen pathway. Three genetic post-testicular diseases have been characterized.

Cystic fibrosis transmembrane conductance regulator mutations: Many autosomal genes are being investigated for possible roles in male factor infertility. Cystic fibrosis transmembrane conductance regulator (*CFTR*) gene, located on chromosome 7,[264] is mutated in 60–90% of patients with congenital bilateral absence of the vas deferens (CBAVD).[1,141] CBAVD is a form of obstructive azoospermia in which there is a disconnection between the epididymis and the ejaculatory duct that causes a functional block to natural fertilization. CBAVD accounts for at least 6% of obstructive azoospermia and approximately 2% of infertility cases.

CFTR gene consists of 190 kb with 27 exons associated with over 1,500 mutations reported so far.[280] The expressed CFTR protein is a glycosylated transmembrane protein that functions as a chloride channel and expressed in epithelial cells of exocrine tissues, such as the lungs, pancreas, sweat glands and vas deferens. Men with CBAVD usually either have two mild mutations in the *CFTR* gene or the combination of a severe mutation and a mild mutation. The common *CFTR* mutations are:

- ΔF508 (three nucleotides that encode the phenylalanine at position 508 are missing in the protein's amino acid sequence). ΔF508 represents 60–70% of the CF mutations in carriers and patients.
- Polymorphisms within intron 8 (5T, 7T). Such polymorphisms reduce the production of the CFTR protein which results in a reduction of the splicing efficiency of the *CFTR* gene.
- The missense R117H mutation in exon 4. It is also related to CBAVD in association with the 5T variant.[270]

Patients with CBAVD owing to *CFTR* mutations are at risk of having both male and female offspring with CF and male offspring with CBAVD. Recent data suggest that azoospermic men with idiopathic obstruction and those presenting the triad composed by chronic sinusitis, bronchiectasis and obstructive azoospermia (Young Syndrome) have an elevated risk for CFTR mutation.[271] Hence, screening for CFTR mutations is recommended to such couples who are ART candidates for determining the risk of transmitting CFTR mutations to the offspring.

ICSI is a useful method of treatment for men with the CFTR mutation as long as the female does not also carry the CFTR mutation.[1] Partners who both carry the mutation should be advised to have PGD to avoid passing the abnormality to their offspring.[141] Nowadays different techniques such as blotting, *in-situ* hybridization, fluorescence *in-situ* hybridization, single strand conformation polymorphism, hetroduplex analysis, PCR, real time PCR followed by direct sequencing have been developed for screening CFTR mutations. Up-to-date information in *CFTR* gene mutations can be found at http://www. genet.sickkids.on.ca/cftr/app, a CFTR mutation database. Direct sequencing for specific mutation or alleles may be advantageous[272] over other methods. PGD has been regarded as a useful tool to identify the presence of CFTR mutations in *in vitro* derived embryos given the fact that mutations have been screened in both male and female partners.

Anti-Mullerian hormone (AMH) and AMH receptor defects: AMH or Mullerian inhibiting substance is essential hormone secreted from fetal Sertoli cells at 7th week of gestation causing regression of Mullerian duct and its derivatives. AMH belongs to transforming growth factor (TGF-B) superfamily and exerts its action through binding with specific membrane bound serine/threonine kinase receptors.[273,274] Persistent Mullerian duct syndrome (PMDS) is characterized by the persistence of female internal reproductive organs (derivatives of Mullerian ducts) inside the male due to either defective AMH or its receptors. The male external genitalia are perfectly normal in this syndrome to differentiate it from other causes Mullerian ducts derivatives persistence, such as testicular dysgenesis are associated with external genital ambiguity.

In PMDS, the Mullerian duct derivatives such as fallopian tubes and uterus are always tightly tethered to the testes.[275] Two clinical variants have been shown: 1) bilateral cryptorchidism in which testes are embedded in the broad ligament of the abnormally persistent uterus and 2) unilateral cryptorchidism in which single testis has dragged the tethered fallopian tube down to the scrotum and the other cryptorchid testis remains in the pelvis in a condition called transverse testicular ectopia.[275] When testes have successfully descended in the scrotum, spermatogenesis may be intact. However, in addition to cryptorchidism, testicular torsion and improper testicular connection to the male seminal ducts due to aplasia of the epididymis or upper part of the vas negatively affect the male reproductive potentials.[276]

Around 85% of PMDS is equally attributed to autosomal recessive (AR) mutations in the gene coding for AMH, mapped to chromosome 19p13.3, and to the AR mutations in the gene coding for its receptor AMHR-II, mapped to chromosome 12(13.q12).[275,276] Knockout mice for gene for AMHR-I usually die in the embryonic life. In 15% of persistent Mullerian defects syndrome, the cause is still unknown.[275]

Young syndrome: Young syndrome is a rare disease and is primarily a constellation of three components: bilateral epididymal obstruction with azoospermia; bronchiectasis and chronic sinusitis. The estimated prevalence is unknown with newly discovered cases are denoted as case reports. Unfortunately, the origin of this disease is also unknown however, childhood exposure to mercury and genetic etiologies have been suggested.[277,278] Its familial incidence in one case and association with medullary sponge kidney in another suggest hereditary background.[279,280] Nevertheless, no definite mutations have been discovered. Male infertility is attributed to bilateral epididymal head dilatation and blockage by expressible amorphous mass, attributed to poor epididymal mucociliary clearance.[278] The diagnosis is by exclusion of two other similar syndromes which are cystic fibrosis (screening for CFTR mutations) and immotile cilia syndrome and is confirmed by prolonged nasal mucociliary clearance of tested material (saccharine).[278] The functional rather than the subtle ultrastructural epididymal and nasal ciliary defects is considered the basic mechanism of the disease and epididymal aspiration revealed motile spermatozoa.[281] Interestingly, epididymal obstruction often occurs in middle age men, therefore previously successful parenthood may be anticipated in such syndrome.[281,282]

Genetic Sperm Functional Defects

CatSper Gene

Recent studies have demonstrated that increased intracellular calcium entry through voltage gated calcium channels (Cation channel of sperm; CatSper1–4) in the principal piece of the sperm flagellum is the prime mechanism for hyperactivation.[283,284] This entry is induced by intracellular alkalinization because of extrusion of H^+ through voltage gated proton pumps, which are also located in the principal piece of the flagellum.[283] Increased intracellular pH and intracellular Ca^+ regulate not only the hyperactivation process but also the AR and the ability of the sperm to fertilize the egg.[283] Interestingly, molecular studies on CatSper ion channel show that it is a novel protein complex composed of 6 subunits. Of these, four are α subunits (CatSper1–4) with calcium-selective pore and two are transmembrane proteins with large extracellular domains, called CatSper beta and CatSper gamma, of unknown functions.[285] For humans, hyperactivation is not well defined as it is for other species, and only a small proportion of the sperm population may be hyperactivated at each time. The extent of hyperactivated motility in a population is positively correlated with the extent of zona binding, the AR, zona-free oocyte penetration and fertilizing capacity *in vitro*. In fact, Avenarius et al.[286] discovered that male patients with mutated *CatSper1* gene are infertile with poor hyperactivation response despite their normal sperm count, morphology and even their initial sperm motility. Furthermore, an animal study on mice concluded that mutation in each of CatSper (1–4) ion channel protein can lead to infertility despite normal semen parameters, normal testicular histology, size and weight.[287] Interestingly, there are two known *CatSper2* gene-related mutations in humans that cause male infertility, termed CatSper-related nonsyndromic male infertility and deafness-infertility syndrome.[288] However, both syndromes are associated with gross semen abnormalities. Further investigation is needed to show the genetic and molecular nature of fertilization in patients with defective hyperactivation response and unexplained infertility. Moreover, minor mutations in human CatSper (1–4) genes are yet to be deciphered in men with unexplained infertility.

Primary Ciliary Dyskinesia and Kartagener's Syndrome

Primary ciliary dyskinesia (PCD) is genetically heterogeneous ciliopathic disorder with autosomal recessive mode of inheritance. It was previously misnomered as immotile cilia syndrome that has been changed to PCD because cilia are motile but in nonsynchronized fashion. PCD is a rare disease with prevalence of 1:15,000–1:60,000 births.[289] The diagnostic clinical features of PCD are chronic sinopulmonary infections and obstructive azoospermia. In 50% of sporadic cases, Situs Inversus is seen and the syndrome is called Kartagener's syndrome.[290] Cilia are characterized by wide array of ultrastructural and functional abnormalities. Specifically, in 80% loss of inner and outer dynein arms underlie the basic mechanism of dysfunctional ciliary motility.[291] In the other 5–10%, loss of ciliary central complex or radial spokes may occur, whereas in 10–20% of cases no ultrastructural defect is seen and dysfunctional nitric oxide (NO) production is detected.[292,293] NO is necessary for ciliary and flagellar movement and its lack due to defective enzymatic synthesis results in immotile cilia.

So far, eight gene mutations, responsible for PCD, have been identified (*DNAII, DNAH5, DNAH11, DNAI2, KTU, RSPH9, RSPH4A* and *TXNDC3*) with *DNAII* and *DNAH5* approximately account for 25% of cases.[290] Selective mutations in *DNAII* and *DNAH5*, mapped to chromosome 9 and 5 respectively, result in abnormal proteins in the ciliary outer dynein arms.[290] Male infertility in this condition is attributed to poor sperm motility and poor epididymal stereocilia function resulting in mucus retention and obstructive azoospermia.

Globozoospermia

Globozoospermia (rounded head sperm) is a rare cause of severe male factor infertility with incidence less than 0.1% among infertile men.[294] Total globozoospermia is characterized by presence of 100% rounded head sperm lacking acrosomal cap. Though ICSI is the treatment of choice for such patients, low fertilization rates have been shown resulting from failure to activate the oocytes.[294] On the other hand, men with partial globozoospermia have variable involvement of sperm and may even be fertile. Several familial case reports support the genetic etiology of this disease however; no specific mode of inheritance has been disclosed. According to our knowledge, three human genetic causes have been reported which are *SPATA16* mutation, *PICK1* and recently discovered *DPY19L2* Deletion.[295] *SPATA16* is spermatogenesis specific gene, mapped to chromosome 3q26, is expressed only in the testes and encodes for protein localized to Golgi apparatus.[296] Homozygous mutations in this gene cause total globozoospermia and even failure of achieving pregnancy by ICSI. *PICK1* is a gene coding for protein interacting with C kinase 1 and its homozygous mutations contribute to total globozoospermia and disordered spermatogenesis.[297] Koscinski et al. recently found that homozygous deletion of 200 kb on chromosome 12, known as *DPY19L2*, accounts for about 20% of men with globozoospermia without alteration in spermatogenesis.[295] In contrast to *SPATA16*, successful pregnancy has been achieved by ICSI.[295]

Genetic Diseases in Individuals with Normal Genotypes in Somatic Cells

This category encompasses a wide array of genetic disorders in infertile men who are otherwise having normal blood karyotype with normal or undeciphered genetic abnormalities.

- Sperm Chromosomal Abnormalities
- Sperm DNA Integrity Defects
- Mitochondrial Genetic Defects
- Epigenetic Disorders

Sperm Chromosomal Abnormalities

Recent application of FISH techniques directly on sperm identifies a subset of infertile men exhibiting a high level of numerical and structural chromosomal abnormalities. Six percent of men with normal somatic cell karyotype are discovered to have sperm chromosomal abnormalities.[226,298,299] Such abnormalities have been shown to be inversely correlated with semen parameters. The frequency of sperm chromosomal aneuploidy (presence of extra or missing chromosome) in infertile men is threefold more than that of controls and it may increase up to tenfold in those with severe oligozoospermia and nonobstructive azoospermia.[300,301] Surprisingly, 3–4% of sperm in fertile men are aneuploid with frequency of 0.1% per chromosome (1-20) and 0.3% for chromosome 21, 22, X, Y.[302,303] These findings pinpoint meiotic errors such as nondisjunction during meiosis I as the causative mechanism for sperm aneuploidy.

Moreover, five studies showed that up to 50–100% incidence of sperm disomy (two pairs of a single chromosome), diploidy (two pairs of all chromosomes) and polyploidy, have been positively correlated with occurrence of sperm morphological abnormalities such as macrocephalic, multinucleated, and multiflagellate sperm.[304–308] The implications of these chromosomal abnormalities include understanding the failure rates of ICSI for men with poor semen quality and practical application of appropriate techniques to detect sperm aneuploidy.

Sperm DNA Integrity Defects

Sperm nuclear genome integrity is vital for the accurate transmission of genetic information to the offspring. Unlike somatic cells, sperm chromatin is tightly packaged due to the presence of protamine, an arginine rich protein. Improper DNA packaging may hinder DNA vulnerable to attacks such as those inflicted by reactive oxygen species (ROS). As a result, sperm DNA integrity is compromised which ultimately impacts the ability of the male gamete to fertilize the oocyte and to form a normal and viable embryo. A small percentage of spermatozoa from fertile men possess detectable levels of DNA damage.[309,310] However, sperm DNA damage is increased in infertile men and approximately 5–15% of such individuals have complete protamine deficiency.[311,312] Sakkas and his colleagues have proposed that spermatozoa with DNA damage initiated and subsequently escaped apoptosis.[313] Sperm nuclear proteins play an important role in chromatin condensation during spermiogenesis. A highly condensed sperm chromatin is essential for maintaining sperm DNA integrity.[314,315] The role of sperm nuclear proteins, the protamines (P) and transitional proteins (TPs) in sperm function has been the focus of many recent studies.[316–319]

Altered sperm P1/P2 ratio leads to abnormal sperm DNA packing and has been reported to be an important cause of male infertility.[320–322] A possible reason for P1/P2 altered ratio is an interrupted post-translation modification or mutation in *PRM/TNP* genes. Although early studies reported rare protamine mutations in association with male infertility, recent observations demonstrated novel mutations and high frequency of SNPs in sperm nuclear protein genes (PRM/TNP).[320–325] Protamine packing of sperm nuclear DNA not only preserves genome integrity that has to be transferred to the offspring without any damage but also helps in various physiological events of the sperm for successful fertilization and embryo development.[326]

DNA damage cannot be analyzed or estimated by conventional cytogenetic or semen analysis. Various tests have been developed to measure sperm DNA damage in the clinical laboratory setting such as sperm chromatin structure assay (SCSA), sperm chromatin dispersion test, transferase-mediated dTUP nick-end labeling (TUNEL), acridine orange test, acidic and basic dye tests (Table 4). Sperm DNA fragmentation index (DFI) is the percentage of spermatozoa with nuclear DNA fragmentation (single and double strand breaks). The cut-off value for DFI measured by TUNEL assay is 19.25%,[327] whereas, the recently established DFI cutoff level of 30.27% measured by SCSA is able to discriminate infertile and fertile men (unpublished data). Infertile men were found to have higher sperm DNA damage compared to fertile controls (Figure 8).

Although it is impossible to treat cytogenetic abnormalities and genetic aberrations, sperm oxidative DNA damage to a large extent can be prevented or decreased. This can be done by lifestyle changes such as quitting smoking, decreasing alcohol intake and exercising, ameliorating food habits by eating antioxidant rich-food and/or treating genital infections and clinical varicocele.

Mitochondrial Genetic Defects

Spermatozoa mitochondria are helically arranged around the mid-piece of sperm and contain 1-2 mt DNA. Mitochondrial DNA codes for 37 genes which regulates oxidative phosphorylation. Mitchondrial DNA is unique and differs from the nuclear DNA with respect of replication, repair mechanism, genome packing and position. However, unlike nuclear DNA mitochondrial DNA is not protected by histones and they are physically associated with the inner mitochondrial membrane, where highly mutagenic oxygen radicals are generated as byproduct of OXPHOS in the respiratory chain.[328,329] The leakage of these free radicals from the respiratory chain makes the mitochondria a major intracellular source of ROS. These unique features are probably the cause of faster accumulation of sequence variations in mitochondrial DNA than in nuclear DNA.[330,331] The PCR amplification of mtDNA has shown a higher incidence of mtDNA deletion in asthenozoospermic patients as compared with unaffected individuals.[332] Recent study by Shamsi et al., 2008 showed that sperm with motility disorders harbored mtDNA mutations and had partially formed or totally dysmorphic and disorganized axonomal apparatus.[333] They also reported that men with idiopathic infertility had low antioxidant levels and increased number of mitochondrial sequence variations. Moreover, it is believed that mtDNA mutation may impair electron transport chain resulting in enhanced production of ROS in mitochondria due to incomplete reduction of oxygen.[334] This excess production of ROS may induce the opening of the membrane permeability transition pore and release of free radicals, cytochrome C and other apoptogenic factors leading to apoptosis. Though mtDNA mutations have been established in various studies, its role as a diagnostic marker in male infertility is still under debate. However, infertility due to mtDNA mutation in men has good prognosis in cases opting for ICSI, as mtDNA is not transmitted to the offspring.

Epigenetic Disorders

Epigenetics refers to regulatory mechanisms of genetic expression that do not affect the basic DNA sequence including functional role of centrosome, DNA methylation, histone modifications, chromatin remodeling, role of RNA transcripts and telomere length. Regions of DNA

Table 4 Sperm DNA integrity methods, principle, merits and demerits

Assay type	Principle	Observation	Measurement	Merits/Demerits
TUNEL	Terminal deoxynucleotidyl transferase-mediated (TdT) deoxyuridine triphosphate (dUTP) nick end labeling assay. TUNEL is a direct quantification of sperm DNA breaks	Sperms are classified as TUNEL positive or negative and expressed as a percentage of the total sperm in the population	Percentage cells with labeled DNA	Can be performed on few sperms. Expensive equipment not required. Thresholds not standardized
SCD	Individual cells immersed in agarose, denatured with acid then lysed	Normal sperm produce halo and sperm which produce a very small halo or no halo at all contain DNA fragmentation	Percentage cells with different grade of halos	Easy and limited clinical data
Acridine orange (AO) test (Microscopy)	Metachromatic shift of AO from green to red fluorescence is used to determine extent of DNA denaturation	Visual interpretation of cells under fluorescent microscopy	Percentage cells with green, red and orange nucleus	Many cells rapidly examined. Expensive equipment is required, time-consuming
COMET	Decondensed sperm are suspended in an agarose gel, subjected to an electrophoretic gradient, stained with fluorescent DNA-binding dye	Low-molecular weight DNA, short fragments of both single-stranded and double-stranded DNA will migrate during electrophoresis giving the characteristic comet tail. High-molecular weight DNA will not migrate and remain in the head of the "comet"	Percentage sperm with long tails (tail length, percentage of DNA in tail)	Sensitive/but labor intensive
SCSA	DNA in sperm with abnormal chromatin structure is more prone to acid or heat denaturation. Using the metachromatic properties of AO, SCSA measures susceptibility of sperm DNA to acid-induced denaturation *in situ* by running the sperm cell suspension using flow cytometry	Metachromatic shift of AO from green to red fluorescence	Calculation of percentage DFI, which is the ratio of the red fluorescence to the sum of red and green fluorescence	Reproducible results. Clinically accepted, Expensive equipment
In situ nick translation	Similar to TUNEL	Identifies single-stranded DNA breaks in a reaction catalyzed by the template-dependent enzyme, DNA polymerase		Simple Lacks sensitivity

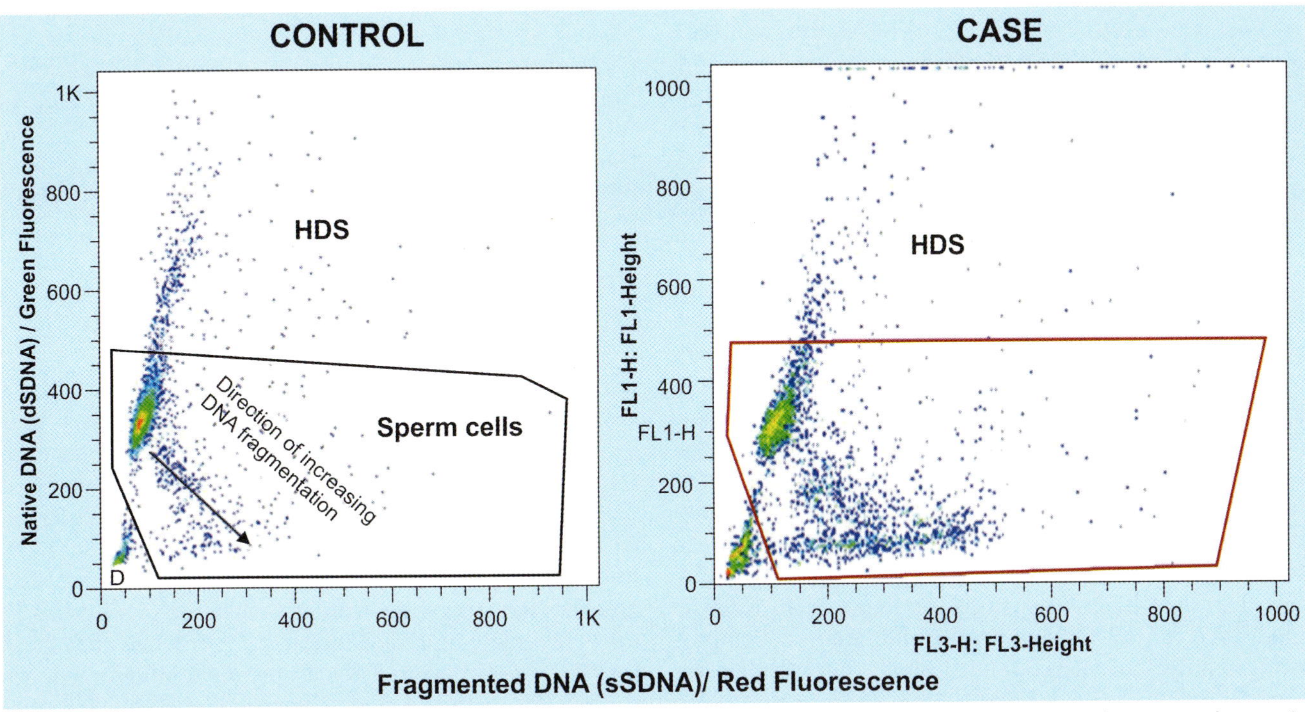

Figure 8 Pseudo-color plot of green versus red fluorescence of sperm DNA treated with acridine orange by sperm chromatin structure assay

HDS: (high DNA stainability) that measure percentage of cells with green fluorescence (normal double stranded DNA)

that are tightly compacted are called heterochromatin and are transcriptionally inactive; conversely, regions that are bound loosely to histones are called euchromatin and are transcriptionally active. The compactness of DNA in a particular region of chromatin is determined by epigenetics; therefore, epigenetic changes play a crucial role in determining which genes are expressed and when in specific cells. Although the genetic code is considered to be static, or the same in every cell for an organism's entire life, the epigenetic code is dynamic and tissue-specific.[335] Therefore, the genetic code defines the permanent imprint of information determining the phenotype and characteristics, whereas the epigenetic code provides a dynamic imprint to finetune the phenotype and characteristics according to environmental and other factors. Alterations in various epigenetic mechanisms result in altered spermatogenesis, poor semen parameters, defective fertilization and even abnormal embryogenesis.

Role of Centrosome: One important contribution that the sperm makes to the embryo is a functional centrosome. The centrosome is involved in the process of fertilization, the separation of chromosomes and cell division.[336] Rawe et al. observed that a patient with abnormal centrosome morphology and sperm aster formation had difficulty in fertilizing oocytes. Furthermore, if a pregnancy was achieved, the fetus was aborted.[337] Sperm harvested from the testicles before maturation may not have a fully functional centrosome, which could lead to problems with the segregation of chromosomes and result in a mosaic or aneuploid embryo.[338,339] Abnormal centrosomes may also be related to the failure of the gametes to unite properly, another error that may cause cleavage arrest.[337]

DNA methylation: Imprinting, the methylation of DNA, determines which genes from the parental and maternal genomes are expressed in the embryo[340] and is critical for normal development.[341] The imprinted regions of DNA are reset every reproductive cycle,[341] which allows novel parental imprints to be established on the germ cells.[342] Imprinting is achieved by the differential marking of DNA regions with histone modifications, methylation, or possibly both, to allow only one copy of a gene to remain active.[343] Kobayashi et al. performed a study examining the fidelity of imprint resetting in infertile males.[341] In fertile men with a normal ejaculate, paternal differentially methylated regions (DMRs) of the DNA should be methylated and the maternal DMRs should be unmethylated. The study found that approximately 14% of infertile patients had abnormalities in the DMRs of the paternal imprint and 21% of the infertile patients had abnormalities in the maternal imprint. Most patients with abnormalities in both imprint regions were oligozoospermic. Additionally, men with abnormally imprinted DMRs had low success rates with ART. It was also discovered that oligozoospermic men may have a higher risk of transmitting imprinting errors to their children.[341] ART could have negative consequences on the imprinting of sperm because it may use sperm that are not yet fully mature and, consequently, their epigenetic code is not established. If the sperm are too immature or abnormal, it is more likely that the offspring could be born with an imprinting disorder.[337] Other defects associated with fertilization by immature sperm are centrosome abnormalities,[344] abnormalities in the sperm's nuclear protein, or an inability to activate the oocyte.[345] The control of methylation may also be a point at which dysregulation could occur. Studies in knockout mice for DNA methyltransferases produced males that were oligozoospermic; however, this has not been replicated in humans.[341] Thus far, studies examining the global methylation patterns of sperm from infertile men have not found significant differences in comparison with normal men, but additional research is necessary to definitively confirm the role of imprinting and epigenetic information in infertility.[346] The correlation between the incidence of imprinting disorders and ART in men with abnormal sperm is a controversial topic. A study by Hartmann et al. found that spermatogonia from infertile men did not have increased imprinting errors in comparison with that of normal men.[347] In contrast, other researchers have asserted that ART, such as ICSI, causes imprinting disorders like Angelman syndrome and Beckwith-Wiedemann syndrome. Angelman syndrome is a rare neurological disorder characterized by cognitive defects, seizures, uncontrolled limb and body movements, spontaneous laughter and difficulties with speech development.[348,349] Two independent groups reported an increased incidence of Angelman syndrome in offspring from ICSI procedures.[350,351] Beckwith-Wiedemann syndrome, also an uncommon disorder, is characterized by large fetal and organ size, hypoglycemia, midline abdominal defects, facial moles and enlarged tongues.[348] Children with Beckwith-Wiedemann syndrome are also at risk for developing tumors.[352] A study by DeBaun et al. reported that the incidence of Beckwith-Wiedemann syndrome was almost 5% in children conceived by ART in comparison with an incidence of less than 1% in the general population.[353] Other studies also reported increased rates of Beckwith-Wiedemann syndrome in ICSI children.[354] However, in consideration of the studies that have not found increased rates of imprinting errors in infertile men, these results are intriguing. Further research into the abnormalities caused by imprinting errors and their patterns of inheritance is needed in this contentious field of research.

Histone modification: Histones are another important contributor to the transmission of epigenetic information. Histone markers signify DNA imprinting control regions during the formation of spermatozoa.[355,356] The transcriptional control of gene expression is regulated by the addition of acetyl, methyl, ubiquitin and phosphate groups to histones.[357] Abnormally modified histones are probable candidates for impeding normal embryogenesis, and their role in the fertility is currently under investigation.[358]

Chromatin remodeling (packaging): Chromatin packaging is an essential step in sperm development, and it is believed that the compacted structure of the chromatin transmits vital instructions to the embryo to guide it through development.[359] During chromatin repackaging, 85% of the histones are replaced by protamines.[311,360,361] In an intermediate step in the replacement process, TPs are inserted into the chromatin structure.[358] Studies in mice revealed that disruption of the genes that code for the TPs—TP1 and TP2 can produce infertile phenotypes.[323,362] Additionally, the functions of the two different human protamines, P1 and P2, have been elucidated. If the mRNA of P1 is translated too early, spermatogenesis is arrested at the spermatid stage and the nucleus condenses prematurely.[363] P2 has been found to be directly related to sperm DNA damage and abnormally packaged chromatin structure.[364] Furthermore, if either of the genes that code for P1 or P2 is mutated, haploinsufficiency, abnormalities in the structure of the chromatin, DNA damage, and infertility can occur.[186] An unequal ratio of P1 and P2 has been observed in infertile men.[312] Men with unequal protamine ratios have decreased semen quality, decreased fertilization ability, and DNA damage.[311,365] Abnormal protamine ratios may also be associated with problems in epigenetic reprogramming and gene imprinting[360] and have been correlated with IVF success and embryo quality.[346] An SNP, G197 T, was found in the gene that codes for P1. This SNP may be a factor that predisposes men to DNA fragmentation and teratozoospermia or to a high prevalence of morphologically abnormal sperm in the ejaculate.[366]

RNA transcripts: The sperm delivers mRNA transcripts to the oocyte upon fertilization, which are needed for the correct development of a functional embryo[358] and which transmit epigenetic information.[359] The fact that these mRNA transcripts are necessary for normal development is emphasized by their presence in zygotes.[367] Furthermore, there is also evidence that the phenotypic characteristics of the embryo might be influenced by the mRNA contributed by the sperm.[367] Studies of the expression profiles of infertile males' mRNA are currently being performed (as discussed in the Novel Technologies section). Micro-RNA (miRNA) is also present in human sperm and in the early embryonic stages.[367] It is possible that miRNA is involved in the control of gene expression in the embryo;[368,369] however, miRNA has been found in high concentrations in the oocyte, so its significance as a sperm contribution still remains controversial.[370]

Telomeres: Telomeres have been also examined as potential candidates for the production of infertile phenotypes. Telomeres protect the genetic information encoded on the chromosome, localize the chromosomes in the nucleus and play a role in DNA replication.[340] Abnormal shortening of the telomeres has been associated with male factor infertility.[371] Hemann et al. performed a study of telomere length in knockout mice for telomerase, the enzyme that maintains the length of telomeres.[372] The results imply that there is a mechanism that degrades spermatocytes with reduced telomere length to prevent their maturation.[372] However, the process is not flawless; Liu et al. discovered spermatocytes that reached meiosis I with shortened telomeres, indicating that they passed the checkpoint without being degraded.[373] Additionally, studies of telomere length in different infertile phenotypes, including nonobstructive and obstructive azoospermic patients and oligozoospermic patients, did not report significant differences in telomerase activity.[374] Thus, the influence of telomere length on male factor fertility must be further elucidated.[340]

IMPORTANCE OF GENETIC TESTING AND COUNSELING

The reasons behind infertility are manifold and a large proportion of cases are still categorized as idiopathic. Genetic testing plays an important role in the evaluation of male infertility not only for diagnosis but also to prevent iatrogenic transmission of the genetic defect to the offspring. Several professional organizations have established recommendations with regard to genetic tests for couples seeking infertility treatment. The European Society of Human Reproduction and Embryology has addressed the issue of "optimal use of infertility diagnostic test and treatments" in the Capri workshop. The Italian community of professionals, supported by international societies, has created guidelines for the appropriate use of genetic tests in infertile couples in 2002. European Molecular Genetics Quality Network has provided elaborated, disease-specific guidelines (www.emgn.org). Here, author recommends various genetic testing in the evaluation of male infertility (Table 5).

ICSI is the only method for many couples with severe male factor infertility due to genetic defects to achieve a live birth. ART success rates may depend on the type of genetic anomaly. Additionally, there is an increased risk of transmitting genetic defects to the offspring. As such, genetic counseling should be a crucial step prior to embark on ART. Genetic anomalies (chromosomal aberrations and AZF microdeletion) comprise an important etiological factor which may lead to poor embryo development and blastocyst formation, and fetal loss. Offspring with genital ambiguity was reported in cases with AZF deletion due to Y chromosome instability. In male offspring from AZF deleted father, AZF deletion status should be determined and parents should be informed about semen cryopreservation.[200] Babies conceived via ART have a higher risk for low birth weight, developmental delay, increased incidence of major and minor congenital malformations like neural tube defects, hypospadias and musculoskeletal disorders and increased incidence of certain cancers.[375] There is also a fourfold increase in incidence of sex chromosomal abnormalities and threefold increase in incidence of structural chromosomal abnormalities.[375] A sixfold increase in the incidence of imprinting defects has also been reported for babies conceived by ART/ICSI.[376] This may be due to retrieval of epigenetically immature germ cells from the testes parental balanced translocations account for the largest percentage of karyotype abnormalities in the fetus.[377] These can result in pregnancy loss because segregation during meiosis results in duplication or deficiency of the chromosome segment. These structural chromosomal anomalies may not have a phenotypic effect on carriers (parents), but result in production of genetically unbalanced gametes, which may result in fetal loss. Studies have shown that the frequency of sex and autosomal chromosomal abnormalities and gene mutation in ART-conceived babies is significantly higher than in babies conceived naturally.[378,379] With recent studies emphasizing the role of oxidative stress (OS) induced DNA damage, men with high DFI should be counseled towards measures aiming to decrease DNA damage, such as lifestyle modifications and varicocele repair, if clinically present.[380]

Genetic counseling is an integral step prior to infertility treatments when any of the partners harbor genetic defects which may be transmitted to the offspring conceived through ART. Counseling these couples prior to assisted conception is strongly encouraged. Such counseling may help prevent the birth of infertile offspring or offspring with increased morbidity and mortality and allow couples to make educated decision

Table 5 Recommendations of various genetic testing based on their phenotypes

Genetic test	Phenotype	Recommendations
Cytogenetic analysis	Severe oligozoospermia Nonobstructive azoospermia	Mandatory Mandatory
Sperm-fluorescent *in situ* hybridization: meiotic segregation analysis	Severe oligozoospermia	Suggested (in cases with mosaicism)
Yq microdeletion analysis	Severe oligozoospermia Nonobstructive azoospermia	Mandatory Mandatory
Cystic fibrosis transmembrane conductance regulator mutation analysis	Congenital bilateral absence of vas deferens	Highly recommended
KAL1 gene mutation analysis	Kallmann's syndrome	Recommended
CAG repeat/AR gene mutation analysis	Androgen insensitivity syndrome	Recommended
Steroid 5alpha-reductase 2(SRD5A2) gene mutation analysis	SRD5A2 deficiency	Recommended
Luteinizing hormone (LH) receptor gene mutation analysis	Pseudohermophroditism, azoospermia, micropenis, delayed puberty and arrest of spermatogenesis	Suggested
Follicle stimulating hormone (FSH) gene mutation analysis	Decreased testicular volume	Suggested
Gonadotropin releasing hormone (GnRH) gene mutation analysis	Low serum LH and FSH levels	Suggested
Protamine/transitional nuclear protein gene mutation analysis	Teratozoospermia or Abnormal P1/P2 ratio	Suggested
Sperm mitochondrial DNA mutation analysis	Asthenozoospermia/Oligozoospermia	Suggested
DAZL/MTHFR mutation analysis	Abnormal sperm parameters	Suggested
Sperm DNA integrity	Idiopathic infertility and recurrent early pregnancy losses	Recommended

regarding than choices to use sperm donor or opt for advanced assisted conception techniques if an abnormal result is revealed.

PREIMPLANTATION GENETIC DIAGNOSIS

Though PGD is not a routine method in the evaluation of male infertility; it is often used to evaluate embryos derived from ART. PGD has a potential role to prevent the transmission of genetic anomalies to the offspring. The technique involves the isolation of one or two cells (blastomere) from a 3-day *in vitro* generated embryo, or multiple cells from a 5-day blastocyst, to perform genetic analysis for aneuploidies or specific mutations by FISH or PCR. PGD is usually recommended for couples having a history of genetic disorders or suspected genetic defects. Infertile males undergoing IVF, such as those with severe sperm defects and KFS individuals with sperm production, may consider PGD analysis as part of their treatment management.

GENETIC TESTS

There are three groups of cytogenetic tests used in andrology to detect genetic diseases: (1) cytogenetic tests that detect chromosomal aneuploidy and structural alterations such as conventional karyotype and FISH technique; b) PCR to detect YCMD and c) specific gene sequencing (mutational analysis of specific gene).

Conventional karyotyping involves the collection of heparinized peripheral blood sample (approximately 5 ml) from the case and isolation of plasma lymphocyte suspension. Sufficient number of lymphocytes with plasma are then transferred into a culture media (RPMI) containing a mitotic stimulator (PHA) and incubated for 72 hours. After 70 hours the cell division is arrested at the metaphase stage by using colchicine. Cells are then subjected to hypotonic treatment (KCl) and fixed with Karnovsky fixative overnight at 4°C. Finally, the cells are spread in a clean grease free wet slide and subjected to GTG banding for karyotyping. The standard protocols are available in various practical guides and should be optimized for respective laboratory conditions.[378] FISH, on the other hand, combines the conventional karyotype approach with molecular techniques by using a fluorescent DNA probe to bind selectively to a specific single stranded chromosomal region (after denaturation) by complimentary base pairing. Such binding is later detected by using fluorescent microscopy. FISH is particularly useful to detect chromosomal aneuploidy and structural abnormalities of specific chromosomes.

Y chromosome microdeletion assay is a PCR-based blood test that detects the presence or the absence of defined STSs and therefore defines by the pattern of presence or absence of any clinically relevant microdeletion region. For specific gene sequencing and mutational analysis "dye terminator sequence" method is performed. This method is high throughput, automated, more efficient and faster than original Sanger method of sequencing. The principle, similar to Sanger's method, depends on premature termination of four separate sequencing reactions, containing all four of the standard deoxynucleotides (dATP, dGTP, dCTP and dTTP) and the DNA polymerase. To each reaction is added only one of the four dideoxynucleotides (ddATP, ddGTP, ddCTP, or ddTTP) which are the chain-terminating nucleotides, lacking a 3′-OH group required for the formation of a phosphodiester bond between two nucleotides, thus terminating DNA strand extension and resulting in DNA fragments of varying length. Then these labeled DNA fragments are separated by gel electrophoresis on a denaturing polyacrylamide-urea gel and read in a specific manner from the shortest to the longest one.

WORK-UP PLAN FOR SPECIFIC GENETIC DIAGNOSIS AND TESTING

Initial evaluation of infertile men usually commences with meticulous history taking and thorough physical examination followed by ordering initial seminal fluid analysis and, if required, endocrine profile testing as well as imaging techniques. In the era of IVF/ICSI, specific genetic diagnosis emerges as diagnostic tool of paramount importance helping the clinicians not only in particularly exploring the specific genetic background of a disease but also in taking the necessary precautions to prevent transmission of the disease to the offspring. History may disclose the cause of infertility and point out to hereditary problem when positive family history of male infertility is reported in the brothers of the proband. Compiling the data from initial evaluation may segregate infertile men with normal looking male genitalia into four major groups based on probability of harboring male fertility related genetic diseases (Figure 9)—for the first group with history and physical examination consistent with cryptorchidism, Noonan syndrome, bilateral anorchia and Prader Willi syndrome, some genetic tests are available, although not routinely used. In the second group, men have normal sperm count; however, their sperm are immotile (PCD), acrosome deficient (globozoospermia) or functionally defective (CatSper gene). In each disease, again there is specific genetic diagnosis that can be used. The third group includes azoospermic men with obvious evidence of seminal ducts obstruction based on physical examination (CBAVD, Young syndrome) and/or imaging techniques (PMDS), requiring testing for CFTR and AMH/AMHR respectively. For the fourth group encompassing men with severe oligozoospermia and nonobstructive azoospermia, exclusion of previous testicular pathologies and history of exposure to gonadotoxins such as radiation and chemotherapy mandates full endocrine evaluation and genetic testing as shown in the algorithm (Figure 9). In contrast, for men with feminized or ambiguous external genitalia, genetic workup , in particular, should consist of karyotype to document the chromosomal gender, pelvic ultrasound to detect persistence of Mullerian structures, electrolyte evaluation to detect salt losing varieties of CAH and lastly hormonal profile (testosterone, DHT, LH, FSH, cortisol, 17-OH progesterone) and AR genetic analysis.

NOVEL TECHNOLOGIES

Adopting a global approach to the examination of novel genes may allow for a more complete understanding of the interaction between genetics and fertility, and may also uncover genes with unknown roles in infertility. This approach may circumvent one of the main problems that geneticists face when relating a genotype to a specific infertility phenotype: the diverse genetic backgrounds of different ethnic groups.[382] Incorporating techniques such as genomics, proteomics, and metabolomics into infertility research could assist in creating a complete portrait of the genes involved in infertility and would allow for improvements of ART for the development of more targeted solutions. Microarrays are valuable tools for the identification of gene expression profiles of infertile phenotypes.[383] Examining the simultaneous expression of genes allows geneticists

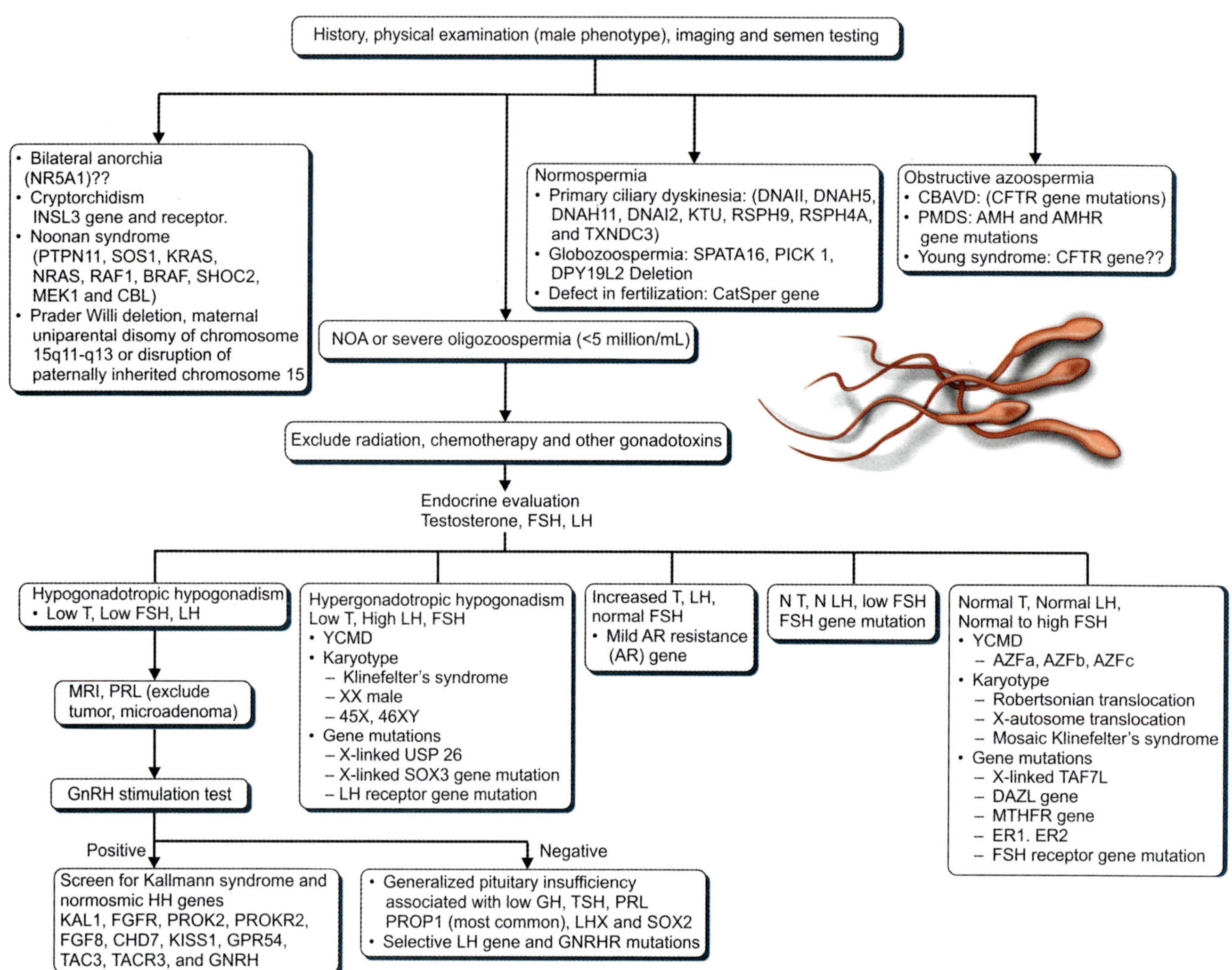

Figure 9 Algorithm for work up plan for specific genetic diagnosis and testing in infertile men with normal male genitalia

CBAVD: congenital bilateral absence of the vas deferens; CFTR: cystic fibrosis transmembrane regulator protein gene; PMDS: persistent Mullerian ducts syndrome; NOA: nonobstructive azoospermia; T: testosterone; FSH: follicular stimulating hormone; LH: luteinizing hormone; MRI: magnetic resonance image; PRL: prolactin; GnRH: gonadotropin releasing hormone; HH: hypogonadotropic hypogonadism; YCMD:Y chromosome microdeletion; GH: growth hormone; TSH: thyroid stimulating hormone; AR: androgen receptor

to determine molecular signatures related to infertile phenotypes.[384] Microarray technology is also useful in the examination of spermatogenesis. An analysis of gene expression over time could be performed to determine the genes that are involved in each stage of the process. Genomic analysis can also be used to determine differentially transcribed genes.[385] An enhanced understanding of transcription regulation could help geneticists discover how different expression patterns impact a patient's fertility.[383] Additionally, microarrays can be used to study the effect of hormones or growth factors on gene expression profiles. In one experiment, T propionate and FSH were administered to mouse testes and the differential expression of genes was measured using microarray analysis.[384] Some advantages of using microarrays are that it is a noninvasive test[386] and it is very effective in studying germ cells because they express 4% of the genome.[387] Disadvantages of genomics are that gene expression can vary between two different samples[382] and infertile patients might have pockets of gene expression that are difficult to detect using microarrays.[388] Ellis et al. performed a study of several different infertile phenotypes that revealed two distinct patterns of gene expression, one related to spermatogenesis and one related to inflammatory activity.[383] They identified functional groups within the gene expression patterns related to spermatid development and motility, DNA synthesis and repair, metabolic functions, and cholesterol and lipid metabolism.[383] The study also discovered a correlation between infertile phenotypes and mRNA expression.[383] Another study of gene expression was performed in teratozoospermic men by Platts et al. which identified characteristic mRNA signatures for teratozoospermic and normospermic men.[383,386] Since the results of microarray studies of gene expression produce variable results, it is necessary to determine global gene expression patterns of RNA samples from the testis before this type of analysis would be clinically relevant. Grouping the expressed genes into functional categories allows for the characterization of a gene expression signature for normal human spermatogenesis that can be used as a baseline marker for diagnosis.[1] Proteomics allows for the determination of protein expression profiles of fertile and infertile men.[389] Proteins are identified with two-dimensional electrophoresis and mass spectrometry techniques, and the results are used to create maps of the proteome.[389] Spermatozoa are ideal for the study of protein expression because they do not have active transcription or translation.[390] Further research in these fields can continue after the sperm proteome is fully defined and the components of seminal plasma are identified.[390] Advances have been made in both of these areas,[391–393] and many new proteins have been identified as a result. The identification of protein biomarkers for male factor infertility will allow for unbiased comparison between fertile and infertile males and will clarify the pathophysiology of the disease.[390] Martinez-Heredia et al. studied asthenozoospermic patients using proteomic techniques. Most of the causes of asthenozoospermia, or abnormally low sperm motility levels, are unknown, even though it is a common infertile phenotype.[389] The study found 17 differentially expressed proteins between the control group and the asthenozoospermic patients. The results were clustered, signifying that results from proteomic studies could possibly be used to characterize or diagnose infertile patients. Subgroupings of functional groups were also determined from the results and were divided into energy production, structure/movement, and intercell signaling. These subgroups could be used to target the underlying causes of asthenozoospermia.[389] An advantageous characteristic of genomic and proteomic technology is that the results can be confirmed through replication using other techniques such as Western blots, flow cytometry and PCR. Without reproducible results, a test is meaningless, especially with multistep procedures like these that may accumulate errors.[384] Another important feature of these testes is that the results provide a definitive characterization of infertile phenotypes.[386] The use of technologies like genomics and proteomics is a step toward creating personalized medical diagnoses by determining individual causes of infertility.[386] Metabolomics is another emerging area of research in the evaluation of the role of genetic factors in male factor infertility. It involves measuring the expression of metabolites, small biomarkers that indicate the functionality of a cell, and characterizing them for certain diseases or physiological states.[394,395] The identification of the human metabolome will reveal the functional phenotype of the system being studied, whether it is a single cell or an entire organism. Mass spectroscopy, nuclear magnetic resonance spectroscopy, and other chromatography methods can be used to create profiles of metabolites. Pathway or cluster analysis is used to determine subsets of metabolites that can be used to quantitatively characterize patients for diagnosis.[393] By identifying differences in the expression of metabolites in infertile phenotypes, new methods of diagnosis and treatment of male factor infertility can be developed that are inexpensive and noninvasive.[394]

So far, metabolomics has been used to identify biomarkers for OS, which signal semen quality.[391] A study performed by Deepinder et al. determined that expression patterns of metabolomic markers for OS in semen were correlated to specific infertile phenotypes with a high level of specificity and sensitivity.[394] This encouraging finding may assist in unraveling the underlying mysteries that still surround many cases of idiopathic male factor infertility. Other future clinical applications of metabolomics are gamete selection (assessing the best sperm to use for ART) and functional genomic testing (screening for aneuploidy and other genetic conditions).[394] Next, efficient clinical methods must be developed to compare standardized metabolomic signatures with patients' personal metabolomic profiles for the creation of individualized fertility care.[396] These novel technologies hold promise for advances in the ways in which information about genetic profiles can aid infertility patients.

REFERENCES

1. Ferlin A, Raicu F, Gatta V, et al. Male infertility: role of genetic background. Reprod Biomed Online. 2007; 14(6):734-45.
2. Jarow JP, Sharlip ID, Belker AM, et al. Best practice policies for male infertility. J Urol. 2002;167:2138-44.
3. Moghissi KS, Wallach EE. Unexplained infertility. Fertil Steril. 1983;39:5-21.
4. Dohle GR, Diemer T, Giwercman A, et al. (2010) European Association of Urology, [Homepage on the internet], Online Guidelines of Male Infertility. [Online] cited on: April 2011, Retrieved from: http://www.uroweb.org/gls/pdf/14_Male_Infertility%202010.pdf.
5. WHO. Manual for the standardized investigation and diagnosis of the infertile couple'. Cambridge University Press; 2000.

6. Meschede D, Lemcke B, Behre HM, et al. Clustering of male infertility in the families of couples treated with intracytoplasmic sperm injection. Hum Reprod. 2000;15(7):1604-8.
7. Gianotten J, Westerveld GH, Leschot NJ, et al. Familial clustering of impaired spermatogenesis: no evidence for a common genetic inheritance pattern. Hum Reprod. 2004;19(1):71-6.
8. van Golde RJ, van der Avoort IA, Tuerlings JH, Kiemeney LA, et al. Phenotypic characteristics of male subfertility and its familial occurrence. J Androl. 2004;25(5):819-23.
9. Inhorn MC, Kobeissi L, Nassar Z, et al. Consanguinity and family clustering of male factor infertility in Lebanon. Fertil Steril. 2009;91(4):1104-9. Epub 2008.
10. Latini M, Gandini L, Lenzi A, et al. Sperm tail agenesis in a case of consanguinity. Fertil Steril. 2004;81(6):1688-91.
11. Dolores J. Look towards the future advances in andrology expected to revolutionize the diagnosis and treatment of infertile men. In: Lipshultz LI, Howards SS, Craig S (Eds). Infertility in the male. UK: Cambridge University Press; 2009. pp. 642-53.
12. Hargreave TB. Genetic basis of male fertility. Br Med Bull; 2000. pp. 650-71.
13. Johnson MH, Everitt BJ. Testicular function in adults. In: MH Johnson, BJ Everitt (Eds). Essential reproduction. Oxford: Blackwell Publishing; 2007. p. 64.
14. Huckins C. The morphology and kinetics of spermatogonial degeneration in normal adult rats: an analysis using a simplified classification of the germinal epithelium. Anat Rec. 1978:190;905-26.
15. Rucker EB, Dierisseau P, Wagner KU, et al. Bcl-x and Bax regulate mouse primordial germ cell survival and apoptosis during embryogenesis. Mol. Endocrinol. 2000:14;1038-52.
16. Matzuk MM, Lamb DJ. Genetic dissection of mammalian fertility pathways. Nat Cell Biol. 2002;4 Suppl:s41-9.
17. Li MW, Xia W, Mruk DD, et al. Tumor necrosis factor {alpha} reversibly disrupts the blood-testis barrier and impairs Sertoli-germ cell adhesion in the seminiferous epithelium of adult rat testes. J Endocrinol. 2006;190(2):313-29.
18. Xia W, Mruk DD, Lee WM, et al. Differential interactions between transforming growth factor-beta3/TbetaR1, TAB1, and CD2AP disrupt blood-testis barrier and Sertoli-germ cell adhesion. J Biol Chem. 2006;281(24):16799-813. Epub 2006.
19. Baudat F, Manova K, Yuen JP, et al. Chromosome synapsis defects and sexually dimorphic meiotic progression in mice lacking Spo11. Mol Cell. 2000:6;989-98.
20. Romanienko PJ, Camerini-Otero RD. The mouse Spo11 gene is required for meiotic chromosome synapsis. Mol Cell. 2000;6:975-87.
21. Yoshida K, Kondoh G, Matsuda Y, et al. The mouse RecA-like gene Dmc1 is required for homologous chromosome synapsis during meiosis. Mol Cell. 1998;1:707-18.
22. Pittman DL, Cobb J, Schimenti KJ, et al. Meiotic prophase arrest with failure of chromosome synapsis in mice deficient for Dmc1, a germlinespecific RecA homolog. Mol Cell. 1998;1: 697-705.
23. Xu X, Toselli PA, Russell LD, et al. Globozoospermia in mice lacking the casein kinase II α' catalytic subunit. Nature Genet. 1999;23:118-21.
24. Barlow C, Hirotsune S, Paylor R, et al. Atm-deficient mice: a paradigm of ataxia telangiectasia. Cell. 1996;86:159-71.
25. Barlow C, Liyanage M, Moens PB, et al. Atm deficiency results in severe meiotic disruption as early as leptonema of prophase I. Development. 1998;125:4007-17.
26. Kneitz B, Cohen PE, Avdievich E, et al. MutS homolog 4 localization to meiotic chromosomes is required for chromosome pairing during meiosis in male and female mice. Genes Dev. 2000;14:1085-97.
27. Edelmann W, Cohen PE, Kane M, et al. Meitoic pachytene arrest in MLH1-deficient mice. Cell.1996;85:1125-34.
28. Edelmann W, Cohen PE, Kneitz B, et al. Mammalian MutS homologue 5 is required for chromosome pairing in meiosis. Nature Genet. 1999;21:123-7.
29. Roest HP, van Klaveren J, de Wit J, et al. Inactivation of the HR6B ubiquitin-conjugating DNA repair enzyme in mice causes male sterility associated with chromatin modification. Cell. 1996; 86:799-810.
30. Xu Y, Ashley T, Brainerd EE, et al. Targeted disruption of ATM leads to growth retardation, chromosomal fragmentation during meiosis, immune defects, and thymic lymphoma. Genes Dev. 1996;10:2411-22.
31. Sassone-Corsi P. Unique chromatin remodeling and transcriptional regulation in spermatogenesis. Science. 2002;296(5576):2176-8.
32. Fuentes-Mascorro G, Serrano H, Rosado A. Sperm chromatin. Arch Androl. 2000;45:215-25.
33. Ward WS. Function of sperm chromatin structural elements in fertilization and development. Mol Hum Reprod. 2010;16:30-6.
34. Sotolongo B, Lino E, Ward WS. Ability of hamster spermatozoa to digest their own DNA. Biol Reprod. 2003;69:2029-35.
35. Martins RP, Ostermeier GC, Krawetz SA. Nuclear matrix interactions at the human protamine domain: a working model of potentiation. J Biol Chem. 2004;279:51862-8.
36. Ajduk A, Yamauchi Y, Ward MA. Sperm chromatin remodeling after intracytoplasmic sperm injection differs from that of in vitro fertilization. Biol Reprod. 2006;75:442-51.
37. Ogura A, Matsuda J, Yanagimachi R. Birth of normal young after electrofusion of mouse oocytes with round spermatids. Proc Natl Acad Sci USA. 1994;91:7460-2.
38. Hammoud SS, Nix DA, Zhang H, et al. Distinctive chromatin in human sperm packages genes for embryo development. Nature. 2009;460:473-8.
39. Ostermeier GC, Goodrich RJ, Diamond MP, et al. Toward using stable spermatozoal RNAs for prognostic assessment of male factor fertility. Fertil Steril. 2005;83:1687-94.
40. Arpanahi A, Brinkworth M, Iles D, et al. Endonuclease-sensitive regions of human spermatozoal chromatin are highly enriched in promoter and CTCF binding sequences. Genome Res. 2009;19:1338-49.

41. Van der Heijden GW, Ramos L, Baart EB, et al. Sperm-derived histones contribute to zygotic chromatin in humans. BMC Dev Biol. 2008;8:34.
42. Shaman JA, Yamauchi Y, Ward WS. The sperm nuclear matrix is required for paternal DNA replication. J Cell Biochem. 2007;102:680-8.
43. Bianco B, Christofolini D, Gava M, et al. Severe oligospermia associated with a unique balanced reciprocal translocation t(6;12)(q23;q24.3): male infertility related to t(6;12). Andrologia. 2011;43(2):145-8. doi: 10.1111/j.1439-0272.2009.01020.x. Epub 2010.
44. Silverman AJ. The gonadotropin-releasing hormone (GnRH) neuronal systems: immunocytochemistry. In: Knobil E, Neill JD (Eds). The Physiology of Reproduction. New York, USA: Raven Press; 1998. pp. 1283-304.
45. Geracioti TD, Strawn JR, Ekhator NN. Neuroregulatory peptides of central nervous system origin: from laboratory to clinic. In: Pfaff DW, Arnold AP, Etgen AM, Fahrbach SE, Rubin RT (Eds). Hormones, Brain and Behavior, 2nd edition. New York, USA: Elsevier Inc. Academic Press; 2009. pp. 2541-96.
46. Schwarting GA, Wierman ME, Tobet SA. Gonadotropin-releasing hormone neuronal migration. Semin Reprod Med. 2007;25(5):305-12.
47. Knobil E. The electrophysiology of the GnRH pulse generator in the rhesus monkey. Journal of Steroid Biochemistry 1989;33:669-71.
48. Van Tijn DA, Schroor EJ, Delemarre-Van de Waal HA, et al. Early assessment of hypothalamic-pituitary-gonadal function in patients with congenital hypothyroidism of central origin. Journal of Clinical Endocrinology and Metabolism. 2007;92:104-9.
49. Layman LC, Reindollar RH. The diagnosis and treatment of pubertal disorders. Adolescent Medicine: State of the Art Reviews. 1994;5:37-55.
50. Bianco SD, Kaiser UB. The genetic and molecular basis of idiopathic hypogonadotropic hypogonadism. Nat Rev Endocrinol. 2009;5(10):569-76. Epub 2009.
51. Pallais JC, Au M, Pitteloud N. Kallmann Syndrome, Genes Review NCBI Bookshelf. Bookshelf US national Library of Medicine, National Institute of Health [homepage on the Internet]. 2011 [cited 2011 May 16]. Available from: US national Library of Medicine, National Institute of Health Web site: http://0-www.ncbi.nlm.nih.gov.library.ccf.org/books/NBK1334/.
52. Dodé C, Hardelin JP. Kallmann syndrome. Eur J Hum Genet. 2009;17(2):139-46. Epub 2008.
53. Behre HM, Nieshelag E, Partsch CJ, et al. Diseases of the hypothalamus and the pituitary gland. In: Nieschlag E, Behre HM, Nieschlag S (Eds). Andrology Male Reproductive Health and Dysfunction, 3rd edition. Germany: Springer Verlag Berlin Heidelberg; 2010. pp. 169-92.
54. Bhagavath B, Podolsky RH, Ozata M, et al. Clinical and molecular characterization of a large sample of patients with hypogonadotropic hypogonadism. Fertil Steril. 2006;85(3):706-13.
55. Trarbach EB. Copy number variation associated with Kallmann syndrome: new genetics insights from genome-wide studies. Asian J Androl. 2011;13(2):203-4. Epub 2010.
56. Iafrate AJ, Feuk L, Rivera MN, et al. Detection of large-scale variation in the human genome. Nat Genet. 2004;36(9):949-51. Epub 2004.
57. Redon R, Ishikawa S, Fitch KR, et al. Global variation in copy number in the human genome. Nature. 2006;444(7118):444-54.
58. Del Castillo I, Cohen-Salmon M, Blanchard S, et al. Structure of the X-linked Kallmann syndrome gene and its homologous pseudogene on the Y chromosome. Nat Genet. 1992;22:305-10.
59. Kim SH, Hu Y, Cadman S, et al. Diversity in fibroblast growth factor receptor 1 regulation: learning from the investigation of Kallmann syndrome. J Neuroendocrinol. 2008;20:141-63.
60. Ballabio A, Andria G. Deletions and translocations involving the distal short arm of the human X chromosome: review and hypotheses. Hum Mol Genet. 1992;1:221-7.
61. Parenti G, Rizzolo MG, Ghezzi M, et al. Variable penetrance of hypogonadism in a sibship with Kallmann syndrome due to a deletion of the KAL gene. Am J Med Genet. 1995;57:476-8.
62. Albuisson J, Pecheux C, Carel JC, et al. Kallmann syndrome: 14 novel mutations in KAL1 and FGFR1 (KAL2). Human Mutation. 2005;25:98-9.
63. Pedersen-White JR, Chorich LP, Bick DP, et al. The prevalence of intragenic deletions in patients with idiopathic hypogonadotropic hypogonadism and Kallmann syndrome. Molecular Human Reproduction. 2008;14: 367-70.
64. Oliveira LM, Seminara SB, Beranova M, et al. The importance of autosomal genes in Kallmann syndrome: genotype phenotype correlations and neuroendocrine characteristics. Journal of Clinical Endocrinology and Metabolism. 2001;86:1532-8.
65. Izumi Y, Tastumi K, Okamoto S, et al. Analysis of the KAL1 gene in 19 Japanese patients with Kallmann syndrome. Endocr J. 2001;48:143-9.
66. Hardelin JP, Levilliers J, Blanchard S, et al. Heterogeneity in the mutations responsible for X chromosome-linked Kallmann syndrome. Hum Mol Genet. 1993;2:373-7.
67. Maya-Nunez G, Zenteno JC, Ulloa-Aguirre A, et al. A recurrent missense mutation in the KAL gene in patients with X-linked Kallmann's syndrome. J Clin Endocrinol Metab. 1998;83:1650-3.
68. Georgopoulos NA, Pralong FP, Seidman CE, et al. Genetic heterogeneity evidenced by low incidence of KAL-1 gene mutations in sporadic cases of gonadotropin-releasing hormone deficiency. J Clin Endocrinol Metab. 1997;82:213-7.
69. Layman LC. Hypogonadotropic hypogonadism. Endocrinol Metab Clin N Am. 2007;36:283-96.
70. Pitteloud N, Meysing A, Quinton R, et al. Mutations in fibroblast growth factor receptor 1 cause Kallmann syndrome with a wide spectrum of reproductive phenotypes. Mol Cell Endocrinol. 2006;254-255:60-9. Epub 2006.

71. Dode´ C, Levilliers J, Dupont JM, et al. Loss-of-function mutations in FGFR1 cause autosomal dominant Kallmann syndrome. Nat Genet. 2003;33:463-5.
72. Groth C, Lardelli M. The structure and function of vertebrate fibroblast growth factor receptor 1. Int J Dev Biol. 2002;46:393-400.
73. Gill JC, Moenter SM, Tsai PS. Developmental regulation of gonadotropin releasing hormone neurons by fibroblast growth factor signaling. Endocrinology. 2004;145:3830-9.
74. Böttcher RT, Niehrs C. Fibroblast growth factor signaling during early vertebrate development. Endocr. Rev. 2005;26:63-77.
75. Pitteloud N, Acierno JS Jr, Meysing A, et al. Mutations in fibroblast growth factor receptor 1 cause both Kallmann syndrome and normosmic idiopathic hypogonadotropic hypogonadism. Proc Natl Acad Sci USA. 2006;103(16):6281-6.
76. Sato N, Katsumata N, Kagami M, et al. Clinical assessment and mutation analysis of Kallmann syndrome 1 (KAL1) and fibroblast growth factor receptor 1 (FGFR1, or KAL2) in 5 families and 18 sporadic patients. J Clin Endocrinol Metab. 2004;89(3):1079-88.
77. Salenave S, Chanson P, Bry H, et al. Kallmann's syndrome: a comparison of the reproductive phenotypes in men carrying KAL1 and FGFR1/KAL2 mutations. J Clin Endocrinol Metab. 2008;93:758-63.
78. Falardeau J, Chung WC, Beenken A, et al. Decreased FGF8 signaling causes deficiency of gonadotropin-releasing hormone in humans and mice. J Clin Invest. 2008;118:2822-31.
79. Trarbach EB, Abreu AP, Silveira LF, et al. Nonsense mutations in FGF8 gene causing different degrees of human gonadotropin-releasing deficiency. J Clin Endocrinol Metab. 2010;95:3491-6.
80. Trarbach EB, Silveira LG, Latronico AC. Genetic insights into human isolated gonadotropin deficiency. Pituitary. 2007;10(4):381-91.
81. Cole LW, Sidis Y, Zhang C, et al. Mutations in Prokineticin 2 and prokineticin receptor 2 genes in human gonadotropin releasing hormone deficiency: molecular genetics and clinical spectrum. Journal of Clinical Endocrinology and Metabolism. 2008;93:3551-9.
82. Vissers LE, van Ravenswaaij CM, Admiraal R, et al. Mutations in a new member of the chromodomain gene family cause CHARGE syndrome. Nature Genetics. 2004;36:955-7.
83. Semple RK, Topaloglu AK. The recent genetics of hypogonadotrophic hypogonadism—novel insights and new questions. Clin Endocrinol (Oxf). 2010;72(4):427-35. Epub 2009.
84. Lalani SR, Safiullah AM, Fernbach SD, et al. Spectrum of CHD7 mutations in 110 individuals with CHARGE syndrome and genotype-phenotype correlation. Am J Hum Genet. 2006;78:303-14.
85. Kim HG, Kurth I, Lan F, et al. Mutations in CHD7, encoding a chromatin-remodeling protein, cause idiopathic hypogonadotropic hypogonadism and Kallmann syndrome. Am J Hum Genet. 2008;83:511-9.
86. Schwarting GA, Raitcheva D, Bless EP, et al. Netrin 1-mediated chemoattraction regulates the migratory pathway of LHRH neurons. Eur J Neurosci. 2004;19:11-20.
87. Bouligand J, Ghervan C, Tello JA, et al. Isolated familial hypogonadotropic hypogonadism and a GNRH1 mutation. N Engl J Med. 2009;360:2742-8.
88. Chan YM, de Guillebon A, Lang-Muritano M, et al. GNRH1 mutations in patients with idiopathic hypogonadotropic hypogonadism. Proc Natl Acad Sci USA. 2009;106(28):11703-8.
89. Bédécarrats GY, Kaiser UB. Mutations in the human gonadotropin-releasing hormone receptor: insights into receptor biology and function. Semin Reprod Med. 2007;25:368-78.
90. Kaiser UB, Dushkin H, Altherr MR, et al. Chromosomal localization of the gonadotropin-releasing hormone receptor gene to human chromosome 4q13.1-q21.1 and mouse chromosome 5. Genomics. 1994;20:506-8.
91. De Roux N, Young J, Misrahi M, et al. A family with hypogonadotropic hypogonadism and mutations in the gonadotropin-releasing hormone receptor. N Engl J Med. 1997;337:1597-602.
92. Layman LC, Cohen DP, Jin M, et al. Mutations in gonadotropin-releasing hormone receptor gene cause hypogonadotropic hypogonadism. Nat Genet. 1998;18:14-5.
93. Costa EM, Bedecarrats GY, Mendonca BB, et al. Two novel mutations in the gonadotropin-releasing hormone receptor gene in Brazilian patients with hypogonadotropic hypogonadism and normal olfaction. J Clin Endocrinol Metab. 2001;86:2680-6.
94. De Roux N, Young J, Brailly-Tabard S, et al. The same molecular defects of the gonadotropin-releasing hormone receptor determine a variable degree of hypogonadism in affected kindred. J Clin Endocrinol Metab. 1999;84:567-72.
95. Caron P, Chauvin S, Christin-Maitre S, et al. Resistance of hypogonadic patients with mutated GnRH receptor genes to pulsatile GnRH administration. J Clin Endocrinol Metab. 1999;84:990-6.
96. Seminara SB, Beranova M, Oliveira LM, et al. Successful use of pulsatile gonadotropin releasing hormone (GnRH) for ovulation induction and pregnancy in a patient with GnRH receptor mutations. J Clin Endocrinol Metab. 2000;85:556-62.
97. Beranova M, Oliveira LM, Bedecarrats GY, et al. Prevalence, phenotypic spectrum, and modes of inheritance of gonadotropin-releasing hormone receptor mutations in idiopathic hypogonadotropic hypogonadism. J Clin Endocrinol Metab. 2001;86:1580-8.
98. Bedecarrats GY, Linher KD, Kaiser UB. Two common naturally occurring mutations in the human gonadotropin releasing hormone (GnRH) receptor have differential effects on gonadotropin gene expression and on GnRH-mediated signal transduction. J Clin Endocrinol Metab. 2003;88:834-43.
99. Pitteloud N, Boepple PA, DeCruz S, et al. The fertile eunuch variant of idiopathic hypogonadotropic hypogonadism: spontaneous reversal associated with a homo-

zygous mutation in the gonadotropin releasing hormone receptor. J Clin Endocrinol Metab. 2001;86:2470-5.
100. Silveira LG, Noel SD, Silveira-Neto AP, et al. Mutations of the KISS1 gene in disorders of puberty. J Clin Endocrinol Metab. 2010;95(5):2276-80. Epub 2010.
101. Messager S, Chatzidaki EE, Ma D, et al. Kisspeptin directly stimulates gonadotropin-releasing hormone release via G protein-coupled receptor 54. Proc Natl Acad Sci USA. 2005;102:1761-6.
102. Topaloglu AK, Reimann F, Guclu M, et al. TAC3 and TACR3 mutations in familial hypogonadotropic hypogonadism reveal a key role for Neurokinin B in the central control of reproduction. Nat Genet. 2009;41:354-8.
103. Guran T, Tolhurst G, Bereket A, et al. Hypogonadotropic hypogonadism due to a novel missense mutation in the first extracellular loop of the neurokinin B receptor. J Clin Endocrinol Metab. 2009;94:3633-9.
104. Gianetti E, Tusset C, Noel SC, et al. TAC3/TACR3 mutations reveal preferential activiation of gonadotropin-releasing hormone release by neurokinin B in neonatal life followed by reversal in adulthood. J Clin Endocrinol Metab. 2010;95:2857-67.
105. Jackson RS, Creemers JW, Ohagi S, et al. Obesity and impaired prohormone processing associated with mutations in the human prohormone convertase 1 gene. Nat Genet. 1997;16:303-6.
106. Muscatelli F, Strom TM, Walker AP, et al. Mutations in the DAX-1 gene give rise to both X-linked adrenal hypoplasia congenita and hypogonadotropic hypogonadism. Nature. 1994;372:672-6.
107. Spratt DI, Carr DB, Merriam GR, et al. The spectrum of abnormal patterns of gonadotropin-releasing hormone secretion in men with idiopathic hypogonadotropic hypogonadism: clinical and laboratory correlations. J Clin Endocrinol Metab. 1987;64:283-91.
108. Smals AG, Kloppenborg PW, van Haelst UJ, et al. Fertile eunuch syndrome versus classic hypogonadotrophic hypogonadism. Acta Endocrinol (Copenh). 1978;87:389-99.
109. Raivio T, Falardeau J, Dwyer A, et al. Reversal of idiopathic hypogonadotropic hypogonadism. N Engl J Med. 2007;357:863-73.
110. Pitteloud N, Acierno JS Jr, Meysing AU, et al. Reversible kallmann syndrome, delayed puberty, and isolated anosmia occurring in a single family with a mutation in the fibroblast growth factor receptor 1 gene. J Clin Endocrinol Metab. 2005;90(3):1317-22. Epub 2004.
111. Burris AS, Rodbard HW, Winters SJ, et al. Gonadotropin therapy in men with isolated hypogonadotropic hypogonadism: the response to human chorionic gonadotropin is predicted by initial testicular size. J Clin Endocrinol Metab. 1988;66(6):1144-51.
112. Dwyer AA, Hayes FJ, Plummer L, et al. The long-term clinical follow-up and natural history of men with adult-onset idiopathic hypogonadotropic hypogonadism. J Clin Endocrinol Metab. 2010;95(9):4235-43. Epub 2010.
113. Jin DK. Systematic review of the clinical and genetic aspects of Prader-Willi syndrome. Korean J Pediatr. 2011;54(2):55-63. Epub 2011.
114. Schmidt H, Schwarz HP. Premature adrenarche, increased growth velocity and accelerated bone age in male patients with Prader-Labhart-Willi syndrome. Eur J Pediatr. 2001;160:69-70.
115. Unanue N, Bazaes R, Iniguez G, et al. Adrenarche in Prader-Willi syndrome appears not related to insulin sensitivity and serum adiponectin. Horm Res. 2007;67:152-8.
116. Kelberman D, Dattani MT. Hypopituitarism oddities: congenital causes. Horm Res. 2007;68(Suppl 5):138-44. Epub 2007.
117. Mendonca BB, Osorio MG, Latronico AC, et al. Longitudinal hormonal and pituitary imaging changes in two females with combined pituitary hormone deficiency due to deletion of A301, G302 in the PROP1 gene. J Clin Endocrinol Metab. 1999;84:942-5.
118. Themmen AP, Huhtaniemi IT. Mutations of gonadotropins and gonadotropin receptors: elucidating the physiology and pathophysiology of pituitary-gonadal function. Endocr Rev. 2000;21(5):551-83.
119. Achermann JC, Weiss J, Lee EJ, et al. Inherited disorders of the gonadotropin hormones. Mol Cell Endocrinol. 2001;179(1-2):89-96.
120. Layman LC, Porto AL, Xie J, et al. FSH beta gene mutations in a female with partial breast development and a male sibling with normal puberty and azoospermia. J Clin Endocrinol Metab. 2002;87:3702-7.
121. Lindstedt G, Nystrom E, Matthews C, et al. Follitropin (FSH) deficiency in an infertile male due to FSHbeta gene mutation. A syndrome of normal puberty and virilization but underdeveloped testicles with azoospermia, low FSH but high lutropin and normal serum testosterone concentrations. Clin Chem Lab Med. 1998;36:663-5.
122. Philip M, Arbelle JE, Segev Y, et al. Male hypogonadism due to a mutation in the gene for the b-subunit of follicle-stimulating hormone. N Engl J Med. 1998;338:1729-32.
123. Díez JJ, Iglesias P, Sastre J, et al. Isolated deficiency of follicle-stimulating hormone in man: a case report and literature review. Int J Fertil Menopausal Stud. 1994;39(1):26-31
124. Layman LC, Lee EJ, Peak DB, et al. Delayed puberty and hypogonadism caused by mutations in the follicle-stimulating hormone beta-subunit gene. N Engl J Med. 1997;337:607-11.
125. Kottler ML, Chou YY, Chabre O, et al. A new FSH mutation in a 29-year-old woman with primary amenorrhea and isolated FSH deficiency: functional characterization and ovarian response to human recombinant FSH. Eur J Endocrinol. 2010;162(3):633-41.
126. Matthews CH, Borgato S, Beck-Peccoz P, et al. Primary amenorrhoea and infertility due to a mutation in the beta-subunit of follicle stimulating hormone. Nat Genet. 1993;5:83-6.
127. Phillip M, Arbelle JE, Segev Y, et al. Male hypogonadism due to a mutation in the gene for the beta-subunit of follicle-stimulating hormone. N Engl J Med. 1998;338:1729-32.
128. Kumar TR, Wang Y, Lu N, et al. Follicle stimulating hormone is required for ovarian follicle maturation but not male fertility. Nat Genet. 1997;15:201-4.

129. Zirkin BR, Awoniyi C, Griswold MD, et al. Is FSH required for adult spermatogenesis? J Androl. 1994;15:27.
130. Tapanainen JS, Aittomaki K, Min J, et al. Men homozygous for an inactivating mutation of the follicle-stimulating hormone (FSH) receptor gene present variable suppression of spermatogenesis and fertility. Nat Genet. 1997;5(2):205-6.
131. Gromoll J, Pekel E, Nieschlag E. The structure and organization of the human follicle stimulating hormone receptor (FSHR) gene. Genomics. 1996;35(2):308-11.
132. Heckert LL, Daley IJ, Griswold MD. Structural organization of the follicle-stimulating hormone receptor gene. Mol Endocrinol. 1992;6(1):70-80.
133. Simoni M, Gromoll J, Hoppner W, et al. Mutational analysis of the follicle-stimulating hormone (FSH) receptor in normal and infertile men: identification and characterization of two discrete FSH receptor isoforms. J Clin Endocrinol Metab. 1999;84:751-5.
134. Ahda Y, Gromoll J, Wunsch A, et al. Follicle-stimulating hormone receptor gene haplotype distribution in normozoospermic and azoospermic men. J Androl. 2005;26:494-9.
135. Weiss J, Axelrod L, Whitcomb RW, et al. Hypogonadism caused by a single amino acid substitution in the beta subunit of luteinizing hormone. N Engl J Med. 1992;326:179-83.
136. Lofrano-Porto A, Barra GB, Giacomini LA, et al. Luteinizing hormone beta mutation and hypogonadism in men and women. N Engl J Med. 2007;357:897-904.
137. Daly AF, Salvi R, Menage J, et al. Identification of a family harboring a novel LH beta-subunit mutation associated with hypogonadism. Abstracts 88th Annu Meet Endocr Soc. Boston; 2006.
138. Rousseau-Merck MF, Misrahi M, Atger M, et al. Localization of the human luteinizing hormone/choriogonadotropin receptor gene (LHCGR) to chromosome 2p21. Cytogenet Cell Genet. 1990;54:77-9.
139. Bertheze`ne F, Forest MG, Grimaud JA, et al. Leydig-cell agenesis: a cause of male pseudohermaphroditism. N Engl J Med. 1976;295:969-72.
140. Foresta C, Garolla A, Bartoloni L, et al. Genetic abnormalities among severely oligospermic men who are candidates for intracytoplasmic sperm injection. J Clin Endocrinol Metab. 2005;90:152-6.
141. Georgiou I, Syrrou M, Pardalidis N, et al. Genetic and epigenetic risks of intracytoplasmic sperm injection method. Asian J Androl. 2006;8:643-73.
142. Ron-El R, Strassburger D, Gelman-Kohan S, et al. A 47, XXY fetus conceived after ICSI of spermatozoa from a patient with non-mosaic Klinefelter's syndrome: case report. Hum Reprod. 2000;15:1804-6.
143. Schiff JD, Palermo GD, Veeck LL, et al. Success of testicular sperm injection and intracytoplasmic sperm injection in men with Klinefelter syndrome. J Clin Endocrinol Metab. 2005;90:6263-7.
144. Staessen C, Tournaye H, Van Assche E, et al. PGD in 47, XXY Klinefelter's syndrome patients. Hum Reprod Update. 2003;9:319-30.
145. Sciurano RB, Luna Hisano CV, Rahn MI, et al. Focal spermatogenesis originates in euploid germ cells in classical Klinefelter patients. Hum Reprod. 2009;24:2353-60.
146. Schweikert HU, Weissbach L, Leyendecker G, et al. Clinical, endocrinological, and cytological characterization of two 46, XX males. J Clin Endocrinol Metab. 1982;54:745-52.
147. Behlke MA, Bogan JS, Beer-Romero P, et al. Evidence that the SRY protein is encoded by a single exon on the human Y chromosome. Genomics. 1993;17:736-9.
148. Abbas NE, Toublanc JE, Boucekkine C, et al. A possible common origin of "Y-negative" human XX males and XX true hermaphrodites. Hum Genet. 1990;84:356-60.
149. Dada R, Ahmed ME, Talwar R, et al. Clinical and Genetic study in a XX (SRY negative) male. Int J Med, 2002.
150. Nieschelag E, Behre H, Wieaker P, et al. Disorders at the testicular level. In: Nieschlag E, Behre HM, Nieschlag S (Eds). Andrology Male Reproductive Health and Dysfunction, 3rd edition. Berlin Heidelberg, Germany; Springer Verlag: 2010. pp. 193-238.
151. Glickman MH, Ciechanover A. The ubiquitin-proteasome proteolytic pathway: destruction for the sake of construction. Physiological Reviews. 2002;82:373-428.
152. Wei L, Shi YC, Cui YX, et al. Mutation of the USP26 gene in spermatogenesis dysfunction. Zhonghua Nan Ke Xue. 2010;16(1):65-7.
153. Stouffs K, Tournaye H, Liebaers I, et al. Male infertility and the involvement of the X chromosome. Hum Reprod Update. 2009;15(6):623-37. Epub 2009.
154. Stouffs K, Lissens W, Tournaye H, et al. Possible role of USP26 in patients with severely impaired spermatogenesis. Eur J Hum Genet. 2005;13:336-40.
155. Paduch DA, Mielnik A, Schlegel PN. Novel mutations in testis-specific ubiquitin protease 26 gene may cause male infertility and hypogonadism. Reprod Biomed Online. 2005;10:747-54.
156. Stouffs K, Lissens W, Tournaye H, et al. Alterations of the USP26 gene in Caucasian men. Int J Androl. 2006;29:614-7.
157. Ravel C, El Houate B, Chantot S, et al. Haplotypes, mutations and male fertility: the story of the testis-specific ubiquitin protease USP26. Mol Hum Reprod. 2006;12:643-6.
158. Kiefer JC. Back to basics: Sox genes. Dev Dyn. 2007;236(8):2356-66.
159. Graves JA. Interactions between SRY and SOX genes in mammalian sex determination. Bioessays. 1998;20:264-9.
160. Graves JA. Evolution of the mammalian Y chromosome and sex-determining genes. J Exp Zool. 1998;281:472-81.
161. Solomon NM, Ross SA, Morgan T, et al. Array comparative genomic hybridisation analysis of boys with X linked hypopituitarism identifies a 3.9 Mb duplicated critical region at Xq27 containing SOX3. J Med Genet. 2004;41:669-78.
162. Solomon NM, Ross SA, Forrest SM, et al. Array comparative genomic hybridisation analysis of boys with X-linked hypopituitarism identifies a 3.9 Mb duplicated

critical region at Xq27 containing SOX3. J Med Genet. 2007;44:e75.
163. Woods KS, Cundall M, Turton J, et al. Over- and underdosage of SOX3 is associated with infundibular hypoplasia and hypopituitarism. Am J Hum Genet. 2005;76:833-49.
164. Raverot G, Lejeune H, Kotlar T, et al. X-linked sex-determining region Y box 3 (SOX3) gene mutations are uncommon in men with idiopathic oligoazoospermic infertility. J Clin Endocrinol Metab. 2004;89(8):4146-8.
165. Weiss J, Meeks JJ, Hurley L, et al. Sox3 is required for gonadal function, but not sex determination, in males and females. Mol Cell Biol. 2003;23:8084-91.
166. Zenaty D, Dijoud F, Morel Y, et al. Bilateral anorchia in infancy: occurence of micropenis and the effect of testosterone. J Pediatr. 2006;149(5):687-91.
167. Philibert P, Zenaty D, Lin L, et al. Mutational analysis of steroidogenic factor 1 (NR5a1) in 24 boys with bilateral anorchia: a French collaborative study. Hum Reprod. 2007;22(12):3255-61.
168. Nora JJ, Nora AH, Sinha AK, et al. The Ullrich-Noonan syndrome (Turner phenotype). American Journal of Diseases of Children. 1974;127:48-55.
169. Tartaglia M, Gelb BD, Zenker M. Noonan syndrome and clinically related disorders. Best Pract Res Clin Endocrinol Metab. 2011;25(1):161-79.
170. Sharland M, Burch M, McKenna WM, et al. A clinical study of Noonan syndrome. Arch Dis Child. 1992;67:178-83.
171. Kelnar CJ. Noonan syndrome: the hypothalamo-adrenal and hypothalamo-gonadal axes. Horm Res. 2009;72(Suppl 2):24-30. Epub 2009.
172. Chang HJ, Clark RD, Bachman H. The phenotype of 45,X/46,XY mosaicism: an analysis of 92 prenatally diagnosed cases. Am J Hum Genet. 1990;46:156-67.
173. Telvi L, Lebbar A, Del Pino O, et al. 45,X/46,XY mosaicism: report of 27 cases. Pediatrics. 1999;104:304-8.
174. Caglayan AO, Demiryilmaz F, Kendirci M, et al. Mixed gonadal dysgenesis with 45,X/46,X,idic(Y)/46,XY,idic(Y) karyotype. Genet Couns. 2009;20(2):173-9.
175. Reynolds N, Cooke HJ. Role of the DAZ genes in male fertility. Reprod Biomed Online. 2005;10:72-80.
176. Schlegel PN. Causes of azoospermia and their management. Reprod Fertil Dev. 2004;16: 561-72.
177. Katagiri Y, Neri QV, Takeuchi T, et al. Y chromosome assessment and its implications for the development of ICSI children. Reprod Biomed Online. 2004;8:307-18.
178. Foresta C, Moro E, Ferlin A. Y chromosome microdeletions and alterations of spermatogenesis. Endocr Rev. 2001;22:226-39.
179. Dohle GR, Halley DJ, Van Hemel JO, et al. Genetic risk factors in infertile men with severe oligozoospermia and azoospermia. Hum Reprod. 2002;17:13-6.
180. de Vries JW, Repping S, Oates R, et al. Absence of deleted in azoospermia (DAZ) genes in spermatozoa of infertile men with somatic DAZ deletions. Fertil Steril. 2001;75:476-9.
181. Peterlin B, Kunej T, Sinkovec J, et al. Screening for Y chromosome microdeletions in 226 Slovenian subfertile men. Hum Reprod. 2002;17:17-24.
182. Krausz C, Forti G, McElreavey K. The Y chromosome and male fertility and infertility. Int J Androl. 2003;26:70-5.
183. Skaletsky H, Kuroda-Kawaguchi T, Minx PJ, et al. The male-specific region of the human Y chromosome is a mosaic of discrete sequence classes. Nature. 2003;423:825-37.
184. Vogt PH. Azoospermia factor (AZF) in Yq11: towards a molecular understanding of its function for human male fertility and spermatogenesis. Reprod Biomed Online. 2005;10:81-93.
185. Ferlin A, Arredi B, Speltra E, et al. Molecular and clinical characterization of Y chromosome microdeletions in infertile men: a 10-year experience in Italy. J Clin Endocrinol Metab. 2007;92:762-70.
186. Nuti F, Krausz C. Gene polymorphisms/mutations relevant to abnormal spermatogenesis. Reprod Biomed Online. 2008;16:504-13.
187. Lardone MC, Parodi DA, Valdevenito R, et al. Quantification of DDX3Y, RBMY1, DAZ and TSPY mRNAs in testes of patients with severe impairment of spermatogenesis. Mol Hum Reprod. 2007;13:705-12.
188. Tyler-Smith C. An evolutionary perspective on Y chromosomal variation and male infertility. Int J Androl. 2008;31:376-82.
189. Brown GM, Furlong RA, Sargent CA, et al. Characterisation of the coding sequence and fine mapping of the human DFFRY gene and comparative expression analysis and mapping to the Sxrb interval of the mouse Y chromosome of the Dffry gene. Hum Mol Genet. 1998;7:97-107.
190. Krausz C, Degl'Innocenti S, Nuti F, et al. Natural transmission of USP9Y gene mutations: a new perspective on the role of AZFa genes in male fertility. Hum Mol Genet. 2006;15:2673-81.
191. Elliott DJ. The role of potential splicing factors including RBMY, RBMX, hnRNPG-T and STAR proteins in spermatogenesis. Int J Androl. 2004;27:328-34.
192. Lavery R, Glennon M, Houghton J, et al. Investigation of DAZ and RBMY1 gene expression in human testis by quantitative real-time PCR. Arch Androl. 2007;53:71-3.
193. Ferlin A, Moro E, Rossi A, et al. The human Y chromosome's azoospermia factor b (AZFb) region: sequence, structure, and deletion analysis in infertile men. J Med Genet. 2003;40:18-24.
194. Vogt PH. Human chromosome deletions in Yq11, AZF candidate genes and male infertility: history and update. Mol Hum Reprod. 1998;4:739-44.
195. Kuroda-Kawaguchi T, Skaletsky H, Brown LG, et al. The AZFc region of the Y chromosome features massive palindromes and uniform recurrent deletions in infertile men. Nat Genet. 2001;29:279-86.
196. Zhang F, Lu C, Li Z, et al. Partial deletions are associated with an increased risk of complete deletion in AZFc: a new insight into the role of partial AZFc deletions in male infertility. J Med Genet. 2007;44:437-44.
197. Arredi B, Ferlin A, Speltra E, et al. Y-chromosome haplogroups and susceptibility to azoospermia factor c microdeletion in an Italian population. J Med Genet. 2007;44:205-8.

198. Siffroi JP, Le Bourhis C, Krausz C, et al. Sex chromosome mosaicism in males carrying Y chromosome long arm deletions. Hum Reprod. 2000;15:2559-62.
199. Jaruzelska J, Korcz A, Wojda A, et al. Mosaicism for 45, X cell line may accentuate the severity of spermatogenic defects in men with AZFc deletion. J Med Genet. 2001;38:798-802.
200. Patsalis PC, Sismani C, Quintana-Murci L, et al. Effects of transmission of Y chromosome AZFc deletions. Lancet. 2002;360:1222-4.
201. Bateson P, Barker D, Clutton-Brock T, et al. Developmental plasticity and human health. Nature. 2004;430:419-21.
202. Lardone MC, Parodi DA, Ebensperger M, et al. AZFc partial deletions in Chilean men with severe spermatogenic failure. Fertil Steril. 2007;88:1318-26.
203. Lin YW, Hsu LC, Kuo PL, et al. Partial duplication at AZFc on the Y chromosome is a risk factor for impaired spermatogenesis in Han Chinese in Taiwan. Hum Mutat. 2007;28:486-94.
204. Ferlin A, Moro E, Garolla A, et al. Human male infertility and Y chromosome deletions: role of the AZF-candidate genes DAZ, RBM and DFFRY. Hum Reprod. 1999;14:1710-6.
205. Yen HW, Jakimiuk AJ, Munir I, et al. Selective alterations in insulin receptor substrates-1, -2 and -4 in theca but not granulosa cells from polycystic ovaries. Mol Hum Reprod. 2004;10:473-9.
206. Reijo R, Lee TY, Salo P, et al. Diverse spermatogenic defects in humans caused by Y chromosome deletions encompassing a novel RNA-binding protein gene. Nat Genet. 1995;10:383-93.
207. Writzl K, Zorn B, Peterlin B. Copy number of DAZ genes in infertile men. Fertil Steril. 2005;84:1522-5.
208. Cram DS, Ma K, Bhasin S, et al. Y chromosome analysis of infertile men and their sons conceived through intracytoplasmic sperm injection: vertical transmission of deletions and rarity of de novo deletions. Fertil Steril. 2000;74: 909-15.
209. Sadeghi-Nejad H, Farrokhi F. Genetics of azoospermia: current knowledge, clinical implications, and future directions. Part II. Y chromosome microdeletions. Urol J. 2007;4:192-206.
210. Mitra A, Dada R, Kumar R, et al. Screening for Y-chromosome microdeletions in infertile Indian males: utility of simplified multiplex PCR. Indian J Med Res. 2008;127:124-32.
211. Schnieders F, Dork T, Arnemann J, et al. Testis-specific protein, Y-encoded (TSPY) expression in testicular tissues. Hum Mol Genet. 1996;5:1801-7.
212. Vodicka R, Vrtel R, Dusek L, et al. TSPY gene copy number as a potential new risk factor for male infertility. Reprod Biomed Online. 2007;14:579-87.
213. Sassone-Corsi P. Transcriptional checkpoints determining the fate of male germ cells. Cell. 1997;88:163-6.
214. Kimmins S, Kotaja N, Davidson I, et al. Testis-specific transcription mechanisms promoting male germ-cell differentiation. Reproduction. 2004;128:5-12.
215. Falender AE, Freiman RN, Geles KG, et al. Maintenance of spermatogenesis requires TAF4b, a gonad-specific subunit of TFIID. Genes Dev. 2005;19:794-803.
216. Akinloye O, Gromoll J, Callies C, et al. Mutation analysis of the X-chromosome linked, testis-specific TAF7L gene in spermatogenic failure. Andrologia. 2007;39:190-5.
217. Stouffs K, Willems A, Lissens W, et al. The role of the testis-specific gene hTAF7L in the aetiology of male infertility. Mol Hum Reprod. 2006;12:263-7.
218. Powell CM. Sex chromosomes and sex chromosome abnormalities. In: Gersen SL, Keagle MB (Eds). The Principles of Clinical Cytogenetics, 2nd edition. New Jersey, USA: Humana Press Inc; 2005. pp. 207-46.
219. Ma S, Yuen BH, Penaherrera M, et al. ICSI and the transmission of Xautosomal translocation: a three-generation evaluation of X ;20 translocation: case Report. Hum. Reprod. 2003;18:1377-82.
220. Sivak LE, Esbenshade J, Brothman AR, et al. Multiple congenital anomalies in a man with (X;6) translocation. Am J Med Genet. 1994;51:9-12.
221. White WM, Willard HF, Van Dyke KL, et al. The spreading of X inactivation into autosomal material of an X; autosome translocation: evidence for a difference between autosomal and X-chromosomal DNA. Am J Hum Genet. 1998;63:20-8.
222. Carrell DT. Contributions of spermatozoa to embryogenesis: assays to evaluate their genetic and epigenetic fitness. Reprod Biomed Online. 2008;16:474-84.
223. Chandley AC, Edmond P, Christie S, et al. Cytogenetics and infertility in man. I. Karyotype and seminal analysis: results of a 5-year survey of men attending a subfertility clinic. Ann Hum Genet. 1975;39:231-54.
224. Elliott DJ, Cooke HJ. The molecular genetics of male infertility. Bioessays. 1997;19:801-9.
225. Therman E, Susman M. Human chromosome: structure, behaviour and effects. New York: Springer-Verlag; 1993.
226. De Braekeleer M, Dao TN. Cytogenetic studies in male infertility: a review. Hum Reprod. 1991;6:245-50.
227. Johnson MD. Genetic risks of intracytoplasmic sperm injection in the treatment of male infertility: recommendations for genetic counseling and screening. Fertil Steril. 1998;70:397-411.
228. Meschede D, Lemcke B, Exeler JR, et al. Chromosome abnormalities in 447 couples undergoing intracytoplasmic sperm injection—prevalence, types, sex distribution and reproductive relevance. Hum Reprod. 1998;13:576-82.
229. Maglott D, Ostell J, Pruitt KD, et al. Entrez Gene: gene-centered information at NCBI. Nucleic Acids Res. 2005;33:D54-8.
230. Tuttelmann F, Rajpert-De Meyts E, Nieschlag E, et al. Gene polymorphisms and male infertility—a meta-analysis and literature review. Reprod Biomed Online. 2007;15:643-58.
231. Teng YN, Lin YM, Lin YH, et al. Association of a single-nucleotide polymorphism of the deleted-in-azoospermia-like gene with susceptibility to spermatogenic failure. J Clin Endocrinol Metab. 2002;87:5258-64.
232. Tung JY, Rosen MP, Nelson LM, et al. Novel missense mutations of the Deleted-in-AZoospermia-Like (DAZL)

gene in infertile women and men. Reprod Biol Endocrinol. 2006;4:40

233. Tung JY, Rosen MP, Nelson LM, et al. Variants in deleted in azoospermia-like (DAZL) are correlated with reproductive parameters in men and women. Hum Genet. 2006;118:730-40.
234. Teng YN, Lin YM, Sun HF, et al. Association of DAZL haplotypes with spermatogenic failure in infertile men. Fertil Steril. 2006;86:129-35.
235. Frosst P, Blom HJ, Milos R, et al. A candidate genetic risk factor for vascular disease: a common mutation in methylenetetrahydrofolate reductase. Nat Genet. 1995;10:111-3.
236. Park JH, Lee HC, Jeong YM, et al. MTHFR C677 T polymorphism associates with unexplained infertile male factors. J Assist Reprod Genet. 2005;22:361-8.
237. Singh K, Singh SK, Sah R, et al. Mutation C677 T in the methylenetetrahydrofolate reductase gene is associated with male infertility in an Indian population. Int J Androl. 2005;28:115-9.
238. Olesen IA, Sonne SB, Hoei-Hansen CE, et al. Environment, testicular dysgenesis and carcinoma in situ testis. Best Pract Res Clin Endocrinol Metab. 2007;21:462-78.
239. Ferlin A, Foresta C. The INSL3-LGR8 hormonal system in humans: testicular descent, cryptorchidism and testicular functions. Curr Med Chem. 2005;10(1):421-30.
240. Zimmermann S, Steding G, Emmen JM, et al. Targeted disruption of the Insl3 gene causes bilateral cryptorchidism. Mol Endocrinol. 1999;13:681-91.
241. Adham IM, Agoulnik AI. Insulin-like 3 signalling in testicular descent. Int J Androl. 2004;27:257-65.
242. Wang PJ, McCarrey JR, Yang F, et al. An abundance of X-linked genes expressed in spermatogonia. Nat Genet. 2001;27:422-6.
243. Lazaros L, Xita N, Kaponis A, et al. Evidence for association of sex hormone-binding globulin and androgen receptor genes with semen quality. Andrologia. 2008;40:186-91.
244. Guarducci E, Nuti F, Becherini L, et al. Estrogen receptor alpha promoter polymorphism: stronger estrogen action is coupled with lower sperm count. Hum Reprod. 2006;21:994-1001.
245. Yoshida R, Fukami M, Sasagawa I, et al. Association of cryptorchidism with a specific haplotype of the estrogen receptor alpha gene: implication for the susceptibility to estrogenic environmental endocrine disruptors. J Clin Endocrinol Metab. 2005;90:4716-21.
246. Galan JJ, Guarducci E, Nuti F, et al. Molecular analysis of estrogen receptor alpha gene AGATA haplotype and SNP12 in European populations: potential protective effect for cryptorchidism and lack of association with male infertility. Hum Reprod. 2007;22:444-9.
247. De Gendt K, Swinnen JV, Saunders PT, et al. A Sertoli cell-selective knockout of the androgen receptor causes spermatogenic arrest in meiosis. Proc Natl Acad Sci USA. 2004;101:1327-32.
248. Galani A, Kitsiou-Tzeli S, Sofokleous C, et al. Androgen insensitivity syndrome: clinical features and molecular defects. Hormones (Athens). 2008;7(3):217-29.
249. Ferlin A, Vinanzi C, Garolla A, et al. Male infertility and androgen receptor gene mutations: clinical features and identification of seven novel mutations. Clin Endocrinol (Oxf). 2006;65:606-10.
250. Mifsud A, Sim CK, Boettger-Tong H, et al. Trinucleotide (CAG) repeat polymorphisms in the androgen receptor gene: molecular markers of risk for male infertility. Fertil Steril. 2001;75:275-81.
251. Tut TG, Ghadessy FJ, Trifiro MA, et al. Long polyglutamine tracts in the androgen receptor are associated with reduced trans-activation, impaired sperm production, and male infertility. J Clin Endocrinol Metab. 1997;82:3777-82.
252. Lundin KB, Giwercman A, Richthoff J, et al. No association between mutations in the human androgen receptor GGN repeat and inter-sex conditions. Mol Hum Reprod. 2003;9:375-9.
253. Rajpert-De Meyts E, Leffers H, Petersen JH, et al. CAG repeat length in androgen-receptor gene and reproductive variables in fertile and infertile men. Lancet. 2002;359:44-6.
254. Yong EL, Loy CJ, Sim KS. Androgen receptor gene and male infertility. Hum Reprod Update. 2003;9:1-7.
255. Dowsing AT, Yong EL, Clark M, et al. Linkage between male infertility and trinucleotide repeat expansion in the androgen-receptor gene. Lancet. 1999;354:640-3.
256. Sharma V, Singh R, Thangaraj K, et al. A novel Arg615Ser mutation of androgen receptor DNA-binding domain in three 46,XY sisters with complete androgen insensitivity syndrome and bilateral inguinal hernia. Fertil Steril. 2011;95(2):804.e19-21.
257. Gottlieb B, Lombroso R, Beitel LK, et al. Molecular pathology of the androgen receptor in male (in)fertility. Reprod Biomed Online. 2005;10(1):42-8.
258. Nenonen H, Bjork C, Skjaerpe PA, et al. CAG repeat number is not inversely associated with androgen receptor activity in vitro. Mol Hum Reprod. 2010;16(3):153-7.
259. Ferlin A, Bartoloni L, Rizzo G, et al. Androgen receptor gene CAG and GGC repeat lengths in idiopathic male infertility. Mol Hum Reprod. 2004;10(6):417-21.
260. Cram DS, Song B, McLachlan RI, et al. CAG trinucleotide repeats in the androgen receptor gene of infertile men exhibit stable inheritance in female offspring conceived after ICSI. Mol Hum Reprod. 2000;6(9):861-6.
261. Stocco DM. StAR protein and the regulation of steroid hormone biosynthesis. Annu Rev Physiol. 2001;63:193-213.
262. Bose HS, Pescovitz OH, Miller WL. Spontaneous feminization in a 46,XX female patient with congenital lipoid adrenal hyperplasia due to a homozygous frameshift mutation in the steroidogenic acute regulatory protein. J Clin Endocrinol Metab. 1997;82:1511-5.
263. Sahakitrungruang T, Soccio RE, Lang-Muritano M, et al. Clinical, genetic, and functional characterization of four patients carrying partial loss-of-function mutations in the steroidogenic acute regulatory protein (StAR). J Clin Endocrinol Metab. 2010;95(7):3352-9. Epub 2010.
264. Metherell LA, Naville D, Halaby G, et al. Nonclassic lipoid congenital adrenal hyperplasia masquerading

as familial glucocorticoid deficiency. J Clin Endocrinol Metab. 2009;94:3865-71.

265. Pang S. The molecular and clinical spectrum of 3b-hydroxysteroid dehydrogenase deficiency disorder. Trends Endocrinol Metab. 1998;9(2)82-6.
266. Müssig K, Kaltenbach S, Maser-Gluth C, et al. Late diagnosis of congenital adrenal hyperplasia due to 21-hydroxylase deficiency. Exp Clin Endocrinol Diabetes. 2006;114(4):208-14.
267. Imperato-McGinley J, Guerrero L, Gautier T, et al. Steroid 5 alpha-reductase deficiency in man. An inherited form of male pseudohermaphroditism. Birth Defects Orig Artic Ser. 1975;11(4):91-103.
268. Leshin M, Griffin JE, Wilson JD. Hereditary male pseudohermaphroditism associated with an unstable form of 5 alpha-reductase. J Clin Invest. 1978;62(3):685-91.
279. Radpour R, Gourabi H, Gilani MA, et al. Molecular study of (TG)m(T)n polymorphisms in Iranian males with congenital bilateral absence of the vas deferens. J Androl. 2007;28:541-7.
270. Uzun S, Gokce S, Wagner K. Cystic fibrosis transmembrane conductance regulator gene mutations in infertile males with congenital bilateral absence of the vas deferens. Tohoku J Exp Med. 2005;207(4):279-85.
271. Bulletin T. Practice Committee of American Society for Reproductive Medicine in collaboration with Society for Male Reproduction and Urology: evaluation of the azoospermic male. American Society for Reproductive Medicine, Fertil Steril. 2008;90(5 Suppl):S74-7.
272. Chillon M, Casals T, Mercier B, et al. Mutations in the cystic fibrosis gene in patients with congenital absence of the vas deferens. N Engl J Med. 1995;332(22):1475-80.
273. Massagué J. TGF-beta signal transduction. Annu Rev Biochem. 1998;67:753-91.
274. Visser JA. AMH signaling: from receptor to target gene. Mol Cell Endocrinol. 2003;211(1-2):65-73.
275. Josso N, Belville C, di Clemente N, et al. AMH and AMH receptor defects in persistent Müllerian duct syndrome. Hum Reprod Update. 2005;11(4):351-6. Epub 2005.
276. Imbeaud S, Belville C, Messika-Zeitoun L, et al. A 27 base-pair deletion of the anti-Müllerian type II receptor gene is the most common cause of the persistent Müllerian duct syndrome. Hum Mol Genet. 1996;5:1269-79.
277. Hendry WF, Levison DA, Parkinson MC, et al. Testicular obstruction: clinicopathological studies. Ann R Coll Surg Engl. 1990;72:396-407.
278. Arya AK, Beer HL, Benton J, et al. Does Young's syndrome exist? J Laryngol Otol. 2009;123(5):477-81. Epub 2009.
279. Teichtahl H, Temple-Smith PD, Johnson JL, et al. Obstructive azoospermia and chronic sinobronchial disease (Young's syndrome) in identical twins. Fertil Steril. 1987;47:879-81.
280. Umeki S, Soejima R, Kawane H. Young's syndrome accompanied by medullary sponge kidney. Respiration. 1989;55:60-4.
281. Handelsman DJ, Conway AJ, Boylan LM, et al. Young's syndrome. Obstructive azoospermia and chronic sinopulmonary infections. N Engl J Med. 1984;310(1):3-9.
282. Meschede D, Dworniczak B, Nieschlag E, et al. Genetic diseases of the seminal ducts. Biomed Pharmacother. 1998;52(5):197-203.
283. Lishko PV, Kirichok Y. The role of Hv1 and CatSper channels in sperm activation. J Physiol. 2010;588 (Pt 23):4667-72.
284. Carlson AE, Burnett LA, Del Camino D, et al. Pharmacological targeting of native CatSper channels reveals a required role in maintenance of sperm hyperactivation. PLoS One. 2009;4:e6844.
285. Wang H, Liu J, Cho KH, et al. A novel, single, transmembrane protein CATSPERG is associated with CATSPER1 channel protein. Biol Reprod. 2009;81:539-44.
286. Avenarius MR, Hildebrand MS, Zhang Y, et al. Human male infertility caused by mutations in the CATSPER1 channel protein. Am J Hum Genet. 2009;84:505-10.
287. Qi H, Moran MM, Navarro B, et al. All four CatSper ion channel proteins are required for male fertility and sperm cell hyperactivated motility. Proc Natl Acad Sci USA. 2007;104:1219-23.
288. Hildebrand MS, Avenarius MR, Smith RJ (2009). CATSPER-related male infertility. Gene Reviews-NCBI Bookshelf. Bookshelf; U.S. National Library of Medicine National Institutes of Health [monograph on the Internet]. Available from: U.S. National Library of Medicine National Institutes of Health, Website: http://0-www.ncbi.nlm.nih.gov.library.ccf.org/books/NBK22925/ [cited May 2011].
289. Afzelius BA. The immotile-cilia syndrome: a microtubule-associated defect. CRC Crit Rev Biochem. 1985;19:63-87.
290. Escudier E, Duquesnoy P, Papon JF, et al. Ciliary defects and genetics of primary ciliary dyskinesia. Paediatr Respir Rev. 2009;10(2):51-4. Epub 2009.
291. Chilvers MA, Rutman AO, Callaghan C. Ciliary beat pattern is associated with specific ultrastructural defects in primary ciliary dyskinesia. J Allergy Clin Immunol. 2003;112:518-24.
292. Chao J, Turner JA, Sturgess JM. Genetic heterogeneity of dynein-deficiency in cilia from patients with respiratory disease. Am Rev Respir Dis. 1982;126:302-5.
293. Fliegauf M, Olbrich H, Horvath J, et al. Mislocalization of DNAH5 and DNAH9 in respiratory cells from patients with primary ciliary dyskinesia. Am J Respir Crit Care Med. 2005;171:1343-9.
294. Dam AH, Feenstra I, Westphal JR, et al. Globozoospermia revisited. Hum Reprod. 2007;13:63-75.
295. Koscinski I, Elinati E, Fossard C, et al. DPY19L2 deletion as a major cause of globozoospermia. Am J Hum Genet. 2011;88(3):344-50.
296. Dam AH, Koscinski I, Kremer JA, et al. Homozygous mutation in SPATA16 is associated with male infertility in human globozoospermia. Am J Hum Genet. 2007;81(4):813-20. Epub 2007.
297. Liu G, Shi QW, Lu GX. A newly discovered mutation in PICK1 in a human with globozoospermia. Asian J Androl. 2010;12(4):556-60. Epub 2010.

298. Egozcue J, Templado C, Vidal F, et al. Meiotic studies in a series of 1100 infertile and sterile males. Hum Genet. 1983;65(2):185-8.
299. Khorram O, Patrizio P, Wang C, et al. Reproductive technologies for male infertility. J Clin Endocrinol Metab. 2001;86(6):2373-9.
300. Bernardini L, Gianaroli L, Fortini D, et al. Frequency of hyper-, hypohaploidy and diploidy in ejaculate, epididymal and testicular germ cells of infertile patients. Hum Reprod. 2000;15:2165-72.
301. Palermo G, Colombero L, Hariprashad J, et al. Chromosome analysis of epididymal and testicular sperm in azoospermic patients undergoing ICSI. Hum Reprod. 2002;17:570-5.
302. Pang M, Hoegerman S, Cuticchia A, et al. Detection of aneuploidy for chromosomes 4, 6, 7, 8, 9, 10, 11, 12, 13, 17, 18, 21, X and Y by fluorescence in-situ hybridization in spermatozoa from nine patients with oligoasthenoteratozoospermia undergoing intracytoplasmic sperm injection. Hum Reprod. 1999;14:1266-73.
303. Griffin DK, Hyland P, Tempest HG et al. Safety issues in assisted reproduction technology: should men undergoing ICSI be screened for chromosome abnormalities in their sperm? Hum Reprod. 2003;18:229-35.
304. Tempest HG, Griffin DK. The relationship between male infertility and increased levels of sperm disomy. Cytogenet Genome Res. 2004;107:83-94.
305. Benzacken B, Gavelle FM, Martin-Pont B, et al. Familial sperm polyploidy induced by genetic spermatogenesis failure: case report. Hum Reprod. 2001;16:2646-51.
306. Devillard F, Metzler-Guillemain C, Pelletier R, et al. Polyploidy in largeheaded sperm: FISH study of three cases. Hum Reprod. 2002;17:1292-8.
307. In't Veld PA, Broekmans FJ, de France HF, et al. Intracytoplasmic sperm injection (ICSI) and chromosomally abnormal spermatozoa. Hum Reprod. 1997;12:752-4.
308. Lewis-Jones I, Aziz N, Sheshadri S, et al. Sperm chromosomal abnormalities are linked to sperm morphological deformities. Fertil Steril. 2003;79:212-5.
309. Spano M, Bonde JP, Hjollund HI, et al. Sperm chromatin damage impairs human fertility. The Danish First Pregnancy Planner Study Team. Fertil Steril. 2000;73(1):43-50.
310. Zini A, Bielecki R, Phang D, et al. Correlations between two markers of sperm DNA integrity, DNA denaturation and DNA fragmentation, in fertile and infertile men. Fertil Steril. 2001;75(4):674-7.
311. Oliva R. Protamines and male infertility. Hum Reprod Update. 2006;12(4):417-35.
312. Carrell DT, Liu L. Altered protamine 2 expression is uncommon in donors of known fertility, but common among men with poor fertilizing capacity, and may reflect other abnormalities of spermiogenesis. J Androl. 2001;22(4):604-10.
313. Sakkas D, Seli E, Manicardi GC, et al. The presence of abnormal spermatozoa in the ejaculate: did apoptosis fail? Hum Fertil (Camb). 2004;7(2):99-103.
314. Giwercman A, Richthoff J, Hjollund H, et al. Correlation between sperm motility and sperm chromatin structure assay parameters. Fertil Steril. 2003;80(6):1404-12.
315. Moskovtsev SI, Willis J, Azad A, et al. Sperm DNA integrity: correlation with sperm plasma membrane integrity in semen evaluated for male infertility. Arch Androl. 2005;51(1):33-40.
316. Tseden K, Topaloglu O, Meinhardt A, et al. Premature translation of transition protein 2 mRNA causes sperm abnormalities and male infertility. Mol Reprod Dev. 2007;74(3):273-9.
317. Hammoud S, Liu L, Carrell DT. Protamine ratio and the level of histone retention in sperm selected from adensity gradient preparation. Andrologia. 2009;41(2):88-94.
318. Haraguchi T, Ishikawa T, Yamaguchi K, et al. Cyclin and protamine as prognostic molecular marker for testicular sperm extraction in patients with azoospermia. Fertil Steril. 2009;91(4 Suppl):1424-6.
319. Tavalaee M, Razavi S, Nasr-Esfahani MH. Influence of sperm chromatin anomalies on assisted reproductive technology outcome. Fertil Steril. 2009;91(4):1119-26.
320. Mengual L, Ballesca JL, Ascaso C, et al. Marked differences in protamine content and P1/P2 ratios in sperm cells from percoll fractions between patients and controls. J Androl. 2003;24(3):438-47.
321. Steger K, Wilhelm J, Konrad L, et al. Both protamine-1 to protamine-2 mRNA ratio and Bcl2 mRNA content in testicular spermatids and ejaculated spermatozoa discriminate between fertile and infertile men. Hum Reprod. 2008;23(1):11-6.
322. Zhang X, San Gabriel M, Zini A. Sperm nuclear histone to protamine ratio in fertile and infertile men: evidence of heterogeneous subpopulations of spermatozoa in the ejaculate. J Androl. 2006;27(3):414-20.
323. Adham IM, Nayernia K, Burkhardt-Gottges E, et al. Teratozoospermia in mice lacking the transition protein 2 (Tnp2). Mol Hum Reprod. 2001;7(6):513-20.
324. Aoki VW, Christensen GL, Atkins JF, et al. Identification of novel polymorphisms in the nuclear protein genes and their relationship with human sperm protamine deficiency and severe male infertility. Fertil Steril. 2006;86(5):1416-22.
325. Cho C, Willis WD, Goulding EH, et al. Haploinsufficiency of protamine-1 or -2 causes infertility in mice. Nat Genet. 2001;28(1):82-6.
326. Nasr-Esfahani MH, Razavi S, Mardani M, et al. Effects of failed oocyte activation and sperm protamine deficiency on fertilization post-ICSI. Reprod Biomed Online. 2007;14(4):422-9.
327. Sharma RK, Sabanegh E, Mahfouz R, et al. TUNEL as a test for sperm DNA damage in the evaluation of male infertility. Urology. 2010;76(6):1380-6. Epub 2010.
328. Venkatesh S, Deecaraman M, Kumar R, et al. Role of reactive oxygen species in the pathogenesis of mitochondrial DNA (mtDNA) mutations in male infertility. Indian J Med Res. 2009;129(2):127-37.
329. Richter C, Suter M, Walter PB. Mitochondrial free radical damage and DNA repair. Biofactors. 1998;7(3):207-8.
330. Wallace DC, Brown MD, Lott MT. Mitochondrial genetics. London: Churchill Livingstone; 1997.

331. Neckelmann N, Li K, Wade RP, et al. cDNA sequence of a human skeletal muscle ADP/ATP translocator: lack of a leader peptide, divergence from a fibroblast translocator cDNA, and coevolution with mitochondrial DNA genes. Proc Natl Acad Sci USA. 1987;84(21):7580-4.
332. Kao S, Chao HT, Wei YH. Mitochondrial deoxyribonucleic acid 4977-bp deletion is associated with diminished fertility and motility of human sperm. Biol Reprod. 1995;52(4):729-36.
333. Shamsi MB, Kumar R, Bhatt A, et al. Mitochondrial DNA mutations in etiopathogenesis of male infertility. Indian J Urol. 2008;24(2):150-4.
334. Tatton WG, Olanow CW. Apoptosis in neurodegenerative diseases: the role of mitochondria. Biochim Biophys Acta. 1999;1410(2):195-213.
335. Li ZX, Ma X, Wang ZH, et al. A differentially methylated region of the DAZ1 gene in spermatic and somatic cells. Asian J Androl. 2006;8:61-7.
336. Sathananthan AH, Ratnasooriya WD, de Silva PK, et al. Characterization of human gamete centrosomes for assisted reproduction. Ital J Anat Embryol. 2001;106:61-73.
337. Rawe VY, Terada Y, Nakamura S, et al. A pathology of the sperm centriole responsible for defective sperm aster formation, syngamy and cleavage. Hum Reprod. 2002;17:2344-9.
338. Palermo G, Munne S, Cohen J. The human zygote inherits its mitotic potential from the male gamete. Hum Reprod. 1994;9:1220-5.
339. Obasaju M, Kadam A, Sultan K, et al. Sperm quality may adversely affect the chromosome constitution of embryos that result from intracytoplasmic sperm injection. Fertil Steril. 1999;72: 1113-5.
340. Emery BR, Carrell DT. The effect of epigenetic sperm abnormalities on early embryogenesis. Asian J Androl. 2006;8:131-42.
341. Kobayashi H, Sato A, Otsu E, et al. Aberrant DNA methylation of imprinted loci in sperm from oligospermic patients. Hum Mol Genet. 2007;16:2542-51.
342. Hajkova P, Erhardt S, Lane N, et al. Epigenetic reprogramming in mouse primordial germ cells. Mech Dev. 2002;117:15-23.
343. Reik W, Dean W, Walter J. Epigenetic reprogramming in mammalian development. Science. 2001;293:1089-93.
344. Sofikitis N, Miyagawa I, Yamamoto Y, et al. Micro- and macro-consequences of ooplasmic injections of early haploid male gametes. Hum Reprod Update. 1998;4:197-212.
345. Kimura Y, Yanagimachi R. Mouse oocytes injected with testicular spermatozoa or round spermatids can develop into normal offspring. Development. 1995;121:2397-405.
346. Aoki VW, Emery BR, Carrell DT. Global sperm deoxyribonucleic acid methylation is unaffected in protamine-deficient infertile males. Fertil Steril. 2006;86:1541-3.
347. Hartmann S, Bergmann M, Bohle RM, et al. Genetic imprinting during impaired spermatogenesis. Mol Hum Reprod. 2006;12:407-11.
348. Lawrence LT, Moley KH. Epigenetics and assisted reproductive technologies: human imprinting syndromes. Semin Reprod Med. 2008;26:143-52.
349. Clayton-Smith J, Laan L. Angelman syndrome: a review of the clinical and genetic aspects. J Med Genet. 2003;40:87-95.
350. De Rycke M, Liebaers I, Van Steirteghem A. Epigenetic risks related to assisted reproductive technologies: risk analysis and epigenetic inheritance. Hum Reprod. 2002;17:2487-94.
351. Cox GF, Burger J, Lip V, et al. Intracytoplasmic sperm injection may increase the risk of imprinting defects. Am J Hum Genet. 2002;71:162-4.
352. Thompson JR, Williams CJ. Genomic imprinting and assisted reproductive technology: connections and potential risks. Semin Reprod Med. 2005;23:285-95.
353. DeBaun MR, Niemitz EL, Feinberg AP. Association of in vitro fertilization with Beckwith-Wiedemann syndrome and epigenetic alterations of LIT1 and H19. Am J Hum Genet. 2003;72:156-60.
354. Maher ER, Brueton LA, Bowdin SC, et al. Beckwith-Wiedemann syndrome and assisted reproduction technology (ART). J Med Genet. 2003;40:62-4.
355. Delaval K, Govin J, Cerqueira F, et al. Differential histone modifications mark mouse imprinting control regions during spermatogenesis. EMBO J. 2007;26:720-9.
356. Reik W. Stability and flexibility of epigenetic gene regulation in mammalian development. Nature. 2007;447:425-32.
357. Martin C, Zhang Y. Mechanisms of epigenetic inheritance. Curr Opin Cell Biol. 2007;19:266-72.
358. Nanassy L, Carrell DT. Paternal effects on early embryogenesis. J Exp Clin Assist Reprod. 2008;5:2.
359. Rousseaux S, Reynoird N, Escoffier E, et al. Epigenetic reprogramming of the male genome during gametogenesis and in the zygote. Reprod Biomed Online. 2008;16:492-503.
360. Aoki VW, Carrell DT. Human protamines and the developing spermatid: their structure, function, expression and relationship with male infertility. Asian J Androl. 2003;5:315-24.
361. Carrell DT, Emery BR, Hammoud S. Altered protamine expression and diminished spermatogenesis: what is the link? Hum Reprod Update. 2007;13:313-27.
362. Yu YE, Zhang Y, Unni E, et al. Abnormal spermatogenesis and reduced fertility in transition nuclear protein 1-deficient mice. Proc Natl Acad Sci USA. 2000;97:4683-8.
363. Lee K, Haugen HS, Clegg CH, et al. Premature translation of protamine 1 mRNA causes precocious nuclear condensation and arrests spermatid differentiation in mice. Proc Natl Acad Sci USA. 1995;92:12451-5.
364. Cho C, Jung-Ha H, Willis WD, et al. Protamine 2 deficiency leads to sperm DNA damage and embryo death in mice. Biol Reprod. 2003;69:211-7.
365. Aoki VW, Moskovtsev SI, Willis J, et al. DNA integrity is compromised in protamine-deficient human sperm. J Androl. 2005;26:741-8.
366. Ravel C, Chantot-Bastaraud S, El Houate B, et al. Mutations in the protamine 1 gene associated with male infertility. Mol Hum Reprod. 2007;13:461-4.
367. Ostermeier GC, Miller D, Huntriss JD, et al. Reproductive biology: delivering spermatozoan RNA to the oocyte. Nature. 2004;429:154.

368. Biermann K, Steger K. Epigenetics in male germ cells. J Androl. 2007;28:466-80.
369. Boerke A, Dieleman SJ, Gadella BM. A possible role for sperm RNA in early embryo development. Theriogenology. 2007;68(Suppl 1):S147-55.
370. Amanai M, Brahmajosyula M, Perry AC. A restricted role for sperm-borne micro RNAs in mammalian fertilization. Biol Reprod. 2006;75:877-84.
371. Zalenskaya IA, Zalensky AO. Telomeres in mammalian male germline cells. Int Rev Cytol. 2002;218:37-67.
372. Hemann MT, Rudolph KL, Strong MA, et al. Telomere dysfunction triggers developmentally regulated germ cell apoptosis. Mol Biol Cell. 2001;12:2023-30.
373. Liu L, Blasco M, Trimarchi J, et al. An essential role for functional telomeres in mouse germ cells during fertilization and early development. Dev Biol. 2002;249:74-84.
374. Fujisawa M, Tanaka H, Tatsumi N, et al. Telomerase activity in the testis of infertile patients with selected causes. Hum Reprod. 1998;13:1476-9.
375. Hansen RS, Laird CD. A new regulatory pathway for fragile X syndrome? Nat Med. 2002;8(11):1204-5.
376. Edwards RG. Genetics, epigenetics and gene silencing in differentiating mammalian embryos. Reprod Biomed Online. 2006;13(5):732-53.
377. Silverstein S, Lerer I, Sagi M, et al. Uniparental disomy in fetuses diagnosed with balanced Robertsonian translocations: risk estimate. Prenat Diagn. 2002;22(8):649-51.
378. Aboulghar H, Aboulghar M, Mansour R, et al. A prospective controlled study of karyotyping for 430 consecutive babies conceived through intracytoplasmic sperm injection. Fertil Steril. 2001;76(2):249-53.
379. Feng C, Wang LQ, Dong MY, et al. Assisted reproductive technology may increase clinical mutation detection in male offspring. Fertil Steril. 2008;90(1):92-6.
380. Dada R, Shamsi MB, Venkatesh S. Attenuation of oxidative stress & DNA damage in varicocelectomy: implications in infertility management. Indian Journal of Medical Research. 2010;(132):728-30.
381. Dada R, Shamsi MB, Venkatesh S (Eds). Genetics of Male Infertility. New Delhi: Jaypee Brothers Medical Publishers (P) Ltd; 2010.
382. Lin YH, Lin YM, Teng YN, et al. Identification of ten novel genes involved in human spermatogenesis by microarray analysis of testicular tissue. Fertil Steril. 2006;86:1650-8.
383. Ellis PJ, Furlong RA, Conner SJ, et al. Coordinated transcriptional regulation patterns associated with infertility phenotypes in men. J Med Genet. 2007;44:498-508.
384. He Z, ChanWY, DymM. Microarray technology offers a novel tool for the diagnosis and identification of therapeutic targets for male infertility. Reproduction. 2006;132:11-9.
385. Shima JE, Mc Lean DJ, Mc Carrey JR, et al. The murine testicular transcriptome: characterizing gene expression in the testis during the progression of spermatogenesis. Biol Reprod. 2004;71:319-30.
386. Platts AE, Dix DJ, Chemes HE, et al. Success and failure in human spermatogenesis as revealed by teratozoospermic RNAs. Hum Mol Genet. 2007;16:763-73.
387. Schultz N, Hamra FK, Garbers DL. A multitude of genes expressed solely in meiotic or postmeiotic spermatogenic cells offers a myriad of contraceptive targets. Proc Natl Acad Sci USA. 2003;100:12201-6.
388. Turek PJ, Ljung BM, Cha I, et al. Diagnostic findings from testis fine needle aspiration mapping in obstructed and nonobstructed azoospermic men. J Urol. 2000;163:1709-16.
389. Martinez-Heredia J, de Mateo S, Vidal-Taboada JM, et al. Identification of proteomic differences in asthenozoospermic sperm samples. Hum Reprod. 2008;23:783-91.
390. Barratt CL. The human sperm proteome: the potential for new biomarkers of male fertility and a transformation in our understanding of the spermatozoon as a machine: commentary on the article,, Identification of proteomic differences in asthenozoospermic sperm samples' by Martinez et-al. Hum Reprod. 2008;23:1240-1.
391. Johnston DS, Wooters J, Kopf GS, et al. Analysis of the human sperm proteome. Ann N YAcad Sci. 2005;1061:190-202.
392. Pilch B, Mann M. Large-scale and high-confidence proteomic analysis of human seminal plasma. Genome Biol. 2006;7:R40.
393. Baker MA, Reeves G, Hetherington L, et al. Identification of gene products present in the Triton X soluble and insoluble fractions of human spermatozoa lysates using LC-MS/ MS analysis. Proteomics Clin Appl. 2007;1:524-32.
394. Deepinder F, Chowdary HT, Agarwal A. Role of metabolomics analysis of biomarkers in the management of male infertility. Expert Rev Mol Diagn. 2007;7:351-8.
395. Hollywood K, Brison DR, Goodacre R. Metabolomics: current technologies and future trends. Proteomics. 2006;6:4716-23.
396. German JB, Hammock BD, Watkins SM. Metabolomics: building on a century of biochemistry to guide human health. Metabolomics. 2005;1:3-9.
397. O'Flynn O'Brien KL, Varghese AC, Agrawal A. The genetic causes of male factor infertility: a review. Fertil Steril. 2010 Jan;93(1):1-12.

3

Female Factor Infertility

SECTION CONTENTS

8

Evaluation and Diagnosis of Female Infertility

Alan S Penzias, Barbara Dube, Robin Irish

CHAPTER CONTENTS

INTRODUCTION

Infertility is not a recent development. Indeed references to infertility, tests for infertility and treatments of infertility can be found in ancient Greek, Egyptian, Arabic, and Hindu texts as well as the Koran and the Bible. Perhaps because reproduction is such a basic human drive, efforts to diagnose and treat infertility have long been a central focus of the obstetrician-gynecologist and more recently, the reproductive endocrinologist.

Advances in science and medicine depend on the formulation of hypotheses then accepting or rejecting them based on critical analysis of data. Sir Peter Medawar, recipient of the 1960 Nobel Prize in Medicine or Physiology, stated "The intensity of conviction that a hypothesis is true has no bearing on whether it is true or not."[1]

As with treatment, theories and hypotheses regarding diagnostic tests of female infertility should be subject to rigorous scientific scrutiny. Each test should be examined by asking two questions: (1) what information am I trying to obtain? and (2) does this test provide that information? Fortunately, good data continues to accrue regarding the reliability and accuracy of diagnostic testing allowing us to rely less on our convictions and belief and more on evidence.

OVARY AND OOCYTE

Assessment of Ovarian Reserve

A fundamental concept in human reproduction is that a woman is born with all of the oocytes that she will ever have. Evidence in mice suggesting the possibility of germ cell repletion[2] has not been corroborated in humans. During the window of fertility between menarche and menopause, numerous studies have demonstrated conclusively, a strong correlation between advancing age, declining fecundity and rising risk of spontaneous pregnancy loss[3-5] (Figures 1 and 2).[6,7] While this information is very useful for understanding populations at risk, a critical question for those providing fertility treatment, is how can we assess the individual reproductive potential of the patient sitting across the desk from us?

Hormonal evaluation of ovarian reserve is based on three central principles: (1) that the serum concentration of pituitary hormones required to initiate follicle growth

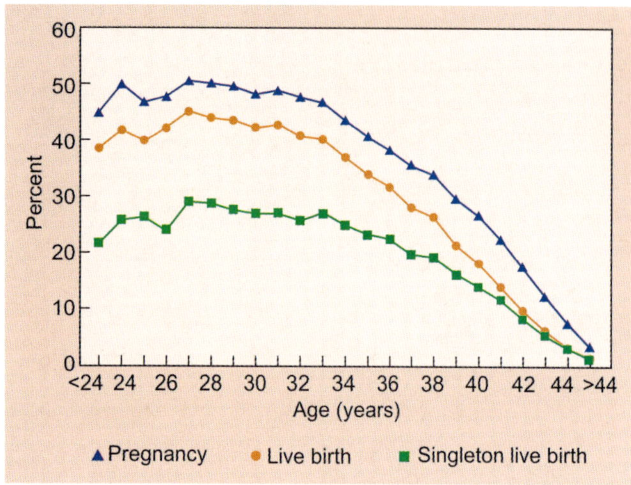

Figure 1 Percentages of ultrasonography assisted reproductive technology cycles using fresh non-donor eggs or embryos that resulted in pregnancies, live births, and singleton live births, by age of woman in 2008[6]

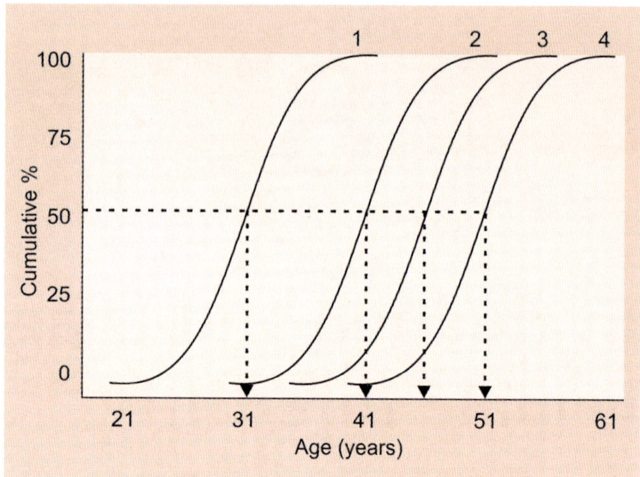

Figure 2 The age variations at the onset of 1. Subfertility (mean age 31 years); 2. sterility (mean age 41 years); 3. climeractic (mean age 46 years); 4. menopause (mean age 51 years)[7]

in a menstrual cycle correlates with oocyte quantity; (2) that serum concentration of hormones produced by the ovary correlates with oocyte quantity, and (3) that oocyte quantity and ovarian reserve correlate with and predict the likelihood of having a baby.

It is challenging, to say the least, to use live birth as an end point. In contrast to simple end points, such as blood pressure, heart rate or total cholesterol level, where variables can be controlled and narrowed to a fine degree allowing cause and effect conclusions, live birth is multidimensional. To begin with, there are two people involved. The prospective father brings to the equation his age, medical comorbidities, lifestyle risk factors, sperm concentration, motility and morphology. The prospective mother must have a functional fallopian tube, structurally sound uterus and receptive endometrium in addition to functional oocytes all with a backdrop of her medical comorbidities and lifestyle risk factors.

Another key concept to grasp is that of attributable risk. For example it is intuitively obvious that a 26-year-old woman with regular menstrual cycles and 1 year of unprotected intercourse without conception is much less likely to be infertile due to low ovarian reserve or poor oocyte quality than a 46-year-old woman with the same history. In the younger woman, the risk of causality attributable to ovarian reserve is very low while in the older woman the risk of causality is very high. If both women present with the identical 'abnormal' cycle day 3 follicle-stimulating hormone (FSH) level, these values must be interpreted differently. This concept is underscored by the widening 95% confidence interval around the mean FSH level spline curve as FSH level rises (Figure 3).[8]

Ultrasound evaluation of the ovaries with determination of the antral follicle count too has the same limitations as serum testing for the same reasons.

The results of numerous studies appear to indicate that ovarian reserve testing is better at predicting oocyte quantity at the time of egg retrieval for *in vitro* fertilization than for the more complex outcome, live birth. This statement applies to all tests of ovarian reserve including ultrasound determination of antral follicle count and serum concentrations of basal FSH, day 10 FSH following a clomiphene citrate challenge test, anti-Müllerian hormone (AMH) and inhibin B.[9-15]

Conclusions

- Patient age, menstrual cycle regularity and length of time without contraception are critical factors that need to be considered when interpreting ovarian reserve tests
- There is no single hormonal value of FSH, AMH, inhibin B or antral follicle count by ultrasound in a woman with regular menstrual cycles that perfectly predicts pregnancy or the inability to ever become pregnant
- In the case of abnormal values (elevated FSH, low AMH, low inhibin B, low antral follicle count) patients can be counseled that their odds of becoming pregnant with their own eggs may be lower than their peers of the same age

- The value of ovarian reserve testing is to have a biological marker beyond age alone that helps to set patient expectations of success

Practical Implications

Patients not seeking immediate pregnancy

- Ovarian reserve testing can serve as a baseline value for future comparison and relative assessment of likelihood of success

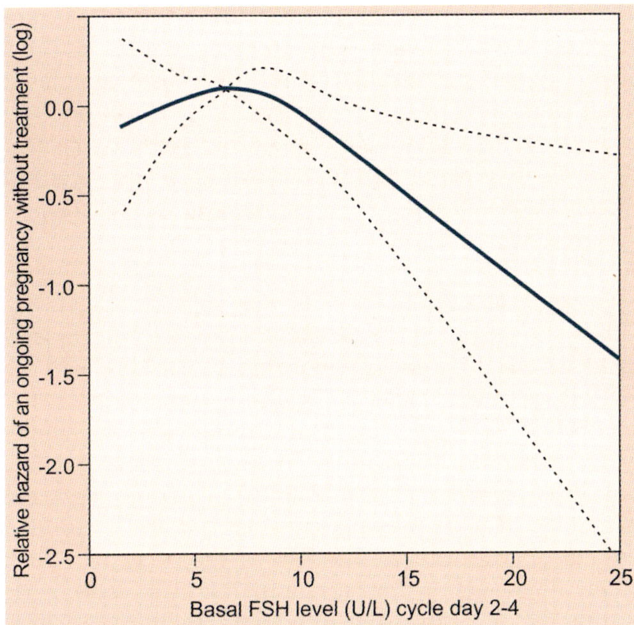

Figure 3 Spline function of basal follicle-stimulating hormone level. This Figure expresses the association between basal follicle-stimulating hormone levels on cycle day 3 versus the relative hazard (fecundity ratio) of a spontaneous ongoing pregnancy. Dotted lines represent 95% confidence interval[8]

- Ovarian reserve tests are not calibrated to predict the future. At the present time, it is not possible to provide long-term reassurance to patients about their future ability to become pregnant

Patients actively seeking pregnancy

- When testing is normal, the patient cannot be counseled that they have a better chance of success than average for age
- In the case of abnormal values (elevated FSH, low AMH, low inhibin B, low antral follicle count), treatment should proceed at the maximum pace and to the maximum level of intervention concordant with the patient's personal limitations in order to maximize the odds of success as time is of the essence

Assessment of Ovulation

In their classic 1968 study, Chiazze et al. (Table 1) studied 30,655 recorded menstrual cycles from 2,316 women. Ninety-five percent of all cycles were between 15 days and 45 days long. When restricted to cycle lengths between 15 days and 45 days, the mean cycles length of the 29,238 cycles was 28.1 days with a standard deviation of 3.95 days. Thus, the range within two standard deviations was established at 20–36 days. Using retrospective analysis of basal body temperature charts, Goldzieher, Henkin and Hamblen established that no ovulatory cycles were under 19 days duration.[16] Thus, the first part of assessment of ovulation begins with the menstrual history.

With multiple technologies available to help assess for ovulation, the natural question is which is the most reliable? Each method, basal body temperature charting, home urinary ovulation predictors and luteal phase progesterone level has its own set of strengths

Table 1 Summary measures by age for 30,655 menstrual cycles experienced by 2,316 women[17]

Summary measure		Age					
All Cycles		*15-19*	*20-24*	*25-29*	*30-34*	*35-39*	*40-44*
No	30,655	5,653	3,320	3,412	6,691	7.414	4.165
Means	29.1	30.5	30.3	29.4	28.8	28.3	28.1
SD	7.49	8.95	8.22	6.54	6.53	6.61	7.71
15-45 Day Cycles							
No	29,238	5,311	3,154	3,286	6,436	7,113	3,938
% of total cycles	95.4	94.0	95.0	96.4	96.2	96.0	94.6
Mean	28.1	29.3	29.1	28.5	28.0	27.3	26.9
SD	3.95	4.74	4.55	6.61	6.45	3.39	3.70

and limitations. Guermandi et al. (Table 2) calculated the sensitivity, specificity and accuracy in predicting or confirming ovulation of these three methods in a population of normal cycling infertile women.

Their results showed that prospective basal body temperature charting nadir is an inaccurate method for predicting ovulation time because ovulation was between 6 days before and 4 days after nadir. However, retrospective basal body temperature chart review that demonstrates a higher average temperature in the second half of the cycle than in the first (biphasic) is still a desirable method, although with low specificity, for the confirmation of ovulation because it is a simple, self-administered test for at-home use by patients.

Further, one midluteal progesterone assessment appears to be highly effective for confirming that ovulation has occurred. For prospective evaluation of ovulation, home urine ovulation predictor kits seem quite reliable with a high degree of sensitivity and accuracy. Finally, endometrial biopsy demonstrating secretory endometrium can confirm ovulation though this method cannot be endorsed in a population of women actively attempting to become pregnant.

CERVIX, UTERUS AND FALLOPIAN TUBES

Postcoital Test

Postcoital test, first described in 1866 by J Marion Sims, as a method of assessing the cervical mucus for the presence of progressively motile sperm was central to the evaluation of infertile female for over 100 years. However, in the modern era, the test does not withstand the scrutiny of evidence-based evaluation. In one of many papers of its kind, Oei et al. (Figure 4) performed a randomized controlled trial that showed no benefit when a group of infertile women treated with ovulation induction using 100 mg clomiphene citrate followed by intrauterine insemination whose evaluation did or did not include the postcoital test were compared. In the intervention group, 38% of women with a normal test result conceived, compared with 34% of those with an abnormal result, a difference that is not significant despite the treatments given for abnormal results.

Uterine Cavity Evaluation

Several methods exist for evaluation of the uterine cavity. The hysterosalpingogram (HSG) is performed using a radiopaque contrast administered through the cervical canal with imaging accomplished by radiography. The saline infusion sonogram uses sonography to evaluate the endometrial cavity after it is filled transcervically with saline. Hysteroscopy offers a direct evaluation of the uterine cavity after distension with liquid media or CO_2. The decision to perform one test over the others may be based on accessibility, cost or patient convenience as they are roughly equivalent in their accuracy (Table 3).

Tubal Patency

Using surgical evaluation as the gold standard, the HSG was compared to saline sonography for the assessment of tubal patency. According to Randolph et al., "Ultrasonography was as accurate (sensitivity 100%, specificity 91%) as HSG (sensitivity 96%, specificity 94%) in demonstrating the presence of tubal patency but less accurate in establishing which tubes were patent".[21] This is because the assessment examined the cul-de-sac prior to the start of the procedure then again afterward. If fluid accumulated in the cul-de-sac during the procedure, the authors were able to conclude that it arrived there through one or both patent fallopian tubes. However, trying to evaluate flow of fluid through a fallopian tube to lateralize tubal patency has proved more challenging. Special materials including the use of opacified flush media or techniques, such as the introduction of air bubbles, for contrast remain in development.

When planning the fertility evaluation, the choice of imaging modality may depend, in part, on the type of treatment that is planned. If the practitioner desires information solely about the endometrial cavity, any of the methods appears to be acceptable. If tubal patency information is critical, hysterosalpingography or saline

Table 2 Reliability of urinary luteinizing hormone, basal body temperature readings, and serum progesterone concent rations in 97 ovulatory cycles confirmed by sonography[18]

	Sensitivity	Specificity	PPV	NPV	Accuracy
Urinary LH	1.0	0.25	0.97	1.0	0.97
BBT chart readings	0.77	0.33	0.94	0.10	0.74
Serum progesteron	0.80	0.71	0.97	0.22	0.79

vaginal or cervical agenesis, intrauterine synechiae (iatrogenic Asherman syndrome, occurring as a result of intrauterine instrumentation, usually in the setting of infection). In the presence of an obstruction, these conditions may present with cyclic pain due to menstrual blood accumulation, as well as hematometra, hematocolpos or both.

HYPOTHYROIDISM AND HYPERPROLACTINEMIA

Hypothyroidism is second as an endocrinologic disorder only to diabetes in prevalence in the United States and it affects mostly women, oftentimes causing amenorrhea. Amenorrhea tends to be a rather late manifestation of hypothyroidism as other symptoms are already present by the time the patient presents to the gynecologist. An elevated thyrotropin-stimulating hormone (TSH) level with depressed free thyroid hormone levels is consistent with hypothyroidism. Timely restoration of normal thyroid hormone values aids in resumption of menstruation.[5]

Hypothyroidism is also linked to hyperprolactinemia; the low thyroid hormone levels stimulate the hypothalamic feedback loop resulting in increased thyroid-releasing hormone (TRH), which in turn stimulates prolactin release. Prolactin subsequently has a direct inhibitory effect on luteinizing hormone (LH) and follicle-stimulating hormone (FSH) secretion, which results in amenorrhea. Patients with elevated prolactin levels also present with galactorrhea, headaches and visual disturbances. Fasting morning prolactin levels higher than 100 ng/mL, where macroprolactinemia has been ruled out, need to be followed up with a brain magnetic resonance imaging (MRI) to rule out pituitary adenomas, the most common cause of hyperprolactinemia. Other causes that need to be ruled out include physiologic hypersecretion (pregnancy, lactation, chest wall stimulation, sleep, stress), hypothalamic-pituitary stalk damage (tumors, empty sella, lymphocytic hypophysitis, adenoma causing stalk compression, granulomas, Rathke's cyst, irradiation, trauma), pituitary hypersecretion (prolactinoma, acromegaly), systemic disorders (chronic renal failure, hypothyroidism, cirrhosis, pseudocyesis, seizures), and drug-induced hypersecretion (dopamine receptor blockers, dopamine synthesis inhibitors, catecholamine depletors, opiates, imipramine, serotonin reuptake inhibitors, calcium channel blockers, histamine receptor antagonists).[6] Treatment options for hyperprolactinemia range from observation with periodic follow-up MRI to evaluate further growth of an adenoma, to treatment with dopamine agonists (bromocriptine and cabergoline) to surgical adenoma excision. In either case, correction of the hormonal aberration should result in resumption of menstrual function.

HYPERGONADOTROPIC HYPOGONADISM

An elevated basal level of FSH is a marker of gonadal failure resulting from lack of negative estrogen feedback from the ovaries. The earliest that gonadal failure can occur is in utero as a result of gonadal agenesis or dysgenesis. Genetic females (46,XX) with gonadal agenesis have primary amenorrhea and incomplete breast development. Normal karyotype genetic females (46,XX) with gonadal dysgenesis usually lack any distinct phenotypic feature. In contrast, 45,X (Turner's syndrome) females with gonadal dysgenesis are characterized by short stature, webbed neck, low hairline, sexual infantilism and of course primary amenorrhea. The gonads of these patients typically contain the normal complement of oocytes by the 18th week of fetal life, but rapidly undergo atresia resulting in very few oocytes at birth and essentially none by puberty.[7] Genetic males (46,XY) with gonadal dysgenesis have non-hormone secreting gonads that need to be removed at diagnosis.

Primary ovarian insufficiency (POI, previously known as premature menopause or premature ovarian failure) is defined as amenorrhea for greater than 4 months and persistent estrogen deficiency occurring prior to age 40 years, and in the presence of two menopausal-range FSH values (separated by at least 1 month). POI affects 1% of women by age 40 years and it is a heterogeneous disorder that occurs through a combination of follicle dysfunction and depletion. Unlike natural menopause, it is not always irreversible, with 5–10% of patients conceiving spontaneously after the diagnosis of POI. Patients with POI are at increased risk of developing cardiovascular disease and osteoporosis, and there is a strong association with other autoimmune disorder, with the most common one being thyroiditis.[8] Patients with POI should be screened for autoimmune conditions by measuring TSH, thyroid and adrenal antibodies, fasting glucose and electrolytes.[9] Adrenal antibodies are positive in up to 4% of patients with POI. These patients should subsequently undergo yearly corticotrophin stimulation test. The use of ovarian antibody testing or ovarian biopsies has not been shown to be specific or beneficial and is thus not warranted.

Although no specific etiology for POI has been identified, there is clearly a genetic component as 10–15% of cases have an affected first-degree relative.[10] A few of the mutations that have been linked to POI involve independent loci on the X chromosome, the inhibin alpha gene and the bone morphogenetic factor 15 gene, as well as additional X chromosomes. Furthermore, 13–26% of women with POI carry the Familial Mental Retardation-1 (*FMR1*) gene premutation.[11] A karyotype and *FMR1* gene mutation screening has therefore become a part of the standard workup for patients who experience POI before age 30 years and/or have a family history of mental retardation.

The diagnosis of POI can be devastating and it should thus be presented in the context of emotional and social support. These patients also have decreased bone mineral density compared to their menstruating cohorts and should thus be treated with estrogen and progestin replacement to decrease the risk of osteoporosis and subsequent fractures. Although large randomized studies are lacking, the recommended regimen consists of 100 mcg of estradiol per day combined with 5–10 mg of cyclic medroxyprogesterone acetate for 12 days each month.

HYPOGONADOTROPIC HYPOGONADISM

Hypothalamic chronic anovulation, also called functional hypothalamic amenorrhea (HA), refers to cessation of menses due to HPG axis down-regulation in the absence of other organic or anatomic causes. Functional hypothalamic disorders are the most common cause of chronic anovulation. In these cases, stress, weight loss, exercise or a combination of these three states act centrally on the hypothalamus to disrupt the pulsatile secretion of GnRH. This in turn down-regulates the HPG axis and leads to a state of estrogen deficiency. One of the modulators of this effect that has been extensively studied is leptin. Leptin is an adipocyte-secreted hormone that regulates the body's basal metabolic rate and energy stores, and has been shown to decrease in response to fasting or in conditions such as anorexia nervosa (AN). Furthermore, when leptin is exogenously replaced in these patients menstrual and hormonal aberrations are corrected.[12] Other hormones that have been implicated in the pathophysiology of HA include ghrelin, neuropeptide Y, β-endorphin, corticotropin-releasing hormone, dopamine and γ-aminobutyric acid (GABA).[13]

The treatment approach for patients with HA begins with the proper identification of the underlying pathology. Adolescents and young adults who are most at risk for developing HA are competitive athletes, especially long-distance runners, anorectics/bulimics, and those suffering from chronic illness (uncontrolled juvenile diabetes, end-stage renal disease, malignancy, immunodeficiency, malabsorption, chronic liver disease).[14] Thorough screening for eating disorders (such as AN and bulimia nervosa), excessive exercising or psychological or physical stressors is essential. Treatment should begin with behavioral modification and change of long-term life patterns. These patients benefit the most from reduction of strenuous activity, less restrictive eating patterns and weight gain. However, such a regimen is very challenging and requires a multidisciplinary approach, involving physicians, nutritionists and psychotherapists. The exact amount of weight gain that will trigger resumption of menstruation has been the topic of controversy[15] and long-term data are lacking. Some studies suggest that the vast majority of patients with the female athlete triad (disordered eating, menstrual disturbances, and osteoporosis) will resume menstruation within 6 months of achieving a weight 90% of their ideal body weight.[16]

Patients with prolonged HA are at increased risk of osteoporosis and stress fractures. In terms of bone health, oral contraceptives, estrogen/progestin combinations and calcium/vitamin D supplementation, in combination with lifestyle changes, have been shown to significantly increase bone mineral density. Bisphosphonates should be avoided in this patient population because of their potential for spontaneous conception and possible teratogenicity. For women desiring fertility, optimal weight should first be achieved and subsequently ovulation can be induced with pulsatile GnRH or injectable gonadotropins (LH and FSH combinations). The use of clomiphene citrate in these hypoestrogenic women has not proven particularly effective and should be avoided as first-line treatment.

A more infrequent cause of chronic anovulation is idiopathic hypogonadotropic hypogonadism (IHH). Normosmic IHH or anosmic IHH (also known as Kallmann syndrome or olfactogenital dysplasia) is a rare genetic disorder that results from an isolated defect in hypothalamic GnRH secretion or in the peripheral action of GnRH (causes by Sheehan syndrome, empty sella turcica, or pituitary gland necrosis). The first mutation identified in IHH involved the cell surface adhesive gene, KAL1, and several others (GNRHR, PCSK1, GPR54, NELF, FGF8, FGFR1, PROK2, PROKR2) have since been described. Men are mostly affected by this disorder (5:1 male-to-female ratio) and they typically present with sexual infantilism, eunuchoid habitus (males) or small ovaries containing almost exclusively primordial follicles (females). Interestingly, these follicles respond readily to treatment with exogenous pulsatile GnRH, which has been successfully used to induce ovulation for over 25 years.[17]

HYPOPITUITARISM

Hypopituitarism refers to the partial or complete loss of hormones from the anterior and/or posterior pituitary. The etiology is often multifactorial, and the disorder can be congenital (idiopathic) or acquired secondary to neurological insult (such as Sheehan syndrome, head injury, neurosurgery, infiltrative disorders and cranial radiotherapy). Patients usually present with weakness, fatigue, lack of libido and cold intolerance. Childhood-onset hypopituitarism is characterized by lack of secondary sexual characteristics, primary amenorrhea and short stature. Thyroid and adrenal function assessment is warranted in these patients. Ovulation induction can be achieved with exogenous pulsatile GnRH or gonadotropins.[18]

POLYCYSTIC OVARY SYNDROME

Polycystic ovary syndrome (PCOS) is a heterogeneous and multifactorial syndrome that affects 5–18% of young females. It is the most common endocrinopathy of reproductive-age women and the most frequent cause of anovulatory infertility. The syndrome was first described by Stein and Leventhal in 1935[19] and its etiology remains largely unknown. Since then, several diagnostic criteria (NIH in 1990, Rotterdam in 2003, Androgen Excess Society in 2006) have been developed and the majority utilizes a combination of the following findings: (1) chronic anovulation, (2) clinical and/or biochemical signs of hyperandrogenism, and/or (3) polycystic ovaries on ultrasound. The typical phenotype of PCOS may include hirsutism and acne, anovulation, obesity, insulin resistance and acanthosis nigricans. Patients with all these phenotypic features may in fact be described as having the HAIR-AN syndrome. Between 10% and 50% of PCOS patients are nonobese, or 'lean PCOS' and their diagnosis is often delayed or missed altogether because they do not exhibit the typical obese PCOS phenotype. PCOS patients typically present seeking fertility treatment or for evaluation of menstrual disturbances.[20]

PCOS is a diagnosis of exclusion. It thus requires the exclusion of other causes of menstrual irregularities and hyperandrogenism (such as non-classical adrenal hyperplasia, Cushing syndrome, and rarely androgen-secreting tumors). The LH/FSH ratio may be elevated, but the diagnosis cannot be confirmed solely based on this finding. The syndrome is characterized by a large number of non-dominant follicles that are part of enlarged, globular ovaries and lead to anovulation. The high insulin levels that result from peripheral insulin resistance act synergistically with LH to increase androgen production from ovarian theca cells. These androgens are then converted within the ovary and in the periphery to estrogen. The negative feedback of estrogen on the pituitary preferentially suppresses FSH preventing adequate folliculogenesis, in spite of a moderately hyperestrogenic environment. In addition, peak estradiol levels required to sensitize the hypothalamus and pituitary and facilitate the LH surge are not achieved. In the long-term, these patients are at increased risk of developing glucose intolerance or overt diabetes, the metabolic syndrome (characterized by abdominal obesity, hypertension, high triglycerides, inflammatory factors and increased levels of thrombophilic factors), as well obstetric risks including pregnancy-induced hypertension and gestational diabetes. Furthermore, chronic anovulation and the associated hyperestrogenic state increase the risk of endometrial hyperplasia and cancer.[21]

The management of PCOS is also multifactorial and it should focus not only on menstrual regulation and/or ovulation induction but also on prevention of endometrial hyperplasia and of long-term health sequelae. Lifestyle changes should be the primary goal, especially in obese, insulin-resistant patients. Counseling and behavioral modification aimed at weight loss or prevention of weight gain, dietary modifications and regular exercise are central in the management of this syndrome. A body weight reduction of 5–10% has been shown to have a significant effect on major psychological, reproductive and metabolic outcomes. Numerous studies have compared the efficacy of different ovulation induction regimens in PCOS with conflicting data. The current consensus supports clomiphene citrate being used at the first-line therapy, followed by the addition of metformin in clomiphene citrate-resistant patients. Other options include injectable gonadotropins, as well as wedge resection of ovaries or laparoscopic ovarian drilling, which are not routinely performed due to their unfavorable risk-benefit ratio.[22]

CONCLUSION

Amenorrhea is an indication of disordered ovulation or outflow obstruction. Once pregnancy is excluded, the four most common causes are ovarian failure, hyperprolactinemia, HA and PCOS. Careful history and physical examination can help decipher the etiology. In addition, useful baseline information can be obtained from serum measurements of human chorionic gonadotropin, TSH, FSH and prolactin. Management of the underlying pathology that is manifesting as amenorrhea is mostly medical, with hormonal replacement or ovulation induction if fertility is desired, and rarely surgical, as is the case in some disorders of outflow obstruction. A multidisciplinary approach to management of these conditions should be utilized to ensure compliance and patient support during this challenging process.

REFERENCES

1. Practice Commitee of the American Society for Reproductive Medicine. Current evaluation of amenorrhea. Fertil Steril. 2008;90(5 Suppl):S219-25.
2. Heiman DL. Amenorrhea. Prim Care. 2009;36(1):1-17.
3. Guerrier D, Mouchel T, Pasquier L, et al. The Mayer-Rokitansky-Kuster-Hauser synrome (congenital absence of uterus and vagina)—phenotypic manifestations and genetic approaches. J Negat Results Biomed. 2006;5:1.
4. Oakes MB, Eyvazzadeh AD, Quint E, et al. Complete androgen insensitivity syndrome—a review. Pediatr Adolesc Gynecol. 2008;21(6):305-10.
5. Hueston Wj. Treatment of hypothyroidism. Am Fam Physician. 2001;64(10):1717-24.
6. Longo DL, Fauci AS, Kasper DL, et al. Harrison's Principles of Internal Medicine, vol. 1. New York: McGraw-Hill; 2012.
7. Hreinsson JG, Otala M, Fridstrom M, et al. Follicles are found in the ovaries of adolescent girls with Turner's sundrome. J Clin Endocrinol Metab. 2002;87(8):3618-2.
8. Nelson LM. Clinical practice. Primary ovarian insufficiency. N Engl J Med. 2009;360(6):606-14.
9. Rebar RW, Connolly HV. Clinical features of young women with hypergonadotropic amenorrhea. Fertil Steril. 1990;53(5):804-10.
10. van Kasteren YM, Hundscheid RD, Smits AP, et al. Familial idiopathic premature ovarian failure: an overrated and underestimated genetic disease? Hum Reprod. 1999;14(10):2455-9.
11. Wittenberger MD, Hagerman RJ, Sherman SL, et al. The FMR1 premutation and reproduction. Fertil Steril. 2007;87(3):456-65.
12. Welt CK, Chan JL, Bullen J, et al. Recombinant human leptin in women with hypothalamic amenorrhea. New Engl J Med. 2004;351(10):987-97.
13. Gordon CM. Functional hypothalamic amenorrhea. N Engl J Med. 2010;363(4):365-71.
14. Warren MP, Goodman LR. Exercise-induced endocrine pathologies. J Endocrinol Invest. 2003;26(9):873-8.
15. Frisch RE, Canick JA, Tulchinsky D. Human fatty marrow aromatizes androgen to estrogen. J Clin Endocrinol Metab. 1980;51(2):394-6.
16. Golden NH, Jacobson MS, Schebendach J, et al. Resumption of menses in anorexia nervosa. Arch Pediatr Adolesc Med. 1997;151(1):16-21.
17. Sykiotis GP, Hoang XH, Avbelj M, et al. Congenital idiopathic hypogonadotropic hypogonadism: evidence of defects in the hypothalamus, pituitary, and tests. J Clin Endocrinol Metab. 2010;95(6): 3019-27.
18. Romero CJ, Nesi-Franca S, Radovick S. The molecular basis of hypopituitarism. Trends Endocrinol Metab. 2009;20(10):506-16.
19. Stein IF, Leventhal ML. Amenorrhea associated with bilateral polycystic ovaries. Am J Obstet Gynecol. 1935;29:181-91.
20. Wilson JF. In the clinic. The polycystic ovary syndrome. Ann Intern Med. 2011;154(3):2-15.
21. Ehrmann DA. Polycystic ovary syndrome. New Engl J Med. 2005;352(12):1223-36.
22. Legro RS, Barnhart HX, Schlaff WD, et al. Clomiphene, metformin, or both for infertiity in the polycystic ovary syndrome. New Engl J Med. 2007;356(6):551-66.

10

Polycystic Ovary Syndrome: Diagnostic Criteria and Treatment in the Anovulatory Patient

Laurel A Stadtmauer

Chapter Contents

INTRODUCTION

Seventy-five years ago, two North American gynecologists, Stein and Leventhal, published the first clear clinical description of what eventually would be known as the polycystic ovary syndrome (PCOS) in women. These patients were usually infertile, obese and hirsute with irregular menstrual cycles, and had large ovaries with multiple peripheral cysts.[1] Despite the advances due to research in this area, the definition of PCOS is still controversial.[2,3] Transatlantic disagreement over the diagnostic features of the PCOS has been reflected in the importance placed by clinicians on the clinical, endocrinologic and ultrasonographic findings at presentation.[4,5] The recommendations of a National Institutes of Health conference on the syndrome approximately 20 years ago indicated that the diagnosis should be made when hyperandrogenism and anovulation coincide with exclusion of other causes, such as late-onset congenital adrenal hyperplasia, Cushing's syndrome and other causes of irregular menstrual cycles.[6] International and European studies have demanded consideration of polycystic morphology as being mandatory for diagnosis. Ultimately, a consensus conference in Rotterdam, the Netherlands in 2003, published a definition of the PCOS that called for the presence of two of three features: polycystic ovary on ultrasonography, anovulation and hyperandrogenism, with the exclusion of other causes.[7,8] However, this definition has not been universally accepted, particularly in the United States, where the role of ultrasonography is debated. This chapter includes recent consensus on etiology and the pathogenesis of the syndrome and will concentrate on the associated infertility in women with PCOS, and the role of obesity and insulin resistance (IR) associated with the syndrome.

PATHOPHYSIOLOGY OF POLYCYSTIC OVARY SYNDROME

Polycystic ovary syndrome is the main cause of anovulatory infertility in women.[9]Approximately, 85–90% of women with oligomenorrhea and up to 30–40% of those with amenorrhoea,[10] and 5–10% of reproductive-aged women[2,9] may have PCOS. The primary abnormality seems to be an excess of androgen production within the ovary that leads to the recruitment of large numbers of small preantral follicles which fails to develop further and forms follicular cysts. Women with PCOS, commonly present in their late teens or early twenties with hirsutism, acne or irregular periods. Even if they ovulate, the chance of conception for those women is reduced because fewer ovulatory events occur in a given time frame.[10,11] The ovarian dysfunction in PCOS is manifested both by an increase in the number of small follicles followed by an arrest in the growth. The accumulation of small follicles gives the typical aspect of multifollicular ovaries at ultrasonography, which is in close relationship with the androgen serum levels. In the androgenized monkey model, the anatomic appearance of ovaries was very close to the one observed in ovaries from women with PCOS, after only 10 days of exposure to androgens.[12] This supports the hypothesis that the increased number of small follicles is due to the trophic effects of androgens. Hyperandrogenism, obesity and IR are all important in the etiology of the disease.

Obesity

Obesity appears to augment anovulation in PCOS through increased peripheral estrogen production [(which interferes with the hypothalamic-pituitary-ovarian axis)/(which exerts negative feedback effect on HPG to produce less FSH)] resulting in elevated luteinizing hormone (LH) levels. Obesity affects follicular maturation,[13] inhibits ovulation and leads to irregular cycles. Obesity increases IR, can significantly contribute to hormonal aberrations[14] and amplify the metabolic[14] and cardiovascular risk,[15] which may be inherently increased in PCOS. Obesity is observed in 35–60% of women with PCOS.[16] Hyperandrogenism also worsens the obesity and is related to the accumulation of fat to central abdominal sites. Women with PCOS have increased abdominal adipose tissue, as depicted in the higher waist-to-hip ratio.[17] This central type obesity is independent of body-mass index (BMI) and related to higher plasma insulin. Due to the high prevalence of impaired glucose tolerance (IGT) and Type 2 diabetes among obese PCOS women with PCOS, the consensus group[18] advocates the screening of obese women (BMI > 27 kg/m^2) with PCOS with an oral glucose tolerance test. Obesity is associated with raised serum insulin, LH and androgens, hypothalamic endorphins and leptin. However, on losing weight, the LH pulse frequency and amplitude and the leptin levels do not appear to alter prior to resumption of menstruation.[19]

Insulin Resistance

In the last 25 years, it has been clear that PCOS is a metabolic disorder associated with IR. The peripheral IR, is similar to that of women with type 2 diabetes mellitus. Insulin-mediated glucose uptake is decreased by 35–40% compared with age- and weight-comparable control women.[20] There is increased basal insulin secretion and decreased hepatic insulin extraction.[21] Normoglycemic women with the syndrome display β-cell compensation that is inadequate for their degree of peripheral insulin resistance.[22,23] Suggesting that they are at high risk of type 2 diabetes.[24]

Indeed, about 40% of obese women with PCOS have IGT after a standard challenge with 75 g oral glucose.[25] Insulin resistance might contribute to hyperandrogenism and gonadotropin abnormalities through several mechanisms. High concentrations of insulin reduce circulating sex hormone binding globulin (SHBG) values, increasing the bioavailability of testosterone[26,27] and might also serve as a cofactor to stimulate adrenal and ovarian androgen biosynthesis, thereby contributing to abnormal gonadotropin concentrations.[28,29] Detectable IR occurs in 50–70% of patients with PCOS.[20]

Insulin might also act directly in the hypothalamus, pituitary gland or both, to regulate gonadotropin release,[30] but the contribution of IR to manifestation of gonadotropin abnormalities in PCOS remains uncertain.[31] Insulin resistance in the disorder is characterized by selective-tissue insulin sensitivity, in which some tissues seem highly resistant and others sensitive. In affected tissues, metabolic pathways are, generally resistant to stimulation by insulin, but mitogenic or steroidogenic pathways are not.[32] The primary cause of PCOS hyperandrogenism is tied into IR not due to hypersecretion of LH alone, the intrinsic effect seems to be a theca interna cell dysfunction or other stimulating influences as insulin or insulin-like growth factor (IGF). Both *in vivo* and *in vitro* data has confirmed that PCOS theca cells hyperrespond to gonadotropins and produce excess androgens escaping their normal downregulation. Prelevic and colleagues[33] supported this theory by demonstrating that suppression of insulin secretion by a somatostatin analogue lowers serum LH and androgens in women with PCOS. Indeed, insulin acts as a 'cogonadotropin' and also amplifies the effects of testosterone by suppressing SHBG. Alternatively, a defect in the IGF system could cause an alteration of the set point for the response of the granulosa cell to FSH. It has been suggested that LH acts on granulosa cells in the presence of insulin, thereby leading to premature luteinization, maturational arrest and excess androgen production.[34]

Acanthosis nigricans is commonly seen. Acanthosis nigricans is a pigmentation that occurs most frequently in the axillae, skin flexures and the nape of the neck, is a marker associated with IR and compensatory increased insulin secretion.[35] It is thought to be present in women with PCOS in 1–3% of cases and may be present more commonly in adolescents with PCOS.[36]

Close to 50% of women with PCOS suffered from the metabolic syndrome.[37] An increase in central fat, hyperinsulinemia, glucose intolerance, increased blood pressure and other isolated features of metabolic syndrome are more common in women with PCOS than they are in the general population. Whether the metabolic syndrome is caused by a feature specific to PCOS or is merely a consequence of adiposity is still unclear. However, there is evidence suggesting that the increased prevalence can be explained by hyperandrogenism seen in women.[38] The prevalence of PCOS of metabolic syndrome in women with PCOS is high among all age groups. This increased prevalence appears to be independent of body weight. Dyslipidemia, particularly decreased HDL cholesterol, and increased triglyceride levels in PCOS are the same lipid profile known to be associated with IR.[39]

Hyperandrogenism

The primary cause of PCOS hyperandrogenism is not due to hypersecretion of LH alone, the intrinsic effect seems to be a theca interna cell dysfunction or other stimulating influences as insulin or IGF.[30] Both *in vivo* and *in vitro*, data has confirmed that PCOS theca cells hyperrespond to gonadotropins and produce excess androgens escaping their normal downregulation.[31] Prelevic and colleagues[33] supported this theory by demonstrating that suppression of insulin secretion by a somatostatin analogue lowers serum LH and androgens in women with PCOS. Indeed, insulin acts as a 'cogonadotropin' and also amplifies the effects of testosterone by suppressing SHBG.

High LH levels have affects on fertility and are shown to decrease pregnancy rates, and lead to high miscarriage rates and poor egg quality.[40-42] In *in vitro* fertilization (IVF), the elevated follicular LH has a detrimental effect on the fertilization rate and pregnancy outcome.[43]

The mechanism for increased miscarriage rates among women with PCOS compared to normal fertile women, is unclear. Pregnant women with PCOS, experience a higher incidence of perinatal morbidity from gestational diabetes, pregnancy-induced hypertension and preeclampsia. Children born of PCOS mothers also show an increased risk of neonatal complications from preterm birth, intra-uterine growth restriction and macrosomia.[44,45]

Oligomenorrhea

The major clinical signs of anovulation, oligomenorrhea or amenorrhea vary in duration, but are generally unambiguous. Oligomenorrhea is defined as less than 8 periods per year, or cycles that are longer than 35 days, and amenorrhea is absence of menstruation for more than 3 months without pregnancy.[46] In PCOS, menstrual dysfunction reflects chronic anovulation and is characterized by irregular and infrequent bleeding that usually occurs from menarche. The pattern of irregular bleeding is a consequence of excessive endometrial proliferation due to unopposed chronic estrogen secretion. The thickened endometrium is prone to superficial sloughing or tissue breakdown in response to persistent secretion or spontaneous decrease in circulating estrogen, respectively. The physiological link between irregular menses and anovulation is related to the persistence of estrogen production arising primarily from extraglandular conversion of androgens to estrogens. It has been assumed that within PCO, granulosa cells generate very little estrogen because there is a lack of mature follicle development.[47]

In the largest series of women with PCOS, Balen et al.[48] reported that of the 1871 women with at least one symptom of PCOS (using the older diagnostic criteria), approximately, 30% had one regular menstrual cycle during their reproductive life, 50% had oligomenorrhea and 20% were amenorrheic. Consequently, the majority of women with PCOS have an abnormal menstrual cycle and the most frequent finding.

Folliculogenesis in Polycystic Ovary Syndrome

The ovarian dysfunction in PCOS is manifested in two ways. There are both increased number of small follicles up to 2–5 mm in diameter and arrest in the development of the antral follicles at 4–7 mm in diameter.[49] This leads to the typical ultrasound appearance (Figure 1). The intra-ovarian hyperandrogenism, which is the fundamental feature of PCOS,[50] is designated as the main culprit for this follicle excess. This effect on folliculogenesis predominates in small follicles, probably due to their richness in androgen receptors.[51]

In the androgenized monkey model, the anatomic appearance of ovaries was very close to the one observed in ovaries from women with PCOS, after only 10 days of exposure to androgens.[12] In line with these experimental data, congenital adrenal hyperplasia, virilizing tumors and exogenous androgen treatment are

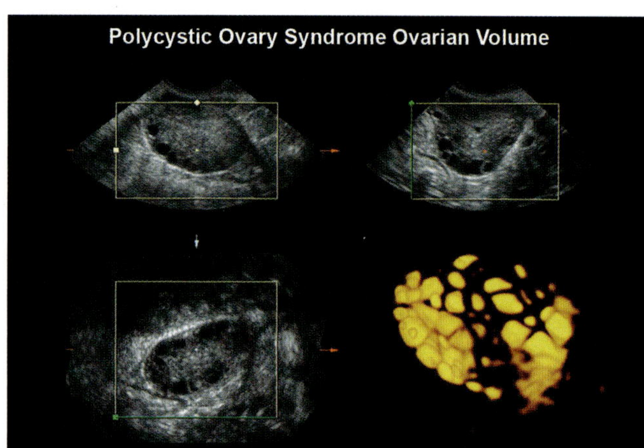

Figure 1 Three-dimensional ultrasound of polycystic ovary syndrome

associated with increased numbers of non-ovulatory antral follicles similar to those seen in women with PCOS.[52] Furthermore, it has been reported that the 2–5 mm follicles number at ultrasound was positively correlated to the serum testosterone and androstenedione levels in patients with PCOS.[53] This supports the hypothesis that the increased number of small follicles is due to the trophic effects of androgens, whether increased locally in the ovary as in PCOS or systemically as in the other conditions. There is also evidence that androgens lead to atresia at a certain point in the development.[54]

Androgen biosynthesis in the human ovary takes place primarily in theca interna cells, whose function is excessive in PCOS. The excess of androgen production can be explained by extra-ovarian, as well as intraovarian factors. Hyperinsulinemia provides another extra-ovarian determinant of hyperandrogenism by enhancing the effects of LH on theca interna cells steroid production. Experimental evidence was recently confirmed by the clinical observation that serum androgen concentrations decrease in women in whom insulin concentrations are lowered with insulin sensitizing agents or by weight loss.[55] The study by Franks and colleagues has shed light on the paradox of insulin multifaceted intracellular behavior, demonstrating that abnormal glucose metabolism is present with significantly impaired insulin-stimulated lactate production by granulosa-lutein cells from women with anovulatory PCOS compared to women with normal ovaries or ovulatory women with PCOS.[56] Notably, these granulosa cells maintained normal steroidogenic output in response to physiological doses of insulin. This finding suggests that the paradox of insulin activity is not only present in the macroenvironment but also in the microenvironment of the ovary.

Recent data about antiMüllerian hormone (AMH) which is produced by granulosa cells, may suggest that it could be implicated in the hyperandrogenism of PCOS. Indeed, the ovarian production of AMH is excessive in PCOS.[57] A positive and significant correlation between AMH and serum testosterone and androstenedione levels in PCOS patients was found, but not in controls.[58] This could suggest a paracrine positive effect of AMH on theca interna cells. However, further experimental studies are required before speculating on implications of AMH in the theca dysregulation of PCOS.

In conclusion, the first follicular abnormality in PCOS is an increased number of early-growing and selectable follicles, which is presumably the consequence of intra-ovarian hyperandrogenism. The accumulation of 2–5 mm follicles gives the typical aspect of multifollicular ovaries at ultrasonography, which is in close relationship with the androgen serum level. Miscarriage rates among women with PCOS are believed to be increased compared to normal fertile women, although supporting evidence is limited. Furthermore, in women with PCOS there is a significantly reduced chance of conception.[59] Studies indicate that in women with PCOS, early miscarriage is a consequence of the failure of the implantation process related to aberrant endometrial beta 3 integrin expression and the failure of the downregulation of the progesterone receptor.[60] Women with PCOS experience a higher incidence of perinatal morbidity from gestational diabetes and pregnancy-induced hypertension. Their offsprings are at increased risk of neonatal complications, such as preterm birth and admission in neonatal intensive care unit.[61,62]

TREATMENT FOR WOMEN WITH POLYCYSTIC OVARY SYNDROME AND INFERTILITY

First-Line Treatment

Fertility treatments for PCOS are focused on ovulation induction. Weight loss is the primary treatment. If not successful, weight increase might induce oligo- or amenorrhea and weight loss can restore ovulation and regular cycles.[63] The beneficial effects of weight loss are consistently shown, in improving menstrual cycle frequency, restoring ovulation and normalizing biochemical indices, particularly, IR.[64] Weight loss can restore ovulation with regular cycles. Due to the high prevalence of IGT and type 2 diabetes among obese PCOS women, screening with an oral glucose tolerance test, as well as liver function testing highly suggested in those with obesity.[63,64] Hypocaloric diets have been shown to modify dyslipidemias in PCOS patients. Recent studies in overweight and obese PCOS patients have suggested that a hypocaloric diet, regardless of its composition, results in weight loss and leptin level reduction along with the improvement of total cholesterol and low-density-lipoprotein levels.[51-65]

Clomiphene citrate (CC), a selective modulator of the estrogen receptor is the first-line treatment for anovulation and leads to an ovulation rate of 60–85% of women with PCOS, however the pregnancy rate is only 30–40%.[45-66] The dose is given at an initial dose of 50 mg per day from days 2–6, 3–7 or 5–9 of the menstrual cycle. The dose can be increased to up to 250 mg per day by increments of 50 until ovulation occurs. To avoid multiple pregnancies, practitioners are strongly advised to monitor ovulation while administering CC by measuring estradiol and progesterone hormone concentrations and/or performing at least one pelvic ultrasound in the midcycle. In a recent randomized controlled trial, CC was found to be very effective in infertile women in terms of ovulation and pregnancy and therefore should be the first medical therapy for treating PCOS related anovulatory infertility.[64-67] It is observed that prolonging CC treatment for more than 6 months did not improve results.[63-66] Clomiphene citrate resistant PCOS can be defined as those who do not ovulate after 6 months of treatment of an appropriate dose or do not conceive after 6 months of ovulatory cycles. In cases of clomiphene resistance, there are several second line treatment choices including aromatase inhibitors, gonadotropin treatment or ovarian drilling. Prior to initiating first or second line treatments, it is important to insist on loss of excess weight and the treatment of any carbohydrate intolerance or diabetes. Obesity appears to augment anovulation in PCOS through increased peripheral estrogen production and insulin production which can worsen the elevated LH levels and interfere with follicular development and ovulation. Al-Azemi et al.[65-68] investigated the effect of obesity on treatment outcome among 270 PCOS patients attending a fertility clinic. Patients were stratified according to BMI (normal-weight: 18–24; overweight: 25–29; obese: 30–34; grossly obese: ≥ 35). Obesity adversely affected the outcome of ovulation induction with CC and gonadotropins. The pregnancy rate and outcome were also adversely affected by obesity. The 2008 consensus conference concluded that patients should lose 5% of their weight before undergoing infertility treatment.[66-69]

Gonadotropin therapy with medications, such as recombinant follicle stimulating hormone, (rFSH) has been recognized as an effective treatment for infertility associated with anovulation in CC resistant women, but its use is limited.[67] Problems with conventional gonadotropin therapy include the need for increased monitoring due to the increased risk of multifollicular development leading to multiple births, as well as the relatively low cycle fecundity.[67,68] The low pregnancy rate of approximately 18–20% per cycle is postulated to be related to either hypersecretion of LH or to premature LH surges. Therefore it is desirable first to try nongonadotropin treatments for clomiphene resistant PCOS women.

Second-Line Treatment: Aromatase Inhibitors

Letrozole has been studied in multiple studies with ovulation induction in women with PCOS and trials show efficacy for increased endometrial thickness, ovulation and pregnancy rates in clomiphene resistant patients. It can be considered a second-line treatment in those women in which a percentage of women will ovulate and get pregnant. Letrozole is an aromatase inhibitor which has been shown to have an ovulation rate of 70–85% and a pregnancy rate of 20–27% per cycle.[70] In CC resistant PCOS patients, ovulation occurs in 54–84% of patients.[71] In addition, trials have shown less of a negative endometrial effect than clomid.[72] Therefore, aromatase inhibitors may be considered in women who are clomiphene resistant prior to gonadotropin treatment.

Second-Line Treatment: Ovarian Drilling

Multiple studies, as well as meta-analysis studies, all show laparoscopic ovarian drilling (LOD) is an effective treatment in ovulation induction and has long-term effects. The mechanism is not entirely understood but it is most likely related to a decline in plasma LH and testosterone and rise in FSH and SHBG with follicle development and ovulation in 80% of cases. Most of the studies have been in CC resistant women and there have been comparisons between gonadotropins and laparoscopic ovarian surgery (LOS). In 50% of cases, adjuvant therapy is required, such as CC after 12 weeks. Multiple randomized controlled trials compared the effectiveness of LOD with gonadotropins for women with CC resistant PCOS showing no difference in live birth rate or ongoing pregnancy.[73,74] LOS achieves unifollicular ovulation with no risks of ovarian hyperstimulation syndrome or high order multiparity and does not require intensive monitoring. A subanalysis study[74] showed that LOD improved reproductive outcome in CC resistant PCOS similarly to metformin with clomiphene treatment with ovulation rates at about 30%, pregnancy rates of 17% and spontaneous abortion rates of 35% and live birth rates of 60%. As randomized controlled trials comparing the effectiveness of LOD to gonadotropin treatment show a comparable improvement on the live birth rates,[75] LOD should be considered, especially in women who have other need for assessment of pelvis, such as pelvic pan.

Metformin Treatment

It has been largely demonstrated that IR contributes to oligoanovulation and infertility.[76,77] In the US, after the study by Legro et al.[64-67] the use of metformin for fertility enhancement in women with PCOS has become controversial due to the lack of benefit in the live birth rate in this large randomized controlled trial (RCT). However, there still remains a place for metformin in ovulation induction. The Legro study[64-67] does not address the metabolic benefits of metformin, as this study was looking strictly at infertility. Metformin has been shown to both, improve IR and reduce levels of intrafollicular androgens by affecting levels of IGFs and IGFBPs.[78] The meta-analysis by Lord[79] indicated that metformin is effective in achieving ovulation alone or combined with clomiphene, and was based on 14 RCTs and a total of 428 women. Since then, there has been another meta-analysis based on 39 RTCs performed between 1996 and 2007 including 1,639 subjects which showed an improvement of metformin in ovulation and pregnancy in women (OR-2.21 compared with placebo for ovulation, and 3.93 metformin and clomiphene compared with clomiphene alone for ovulation and 1.58 for pregnancy).[80] Their meta-analysis concluded that there is a benefit in ovulatory rates and pregnancy rates but not live birth rates. The discrepancy in the results of multiple studies may be due to the type of PCOS women especially related to the BMI and whether or not they had IR. It may also be due to some of the undesirable effects of CC causing an increase in ovulation of multiple follicles verses a single follicle growth in metformin, consistent with the multiparity rate of 6% in clomid. In addition, metformin is a drug that affects insulin concentrations. The action of metformin is slow and gradual and it may take up to 6 months to improve ovulation.[80] CC works more rapidly. Therefore, it is not unexpected to find that cumulative 6 months live births rates to be different in the two groups. A recent analysis of RCTs has shown benefits of metformin in lean PCOS women and less with obese PCOS.[81] The authors concluded that BMI is an important prognostic factor in response to metformin for women with ovulation dysfunction related to PCOS, suggesting that women with a lower BMI may respond better to metformin treatment versus placebo amongst women with BMI more than 32 kg/m^2. The previous studies comparing metformin with CC differ in the patient inclusion criteria, ethnic background, methods of measuring insulin sensitivity, as well as the BMI of the patients and dose and length of treatment of metformin, making comparisons difficult. The majority of these studies showing no improvement of metformin on the insulin sensitivity or hyperandrogenemia were in severely obese women. The incidence of IR is known to differ in obese verses lean PCOS patients.[82,83] In addition, when comparing studies, there is no consensus as to the most accurate measurement of insulin sensitivity. The hyperinsulinemic-euglycemic clamp technique is still regarded as the gold standard diagnostic test for IR. However, its routine use in clinical setting is not practical. Other indices such as fasting insulin, fasting glucose, fasting glucose-to-insulin ratio, IVGTT, HOMA and QUICKI have also been used but there is no direct comparison of their sensitivities and specificities so far.[84] With the inconsistency among clinical studies on whether IR was documented and how it was documented among PCOS patients, it is difficult to conclude whether there is a relationship between the effect of metformin and the amount of IR but the effect is related to the BMI of the subjects. This is consistent with two[79,81] recent publications showing that metformin is equivalent to CC as a first line drug for ovulation induction in lean women.

In summary, although the Legro trial[64-67] was the largest prospective randomized study, the biggest concern with the conclusions is that the mean BMI of women participating in the study was 35 kg/m^2. In addition, the trial did not have adequate power to show statistical significant differences in live birth rates in the combination treatment (45%) compared to metformin (30%). Therefore, combination of metformin with clomid may lead to increased ovulation and pregnancy rates in selected groups of patients.

Second-Line Treatment Gonadotropins

Gonadotropin treatment is very effective in ovulation induction but has a high cost and increased risk in multiple follicle development and ovarian hyperstimulation syndrome (OHSS). The recommended starting dose is 37.5–50 IU/day. The duration should not exceed six ovulatory cycles.[85] Low dose regimens are used: the step-up or step-down treatments.[86] Both have high rates of multifollicular development, significantly high hyperstimulation rate and intense ovarian monitoring to reduce complications. Several studies showed the very low dose recombinant FSH step up protocol was successful in reducing the risks related to gonadotropins administration in PCOS.[86,87]

Metformin with Gonadotropins

Administration of metformin has been shown to improve ovarian response to exogenous gonadotropin in women with clomiphene-resistant PCOS.[88] In the DeLeo et al. study, metformin showed a more orderly growth of follicles leading to improved reduction in the multi-follicular development, decreasing the ovarian hyperstimulation rate. The authors'study in IVF showed that metformin also increased the mono-ovulatory cycles and reduced days of stimulation and the number of cancelled cycles due to hyper response.[89] There appears to be a shift in follicle size, reducing the number of small cohort follicles. In addition, there was improvement in reproductive outcomes after coasting and improvement in embryology parameters including oocyte maturity and embryo quality. This led to improvements in pregnancy rates. However, these results are not consistent with other studies, including RCTs which did not show any benefit of metformin on IVF outcomes in women with PCOS.[90,91] Again discrepancies may be due to large number of obese women, a too short pretreatment period with metformin, possible differences between immediate release and extended release preparations of metformin and outcomes measured.

The most recent RCT, Kjøtrød et al.[92] have published a multicenter double-blind RCT of the use of metformin as an adjuvant to PCOS, in a thin population of women starting (thin) 3 months prior to IVF. This trial suggests a benefit to metformin but the use of intention to treat analysis showed the benefit was due to increased pregnancies in the metformin pretreatment phase with no statistical differences in pregnancies from the IVF treatment. Therefore, there is still not sufficient evidence to make the treatment standard of care.

Use of Gonadotropin-Releasing Hormone Antagonist in Ovulation Induction

There is a benefit in the addition of a gonadotropin-releasing hormone (GnRH) antagonist to the ovulation induction (OI) protocol. Recently, developed third generation GnRH antagonists, such as Ganirelix® and Cetrorelix®, are devoid of the side effects associated with earlier generation compounds.[93] By competitively inhibiting endogenous GnRH, the GnRH antagonists produce an immediate and rapid decrease in LH and FSH levels without a 'flare-up' effect. Their administration in the late follicular phase prevents (or interrupts) an LH surge.[94,95] These compounds have been used in OI and in IVF.

In OI only two RCT has been published as related to their use as adjuvants in controlled ovarian hyperstimulation/intrauterine insemination cycles in PCOS patients. The first publication[96] showed the antagonist was beneficial in reducing premature luteinization rates, multifollicular development and cancellation rates but did not affect pregnancy rates.

The authors performed a prospective and randomized clinical study to evaluate the efficacy of the GnRH antagonist, (Ganirelix®) when used as adjuvant to gonadotropin stimulated cycles in PCOS patients.[97] The study also compared its commencement in an individualized manner (leading follicles at or greater than 13 mm in diameter), with commencement on day 1 of the cycle. The authors found that the addition of the GnRH antagonist to gonadotropins in a flexible protocol based on follicle size lead to increased pregnancy rates in ovulation induction by inhibiting the premature surges seen commonly in these women with pregnancy rates and live birth rates of 32%.

Third-Line Treatment: *In Vitro* Fertilization-Use of Gonadotropin-Releasing Hormone Antagonist Protocol

Many PCOS women are receiving IVF as a primary treatment and the role of ovulation induction with CC, low dose FSH and ovarian drilling sometimes seen to be forgotten. Besides the increase in cost, IVF has higher risk of OHSS and prevention is crucial. In 2006, a systematic review of large RCTs comparing the GnRH agonist and GnRH antagonist protocol in women with PCOS showed that the GnRH antagonist protocol resulted in equivalent pregnancy results to those obtained with GnRH agonist.[98] The antagonists had the advantage of decreasing the amount of gonadotropins used and shortened the period of stimulation.

In addition,this systematic review showed decrease in OHSS. This may be due to lower estradiol levels, less antral follicles (small) developing and less total gonadotropins used. In addition, there is the opportunity to trigger with agonist, lowering OHSS further.[99] In the recent updated Cochrane review,[100] Al-Inanyet et al. demonstrated that the use of antagonist is associated with a large reduction of OHSS and similar pregnancy and live birth rates. The rate of severe OHSS is shown to be significantly lower in PCOS patients. In addition there are studies using GnRH agonist trigger also decreasing the rate of OHSS.[101]

In vitro fertilization treatment is a less efficient process in the context of PCOS in terms of pregnancy rate per oocyte retrieved as it yields more oocytes to be inseminated and fertilized but lower fertilization rates and oocyte quality. However, the final outcomes of IVF treatment, including pregnancy, live birth and miscarriage rates, per embryo transfer cycle appear to be similar among PCOS and non-PCOS patients, but lower in obese patients matched for age.[102,103] Existing evidence suggests that irrespective of PCOS status and insulin resistance, BMI may play a key role in IVF treatment success. More specifically, obese women may have a lower chance of becoming pregnant and a higher

Table 1 The recommendation for treatment of CC resistant women with polycystic ovary syndrome

- **Clomiphene citrate** is more effective in rapid establishment of pregnancy than metformin. Further evaluation of the aromatase inhibitors for first line treatment is warrented.
- **Treatment with metformin** should be considered in **lean** women with PCOS as well as those with metabolic disturbances, as lean patients are most likely to benefit from therapy.
- There is a place for **laparoscopic ovarian drilling** in women who are resistant to CC, those who need evaluation of the pelvis, or those with very elevated testosterone or LH levels.
- **In ovulation induction, gonadotropins** should not be used routinely due the expense of intensive monitoring, risk of OHSS, multiple births and lower pregnancy rates.
- For the gonadotropin cycles, use of **GnRH antagonists** in a flexible protocol in conjunction with gonadotropins appears to improve pregnancy rates with low risks of multiple births with a low and slow step-up protocol.
- **IVF** is a very highly successful option if the above strategies fail, however **OHSS** risks are high and success of cycle is BMI related.
- **The GnRH antagonist protocol** is preferred for ovarian stimulation in PCOS to reduce risk of OHSS and allows options of using a **GnRH agonist trigger.**

chance of miscarriage after an IVF treatment. Clinical studies have also shown that 35–65% of PCOS patients are obese.[104-107] Since high BMI and PCOS diagnosis can influence IVF differently, future studies should examine the effect of obesity related effects separate from the effects of PCOS, Given the link between PCOS, IR and infertility, prospective cohort studies are needed to examine how PCOS can influence post-IVF health outcomes of women and their newborn infants.

CONCLUSION

The recommendation for treatment of CC resistant women with PCOS are summarized in Table 1.[108]

REFERENCES

1. Stein I, Leventhal M. Amenorrhoea associated with bilateral polycystic ovaries. Am J Obstet Gynecol. 1935;29:181-5.
2. Franks S. Assessment and management of anovulatory infertility in polycystic ovary syndrome. Endocrinol Metab Clin North Am. 2003;32:639-51.
3. Richardson MR. Current perspectives in polycystic ovary syndrome. Am Fam Physician. 2003;68:697-704.
4. Azziz R. Controversy in clinical endocrinology: diagnosis of polycystic ovarian syndrome: the Rotterdam criteria are premature. J Clin Endocrinol Metab. 2006;91:781-5.
5. Franks S. Controversy in clinical endocrinology: diagnosis of polycystic ovarian syndrome: in defense of the Rotterdam criteria. J Clin Endocrinol Metab. 2006; 91:786-9.
6. Zawadzki JK, Dunaif AD. Diagnostic criteria for polycystic ovary syndrome: towards a rationale approach. In: Dunaif A, Givens JR, Haseltine FP, Merriam GR, (Eds). Polycystic Ovary Syndrome. Boston: Blackwell Scientific Publications; 1992:377-84.
7. Rotterdam ESHRE/ASRM-Sponsored PCOS Consensus Workshop Group. Revised 2003 consensus on diagnostic criteria and long-term health risks related to polycystic ovary syndrome. Fertil Steril. 2004;81:19-25.
8. Rotterdam ESHRE/ASRM-Sponsored PCOS Consensus Workshop Group. Revised 2003 consensus on diagnostic criteria and long-term health risks related to polycystic ovary syndrome. Hum Reprod. 2004;19:41-7.
9. Norman RJ, Dewailly D, Legro RS, et al. Polycystic ovary syndrome. Lancet. 2007;370:685-97.
10. Goldzieher JW, Green JA. The polycystic ovary. Clinical and histologic features. J Clin Endocrinol Metab. 1962;22:325-38.
11. Hamilton-Fairly D, Taylor A. Anovulation. BMJ. 2006;327:546-9.
12. Vendola KA, Zhou J, Adesanya OO, et al. Androgens stimulate early stages of follicular growth in the primate ovary. J Clin Invest. 1998;101:2622-9.
13. Ehrmann DA. Polycystic ovary syndrome. N Engl J Med. 2005;352:1223-36.
14. Diamanti-Kandarakis E, Christakou C, Kandarakis H. Polycystic ovarian syndrome: the commonest cause of hyperandrogenemia in women as a risk factor for metabolic syndrome. Minerva Endocrinol. 2007;32:35-47.
15. Kousta E, Tolis G, Franks S. Polycystic ovary syndrome. Revised diagnostic criteria and long-term health consequences. Hormones (Athens). 2005;4:133-47.
16. Legro RS, Kunselman AR, Dunaif A. Prevalence and predictors of dyslipidemia in women with polycystic ovary syndrome. Am J Med. 2001;111:607-11.
17. Dahlgren E, Johansson S, Lindstedt G, et al. Women with polycystic ovary syndrome wedge resected in 1956 to 1965: a long-term follow-up focusing on natural history and circulating hormones. Fertil Steril. 1992;57:505-13.
18. Stadtmauer L. The significance of the first Latin American Consensus on polycystic ovary syndrome. Int J ClinPrac. 2010;64:536-40.

19. Lecke SB, Mattei F, Morsch DM, et al. Abdominal subcutaneous fat gene expression and circulating levels of leptin and adiponectin in polycystic ovary syndrome. Fertil Steril. 2011;95(6):2044-9.
20. Dunaif A. Insulin resistance and the polycystic ovary syndrome: mechanism and implications for pathogenesis. Endocr Rev. 1997;18:774-800.
21. Ehrmann DA, Sturis J, Byrne MM, et al. Insulin secretory defects in polycystic ovary syndrome. Relationship to insulin sensitivity and family history of non-insulin-dependent diabetes mellitus. J Clin Invest. 1995;96:520-7.
22. Dunaif A, Finegood DT. Beta-cell dysfunction independent of obesity and glucose intolerance in the polycystic ovary syndrome. J Clin Endocrinol Metab. 1996;81:942-7.
23. Kahn SE, Prigeon RL, McCulloch DK, et al. Quantification of the relationship between insulin sensitivity and beta-cell function in human subjects. Evidence for a hyperbolic function. Diabetes. 1993;42:1663-72.
24. Ovalle F, Azziz R. Insulin resistance, polycystic ovary syndrome, and type 2 diabetes mellitus. Fertil Steril. 2002;77:1095-105.
25. Diamanti-Kandarakis E, Papavassiliou AG. Molecular mechanisms of insulin resistance in polycystic ovary syndrome. Trends Mol Med. 2006;12:324-32.
26. Nestler JE, Powers LP, Matt DW, et al. A direct effect of hyperinsulinemia on serum sex hormone-binding globulin levels in obese women with the polycystic ovary syndrome. J Clin Endocrinol Metab. 1991;72:83-9.
27. Pugeat M, Crave JC, Elmidani M, et al. Pathophysiology of sex hormone binding globulin (SHBG): relation to insulin. J Steroid Biochem Mol Biol. 1991;40:841-9.
28. Azziz R, Ehrmann DA, Legro RS, et al. Troglitazone decreases adrenal androgen levels in women with polycystic ovary syndrome. Fertil Steril. 2003;79:932-7.
29. Nestler JE, Jakubowicz DJ. Decreases in ovarian cytochrome P450c17 alpha activity and serum free testosterone after reduction of insulin secretion in polycystic ovary syndrome. N Engl J Med. 1996;335:617-23.
30. Willis D, Mason H, Gilling-Smith C, et al. Modulation by insulin of follicle-stimulating hormone and luteinizing hormone actions in human granulosa cells of normal and polycystic ovaries. J Clin Endocrinol Metab. 1996;81(1):302-9.
31. Adashi EY, Hsueh AJ, Yen SS. Insulin enhancement of luteinising hormone and follicle-stimulating hormone release by cultured pituitary cells. Endocrinol. 1981;108:1441-9.
32. Norman RJ, Dewailly D, Legro RS, et al. Polycystic ovary syndrome. Lancet. 2007;370:685-97.
33. Prelevic G, Wurzburger M, Balint-Peri C, et al. Inhibitory effect of sandostatin on secretion of luteinising hormone and ovarian steroids in polycystic ovary syndrome. Lancet. 1990;336:900-3.
34. Balen AH. The pathophysiology of polycystic ovary syndrome: trying to understand PCOS and its endocrinology. Best Pract Res Clin Obstetr Gynecol. 2004; 18:685-706.
35. Schwartz RA. Acanthosis nigricans. J Am Acad Dermatol. 1994;31:1-19.
36. Orio F, Palomba S, Spinelli L, et al. The cardiovascular risk of young women with polycystic ovary syndrome: an observational, analytical, prospective case-control study. J Clin Endocrinol Metab. 2004;89:3696-701.
37. Alberti KG, Zimmet P, Shaw J. The metabolic syndrome–a new worldwide definition. Lancet. 2005;366:1059-62.
38. Apridonidze T, Essah PA, Iuorno MJ, et al. Prevalence and characteristics of the metabolic syndrome in women with polycystic ovary syndrome. J Clin Endocrinol Metab. 2005;90:1929-35.
39. Essah PA, Nestler JE. The metabolic syndrome in polycystic ovary syndrome. J Endocrinol Invest. 2006; 29:270-80.
40. Loumaye E, Vankriken L, Depreester S, et al. Hormonal changes induced by short-term administration of gonadotropin-releasing hormone agonist during ovarian hyperstimulation for in vitro fertilization and their consequences for embryo development. Fertil Steril. 1989;51:105-11.
41. Homburg R, Armar NA, Eshel A, et al. Influence of serum luteinizing hormone concentration on ovulation, conception and early pregnancy loss in polycystic ovary syndrome. Br Med J. 1988;297:1024-6.
42. Balen AH, Tan SL, Jacobs HS. Hypersecretion of luteinising hormone: a significant cause of infertility and miscarriage. Br J Obstet Gynaecol. 1993;100:1082-9.
43. Tarlatzis BC, Grimbizis G, Pournaropoulos F, et al. The prognostic value of basal luteinizing hormone: follicle-stimulating hormone ratio in the treatment of patients with polycystic ovarian syndrome by assisted reproduction techniques. Hum Reprod. 1995;10:2545-9.
44. Boomsa CM, Fauser BC, Macklon NS. Pregnancy complications in women with polycystic ovary syndrome. Semin Reprod Med. 2008;26:72-84.
45. Legro RS. Pregnancy considerations in women with polycystic ovary syndrome. Clin Obstet Gynecol. 2007;50:295-304.
46. Norman RJ, Dewailly D, Legro RS, et al. Polycystic ovary syndrome. Lancet. 2007;370:685-97.
47. Erickson GF, et al. The effects of insulin and insulin-like growth factors-I and -II on estradiol production by granulosa cells of polycystic ovaries. J Clin Endocrinol Metab. 1990;70:894-902.
48. Balen AH, Conway GS, Kaltsas G, et al. Polycystic ovary syndrome: the spectrum of the disorder in 1741 patients. Hum Reprod. 1995;10:2107-11.
49. Jonard S, Dewailly D. The follicular excess in polycystic ovaries, due to intra-ovarian hyperandrogenism, may be the main culprit for the follicular arrest. Hum Reprod Update. 2004;10:107-17.
50. Strauss JF, Dunaif A. Molecular mysteries of polycystic ovary syndrome. Mol Cell Endocrinol. 1999;13:800-5.
51. Weil SJ, Vendola K, Zhou J, et al. Androgen receptor gene expression in the primate ovary: cellular localization, regulation, and functional correlations. J Clin Endocrinol Metab. 1998;83:2479-85.

52. Quezada S, Pache TD, Hop WC, et al. 17β-Oestradiol, androstendione and inhibin levels in fluid from individual follicles of normal and polycystic ovaries, and in ovaries from androgen treated female to male transsexuals. Clin Endocrinol (Oxf). 1992;36:565-71.
53. Avellaira C, Johnson MC, Gabler F, et al. Evaluation of steroid receptors, coregulators, and molecules associated with uterine receptivity in secretory endometria from untreated women with polycystic ovary syndrome. Fertil Steril. 2006;85(4):1017-26.
54. Jonard S, Robert Y, Cortet-Rudelli C, et al. Ultrasound examination of polycystic ovaries: it is worth counting the follicles? Hum Reprod. 2003;18:598-603.
55. Dunaif A. Insulin resistance and the polycystic ovarian syndrome: mechanism and implications for pathogenesis. Endocr Rev. 1997;18:774-800.
56. Franks S, Gharani N, Waterworth D, et al. The genetic basis of polycystic ovary syndrome. Hum Reprod. 1997;12:2641-48.
57. Fallat ME, Siow Y, Marra M, et al. Müllerian inhibiting substance in follicular fluid and serum—a comparison of patients with tubal factor infertility, polycystic ovarian syndrome and endometriosis. Fertil Steril. 1997;962-5.
58. Jakimiuk AJ, Jakowicki JA, Magoffin DA. Follicular development in polycystic ovary syndrome. Assist Reprod Rev. 1997;7:54-7.
59. Homburg R, Armar NA, Eshel A, et al. Influence of serum luteinizing hormone concentrations on ovulation, conception and early pregnancy loss in polycystic ovary syndrome. Br Med J. 1988;297:1024-6.
60. Quezada S, Avellaira C, Johnson MC, et al. Evaluation of steroid receptors, coregulators, and molecules associated with uterine receptivity in secretory endometria from untreated women with polycystic ovary syndrome. Fertil Steril. 2006;85(4):1017-26.
61. Boomsa CM, Fauser BC, Macklon NS. Pregnancy complications in women with polycystic ovary syndrome. Semin Reprod Med. 2008;26:72-84.
62. Legro RS. Pregnancy considerations in women with polycystic ovary syndrome. Clin Obstet Gynecol. 2007;50:295-304.
63. Gambineri A, Pelusi C, Vicennati V, et al. Obesity and the polycystic ovary syndrome. Inter J Obesity Rel Metab Disor. 2002;26:883-96.
64. Motta AB. Report of the International symposium: Polycystic Ovary Syndrome: First Latin-American Concensus. Int J Clin Prac. 2010;64:544-57.
65. Stamets K, Taylor DS, Kunselman A, et al. A randomised trial of the effects of two types of short-term hypocaloric diets on weight loss in women with polycystic ovary syndrome. Fertil Steril. 2004;81:630-7.
66. Guzick DS. Ovulation induction management of PCOS. Clin obstet gynecol. 2007;50:255-67.
67. Legro RS, Barnhart HX, Schlaff WD et al. Clomiphene, metformin, or both for infertility in the polycystic ovary syndrome. N Engl J Med. 2007;356:551-66.
68. Al-Azemi M, Omu FE, Omu AE. The effect of obesity on the outcome of infertility management in women with polycystic ovary syndrome. Arch gynecol obstet. 2004;270:205-10.
69. Thessalonki ESHRE/ASRM sponsored PCOS Consensus Workshop Group. Consensus on infertility treatment related to polycystic ovary syndrome. Fertil Steril. 2008;89:505-22.
70. Ganesh A, Goswani SK, Chattopadhyay R, et al. Comparisons of letrozole with continuous gonadotropins and clomiphine-gonadotropin combination for ovulation induction in 1387 PCOS women after clomiphene cirate failure; a randomized prospective clinical trial. J Assist Reprod Genet. 2009;25:19-24.
71. Casper RF. Aromatase inhibitors in ovarian stimulation. J Steriod Biochem Mol Biol. 2007;106:71-5.
72. Eckmann KR, Kockler DR. Aromatase inhibitors for ovulation and pregnancy in polycystic ovary syndrome. Ann Pharmacather. 2009;43:1338-46.
73. Gjonnaess H. Polycystic ovarian syndrome treated by ovarian electrocautery through the laparoscope. Fertil Steril. 1984;41:20-5.
74. Bayram N, van Wely M, Kaaijk EM, et al. Using an electrocautery strategy or recombinant follicle stimulating hormone to induce ovulation in polycystic ovary syndrome; randomized controlled trial. BMJ. 2004;328:192-4.
75. Palomba S, Orio F, Falbo A, et al. Metformin administration and laparoscopic ovarian drilling improved ovarian response to clomiphene citrate (CC) in oligo-anovulatory CC-resistant women with polycystic ovary syndrome. Clin Endocrinol. 2005;62:631-5.
76. Ehrmann DA, Sturis J, Byrne MM, et al. Insulin secretory defects in polycystic ovary syndrome. Relationship to insulin sensitivity and family history of non-insulin-dependent diabetes mellitus. J Clin Invest. 1995;96:520-7.
77. Dunaif A, Finegood DT. Beta-cell dysfunction independent of obesity and glucose intolerance in the polycystic ovary syndrome. J Clin Endocrinol Metab. 1996;81:942-7.
78. Stadtmauer LA, Toma SK, Riehl RM, et al. Metformin treatment of patients with polycystic ovary syndrome undergoing in vitro fertilization improves outcomes and is associated with modulation of the insulin-like growth factors. Fertil Steril. 2001;75:505-9.
79. Lord JM, Flight IH, Normal RJ. Metformin in polycystic ovary syndrome; systematic review and meta-analysis. BMJ. 2003;327:951-3.
80. Creanga AA, Bradley HM, McCormick C, et al. Use of metformin in polycystic ovary syndrome: a meta-analysis. Obstet Gynecol. 2008;111:959-68.
81. Johnson NP, Bontekow S, Stewart AW. Analysis of factors predicting success of metformin and clomiphene treatment for women with infertility owing to PCOS-related ovulation dysfunction in a randomized controlled trial. Aust NZ J Obstet Gyneaecol. 2011;51:252-6.
82. Fedoresac P, Dale PO, Storeng R, et al. The impact of obesity and insulin resistance on the outcome of ICSI in women with polycystic ovarian syndrome. Hum Reprod. 2001;16:1086-91.

83. Dunaif A. Insulin resistance and the polycystic ovary syndrome: mechanism and implications for pathogenesis. Endocr Rev. 1997;18:774-800.
84. Antuna-Puente B, Disse E, Rabasa-Lhoret R, et al. How can we measure insulin sensitivity/resistance? Diabetes Metab. 2011;37(3):179-88.
85. Phillips WR. Polycystic ovary syndrome and ovulation induction. Obstet Gynecol Clin North Am. 2001;28:165-82.
86. Homburg R. Management of infertility and prevention of ovarian hyperstimulation in women with polycystic ovary syndrome. Best Pract Res. 2004;18:773-88.
87. Nugent D, Vandekerckhove P, Hughes E, et al. Gonadotropin therapy for ovulation induction in subfertility associated with polycystic ovary syndrome. Cochrane Database Syst Rev. 2000;CD000410.
88. De Leo V, La Marca A, Ditto A, et al. Effects of metformin on gonadotropin-induced ovulation in women with polycystic ovary syndrome. Fertil Steril. 1999;72:282-5.
89. Stadtmauer LA, Toma SK, Riehl RM, et al. Impact of metformin therapy on ovarian stimulation and outcome in 'coasted' patients with polycystic ovary syndrome undergoing in-vitro fertilization. Reprod Biomed Online. 2002;5:112-6.
90. Yarali H, Yildiz BO, Demirol A, et al. Co-administration of metformin during rFSH treatment in patients with clomiphene citrate-resistant polycystic ovarian syndrome: a prospective randomized trial. Hum Reprod. 2002;17:289-94.
91. Onalan G, Pabuccu R, Goktolga U, et al. Metformin treatment in patients with polycystic ovary syndrome undergoing in vitro fertilization: a prospective randomized trial. Fertil Steril. 2005;84:798-801.
92. Kjøtrød SB, Carlsen SM, Rasmussen PE, et al. Use of metformin before and during assisted reproductive technology in non-obese young infertile women with polycystic ovary syndrome: a prospective, randomized, double-blind, multi-centre study. Hum Reprod. 2011;26(8):2045-53.
93. Kenisberg D, Littman BA, Hodgen GD. Medical hypophysectomy: I. Dose-response using a gonadotropin-releasing hormone antagonist. Fertil Steril. 1984;42:112-5.
94. Leroy I, d'Acremont MF, Brailly-Tabard S, et al. A single injection of a LH-RH-a (cetrorelix) postpones the LH surge: further evidence for the role of LH-RH during the LH surge. FertilSteril. 1994;62:461-7.
95. Oberye JJ, Mannaerts BM, Huisman JA, et al. Pharmacokinetic and pharmacodynamic characteristics of ganirelix (Antagon). Part II. Dose-proportionality and gonadotropin suppression after multiple doses of ganirelix in healthy female volunteers. Fertil Steril. 1999;72:1006-12.
96. Elkind-Hirsch KE, Webster BW, Brown CP, et al. Concurrent ganirelix and follitropin-beta therapy is an effective and safe regimen for ovulation induction in women with polycystic ovary syndrome. Fertil Steril. 2003;79:603-7.
97. Stadtmauer L, Sarhan A, Duran H, et al. The impact of a gonadotropin-releasing hormone antagonist on gonadotropin ovulation induction cycles in women with polycystic ovarian syndrome: a prospective randomized study. Fertil Steril. 2011;95:216-20.
98. Griesinger G, Diedrich K, Tarltzis BC, et al. GnRH-antagonists in ovarian stimulation for IVF in patients with poor response to gonadotrophins, polycystic ovary syndrome, and risk of ovarian hyperstimulation: a meta-analysis. Reprod Biomed Online. 2006;13(5):628-38.
99. Lainas RG, Sfontouris IA, Zorzovilis IZ, et al. Flexible GnRH antagonist protocol versus GnRH long agonist protocol in patients with polycystic ovary syndrome treated for IVF: A prospective randomised controlled trial (RTC). Hum Reprod. 2010;25(3):683-9.
100. Al-Inany HG, Abou-Setta AM, Alboulghar M. Gonadotrophin-releasing hormone antagonists for assisted conception. Cochrane Database Syst Rev. 2006;3:CD001750.
101. Tehranihejad ES, Nasiri R, Rashidi B, et al. Comparison of the GnRH antagonist with long GnRH agonist protocol after OCP pretreatment in PCOS patients. Arch Gynecol Obstet. 2010;282:319-25.
102. Beydoun HA, Stadtmauer L, Beydoun MA, et al. Polycystic ovary syndrome, body mass index and outcomes of assisted reproductive technologies. Reprod Biomed Online. 2009;18:856-63.
103. Beydoun HA Stadtmauer L, Zhao Y, et al. Impact of polycystic ovary syndrome on selected indicators of in vitro fertilization and intracytoplasmic sperm injection treatment success. J Womens Health (Larchmt). 2009;18:717-23.
104. Al-Azemi M, Omu FE, Omu AE. The effect of obesity on the outcome of infertility management in women with polycystic ovary syndrome. Arch Gynecol Obstet. 2004;270:205-10.
105. Fedorcsak P, Storeng R, Dale PO, et al. Obesity is a risk factor for early pregnancy loss after IVF or ICSI. Acta Obstet Gynecol Scand. 2000;79:43-8.
106. Lashen H, Ledger W, Bernal AL, et al. Extremes of body mass do not adversely affect the outcome of superovulation and in vitro fertilization. Hum Reprod. 1999;14:712-5.
107. Fedorcsak P, Dale PO, Storeng R, et al. The impact of obesity and insulin resistance on the outcome of IVF or ICSI in women with polycystic ovarian syndrome. Hum Reprod. 2001;16:1086-91.
108. Stadtmauer L, Oehninger S. Management of infertility in women with polycystic ovary syndrome: a practical guide. Treat Endocrinol. 2005;4:279-92.

11

Endometriosis and Infertility

Albert L Hsu

CHAPTER CONTENTS

INTRODUCTION

Endometriosis is a benign gynecological disorder which often presents with pain and infertility. It is defined by endometrial glands and stroma outside of the endometrial cavity, typically on the pelvic organs or pelvic peritoneum. The three primary types of endometriosis are: superficial peritoneal lesions, ovarian endometriomas and deep infiltrating endometriosis.

Theories of the etiology of endometriosis include retrograde menstruation, coelomic metaplasia, hematogenous and lymphatic spread and direct implantation. Genetic and immunologic factors likely also play a role. Endometriosis is an estrogen-dependent, progesterone-resistant inflammatory disease. This chapter will focus on the potential mechanisms and treatment of endometriosis-associated infertility; a full discussion of the management of endometriosis-associated pain is beyond the scope of this chapter.

EPIDEMIOLOGY

Endometriosis affects 6–10% of women of reproductive age,[1] 5–21% of women with pelvic pain[2] and up to 50% of women with pain and/or infertility.[1,2] Risk factors for endometriosis include prolonged exposure to estrogen (obesity, early menarche, short cycle lengths, late menopause, nulliparity), lower body mass index, exposure to endocrine-disrupting chemicals and anatomic distortions (such as, Müllerian anomalies and exposure to diethylstilbestrol *in utero*).[2,3]

Childbearing, lactation and treatment with progestin-based therapies appear to be protective.[2] There is also an increased prevalence of rheumatoid arthritis, systemic lupus erythematosus and thyroid disorders among patients with endometriosis compared with the general population.[2] Family and genetic studies suggest a multifactorial inheritance pattern, with a 4–8-fold increased risk in first-degree relatives of patients with endometriosis.[3,4]

DIAGNOSIS

Endometriosis pain can present as dysmenorrhea, dyspareunia or dyschezia. Other bowel and bladder symptoms may include constipation, diarrhea, hematochezia and cyclic urinary frequency or urgency. In patients with pain for whom endometriosis is suspected, a full evaluation is necessary to rule out other pain syndromes, including painful bladder syndrome, irritable bowel syndrome, inflammatory bowel disease, myofascial pain, fibromyalgia and migraines. Because endometriosis is often a diagnosis of exclusion, there is frequently a significant delay between the onset of symptoms and definitive diagnosis.[5]

A pelvic mass, rectovaginal nodules and immobile pelvic organs may suggest endometriosis. However, the suspicion of endometriosis is insufficient for diagnosis, and an evaluation to rule out leiomyomata, adenomyosis, ovarian cysts and pelvic inflammatory disease is necessary. No serum marker has yet been found to diagnose endometriosis with adequate sensitivity and specificity. While imaging with pelvic ultrasound or MRI may confirm an endometriotic cyst or deep infiltrating endometriosis and help guide surgical therapy, these imaging techniques do not identify peritoneal implants or adhesions.

The gold standard for the diagnosis of endometriosis is visual inspection by laparoscopy, preferably with histologic confirmation.[5] Although visualization without biopsy has been considered to be acceptable to diagnose endometriosis in the past, one meta-analysis of the visual diagnosis of endometriosis indicates that a positive finding of endometriosis on laparoscopy is only 50% accurate.[6] In addition, biopsy of normal-appearing peritoneum has also diagnosed endometriosis in 11% of women (5 out of 47) with macroscopic evidence of endometriosis and 6% of women (3 out of 53) with no visible lesions on laparoscopy.[7]

INFERTILITY

The exact relationship between endometriosis and infertility remains unclear, especially as surgical findings often do not correlate with infertility, nor predict therapeutic response.[3,8] D'Hooghe has reported a 4% prevalence of endometriosis in fertile women, compared with 33% in infertile women.[8] Some studies have reported no adverse impact of endometriosis on *in vitro* fertilization (IVF) outcomes, as compared with tubal factor controls.[9,10] However, a meta-analysis of 22 studies has demonstrated a lower chance of pregnancy for endometriosis patients compared with patients who have tubal disease (odds ratio 0.56; 95% CI 0.44-0.70).[11] The reasons for this decreased fertility in patients with endometriosis are unclear, but may include anatomical distortion, the toxic influence of peritoneal fluid, decreased oocyte or embryo quality, defective endometrial receptivity or diminished ovarian reserve.[1,12]

The distortion of pelvic anatomy by severe endometriosis may reduce fertility mechanically by inhibiting oocyte release from the ovary or impeding ovum transport.[12] Inflammatory changes stimulated by peritoneal fluid may also be detrimental to fertility; the peritoneal fluid of women with endometriosis has been found to be toxic to mouse embryos.[13] This peritoneal fluid has a high concentration of proteases, prostaglandins and activated macrophages, which may have adverse effects on the oocyte, sperm or embryo.[12] Defective endometrial receptivity may also be a feature of endometriosis, possibly mediated by overexpression of aromatase and elevated estradiol levels, by abnormal integrin expression, by defective homeobox genes, by the presence of antiendometrial antibodies or by the absence of varying glutathione peroxidase levels.[14]

Studies of oocyte donors suggest a trend for lower pregnancy rate and implantation rate in women undergoing controlled ovarian hyperstimulation when using oocyte donors with endometriosis instead of donors without endometriosis.[15] Conversely, when women with endometriosis receive fresh donor oocytes, their implantation rate and pregnancy rate are similar to those of patients in other diagnostic groups.[16,17] This suggests that endometriosis may affect the oocyte or embryo, rather than the endometrium.[18]

Finally, diminished ovarian reserve has been observed in patients who have had laparoscopic cystectomy for endometriomas. In one study, women with endometriosis who had undergone previous surgery responded with lower oocyte yields, lower peak E2 levels and higher cancellation rate compared with tubal factor control subjects.[19] In another study, the number of dominant follicles and eggs retrieved from ovaries previously treated for unilateral endometriomas was found to be significantly less than the normal contralateral ovaries in the same patients.[20] In a similar study, follicular response was significantly reduced in post-cystectomy ovaries compared with normal ovaries in natural cycles (0.30 vs 1.00 follicles per cycle) and in clomiphene citrate-stimulated cycles (0.87 vs 1.27 follicles per cycle).[21] Thus, while patients with endometriosis may not inherently have diminished ovarian reserve, iatrogenic damage from inadvertent removal of ovarian cortex may compromise ovarian function during surgical management of endometriosis.[22]

Treatment of Infertility

Given that infertility is a multifactorial condition, it is important to test and exclude other sources of infertility in treating couples with endometriosis. These tests include a semen analysis to diagnose male factor infertility; assessment of ovarian reserve with tests, such as follicle-stimulating hormone, anti-Müllerian hormone or antral follicle count; and an evaluation of the uterine cavity and tubes for Müllerian anomalies, intrauterine filling defects and blocked or damaged fallopian tubes. Treatment must also be individualized depending on age, concomitant symptoms, insurance coverage and patient preferences.

In vitro fertilization is the most effective treatment for endometriosis-associated infertility,[5] but may be cost prohibitive. Expectant management for 1–25 months has enabled approximately 50% of women with mild endometriosis to conceive, compared with 25% of women with moderate endometriosis and no women with severe disease.[23] In a meta-analysis of 25 randomized controlled trials and cohort studies, ovulation suppression with danazol or gestrinone or medroxyprogesterone acetate has shown no benefit compared with placebo.[24]

Regarding surgical management of infertility in patients with minimal-to-mild endometriosis, two large randomized controlled studies have shown contradictory results. Marcoux has studied 341 women in Canada with minimal or mild endometriosis, finding that women who had resection or ablation of endometriosis had a higher chance of pregnancy than women who had diagnostic laparoscopy alone (30.7% vs 17.7%, P = 0.006).[25] On the other hand, Parazzini has studied 101 women in Italy with minimal or mild endometriosis, finding no difference in conception (24% vs 29%) or live birth rate (20% vs 22%) in women who had resection/ablation of endometriosis compared with diagnostic laparoscopy alone.[26] A meta-analysis of these two studies suggests a slight benefit for laparoscopic ablation or resection of endometriosis compared with diagnostic laparoscopy alone.[27]

While there may be some benefits of surgery for mild-to-moderate endometriosis, surgical management of severe endometriosis carries a risk of ovarian damage.[22] Given this concern, it may be reasonable to restrict surgery for suspected endometriosis to patients with pain, hydrosalpinges and very large endometriomas.[28] While there may be benefit to laparoscopic treatment of endometriosis after multiple failures of IVF,[29] repeat surgery for endometriosis-associated pelvic pain results in half the pregnancy rate after primary surgery.[30]

Hormonal suppression in conjunction with surgery for endometriosis has not been shown to decrease the recurrence of pain or infertility. Superovulation and intrauterine insemination also likely confer a higher chance of pregnancy than laparoscopic treatment of mild endometriosis.[31] Long luteal suppression with gonadotropin-releasing hormone analogs before gonadotropins improves outcomes compared with cycles using shorter courses of luteal suppression.[32]

In the context of infertility, the management of asymptomatic endometriomas is unclear. For patients with endometriomas who present with pain and infertility, it may be reasonable to laparoscopically excise these ovarian lesions, especially since recurrence is frequent if the endometrioma is drained by aspiration. However, thermal injury to the ovary during surgery can damage ovarian reserve, and there appears to be little to no benefit in removing endometriomas prior to IVF.[33,34] Interestingly, the presence of an endometrioma has been associated with a lower embryo quality and implantation rate compared with patients, who had simple ovarian cysts. While this suggests that the endometrioma itself caused an adverse effect rather than the space-occupying effect of the cyst, there was no difference in pregnancy rate.[35]

FUTURE DIRECTIONS

Adamson and Pasta have recently proposed and validated a staging system for surgically confirmed patients with endometriosis attempting conception without IVF.[36] Their 'endometriosis fertility index' predicts pregnancy rate based on surgical factors and patient demographics (including age, years of infertility and prior pregnancies). This fertility index awaits further validation by other investigators, but may help predict outcomes in patients with endometriosis and infertility. Others are seeking nonsurgical means to diagnose endometriosis, as well as the use of immunomodulators, hormonal suppression and cyclo-oxygenase-2 inhibitors to eliminate the need for surgical treatment of endometriosis.[37]

REFERENCES

1. Giudice LC, Kao LC. Endometriosis. Lancet. 2004;364:1789-99.
2. McLeod BS, Retzloff MG. Epidemiology of endometriosis: an assessment of risk factors. Clin Obstet Gynecol. 2010;53(2):389-96.
3. Giudice LC. Clinical practice. Endometriosis. N Engl J Med. 2010;362:2389-98.
4. Hansen KA, Eyster KM. Genetics and genomics of endometriosis. Clin Obstet Gynecol. 2010;53(2):403-12.
5. Kennedy S, Bergqvist A, Chapron C, et al. ESHRE guideline for the diagnosis and treatment of endometriosis. ESHRE Special Interest Group for Endometriosis and Endometrium Guideline Development Group. Hum Reprod. 2005;20:2698-704.
6. Wykes CB, Clark TJ, Khan KS. Accuracy of laparoscopy in the diagnosis of endometriosis: a systematic quantitative review. BJOG. 2004;111:1204-12.
7. Balasch J, Creus M, Fabregues F, et al. Visible and nonvisible endometriosis at laparoscopy in fertile and infertile women and in patients with chronic pelvic pain: a prospective study. Hum Reprod. 1996;11(2):387-91.

8. D'Hooghe TM, DeBrock S, Hill JA, et al. Endometriosis and subfertility: is the relationship resolved? Semin Reprod Med. 2003;21:243-54.
9. Olivennes F, Feldberg D, Liu HC, et al. Endometriosis: a stage by stage analysis–the role of in vitro fertilization. Fertil Steril. 1995;64:392-8.
10. Gibbons WE. Management of endometriosis in fertility patients. Fertil Steril. 2004;81(5):1204-5.
11. Barnhart K, Dunsmoor-Su R, Coutifaris C. Effect of endometriosis on in vitro fertilization. Fertil Steril. 2002; 77:1148-55.
12. Bulletti C, Coccia ME, Battistoni S, et al. Endometriosis and infertility. J Assist Reprod Genet. 2010;27:441-7.
13. Morcos RN, Gibbons WE, Findley WE. Effect of peritoneal fluid on in vitro cleavage of 2-cell mouse embryos: possible role in infertility associated with endometriosis. Fertil Steril. 1985;44:678-83.
14. Garrido N, Navarro J, Garcia-Velasco J, et al. The endometrium versus embryonic quality in endometriosis-related infertility. Hum Reprod Update. 2002; 8(1):95-103.
15. Katsoff B, Check JH, Davies E, et al. Evaluation of the effect of endometriosis on oocyte quality and endometrial environment by comparison of donor and recipient outcomes following embryo transfer in a shared oocyte program. Clin Exp Obstet Gynecol. 2006;33(4):201-2.
16. Sung L, Mukherjee T, Takeshige T, et al. Endometriosis is not detrimental to embryo implantation in oocyte recipients. J Assist Reprod Genet. 1997;14(3):152-6.
17. Pellicer A, Navarro J, Bosch E, et al. Endometrial quality in infertile women with endometriosis. Ann N Y Acad Sci. 2001;943:122-30.
18. Garcia-Velasco JA, Arici A. Is the endometrium or oocyte/embryo affected in endometriosis? Hum Reprod. 1999;14(Suppl 2):77-89.
19. Matalliotakis I, Cakmak H, Mahutte N, et al. Women with advanced-stage endometriosis and previous surgery respond less well to gonadotropin stimulation, but have similar IVF implantation and delivery rates compared with women with tubal factor infertility. Fertil Steril. 2007;88(6):1568-72.
20. Ho HY, Lee RK, Hwu YM, et al. Poor response of ovaries with endometrioma previously treated with cystectomy to controlled ovarian hyperstimulation. J Assist Reprod Genet. 2002;19:507-11.
21. Loh FH, Tan AT, Kumar J, et al. Ovarian response after laparoscopic ovarian cystectomy for endometriotic cysts in 132 monitored cycles. Fertil Steril. 1999;72(2):316-21.
22. Feinberg EC, Levens ED, DeCherney AH. Infertility surgery is dead: only the obituary remains? Fertil Steril. 2008;89(1):232-6.
23. Olive DL, Stohs GF, Metzger DA, et al. Expectant management and hydrotubations in the treatment of endometriosis-associated infertility. Fertil Steril. 1985;44:35-41.
24. Hughes EG, Fedorkow DM, Collins JA. A quantitative overview of controlled trials in endometriosis-associated infertility. Fertil Steril. 1993;59:963-70.
25. Marcoux S, Maheux R, Berube S. Laparoscopic surgery in infertile women with minimal or mild endometriosis. Canadian Collaborative Group on Endometriosis. N Engl J Med. 1997;337:217-22.
26. Parazzini F. Ablation of lesions or no treatment in minimal-mild endometriosis in infertile women: a randomized trial. Gruppo Italian per lo Studio dell'Endometriosi. Hum Reprod. 1999;14(5):1332-4.
27. Jacobson TZ, Barlow DH, Koninckx PR, et al. Laparoscopic surgery for subfertility associated with endometriosis. Cochrane Database Syst Rev. 2002;(4):CD001398.
28. De Ziegler D, Borghese B, Chapron C. Endometriosis and infertility: pathophysiology and management. Lancet. 2010;376:730-8.
29. Littman E, Giudice L, Lathi R, et al. Role of laparoscopic treatment of endometriosis in patients with failed in vitro fertilization cycles. Fertil Steril. 2005;84(6):1574-8.
30. Berlanda N, Vercellini P, Fedele L. The outcomes of repeat surgery for recurrent symptomatic endometriosis. Curr Opin Obstet Gynecol. 2010;22:320-5.
31. Grow DR, Hsu AL. Endometriosis, Part 2: Surgery for symptom relief and infertility. The Female Patient. 2006;31(11):62-8.
32. Lessey BA. Medical management of endometriosis and infertility. Fertil Steril. 2000;73:1089-96.
33. Garcia-Velasco JA, Mahutte NG, Corona J, et al. Removal of endometriomas before in vitro fertilization does not improve fertility outcomes: a matched, case-control study. Fertil Steril. 2004;81:1194-7.
34. Somigliana E, Vercellini P, Vigano P, et al. Should endometriomas be treated before IVF-ICSI cycles? Hum Reprod Update. 2006;12(1);57-64.
35. Kumbak B, Kahraman S, Karlikaya G, et al. In vitro fertilization in normoresponder patients with endometriomas: comparison with basal simple ovarian cysts. Gynecol Obstet Invest. 2008;65(3):212-6.
36. Adamson GD, Pasta DJ. Endometriosis fertility index: the new, validated endometriosis staging system. Fertil Steril. 2010;94(5):1609-15.
37. Gupta S, Goldberg JM, Aziz N, et al. Pathogenic mechanisms in endometriosis-associated infertility. Fertil Steril. 2008;90(2):247-57.

12

Recurrent Pregnancy Loss

John C Petrozza, Aleksandar Stanic, Annemarie E Fogerty

Chapter Contents

INTRODUCTION

Early pregnancy loss is a frustrating and sad experience for both, the patient and the physician. Unfortunately, early pregnancy loss is the most common complication of human gestation, occurring in as many as 75% of all women trying to conceive. Most of these losses are unrecognized and occur before or with the next expected menses. Of those that are recognized, 15–20% results in spontaneous abortions (SABs) or ectopic pregnancies. Approximately, 5% of couples trying to conceive have two consecutive miscarriages, and approximately, 1% of couples have three or more consecutive losses.

Early pregnancy loss is defined as the termination of pregnancy before 20 weeks' of gestation or with a fetal weight of less than 500 g. Most investigators agree that both ectopic and molar pregnancies should not be included in the definition. Table 1 provides specific definitions.

INCIDENCE

Most studies demonstrate a spontaneous miscarriage rate of 10–15%. However, the actual rate of early pregnancy loss is close to 50% because of the high number of chemical pregnancies that are not recognized in the 2–4 weeks after conception. Most of these pregnancy failures are due to gamete failure (e.g. sperm or oocyte dysfunction). In a classic study by Wilcox et al. in 1988, 221 women were followed up during 707 total menstrual cycles. A total of 198 pregnancies occurred. Of these, 43 (22%) were lost before the onset of menses, and another 20 (10%) were clinically recognized losses.[1]

The likelihood for SAB increases with each successive miscarriage. Data from various studies indicate that after one SAB, the baseline risk of a couple having

Table 1 *Early pregnancy loss terms and definitions

Term	Definition
Chemical pregnancy	Loss of a biochemically evident pregnancy
Early pregnancy loss	Abortion in the 1st trimester, loss of a histologically recognized pregnancy, or loss based on the presence of a gestation on ultrasound
SAB	Loss before 20 weeks gestation, as based on last menstrual period
Habitual or recurrent abortion	2 or more consecutive, unexplained SABs
Stillbirth	Loss after 20 weeks gestation

*American Society for Reproductive Medicine. Practice Committee Report redefined recurrent pregnancy loss (RPL), as above, in January, 2008.

another SAB is approximately 15%. However, if two SABs occur, the subsequent risk increases to approximately 30%. The rate is higher for women who have not had at least one live born infant. Several groups have estimated that the risk of pregnancy loss after three successive abortions is 30–45%, which is comparable to the risk in those who had two SABs. This data prompted a controversy regarding the timing of diagnostic evaluation with many specialists preferring to begin after two losses rather than three.

ETIOLOGY

The etiology of early pregnancy loss is varied and often controversial. More than one etiologic factor is often present. The most common causes of recurrent miscarriages are as follows:

Genetic Causes

- Aneuploidy
- Somatic
- Sex chromosome
- Mendelian disorders
- Multifactorial disorders
- Parental chromosomal abnormalities (translocations)
- Chromosomal inversions.

Immunologic Causes

- Autoimmune causes
- Alloimmune causes.

Anatomic Causes

- Uterine Müllerian anomaly
  - Uterine septum (the anomaly most commonly associated with pregnancy loss)
  - Hemiuterus (unicornuate uterus)
  - Bicornuate uterus
- Diethylstilbestrol-linked condition
- Acquired defects (e.g. Asherman syndrome)
- Incompetent cervix
- Leiomyomas
- Uterine polyps.

Infectious Causes

Environmental Causes

- Smoking
- Excessive alcohol consumption
- Caffeine.

Endocrine Factors

- Diabetes mellitus
- Antithyroid antibodies
- Luteal phase deficiency.

Hematologic Disorders

The gestational age at the time of SAB can provide clues about the cause. For example, nearly 70% of SABs in the first 12 weeks are due to chromosomal anomalies. However, losses due to antiphospholipid syndrome (APS) and cervical incompetence tend to occur after the first trimester. For many patients, a comprehensive evaluation does not reveal a specific cause and in some cases may tease out a nonspecific finding or lead to unnecessary treatment.

Genetic Causes

Prevalence and Types

Most spontaneous miscarriages are caused by an abnormal (aneuploid) karyotype of the embryo. At least, 50% of all first trimester SABs are cytogenetically abnormal. This figure does not include abnormalities caused by single genetic disorders, such as Mendelian disorders or mutations at several loci. Some examples that may not be detected by evaluating karyotypes are polygenic or multifactorial disorders.

The highest rate of cytogenetically abnormal concept occurs earliest in gestation with rates declining after the embryonic period (> 30 mm crown-rump length). The rate of normal (euploid) and abnormal (aneuploid) abortuses increases with maternal age.

Recurrent miscarriage may result from two types of chromosomal abnormalities: (1) the recurrence of a numerical abnormality (aneuploidy) in the embryo, which is usually not inherited or; (2) a structural abnormality derived from one parent.

Aneuploidy: Cytogenetically abnormal embryos are usually aneuploid because of sporadic events, such as meiotic nondisjunction or polyploid from fertilization abnormalities.

Autosomal trisomy: Autosomal trisomy is involved in 50% of the cytogenetically abnormal abortuses in the first trimester. It may arise *de novo* because of meiotic nondisjunction during gametogenesis in parents with a normal karyotype. Autosomal trisomy results from maternal meiosis I errors (either complete trisomies or monosomies).

Specific trisomies: Trisomy 16, which accounts for 30% of all trisomies is the most common. Viable trisomies have been observed for chromosomes 13, 16, and 21. Approximately, one-third of fetuses with down syndrome (trisomy 21) survive to term.

Autosomal monosomies: Autosomal monosomies are rarely, if ever, observed.

Monosomy X (Turner's syndrome): Turner's syndrome is frequently observed and is the most common chromosomal abnormality observed in SABs. Turner's syndrome accounts for 20–25% of cytogenetically abnormal abortuses.

Triploidy and tetraploidy: Triploidy and tetraploidy are related to abnormal fertilization and are not compatible with life. Triploidy is found in 16% of abortions, with fertilization of a normal haploid ovum by two sperm (dispermy) as the primary pathogenic mechanism. Tetraploidy occurs in approximately 8% of chromosomally abnormal abortions resulting from failure of an early cleavage division in an otherwise normal diploid zygote.

Parental chromosomal abnormalities: Structural chromosomal abnormalities occur in approximately 3% of cytogenetically abnormal abortuses.[2]

- These abnormalities are thought to be the most commonly inherited from the mother.
- Structural chromosomal problems found in men often lead to low sperm concentrations, male infertility and therefore, a reduced likelihood of pregnancy and miscarriage.

Translocations are the most common types of structural abnormalities and can be balanced or unbalanced. Slightly more than one half of unbalanced rearrangements result from abnormal segregation of Robertsonian translocations (when two acrocentric chromosomes fuse near the centromere region with loss of the short arms) and the rest arise *de novo* during gametogenesis.

In reciprocal translocations, there is an exchange of material between nonhomologous chromosomes. The offspring created from parental gametes with the abnormality may have normal or carrier karyotypes. Adjacent segregation results in unbalanced distribution of the chromosomes involved in the translocation, leading to partial trisomy for one chromosome and partial monosomy for the other chromosome. The severity of the phenotype depends on the chromosomes involved and on the positions of their breakpoints.

Other structural rearrangements, such as inversions or ring chromosomes are relatively rare. These chromosomal abnormalities can be associated with congenital malformations and mental retardation, as well as SAB.

Genetic Abnormalities/Mendelian Disorders

Certain genetic mutations, such as the autosomal dominant disorder leading to myotonic dystrophy, may predispose a patient to infertility or even miscarriage. The cause of the abortion in this disease is unknown, but it may be related to abnormal gene interactions combined with disordered uterine function and implantation defects.

Other presumed autosomal dominant disorders associated with SAB include lethal skeletal dysplasias, such as, thanatophoric dysplasia and type II osteogenesis imperfecta.

Maternal disease associated with increased fetal wastage includes connective tissue disorders, such as Marfan syndrome, Ehlers-Danlos syndrome, homocystinuria and pseudoxanthoma elasticum.

Hematologic abnormalities associated with RPL include dysfibrinogenemia, factor XIII deficiency, congenital hypofibrinogenemia and afibrinogenemia and sickle cell anemia.

Women with sickle cell anemia are at increased risk for fetal loss possibly because of placental bed microinfarcts.

Management

For couples who have had a SAB due to a suspected genetic cause, the standard of care is to offer genetic counseling. Because advanced age increases the risk of an abnormal karyotype in a conceptus, amniocentesis is routinely offered for all pregnant women of advanced maternal age, which is defined as women older than 35 years. A woman's risk of having an aneuploid fetus is 1 per 80 when she is older than 35 years; this is far greater than the risk of fetal loss after amniocentesis which is 1 per 200.

A study by Warburton et al. indicated that routine karyotype analysis after one miscarriage is not cost-effective or prognostic.[3] However, after two SABs, analysis of the abortuses is useful. In 1990, Drugan et al. examined 305 women with two or more miscarriages and found an increased risk for fetal aneuploidy in these couples

with chorionic villus sampling or amniocentesis.[4] Thus, although controversial, couples with recurrent miscarriage may consider karyotype evaluation by means of amniocentesis, chorionic villus sampling or early first trimester screening during a subsequent pregnancy. In addition, some experts recommend karyotpe analysis of any products of conceptions in women with two prior miscarriages because the presence of an aneuploid fetus is associated with a better chance for a subsequent successful pregnancy.[5] Array comparative genomic hybridization may complement regular karyotype evaluation of products of conception, as this may eliminate maternal cell contamination and screen for smaller chromosomal abnormalities. However, genomic hybridization cannot identify balanced translocations.[6]

Because karyotype analysis does not help in detecting abnormalities caused by single gene mutations or mutations at several loci (small structural deletions and rearrangements), different techniques, such as fluorescence *in situ* hybridization (FISH), are being used to complement standard cytogenetics. If a parental chromosome abnormality is found, this should be the starting point for familial testing, and proper family counseling is recommended. If an increased risk for future pregnancies is identified, all alternatives should be discussed, including foregoing any attempts at further conception, adopting, trying to conceive again with early prenatal testing, using donor gametes or performing preimplantation genetic diagnosis (PGD).

The concept of preimplantation genetic screening (PGS) has been utilized recently. This involves using FISH to screen the removed blastomere for aneuploidy in older women and in those with recurrent SABs. Preimplantation genetic screening and FISH can be used to accurately detect common aneuploidies accounting for 70% of aneuploidic first trimester losses (chromosomes 13, 15, 16, 17, 18, 21, X and Y), but these methods are criticized for their inability to detect all chromosomal abnormalities. Theoretically, selection of chromosomally normal embryos for uterine transfer increases the likelihood for implantation, but the reports in the literature have been conflicting in regards to the efficacy of PGS in this setting.

In 2006, a retrospective analysis by Munne et al. of women older than 40 years showed a decrease in the SAB rates from 40–22% in the group that underwent PGD.[7] However, efficacy of PGS in decreasing SAB rates was challenged in other studies.

A randomized trial of 408 women of advanced maternal age undergoing a total of 836 cycles concluded that the ongoing pregnancy rate, as well as live birth rate, was significantly lower in the women assigned to the PGS group compared with those without PGS.[8] The authors theorized the possibility that biopsy of a blastomere on day 3 hampers the potential of an embryo to successfully implant. Another reason for their result could be the flaws inherent in the FISH procedure, such as, inability to detect aneuploidy in all chromosomes or examining mosaic cells.

Based on the practice guidelines published in Fertility and Sterility in 2007 and 2008, available evidence does not support the use of PGS to increase live birth rates in women of advanced maternal age.[9]

Also, available evidence does not currently support the use of PGS for chromosomally normal patients with RPL because it does not improve ongoing pregnancy or live birth rates and does not decrease miscarriage rates in such women.[10] In fact, for women with a known balanced translocation, there is up to 70% chance of a live born with no intervention at all.[11] The chance of having a live born baby with a translocation is typically less than 1%, which questions the benefit of PGD. However, couples in whom pregnancy loss can be attributed to a balanced translocation may desire specific genetic testing by PGD, for which careful counseling must be performed to ensure that the patient is completely aware of the limitations with this technology.

Reported disadvantages of PGD include misdiagnosis of chromosomal normality, possible lowering of implantation rates with embryonic biopsy and poor suitability of tested embryos for cryopreservation. The use of array comparative genomic hybridization, with its finer resolution and ability to screen all chromosomes, may improve the success of PGS, but adequate trials are still lacking in women with RPL.

Anatomic Causes

Anatomic uterine defects are known to cause obstetric complications, including RPL, preterm labor and delivery and malpresentation, although many women with such defects may have uncomplicated pregnancies. Most commonly, the complications result from impaired vascularization and fetal growth restriction.

The incidence of uterine anomalies is estimated to be 1 per 200–600 women, depending on the method used for diagnosis. When manual exploration is performed at the time of delivery, uterine anomalies are found in approximately 3% of women. However, uterine abnormalities are present in approximately 27% of women with a history of pregnancy loss.

Uterine Müllerian Anomalies

The most common uterine defects include septate, unicornuate, bicornuate and didelphic uteri. Of these, the unicornuate uterus is least common, but can result in malpresentation and fetal growth restriction. The highest rate of reproductive losses are found in bicornuate uteri (47%) compared with unicornuate uteri (17%), but both are frequently associated with second trimester loss and preterm delivery. Women with unicornuate and didelphic uteri have the highest rate of abnormal deliveries, while women with uterine septa have a 26% risk of reproductive loss.

In addition to Müllerian anomalies, other anatomic causes of RPL to consider for include diethylstilbestrol exposure related anomalies, Asherman syndrome, incompetent cervix, leiomyomas and uterine polyps.

Controversies exist among these listed uterine anatomic abnormalities as causes for pregnancy loss. They are suggested but not scientifically proved potential causes.

Management

Accurate diagnosis of Müllerian anomalies is essential. Imaging studies of choice include hysteroscopy, hysterosalpingography, sonohysterograms and vaginal ultrasonography. Findings may be confirmed with MRI. Three dimensional ultrasonography and sonohysterography are becoming more pronounced in evaluating these abnormalities, and are much more cost effective than MRI. For instance, a banana-shaped cavity with a single fallopian tube is the most common finding in a unicornuate uterus. Prophylactic cervical cerclage should be considered in patients with a unicornuate uterus. Some authors support expectant management in these patients with serial assessments of cervical lengths by using digital and ultrasonographic examinations.

Surgical correction of uterine anatomic abnormalities has not been shown to benefit pregnancy outcomes in a prospective controlled trial. In fact, most women with bicornuate or unicornuate uteruses have good obstetrical outcomes and surgical repairs of these anomalies are either impossible or quite invasive. However, data from multiple uncontrolled retrospective reviews have suggested that resection of the uterine septum increases live born delivery rates (70–85%).[12,13] For this reason, and the fact that is difficult, if not impossible to set up a proper controlled study, it is not unreasonable to consider transection of a uterine septum in patients with recurrent miscarriage. In women who have never been pregnant, the incidental finding of a uterine septum can be quite worrisome for a young woman. Although there is a high likelihood for a successful pregnancy without surgery, the data is quite sparse, especially with large septums.[14] The decision to repair the septum should be considered carefully and with careful consideration of the patient's history.

Uterine Fibroids

Fibroids, especially those that are submucosal are associated with an increased risk of miscarriage.[15] The value of myomectomy in these situations of recurrent miscarriage is uncertain and supported only by data comparing results of pre- and post-surgery. Once again, data to support the benefit myomectomy will be difficult to obtain due to the inherent issues with designing a proper, controlled study. As with septums, the decision to repair the uterus should be considered carefully and with complete understanding from the patient of all potential risks and benefits.

Infectious Causes

The theory that microbial infections can cause miscarriage has been presented in the literature as early as 1917 when DeForest et al. observed recurrent abortions in women exposed to farm animals with brucellosis. Numerous organisms have been implicated in sporadic causes of miscarriage, but common microbial causes of RPL have not been confirmed. In fact, infection is viewed as a rare cause of recurrent miscarriage. A recent review failed to show sufficient evidence for the notion that any type of infection can be identified as a causal factor for recurrent miscarriage. Most patients with a history of recurrent miscarriage do not benefit from an extensive infection workup. More recently, some interesting information regarding the impact of human papillomavirus on adverse reproductive outcomes raised some interesting concerns, but as of yet, screening for this virus is not indicated.[16]

Environmental Causes

Environmental causes of human malformation account for approximately 10% of malformations, and less than 1% of all human malformations are related to exposures to prescription drugs, chemicals or radiation.

Isotretinoin (Accutane)

Isotretinoin is a retinoic acid used to treat severe acne and is associated with SAB.

Anesthetic Gases

The relationship between exposure to trace concentrations of waste anesthetic gases in the operating room and the possible development of adverse health effects has been a concern for many years.[17] However, the studies that did show an increased incidence of miscarriage and congenital anomalies had many flaws. A meta-analysis from 1997 pooled data from 19 reports and concluded that in the pre-scavenging era, the relative risk (RR) of SAB from exposure to anesthetic gas was 1.9. Since then, most operating rooms use ventilation systems to minimize occupational exposure to the gases.[18]

Tobacco

Maternal exposure to tobacco and its effect on reproductive outcomes has been the subject of many studies. Cigarette smoke contains hundreds of toxic compounds. Nicotine is thought to reduce placental and fetal circulation through its vasoactive actions. Carbon monoxide depletes both fetal and maternal oxygen supply, and lead is a known neurotoxin. Despite the many harmful effects to a woman's health, maternal smoking appears to only slightly increase the risk of SABs.

Alcohol

Maternal exposure to excess alcohol has been reported to be associated with an increased risk for SAB.

Coffee Consumption

Coffee consumption has been the subject of much debate since the 1980s. Studies have demonstrated conflicting results, some find that moderate coffee consumption (< 350 mg/d) is not related to the risk of SABs,[19] whereas others claim that the risk of SAB increases even at this level of exposure.[20]

In 2008, a large cohort study of 1063 patients by Weng et al. demonstrated that caffeine consumption had a dose-dependent increase in the risk of miscarriage at all levels of consumption. Patients with caffeine intake of less than 200 mg/d were 1.42 times more likely to have an early miscarriage, whereas in those with intake of 200 mg/d or greater, the risk increased to 2.23 times compared with patients with no caffeine use. In addition, the magnitude of the association appeared to be stronger among women without a history of miscarriage than that among women with such a history.[21]

Endocrine Causes

Ovulation, implantation and the early stages of pregnancy depend on an intact maternal endocrine regulatory system. Most attention was historically directed at maternal systemic endocrine disorders, luteal phase abnormalities and hormonal events that follow conception, particularly progesterone levels in early pregnancy.

Diabetes Mellitus

Women with diabetes mellitus who have good metabolic control are no more likely to miscarry than women without diabetes. However, women with poorly controlled diabetes, as evidenced by high glycosylated Hg A1c levels in the first trimester, are at a significantly increased risk of both miscarriage and fetal malformation. The SAB rate increases 2–3 fold in these women compared with the general population. Screening for occult diabetes in asymptomatic women is not necessary unless the patients present with an elevated random glucose level or exhibits other clinical signs of diabetes mellitus or if there is an unexplained loss in the second trimester.

Thyroid Dysfunction

No direct evidence suggests that thyroid disease is associated with recurrent miscarriages. However, the presence of antithyroid antibodies (two thyroid antigens: thyroglobulin and thyroid peroxidase) may represent a generalized autoimmune abnormality, which could be a contributing factor in miscarriages. Screening for thyroid disease is not useful unless the patient is symptomatic.

Low Progesterone Levels

Progesterone is the principal factor responsible for the differentiation of proliferative endometrium to secretory, rendering the endometrium receptive to embryo implantation. Since Allen and Corner published their classic results on physiologic properties of the corpus luteum in 1929, low progesterone levels have been assumed to be associated with miscarriage.

Luteal support remains critical till approximately 7 weeks' gestation, at which time the placental trophoblast has acquired enough steroidogenic ability to support the pregnancy. Miscarriage results in patients whom the corpus luteum is removed before 7 weeks. If progesterone is given to these patients, the pregnancy is salvaged. Recent experience with RU486 (an antiprogestin) has shown that this treatment can effectively terminate a pregnancy up to 56 days from the last menstrual period.

Luteal Phase Defects

In 1943, Jones first discussed the concept of insufficient luteal progesterone resulting in either infertility or early pregnancy loss. This disorder was defined as inadequate endometrial maturation resulting from a qualitative or quantitative disorder in corpus luteal function. Methods used to diagnose luteal phase defects (LPDs) include records of basal body temperature, evaluation of progesterone concentrations and histologic dating of endometrial biopsy specimens.

The criterion standard in diagnosis of LPD is the histological characteristics of a luteal phase endometrial biopsy being more than 2 days behind the findings expected in a normal cycle. However, substantial inter and intraobserver discrepancies occur even when the standard histologic criterion is applied, which has lead to the controversy surrounding this disorder. Furthermore, although LPD have been reported in 23–60% of women with recurrent miscarriage, as many as 31% of normally fertile women have an LPD according to the results from serial endometrial biopsy procedures. However, since no reliable method is available to diagnose this disorder, controversy exists regarding both, the definition and the diagnosis itself. An additional factor that accounts for many of the discrepancies in the literature is the frequent use of the patient's subsequent menses as a reference point for determining when she had ovulated, which assumes a normal 28 days cycle.

In one of the few prospective studies on this subject, endometrial biopsy was performed in women with three or more consecutive miscarriages. The pathologist then accurately dated the biopsy samples using luteinizing hormone (LH) assays to pinpoint the time of ovulation. Luteal phase defects were believed to be the cause in 17% of these recurrent miscarriages. The authors also examined luteal phase serum progesterone levels and noted that they were normal in the women with LPD. Thus, luteal phase deficiency was most likely the result of an abnormal response of the endometrium to progesterone rather than a subnormal production of progesterone by the corpus luteum. This finding is corroborated by other studies, showing that as many as 50% of women with histologically defined LPD have normal serum progesterone levels.

The physician must be selective in deciding who should be screened for LPD, since there is no definitive treatment to make a difference in pregnancy outcomes. Only one randomized trial has shown that treatment with progesterone supplementation has a beneficial effect on pregnancy outcomes,[22] while most other studies failed to demonstrate that any type of support (e.g. progesterone, human chorionic gonadotropin) results in a significant difference.

So, although it is known that postimplantation failure or an early nonviable pregnancy are associated with low serum progesterone levels, there is no evidence that progesterone supplementation in patients with LPD would restore the normal hormonal profile. Therefore, one approach is to screen only patients with either a history of recurrent miscarriages or recurrent failures with infertility therapy. In addition, the best accuracy is achieved if the same pathologist reviews the histologic findings and if the day of ovulation is based on LH levels rather than subsequent menses.

Polycystic Ovarian Syndrome

The risk of recurrent miscarriage appears to be higher in women with polycystic ovarian syndrome (PCOS).[23] However, rates of miscarriage do not appear to be higher in women with PCOS who conceive after ovulation induction compared to women without the syndrome.[24] Furthermore, suppressing LH with gonadotropin-releasing hormone agonist did not improve live born rates in women with PCOS.[24] Data is lacking regarding the benefit of an insulin sensitizer, such as metformin, in reducing recurrent miscarriage in women with PCOS, although its use has not been shown to reduce isolated miscarriages in women with the disease.[25]

Endocrine Modulation of Decidual Immunity

The transformation of endometrium to decidua affects all cell types present in the uterine mucosa. These morphologic and functional changes facilitate implantation, but they also help to control trophoblast migration and prevent over invasion in maternal tissue. Attention focuses on the interaction between the extravillous trophoblast and the leukocyte populations infiltrating the uterine mucosa. Most of these cells are large granular lymphocytes (LGLs) and macrophages; few T and B cells are present. The LGL population is unusual, staining strongly for natural killer (NK) cell marker CD56, but the cells do not express the CD16 and CD3 NK markers. Natural killer cells with this distinct phenotype are found in high numbers, primarily in the progesterone-primed endometrium of the uterus. The number of CD56 cells, which is low in the proliferative phase endometrium, increases in the midluteal phase and peaks in the late secretory phase, suggesting that recruitment of LGLs is under hormonal control.

Progesterone is essential in this process because LGLs are not found before menarche, after menopause or in conditions associated with unopposed estrogen (e.g. endometrial hyperplasia, carcinoma). In women who have undergone oophorectomy, LGLs appear only after treatment with both estrogen and progesterone. The increase in the number of NK cells at the implantation site in the first trimester suggests their role in pregnancy maintenance. They preferentially kill target cells with little or no human leucocyte antigen (HLA) expression. The extravillous trophoblast (which expresses modified forms of 1 HLA) is resistant to lysis by decidual NK cells under most circumstances, allowing the invasion needed for normal placentation. These CD56 cells probably differentiate *in utero* from precursor cells because serum levels are negligible.

The only cytokine that has been able to induce proliferation of these cells is interleukin-2 (IL-2). Interleukin-2 also transforms NK cells into lymphokine-activated killer (LAK) cells, which can lyse first trimester trophoblast cells *in vitro*. As expected, IL-2 has not been found *in vivo* at uterine implantation sites; otherwise, stimulation of decidual NK cells would cause widespread destruction of the trophoblast. Trophoblast HLA expression is increased by interferon, a phenomenon that may offer protection from LAK cell lysis. Therefore, equilibrium exists between the level of HLA expression on the trophoblast and the amount of lymphokine activation of NK cells, leading to the concept of fine regulation of trophoblast invasion.

IMMUNE PATHOPHYSIOLOGY OF RECURRENT PREGNANCY LOSS

Immunology of the Feto-placental Unit in Recurrent Pregnancy Loss

Achievement of a successful reproductive cycle in humans from conception to birth requires transfer of large amounts of maternal resources to the immunologically foreign developing fetus while assuring safety from immunological attack. The immune tolerance of the developing semi-allogeneic fetus is particularly tricky in humans, as we have the most invasive form of haemochorial placentation amongst eutherian mammals.[26] Consequently, the coexistence and cooperation of specialized immune cells in the transformed uterine endometrium underlying the placenta (termed the decidua) with invading trophoblasts is essential for successful pregnancy outcome. Disturbances of proper placentation are hypothesized to play a major role in RPL and pregnancy complications, such as pre-eclampsia and intrauterine growth restriction. In contrast to the essential role of immune interactions at the placental surface, anti-embryonic adaptive immune responses have been very difficult to demonstrate.

Microanatomy

Placenta in mammalian species is highly diverse in both shape and microanatomy. From an immunological perspective, the key difference between different mammals is the depth of invasion of placental cytotrophoblasts, ranging from no invasion in epitheliochorial placentation to extensive invasion in human hemochorial placentation. In humans, extravillous trophoblasts penetrate into the uterine epithelium and participate in the decidualization of the endometrium. Furthermore, extravillous cytotrophoblasts infiltrate the inner one-third of the myometrium to directly remodel the endothelium of spiral arteries and remove part of the muscular media of these vessels. This remodeling allows lowering of the vascular resistance in the decidual bed, resulting in low-pressure, high-volume dependent flow.

Antigen Presentation

The syncytiotrophoblasts bathed in maternal blood and extravillous cytotrophoblasts in the decidua are, therefore, at the forefront of the feto-maternal immune boundary. The tolerance of the maternal immune system to the fetus is a combination of cytotrophoblast stealth and active regulation by the maternal lymphocytes. Syncytiotrophoblast does not express any major histocompatibility complex molecules (MHC), contributing to immune neutrality of the placental surface as neither cytotoxic nor helper T cells are able to recognize and kill cells not expressing MHC. Extravillous cytotrophoblasts also have a highly restricted expression of MHC molecules, with only HLA-G, HLA-E and HLA-C, but not HLA-A or HLA-B expressed.[27-29] As the HLA-A and HLA-B are the major contributors to transplant allograft rejection, invading cytotrophoblasts are thus protected from local uterine T cells.

Cellular Phenotype

Specialized local microenvironment in the decidua is exemplified by its cellular composition. Approximately, 40% of all cells in the decidua are maternal immune cells.[30,31] Most of these (50–70%) are CD56 (bright) CD16 (negative) uterine Natural Killer (uNK) cells, then macrophages, dendritic cells, regulatory and helper $CD4^+$ T cells, and a few $CD8^+$ T cells and NKT cells.[30-32] Unlike peripheral CD56 (dim) $CD16^+$ NK cells, which are highly cytotoxic, the uNK cells have a decreased cytotoxicity and a higher cytokine secretion capability.[33] Moreover, uNK cells have been demonstrated to directly interact with cytotrophoblasts and assist and direct their remodeling of the spiral arteries in the decidua via secretion of IL-8, IIP-10 and possible vascular endothelial growth factor and placental growth factor.[34] Consequently, not only uNK cells are not cytotoxic to invading cytotrophoblasts, but they actively support and regulate their decidual invasion and remodeling.[33-35] Similarly, the decidual $CD14^+$ macrophages (alternatively termed decidual $CD14^+$ myelomonocytic cells[36]) can be activated to secrete IL-8 by HLA-G mediated activation of its receptor LILRB1.[37] Additionally, they produce indoleamine 2,3-dioxygenase (IDO),[38] a key enzyme required for T cell tolerance to the fetus. This community of cytotrophoblasts, uNK cells and macrophages attracts specific fetal alloimmune regulatory $CD4^+$ T[39] (Treg) cells to the feto-maternal interface via hCG,[40] and via IDO induces local Treg cells.[36] Additionally, pregnant state increases global Treg number independent of alloimmune expansion.[41] Consistent with their important role in fetal alloimmune tolerance, Treg depletion results in rejection of allogeneic, but not syngeneic, feti and pregnancy failure.[41] Uterine dendritic cells also contribute to the feto-tolerant environment in the presence of uNK cells and cytotrophoblasts by abolishing IL-12 production,[42] increasing IL-10 secretion[43] and promoting Th2-type responses.[44]

Cytokines

Secretion of cytokines and other mediators from all participating cells in the decidua is critical for pregnancy from implantation to birth. Even embryos secrete a plethora of cytokines (e.g. IL-1, IL-6, IL-8 and IP-10 amongst others).[45-47] As noted above, uNK cells are critical in decidualization, and in mouse models, uNK inducers IL-12, IL-15 and IL-18 are critical to decidual remodeling.[48-50] On a global level, maternal Th1-skew of CD4 T cells has been associated with RPL.[51,52] Similarly, in mouse models of RPL, administration of IL-2, TNF-α or IFN-γ can increase fetal loss rates.[53] Overall, it appears that induction of global maternal inflammatory responses, either via intrinsic skew of helper T cells or via induction of inflammatory cytokines from antigen presenting cells by toll-like receptor activation,[54-57] is strongly associated with fetal loss.

In summary, the decidua is a highly collaborative environment wherein both maternal and fetal cells collaborate in building a conducive microenvironment for efficient nutrient transfer to meet the very high metabolic demands of the developing human fetus. Furthermore, in contrast to the prior paradigm in the field which stressed the competition between fetal and maternal cells in uterine remodeling, the maternal immune cells not only actively ignore fetal cells, but also participate in the adaptation of uterine vasculature for the demands of pregnancy.

Immune Syndromes Associated with Recurrent Pregnancy Loss

The complexity of feto-maternal immune interface exposes this system to failure when the maternal immune system or presumably the fetal cytotrophoblasts are altered physiology. Autoimmune disorders in the mother can consequently alter the local immune balance and result in pregnancy failure.

Antiphospholipid Antibody Syndrome

Amongst women with RPL, between 9% and 17% are found to have antiphospholipid antibodies (APLAs),[58,59] either in isolation or as a component of APS[60] Antiphospholipid syndrome diagnostic criteria, revised in 2006, include clinical and laboratory criteria. Clinical criteria include inflammation-related vascular thrombosis or pregnancy morbidity (RPL, intrauterine fetal death and preterm birth due to eclampsia or severe preeclampsia).[60] Laboratory criteria include the presence of lupus anticoagulant, anticardiolipin antibody or anti-β2 glycoprotein 1 (β2GPI) antibodies measured twice, 12 weeks apart. Clinical use of other APLAs, such as anti-annexin V, anti-phosphatidylserine (anti-PS), anti-phosphatidylethanolamine (anti-PE) and others is currently controversial. It should be noted that the term 'lupus anticoagulant' describes antibodies directed against a variety of targets, including β2GPI, cardiolipins, other phospholipids or proteins, which demonstrate ability to interfere with coagulation testing.

The anti-cardiolipin-β2GPI antibodies are the most well studied and most strongly associated with RPL.[61,62] Antibodies directed against cardiolipin are almost always directed against β2GPI as well, and for clinical purposes, testing for either identifies the same antibody repertoire.[63] Animal models provide support for a direct role of anti-β2GPI antibodies in RPL as their passive transfer or active induction in mice causes fetal loss.[64-72] Mechanism of fetal loss mediated by anti-β2GPI antibodies seems to be complex and multifactorial. Placental thrombosis has been implicated when transferring antibodies into already pregnant mice.[69] Thrombosis in the APLA-affected placenta is thought to be secondary to tissue factor release.[73-76] Furthermore, embryo implantation is impaired upon exposure to anti-β2GPI antibodies.[77] Secretion of human chorionic gonadotropin from trophoblasts is diminished in the presence of anti-β2GPI antibodies,[78] likely due to defective decidual invasion by the cytotrophoblast.[79] Finally, and possibly most importantly, anti-β2GPI antibodies recruit complement *in vivo* and cause inflammation exemplified by increased TNF-α level, as well as direct fetal damage.[80,81]

As noted above, clinical utility of anti-PE, anti-PS, and anti-annexin V antibodies is currently unclear, however, there is a significant amount of data supporting their pathogenic role in RPL. These antibodies are inter-related, as Annexin V binds exposed membrane phospholipids, especially PS, which is critical to shield it from circulating procoagulant proteins, as exposed PS activates the coagulation cascade.[82-84] Antibodies to Annexin V disrupt its anticoagulant activity[85] and are associated with RPL and implantation failure.[86,87] Unlike most other tissues utilize flippases (aminophospholipid translocases) to remove PS from the outer leaflet and confine it in the inner leaflet of cell membranes,[88] developing trophoblasts express PS on their cell surface.[89-91] Consequently, it is no surprise that presence of anti-PS antibodies is associated with RPL.[92,93] Anti-PS antibodies have been found to increase the apoptosis of rat trophoblasts[94] and exert strong cytotoxicity against mouse trophoblasts.[95] In contrast to PS, PE is found on both outer and inner leaflets of cell membranes.[96] Antibodies to PE have also been found in women with RPL,[93] but their role is less clear. Interestingly, and exemplifying the inter-relatedness of APLA antibodies, the native β2GPI also binds PS and is critical to efficient clearance of PS-expressing cells by phagocytes.[96-98] A variety of non-classical APLA antibodies have been recently described, but their role in RPL has not been described.

Systemic Lupus Erythematosus

Unlike APLA syndrome, systemic lupus erythematosus (SLE) is not associated with early RPL (early first trimester), rather patients affected have a high incidence of second and third trimester pregnancy loss and complications, such as intrauterine growth restriction, pre-eclampsia, preterm labor and intrauterine fetal demise.[99] It should be noted that the lack of association of SLE with RPL is only in the setting of no APLAs, as these antibodies are commonly found in association with SLE. In the Hopkins Lupus Cohort, only 28% of SLE patients were negative for all three major APLA classes (lupus anticoagulant, anticardiolipin, anti-β2GPI).[100]

Complications of pregnancy associated with SLE are dependent on the presence and activity of SLE before pregnancy, and especially the diagnosis of lupus nephritis. Fetal loss rates are associated with disease activity, as patients with inactive SLE have been reported to have a rate of 8–12%, compared with 25–52% in those with active disease.[101] Systemic lupus erythematosus activity is significantly associated with pre-eclampsia,[99,102] and with those who have active renal disease, it has been reported to be 30–66%.[76,103] Additionally, presence of SLE-related hypertension prior to pregnancy carries the odds ratio of 23 for fetal loss. Consequently, it has been argued that to minimize risk during pregnancy, SLE should be treated and be inactive for at least six months prior to conception.

Presence of antinuclear antibodies (ANA), with or without concurrent SLE, has been also associated with RPL. This observation is confounded by the finding that as many as 10–30% of apparently, normal individuals have at least a low titer of these antibodies.[104,105] It is therefore not surprising that studies have been conflicting with some showing increased prevalence of ANA antibodies in women with RPL,[106,107] while others do not.[108,109] Consequently, at this time, routine and independent evaluation of ANA antibodies is not recommended, as further studies are required to determine their role in both the pathophysiology and diagnosis of RPL.

Alloimmune Abnormalities

Inappropriate immune rejection of fetal antigens has been suggested to be a factor behind a subset of miscarriages. However, to date, there is insufficient solid experimental evidence to support this hypothesis. This is in part due to efficient masking of fetal antigen presentation at the feto-maternal interface as described above. Additionally, studies of highly inbred human populations suggested higher rate of miscarriage and RPL, however, no evidence for immune etiology has been demonstrated. Finally, the majority of mouse strains used in research are highly inbred and homozygous at the MHC loci, without the evidence of maternal rejection of these syngeneic feti. On the other hand, particular combinations of HLA-C loci and NK cells expressed killer Ig-like receptors associated with pre-eclampsia and possibly very early fetal losses, presumably due to disordered uNK-mediated decidual remodeling.[110]

Thrombophilia in Recurrent Pregnancy Loss

Changes during normal pregnancy promote coagulation, decrease anticoagulation and inhibit fibrinolysis.[111,112] Specifically, there is a marked increase in coagulation factors II, VII, VIII, IX, X and von Willebrand factor. There is also a decrease of physiologic anticoagulants, with protein S levels falling to 40–60% starting in the first trimester and remaining decreases for 3 months postpartum. This change is attributed to an estrogen-induced decrease in total protein S and an increase in C4b, which binds protein S. The combined impact of decreased protein S and increased factor VIII leads to increased resistance to activated protein C. The combination of hematologic, anatomic and immunologic changes in pregnancy increases the risk of venous thrombosis by 4–5 fold.[113,114] Whether or not an underlying hematologic disorder that may potentiate the natural gestational changes can similarly increase the risk for RPL remains an area of debate.

The most established association with RPL and maternal thrombophilia is with APS, as discussed above. This is a complex disorder that predisposes to venous and arterial clots, as well as pregnancy complications. The criteria for diagnosis include both laboratory and clinical findings. Specifically, the presence of APLAs (lupus anticoagulant, B2 glycoprotein or anticardiolipin antibodies) must be demonstrated to be persistently positive on two laboratory measures separated by 12 weeks. Qualifying clinic events include any venous or arterial thrombosis without other obvious cause or a pregnancy complication, defined as three pregnancy losses before 10 weeks or one event after 10 weeks (pregnancy loss, intrauterine growth retardation from placental insufficiency, severe pre-eclampsia or eclampsia).[115] An initial hypothesis was that pregnancy complications result from clotting of the placental microvessels. This was the rationale for using anticoagulation strategies in attempt to increase live birth rate in mothers with APS.

Two meta-analyses examined the role of heparin and aspirin (ASA) versus aspirin alone in women with APS.[116,117] Both meta-analyses identified randomized controlled trials involving RPL and APS. In each meta-analysis, five trials were examined and greater than

300 patients were included. The two meta-analyses differed by only one of the trials included and both unfractionated heparin (UFH) and low molecular weight heparin (LMWH) were used. The first meta-analysis[116] reported a live birth rate of 74% in the ASA/heparin group versus 55% in the ASA alone group. The number needed to treat (NNT) in the ASA/heparin combination group for one live birth was 5.6. Although all included trials were identified as randomized, two received low Jadad scores given lack of detail provided regarding the randomization design or for randomization via alternating assignment to the two groups,[118,119] such that enrolling providers would know the destined group of a potential subject prior to enrollment.

The second meta-analysis[117] yielded similar results with improved live birth rates in the combination group. The calculated live birth rate was 81% in the combination group versus 64% in the ASA only group. The data in this meta-analysis was presented in odds ratios (ORs) and stratified by whether UFH or LMWH was used. The OR for a poor outcome in the LMWH/ASA group was 0.7, whereas the OR was 0.26 in the UFH/ASA combination group. The NNT in the UFH/ASA group to prevent a clinical event was four. To note, neither combination was shown to prevent late term losses.

The reason for the disparity in effectiveness between LMWH and UFH is not clear. Many women were enrolled late in term and thus earlier losses may have been missed. There was a low titer threshold of antibody level allowed, thus many included women may not have met traditional criteria for APS and may therefore have been destined for a better outcome. One of the trials using LMWH in this meta-analysis[120] also included inherited thrombophilia and positive ANA as inclusion criteria, which is not part of the criteria for an APS diagnosis.

Despite these critiques, these two meta-analyses established the role for the combination of heparin and aspirin in pregnant women with APS. Compared to UFH, LMWH provides more reliable dosing and with rare exception, does not require active monitoring. As such, LMWH is preferred over UFH for gestational management of APS. The majority of trials in these meta-analyses used prophylactic dosing of heparin and ASA 81 mg daily, although treatment doses of heparin was also used. The appropriate dosing of the heparin is an individualized case-based assessment based on a woman's past medical and obstetric history.

The results of these trials invite consideration about the function of heparin and aspirin in preventing pregnancy loss in women with APS. Hypotheses have included that heparin assists trophoblasts in facilitating implantation. Another theory is that heparin binds to ALPA and renders them biologically inactive.[121] One study[122] hypothesized that heparin reduces complement activation. This study used a mouse model of APS by passive transfer of human APLAs. The proposal was that APLAs target placenta and deciduas, thereby activating the complement cascade. This activation in turn recruits inflammatory cells and accelerates local alternative pathway activation and creates a pro-inflammatory amplification loop that enhances C3.

In this study, the APLA mouse model was demonstrated to have significantly higher levels of plasma C3a than the normal host model. Immunohistochemical analyses of deciduas from day 8 pregnant mice were also examined. Interestingly, the mice treated with UFH or LMWH both showed complement levels similar to the normal host, whereas mice treated with the anticoagulants fondaparinux or hirudin (a direct thrombin inhibitor) had complement levels similar to untreated APLA mice. In addition, the deciduas examination of the normal host model and the APLA mice treated with UFH and LMWH, all demonstrated preserved embryo; alternatively, the untreated APLA mice and those treated with fondaparinux or hirudin, all revealed embryo destruction.

This finding would suggest that the benefit of heparin in increasing the live birth rate in APS is not strictly that of an anticoagulant and that the pathophysiology of pregnancy loss is not solely a clotting problem. These issues have been evaluated when investigating the association of the inherited thrombophilias and pregnancy loss. The inherited thrombophilias included factor V Leiden (FVL) mutation, prothrombin gene mutation (PGM) and deficiencies of antithrombin, protein C and S. Patients with these syndromes have increased risk of venous clotting. Their role in pregnancy loss and complications has been controversial.

An early publication about risk assessment was a case-controlled study of over 500 women with inherited thrombophilia and a collective 1,500 pregnancies compared to controls.[123] There was a statistically significant increase in still birth, defined as loss greater than 34 weeks gestation, in women with an inherited thrombophilia. Miscarriage did not differ between the two groups. Another publication was a meta-analysis of 31 studies[124] that found a strong association with inherited thrombophilia and miscarriage at greater than 10 weeks and late non-recurrent events, but not for miscarriages in early weeks.

Another cohort study[125] parsed out the likelihood of an adverse pregnancy outcome and thrombophilia by weeks' gestation. Similar to earlier publications, the study demonstrated no significant association with maternal thrombophilia and miscarriage less than

10 weeks' gestation, but an OR of greater than 1.5 for miscarriages after 10 weeks. The association of thrombophilia and miscarriage was even stronger in miscarriages occurring at greater than 14 weeks with an OR of about 3.5. As placental vessels do no typically form until gestational week 10, this association is compatible with a pathophysiologic explanation that miscarriage in a woman with thrombophilia may result from a clotting event involving the placental microvessels.

The first prospective study of inherited thrombophilia and pregnancy loss was published in 2004.[122] It included 160 patients with a history of miscarriage at greater than 10 weeks of gestation and documented FVL mutation, PGM or protein S deficiency. Included women were randomized to receive the LMWH, enoxaparin, at 40 mg subcutaneously daily or ASA 100 mg daily after week 8. The group receiving LMWH had a significantly higher live birth rate of 86% compared to the group receiving ASA, who had a live birth rate of 29%. Potential limitations of this trial included the absence of a placebo arm and a lower live birth rate in the ASA group than had been previously reported. Nonetheless, the results rendered enthusiasm for using LMWH in women with inherited thrombophilia and history of miscarriage. The degree of benefit seen with use of LMWH has not been confirmed or disputed in subsequent trials or any with a placebo arm.

Other trials have shown that the likelihood of a successful pregnancy following a loss for women with inherited thrombophilia rivals that of non-thrombophilia carriers and is overall quite favorable. One trial studied pregnancy outcomes in women who were identified as first degree family members of probands with either FVL and documented venous thromboembolism (VTE), or PGM and persistent elevation of factor VIII, hyperhomocysteinuria, VTE or premature atherosclerosis.[126] Identified women over the age of 14 were screened and about half were confirmed to be a thrombophilia carrier (isolated heterozygote, compound heterozygote or homozygote for FVL or PGM). Pregnancies where heparin was used were excluded for evaluation. Of the 1,049 women with at least one pregnancy, the live birth rate for the first pregnancy was 87% for thrombophilia carriers and 91% for non-carriers. Thirteen percent of carriers had a first pregnancy loss (9% early and 4% late) versus 9% of non-carriers who had a first pregnancy loss (7% early and 2% late). The RR for an initial pregnancy loss in a thrombophilia carrier was 1.5 total, 1.4 for early loss and 2.1 for late loss.

There were 93 women in the trial with a first pregnancy loss who became pregnant a second time, 58 thrombophilia carriers and 35 non-carriers. Collectively, these women had a 75% live birth rate in the second pregnancy, 74% in carriers versus 77% in non-carriers. Results between the groups were essentially the same if the first pregnancy loss was early: live birth rate of 77% in the carrier group and 76% in the non-carrier group. There were only 29 women with a second pregnancy after a late loss in the first pregnancy, 19 in the carrier group and 10 in the non-carrier group. The live birth rate in the second pregnancy following a first pregnancy loss after 12 weeks was 68% in the thrombophilia carrier group versus 80% in non-carriers. The second pregnancy losses in this group were evenly distributed between early and late losses. The overall small number of women with a late first pregnancy loss who achieved a second pregnancy limits the general applicability of these findings and may minimize a more significant difference. Arguably, these findings trend with what was seen in the aforementioned randomized trial[122] where women with an inherited thrombophilia and pregnancy loss after 10 weeks were shown to benefit from use of heparin in a subsequent pregnancy.

Three more recent randomized trials revisited the potential benefit of heparin and/or ASA in women with RPL.[127-129] To note, two[127,128] of these trials excluded women with APS and the third[129] included only a small number of women with APLAs. Thus, the results have not changed current practices in treating pregnant women with APS.

The first publication, the ALIFE trial,[102] was a placebo-controlled randomized design with three arms. Women with a history of RPL received either the combination of LMWH and ASA, ASA alone or placebo. In total, 16% of these women had an inherited thrombophilia. The second publication, the SPIN trial,[103] randomized women to receive the combination of LMWH and ASA versus clinical surveillance. Less than 3% of included women harbored an inherited thrombophilia. The final publication, the HABENOX trial,[129] randomized women to either LMWH and placebo, LMWH and ASA 100 mg daily or ASA 100 mg daily alone. In total, 23.8–25% of included women had an identified thrombophilia, both inherited and acquired.

The results of these trials are shown in the Figure 1. As is evident, there was no statistically significant benefit to heparin, ASA or the combination in any trial. All regimens were well tolerated from a safety standpoint. There were potential limitations in these trials, including slower than expected enrollment[103,129] and use of LMWH was not blinded.[102] That said, these collective findings would suggest that there is no role for the standard use of heparin or ASA in women with RPL and no underlying thrombophilia. Given the exclusion of women with APS and the low number of enrolled women with inherited thrombophilia, however, the

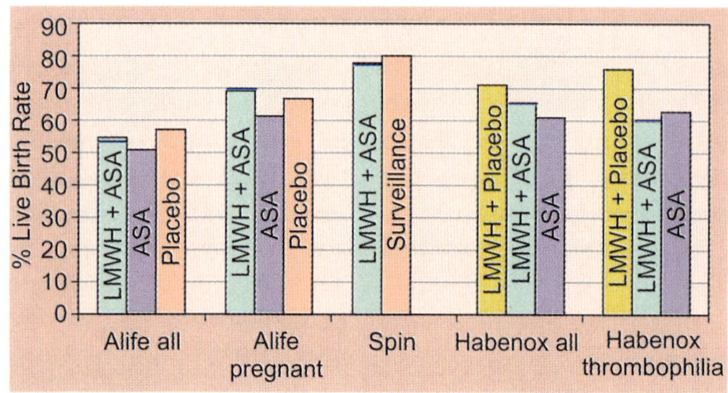

Figure 1 Live birth rates in women with history of RPL randomized to various treatment arms. ALIFE trial[127], SPIN trial[128], HABENOX trial[129]

Abbreviations: LMWH, low molecular weight heparin; ASA, aspirin

Table 2 Treatment guidelines for women with recurrent pregnancy loss

Results of evaluation of RPL	Recommendation
No identified thrombophilia	No benefit of heparin or ASA
APLAS diagnosed[1]	Heparin and ASA have shown benefit
Inherited thrombophilia[2] identified	History of pregnancy losses <10 weeks - No benefit of heparin or ASA History of pregnancy losses >10 weeks - Potential benefit of prophylactic doses of LMWH

1. Defined as both persistent presence of APLAs (lupus anticoagulant, anticardiolipin antibodies and B2 glycoprotein antibodies) over 12 weeks and either 3 pregnancy losses at less than 10 weeks or one pregnancy morbid event after 10 weeks (loss, premature delivery due to placental insufficiency, severe pre-eclampsia or eclampsia)
2. Inherited thrombophilia defined as FVL, PGM, deficiency of AT, protein C or protein S

APLAs: antiphospholipid antibodies; ASA: aspirin; LMWH: low molecular weight heparin; RPL: recurrent pregnancy loss

same cannot be concluded about the potential benefit of heparin in these populations.

The clinical approach to women with APS has been previously discussed and use of heparin and ASA has been shown to improve pregnancy outcomes. The recent randomized trials of women with RPL demonstrate that heparin and ASA do not appear to benefit women without an underlying thrombophilia. The ideal placebo-controlled trial including only women with an inherited thrombophilia and history of late pregnancy loss has not been conducted and some have argued that based on currently available data, it would be unethical to enroll in such a trial. The data currently available to inform on the management of women with inherited thrombophilia and a history of late pregnancy loss suggest a trend toward decreased live birth rate in thrombophilia carriers compared to non-carriers in an untreated population[126] and a benefit to use of heparin compared to ASA.[122]

To summarize, two or more consecutive losses will affect about 2–5% of reproductive aged women and three or more consecutive losses will affect about 1%. Given the emotional distress involved, there is an obvious desire to identify and potentially treat the underlying etiology. Unfortunately, in the majority of cases, a cause will not be identified. Fortunately, studies have shown that the possibility for a subsequent successful pregnancy remains, even without specific medical intervention. The approach in managing RPL should start with evaluating for a possible underlying etiology, including chromosomal assessments of the fetus and parents, placenta evaluation if available and screening for maternal thrombophilia. An individualized treatment plan for a woman with history of RPL should be developed based on careful review of the circumstances and timing of her pregnancy losses and the subsequent data collected. Any potential benefit of treatment should also be balanced with an assessment of the potential risks and morbidity introduced by use of heparin.

Treatment recommendations are summarized in Table 2. If a woman has no identified thrombophilia, use of heparin and/or ASA in pregnancy is discouraged. Women with APS should receive heparin and ASA in pregnancy. Women with inherited thrombophilia should be further classified as having had early or late pregnancy losses. In women with inherited thrombophilia and a history of early losses, even when recurrent, there is no sufficient data to support the use of heparin or ASA. However, women with inherited thrombophilia and history of late pregnancy losses have been shown to benefit from the use of prophylactic heparin in a subsequent pregnancy.

REFERENCES

1. Wilcox AJ, Weinberg CR, O'Connor JF, et al. Incidence of early loss of pregnancy. N Engl J Med. 1988;319:189-94.
2. Sierra S, Stephenson M. Genetics of recurrent pregnancy loss. Semin Reropd Med. 2006;24:17-24.

3. Warburton D. Reproductive loss: how much is preventable? N Engl J Med. 1987;316:158-60.
4. Drugan A, Koppitch FC, Williams JC , et al. Prenatal genetic diagnosis following recurrent early pregnancy loss. Obstet Gynecol. 1990;75:381-4.
5. Carp H, Toder V, Aviram A, et al. Karyotype of the abortus in recurrent miscarriage. Fertil Steril. 2001;75:678-82.
6. Branch DW, Gibson M, Silver RM. Clinical practice. Recurrent miscarriage. N Engl J Med. 2010;363:1740-7.
7. Munne S, Fischer J, Warner A, et al. Preimplantation genetic diagnosis significantly reduces pregnancy loss in infertile couples: a multicenter study. Fertil Steril. 2006;85:326-32.
8. Twisk M, Haadsma ML, van Der Veen F, et al. Preimplantation genetic screening as an alternative to prenatal testing for Down syndrome: preferences of women undergoing in vitro fertilization/intracytoplasmic sperm injection treatment. Fertil Steril. 2007;88:804-10.
9. Practice Committee of Society for Assisted Reproductive Technology; Practice Committee of American Society for Reproductive Medicine. Preimplantation genetic testing: a Practice Committee opinion. Fertil Steril. 2007;88:1497-504.
10. Practice Committee of Society for Assisted Reproductive Technology; Practice Committee of American Society for Reproductive Medicine. Preimplantation genetic testing: a Practice Committee opinion. Fertil Steril. 2008;90:S136-43.
11. Staessen C, Platteau P, Van Assche E, et al. Comparison of blastocyst transfer with or without preimplantation genetic diagnosis for aneuploidy screening in couples with advanced maternal age: a prospective randomized controlled trial. Hum Reprod. 2004;19:2849-58.
12. Heinonen PK. Reproductive performance of women with uterine anomalies after abdominal or hysteroscopic metroplasty or no surgical treatment. J Am Assoc Gynecol Laparosc. 1997;4:311-7.
13. Valli E, Vaquero E, Lazzarin N, et al. Hysteroscopic metroplasty improves gestational outcome in women with recurrent spontaneous abortion. J Am Assoc Gynecol Laparosc. 2004;11:240-4.
14. Heinonen PK. Complete septate uterus with longitudinal vaginal septum. Fertil Steril. 2006;85:700-5.
15. Klatsky PC, Tran ND, Caughey AB, et al. Fibroids and reproductive outcomes: a systematic literature review from conception to delivery. Am J Obstet Gynecol. 2008;198:357-66.
16. Perino A, Giovannelli L, Schillaci R, et al. Human papillomavirus infection in couples undergoing in vitro fertilization procedures: impact on reproductive outcomes. Fertil Steril. 2011;95:1845-8.
17. McGregor DG. Occupational exposure to trace concentrations of waste anesthetic gases. Mayo Clin Proc. 2000;75:273-7.
18. Boivin JF. Risk of spontaneous abortion in women occupationally exposed to anaesthetic gases: a meta-analysis. Occup Environ Med. 1997;54:541-8.
19. Savitz DA, Chan RL, Herring AH, et al. Caffeine and miscarriage risk. Epidemiology. 2008;19:55-62.
20. Dlugosz L, Belanger K, Hellenbrand K, et al. Maternal caffeine consumption and spontaneous abortion: a prospective cohort study. Epidemiology. 1996;7:250-5.
21. Weng X, Odouli R, Li DK. Maternal caffeine consumption during pregnancy and the risk of miscarriage: a prospective cohort study. Am J Obstet Gynecol. 2008;198:279.e1-8.
22. Balasch J, Vanrell JA, Marquez M, et al. Dehydrogesterone versus vaginal progesterone in the treatment of the endometrial luteal phase deficiency. Fertil Steril. 1982;37:751-4.
23. Clifford K, Rai R, Watson H, et al. Does suppressing luteinising hormone secretion reduce the miscarriage rate? Results of a randomised controlled trial. BMJ. 1996;312:1508-11.
24. Legro RS, Barnhart HX, Schlaff WD, et al. Clomiphene, metformin, or both for infertility in the polycystic ovary syndrome. N Engl J Med. 2007;356:551-66.
25. Palomba S, Falbo A, Orio F Jr, et al. Effect of preconceptional metformin on abortion risk in polycystic ovary syndrome: a systematic review and meta-analysis of randomized controlled trials. Fertil Steril. 2009;92:1646-58.
26. Moffett A, Loke C. Immunology of placentation in eutherian mammals. Nat Rev Immunol. 2006;6:584-94.
27. King A, Allan DS, Bowen M, et al. HLA-E is expressed on trophoblast and interacts with CD94/NKG2 receptors on decidual NK cells. Eur J Immunol. 2000;30:1623-31.
28. Apps R, Murphy SP, Fernando R, et al. Human leucocyte antigen (HLA) and expression of primary trophoblast cells and placental cell lines, determined using single antigen beads to characterize allotype specificities of anti-HLA antibodies. Immunolo. 2009;127:26-39.
29. Blaschitz A, Hutter H, Dohr G. HLA Class I protein expression in the human placenta. Early Pregnancy. 2001;5:67-9.
30. Moffett-King A. Natural killer cells and pregnancy. Nat Rev Immunol. 2002;2:656-63.
31. Tabiasco J, Rabot M, Aguerre-Girr M, et al. Human decidual NK cells: unique phenotype and functional properties—a review. Placenta. 2006;27 (Suppl A):S34-9.
32. Manaster I, Mandelboim O. The unique properties of uterine NK cells. Am J Reprod Immunol. 2010;63:434-44.
33. King A, Jokhi PP, Burrows TD, et al. Functions of human decidual NK cells. Am J Reprod Immunol. 1996;35:258-60.
34. Hanna J, Goldman-Wohl D, Hamani Y, et al. Decidual NK cells regulate key developmental processes at the human fetal-maternal interface. Nat Med. 2006;12:1065-74.
35. El Costa H, Tabiasco J, Berrebi A, et al. Effector functions of human decidual NK cells in healthy early pregnancy are dependent on the specific engagement of natural cytotoxicity receptors. J Reprod Immunol. 2009;82:142-7.
36. Vacca P, Cantoni C, Vitale M, et al. Crosstalk between decidual NK and CD14+ myelomonocytic cells results in induction of Tregs and immunosuppression. Proc Natl Acad Sci USA. 2010;107:11918-23.

37. Li C, Houser BL, Nicotra ML, et al. HLA-G homodimer-induced cytokine secretion through HLA-G receptors on human decidual macrophages and natural killer cells. Proc Natl Acad Sci USA. 2009;106:5767-72.
38. Heikkinen J, Mottonen M, Komi J, et al. Phenotypic characterization of human decidual macrophages. Clin Exp Immunol. 2003;131:498-505.
39. Tilburgs T, Roelen DL, van Der Mast BJ, et al. Evidence for a selective migration of fetus-specific CD4+CD25bright regulatory T cells from the peripheral blood to the decidua in human pregnancy. J Immunol. 2008;180:5737-45.
40. Schumacher A, Brachwitz N, Sohr S, et al. Human chorionic gonadotropin attracts regulatory T cells into the fetal-maternal interface during early human pregnancy. J Immunol. 2009;182:5488-97.
41. Aluvihare VR, Kallikourdis M, Betz AG. Regulatory T cells mediate maternal tolerance to the fetus. Nat Immunol. 2004;5:266-71.
42. Blois SM, Barrientos G, Garcia MG, et al. Interaction between dendritic cells and natural killer cells during pregnancy in mice. J Mol Med (Berl). 2008;86:837-52.
43. Blois SM, Alba Soto CD, Tometten M, et al. Lineage, maturity, and phenotype of uterine murine dendritic cells throughout gestation indicate a protective role in maintaining pregnancy. Biol Reprod. 2004;70:1018-23.
44. Miyazaki S, Tsuda H, Sakai M, et al. Predominance of Th2-promoting dendritic cells in early human pregnancy decidua. J Leukoc Biol. 2003;74:514-22.
45. Austgulen R, Arntzen KJ, Vatten LJ, et al. Detection of cytokines (interleukin-1, interleukin-6, transforming growth factor-beta) and soluble tumour necrosis factor receptors in embryo culture fluids during in vitro fertilization. Hum Reprod. 1995;10:171-6.
46. Borgatti M, Rizzo R, Canto MB, et al. Release of sICAM-1 in oocytes and in vitro fertilized human embryos. PLoS One. 2008;3:e3970.
47. Kita M, Tanaka K, Shinmura K, et al. [Expression of cytokines and interferon-related genes in the mouse embryo]. C R Seances Soc Biol Fil. 1994;188:593-600.
48. Croy BA, Esadeg S, Chantakru S, et al. Update on pathways regulating the activation of uterine Natural Killer cells, their interactions with decidual spiral arteries and homing of their precursors to the uterus. J Reprod Immunol. 2003;59:175-91.
49. Croy BA, He H, Esadeg S, et al. Uterine natural killer cells: insights into their cellular and molecular biology from mouse modelling. Reproduction. 2003;126:149-60.
50. Croy BA, Luross JA, Guimond MJ, et al. Uterine natural killer cells: insights into lineage relationships and functions from studies of pregnancies in mutant and transgenic mice. Nat Immun. 1996;15:22-33.
51. Kwak-Kim JY, Chung-Bang HS, Ng SC, et al. Increased T helper 1 cytokine responses by circulating T cells are present in women with recurrent pregnancy losses and in infertile women with multiple implantation failures after IVF. Hum Reprod. 2003;18:767-73.
52. Polgar K, Hill JA. Identification of the white blood cell populations responsible for Th1 immunity to trophoblast and the timing of the response in women with recurrent pregnancy loss. Gynecol Obstet Invest. 2002;53:59-64.
53. Chaouat G, Menu E, Clark DA, et al. Control of fetal survival in CBA x DBA/2 mice by lymphokine therapy. J Reprod Fertil. 1990;89:447-58.
54. Zhang J, Wei H, Wu D, et al. Toll-like receptor 3 agonist induces impairment of uterine vascular remodeling and fetal losses in CBA x DBA/2 mice. J Reprod Immunol. 2007;74:61-7.
55. Koga K, Mor G. Expression and function of toll-like receptors at the maternal-fetal interface. Reprod Sci. 2008;15:231-42.
56. Abrahams VM, Aldo PB, Murphy SP, et al. TLR6 modulates first trimester trophoblast responses to peptidoglycan. J Immunol. 2008;180:6035-43.
57. Abrahams VM. Pattern recognition at the maternal-fetal interface. Immunol Invest. 2008;37:427-47.
58. Yetman DL, Kutteh WH. Antiphospholipid antibody panels and recurrent pregnancy loss: prevalence of anticardiolipin antibodies compared with other antiphospholipid antibodies. Fertil Steril. 1996;66:540-6.
59. Rai RS, Regan L, Clifford K, et al. Antiphospholipid antibodies and beta 2-glycoprotein-I in 500 women with recurrent miscarriage: results of a comprehensive screening approach. Hum Reprod. 1995;10:2001-5.
60. Miyakis S, Lockshin MD, Atsumi T, et al. International consensus statement on an update of the classification criteria for definite antiphospholipid syndrome (APS). J Thromb Haemost. 2006;4:295-306.
61. Lee RM, Emlen W, Scott JR, et al. Anti-beta2-glycoprotein I antibodies in women with recurrent spontaneous abortion, unexplained fetal death, and antiphospholipid syndrome. Am J Obstet Gynecol. 1999;181:642-8.
62. Carp HJ. Antiphospholipid syndrome in pregnancy. Curr Opin Obstet Gynecol. 2004;16:129-35.
63. Galli M, Comfurius P, Maassen C, et al. Anticardiolipin antibodies (ACA) directed not to cardiolipin but to a plasma protein cofactor. Lancet. 1990;335:1544-7.
64. Branch DW, Dudley DJ, Mitchell MD, et al. Immunoglobulin G fractions from patients with antiphospholipid antibodies cause fetal death in BALB/c mice: a model for autoimmune fetal loss. Am J Obstet Gynecol. 1990;163:210-6.
65. Bakimer R, Fishman P, Blank M, et al. Induction of primary antiphospholipid syndrome in mice by immunization with a human monoclonal anticardiolipin antibody (H-3). J Clin Invest. 1992;89:1558-63.
66. Garcia CO, Kanbour-Shakir A, Tang H, et al. Induction of experimental antiphospholipid antibody syndrome in PL/J mice following immunization with beta 2 GPI. Am J Reprod Immunol. 1997;37:118-24.
67. Blank M, Cohen J, Toder V, et al. Induction of anti-phospholipid syndrome in naive mice with mouse lupus monoclonal and human polyclonal anti-cardiolipin antibodies. Proc Natl Acad Sci USA. 1991;88:3069-73.

68. Suzuki T, Takabayashi K, Ichikawa K, et al. Effects of monoclonal anticardiolipin antibody on pregnant mice. J Rheumatol. 1996;23:83-6.
69. Piona A, La Rosa L, Tincani A, et al. Placental thrombosis and fetal loss after passive transfer of mouse lupus monoclonal or human polyclonal anti-cardiolipin antibodies in pregnant naive BALB/c mice. Scand J Immunol. 1995;41:427-32.
70. Blank M, Waisman A, Mozes E, et al. Characteristics and pathogenic role of anti-beta2-glycoprotein I single-chain Fv domains: induction of experimental antiphospholipid syndrome. Int Immunol. 1999;11:1917-26.
71. Blank M, Faden D, Tincani A, et al. Immunization with anticardiolipin cofactor (beta-2-glycoprotein I) induces experimental antiphospholipid syndrome in naive mice. J Autoimmun. 1994;7:441-55.
72. Gharavi AE, Vega-Ostertag M, Espinola RG, et al. Intrauterine fetal death in mice caused by cytomegalovirus-derived peptide induced aPL antibodies. Lupus. 2004;13:17-23.
73. Kornberg A, Blank M, Kaufman S, et al. Induction of tissue factor-like activity in monocytes by anti-cardiolipin antibodies. J Immunol. 1994;153:1328-32.
74. Rand JH, Wu XX, Andree HA, et al. Pregnancy loss in the antiphospholipid-antibody syndrome—a possible thrombogenic mechanism. N Engl J Med. 1997;337:154-60.
75. Redecha P, Franzke CW, Ruf W, et al. Neutrophil activation by the tissue factor/Factor VIIa/PAR2 axis mediates fetal death in a mouse model of antiphospholipid syndrome. J Clin Invest. 2008;118:3453-61.
76. Redecha P, Tilley R, Tencati M, et al. Tissue factor: a link between C5a and neutrophil activation in antiphospholipid antibody induced fetal injury. Blood. 2007;110:2423-31.
77. Sthoeger ZM, Mozes E, Tartakovsky B. Anti-cardiolipin antibodies induce pregnancy failure by impairing embryonic implantation. Proc Natl Acad Sci USA. 1993;90:6464-7.
78. Shurtz-Swirski R, Inbar O, Blank M, et al. In vitro effect of anticardiolipin autoantibodies upon total and pulsatile placental hCG secretion during early pregnancy. Am J Reprod Immunol. 1993;29:206-10.
79. Sebire NJ, Fox H, Backos M, et al. Defective endovascular trophoblast invasion in primary antiphospholipid antibody syndrome-associated early pregnancy failure. Hum Reprod. 2002;17:1067-71.
80. Holers VM, Girardi G, Mo L, et al. Complement C3 activation is required for antiphospholipid antibody-induced fetal loss. J Exp Med. 2002;195:211-20.
81. Salmon JE, Girardi G. Antiphospholipid antibodies and pregnancy loss: a disorder of inflammation. J Reprod Immunol. 2008;77:51-6.
82. Swairjo MA, Concha NO, Kaetzel MA, et al. Ca (2+)-bridging mechanism and phospholipid head group recognition in the membrane-binding protein annexin V. Nat Struct Biol. 1995;2:968-74.
83. Bevers EM, Comfurius P, van Rijn JL, et al. Generation of prothrombin-converting activity and the exposure of phosphatidylserine at the outer surface of platelets. Eur J Biochem. 1982;122:429-36.
84. Williamson P, Bevers EM, Smeets EF, et al. Continuous analysis of the mechanism of activated transbilayer lipid movement in platelets. Biochemistry. 1995;34:10448-55.
85. Rand JH. Antiphospholipid antibody-mediated disruption of the annexin-V antithrombotic shield: a thrombogenic mechanism for the antiphospholipid syndrome. J Autoimmun. 2000;15:107-11.
86. Rand JH, Wu XX, Guller S, et al. Reduction of annexin-V (placental anticoagulant protein-I) on placental villi of women with antiphospholipid antibodies and recurrent spontaneous abortion. Am J Obstet Gynecol. 1994;171:1566-72.
87. Matsubayashi H, Arai T, Izumi S, et al. Anti-annexin V antibodies in patients with early pregnancy loss or implantation failures. Fertil Steril. 2001;76:694-9.
88. Seigneuret M, Devaux PF. ATP-dependent asymmetric distribution of spin-labeled phospholipids in the erythrocyte membrane: relation to shape changes. Proc Natl Acad Sci USA. 1984;81:3751-5.
89. Leventis PA, Grinstein S. The distribution and function of phosphatidylserine in cellular membranes. Annu Rev Biophys. 2010;39:407-27.
90. McIntyre JA. Antiphospholipid antibodies in implantation failures. Am J Reprod Immunol. 2003;49:221-9.
91. Tait JF, Gibson D. Phospholipid binding of annexin V: effects of calcium and membrane phosphatidylserine content. Arch Biochem Biophys. 1992;298:187-91.
92. Ulcova-Gallova Z, Krauz V, Novakova P, et al. Anti-phospholipid antibodies against phosphatidylinositol, and phosphatidylserine are more significant in reproductive failure than antibodies against cardiolipin only. Am J Reprod Immunol. 2005;54:112-7.
93. Matsubayashi H, Sugi T, Arai T, et al. Different antiphospholipid antibody specificities are found in association with early repeated pregnancy loss versus recurrent IVF-failure patients. Am J Reprod Immunol. 2001;46:323-9.
94. Matalon ST, Shoenfeld Y, Blank M, et al. Antiphosphatidylserine antibodies affect rat yolk sacs in culture: a mechanism for fetal loss in antiphospholipid syndrome. Am J Reprod Immunol. 2004;51:144-51.
95. Di Simone N, Meroni PL, De Papa N, et al. Antiphospholipid antibodies affect trophoblast gonadotropin secretion and invasiveness by binding directly and through adhered beta2-glycoprotein I. Arthritis Rheum. 2000;43:140-50.
96. Balasubramanian K, Schroit AJ. Aminophospholipid asymmetry: A matter of life and death. Annu Rev Physiol. 2003;65:701-34.
97. Chonn A, Semple SC, Cullis PR. Beta 2 glycoprotein I is a major protein associated with very rapidly cleared liposomes in vivo, suggesting a significant role in the immune clearance of "non-self" particles. J Biol Chem. 1995;270:25845-9.
98. Balasubramanian K, Chandra J, Schroit AJ. Immune clearance of phosphatidylserine-expressing cells by

phagocytes. The role of beta2-glycoprotein I in macrophage recognition. J Biol Chem. 1997;272:31113-7.
99. Petri M, Allbritton J. Fetal outcome of lupus pregnancy: a retrospective case-control study of the Hopkins Lupus Cohort. J Rheumatol. 1993;20:650-6.
100. Petri M. Update on anti-phospholipid antibodies in SLE: the Hopkins' Lupus Cohort. Lupus. 2010;19:419-23.
101. Yan Yuen S, Krizova A, Ouimet JM, et al. Pregnancy Outcome in Systemic Lupus Erythematosus (SLE) is Improving: Results from a Case Control Study and Literature Review. Open Rheumatol J. 2008;2:89-98.
102. Moroni G, Ponticelli C. The risk of pregnancy in patients with lupus nephritis. J Nephrol. 2003;16:161-7.
103. Kwok LW, Tam LS, Zhu T, et al. Predictors of maternal and fetal outcomes in pregnancies of patients with systemic lupus erythematosus. Lupus. 2011;20:829-36.
104. Bagnasco M, Grassia L, Pesce G. The management of the patient with unexpected autoantibody positivity. Autoimmun Rev. 2007;6:347-53.
105. Ticconi C, Rotondi F, Veglia M, et al. Antinuclear autoantibodies in women with recurrent pregnancy loss. Am J Reprod Immunol. 2010;64:384-92.
106. Harger JH, Rabin BS, MArchese SG. The prognostic value of antinuclear antibodies in women with recurrent pregnancy losses: a prospective controlled study. Obstet Gynecol. 1989;73:419-24.
107. Xu L, Chang V, Murphy A, et al. Antinuclear antibodies in sera of patients with recurrent pregnancy wastage. Am J Obstet Gynecol. 1990;163:1493-7.
108. Ruiz JE, Cubillos J, Mendoza JC, et al. Autoantibodies to phospholipids and nuclear antigens in non-pregnant and pregnant Colombian women with recurrent spontaneous abortions. J Reprod Immunol. 1995;28:41-51.
109. Shoenfeld Y, Carp HJ, Molina V, et al. Autoantibodies and prediction of reproductive failure. Am J Reprod Immunol. 2006;56:337-44.
110. Hiby SE, Apps R, Sharkey AM, et al. Maternal activating KIRs protect against human reproductive failure mediated by fetal HLA-C2. J Clin Invest. 2010;120:4102-10.
111. Hellgren M. Hemostasis during normal pregnancy and puerperium. Semin Thromb Hemost. 2003;29:125-30.
112. Lockwood CJ. Pregnancy-associated changes in the hemostatic system. Clin obstet Gynecol. 2006;49:836-43.
113. Heit JA, Kobbervig CE, James AH, et al. Trends in the incidence of venous thromboembolism during pregnancy or postpartum: a 30-year population-based study. Ann Intern Med. 2005;143:697-706.
114. James AH, Jamison MG, Brancazio LR, et al. Venous thromboembolism during pregnancy and the postpartum period: incidence, risk factors, and mortality. Am J Obstet Gynecol. 2006;194:1311-5.
115. Swadzba J, Iwaniec T, Szczeklik A, et al. Revised classification criteria for antiphospholipid syndrome and the thrombotic risk in patients with autoimmune diseases. J Thromb Haemost. 2007;5:1883-9.
116. Mak A, Cheung MW, Cheak AA, et al. Combination of heparin and aspirin is superior to aspirin alone in enhancing live births in patients with recurrent pregnancy loss and positive anti-phospholipid antibodies: a meta-analysis of randomized controlled trials and meta-regression. Rheumatology (Oxford). 2010;49:281-8.b
117. Ziakas PD, Pavlou M, Voulgarelis M. Heparin treatment in antiphospholipid syndrome with recurrent pregnancy loss: a systematic review and meta-analysis. Obstet Gynecol. 2010;115:1256-62.
118. Franklin RD, Kutteh WH. Antiphospholipid antibodies (APA) and recurrent pregnancy loss: treating a unique APA positive population. Human Reprod. 2002;17:2981-5.
119. Kutteh WH. Antiphospholipid antibody-associated recurrent pregnancy loss: treatment with heparin and low-dose aspirin is superior to low-dose aspirin alone. Am J Obstet Gynecol. 1996;174:1584-9.
120. Laskin CA, Spitzer KA, Clark CA, et al. Low molecular weight heparin and aspirin for recurrent pregnancy loss: results from the randomized, controlled HepASA Trial. J Rheumatol. 2009;36:279-87.
121. Ermel LD, Marshburn PB, Kutteh WH. Interaction of heparin with antiphospholipid antibodies (APA) from the sera of women with recurrent pregnancy loss (RPL). Am J Reprod Immunol. 1995;33:14-20.
122. Gris JC, Mercier E, Quere I, et al. Low-molecular-weight heparin versus low-dose aspirin in women with one fetal loss and a constitutional thrombophilic disorder. Blood. 2004;103:3695-9.
123. Preston FE, Rosendaal FR, Walker ID, et al. Increased fetal loss in women with heritable thrombophilia. Lancet. 1996;348:913-6.
124. Rey E, Kahn SR, David M, et al. Thrombophilic disorders and fetal loss: a meta-analysis. Lancet. 2003;361:901-8.
125. Roque H, Paidas MJ, Funai EF, et al. Maternal thrombophilias are not associated with early pregnancy loss. Thromb Haemost. 2004;91:290-5.
126. Coppens M, Folkeringa N, Teune MJ, et al. Outcome of the subsequent pregnancy after a first loss in women with the factor V Leiden or prothrombin 20210A mutations. J Thromb Haemost. 2007;5:1444-8.
127. Kaandorp SP, Goddijn M, van Der Post JA, et al. Aspirin plus heparin or aspirin alone in women with recurrent miscarriage. N Engl J Med. 2010;362:1586-96.
128. Clark P, Walker ID, Langhorne P, et al. SPIN (Scottish Pregnancy Intervention) study: a multicenter, randomized controlled trial of low-molecular-weight heparin and low-dose aspirin in women with recurrent miscarriage. Blood. 2010;115:4162-7.
129. Visser J, Ulander VM, Helmerhorst FM, et al. Thromboprophylaxis for recurrent miscarriage in women with or without thrombophilia. HABENOX: a randomised multicentre trial. Thromb Haemost. 2011;105:295-301.

13

Cancer and Fertility Drugs

Shvetha M Zarek, Anil K Dubey

Chapter Contents

INTRODUCTION

Although nulliparity and infertility are thought to be risk factors for ovarian, breast and endometrial cancer, the effect of fertility treatment on cancer risk is not well characterized. Cellular exposure to hormones is known to proliferation that leads to an increased risk of cancer. Ovarian stimulation with fertility drugs like exogenous gonadotropins increased estradiol levels; however, whether these increases in hormone levels increase cancer risk has not been elucidated in this chapter.

Early studies have indicated that drugs causing ovarian stimulation could cause an increase in ovarian cancer risk. Subsequent studies demonstrated that fertility medicines do not increase the ovarian risk and although some studies showed a possible increased risk in nulligravid women. Effects of fertility drugs and breast cancer demonstrate conflicting results. However, increased risk of endometrial cancer related to clomiphene usage has been demonstrated. As women exposed to fertility drugs become older and longer follow up is possible, the authors will be able to further elucidate the effect of fertility drugs on cancer risk.

MECHANISM OF ACTION OF HORMONES IN CANCER

Estrogens control the transcription of an extensive and diverse set of genes. Indeed, microarray studies show that the hormone modulates hundreds of genes in numerous cell lines and tissues. Complicating matters is that the precise response to estrogen depends upon the relative ratio of the two estrogen receptor (ER) subtypes, as well as the length and strength of estrogen exposure and the presence or absence of various coregulators.[1] Among the many actions of estrogen is its tumorigenic capacity. Estrogen plays a significant role in the genesis and maintenance of gynecologic cancers.

The role of estrogen signaling in breast cancer has been the most studied of the gynecologic cancers, although studies are emerging and examining its role in other tumor pathologies. Estrogen's mechanism of action appears to be similar across all tumor types, with various idiosyncrasies specific to the particular cancer.

In the breast, estrogen mediates its carcinogenic effect via estrogen metabolism and signaling through the estrogen receptor.[2] Estradiol (E2) is broken down by cytochrome P450 enzymes (predominantly 1A1, 1A2, 3A, and 1B1) to catechol or quinone metabolites. The catechols are further metabolized by catechol O-methyltransferase (COMT) to 2- or 4-methoxycatechol and can covalently bind to proteins and DNA. The quinones undergo additional processing by P450 enzymes to become 2, 3- or 3, 4-quinones, which form stable DNA adducts or depurinating DNA adducts, respectively. These processes ultimately result in oxidative DNA damage, gene mutation, neoplastic transformation and tumor development.

The ER is the intracellular receptor for estrogens. It exists as a homo- or heterodimer of the alpha and beta subtypes and is found both in the nucleus and nonnuclear subcellular fractions, such as the plasma membrane and mitochondria. ERα and ERβ are virtually identical in their DNA-binding domains (> 95% homology) but differ quite a bit in their ligand binding domain (approximately 50% homology). There are also differences in the activation domains of ERα and ERβ such that they recruit different proteins to the transcription complex. The inconsistent effects of various natural and synthetic estrogens and selective estrogen receptor modulators (SERMs) across tissues can be attributed to the differences between ERα and ERβ ligand binding domains, activation domains and their relative expression in a given tissue. Indeed, ERα promotes cell proliferation while ERβ appears to possess antiproliferative properties.[3]

The classical mechanism of action of estrogen signaling involves nuclear estrogen receptors, which dimerize (ERα-ERα, ERα-ERβ, or ERβ-ERβ) following binding of the estrogen to the ER. The dimers then bind to estrogen response elements (EREs; consensus sequence: GGTCANNNTGACC) in the regulatory regions of estrogen-responsive genes. This ER-ERE complex recruits various transcription factors, coactivators, and corepressors which finally influence gene expression.

Just as ERα and ERβ can homo- or heterodimerize with each other, they can also bind to other activators, such as Sp1 and AP-1. This interaction explains how estrogens can influence expression of genes that lack a consensus ERE.[4] Such interactions further demonstrate how ERα and ERβ signaling can result in diverse outcomes.

Estrogen receptors are also present in the mitochondria and plasma membrane. Mitochondrial DNA suggests sequences to which ERs can bind and estrogen has been shown to increase the mitochondrial DNA transcription. Estrogen receptors on the plasma membrane are linked to the ras-MAPK cascade, as well as increasing cAMP levels within the cell. Activation of these pathways simultaneously increase cellular proliferation and inhibit apoptosis. The nongenomic effects of ER signaling can enhance the effect of other proliferation-inducing pathways, including the epidermal growth factor receptor and insulin-like growth factor-1 receptor pathways.[2]

At least with respect to ERα, it is easy to imagine a situation where estrogen metabolism and ER signaling combine to form a perfect storm for tumorigenesis. Enzymatic breakdown of E2 leads to DNA damage, increasing the chance of cancer-causing mutations. Receptor-mediated estrogen signaling induces the cell to proliferate while inhibiting apoptosis, also creating more chances for genetic mutations caused by copying errors of DNA polymerase replication. Furthermore, the enhanced proliferative capacity of cells exposed to elevated estrogen levels provides the opportunity for the population of cells with cancer-causing mutations to increase.

As in the breast, ovarian cells are susceptible to direct genotoxic effects of estrogen.[5] Also, ER signaling promotes growth of normal and malignant ovarian surface epithelium. The mitogenic effects of estrogens in ovarian surface epithelium appear to be mediated by activation of the IL-6/STAT3 pathway. Whereas ERβ is the predominant isoform of ER in normal ovarian tissue, progression to ovarian cancer shows an increase of ERα, both at the mRNA and protein levels.[6] This finding may be in dispute, though, as at least one group has seen a decrease of ERα mRNA with no disclosed change in ERβ levels.[5]

ERα is the predominant ER subtype in the uterus. There is a decrease in the ERα:ERβ ratio as the endometrium shifts from normal or grade 1 to grade 3 lesions. It is unclear what the significance of the altered ratio is. Although ERα in general is downregulated in endometrial carcinomas, there is an increase in the exon 5 splice variant of ERα, which is not present in normal endometrium. This splice variant shows constitutively active transcription of ER-dependent genes, even in the absence of estrogen.[7] The constitutive activity of the exon 5 splice variant may compensate for the decrease in ERα expression in endometrial carcinoma.

In contrast to the complicated expression profile of ERα and ERβ in uterine cancer, the function of the two ER isotypes is relatively straightforward with respect to colon cancer. In the normal colon, ERβ is the predominant ER subtype. Hormone dependent colon cancers show an inverse relation between tumor progression and ERβ expression.[8] Enhanced ERβ signaling may be pro-apoptotic with the field disagreeing on an exact mechanism. Perhaps there is an upregulation in BAXα gene, or a shift in the ratio of Bcl-2 to BAXα. There may be an upregulation in p53 signaling as well.[8]

BIOLOGIC PLAUSABILITY

Continued ovulation has been proposed as one of the primary causes of epithelial ovarian cancer with promotion of carcinogenesis via the regular damage and subsequent repair to the ovarian epithelium.[9,10] The proliferation of epithelial ovarian cells during each ovulation is thought to promote mutagenesis. The theory of incessant ovulation is supported by known risks factor, such as nulliparity.[11,12] Parity and ovarian cancer risk are inversely related and pregnancy is thought to reduce ovarian cancer risk by 30–60%. As more women delay childbearing, there is a concomitant increase in women diagnosed with infertility. As such, there has been a rapid increase in the usage of ovarian stimulating drugs like gonadotropins and clomiphene citrate. Ovarian stimulation is thought to be a risk factor for cancer, increasing levels of estradiol and progesterone, which have been implicated in the growth of gynecological cancers.[13-16]

Oral contraceptive use provides protection against ovarian cancer, adding support to the theory of incessant ovulation.[16] For users of oral contraceptives for five years or longer, their risk is reduced to more than 50%. This effect is seen for at least 10 years. The Cancer and Steroid Hormone Study suggested that women with a family history of ovarian cancer and 10 years of oral contraceptives reduce their risk to the levels lower than those of women with no family history of ovarian cancer who never used oral contraceptives.[16-20]

CLINICAL DATA

Ovarian Cancer

Ovarian cancer remains the leading cause of gynecologic cancer mortality in the United States. One in 72 women will be diagnosed with the disease and 1 in 100 will die from the disease.[9-11] A major risk factor for epithelial ovarian cancer is age, making it a disease of perimenopausal and postmenopausal women. More than 80% of disease is found in women over the age of forty.[9-11]

In the early 1990s, a number of case control studies were published that looked at the risk of ovarian cancer and fertility treatment. These studies allowed for a meta-analysis by Whittemore et al. that compiled data from 12 cases of control studies looking at ovarian cancer risk in the infertility population. In this meta-analysis a 2.8 odds ratio (OR 2.8, 95% CI 1.3–6.1) was seen with self-reported use of fertility medication and development of ovarian cancer. In addition, the study seemed to suggest that pregnancy even after fertility treatment was beneficial in preventing ovarian cancer. Women who took fertility drugs and did not get pregnant had a much higher risk of developing cancer (OR 27.0, 95% CI 2.3–315.6). Infertile women who did get pregnant, had no increased risk of developing ovarian cancer (OR 1.4, 95% CI 0.52–3.6).[21] This study was heavily criticized for its limited numbers. In a large 1994 retrospective cohort study of 3,837 women, Rossing et al. looked specifically at clomiphene citrate use which was associated with an adjusted 2.3-fold increased risk (95% CI 0.5–11.4), based on nine cases of cancer. But use of clomiphene for less than one year was not associated with increased risk. On the basis on these observations, many practitioners, including the latest Cochrane review, implicated a greater than year long use of clomiphene with an increased risk of ovarian cancer.[22]

After the release of these two early and alarming studies, multiple studies went on to find no increased risk of ovarian cancer. Ness et al. in 2002 conducted a meta-analysis of 1,060 cases and 1,337 controls and showed no statistically significant risk, although increased risk was seen in nulligravid women after fertility drug use after adjustment was done for types of infertility[23]

Modan et al. was able to report on a much larger population. A cohort of 2,496 infertile women were followed over a span of 10 years from 1964–1974. Twelve ovarian tumors were detected. The authors reported a standardized incidence ratio of 1.6 (95% CI 0.8–2.9) and concluded that ovulation induction drugs did not appear to increase the risk of ovarian cancer.[24]

Brinton et al., published a much larger study of 12,193 infertile women with a median follow-up period of 18.8 years. The results showed no correlation between use of clomiphene (SIR 0.8, 95% CI 0.4–1.5) and/or gonadotropin (SIR 1.1, 95% CI 0.4–2.8) and ovarian cancer had been established.[25] In addition, refuting Rossing et al. no correlation was seen with duration of treatment.

One of the largest most recent groups to examine was Jensen et al. in 2009. In this study, 54,362 infertile women with a median follow-up of 16 years were studied and no overall increase of risk of ovarian cancer after any use of gonadotropins (RR 0.83, 95% CI 0.50–1.37), clomiphene citrate (RR 1.14, 95% CI 0.79–1.64), human chorionic gonadotropin (RR 0.89, 95% CI 0.62–1.29) or gonadotropin releasing hormone analogs (RR 0.80, 95% CI 0.42–1.51) was found. Furthermore, the risk was not related to the number of cycles use, length of follow-up or parity (Tables 1 to 4).[26]

However, there remain conflicting results. In a recent meta-analysis by Kashyap et al., 28 women diagnosed with ovarian cancer had a significantly higher odds

Table 1 Rate ratios for ovarian cancer according to reproductive factors

Variable	No. of cases/No. in subcohort	Rate ratio (95% CI)
Parity:		
Nulliparous	85/425	1.00
Parous	71/816	0.45 (0.32-0.63)
No. of births:		
1	44/388	0.55 (0.38-0.82)
2	22/323	0.36 (0.22-0.60)
≥3	5/105	0.28 (0.11-0.71)
Per additional birth among parous women	–	0.68 (0.47-0.99)
Maternal age at birth of first child (years):		
<25	23/246	0.51 (0.31-0.83)
25-29	22/236	0.51 (0.31-0.84)
≥30	27/334	0.41 (0.26-0.65)
Per 5 years older among parous women	–	0.95 (0.77-1.16)
Maternal age at birth of last child (years):		
<30	36/270	0.69 (0.45-1.04)
30-35	23/324	0.38 (0.23-0.63)
≥35	13/220	0.32 (0.17-0.58)
Per 5 years older among parous women		0.89 (0.73-1.09)

Note: All analyses stratified according to calendar year (in categories) and age at start of follow-up (in categories) All rate ratios (except parity) adjusted for parity (nulliparous/parous) and number of additional births (linear)

Source: Jensen A, Sharif H, Frederiksen K, et al. Use of fertility drugs and risk of ovarian cancer: Danish Population Based Cohort Study. BMJ. 2009;338:b249

ratio of exposure to fertility drugs when they compared to normal controls (OR 1.52, 95% CI 1.18–1.97). This was a meta-analysis of seven case-control and three cohort studies. However, when participants with ovarian cancer were compared to infertile controls for exposure to infertility medications the OR (0.99, 95% CI 0.67–1.45) was not elevated.[27]

A few case reports delve into the relation of fertility drugs and particular histological subtypes of ovarian cancer. These case reports connect fertility drugs with clear-cell carcinoma, germ-cell malignant tumors. *In vitro* models demonstrate that gonadotropins may be related to Granulosa-cell tumors.[28,29] However, a Finnish study reported a reduction in the frequency of granulosa-cell carcinomas of the ovary in women taking drugs for fertility treatment.[30]

Still others have associated with the use of infertility drugs to ovarian borderline carcinomas, with a relative risk of three to four as compared to the general population. Cusido et al. conducted a recent case control study of 42 women with borderline ovarian tumors and 257 women with benign ovarian pathology, reported that ovulation induction treatment does not increase development of borderline ovarian tumors.[31]

Breast Cancer

Breast cancer is the most common malignancy in women in developed countries, accounting for 30–35% of all malignancies in females. A number of studies show that one of the risk factors for breast cancer is exogenous and endogenous hormones with a noted effect of ovulation on breast cancer risk.[32] A case-control study of over 4,500 breast cancer cases by Burkman et al. found no association of risk related to use of clomiphene. However, there was some indication of a risk elevation among women with long-term use of menopausal gonadotropins which was associated with RR ranging from 2.7–3.8.[33] Rossing et al. found a nonsignificant reduction in risk of invasive and *in situ* breast cancer (adjusted RR 0.5, 95% CI 0.2–1.2).[34] Tamoxifen, a selective estrogen receptor modulator, is used in the treatment of breast cancer and clomiphene citrate belongs in the same family of medications. The Nurses Health Study demonstrated a reduced risk of breast cancer which showed a RR of 0.40 (95% CI 0.2–0.7) associated with use of clomiphene among women treated for ovulatory infertility. Ten or more months of treatment resulted in a further reduction with a RR of 0.25 (95% CI 0.09–0.75) when compared with nonexposed women.[35]

Table 2 Rate ratios for ovarian cancer according to use of fertility drugs

Variables	No. with ovarian cancer/No. in subcohort				Adjusted rate ratio (95% CI)			
	Gonado-trophins*	Clomifene citrate	hCG	GnRH	Gonadotro-phins*	Clomifene citrate	hCG	GnRH
Use:								
Never	130/1057	98/824	107/828	141/1131	1.00	1.00	1.00	1.00
Ever	26/184	58/417	49/413	15/110	0.83 (0.50-1.37)	1.14 (0.79-1.64)	0.89 (0.62-1.29)	0.80 (0.42-1.51)
No. of cycles:								
1-4	18/130	35/226	31/232	14/100	0.74 (0.41-1.33)	1.27 (0.83-1.94)	0.96 (0.62-1.48)	0.81 (0.42-1.56)
5-9	7/46	15/117	13/121	1/10	1.09 (0.49-2.44)	1.03 (0.57-1.86)	0.86 (0.47-1.57)	0.68 (0.09-5.38)
≥10	1/8	8/74	5/60	0/0	0.96 (0.09-10.30)	0.92 (0.42-2.02)	0.70 (0.28-1.80)	–
Time since first use (years):								
<5	8/3	8/3	9/3	5/1	0.67 (0.29-1.54)	0.80 (0.32-1.99)	0.78 (0.35-1.75)	0.72 (0.28-1.89)
5-9	12/33	17/14	16/26	8/32	1.12 (0.58-2.21)	1.48 (0.80-2.73)	1.22 (0.67-2.23)	0.99 (0.43-2.33)
10-14	5/77	13/77	10/81	2/57	0.80 (0.29-2.18)	0.99 (0.53-1.87)	0.83 (0.43-1.62)	0.60 (0.13-2.70)
≥15	1/71	20/323	14/303	0/20	0.44 (0.06-3.14)	1.18 (0.70-1.99)	0.78 (0.43-1.42)	–

Note: All analyses stratified according to calendar year (in categories) and age at start of follow-up (in categories). Rate ratios adjusted for parity (nulliparous or parous) and number of additional births (linear). hCG: human chorionic gonadotropin; GnRH: gonadotropin releasing hormone

*Follicle stimulating hormone and human menopausal gonadotropins.

Source: Jensen A, Sharif H, Frederiksen K, et al. Use of fertility drugs and risk of ovarian cancer: Danish Population Based Cohort Study. BMJ. 2009;338:b249

In a large cohort study from France, involving 92,555 women and 2,571 invasive breast cancers, there was no evidence of an increased risk of breast cancer. However, an increased risk with fertility treatment was seen among women with a family history of breast cancer (RR 2.32–2.77).[36]

Two epidemiological IVF studies did not find differences in risk between exposed and unexposed subjects. In Venn et al. however, an approximately two-fold increased risk of breast cancer was seen within a year of treatment. This finding has not been seen in subsequent studies.[37,38]

The most recent large scale study was conducted in 2007 by Jensen et al. This study was comprised of 54,362 women with infertility problems referred to all Danish fertility. Three hundred and thirty-one invasive breast cancers were diagnosed with follow-up until 1998. No increased risk was seen after use of gonadotropins, clomiphene, human chorionic gonadotropin or gonadotropin-releasing hormone. However, progesterone increased breast cancer risk (RR 3.36, 95% CI 1.3–8.6). No effect of number of cycles of use or years since first use of fertility drug was seen. The conclusion was that no strong relationship between breast cancer risk and use of fertility drugs.[39]

Endometrial Cancer

In many developed nations, cancer of the corpus uteri is about as frequent as ovarian cancer, comprising 6% of all new cancers. Risk factors for endometrial cancer are nulliparity, late age menopause, obesity, polycystic ovary syndrome, and presence of estrogen-secreting

Table 3 Rate ratios for ovarian cancer in nulliparous and parous women according to use of fertility drugs

Fertility drug and use	Nulliparous women		Parous women		Interaction (P value)
	No. with ovarian cancer/No. in subcohort	Rate ratio (95% CI)	No. with ovarian cancer/No. in subcohort	Rate ratio (95% CI)	
Gonadotrophins*:					
Never	68/351	1.00	62/706	1.00	
Ever	17/74	0.85 (0.44-1.64)	9/110	0.89 (0.43-1.83)	0.93
Clomifene citrate:					
Never	50/276	1.00	48/548	1.00	
Ever	35/149	1.28 (0.79-2.07)	23/268	1.04 (0.61-1.78)	0.56
hCG:					
Never	57/285	1.00	50/543	1.00	
Ever	28/140	0.95 (0.57-1.58)	21/273	0.87 (0.51-1.49)	0.81
GnRH:					
Never	75/369	1.00	66/762	1.00	
Ever	10/56	0.71 (0.32-1.54)	5/54	1.09 (0.41-2.91)	0.48

Note: All analyses stratified according to calendar year (in categories) and age at start of follow-up (in categories). Rate ratios adjusted for parity (nulliparous or parous) and number of additional births (linear). hCG: human chorionic gonadotropins; GnRH: gonadotropin releasing hormone

*Follicle stimulating hormone and human menopausal gonadotropins

Source: Jensen A, Sharif H, Frederiksen K, et al. Use of fertility drugs and risk of ovarian cancer: Danish Population Based Cohort Study. BMJ. 2009;338:b249

malignancies. Anovulatory menstrual cycles have a prolonged follicular phase, resulting in prolonged exposure to estrogen or progesterone and increasing the risk of endometrial cancer.

Modan et al. found a significant two-fold increase in risk with fertility drugs after a 20-year follow-up of about 21 cases of endometrial cancer.[40] A cohort study by Althuis et al. found a nonsignificant increase in endometrial cancer associated with the use of clomiphene. Increases in risk were seen with patients on higher dosages or exposure or longer follow-up periods. Nulligravid and obese women had more effects of the drugs with women (RR of 3.5 and 6, respectively).[41] Long term follow-up is needed for these cases. Ron et al. showed no increased risk after a 12 year follow-up but a SIR of 6.8 only after 21 years of follow-up was demonstrated. Most studies demonstrate an increased risk of endometrial cancer in infertile women with a possible effect of fertility treatment.[42]

Melanoma

The effect of fertility drugs on the development of cutaneous melanoma is unclear. In Klip et al. a total of 34 melanomas were observed during follow-up, with differences in melanoma risk in patients who had fertility treatment and controls.[38]

A cohort study by Rossing et al. found no overall increase in melanoma risk with drug use, but a nonsignificant increase in risk when 12 or more cycles of clomiphene (RR 2.2, 95% CI, 0.5–10.2) and hCG (1.7, 95% CI, 0.5–6.2) were given.[38] Venn et al., found no overall risk with fertility treatment.[37]

The most recent study by Hannibal et al. studied a cohort of 54,362 women. One hundred and twelve malignant melanomas were identified during follow-up through 2,000. Use of all fertility drugs did not increase melanoma risk. However, a significant increase in parous women was seen with the use of gonadotropins (RR = 2.29; 95%CI: 1.16–4.52) or GnRH (RR = 3.26; 95%

Table 4 Rate ratios for histological subgroups of ovarian cancer according to use of fertility drugs

Fertility drugs and use	No. with ovarian cancer/No. in subcohort					Adjusted rate ratio (95% CI)				
	Serous	Mucinous	Endometrioid	Clear cell	Other	Serous	Mucinous	Endometrioid	Clear cell	Other
Gonadotropins*:										
Never	72/1057	9/1057	21/1057	6/1057	22/1057	1.00	1.00	1.00	1.00	1.00
Ever	18/184	3/184	2/184	2/184	1/184	1.04 (0.57-1.90)	1.14 (0.33-3.99)	0.74 (0.19-2.93)	1.59 (0.34-7.55)	0.57 (0.14-2.28)
Clomifene citrate:										
Never	48/824	9/824	19/824	4/824	18/824	1.00	1.00	1.00	1.00	1.00
Ever	42/417	3/417	4/417	4/417	5/417	1.67 (1.07-2.61)	0.60 (0.18-2.08)	0.68 (0.27-1.67)	1.62 (0.55-4.74)	0.70 (0.29-1.73)
hCG:										
Never	54/828	8/828	18/828	6/828	21/828	1.00	1.00	1.00	1.00	1.00
Ever	36/413	4/413	5/413	2/413	2/413	1.29 (0.83-2.01)	0.61 (0.20-1.79)	0.68 (0.28-1.67)	0.44 (0.10-1.92)	0.24 (0.08-0.79)
GnRH:										
Never	80/1131	11/1131	22/1131	6/1131	22/1131	1.00	1.00	1.00	1.00	1.00
Ever	10/110	1/110	1/110	2/110	1/110	0.93 (0.44-1.98)	1.47 (0.26-8.21)	0.75 (0.13-4.38)	2.89 (0.54-15.54)	1.14 (0.27-4.85)

Note: All analyses stratified according to calendar year (in categories) and age at start of follow-up (in categories). Rate ratios adjusted for parity (nulliparous and parous) and number of additional births (linear). hCG: human chorionic gonadotropins; GnRH: gonadotropin releasing hormone

*Follicle stimulating hormone and human menopausal gonadotropins

Source: Jensen A, Sharif H, Frederiksen K, et al. Use of fertility drugs and risk of ovarian cancer: Danish Population Based Cohort Study. BMJ. 2009;338:b249

CI: 1.50–7.09) associated with a significant increased risk. No association was seen with the number of cycles.

CONCLUSION

Although there are some studies that demonstrate an increased risk of cancer after the use of fertility drugs, there are also many studies that do not show an increased risk, but do support that nulliparous and infertile women are already at a higher risk of gynecologic cancers, particularly ovarian cancer. In counseling a patient, it is important to discuss the heterogeneity in the findings, but also discuss that there may be risk related to use of the fertility drugs that is also related to duration of exposure.

REFERENCES

1. Tang S, Han H, Bajic VB. ERGDB: Estrogen Responsive Genes Database. Nucleic Acids Res. 2004;32:D533-6.
2. Yager JD, Davidson NE. Estrogen carcinogenesis in breast cancer. N Engl J Med. 2006;354(3):270-82.
3. Vivar OI, Zhao X, Saunier EF, et al. Estrogen receptor beta binds to and regulates three distinct classes of target genes. J Biol Chem. 2010;285(29):22059-66.
4. Loose-Mitchell DS, Stancel GM. Estrogens and Progestins. In: Hardman JG, Limbird LE, (Eds). Goodman & Gilman's The Pharmacological Basis of Therapeutics, 10th edition., New York: McGraw-Hill; 2001. pp. 1597-634.
5. Ho SM. Estrogen, progesterone and epithelial ovarian cancer. Reprod Biol Endocrinol. 2003;1:73-80.
6. Jazaeri AA, Nunes KJ, Dalton MS, et al. Well-differentiated endometrial adenocarcinomas and poorly differentiated mixed Mullerian tumors have altered ER and PR isoform expression. Oncogene. 2001;20(47):6965-9.
7. Doll A, Abal M, Rigau M, et al. Novel molecular profiles of endometrial cancer-new light through old windows. J Steroid Biochem Mol Biol. 2008;108(3-5):221-9.
8. Kennelly R, Kavanagh DO, Hogan AM, et al. Oestrogen and the colon: potential mechanisms for cancer prevention. Lancet Oncol. 2008;9(4):385-91.
9. Jemal A, Siegel R, Ward E, et al. Cancer Statistics, 2009. CA Cancer J Clin. 2009;59:225-49.
10. Berek J. Epithelial ovarian cancer. In: Berek JS, Hacker NF, (Eds). Practical Gynecologic Oncology, 4th edition. Philadelphia: Lippincott Williams & Wilkins; 2005. pp. 443-509.
11. Ozols R, Rubin S, Thomas G, et al. In: Hoskins W, et al. (Eds). Principles and Practice of Gynecologic Oncology, 4th edition. Philadelphia: Lippincott Williams & Wilkins; 2005. pp. 895-987.
12. Fathalla MF. Incessant ovulation-a factor in ovarian neoplasia? Lancet. 1971;2(7716):163.
13. Greene MH, Clark JW, Blayney DW. The epidemiology of ovarian cancer. (Review). Semin Oncol.1984;11(3): 209-26.
14. Pelucchi C, Galeone C, Talamini R, et al. Lifetime ovulatory cycles and ovarian cancer risk in 2 Italian case-control studies. Am J Obstet Gynecol.2007;196(1):83.e1-83.e7.
15. Franceschi S, La Vecchia C, Booth M, et al. Pooled analysis of 3 European case-control studies of ovarian cancer: II. Age at menarche and at menopause. Int J Cancer.1991;49(1):57-60.
16. La Vecchia C. Oral contraceptives and ovarian cancer: an update, 1998–2004. (Review). Eur J Cancer Prev. 2006;15(2):117-24.
17. Franceschi S, Parazzini F, Negri E, et al. Pooled analysis of 3 European case-control studies of epithelial ovarian cancer: III. Oral contraceptive use. Int J Cancer. 1991;49(1):61-5.
18. Gross TP, Schesseleman JJ. The estimated effect of oral contraceptive use on the cumulative risk of epithelial ovarian cancer. Obstet Gynecol. 1994;83(3):419-24.
19. Rosenblatt KA, Thomas DB. Lactation and the risk of epithelial ovarian cancer. The WHO Collaborative Study of Neoplasia and Steroid Contraceptives. Int J Epidemiol.1993;22(2):192-7.
20. Gwinn ML, Lee NC, Rhodes PH, et al. Pregnancy, breast feeding, and oral contraceptives and the risk of epithelial ovarian cancer. J Clin Epidemiol. 1990;43(6):559-68.
21. Whittemore AS, Harris R, Itnyre J. Characteristics relating to ovarian cancer risk: collaborative analysis of 12US case-control studies. II. Invasive epithelial ovarian cancers in white women. Collaborative Ovarian Cancer Group. Am J Epidemiol. 1992;136:1184-203.
22. Rossing MA, Daling JR, Weiss NS, et al. Ovarian tumors in a cohort of infertile women. N Engl J Med. 1994;331:771-6.
23. Ness RB, Cramer DW, Goodman MT, et al. Infertility, fertility drugs, and ovarian cancer: a pooled analysis of case-control studies. American Journal of Epidemiology. 2004;155:217-24.
24. Modan B, Ron E, Lerner-Geva L, et al. Cancer incidence in a cohort of infertile women. Am J Epidemiol. 1998;147:1038-42.
25. Brinton LA, Lamb EJ, Moghissi KS, et al. Ovarian cancer risk after the use of ovulation-stimulating drugs. Obstetrics and Gynecology. 2004;103:1194-203.
26. Jensen A, Sharif H, Frederiksen K, et al. Use of fertility drugs and risk of ovarian cancer: Danish Population Based Cohort Study. BMJ. 2009;338:b249.
27. Kashyap S, Moher D, Fung MF, et al. Assisted reproductive technology and the incidence of ovarian cancer: a meta-analysis. Obstet. Gynecol. 2004;103:785-94.
28. Tennent BJ, Shultz KL, Sundberg JP, et al. Ovarian granulosa cell tumorigenesis in SWR-derived F1 hybrid mice: preneoplastic follicular abnormality and malignant disease progression. Am J Obstet Gynecol. 1990;163:625-34.

29. Hahlin M, Crona N, Knutsson F, et al. Human granulosa cell tumor: stimulation of steroidogenesis by gonadotropins in vitro. Gynecol Oncol. 1991;40:201-06.
30. Unkila-Kallio LA, Leminen A, Tiitinen A, et al. Nationwide data on falling incidence of ovarian granulosa cell tumours concomitant with increasing use of ovulation inducers. Hum Reprod. 1998;13:2828-30.
31. Cusidó M, Fábregas R, Pere BS, et al. Ovulation induction treatment and risk of borderline ovarian tumors. Gynecol Endocrinol. 2007;23:373-6.
32. Bernstein L. Epidemiology of endocrine-related risk factors for breast cancer. J Mammary Gland Biol Neoplasia. 2002;7(1):3-15.
33. Burkman RT, Tang MT, Malone KE, et al. Infertility drugs and the risk of breast cancer: findings from the National Institute of Child Health and Human Development Women's Contraceptive and Reproductive Experiences Study. Fertility and Sterility. 2003;79:844-S51.
34. Rossing MA, Daling JR, Weiss NS, et al. Risk of breast cancer in a cohort in infertile women. Gynecologic Oncology. 1996;60:3-7.
35. Terry KL, Willett WC, Rich-Edwards JW, et al. A prospective study of infertility due to ovulatory disorders, ovulation induction, and incidence of breast cancer. Archives of Internal Medicine. 2006;166:2484-9.
36. Giiuthier E, Paoletti X, Clavel-Chapelon F. Breast cancer risk associated with being treated for infertility: results from the French E3N eohort study. Human Reproduction. 2004;19:2216-21.
37. Venn A, Watson L, Bruinsma F, et al. Risk of cancer after use of fertility drugs with in vitro fertilisation. Lancet. 1999;554:1586-90.
38. Klip H, Burger C van Leeuwen F, et al. Risk of hormone-related cancers after ovarian stimulation for in vitro fertilisation in a cohort of 25.152 women. 2002 PrintPartners Ipskamp B V, Enschede. The Netherlands. p. 27
39. Jensen A, Sharif H, Svare EI, et al. Risk of breast cancer after exposure to fertility drugs: results from a large Danish cohort study. Cancer Epidemiol Biomarkers Prev. 2007;16:1400-7.
40. Modan B, Ron E, Lerner-Geva L, et al. Cancer incidence in a cohort of infertile women. Am J Epidemiol. 1998;147:1038-42.
41. Althuis MD, Moghissi KS, Westhoff CL, et al. Uterine cancer after use of clomiphene citrate to induce ovulation. Am J Epidemiol. 2005;161:607-15.
42. Ron E, Lunenfeld B, Menczer J, et al. Cancer incidence in a cohort of infertile women. Am J Epidemiol. 1987;125:780-90.

14

Unexplained Infertility

Ioanna Athanasiadis, Anil K Dubey

CHAPTER CONTENTS

INTRODUCTION

Infertility is the failure of a couple to conceive after 1 year of unprotected intercourse without contraception. The issue of infertility requires a thorough evaluation of the two separate individuals to determine a cause for their problem. The most common factors involved in causing infertility include male factor (35%), ovulatory dysfunction (15%), tubal disease (20%), endometriosis (10%) and cervical factors (5%).[1]

In approximately, 15% of couples, an evaluation of infertility will reveal no abnormal result and these couples will be described as having unexplained infertility.[2] Currently, a thorough evaluation consists of assessing tubal patency, documenting ovulation and a normal ovarian reserve, adequate sperm production, and a normal uterine cavity. Historically, a positive postcoital test and 'in phase' endometrial dating also would have been required, but no longer. However, even an extensive set of diagnostic tests cannot reveal all the possible underlying causes of infertility.

POSSIBLE ETIOLOGIES OF UNEXPLAINED INFERTILITY

Several possibilities have been suggested to explain the failure to conceive in couples with unexplained infertility. These couples may simply represent the lower extreme of the normal distribution of fertility. However, others have suggested that these couples may have functional abnormalities in oocyte and/or sperm function, fertilization or embryo development that is not readily detected by the currently available diagnostic tests.

In the literature, it has been reported that there may be subtle changes in follicular development, ovulation and the luteal phase in women who have otherwise no identifiable cause for infertility.[3,4] Elevated titers of autoantibodies to the zona pellucida have been observed in patients with unexplained infertility when compared with those who had a known cause of infertility and their healthy counterparts.[5] Guzick et al. reported that, in the unexplained infertile couple, the male partner's semen analysis showed sperm motility and concentration at the lower end of the normal range.[6]

Unexplained infertility may be a result of an undiscovered defect in fertilization, implantation and embryo development. In a study done by Hull et al. couples with unexplained infertility treated with *in vitro* fertilization (IVF) showed decreased oocyte fertilization and embryo cleavage rate as compared to couples with tubal factor infertility, 52% and 60% respectively.[7]

PROGNOSIS OF UNEXPLAINED INFERTILITY

The prognosis for couples with unexplained infertility seems to be dependent upon the possibility that an unidentifiable cause of infertility will correct itself over time. Overall, infertility has a significant spontaneous cure rate that varies with the age of the female partner, duration of infertility, past obstetrical history and the cause of infertility. The average cycle fecundity in untreated women with unexplained infertility is about 2–4% or about 80–90% lower than in normal fertile couples (20–25%).[8] Without treatment, the probability for achieving a live birth decreases with increasing age and duration of infertility. Overall, the likelihood of conceiving without treatment declines by approximately 5% for each additional year of the female partner's age and by 15–25% for each subsequent year of infertility.[9] Couples who have conceived before generally have a better prognosis than those who have never achieved pregnancy. Table 1 shows the effect on prognosis in terms of the duration of infertility together with the effect of a prior pregnancy as suggested by Collins et al.[10]

This was further shown in a study performed by Evers. After 3 years of infertility, the likelihood of a spontaneous pregnancy falls to approximately 40% and after 5 years, the likelihood falls to 20% of what it was when the couple began efforts to conceive.[11]

Table 1 Effect on prognosis suggested by Collins et al.

Unexplained infertility (number of couples)	Cumulative pregnancy Rate (%)	
Primary infertility	12 months	36 months
Duration < 36 months (131)	40 ± 9	62 ± 14
Duration ≥ 36 months (89)	13 ± 8	40 ± 19
Secondary infertility (both duration groups)	46 ± 16	65 ± 19

CLINICAL EVALUATION TO DIAGNOSE UNEXPLAINED INFERTILITY

In order to diagnose a couple with unexplained infertility, the minimum evaluation includes a normal semen analysis, a normal uterine cavity and tubal patency as demonstrated by hysterosalpingogram and/or laparoscopy and confirmation of ovulation with a normal ovarian reserve.

The use of diagnostic laparoscopy remains controversial in the evaluation of couples with unexplained infertility. Although laparoscopy can detect tubal disease and endometriosis that may not have been apparent on transvaginal imaging or hysterosalpingogram, it is unlikely that diagnostic laparoscopy alone will determine the cause of previously unexplained infertility in an asymptomatic patient with an otherwise normal work-up. This becomes particularly true if a clinician does not consider minimal or mild endometriosis as a major cause of infertility. The Canadian Collaborative Group on Endometriosis performed a large multicenter randomized controlled trial on 341 infertile women with minimal and mild endometriosis diagnosed by laparoscopy. These women were randomly assigned to undergo resection or ablation of endometriosis or diagnostic laparoscopy alone. Of the women who were surgically treated, approximately, 30% became pregnant versus only 17% in the control group.[12] A study by Parazzini, however, showed no difference in conception rates in women who were treated with laparoscopy when compared to those who did not undergo surgery.[13]

It is currently recommended that a transvaginal ultrasound examination be used as a method of infertility evaluation instead of diagnostic laparoscopy. This imaging modality is useful in detecting significant endometriomas and uterine abnormalities (myomas, polyps) that have been proven to negatively affect fertility, consistently in the literature.

Some apparent causes of infertility may change over a period of time and not necessarily be detected, if specific diagnostic tests are not repeated. The question as to whether or not previously normal examinations should be repeated arises in the situation of couples with persistent unexplained infertility. There have been no studies showing any benefit in repeating a tests unless a new exposure factor arises. Only if the results of the initial workup are unavailable, incomplete or outdated, should a new workup be initiated in the same couple. Additionally, there is no utility in repeating diagnostic laparoscopy in an otherwise healthy female with a previously normal pelvis. It may, however, be performed if a clinician suspects a substantial increase in the patient's risk of newly developed endometriosis, tubal disease or other infertility-associated pathology based on the patient's symptoms.

TREATMENT OF UNEXPLAINED INFERTILITY

The treatment of couples with unexplained infertility presents a very unique dilemma. Since there is no identifiable abnormality that can be corrected, all methods of treatment for these couples are empirical. Several proposed treatments for unexplained infertility include expectant management, intrauterine insemination (IUI), ovarian superovulation (clomiphene citrate, gonadotropins), ovarian stimulation combined with IUI and IVF.

Expectant Management

It has been shown that 1–3% of couples with unexplained infertility treated expectantly become pregnant each month.[11] Therefore, the focus of fertility treatment of this group of patients should be to increase the pregnancy rate above this baseline fecundity. The age of the female partner, however, does influence the pregnancy rate in the unexplained infertile couple that is being expectantly managed.[14] Steures et al. randomly assigned subfertile couples with a good prognosis (young age, no tubal disease, normal semen analysis) to either undergo 6 months of expectant management or IUI with controlled ovarian hyperstimulation (COH). Thirty-three percent of women in the treatment group conceived within 6 months as compared to 32% in the expectant management group.[15] This data suggests that expectant management may be a feasible option for couples with unexplained infertility in whom the female partner is young without any concern for ovarian aging and possible oocyte depletion. However, more aggressive treatment options should be offered to older women in whom the decline of ovarian function is likely to lead to a cause of infertility.

Intrauterine Insemination

Intrauterine insemination is a procedure that involves washing a semen specimen, concentrating the sperm in a small amount of media and injecting it directly into a patient's uterine cavity through the cervix to facilitate fertilization. Although IUI has been proven to improve the pregnancy rate in couples when combined with either clomiphene citrate (CC) or gonadotropins, its use alone in couples with unexplained infertility may be an effective treatment modality.

Kirby et al. performed a randomized clinical trial that compared IUI with timed intercourse in 73 couples with unexplained infertility. The timed intercourse was 40 hours after the detection of a rise in the serum luteinizing hormone (LH). The pregnancy rates in these couples were 4.1% in the IUI group and 2.4% in the timed intercourse group; a difference that was not statistically significant.[16] Subsequently, a large clinical trial sponsored by the National Institutes of Health was performed to further evaluate the efficacy of IUI alone in the couple with unexplained infertility.[6] This study included 932 couples, who were randomly assigned to undergo intracervical insemination of sperm (ICI), IUI, superovulation with gonadotropins plus ICI and superovulation plus IUI. The ICI group was intended to serve as a control that would represent natural intercourse. Table 2 summarizes the results of this study.

Based on the results of this study, IUI alone is almost twice as likely to result in pregnancy than timed intercourse, as represented by the ICI group. It is evident that superovulation with IUI is superior to IUI alone and this will be discussed later in the chapter.

Clomiphene Citrate Therapy

Although clomiphene citrate (CC) is an effective treatment of infertility secondary to anovulation, ovarian stimulation has been proposed as a treatment option for couples with unexplained infertility as well. Several trials have evaluated the efficacy of CC combined with intercourse in couples with unexplained infertility.

A double blind randomized trial compared empiric CC treatment (100 mg on cycle days 5–9) with placebo in 148 couples with unexplained infertility over a 4 months period. There were no pregnancies in the placebo group during this time frame whereas the CC treatment group had a significantly better pregnancy rate at 19%.[17] Harrison et al. performed a study involving CC treatment with ovulation triggered by human chorionic

Table 2 National Institute of Health's evaluation on efficacy of ICI and IUI

Treatment	Number of couples	Number of pregnancies	Pregnancy rate per couple (%)
ICI	233	23	10
IUI	234	42	18
Gonadotropins + ICI	234	44	19
Gonadotropins + IUI	231	77	33

gonadotropin. They report a 3.1% pregnancy rate per cycle in the treated group and a 0.6% rate in the control group ($P < 0.04$).[18] Glazener et al. also showed a significant improvement in conception with the use of CC in 118 couples with unexplained infertility. These patients were treated with CC 100 mg for up to 3 months. Pregnancies occurred in 24 of 295 cycles (8.1%) in the CC group and in 15 of 295 (5.1%) of the placebo cycles. The 3 months cumulative conception rate was increased by approximately 53% when CC was used in these patients. In fact, women with infertility lasting more than 3 years seemed to benefit most, with a 3 months conception rate increasing from 2.9% to 14.4%.[19]

However, one trial showed that CC was ineffective in treating unexplained infertility. Eighteen patients received CC 50 mg and were compared with 15 control patients. The pregnancy rate per patient was significantly decreased for those women receiving CC [four out of eighteen (22.2%)] than in the spontaneous group [eleven out of fifteen (73.3%)].[20] Additionally, a Cochrane meta-analysis of two randomized trials treating women with unexplained infertility with CC therapy found no evidence that CC alone was more beneficial than placebo or no treatment at all.[21] Therefore, despite early data, the overall effect of CC therapy alone may not be as efficacious for this group of patients as previously thought.

Clomiphene Citrate and Intrauterine Insemination

Numerous studies have examined the efficacy of CC with IUI as a treatment modality for couples with unexplained infertility. Superovulation with CC combined with IUI to place a large number of normal sperm within the uterus may treat mild undetectable abnormalities in ovulation and sperm function. In a randomized clinical trial by Deaton, 67 couples with unexplained infertility underwent 298 treatment cycles with either observation alone or with CC and IUI. The pregnancy rate among couples treated with clomiphene plus IUI was 9.5% (14/1148 cycles) versus 3.3% (5/150) among those using timed intercourse.[22]

In a review of eight separate studies that included 932 cycles in couples with unexplained infertility, the combined pregnancy rates per cycle initiated were 3.8% with IUI alone, 5.6% with CC and 8.3% with CC/IUI.[8] A randomized crossover trial in 1994 involved 26 couples with unexplained infertility observed an even greater efficacy for CC/IUI compared with IUI alone. Among this group, there was one pregnancy in 20 cycles (PR 5% per cycle) in the IUI alone group, compared with 6 pregnancies in 23 cycles (PR 26.1%) in the CC/IUI group.[23]

However, in 2004, Agarwal et al. showed that combined CC/IUI did not improve conception rates in couples with unexplained infertility. In this trial, 140 couples underwent 556 cycles of either COH with clomiphene alone plus timed intercourse or CC combined with IUI. The pregnancy rate and cycle fecundity rate was 18% and 3.4% after CC/IUI compared to a pregnancy rate and cycle fecundity rate of 41% and 8.8% after CC/timed intercourse. This difference, however, was not statistically significant and was also flawed secondary to the loss of 30 couples to follow up.[24]

Custers et al. performed a multicenter retrospective cohort study of couples who underwent 15,303 IUI cycles in order to determine the maximum number of IUI cycles that should be performed for patients with unexplained infertility.[25] In 70% of cycles, the patients underwent COH (51% CC, 19% gonadotropins) in addition to IUI. The cumulative ongoing pregnancy rates after cycle numbers 3, 6, and 9 were 18%, 30% and 41%, respectively. The results of this study suggests that conducting up to nine cycles of COH plus IUI may be a reasonable treatment option for couples with unexplained infertility.

The age of the female partner, however, must be considered when deciding on the number of cycles that will be administered to a couple before moving on to another treatment option. Dovey et al. performed a retrospective study in over 1,700 infertile patients to determine the effect that age has on the efficacy of CC combined with IUI. Table 3 summarizes their results.

The success rate of CC and IUI is greater in younger patients with unexplained infertility than in their older counterparts. In this study, there were no pregnancies reported in women older than 41-year old beyond the fourth cycle. Additionally, there is a sharp decline in the pregnancy rate in women over the age of 42. Therefore, it is suggested that CC plus IUI should not be a preferred method of treatment in older women (age > 42) with unexplained infertility.[26]

Gonadotropin Therapy

A literature review of numerous studies suggests that empiric gonadotropin therapy can be an effective

Table 3 Result of study performed by Dovey et al.

Age (years)	Number of patients	Number of cycles	Cumulative pregnancy rate
< 35	983	2351	24.2%
35-37	422	947	18.5%
38-40	265	614	15.1%
41-42	81	166	7.4%
> 42	55	120	1.8%

treatment for unexplained infertility. This becomes especially true when combined with IUI.[8] This method of treatment seems to be appropriate in those patients who do not conceive with CC therapy. Aboulghar et al. found that the pregnancy rate per patient was improved when gonadotropin therapy plus IUI (PR 34.7%) was used as treatment versus expectant management (PR 8.9%).[27]

Studies have shown that combining IUI with gonadotropin injections was more effective in treating couples with unexplained infertility than either treatment alone. Serhal et al. performed a study that included 62 couples who were randomly assigned to undergo IUI alone, gonadotropin therapy alone or gonadotropins plus IUI. The pregnancy rate per cycle was 2.2% for IUI alone, 6.1% for gonadotropins alone and 26% for gonadotropins plus IUI.[28] As mentioned previously, a randomized controlled trial sponsored by the NIH assigned couples with unexplained infertility to receive ICI, IUI, follicle-stimulating hormone (FSH) injections plus ICI or FSH injections plus IUI. The FSH plus ICI and FSH plus IUI groups were more effective than the control groups, with pregnancy rates per cycle of 4% and 9%, respectively.[6] Additionally, Chung et al. performed a study in which 100 patients were randomized to ovulation induction with gonadotropins with or without IUI. They showed that superovulation with IUI was superior to superovulation with timed intercourse in terms of both improved cycle fecundity (21.8% and 8.5%), and cumulative ongoing pregnancy rate (42% and 20%).[29]

Several studies have been aimed to compare fertility rates in unexplained infertility patients receiving CC with those undergoing gonadotropin therapies. Karlström et al. reported that a combination of gonadotropins with IUI had higher cycle fecundity (19%) as compared with CC/IUI (4%).[30] Furthermore, a Cochrane review of 43 trials involving 3,957 women suggested that women undergoing IUI had significantly improved pregnancy rates when superovulation was achieved with gonadotropins rather than CC (OR 1.8, 95% CI 1.2–2.7).[31]

Researchers and clinicians suggest that couples with unexplained infertility should not undergo more than three cycles of gonadotropin injections plus IUI since most pregnancies with this treatment modality will occur within the first three cycles. In 2001, Aboulghar et al. showed that the cycle fecundity decreased after three cycles of gonadotropins/IUI to 5.6% from 16.4%.[32] The authors recommend that couples who fail to become pregnant after three cycles of superovulation/IUI should be offered IVF.

Reindollar et al. recently published the fast track and standard treatment (FASTT) trial to evaluate the optimal method of treatment of unexplained infertility.[33] This was a trial that compared treatment outcomes in couples randomly assigned to receive 3 cycles of CC/IUI, 3 cycles of FSH/IUI and up to 6 cycles of IVF versus an accelerated treatment strategy that omitted the three cycles of FSH/IUI. Couples in the accelerated arm of this trial required less time to achieve a pregnancy (median time 8 months vs. 11 months in the conventional arm). These couples also required fewer treatment cycles to achieve pregnancy and had a significantly lower total charge per delivery than those couples undergoing conventional treatment. Cumulative pregnancy rates were also improved using the accelerated strategy (Table 4) without increasing the incidence of multiple gestations.

The major concern with using gonadotropin therapy for treatment of infertility is the increase in the rates of multiple gestations. According to the National Center for Health Statistics,[34] the annual number of twin births increased 70% from 1980 through 2004, whereas the number of triplet and higher-order multiple births increased by more than 400% until peaking in 1998, after which it has decreased by 24% until 2008. It is estimated that one-third of these birth are spontaneous and that two-thirds are the direct result of assisted reproductive technology.[35] In an effort to decrease the number of multiples in each pregnancy, the American Society of Reproductive Medicine published guidelines on the number of embryos to transfer during IVF.[36] Due to the risk of multiple gestation and the improved pregnancy rates with IVF, many authorities suggest that gonadotropin therapy, with or without IUI, should be used very cautiously in the treatment of couples with unexplained infertility.

In Vitro Fertilization

In vitro fertilization has been shown to be the treatment modality that results in the highest pregnancy rate per cycle in a shorter time frame for couples with unexplained infertility. In the Centers for Disease Control and Prevention (CDC) report on assisted reproductive technology results for 2008, the live birth rate among women with unexplained infertility undergoing IVF was 33.4%.[37] Hughes et al. randomly assigned women

Table 4 Pregnancy rates using the accelerated strategy

Time (months)	Cumulative pregnancy rate (conventional arm)	Cumulative pregnancy rate (accelerated arm)
6	31.9%	43.2%
9	43.8%	54.7%
12	55.4%	65.4%

with unexplained infertility to receive either IVF or have expectant management for a period of 90 days. The live birth rates were significantly higher in couples undergoing IVF (29%) versus no treatment (1%).[38]

There have been studies that aimed to compare IVF with other treatment options for couples with unexplained infertility. In one trial, 258 couples were randomized to receive IUI only, gonadotropins and IUI, or IVF. The pregnancy rate per cycle was higher in the IVF group (12.2%) than in the IUI alone (7.4%) and gonadotropin/IUI (8.7%). However, the cumulative pregnancy rate was not significantly better than that for the IUI groups (P=0.09).[39] A cohort study by Aboulghar et al. included 485 patients, who were initially treated with a maximum of three cycles of gonadotropin injections. Those who did not conceive were then treated with IVF. The pregnancy rate per cycle more than doubled when couples with unexplained infertility were treated with IVF when compared to those receiving gonadotropins/IUI (37% and 16%, respectively).[40]

Despite data supporting the use of IVF in the unexplained infertile couple, a Cochrane review of ten randomized trials comparing IVF with expectant management, CC alone, gonadotropins alone or IUI with ovarian stimulation reveals that larger trials comparing all of these treatment modalities are required to establish the effectiveness of IVF in this patient population.[41]

CONCLUSION

After a couple has completed their infertility evaluation and has been determined to have unexplained infertility, it is essential that these patients be counseled appropriately regarding their prognosis and treatment options. It is imperative that the physician takes into account the duration of infertility, the female partner's age and possibly ovarian reserve and previous obstetrical history prior to offering specific treatment recommendations. Expectant management may be appropriate for couples where the female partner is less than 32 years old. However, empiric treatment should be offered to those female patients older than 37 years old. It is usually proposed that conservative efforts be offered to these couples before initiating IVF, although recent trials have shown improved outcomes with a more accelerated approach.[33] Couples who decide to undergo treatment should be thoroughly counseled regarding their management options, relative costs, prognosis and risks, particularly multiple gestation and ovarian hyperstimulation, in order for them to select the most appropriate treatment plan that best achieves their goals.

REFERENCES

1. Collins JA, Crosignani PG. Unexplained infertility: a review of diagnosis, prognosis, treatment efficacy and management. Int J Gynaecol Obstet. 1992;39:267-75.
2. Guzick DS, Grefenstette I, Baffone K, et al.Infertility evaluation in fertile women: a model for assessing the efficacy of infertility testing, Hum Reprod.1994;9:2306-10.
3. Leach RE, Moghissi KS, Randolph JF, et al. Intensive hormone monitoring in women with unexplained infertility: evidence for subtle abnormalities suggestive of diminished ovarian reserve. Fertil Steril. 1997;68:413-20.
4. Blacker CM, Ginsburg KA, Leach RE, et al. Unexplained infertility: evaluation of the luteal phase; results of the National Center for Infertility Research at Michigan. Fertil Steril. 1997;67:437-42.
5. Singh J, Mhaskar AM. Enzyme-linked immunosorbent determination of autoantibodies to zona pellucida as a possible cause of infertility in women. J Immunol Methods. 1985;79:133-41.
6. Guzick DS, Carson SA, Coutifaris C, et al. Efficacy of superovulation and intrauterine insemination in the treatment of infertility. National Cooperative Reproductive Medicine Network. N Engl J Med. 1999;340:177-83.
7. Hull MG. Effectiveness of infertility treatments: choice and comparative analysis. Int J Gynaecol Obstet. 1994;47:99-108.
8. Guzick DS, Sullivan MW, Adamson GD, et al. Efficacy of treatment for unexplained infertility, Fertil Steril. 1998;70:207-13.
9. Collins JA, Burrows EA, Wilan AR. The prognosis for live birth among untreated infertile couples. Fertil Steril. 1995;64:22-8.
10. Collins JA, So Y, Wilson EH, et al. Clinical factors affecting pregnancy rates among infertile couples. Can Med Assoc J. 1984;130:269-73.
11. Evers JL. Female subfertility. Lancet. 2002;360:151-9.
12. Marcoux S, Maheux R, Bérubé S. Laparoscopic surgery in infertile women with minimal or mild endometriosis.Canadian Collaborative Group on Endometriosis. N Engl J Med. 1997;337:217-22.
13. Parazzini F. Ablation of lesions or no treatment in minimal-mild endometriosis in infertile women: a randomized trial. Gruppo Italiano per lo Studio dell' Endometriosi. Hum Reprod.1999;14:1332-4.
14. Hull MG, Glazener CM, Kelly NJ, et al. Population study of causes, treatment, and outcome of infertility. Br Med J (Clin Res Ed). 1985;291:1693-7.
15. Steures P, van der Steeg JW, Hompes PG, et al. Intrauterine insemination with controlled ovarian hyperstimulation versus expectant management for couples with unexplained subfertility and an intermediate prognosis: a randomized clinical trial. Lancet. 2006;368:216-21.
16. Kirby CA, Flaherty SP, Godfrey BM, et al. A prospective trial of intrauterine insemination of motile spermatozoa versus timed intercourse. Fertil Steril. 1991;56:102-7.

17. Fisch P, Casper RF, Brown SE, et al. Unexplained infertility: evaluation of treatment with clomiphene citrate and human chorionic gonadotropin. Fertil Steril. 1989;51:828-33.
18. Harrison RF, O'Moore RR. The use of clomiphene citrate with and without human chorionic gonadotropin. Ir Med J. 1983;76:273-4.
19. Glazener CM, Coulson C, Lambert PA, et al. Clomiphene treatment for women with unexplained infertility: placebo-controlled study of hormonal responses and conception rates. Gynecol Endocrinol. 1990;4:75-83.
20. Fujii S, Fukui A, Fukushi Y, et al. The effects of clomiphene citrate on normally ovulatory women. Fertil Steril. 1997;68:997-9.
21. Hughes E, Collins J, Vandekerckhove P. Clomiphene citrate for unexplained subfertility in women. Cochrane Database Syst Rev. 2000;CD000057.
22. Deaton JL, Gibson M, Blackmer KM, et al. A randomized, controlled trial of clomiphene citrate and intrauterine insemination in couples with unexplained infertility or surgically corrected endometriosis, Fertil Steril. 1990;54:1083-8.
23. Arici A, Byrd W, Bradshaw K, et al. Evaluation of clomiphene citrate and human chorionic gonadotropin treatment: a prospective, randomized, crossover study during intrauterine insemination cycles, Fertil Steril. 1994;61:314-8.
24. Agarwal S, Mittal S. A randomised prospective trial of intrauterine insemination versus timed intercourse in superovulated cycles with clomiphene. Indian J Med Res. 2004;120:519-22.
25. Custers IM, Steures P, Hompes P, et al. Intrauterine insemination: how many cycles should we perform? Hum Reprod. 2008;23:885-8.
26. Dovey S, Sneeringer RM, Penzias AS. Clomiphene citrate and intrauterine insemination: analysis of more than 4100 cycles. Fertil Steril. 2008;90:2281-6.
27. Aboulghar MA, Mansour RT, Serour GI, et al. Ovarian superstimulation and intrauterine insemination for the treatment of unexplained infertility. Fertil Steril. 1993;60:303-6.
28. Serhal PF, Katz M, Little V, et al. Unexplained infertility--the value of Pergonal superovulation combined with intrauterine insemination. Fertil Steril. 1988;49:602-6.
29. Chung CC, Fleming R, Jamieson ME, et al. Randomized comparison of ovulation induction with and without intrauterine insemination in the treatment of unexplained infertility. Hum Reprod. 1995;10:3139-41.
30. Karlström PO, Bergh T, Lundkvist O. A prospective randomized trial of artificial insemination versus intercourse in cycles stimulated with human menopausal gonadotropin or clomiphene citrate. Fertil Steril. 1993;59:554-9.
31. Cantineau AE, Cohlen BJ, Heineman MJ. Ovarian stimulation protocols (anti-estrogens, gonadotropins with and without GnRH agonists/antagonists) for intrauterine insemination (IUI) in women with subfertility. Cochrane Database Syst Rev. 2007;CD005356.
32. Aboulghar M, Mansour R, Serour G, et al. Controlled ovarian hyperstimulation and intrauterine insemination for treatment of unexplained infertility should be limited to a maximum of three trials. Fertil Steril. 2001;75:88-91.
33. Reindollar RH, Regan MM, Neumann PJ, et al. A randomized clinical trial to evaluate optimal treatment for unexplained infertility: the fast track and standard treatment (FASTT) trial. Fertil Steril. 2010;94:888-99.
34. Martin JA, Hamilton BE, Sutton PD. Births: final data for 2008. Natl Vital Stat Rep. 2010;58:1-85.
35. Jones HW, Schnorr JA. Multiple pregnancies: a call for action. Fertil Steril. 2001;75:11-3.
36. Practice Committee of the American Society for Reproductive Medicine; Practice Committee of the Society for Assisted Reproductive Technology. Guidelines on number of embryos transferred. Fertil Steril. 2009; 92:1518-9.
37. 2008 Assisted Reproductive Technology Success rates. National Summary and Fertility Clinic Reports 2008. [Online] Available from www.cdc. gov/ART/ART 2008. [Accessed August 2011].
38. Hughes EG, Beecroft ML, Wilkie V, et al. A multicenter randomized controlled trial of expectant management versus IVF in women with Fallopian tube patency. Hum Reprod. 2004;19:1105-9.
39. Goverde AJ, McDonnell J, Vermeiden JP, et al. Intrauterine insemination or in vitro fertilization in idiopathic subfertility and male subfertility: a randomised trial and cost-effectiveness analysis. Lancet.2000;355:13-8.
40. Aboulghar MA, Mansour RT, Serour GI, et al. Management of long-standing unexplained infertility: A prospective study. Am J Obstet Gynecol. 1999;181:371-5.
41. Pandian Z, Bhattacharya S, Vale L, et al. In vitro fertilization for unexplained subfertility. Cochrane Database Syst Rev. 2005;(2):CD003357.

15

Reproductive Surgery: Technique and Reproductive Outcomes

Molina B Dayal, Nadim Hawa, Gaby Moawad

Chapter Contents

INTRODUCTION AND BACKGROUND

Progress in medicine frequently follows innovations and improvements in technology. The technique of microsurgery with microscopes or surgical loupes was first developed in the 1970s and widely practiced through the 1990s. Assisted reproductive technology (ART), specifically *in vitro* fertilization (IVF), developed concurrently in the 1980s as laparoscopy, followed shortly by advances in hysteroscopy. Since then, both IVF and laparoscopy/hysteroscopy have matured to be state-of-the-art technologies used to treat a variety of disorders related to infertility.

The use of laparoscopic and hysteroscopic access for reproductive surgery is now considered a standard surgical practice. The advantages of laparoscopic access as opposed to conventional laparotomy include shortened postoperative hospital stay and recovery, reduced postoperative discomfort, frequently lesser costs and the ensuing medical and cosmetic gains associated with the avoidance of a laparotomy. Many complex gynecological procedures can now be successfully performed by laparoscopy.

In the 1970s, hysteroscopy was purely diagnostic with its clinical indications being limited. Since then, hysteroscopy has evolved and its impact on reproductive surgery has been radical. As hysteroscopy provides a means for surgical access into the uterus, it greatly simplified many procedures that previously required a laparotomy and a hysterotomy to access the uterine cavity, such as lysis of severe intrauterine synechiae, metroplasty for a septate uterus and excision of symptomatic submucosal/intracavitary myomas. Hysteroscopy, thus, radically simplified these procedures and reduced their associated morbidity.

Both laparoscopic and hysteroscopic surgery are considered minimally invasive surgery. However, minimal only refers to access, neither to the level of skill required nor to the incidence of complications. Proper technique and vigilance are of utmost importance in maintaining safety and decreasing the likelihood of complications. Neither the use of minimal access nor technical feasibility is an indication for surgical intervention as all surgical procedures are undertaken for the benefit of the patient.

This chapter is divided into three separate, yet related sections: (1) surgical principles; (2) brief overviews of laparoscopy and hysteroscopy and; (3) a summary of reproductive surgical techniques and their associated fertility outcomes for a variety of conditions that challenge the reproductive surgeon.

SURGICAL PRINCIPLES

Preoperative Evaluation

The preoperative evaluation of all gynecologic patients addresses issues that may potentially affect them during their surgery and recovery and is essential in achieving successful surgical results. The goals of the preoperative evaluation are to decrease surgical morbidity, evaluate and optimize the patient's medical status, assist the planning of anesthesia, reduce patient anxiety and obtain informed consent.[1] To accomplish these goals, the gynecologic surgeon reviews the patient's history and performs a physical examination, gathers information required to plan surgery, optimizes health status and educates the patient about expectations from the procedure and during the recovery period.

A complete history and physical examination are the most critical aspects in the preoperative evaluation of women. These provide the surgeon, a thorough understanding of the gynecologic problem and ultimately lead to a more accurate diagnosis, correct selection of preoperative testing and the most suitable surgical plan to manage the problem. Proper preoperative history taking includes an accurate and detailed menstrual history with special attention to discrepancies between menstrual dates and pelvic findings in a woman of reproductive age (which may warrant a pregnancy test). Reproductive history including previous pregnancies and their complications, marital history, urologic history, endocrine history, gastrointestinal tract history and musculoskeletal history are important to document, as many diseases can mimic symptoms of gynecologic origin. A history of prior abdominal surgery, disease or radiation therapy should be determined, as this history is associated with intra-abdominal adhesions and anatomic alterations that may impact the surgery. A thorough physical examination beyond the lower abdomen and pelvis is also required.

The preoperative laboratory assessment is limited to those tests that could alter surgical outcome based on current evidence from both prospective and retrospective studies. They are selected based on the patient's individual history and physical examination and not a routine panel for all patients.[2]

Educating a woman and her family preoperatively can often prevent postoperative misunderstandings. Obtaining informed consent from the patient ensures that the patient makes a voluntary, educated decision to proceed with a procedure with a good understanding of its rationale, its indications, expected benefits, alternatives and the expected course of the condition without surgical intervention. The discussion also includes possible complications and steps to prevent them, possible need for transfusion of blood products and alternatives to transfusion, potential unexpected findings at surgery and proper documentation of the discussion.[3,4] In cases where the patient refuses to consent to the recommended intervention, the chart should document the explanation for the need for treatment, a description of the consequences of declining it and the reasons for the patient's refusal.[5]

Preoperative Preparation

Once the patient is adequately anesthetized in the operating room, preoperative preparation begins. The pubic or abdominal hair is trimmed, followed by a careful bimanual pelvic exam by the surgeon. The perineum and vagina are then cleansed with a sponge soaked in surgical soap or a povidone-iodine solution, followed by the abdominal preparation. The abdomen is cleansed with a 5-minute scrub using a povidone-iodine solution or with a four-round application of a povidone-iodine gel sponge stick.[6,7]

Microsurgical principles are used with all types of minimally invasive surgery. Microsurgery entails surgery under magnification, thus minimizing peritoneal trauma and/or tissue damage; the goal of this technique is to limit or even prevent the formation of postoperative adhesions.

Tissue damage can be minimized in the following manner:[8]

- Delicately handling tissues
- Limiting the use of electrical/laser energy
- Irrigating the peritoneal cavity with heparinized LR solution, thus providing constant moisture to the serosa and preventing tissue desiccation
- Limiting foreign body exposure
- Ensuring scrupulous hemostasis
- Limiting lateral tissue damage
- Completely removing injured tissue
- Carefully dissecting proper tissue plane cleavage
- Exactly reapproximating tissue planes

- Using magnification with fine microsurgical instruments and suture material to ensure the above principles are adhered to
- Thoroughly irrigating the peritoneal cavity with complete removal of foreign body, blood, and/or debris.

LAPAROSCOPY: AN OVERVIEW

Laparoscopy, with the introduction of high definition technology, provides inherent magnification with its technology. Laparoscopy provides excellent visualization due to camera resolutions of 250,000–380,000 pixels with high-definition flat panel monitors. Clear images are obtained by bringing the camera close to operative field. Other advantages of laparoscopy include elimination of the theoretical introduction of lint by not using sponges and a reduction in venous oozing form pneumoperiteum pressure. By introducing warmed humidified gas for insufflation, desiccation of the peritoneal cavity lining can be also minimized.

The laparoscope is used as an essential diagnostic and therapeutic operative tool. The patient is placed in a supine or dorsal lithotomy position with the patient's legs placed in Allen stirrups. The knees should be deflexed to avoid stretching of the femoral nerve.[9] The buttocks should be a few centimeters beyond the edge of the table to allow uterine manipulation. A bladder catheter is inserted to prevent bladder distention, thereby decreasing the risk of bladder perforation and facilitating visualization of pelvic structures.

Contemporary laparoscopy equipment consists of an imaging system comprising of a telescope (laparoscope) and video camera system, an abdominal insufflation system and specialized surgical instruments. Laparoscopes range in size from 1.8–12 mm in diameter with lenses available in varying viewing angles. Most gynecologic surgeons prefer the 0° lens, as it provides a panoramic view of the pelvis. Angled lenses help in evaluating the anterior abdominal wall or operating around masses. Similar to hysteroscopes, operative laparoscopes are equipped with a central channel that allows laser, electrosurgical or mechanical instruments to be introduced into the abdomen. The abdominopelvic cavity is illuminated with a light source inserted through the laparoscope with a fiberoptic cable.

Insufflation systems expand the abdominopelvic cavity with gas to optimize visualization. Insufflation may be achieved with a Veres needle or the Hassan trocar, filtered tubing, an insufflator and gas tanks. Insufflation tubing with a 0.3-micron filter is recommended to prevent intraperitoneal contamination with bacteria, microparticles and debris from the insufflator and gas tank.[8]

A Veres needle, direct trocar insertion and open laparoscopy are used to create a pneumoperitoneum. Most gynecologic surgeons use carbon dioxide, as it is rapidly absorbed by blood. Because carbon dioxide causes pain upon conversion to carbonic acid, some surgeons prefer using nitrous oxide or helium. Other surgeons use heated or hydrated gas to avoid hypothermia during laparoscopy.[10]

Trocars and sleeves are important to puncture the abdominal wall for placement of the laparoscope and surgical instruments. Trocar sleeves range from 2–15 mm in diameter and are available as reusable and disposable systems. Uterine manipulators or cannula modify the position of the uterus to improve visualization of and access to pelvic structures. The use of uterine cannulas is contraindicated in the event that a patient has no uterus, has anatomic distortions that prevent visualization of the cervix, is a prepubescent female, or an intrauterine pregnancy is suspected. A sponge stick or examining hand may be positioned in the vagina in the absence of the uterus or if pregnant.

Grasping forceps are used to manipulate tissue and come in a variety of types with different specializations. There are broad, flat forceps and finer forceps used to handle more delicate tissue. Toothed forceps apply traction on tissue, such as ovarian cysts or leiomyomas that need to be removed. Forceps with pointed ends are used for tissue dissection and surgical plane development. A disposable Babcock-type atraumatic grasper with a ratcheted scissors handle is useful in handling adnexal structures.

Many devices have been created to facilitate laparoscopic suturing and stapling. Laparoscopic suturing uses stock suture, which is usually 36–48 inches in length. Needle drivers are used to drive needles through tissue, and knots may be tied outside the laparoscopic port (extracorporeal knot) or within the body (intracorporeal knot). The prettied loop is the simplest laparoscopic ligature to tie. The Roeder loop can also be applied using standard suture. To simplify laparoscopic suturing, the endoswitch instrument is used, which uses a preloaded needle and passes suture through tissue up to 2 cm thick by closing a handle and a toggle switch. The endo-GIA is used as a stapling device for securing and dividing tissue by laying 6 staggered rows of staples, 3 cm in length and 1 cm in width.

Special instruments have been designed to achieve hemostasis while preventing thermal damage. Endoscopic vascular clips and the harmonic scalpel, for example, are safe to use near vital structures. The harmonic scalpel uses vibration at the rate of 55,000 cycles per second as an energy source to break hydrogen bonds in tissue, resulting in cutting or coagulation of vessels. Monopolar and bipolar electrosurgical instruments can also be used to obtain hemostasis.

Suction and irrigation are essential for all types of laparoscopic surgery. Irrigation is important to remove debris, visualize a bleeding source and to dissect and create tissue planes (hydrodissection). Many types of suction instruments have been designed that are adequate for removal of irrigation fluid or intraperitoneal air and smoke. A large-bore device is best for removal of blood clots when brisk bleeding is encountered and also for passing laser fiber.

Tissue morcellators are used to reduce large masses into smaller fragments to assist with tissue removal. Manual and automatic morcellators can be used. Automatic morcellators are more effective and time-efficient in removing large amounts of tissue but are more expensive than manual morcellators. To facilitate tissue removal, tissue dilators are used for stretching a 10 mm port to a 20 mm port. Furthermore, a corkscrew device can be screwed into leiomyomas to remove them through a colpotomy incision or through a mini-laparotomy incision.

HYSTEROSCOPY: AN OVERVIEW

A hysteroscope is a telescope that is inserted through the vagina and cervix and into the uterus to visualize the endometrial cavity, as well as the tubal ostia, endocervical canal, cervix and vagina. Operative hysteroscopes are used to remove endocervical or endometrial lesions or to perform an endometrial ablation or resection. Some operative hysteroscopes use electrocautery; lasers are rarely used in modern hysteroscopic procedures. The three types of operative hysteroscopes are operative sheath with instruments inserted through channels or fixed to the sheath, electrocautery resectoscope and hysteroscopic morcellator. Diagnostic hysteroscopes allow direct visual observation and accurate localization of pathology; hysteroscopic scissors, biopsy forceps and graspers can be passed through the diagnostic hysteroscope as a means to sample the area to obtain the most accurate results.

There are many different sizes and types of hysteroscopes. Most hysteroscopes are rigid, but scopes less than 5 mm in caliber may also be semi-rigid or flexible. Rigid hysteroscopes include an outer sheath which enables space for the telescope, distending media and operative tools. Rigid hysteroscopes offer superior optical quality and cost effectiveness than flexible ones, but they may cause more intraoperative pain. Flexible hysteroscopes are particularly useful for diagnostic or operative procedures in women with an irregularly shaped uterus, as the distal tip can be deflected upward or downward. A light source is introduced through the hysteroscope by a fiberoptic cable which allows transmission of bright light without the transmission of significant heat.

Hysteroscopy is performed using a distending medium to provide a global view of the endometrial cavity. The most commonly used distending media are low viscosity fluids and carbon dioxide. The low viscosity fluids include electrolyte-rich media and electrolyte-poor media. The electrolyte-containing media include the isotonic fluids, normal saline and lactated Ringer's solution and are used in bipolar electrosurgical procedures and with mechanical and laser energy. This prevents imbalances in electrolytes and osmolarity associated with nonconductive solutions. Isotonic fluids cannot be used with monopolar electrocautery because they conduct electric current. The electrolyte-poor media are 5% dextrose, 1.5% glycine, 3% sorbitol and 5% mannitol and are used with monopolar energy systems. For operative procedures that use monopolar electrosurgical instruments, a nonconductive fluid is required to avoid thermal injury. While diagnostic procedures can be performed using either carbon dioxide or normal saline, normal saline is associated with decreased pain, increased satisfaction, better visualization and decreased operative time.[11,12]

TREATMENT OF SPECIFIC REPRODUCTIVE DISORDERS AS APPLIED TO FERTILITY

DISORDERS OF THE UTERUS

Uterine Myomas

Advances in medicine have provided numerous conservative options for the management of symptomatic uterine myomas. Myomectomy, however, remains the standard therapy for women desiring fertility and/or uterine conservation.

Evidence of a cause-and-effect relationship between fibroids and subfertility is lacking. Therefore, in patients with infertility and myomas, the entire fertility investigation should be completed [including a hysterosalpingogram (HSG), a study of ovarian reserve levels of anti-Müllerian hormone (AMH) and early follicular follicle stimulating hormone (FSH) and estradiol and a semen analysis], in order to exclude other contributing causes for their infertility. In the presence of decreased ovarian reserve, the postoperative fertility results are poor. In these women, the preoperative and postoperative treatment strategy of IVF with autologous or donated eggs should be carefully discussed.

Multiple mechanisms by which myomas may affect fertility have been proposed. These mechanisms include: (1) interference with sperm transport or access by anatomic distortion of the cervix; (2) deforming the endometrial cavity which may impact implantation and/or alter normal endometrial development; (3) altering uterine contractility and; (4) obstructing the tubal ostia.[13,14]

Preoperative detection and evaluation of myomas should be particularly meticulous, as this assessment dictates the appropriate route of surgical intervention. The preoperative evaluation must include an abdominal and transvaginal ultrasonography, and/or abdominal/pelvic MRI to better characterize the number, size and location of each myoma. The uterine cavity can be further evaluated with the use of hysterosonography, thus determining the extent of submucosal or endometrial cavity involvement.

Difficulties with laparoscopic myomectomy increase with myoma size. While the upper size limit that can be safely removed with the laparoscopic technique is controversial, surgical feasibility is mostly dependent on the characteristics of the myomas (i.e. location, depth of penetration) and the patient (i.e. bodymass index, pelvic adhesions and prior pelvic surgeries). Subserosal and intramural myomas are indications for elective operative laparoscopy. Although the ablation of an entirely submucous myoma must be performed by operative hysteroscopy when its diameter is less than 4–5 cm, cases of deep intramural myoma with a submucosal component are difficult to treat hysteroscopically, and may require repeat procedures. Medium sized (4–7 cm) myomas involving the uterine cavity can be easily treated with a laparoscopic or open approach. Those myomas that are completely transmural (submucous myoma reaching the serosa) should also be treated by laparoscopy or an open procedure. Myomas situated in the broad ligament or at the uterine isthmus can also be treated by operative laparoscopy or laparotomy.

Laparoscopy Versus Laparotomy

Multiple studies comparing laparoscopic myomectomy with abdominal myomectomy have been published. The first prospective randomized study comparing these two approaches was published by Mais et al. in 1996.[15] Forty patients were equally divided between surgical approaches. Compared to abdominal myomectomy, laparoscopic myomectomy provided less postoperative pain and a shorter recovery time.

A few years later, Seracchioli et al.[16] published a study where 131 patients were randomly assigned to laparotomy or laparoscopic myomectomy. All patients had at least one intramural myoma measuring 5 cm in mean diameter and both groups were comparable across most clinical parameters. The incidence of postoperative fever and a drop in hemoglobin level was greater and more pronounced in the laparotomy group. The duration of hospital stay was significantly shorter in the laparoscopic group. No significant difference was noted between groups with regards to pregnancy outcome. No cases of uterine rupture were observed in either group.

Surgical Technique

Prior to the start of a laparoscopic myomectomy, many surgeons advocate the instillation of a dilute dye (either indigo carmine or methylene blue) into the endometrial cavity. According to Dubuisson et al.[17] staining the endometrium provides a boundary for removing myomas close to the endometrial cavity and allows for optimal closure of the myometrium, preventing inadvertent closure of/entry into the cavity. A uterine manipulator should also be inserted into the endometrial cavity to provide a means to better access of the myomas.

Successful and safe laparoscopic myomectomy depends upon the proper positioning of the operative trocars. Trocar placement is dependent upon, other variables, the size of the uterus, the number, location and size of the myomas. A general rule is to place one trocar approximately 3 cm above the uterine fundus (10 mm), one 5 mm trocar in left lower quadrant and a third 5 mm trocar in the right lower quadrant. Placement of trocars in this fashion allows for quick and easy operation of the operative forceps.[18]

Instrumentation is variable amongst surgeons but the principles integral to the successful completion of a laparoscopic myomectomy remain similar. The four principle steps of a myomectomy include hysterotomy, enucleation, suture of the myomectomy site and extraction of the myoma from the surgical field.[19]

The initial incision into the uterus or hysterotomy must be strategically placed as the remainder of the surgery is dependent on its location. Either a longitudinal or a transverse hysterotomy can be made (Figure 1).

Many surgeons advocate a transverse incision as the arteries and arterioles within the myometrium run in a transverse direction. Dilute vasopressin can also be used prior to hysterotomy to improve hemostasis during the procedure. Enucleation involves firmly grasping the myoma and resecting it from its capsule using scissors or an energy source (Figure 2).

The myometrial defect can either be repaired with continuous or interrupted suture/knots, tied either

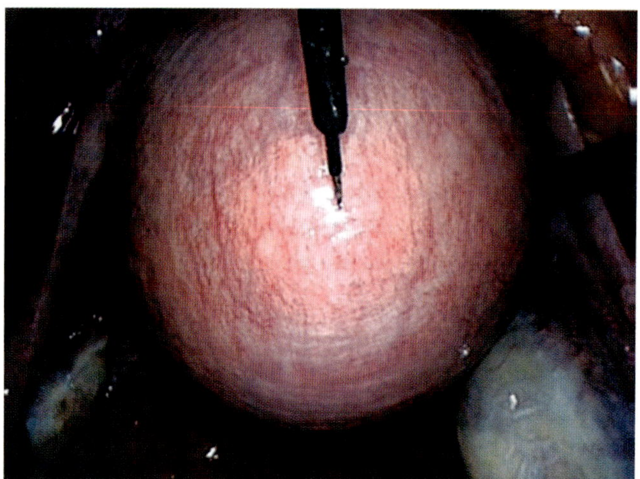

Figure 1 Vertical incision across posterior intramural myoma

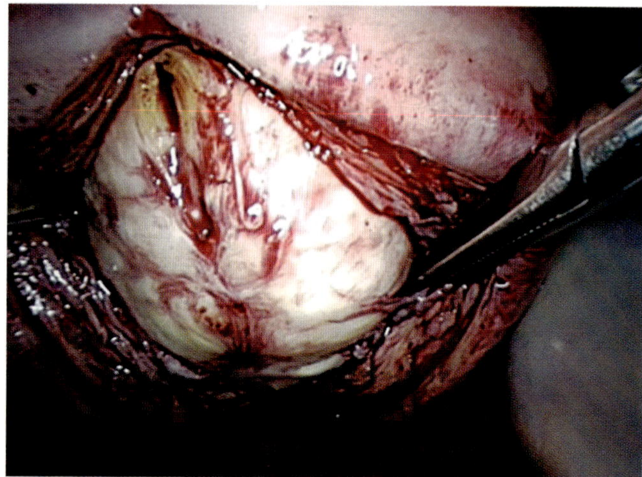

Figure 2 Enucleation of myoma

intracorporally or extracorporally. In addition, the defect is closed in either multiple or single layers depending on the size of the defect. Once the defects are repaired, the surgical specimens must then be removed. While a posterior culdotomy incision was the classic method to remove surgical specimens, a laparoscopic tissue morcellator is now used to remove cylinders of tissue in a systematic manner.

Fertility

The role of surgical procedures in the infertile woman has been heavily debated.[20] When women with subserosal fibroids have been examined in comparison with women without fibroids, no difference is observed for any outcome measure. Women with intramural fibroids appear to have significantly lower clinical pregnancy rate [relative risk (RR) 0.81, 95% CI 0.70–0.94], implantation rate (RR 0.68, 95% CI 0.59–0.80), and ongoing pregnancy/live birth rate (RR 0.70, 95% CI 0.58–0.85) and significantly higher spontaneous abortion (SAB) rate (RR 1.75, 95% CI 1.23–2.49) compared to women without fibroids. However, when the analysis is limited to studies using a hysteroscopy to assess the uterine cavity in all subjects, only the difference in implantation rate remains statistically significant (clinical pregnancy rate RR 0.85, 95% CI 0.67–1.07; implantation rate RR 0.71, 95% CI 0.55–0.93).

If fibroid removal is beneficial, myomectomy subjects would be expected to have higher pregnancy rate and lower abortion rate than those with fibroids in place. However, in a recent meta-analysis,[20] clinical pregnancy (RR 3.77, 95% CI 0.47–30.14), ongoing pregnancy/livebirth rate (RR 1.67, 95% CI 0.75–3.72) and miscarriage rate (RR 0.76, 95% CI 0.30–1.94) are not better in those individuals who underwent myomectomy for an intramural fibroid compared to those that were expectantly managed. Intramural fibroids (> 4 cm in mean diameter) that encroach the uterine cavity appear to decrease fertility, however the benefit of surgical intervention even for these large lesions at this time is unclear.[21] Therefore, no conclusive evidence currently exists for a beneficial effect on fertility of surgical intervention for intramural or subserous fibroids.

Reproductive outcomes are similar between laparoscopic and abdominal myomectomies.[22] Subserosal fibroids do not affect fertility outcomes, and removal does not confer benefit.[23-25] The main concern surrounding pregnancy following a laparoscopic myomectomy is the risk of uterine rupture. Although multiple case reports have reported incidences of uterine rupture in the third trimester, prior to the onset of labor or entirely unremarkable (i.e. safe) pregnancies, the true risk of uterine rupture following either surgical technique is unknown as elective cesarean sections are often performed.[26,27]

The underlying cause for uterine rupture has been thought to be secondary to inadequate or absent suturing of the myometrial defect after enucleation of a myoma. Given the difficulty in suturing laparoscopically, many speculated that laparoscopic myomectomy would increase the likelihood of uterine rupture. Thus far, the body of published evidence suggests that the risk of uterine rupture following laparoscopic myomectomy is no worse than the approach with laparotomy.[27-29] Regardless of the approach, it is recommended that patients delay attempts at conception for 6 months after having an open or laparoscopic myomectomy.

Hysteroscopy

Operative hysteroscopy is the surgical treatment of choice for submucosal myomas. The proper preoperative assessment of submucosal myomas is essential for performing a safe and complete performance of a hysteroscopic myomectomy. A sonohysterogram or 3D sonogram can be used to evaluate the degree of endometrial cavity involvement and depth of myometrial penetration.

Surgical Technique

An operative hysteroscope is used in conjunction with a fluid management apparatus. Operative hysteroscopy requires distention of the uterine cavity with fluid media; the instillation of media also provides for better visualization of the cavity as it continuously irrigates the operative field.

Resection of a submucosal myoma (Figures 3 and 4) can be used with monopolar current in a cutting loop using mannitol or sorbitol as distention media or with a bipolar cutting loop (Versapoint) using normal saline as the distention media. Both methods use the same operative technique. The Versapoint system has the added advantage of decreasing the risk of fluid-associated complications.

Once an appropriate balance of irrigation inflow and outflow (suction) has been achieved, the uterine cavity will distend. Maintaining an adequate flow of media will provide continuous irrigation of the operative field by removing blood and debris. Resection begins at the apex of the myoma and progresses longitudinally along the length of the myoma. Resection is continued until the myometrium is visualized. During the resection, it is imperative that the loop electrode is activated only while withdrawing the loop, thus decreasing the risk of uterine perforation and visceral injury. In addition, the net fluid deficit should be monitored at all times with the operative procedure being terminated if fluid deficits reach approximately 1,000 cc of nonelectrolyte solution or 2,500 cc of normal saline.[30] The procedure should be terminated if visualization is suboptimal given the increased risk of uterine perforation.

Fertility

The first evaluation of a series of 60 women undergoing hysteroscopic myomectomy was published in1990.[31] Of the 60 women, 24 desired pregnancy and had no other identifiable cause for infertility. Sixteen (66%) women became pregnant during the first 8 months after the return of regular menstruation. No miscarriages or premature labor occurred in these women; one cesarean section was necessary because of fetal distress.

Fertility outcomes for women undergoing surgical intervention for submucosal myomas are contradictory. Hysteroscopic submucosal myomectomy has proven capable of increasing fertility rate in some studies, although this statement may not apply to type 2 submucous myomas.[21] Review of current evidence by a recent meta-analysis suggests that fertility outcomes are decreased in women with submucosal fibroids (RR for clinical pregnancy 0.363; 95% CI 0.18–0.74), and removal may confer benefits.[20] Compared to those patients that were expectantly managed, those patients with submucosal fibroids who underwent myomectomy had higher clinical pregnancy rate (RR for clinical pregnancy 2.03, 95% CI 1.08–3.83), but all other reproductive outcomes (ongoing pregnancy/live birth rate and miscarriage rate) were not significantly better (RR for ongoing pregnancy/livebirth rate 2.65, 95% CI 0.92–7.66; RR for SAB 0.77, 95% CI 0.36–1.66). Many concerns have been raised about resecting large endometrial surface areas when

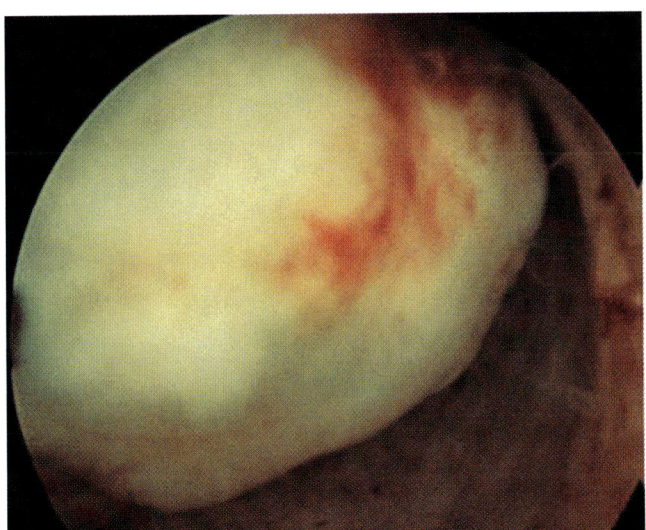

Figure 3 Hysteroscopic visualization of a submucosal myoma

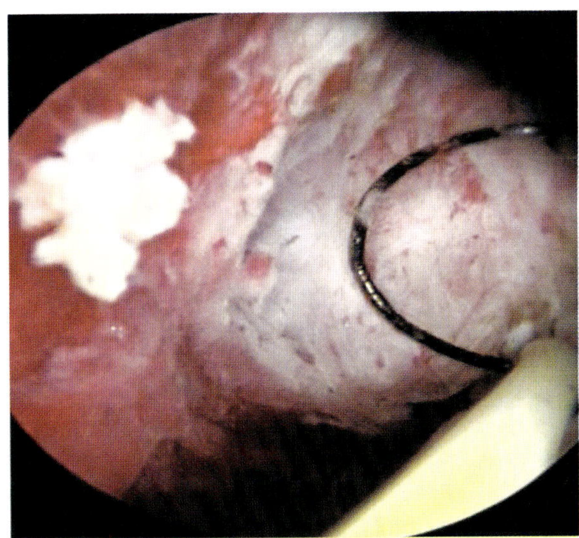

Figure 4 Resection of a submucosal myoma with a resectoscope

managing submucosal myomas. However, one study has shown that hysteroscopic myomectomy[32] appears to enhance fertility despite resection of a large filling defect.

Endometrial Polyps

Operative hysteroscopy (Figures 5 and 6) is the surgical treatment of choice for endometrial polyps. A sonohysterogram or 3D sonogram can be used to evaluate the number and size of each endometrial polyp.

Surgical Technique

A slender rigid hysteroscope with channels for instrument insertion or an operative hysteroscope can be used to remove polyps. Often times, normal saline can be used with hysteroscopic scissors for removal of polyps. Otherwise, resection of an endometrial polyp can be performed with a cutting loop using monopolar current, using mannitol or sorbitol as distention media or with a bipolar cutting loop (Versapoint) using normal saline as the distention media. Using the slender hysteroscope with scissors is the method of choice and has the added advantage of decreasing the risk of fluid-associated complications. Regardless of the method chosen, each endometrial polyp should be excised from its base thus leaving a smooth contour to the endometrial cavity. On occasion, thickened and polypoid-like endometrium can be smoothened with a vacuum suction device; this provides a means of removing the most superficial aspect of the endometrial lining and reduces the chance of developing intrauterine synechiae as no sharp curettage is performed.

Fertility

Multiple studies have been attempted to characterize the impact of endometrial polyps on fertility. In one large study of 215 patients with otherwise unexplained infertility, patients were randomly allocated to one of two pretreatment groups with hysteroscopic polypectomyperformed in the study group while diagnostic hysteroscopy was being performed in the control group.[33] The total pregnancy rate and time for success in both groups after four intrauterine insemination (IUI) cycles were compared by means of contingency tables and life-table analysis. A total of 93 pregnancies occurred, 64 in the study group and 29 in the control group. Women in the study group had a better possibility of becoming pregnant after polypectomy with a RR of 2.1 (95% confidence interval 1.5–2.9). Pregnancies in the study group were obtained before the first IUI in 65% of the cases. These findings suggest that hysteroscopic polypectomy before IUI might be an effective measure. Others have noted an increase, albeit statistically nonsignificant, in spontaneous pregnancy and delivery rate in women with unexplained infertility, after hysteroscopic polypectomy. In one such study, no difference was noted between rate for polyps less than 1 cm or more than 1 cm in size.[34] While in contrast, a meta-analysis of randomized controlled trials suggested that hysteroscopic removal of endometrial polyps with a mean diameter of more than 15 mm detected by ultrasound doubles the pregnancy rate when compared with diagnostic hysteroscopy and polyp biopsy in patients undergoing IUI, starting 3 months after the surgical intervention [RR = 2.3; 95% confidence interval (CI): 1.6–3.2].[35]

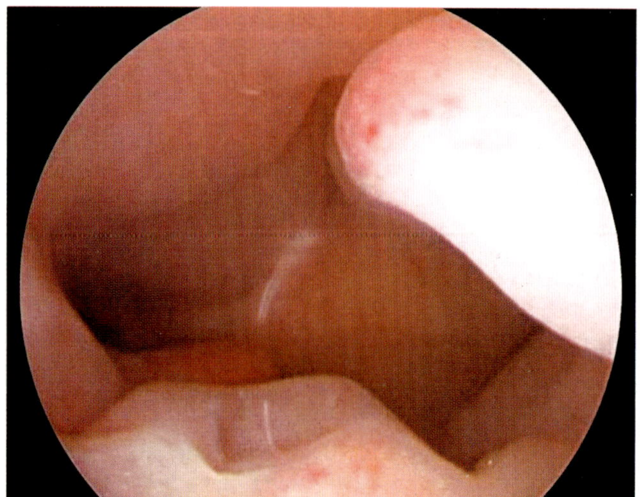

Figure 5 Hysteroscopic appearance of multiple polyps

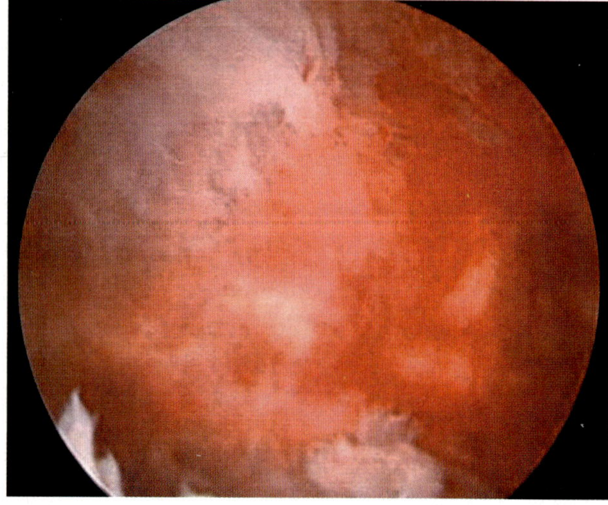

Figure 6 Hysteroscopic appearance of cavity after vacuum curettage of endometrial polyps

Intrauterine Synechiae

Intrauterine adhesions have been related to recurrent pregnancy loss, infertility and menstrual disorders, such as hypomenorrhea or amenorrhea. In 1948, Asherman described 'amenorrhea traumatica' as amenorrhea secondary to intrauterine adhesions, following curettage for incomplete or missed abortion and postpartum hemorrhage.[36] Findings of intrauterine adhesions in the setting of associated symptoms is thus termed 'Asherman Syndrome'.

Infection (endometritis) rarely causes adhesions, except in cases of severe pelvic inflammatory disease (PID) or tuberculous endometritis. The vast majority (> 90%) of intrauterine adhesions develop after curettage.[37] The most important factor in the development of intrauterine adhesions is traumatic curettage or manipulation of the endometrium during the postpartum or postabortal period. Denudation of the basalis layer and exposure of the muscularis layer produce adhesions by coaptation of the opposing uterine walls.

Diagnosis

Intrauterine synechiae should be suspected in amenorrheic women with abiphasic basal body temperature curve and no withdrawal bleed from a progestin challenge and/or estrogen/progestin challenge, especially in the setting of a past history of a postpartum or postabortal curettage. Hysterosalpingography (Figure 7) or sonohysterography can be used as accurate screening methods in the diagnosis of intrauterine adhesions.

Adhesions are suggested by radiographic filling defects. Hysteroscopyconfirms the presence of intrauterine adhesions and allows definitive surgical treatment.

The American Fertility Society (AFS) has proposed a classification of intrauterine adhesions based on findings upon hysterosalpingography and hysteroscopy and correlation with menstrual patterns. The AFS classifications of adnexal adhesions, distal tubal occlusion, tubal occlusion secondary to tubal ligation, tubal pregnancies, Müllerian anomalies and intrauterine adhesion are three stages of disease: stage I (mild), stage II (moderate) and stage III (severe). The stage of disease is determined by the extent of the endometrial cavity involved (adhesions throughout the uterus or just in a small area), the type of adhesions (filmy or dense) and the menstrual pattern.

Surgical Technique

Blind transection of intrauterine adhesions by dilatation does not provide accurate and precise treatment. Hysteroscopy remains the standard operative approach for the treatment of intrauterine synechiae. Thin or filmy endometrial adhesions are often easily transected by atraumatically pushing with the tip of the hysteroscopic sheath. Dense adhesions require lysis (Figure 9). The surgical treatment of intrauterine adhesions consists of dividing the adhesions mechanically with hysteroscopic scissors, or using electrosurgery and/or fiberoptic lasers. The gynecological resectoscope with a modified knife electrode has been used to divide adhesions electrosurgically. Fiberoptic lasers, such as the argon, krypton (KTP)/532, and neodymium: yttrium-aluminum-garnet (Nd : YAG) laser with sculpted or extruded fibers have also been used.

Regardless of the technique employed, the goal of surgery remains the same: to recreate the normal endometrial cavity appearance and volume. Adhesions should

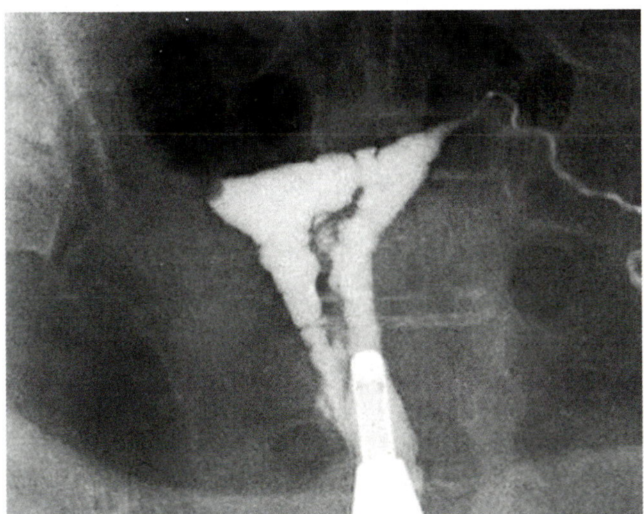

Figure 7 Hysterosalpingogram (HSG) of intrauterine synechiae

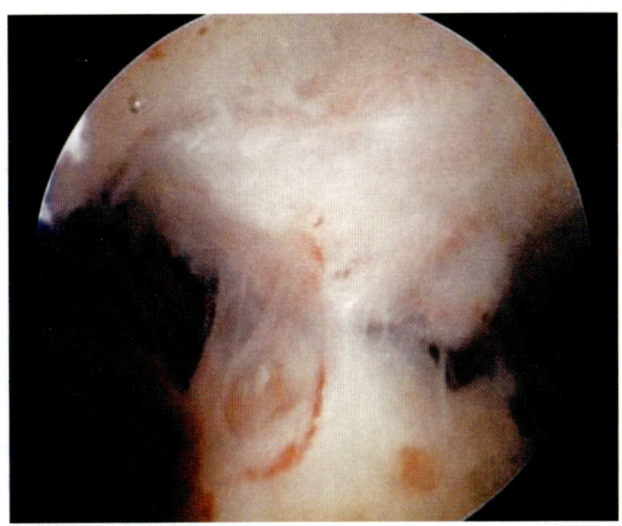

Figure 8 Midline intrauterine synechiae

be transected in the middle, in an area equidistant from anterior and posterior walls. In the manner, the already damaged endometrium will not be further traumatized. The remaining anterior and posterior adhesion 'stumps' retract and the uterine cavity distends, providing a panoramic view. Adhesions located at the lateral margins of the endometrial cavity may be difficult to divide, especially if the adhesions are fibromuscular or composed of connective tissue. For uterine adhesions obliterating the entire endometrial cavity, the procedure should be performed with intraoperative transabdominal ultrasound. Hysteroscopic assessment of the uterine cavity should begin at the internal cervical os with adhesiolysis being performed at that location, if indicated. As adhesions are divided and the uterine cavity begins to open, the hysteroscope is advanced to the fundus so that both tubal ostia can be visualized. Occasionally, increasing the inflow pressure of the distention media can further facilitate the adhesiolysis by distending the uterine cavity. However, although theplane of dissection is better exposed, increasing the inflow pressure can lead to excessive fluid intravasation if prolonged. For this reason, the use of hysteroscopic scissors with normal saline as distention media is optimal.

Postoperative Care

Once the synechiae have been resected, placing an intrauterine balloon to prevent apposition of the endometrial surfaces for 3–5 days is advisable to prevent a recurrence of adhesions. The patient should receive prophylactic antibiotics and uterine relaxants (e.g. ibuprofen) during these 3–5 days to prevent infection and balloon expulsion, respectively. The patient should be prescribed high-dose estradiol (2 mg qd for 21 d) followed by medroxyprogesterone (10 mg qd for 10 d). A postoperative sonohysterogram should be performed 1–2 months later. In many instances, more than one hysteroscopy is required for total resection of dense intrauterine synechiae.

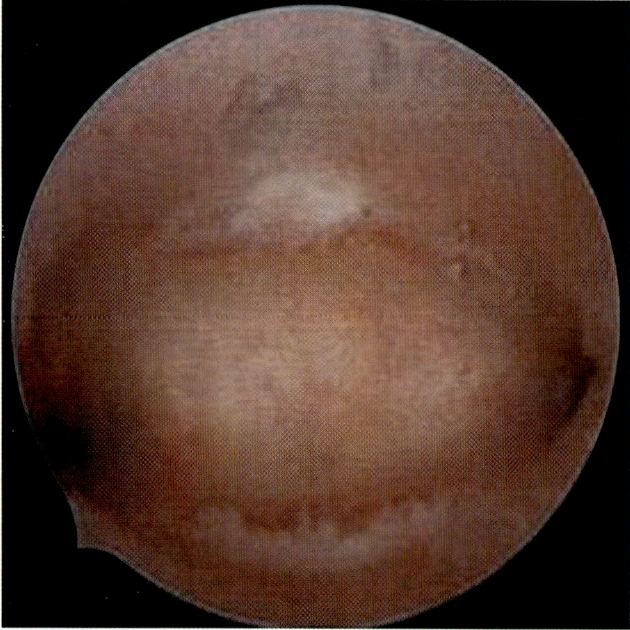

Figure 9 Endometrial cavity after lysis of adhesions

Fertility

Randomized controlled studies on hysteroscopic treatment of intrauterine adhesions are lacking. Multiple series have suggested success rate for correction of menstrual disorders and/or pregnancy of 74–94%.[38] While the results appear reassuring, it is very difficult to compare these series because the results have neither been evaluated according to severity of adhesive disease nor have been assessed according to comparable outcomes.

Uterine Septum

A septate uterus is the most common Müllerian fusion defect with an estimated incidence in the general population of 1.8%.[39] This anomaly results from a failure of lateral fusion of the two Müllerian ducts, a condition which may be obstructive or nonobstructive. Failure of fusion of the Müllerian ducts occurs to varying degrees, as partial (Figures 10 and 11) or complete (Figures 12 and 13).

Surgical Technique

Hysteroscopy remains the standard operative approach for the treatment of both partial and complete uterine septate (Figures 14 and 15). Various instruments, including hysteroscopic scissors, resectoscope or lasers can be used for resection of the septum. In many cases, hysteroscopic scissors provide enough pressure to resect uterine septate. Regardless of the technique employed, the goal of surgery remains the same: to recreate the normal endometrial cavity appearance and volume. The uterine septum should be transected in the middle, in an area equidistant from anterior and posterior walls. In the manner, the cut edges of the septum will retract in both the anterior and posterior directions. In addition, the surgeon should always be able to visualize the right and left cornual regions or tubal ostia completely, and keep the septum in view at all times. Concurrent laparoscopy or transabdominal sonography at the time of hysteroscopic resection is recommended to reduce the likelihood of uterine perforation and to determine if further resection is indicated. Intraoperative transabdominal sonography is the preferred approach as this avoids an invasive laparoscopic procedure and improves recovery time. The procedure should be stopped when

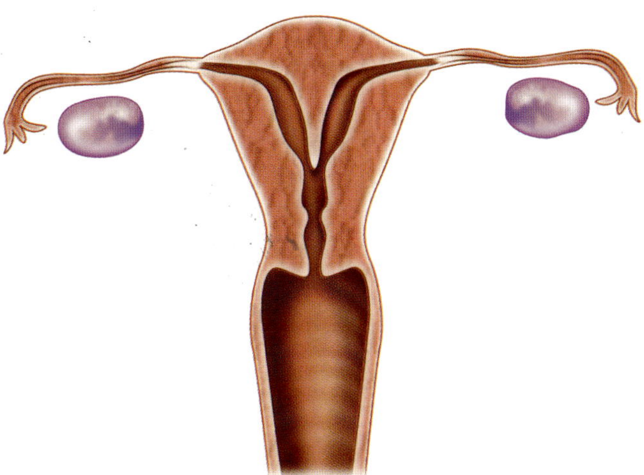

Figure 10 Schematic depiction of a partial uterine septum

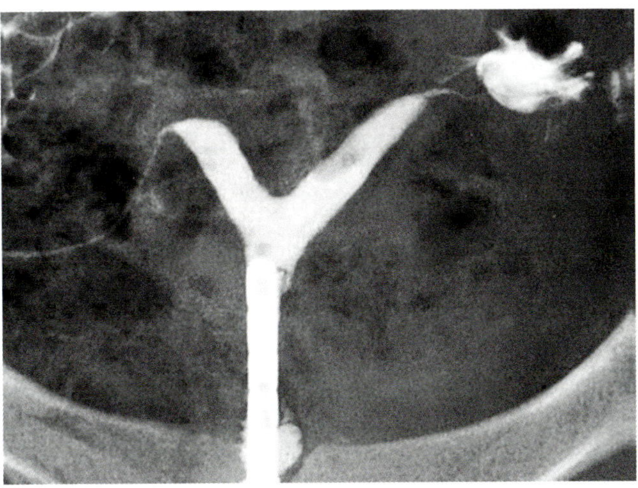

Figure 11 Partial uterine septum as noted with hysterosalpingogram (HSG)

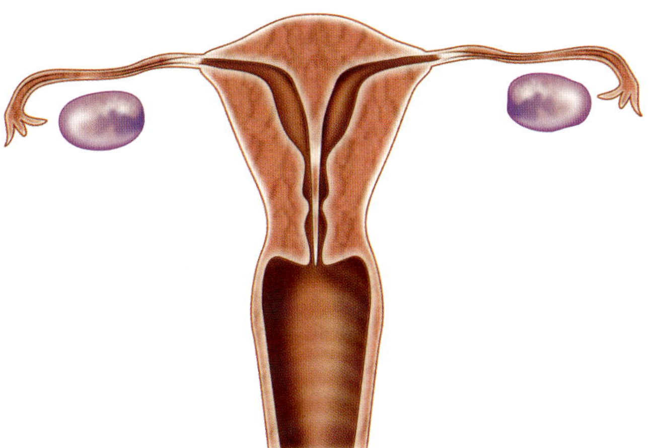

Figure 12 Schematic depiction of a complete uterine septum

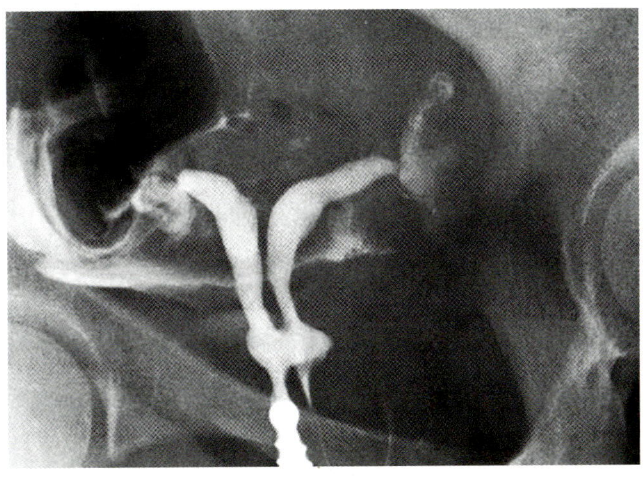

Figure 13 Complete uterine septum as noted with hysterosalpingogram (HSG)

the area between the tubal ostia is a straight line, where the location of both tubal ostia is symmetrical. Having a residual septum of less than 1 cm after hysteroscopic metroplasty does not impair reproductive outcome and therefore does not require a repeat surgical procedure.[40] Because the septum is poorly vascularized, bleeding is usually minimal with this procedure.

Postoperative Management

Multiple techniques for reducing the likelihood of intrauterine synechiae have been proposed. These include the insertion of an intrauterine devices, insertion of a pediatric Foley catheter, hormone supplementation with a 2–3 week course of high dose estrogen (Estrace 2 mg qd for 14–21 days) followed by a progestin withdrawal (Provera 10 mg qd for 10 days), repeat office hysteroscopy at 1 month intervals to lyse adhesions or expectant management.[41-43] Almost all agree that a follow-up examination with a sonohysterogram or office hysteroscopy should be performed 1–2 months after the operation, irrespective of the postoperative management to assess the integrity of the endometrial cavity.

Fertility

It is not clear why uterine anomalies are associated with reproductive failure. According to histological observations, the septum has been described as 'fibroelastic tissue'[44] that can have defective endometrial development indicating reduced sensitivity to steroid hormones. Another hypothesis that could explain reproductive

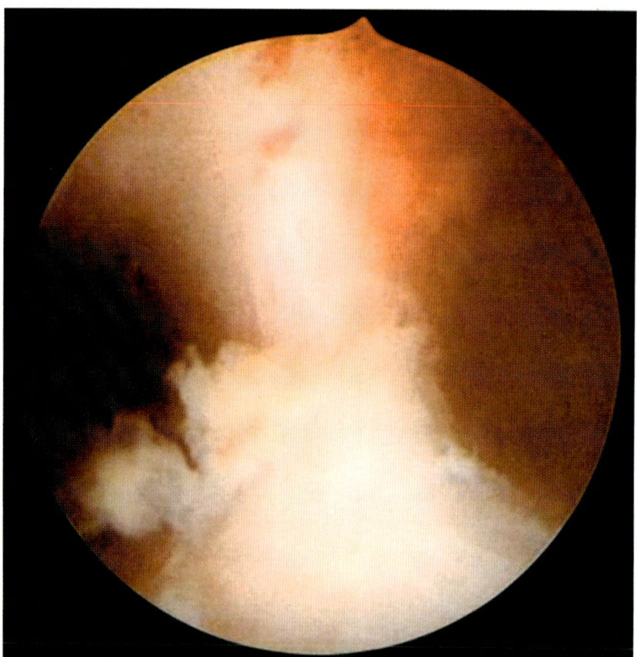

Figure 14 Partial uterine septum before septoplasty

Figure 15 Endometrial cavity after septoplasty

failure is that spontaneous miscarriage may be the result of a poor blood supply to the septum, leading to poor implantation dynamics.[45]

In a literature review, Homer et al. reported data from several series that compared the outcomes of pregnancies before and after hysteroscopic metroplasty in patients with a septate uterus. The miscarriage rate, preterm delivery rate and term delivery rate were 88%, 9% and 3%, respectively, before surgery, and 14%, 6% and 80% after hysteroscopic metroplasty.[46] Several others have corroborated these results of significantly reducing the rate of pregnancy wastage and increasing livebirth rate.[47-49]

DISORDERS OF THE PELVIC PERITONEUM AND OVARY (ENDOMETRIOSIS)

Endometriosis is a benign gynecological disease defined by the presence of endometrial glands and stroma out of the uterine cavity (Figure 16).

The disease exhibits a wide spectrum of clinical symptoms, such as pelvic pain and infertility and has a tendency to progress and recur.

While complete resolution of endometriosis is not possible, therapy has the three main objectives of reducing pain, improving the likelihood of pregnancy and to delay recurrence. Medical and/or surgical therapy can be proposed for endometriosis. However, the efficacy of medical and surgical treatment of endometriosis-associated infertility and pelvic pain continues to be a source of debate and controversy. Surgical intervention and outcome is discussed here while the broad topic of endometriosis is covered in another chapter of this textbook.

Surgical Technique

Three different laparoscopic techniques exist for the surgical management of endometriosis: laser vaporization, excision and coagulation.

Laser Vaporization

A CO_2 laser with a power setting of 40–50W is used to vaporize peritoneal endometriosis. In this manner, endometriosis can be effectively 'debulked'. If a lesion is overlying a vital structure (i.e. ureter, bladder, small or large bowel or blood vessels), retroperitoneal injection of fluid or hydrodissection can provide an extra tissue layer for attempts at vaporization of the lesions. Hydrodissection allows a 100–200 μm depth of vaporization, thus substantially limiting the depth of laser penetration. The endometriotic implant is considered vaporized when bubbling of old blood or peritoneal fat is noted.

Excision

Another technique for removal of peritoneal endometriosis is excision with scissors. The lesion is grasped with forceps and then, using scissors, the peritoneum and endometriotic lesion are excised and removed from the pelvis. Care is taken to remove all the lesions in their entirety and to have wide borders between the lesions and normal peritoneum. Major disadvantages of this technique include possible excessive removal of normal peritoneum and possible development of postoperative adhesions. In general, the risk of adhesion development is higher with excisional therapy than with laser vaporization.

Coagulation

Coagulation with bipolar forceps is another technique for surgically treating endometriosis. This technique is infrequently used due to the observation that thermal damage appears to be greater with CO_2 laser and the uncertainty of complete lesion destruction, theoretically increasing the risk of recurrent disease.

Data regarding the superiority of one technique over another are scant as direct comparisons between techniques have not been investigated.

The optimal surgical intervention for endometriomas is controversial as some advocate wedge resection while others recommend cyst stripping (Figures 17 to 19) or cyst drainage with and without ablation of the internal cyst wall. In general, drainage without ablation results in a higher reoperation rate compared to cystectomy.[50] While, in theory, drainage and ablation of an endometrioma may preserve more functional ovarian tissue, studies of ovarian response to gonadotropins after cystectomy have countered that theory.[51,52] The recurrence risk of endometriomas after cystectomy is 7%.[53]

Removal of an endometrioma is initiated by longitudinally incising the ovarian cortex overlying the cyst. An attempt is made to have the incision located opposite to the ovarian hilus so that healthy ovary can appose the tubal fimbria. The cyst contents are then drained with a suction cannula and the cyst cavity is irrigated. After inspecting the cavity, the normal ovarian cortex is stabilized with atraumatic graspers and the edge of the cyst wall is firmly held and stripped from the underlying normal tissue. Hydrodissection can be used to better separate the cyst wall from normal ovarian tissue. Residual cyst tissue can be fulgurated. The ovarian defect is left to seal and heal spontaneously (Figures 17 to 19).

Fertility

In infertile women presenting with minimal or mild endometriosis (AFS classification), laparoscopic 'destruction' was initially thought to be the first line of therapy.[54] In a study by Marcoux, 341 women with unexplained infertility underwent diagnostic laparoscopy with findings of

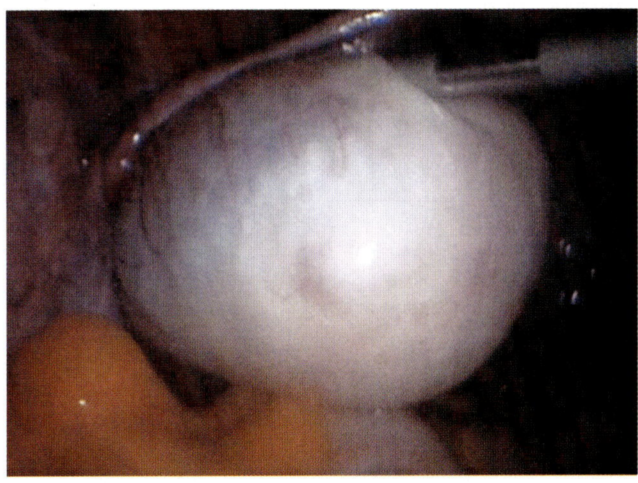

Figure 17 Laparoscopic appearance of a left-sided endometrioma

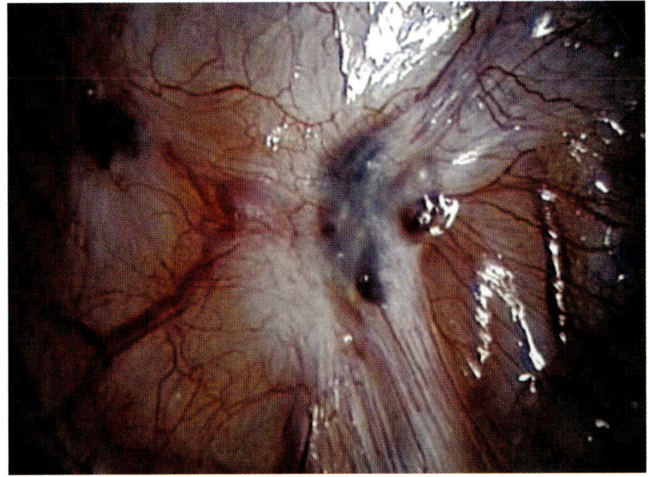

Figure 16 Laparoscopic appearance of black endometriotic foci

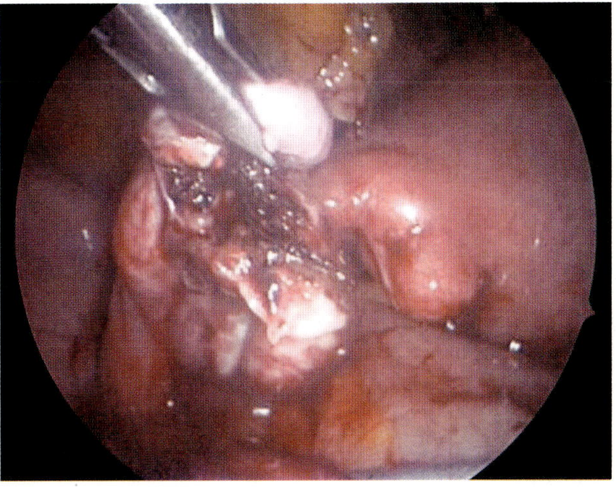

Figure 18 Incision of endometrioma with cystectomy in progress

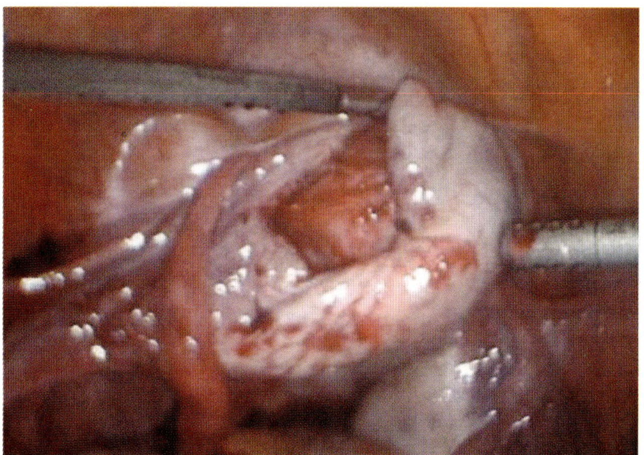

Figure 19 Left ovary after complete endometriotic excision

minimal or mild endometriosis randomized to expectant management or excision/ablation of disease. Women were followed for 36 weeks postoperatively to assess for pregnancy. Twenty-one percent of women with surgically treated endometriosis achieved an ongoing pregnancy compared to 17% of those expectantly managed (no ablation of their endometriosis). The treatment effect was 0.12, with a number needed to treat of 9 (9 women with minimal or mild disease would have to undergo surgical treatment for one additional pregnancy). Based upon an established prevalence of endometriosis of approximately 30% in an infertile population, the number of laparoscopies required for one additional pregnancy would be 25. Furthermore, the improvement in pregnancy rate, as well as the number needed to treat is greater with controlled ovarian hyperstimulation (COH) and IUI, with the advantage of COH/IUI being the avoidance of an invasive procedure.

No published trial comparing surgical treatment with expectant management for moderate to severe endometriosis exists. However, many publications examining the likelihood of pregnancy with severe disease to be near zero with either expectant management or surgery. There is little or no benefit of surgical intervention for women with moderate to severe endometriosis.[55]

DISORDERS OF THE FALLOPIAN TUBE

Hydrosalpinx

Disease or damage to the fallopian tubes accounts for 25–30% of cases of infertility. Infertility is caused by impaired ovum/embryo transport due to fimbrial damage and/or adnexal adhesions. Furthermore, the risk of ectopic pregnancy is also increased. Factors responsible for tubal disease can include PID, pelvic surgery, and endometriosis; in some cases, the cause is unknown.

Treatments for infertility caused by tubal disease include reconstructive surgery or IVF. *In vitro* fertilization is the only treatment available for severely damaged, inoperable fallopian tubes and for situations where tubal disease is concurrent with another fertility factor. *In vitro* fertilization may also be considered if the woman is of advancing maternal age so that the maximum potential for treatment success is attainable. Reconstructive tubal surgery, however, should be considered in some selected individuals.

Patient Selection

The gold standard for evaluating the patency of tubes is diagnostic laparoscopy. However, given the invasive nature of a laparoscopy, an HSG often serves a useful initial procedure for evaluating the fallopian tubes.

Compared to laparoscopy, the HSG has moderate sensitivity (ability to detect patency when the tubes are open) but relatively high specificity. In other words, when an HSG suggests that both tubes are proximally occluded, there is a small likelihood that the tubes really are open.[56] However, if the HSG demonstrates patency, there is little chance that the tubes are blocked. The diagnosis of distal tubal occlusion is generally accurate but proximal tubal occlusion may be the result of uterine contractions or catheter placement as opposed to true pathologic obstruction. A recent review estimated the sensitivity and specificity of HSG in detecting any tubal pathology to be 53% and 87%, respectively. For bilateral tubal disease, the sensitivity and specificity were noted to be 46% and 95%, respectively.[57]

The cause of tubal disease must be taken into consideration when determining the prognosis for successful surgery. Successful surgical outcomes depend on whether tubal disease is due to intrinsic (from ascending infection or salpingitis isthmica nodosa) or extrinsic (previous pelvic surgery, endometriosis) causes. The location, type and degree of tubal injury impact the chance of surgical success. According to Schlaff et al. the presence of tubal rugae on HSG, the absence or presence of small hydrosalpinges (less than 15 mm in diameter), the absence of significant pelvic adhesions and the presence of fimbriae during laparoscopy were all associated with good prognosis following tubal reconstructive surgery.[58]

For many infertile couples, a several-month postoperative trial at spontaneous conceiving is undesirable and unwise. Therefore, patient selection for surgical treatment of infertility must be individualized and carefully considered.

Surgical Technique

Distal tubal obstruction is found to be the culprit of tubal disease in the majority of cases (Figure 20). Various techniques of treating or bypassing tubal disease include either open or laparoscopic surgery, namely salpingectomy or salpingostomy, or ART. Fimbrioplasty is performed in situations where patients have patent fallopian tubes whereas salpingostomy is performed with occluded tubes. Many times, patients have pelvic adhesions and phimosis of the fimbriated end of the fallopian tube.

Fimbrioplasty

Fimbrioplasty is reconstruction of the tubal fimbriae or infundibulum where fimbrial agglutination or partial distal tubal occlusion exists. The technique of fimbrioplasty is the same regardless of whether the procedure is performed via an open incision or a laparoscopic approach.

A small opening is usually present at the distal end of the tube which can be easily visualized with transcervical chromopertubation. If the opening is covered by fibrous tissue, this tissue must be excised to gain access to the fimbriae (Figure 21). Agglutination can be corrected by inserting either a mosquito forceps or alligator forceps with its jaws closed followed by opening its jaws and withdrawing the forceps multiple times. The direction in which the jaws are opened should be varied in order to optimize the deagglutination. Bleeding is usually minimized with a gentle technique.

In some instances, the ampullary portion of the tube distends with minimal efflux of dye solution. In this situation, it is necessary to longitudinally incise the tube along its antimesosalpingeal border to the fimbriated end. The incision is made electrosurgically with a microelectrode or mechanically with microsurgical scissors. The edges of the two flaps can be folded back with electrosurgery by desiccating the serosal margins of the flaps, causing them to fold backward, away from the fimbriae.

Salpingostomy (Neosalpingostomy)

Salpingostomy or neosalpingostomy is the creation of a new opening in a tube with an occluded distal hydrosalpinx. The new stoma (opening) can be located at the terminal end of the tube or at the ampullary or isthmic portions of the tube. Ampullary and isthmic neosalpingostomies, however, have little clinical applicability as the likelihood of pregnancy with limited tubal length is extremely low.

It is important that all pelvic and periadnexal adhesions are lysed prior to undertaking an attempt of neosalpingostomy. This method ensures that the new opening will be placed at an appropriate location, at the distal-most portion of the tube. Once the salpingo-ovariolysis is completed and the tube is completely free, the tube is distended with transcervical chromopertubation. An avascular area is identified at the distal-most aspect of the fallopian tube and a cruciate area is cauterized and then incised using microelectrode/microsurgical scissors. (Figure 22) The central avascular point is then entered with the incision being extended in a cruciate fashion.

In this manner, the new opening forms a new fimbria-ovary relationship. Bleeding is controlled with careful desiccation using a microelectrode. Once a reasonable sized stoma is attained, the flaps created in the process are secured by desiccating their serosal surface which allows them to fold back upon themselves.

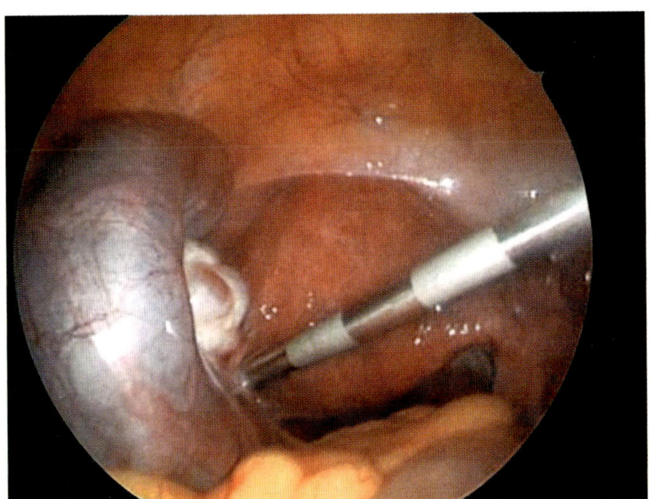

Figure 20 Left sided hydrosalpinx

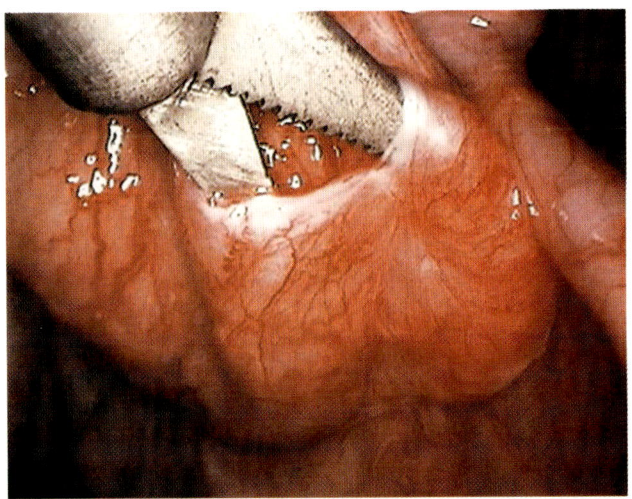

Figure 21 Deagglutination of fimbriated end of fallopian tube

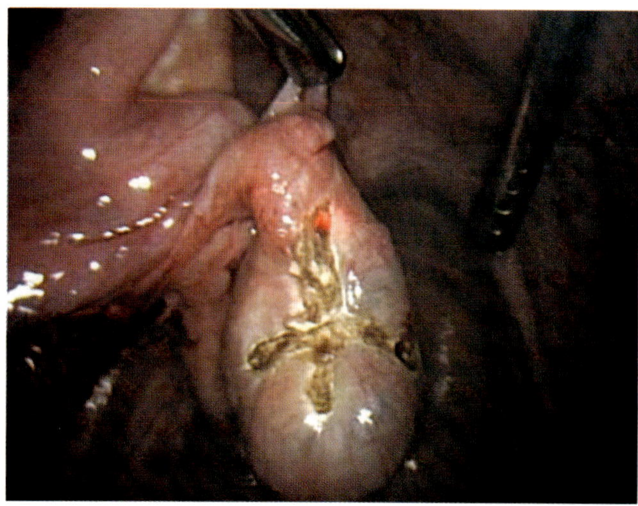

Figure 22 A cruciate incision is made with electrocautery

Fertility

Of variables being ascertained in studies, outcome or end results are clinically the most important and yet often the most difficult to compare between studies. Without question, the only meaningful method of evaluating end results is to assess cumulative pregnancy rate per month of year of exposure (similar to a life-table analysis) or the evaluation of pregnancy rate per menstrual cycle. Despite this, most studies will present data as the percentage of patients who are pregnant after some arbitrary amount of time. Furthermore, studies comparing surgical versus ART can be difficult as pregnancy rate after surgery are calculated as cumulative pregnancy rate per unit of time, typically 1–5 years while success after IVF is expressed per cycle initiated or per embryo transfer.

In women with distal tubal disease, the probability of conceiving on a monthly basis decreases as the severity of hydrosalpinges increases. The type and extent of pelvic disease, the thickness of the tubal wall and the appearance of the tubal mucosa all impact the chance of pregnancy.

Twenty-five percent of cases have mild distal tubal disease. Long-term livebirth rate after surgical treatment ranges from 39–59% (approximately 5% per month probability of pregnancy) with an associated ectopic pregnancy rate of 4–10%.[59,60] The outcome for patients with severe distal tubal disease (>50% of patients) is significantly worse with an overall pregnancy rate of less than 15% which equates to a monthly fecundability rate of 1–2%.[60]

The role of reconstructive tubal surgery in a woman of advanced maternal age is limited. Given the low monthly chance of pregnancy following surgery in the setting of an already reduced fecundability in a woman of advanced maternal age, IVF is the better treatment option. In contrast, reconstructive surgery for a young woman with minimal tubal disease is a reasonable option.

In many studies, the operating technique is the variable being studied. However, due to individual variability of pelvic adhesive and/or tubal disease, operative results within and between operative techniques may not be comparable.

After Fimbrioplasty

In general, results of fimbrioplasty are difficult to distinguish from other tubal corrective surgeries as this procedure tends to be included as a method of salpingostomy. In one series of 40 patients who underwent microsurgical fimbrioplasty authored by Patton et al. 63% (n=25) of patients had intrauterine pregnancies and 5% (n=2) had ectopic pregnancies after 2 years of follow-up.[61] Other series have reported an ectopic pregnancy rate ranging between 5–12.9% after 18 months of follow-up.[62,63] In most cases, approximately half of the patients never conceived in the interval of time studied. No randomized controlled trials for fimbrioplasty versus other methods of tubal reconstructive surgery have been done.

After Neosalpingostomy

The major determinants of outcome from neosalpingostomy are the degree of pre-existing tubal damage and the extent and type of periadnexal adhesions. In cases of mild tubal damage, the reported live birth rate ranges from 40–60%. Live birth rate are reported to be less than 20% in cases where severely damaged tubes exist.

SECOND OPERATIONS

In general, patients who fail to conceive after primary tubal reconstructive surgery have severely limited success with repeat surgical procedures. In these cases, ART is strongly indicated.

Salpingectomy

While the surgeon should be as conservative as possible, he or she should consider that the patient is better served with a single well-functioning fallopian tube than with two defective tubes, which elicits an increased risk for ectopic pregnancy or recurrence of pelvic adhesions. If the fallopian tubes are beyond repair, bilateral salpingectomy is recommended in preparation for IVF.

Surgical Technique

A salpingectomy can be performed as either an open or laparoscopic procedure. Endoscopic staplers, endocoagulation, bipolar cautery and endoscopic ligatures can be used as methods of performing a laparoscopic salpingectomy. One simple laparoscopic method included cauterization of the tubo-ovarian ligament first with bipolar cautery followed by sharp transection of the tube with scissors. The mesosalpinx is also cauterized and transected in a similar manner, staying as close as possible to the length of the tube so as to not impact the vascular supply. The proximal tube is then cauterized and transected leaving approximately 1 cm of non-diseased interstitial tube, if possible. The specimen is then removed with an endoscopic bag through a 12 mm port.

Fertility

Many investigators have reported the possible deleterious impact of hydrosalpinges on IVF outcome.[64] The detrimental effect on IVF is thought to be secondary to a mechanical 'washing' out of the endometrial cavity, which can therefore impact the success of an embryo transfer. In addition, it is theorized that direct flow of hydrosalpingeal fluid into the uterine cavity occurs which exposes the endometrium and the embryo to potentially toxic fluid, thus detrimentally affecting the endometrium and developing embryo. This negative impact is most evident when hydrosalpinges are sizeable enough to be visualized on transvaginal sonogram.[64,65] Some have suggested a beneficial impact of removing hydrosalpinges in patients with repeated IVF failures. In a study by Strandell et al. a total of 186 women underwent 452 IVF cycles. Among the 77 women randomized to no surgical intervention, 24 underwent salpingectomy after one or two failed cycles. Cumulative results were analyzed by Cox regression, taking into account the number of cycles per patient and the presence of a salpingectomy after a previous transfer. Salpingectomy implied a significant increase in birth rate (hazard ratio 2.1, 95% CI 1.6–3.6, P = 0.014). Within the subgroup of patients with ultrasound-visible hydrosalpinges, the birth rate was even higher (hazard ratio 3.8, 95% CI 1.5–9.2, P = 0.004). Implantation rate was significantly higher in patients who had undergone salpingectomy (27.2% versus 20.2, P = 0.03) and, in the subgroup of patients with ultrasound-visible hydrosalpinges, the difference was even larger (30.3% versus 17.1%, P = 0.003).

Thus, surgical treatment should be considered for all women with hydrosalpinges prior to IVF treatment. In cases of sonographically apparent hydrosalpinges, a salpingectomy, rather than a salpingostomyis the preferred route of treatment. Some couples, however, may prefer a salpingostomy which offers some potential of a spontaneous pregnancy.

Another method of possibly reducing the negative impact of a hydrosalpinx is to occlude the proximal (corneal) end of the affected fallopian tube. In a Cochrane review, five randomized controlled trials involved 646 women, provides evidence that laparoscopic tubal occlusion is a reasonable alternative to laparoscopic salpingectomy in improving IVF pregnancy rate in women with hydrosalpinges.[66] Four randomized controlled studies assessed salpingectomy versus no treatment, two also included a tubal occlusion arm and one trial assessed aspiration versus no treatment. No trials reported on the primary outcome of live birth. The odds of ongoing pregnancy (OR 2.14, 95%CI 1.23–3.73) and of clinical pregnancy (OR 2.31, 95%CI 1.48–3.62) were increased with laparoscopic salpingectomy for hydrosalpinges prior to IVF compared to expectant management. Laparoscopic occlusion of the fallopian tube versus no intervention did not increase the odds of ongoing pregnancy significantly (OR 7.24, 95%CI 0.87–59.57) but the odds of clinical pregnancy (OR 4.66, 95%CI 2.47–10.01) had sufficient power to show a significant increase. Comparison of tubal occlusion to salpingectomy did not show a significant advantage of either surgical procedure in terms of ongoing pregnancy (OR 1.65, 95%CI 0.74–3.71) or clinical pregnancy (OR 1.28, 95%CI 0.76–2.14). No significant differences were seen in adverse effects of surgical treatments in any study. Aspiration of tubal contents did not confer any benefit over expectant management.

Prior Tubal Ligation

Tubotubal anastomoses refer to any anastomoses performed along the length of the tube to treat occlusive disease. The principles of microsurgery are most applied to this type of reproductive surgery. Tubotubal anastomoses are typically utilized to reverse a prior tubal sterilization rather than to repair an occluded, diseased tube. Depending on the segments being reapproximated, tubotubal anastomoses can be intramural-isthmic, intramural-ampullary, isthmic-isthmic, isthmic-ampullary or ampullary-infundibular.

Technique

Access can be achieved with laparotomy, minilaparotomy or laparoscopy. For open procedures, the side of interest is elevated with the use of pads soaked in irrigation solution. The contralateral side is left in its natural position. For laparoscopic procedures, the mesosalpinx under the site of anastomoses can be injected with dilute vasopressin to aid in hemostasis.

The principles for anastomoses are the same regardless of the approach. The proximal tubal segment is first distended by transcervical chromopertubation with methylene blue allowing for identification of the site of occlusion and providing easy visualization of the tubal lumen for anastomoses. The tube is then sharply transected at the occluded end. The incision should stop at the mesosalpinx to avoid damage to the tubal vasculature. The blue dye should easily escape from the previously occluded tubal segment. The cut surface is then examined under magnification to ensure normal muscular and mucosal architecture are present. If scar tissue is present, it can be lysed or the tube can be further proximally transected. Hemostasis can be achieved with precise electro desiccation; desiccation of the tubal epithelium should be avoided as this will impact future tubal function. Attention is now turned to the distal site of occlusion. Before transection, the tube is distended from the fimbriated end thus allowing better visualization of the distal occluded stump. The occluded segment is then sharply transected providing visualization of the dye. As previously described, the transected portion is then evaluated for anastomoses.

The tubal segments are reapproximated in two layers, the first of which joins the epithelium and muscularis, and the second joins the serosa. Eight to zero Vicryl on a taper-cut needle is used for reapproximation. The first suture of the epithelium and muscularis is always placed at the mesosalpingeal border (6 O'clock position) to ensure proper alignment of the tubal mucosa. (Figure 23)

The knot is tied peripherally. Once the 6 O'clock position suture is tied, three additional sutures are placed to appose the inner layer, typically at the 3, 9 and 12 O'clock positions (Figure 24). These can be done in an interrupted or a continuous fashion. If performed in a continuous fashion, the suture should be cut at the 3, 9 and 12 O'clock positions such that individual knots can be tied.

After approximation of the inner layer, chromopertubation should demonstrate tubal patency and tight anastomoses. The serosa is then joined with interrupted sutures in a circumferential fashion (3–4 sutures) followed by repair of the defect within the underlying mesosalpinx.

If significant disparity between tubal lumen is present (i.e. in isthmic-ampullary anastomoses), anchoring stitches should be placed at the 6 and 12 O'clock positions to provide easier approximation.

Laparoscopic anastomoses may require the placement of only two sutures, one at the 6 O'clock position and the second at the 12 O'clock position.

Fertility

Factors that affect outcome include the type of prior sterilization, the site of anastomoses, the length of the reconstructed tube, single versus double anastomoses, the extent and nature of surrounding adhesive disease, age of the patient, the length of time since the sterilization, the status of other fertility factors (specifically male partner) and the technique used. Therefore, the success of tubotubal anastomoses depends on patient selection and surgical technique.

In general, multiple series report live birth rate between 40–80% with an ectopic pregnancy rate of less than 2–12.5%. Several reports of laparoscopic anastomoses have been published. The largest one of 202 cases followed patients for 12 months. Seventy-seven (n=154) achieved intrauterine pregnancies of which 25 had pregnancy losses; five patients had an ectopic pregnancy.[67]

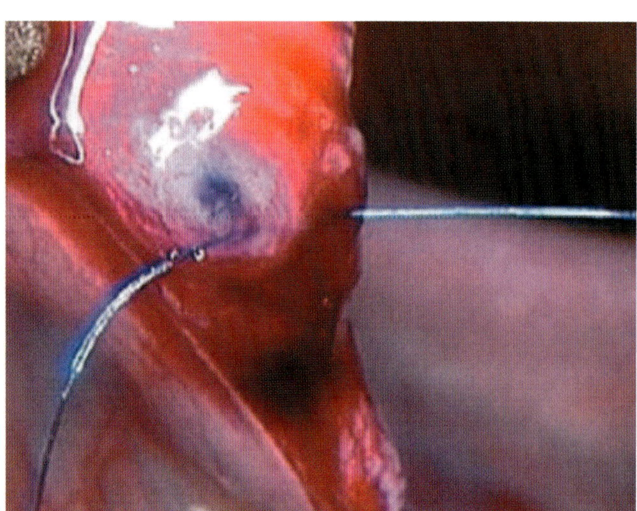

Figure 23 Suture placed at 6 O'clock position

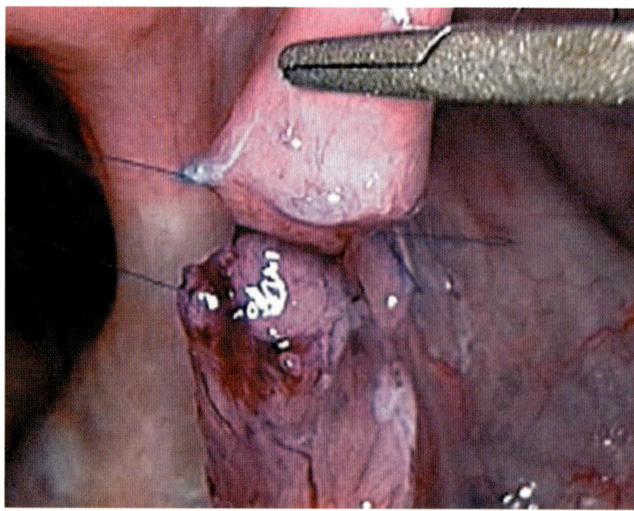

Figure 24 Suture placed at 12 O'clock position

These results are similar to those found after open anastomoses.[68]

RECENT ADVANCES IN REPRODUCTIVE SURGERY

Robotically Assisted Reproductive Surgery

Robotic surgery, also known as computer assisted surgery or robot-assisted surgery was initially developed to overcome limitations of minimally invasive surgery. Instead of directly moving the instruments with his/her hands, the surgeon uses a computer console to manipulate the instruments attached to multiple robot arms. The computer translates the surgeon's movements which are then carried out on the patient by the robot. The console is located in the same operating room as the patient, but physically separated from the operative workspace or in another place. Since the surgeon does not need to be in the immediate location of the patient while the operation is being performed, it can be possible for specialists to perform remote surgery on patients.

The da Vinci Surgical System comprises three components: a surgeon's console, a patient-side robotic cart with four arms manipulated by the surgeon (one to control the camera and three to manipulate instruments) and a high-definition 3D vision system. Articulating surgical instruments are mounted on the robotic arms which are introduced into the body through cannulas. Although the telesurgical robot was originally intended to facilitate remotely performed surgery in battlefield and other remote environments, it turned out to be more useful for minimally invasive on-site surgery.

The da Vinci senses the surgeon's hand movements and translates them electronically into scaled-down micromovements to manipulate the tiny proprietary instruments. It also detects and filters out any tremors in the surgeon's hand movements, so that they are not duplicated robotically. The camera used in the system provides a true stereoscopic picture transmitted to a surgeon's console. The da Vinci system is approved by the Food and Drug Administration (FDA) for a variety of surgical procedures including surgery for prostate cancer, hysterectomy and mitral valve repair. Robotic surgery in gynecology is one of the fastest growing fields of robotic surgery. This includes the use of the da Vinci surgical system in benign gynecology and gynecologic oncology. Robotic surgery can be used to treat fibroids, abnormal periods, endometriosis, ovarian tumors and female cancers. Using the robotic system, gynecologists can perform hysterectomies, myomectomies and lymph node biopsies.

Advantages and Disadvantages

Major advances aided by surgical robots have been remote surgery, minimally invasive surgery and unmanned surgery. Some major advantages of robotic surgery are precision, miniaturization, smaller incisions, decreased blood loss, less pain and quicker healing time. Further advantages are articulation beyond normal manipulation and three-dimensional magnification, resulting in improved ergonomics. Robotic techniques are also associated with reduced duration of hospital stays, blood loss, transfusions and use of pain medication.[69]

Additional surgical training is needed to operate the system.[70] Surgeons report that, although the manufacturers of such systems provide training on this new technology, the learning phase is intensive and surgeons must operate on 12–18 patients before they adapt. Moreover during the training phase, minimally invasive operations can take up to twice as long as traditional surgery, leading to operating room tie ups and surgical staff keeping patients under anesthesia for longer periods.

While the use of robotic surgery has become an item in the advertisement of medical services, critics point out that studies that indicate that long-term results are superior to those after laparoscopic surgery are lacking.[71] The robotic system does not come cheap and has a learning curve. Data is absent that proves the increased costs can be justified. In medical literature, very experienced surgeons tend to publish their results with robotic systems. However, these may not be representative of surgeons with lesser experience.[71]

Office Hysteroscopy

Since the early 1990s, new scopes with diameters ranging between 1.2 mm and 3 mm have been developed, thus providing a maximum outer sheath diameter equal to or less than 5 mm for operative procedures. These miniaturized hysteroscopes can therefore be inserted into a uterine cavity without the need for cervical dilation. Furthermore, these scopes can be used for directed biopsies within the uterine cavity. Many of these office hysteroscopes are oval in shape thus allowing an atraumatic entry into the uterine cavity. Because sensitive innervation in the uterus begins from the myometrium and the endometrium or any fibrotic tissue are not similarly innervated, a hysteroscopic procedure can be performed without any analgesia/anesthesia, provided that some steps for avoiding patient discomfort are respected. Distention of the uterus can be attained either with an electronic suction-irrigation pump (Storz) that can maintain a constant, intrauterine pressure around 30–40 mm Hg, or with a pressurized intravenous fluid bag. These methods control the rate of distention that is necessary to avoid overdistention and patient discomfort. These improvements in technology now enable reproductive surgeons to perform many diagnostic and operative procedures in an office setting, without significant patient discomfort, thus eliminating the need for anesthesia.

CONCLUDING THOUGHTS

Enormous progress has been made in the field of ART, allowing its success in treating thousands of couples worldwide. In a parallel fashion, minimally invasive surgery with both laparoscopy and hysteroscopy, have significantly advanced in their safety and successful application. While one treatment strategy may be more successful in achieving pregnancy in some instances, the optimal treatment of a woman or couple with infertility oftentimes requires surgery complementing ART. Indeed both techniques will continue to concurrently evolve as distinct yet symbiotic treatment strategies, thus enhancing the likelihood of pregnancy in patients facing complex fertility problems.

REFERENCES

1. Fischer SP. Cost-effective preoperative evaluation and testing. Chest. 1999;115:96S-110S.
2. Blery C, Charpak Y, Szatan M, et al. Evaluation of a protocol for selective ordering of preoperative tests. Lancet. 1986;1:139-41.
3. ACOG Committee on Ethics. ACOG Committee Opinion No. 439: Informed consent. Obstet Gynecol. 2009;114:401-8.
4. Abed H, Rogers R, Helitzer D, et al. Informed consent in gynecologic surgery. Am J Obstet Gynecol. 2007;197:674.e1-5.
5. ACOG Committee on Professional Liability. ACOG Committee Opinion No. 306. Informed refusal. Obstet Gynecol. 2004;104:1465-6.
6. Wenzel RP. Minimizing surgical-site infections. N Engl J Med. 2010;362:75-7.
7. Culligan PJ, Kubik K, Murphy M, et al. A randomized trial that compared povidone iodine and chlorhexidine as antiseptics for vaginal hysterectomy. Am J Obstet Gynecol. 2005;192:422-5.
8. TeLinde's. Operative Gynecology. In: Rock JA and Jones HW III (Eds), 9th edition. Philadelphia: Lippincott Williams and Wilkins; 2003.
9. Bradshaw AD, Advincula AP. Optimizing patient positioning and understanding radiofrequency energy in gynecologic surgery. Clin Obstet Gynecol. 2010;53:511-20.
10. Cooper NA, Smith P, Khan KS, et al. A systematic review of the effect of the distension medium on pain during outpatient hysteroscopy. Fertil Steril. 2011;95:264-71.
11. Pellicano M, Guida M, Zullo F, et al. Carbon dioxide versus normal saline as a uterine distension medium for diagnostic vaginoscopic hysteroscopy in infertile patients: a prospective, randomized, multicenter study. Fertil Steril. 2003;79:418-21.
12. Cooper NA, Smith P, Khan KS, et al. A systematic review of the effect of the distension medium on pain during outpatient hysteroscopy. Fertil Steril. 2011;95:264-71.
13. The Practice Committee of the American Society for Reproductive Medicine, Myomas and Reproductive Function, Fertil Steril. 2004;82:S111.
14. Sylvestre C, Child TJ, Tulandi T, et al. A prospective study to evaluate the efficacy of two- and three-dimensional sonohysterography in women with intrauterine lesions. Fertil Steril. 2003;79:1222-5.
15. Mais V, Ajossa S, Guerriero S, et al. Laparoscopic versus abdominal myomectomy: a prospective randomized trial to evaluate benefits in early outcome. Am J Obstet Gynecol. 1996;174:654-8.
16. Seracchioli R, Rossi S, Govoni F, et al. Fertility and obstetric outcome after laparoscopic myomectomy of large myomata: a randomized comparison with abdominal myomectomy. Hum Reprod. 2006;15:2663-8.
17. Dubuisson JB, Lecuru F, Foulot H, et al. Myomectomy by laparoscopy: a preliminary report of 43 cases. Fertil Steril. 1991;56:827-30.
18. Koh CH, Janik GM. Laparoscopic microsurgical tubal anastomosis: difficulties and pitfalls. In: Corfman RS, Diamond MP, DeCherney A(Eds). Complications of Laparoscopy and Hysteroscopy, 2nd edition. Malden MA: Blackwell Science; 1997.
19. Dubuisson JB, Fauconnier A, Babaki-Fard K, et al. Laparoscopic myomectomy: a current view. Hum Reprod Update. 2000;6:588-94.
20. Pritts EA, Parker WH, Olive DL. Fibroids and infertility: an updated systematic review of the evidence. Fertil Steril. 2009;91:1215-23.
21. Oliveira FG, Abdelmassih VG, Diamond MP, et al. Impact of subserosal and intramural uterine fibroids that do not distort the endometrial cavity on the outcome of in vitro fertilization-intracytoplasmic sperm injection. Fertil Steril. 2004;81:582-7.
22. Dubuisson JB, Chapron C, Fauconnier A. Laparoscopic myomectomy. In: Sutton C, Diamond MP (Eds). Endoscopic Surgery for Gynecologists, 2nd edition. London: WB Saunders; 1998.
23. Pritts EA, Parker WH, Olive DL. Fibroids and infertility: an updated systematic review of the evidence. Fertil Steril. 2009; 91:1215-23.
24. Casini ML, Rossi F, Agostini R, et al. Effect of the position of fibroids on fertility. Gynecol Endocrinol. 2006; 22:106-9.
25. Shokeir T, El-Shafei M, Yousef H, et al. Submucous myomas and their implications in the pregnancy rate of

patients with otherwise unexplained primary infertility undergoing hysteroscopic myomectomy: a randomized matched control study. Fertil Steril. 2010;94:724.
26. Hockstein S. Spontaneous uterine rupture in the early third trimester after laparoscopically assisted myomectomy. A case report. J Reprod Med. 2000;45:139-41.
27. Dubuisson JB, Fauconnier A, Deffarges JV, et al. Pregnancy outcome and deliveries following laparoscopic myomectomy. Hum Reprod. 2000;15:869-73.
28. Dessolle L, Soriano D, Poncelet C, et al. Determinants of pregnancy rate and obstetric outcome after laparoscopic myomectomy for infertility. Fertil Steril. 2001;76:370-4.
29. Seinera P, Farina C, Todros T. Laparoscopic myomectomy and subsequent pregnancy: results in 54 patients. Hum Reprod. 2000;15:1993-6.
30. Loffler FD, Bradley LD, Brill AI, et al. Hysteroscopic fluid monitoring guidelines. J Am Assoc Gynecol Laparosc. 2000;7:167.
31. Donnez J, Gillerot S, Bourgonjon D, et al. Neodymium: YAG laser hysteroscopy in large submucous fibroids. Fertil Steril. 1990;54:999-1003.
32. Varasteh NN, Neuwirth RS,Levin B, et.al.Pregnancy rate after hysteroscopic polypectomy and myomectomy in infertile women. Obstet Gynecol.1999;94:168-71.
33. Pérez-Medina T, Bajo-Arenas J, Salazar F, et al. Endometrial polyps and their implication in the pregnancy rate of patients undergoing intrauterine insemination: a prospective, randomized study. Hum Reprod. 2005;20:1632-5.
34. Stamatellos I, Apostolides A, Stamatopoulos P, et al. Pregnancy rate after hysteroscopic polypectomy depending on the size or number of the polyps. Arch Gynecol Obstet. 2008;277:395-9.
35. Bosteels J, Weyers S, Puttemans P, et al.The effectiveness of hysteroscopy in improving pregnancy rate in subfertile women without other gynaecological symptoms: a systematic review. Hum Reprod Update. 2010;16:1-11.
36. Asherman JG. Amenorrhoea traumatica (atretica). J Obstet Gynaecol Br Emp. 1948;55: 23-30.
37. Schenker JG, Margalioth EJ. Intrauterine adhesions: an updated appraisal. Fertil Steril. 1982;37:593-610.
38. American Fertility Society. The American Fertility Society classifications of adnexal adhesions, distal tubal occlusion, tubal occlusion secondary to tubal ligation, tubal pregnancies, müllerian anomalies and intrauterine adhesion. Fertil Steril. 1988;49:944-55.
39. Ashton D, Amin HK, Richart RM, et al. The incidence of symptomatic uterine anomalies in women undergoing transcervical tubal sterilization. Obstet Gynecol. 1988;72:28-30.
40. Fedele L, Bianchi S, Marchini M, et al. Residual uterine septum of less than 1 cm after hysteroscopic metroplasty does not impair reproductive outcome. Hum Reprod. 1996;11:727-9.
41. DeCherney AH, Russell JB, Graebe RA, et al. Resectoscopic management of müllerian defects. Fertil Steril. 1986;45:726-8.
42. Perino A, Mencaqlia L, Hamou J, et al. Hysteroscopy for metroplasty of uterine septa: report of 24 cases. Fertil Steril. 1987;48:321-3.
43. Hamou J. Electroresection of fibroids. In: Sutton C, Diamond M(Eds). Endoscopic Surgery for Gynaecologists. London: WB Saunders; 1993.
44. Fedele L, Bianchi S. Hysteroscopic metroplasty for the septate uterus. Obstet Gynecol Clin North Am. 1995;22:473-8.
45. Burchell RC, Creed F, Rasoulpour M, et al. Vascular anatomy of the human uterus and pregnancy wastage. Br J Obstet Gynaecol. 1978;85:698-706.
46. Homer HA, Li TC, Cooke ID. The septate uterus: a review of management and reproductive outcome. Fertil Steril. 2000;73:1-14.
47. Hickok LR. Hysteroscopic treatment of the uterine septum: a clinician's experience. Am J Obstet Gynecol. 2000;182:1414-20.
48. Patton P, Novy MJ, Lee DM, et al. The diagnosis and reproductive outcome after surgical treatment of the complete septate uterus, duplicated cervix and vaginal septum. Am J Obstet Gynecol. 2004;190:1669-75.
49. Litta P, Pozan C, Merlin F, et al. Hysteroscopic metroplasty under laparoscopic guidance in infertile women with septate uteri: follow-up of reproductive outcome. J Reprod Med. 2004;49:274-8.
50. Hemmings R, Bissonnette F, Bouzayen R. Results of laparoscopic treatments of ovarian endometriomas: laparoscopic ovarian fenestration and coagulation. Fertil Steril. 1998;70:527-9.
51. Loh FH, Tan AT, Kumar J, et al. Ovarian response after laparoscopic ovarian cystectomy for endometriotic cysts in 132 monitored cycles. Fertil Steril. 1999;72:316-21.
52. Canis M, Pouly JL, Tamburro S, et al. Ovarian response during IVF-embryo transfer cycles after laparoscopic ovarian cystectomy for endometriotic cysts > 3 cm in diameter. Hum Reprod. 2001;16:2583-6.
53. Busacca M, Marana R, Caruana P, et al. Recurrence of ovarian endoemetrioma after laparoscopic excision. Am J Obstet Gynecol. 1999;180:519-23.
54. Marcoux S, Maheux R, Berube S. Laparoscopic surgery in infertile women with minimal or mild endometriosis. Canadian collaborative group on endometriosis. N Engl J Med. 1997;337:217-22.
55. Olive D, Pritts E. The treatment of endometriosis: a review of the evidence. Ann N Y Acad Sci.2002;955:360-72.
56. Swart P, Mol BW, van der Veen F, et al. The accuracy of hysterosalpingography in the diagnosis of tubal pathology: a meta-analysis. Fertil Steril. 1995;64:486-91.
57. Broeze KA, Opmeer BC, Van Geloven, et al. Are patient characteristics associated with the accuracy of hysterosalpingography in diagnosing tubal pathology? An individual patient data meta-analysis. Human Reprod Update. 2010;17:293.
58. Schlaff WD, Hassiakos DK, Damewood MD, et al. Neosalpingostomy for distal tubal obstruction:

prognostic factors and impact of surgical technique. Fertil Steril. 1990;54:984-90.

59. Boer-Meisel ME, te Velde ER, Habbema JD, et al. Predicting the pregnancy outcome in patients treated for hydrosalpinx: a prospective study. Fertil Steril. 1986;45:23-9.
60. Winston RM, Margara RA. Microsurgical salpingostomy is not an obsolete procedure. Br J Obstet Gynaecol. 1991;98:637-42.
61. Patton PE, Williams TJ, Coulam CB. Results of microsurgical reconstruction in patients with combined proximal and distal tubal occlusion: double obstruction. Fertil Steril. 1987;48:670-4.
62. Gomel V, Swolin K. Salpingostomy: microsurgical technique and results. Clin Obstet Gynecol. 1980; 23(4):1243-58.
63. Dubuisson JB, Bouquet de Joliniere J, Aubriot FX, et al. Terminal tuboplasties by laparoscopy: 65 consecutive cases. Fertil Steril. 1990;54:401-3.
64. Strandell A, Waldenstrom U, Nilsson L, et al. Hydrosalpinx reduces in vitro fertilization/embryo transfer pregnancy rate. Hum Reprod. 1994;9:861-3.
65. Andersen AN, Yue Z, Meng FJ, et al. Low implantation rate after in vitro fertilization in patients with hydrosalpinges diagnosed by ultrasonography. Hum Reprod. 1994;9:1935-8.
66. Johnson N, van Voorst S, Sowter MC, et al. Surgical treatment for tubal disease in women due to undergo in vitro fertilisation. Cochrane Database Syst Rev. 2010;20;CD002125.
67. Yoon TK, Sung HR, Kang HG, et al. Laparoscopic tubal anastomoses: fertility outcome in 202 cases. Fertil Steril. 1999;72:1121-6.
68. Cha SH, Lee MH, Kim JH, et al. Fertility outcome after tubal anatomoses by laparoscopy and laparotomy. J Am Assoc Gynecol Laparosc. 2001;8:348-52.
69. Estey EP. Robotic prostatectomy: the new standard of care or a marketing success? Can Urol Assoc J. 2009;3:488-90.
70. Finkelstein J, Eckersberger E, Sadri H, et al. Open versus laparoscopic versus robot-assisted laparoscopic prostatectomy: the European and US experience. Rev Urology. 2010;12:35-43.
71. Gina Kolata. "Results Unproven, Robotic Surgery Wins Converts". The New York Times, 2010.

16

The Molecular and Genetic Basis of Infertility

Karenne N Fru, Kimberly S Moon, James H Segars

Chapter Contents

INTRODUCTION

The known genetic causes of infertility are diverse and expanding. Mechanisms for genetic alterations include aneuploidies, insertions, deletions, inversions, duplications, translocations (balanced and unbalanced), fragile sites, repetitive elements and various complex rearrangements of chromosomes (Table 1). Some genetic alterations are detectable at the chromosomal level but others require sophisticated molecular detection techniques, such as comparative genomic hybridization (CGH),[1] polymerase chain reaction (PCR) based strategies[2] or paired-end sequencing techniques.[3] This chapter summarizes current knowledge of the molecular and genetic changes that are known to be associated with human infertility. Where necessary, studies in nonhuman species are cited when studies in humans are not available.

MOLECULAR AND GENETIC MECHANISMS INVOLVED IN INFERTILITY

Chromosomal Number Abnormalities

The entirety of the human genome compactly resides in 46 chromosomes. Defects in cellular replication and germ cell errors may result in abnormalities of chromosome number known as aneuploidies (Table 1). These may consist of additions of chromosome copies, such as trisomy (three copies) or conversely, omission of a chromosome resulting in a monosomy. A clinically significant abnormality of chromosome number that results in male infertility is Klinefelter syndrome. The estimated incidence is 1 in 500 and it is the most common chromosomal abnormality associated with male infertility. First described in 1942 by Dr Klinefelter as a karyotype of 47,XXY and a phenotype of tall stature, failure to develop male secondary sex characteristics and infertility, it encompasses a broad definition and includes a number of variants including increased X chromosome copies (48,XXXY), mosaics (46,XY/47,XXY) and Klinefelter variants, such as an additional isochromosome Xq.[4]

Deletions of the X chromosome resulting in a 45,X karyotype (Turner syndrome) result in gonadal failure.

Table 1 Genetic mechanisms involved in infertility

Mechanism	Definition	Example
Aneuploidy	An abnormal number of chromosomes (monosomy or trisomy for example)	Klinefelter's Syndrome Turner's Syndrome
Gene Deletion	Partial or complete absence of a gene	Yq microdeletion
Gene Mutation	A permanent alteration in the genomic sequence ranging from one to many nucleotides	NROB1 mutation
Gene Premutation	An expansion of nucleotide repeats on a gene	FMR1 premutation
CNVs	A variation in the copy number of portions of the genome ranging from one kilobase to several megabases	TSPY1 gene
SNPs	A DNA sequence variation in a single nucleotide that occurs with appreciable frequency in a population	D19S884
miRNAs	Small non-coding RNAs that regulate the stability and translation of mRNA	
Epigenetics	Chromosomal changes that do not alter the DNA sequence including methylation and acetylation	

In the event of mosaicism, 45,X and 46,XY will result in absent pubarche and menarche.[5] These patients typically demonstrate hypergonadotropic hypogonadism. If puberty is attained, menopause typically occurs before age 40 (premature ovarian insufficiency). Another defining feature is short stature possibly regulated by the pseudoautosomal homeobox containing osteogenic or short stature homeobox gene, although neither have been definitively linked to Turner syndrome. Partial deletions of the X chromosome also result in ovarian failure or menstrual dysregulation (Xp11) and even more distal deletions (Xp21) may result in secondary amenorrhea and infertility. Similarly, proximal Xq deletions result in a more severe phenotype than distal deletions. This may be due to deletion of genes like POF1 region Xq26-q28, POF2 region Xq13.3-q22 (containing Diaphanous; DIAPH2)[6]

Gene Deletion

As cells undergo meiosis, an entire gene might be deleted. Rarely is the deleted region large enough to be detected by karyotypic analysis. More typically, deletions associated with infertility are in the category of microdeletions, which require a higher resolution analysis for detection. The most thoroughly characterized infertility-associated microdeletions are on the long arm of chromosome Y resulting in a phenotype of azospermia and are therefore termed as azoospermia factor (AZF). Three distinct areas of deletion have been described; proximal AZFa, middle AZFb and distal AZFc on Yq11.[7,8] Such deletions present in a variety of phenotypes, discussed in more detail below.

Gene Mutation

Genetic material is organized along the chromosome so that regions coding for proteins are interspersed with non-coding regions, which may nonetheless be important for proper transcription. Genes are coded by trinucleotide sequences referred to as codons, each corresponding to a specific amino acid. A mutation refers to any change in the DNA sequence. Mutations come in various forms. Single base substitutions include sense mutations which do not alter the ability of the gene to be transcribed into mRNA although function of the final protein may be altered, and missense mutations, which typically result in truncated gene product downstream of the mutation site.

The orphan nuclear receptor DAX1 (NROB1), which causes X-linked adrenal hypoplasia congenita (AHC) is an example of a genetic mutation that impacts fertility. This disorder presents with primary adrenal failure, hypogonadotropic hypogonadism and azoospermia.[9] The associated azoospermia is not reversible with gonadotropin therapy suggesting a direct effect on spermatogenesis. Studies to link the DAX1 gene mutation to patients with non-obstructive azoospermia and normal hormonal parameters have been unsuccessful.[10,11] This mutation may be limited to the context of AHC.

Gene Premutation

On occasion, there is a dose-dependent genetic effect to a mutation as is the case with fragile X mental retardation 1 gene (FMR1) whereby a trinucleotide CGG repeat accumulates in the promoter region. A normal gene carries about 30 repeats, while in cases of fragile X syndrome there are more than 200 copies.[12] The premutation, therefore, refers to any intermediary phenotype with 55–200 copies of the CGG repeat. The expanded sequence of repeats results in DNA hypermethylation such that the gene is silenced in the full mutant with low or undetectable FMR protein (FMRP).[13] The fragile X phenotype is due to loss of FRMP, which acts as a translation suppressor[14] binding up to 4% of the mRNA in the mammalian brain.[15]

Copy Number Variant

Copy number variants (CNVs) refer to structural variations in chromosomes resulting in alternate quantities or 'dosing' of genetic material. This is best exemplified on the Y chromosome where the long arm (Yq) is not involved in homologous recombination with the X chromosome but is subject to multiple repeated sequences (segmental duplications, SDs). This area of the Y chromosome carries the testis determining area (SRY), as well as the AZF regions. The deletions or duplications that occur in the AZF region are typically the result of nonallelic homologous recombination.[16]

Another gene affected by CNVs is the TSPY1 gene, located on the Y chromosome (Yp). TSPY1 is a member of the TSPY1/SET/NAP-1 superfamily. These genes are expressed in the cytoplasm of spermatogonia and function as activators of replication.[17,18] TSPY1 is a multi-copy gene arranged in tandem array of 20.4kb proximal repeats and one active distal copy. The median copy number ranged from 29–32 in two studies.[19,20] Whereas, increased copy number has been implicated in defective spermatogenesis and male infertility,[21] low copy number has not been associated with any known adverse effects.

Single Nucleotide Polymorphism

A single nucleotide polymorphism (SNP) is a DNA sequence variation in a single nucleotide within the gen that occurs with an appreciable frequency within a population. An association has been found with polycystic ovary syndrome (PCOS) and a dinucleotide repeat (GT) polymorphism D19S884, located within intron 55 of the fibrillin-3 gene (FBN3, NM_032447). Fibrillin-3 is an extracellular matrix protein and has been localized to the ovary; however, studies have not clarified a mechanistic role for fibrillin-3 in PCOS.[22]

Emerging Mechanisms

Micro-RNAs (miRNAs) are being increasingly recognized as another genetic factor in controlling translation and therefore protein expression in cells. MiRNAs are small (20–30 nucleotide) non-coding RNAs comprising 1–4% of mammalian genes.[23] They are derived from pre-miRNA hairpin loops that undergo cytoplasmic cleavage by the highly conserved RNAse III enzyme Dicer yielding single stranded products. These miRNAs bind to target mRNA sequences: (1) preventing transcription by partial complementary RNA annealing,[24] (2) direct mRNA cleavage,[25] (3) mRNA target for decay by deadenylation[26] or conversely, positive targeting of gene promoters.[27]

Epigenetics refers to changes in chromosomes that do not alter the DNA sequence and are stably heritable.[28] These changes include post-translational modifications to DNA-associated histones (methylation, phosphorylation, acetylation, glycosylation, ubiquitination, sumoylation, adenosine diphosphate ribosylation, biotinylation and carbonylation), as well as DNA methylation and nucleosome packing.[29,30] DNA methylation is maintained by the action of DNA methyltransferases (DNMT1)[31-33] ensuring mitotic inheritance while DNMT3A and DNMT3B are responsible for *de novo* DNA methylation.[34] Methylation may cause transcriptional repression through differentially methylated regions in the promoters of silenced genes compared to actively transcribed genes.[35,36] More globally, chromatin can be variably condensed or uncondensed depending on stimuli, such as transcriptional repressors, functional RNAs or accessory factors.[37] Alterations in chromatin condensation affect gene expression; condensed chromatin packaging leads to diminished transcription and uncondensed chromatin promotes gene transcription.[38]

GENES AFFECTING GAMETES/GAMETOGENESIS

Genes Affecting the Ovary/Oogenesis

The human ovary is a dynamic organ with the follicle as its functional unit. Oocyte number, which is determined by birth in the human, continues to decline secondary to atresia or ovulation. An estimated 400 oocytes are ovulated over a woman's reproductive lifetime. The oocyte destined for ovulation is selected out of a cohort recruited with each menstrual cycle by careful orchestration of pituitary gonadotrophs and paracrine effects of follicle-derived steroid hormones. Follicle-stimulating hormone (FSH)-independent growth of the follicles is mediated by two members of the transforming growth factor β (TGF-β) family. These are growth differentiation factor-9 (GDF9) and bone morphogenic protein 15 (BMP15). Mouse studies on GDF9 null animals demonstrated smaller ovaries, no maturation beyond the single layer follicle stage and an absent theca lutein layer.[39] These effects lead to infertility but importantly GDF9 add-back improved ovarian weight and follicle progression.[40] Mutations of the GDF9 receptor BMPR2 present on granulosa cells has been implicated in pulmonary hypertension,[41] but not ovarian dysgenesis.

Follicle-stimulating hormone receptor (FSHR) is important in follicular development in females. Several mutations of the FSHR have been documented in women with primary amenorrhea.[42,43] Compared to mutations in the FSH beta subunit (FSH-β), the phenotype is milder. Similarly, mutations in the luteinizing hormone receptor (LHR) have been reported with normal breast development and amenorrhea or anovulation.[44,45] Serum LH may be normal or elevated but without elevation of testosterone or evidence of hirsuitism.

Even when ovarian architecture and function are grossly normal, the oocyte may fail to develop normally. Oocyte maturation is achieved by reinitiation of meiosis I signaled by germinal vesicle breakdown and terminates in metaphase II (MII) at which point the oocyte is typically capable of fertilization. Any disruption in the oocyte derived factors central to this process will result in oocyte maturation failure with arrest at germinal vesicle (GV), MI or MII.[46] For example, failure to activate maturation promoting factor, a heterodimer of cyclin dependent kinase 1 (Cdk1) and cyclin B, results in GV arrest (proposed oocyte maturation failure type 1). While 8.6–15.2% of patients with infertility produce at least one meiotically incompetent oocyte[47,48] some patients demonstrate oocyte maturation failure that is profound at ART. Target genes affecting progression of the oocyte through meiosis are currently being investigated in mice with implications for explaining human infertility, (such as Cdc25b,[49] Pde3a,[50] MIh1,[51] Smc1 beta,[52] and Mih3[53]).

Genes Affecting Testis/Spermatogenesis

Yq Microdeletions

Azoospermia factor microdeletions are found in 10–15% of men with idiopathic severe oligospermia and azoospermia[54] and 7–8% of infertile men.[55,56] The highest frequency is found in men with the lowest sperm concentrations[57] but not all men with AZF microdeletions are infertile.[56]

The AZF locus is located on the long arm of the Y chromosome (Yq) and consists of at least three regions: AZFa, AZFb and AZFc from proximal to distal Yq.[57] Of these, AZFc deletions are the most common (60%), while the AZFb and AZFa regions comprise about 16% and 5% of the total deletions, respectively, the rest being constituted of deletions involving more than one region.[55] The three regions were originally subdivided by association of specific phenotypes to deletion intervals.[7] One-third of men with deletions involving only the AZFc region have severe oligospermia and, in those with azoospermia, many have sperm recoverable by sperm extraction techniques. Deletions involving the entire AZFa or AZFb regions are associated with a poorer prognosis for sperm retrieval.[58] In most cases, AZF microdeletions will be inherited by male offspring.[59]

Azoospermia factor-encoded transcripts appear to play a role in sperm production, however, despite knowledge of the gene content of these regions the contribution of each AZF region to the molecular mechanisms involved in male fertility has yet to be clarified. AZFa deletions occur with homologous recombination between the retroviral sequences HERVyq1 and HERVyq2.[60] The entire AZFa region includes two single copy genes, *USP9Y* and *DDX3Y*. The phenotype associated with *USP9Y* deletion is variable, ranging from azoospermia to normal spermatogenesis.[61] Little is known about the phenotype of the *DDX3Y* deletion. AZFb deletion is the result of homologous recombination between palindromes P5 and proximal P1 (6.2Mb),[8] while the AZFc deletion removes 3.5Mb with recombination of the regions between b2 (Palindrome P3) and b4 (Palindrome P1).[62] It is now known that there is overlap between the AZFb and AZFc regions at P1 and both contain large segments of duplicated sequence. A complete AZFb deletion involves a large number of Y genes and causes meiotic arrest.[63] The AZFc region encodes deleted in azoospermia (DAZ) gene present in four copies (DAZ1, DAZ2, DAZ3, DAZ4). DAZ belongs to a family of genes, including BOULE (chromosome 2) and DAZL (DAZ like; chromosome 3), that are germ cell specific and encode testis-specific RNA binding proteins.[64] *CDY1*, a two copy gene coding for histone acetyltransferases, is likely to be involved in spermatogenic histone replacement and DNA transcription.[65] Other genes coded for AZFc are not as well characterized (*BPY2, TTTY3, TTTY4, TTTY17, CSP4LY* and *GOLGA2LY*). Partial deletions of the AZFc region exist particularly the gr/gr deletion.[66] This deletion removes 2 DAZ copies, one *CDY1* copy and one *BPY1* copy. This has been shown to decrease sperm count even in normospermic carriers[67] and is a risk factor for oligospermia and spermatogenic impairment.

Gonadotropin Receptor Gene Mutations

Mutations in gonadotropin receptors have negative consequences for male fertility. For example, *FSHR* gene mutations have been documented in men.[68,69] These men may progress normally through puberty and have normal testosterone levels but the testes are small and sperm concentrations range from normal to severe oligospermia.[68]

By contrast, LHR gene mutations result in a more severe phenotype in the male. This can range from severe feminization with a blind-ending vagina without Müllerian-derived structures (uterus, fallopian tubes) to a milder phenotype of descended testes and micropenis. With LHR gene mutations, FSH levels are normal and LH levels are elevated. In this condition, biopsy of the testes demonstrates absent germ cells and reduction in Leydig cells.[70]

GENES AFFECTING THE EMBRYO

Maternal Effect Genes

Maternal effect genes are involved with the maternal-to-zygotic transition.[71] The fertilized egg is transcriptionally silent prior to embryonic genome activation. Instead, maternally derived mRNA accumulates in growing oocytes and the associated proteins subsequently regulate development in the early preimplantation embryo.[72] Extrapolating from studies in *Xenopus laevis* and *Drosophila melanogaster*,[73,74] Tong et al.[75] were among the first to identify a maternal-effect gene in the mouse. 'Mater' (maternal antigen that embryos require) is a single copy, oocyte-specific gene. When *Mater*-null females were mated with normal males no offspring resulted, while *Mater*-null males were reproductively competent when mated with normal females. The *Mater*-null females were phenotypically normal, produced ova and underwent normal ovarian development, oocyte maturation, ovulation, and fertilization but development of embryos failed to proceed beyond the two-cell stage.[75] A number of other murine maternal-effect genes have been identified including *Zar1*,[76] *Stella/Pgc7/Dppa3*,[77] *Npm2*,[78] *Hsf1*,[79] *Ooep/Ces6/Moep19/Floped*,[80,81] *Padi6*,[82] *Filia*,[81] *Tle6*,[81] and *Trim24/Tif1α*.[83] As with *Mater*-mutant mice, phenotypic infertility in homozygous mutants of the above genes was attributed to developmental arrest in the cleavage stage of embryo development. Human homologues have been characterized for some of these maternal-effect genes (*Mater*, *Floped*, *Tle6*, *Filia*, *Padi6* and *Stella*)[72,77,81,84] but less is known about their function in human embryonic development.

Imprinting Disorders

As assisted reproductive technologies (ART) have gained popularity, concern has remained over the potential consequences of ART on non-DNA altering changes to the embryonic genome (epigenetics). Genomic imprinting is the process of introducing functional differences in the maternal or paternal alleles, most commonly by DNA methylation or histone modifications, resulting in monoallelic gene expression.[85,86] Higher rates of rare imprinting disorders, mainly Beckwith-Wiedemann Syndrome (BWS) and Angelman Syndrome (AS), have been reported in offspring conceived by ART when compared to the general population.[86-88] Angelman syndrome has a prevalence of 1 in 15,000 live births in the general population and less than 5% of cases are due to imprinting defects at 15q11–13.[89] Of the AS offspring born after ART, the proportion of cases with imprinting defects is much higher, up to 25% in one cohort,[90] which raised concern for over-representation in this population. Beckwith-Wiedemann syndrome is an imprinting disorder with defects mapping to 11p15. Beckwith-Wiedemann syndrome has a reported prevalence of 1 in 13,700 live births in the general population but as high as 1 in 1,524 live births after ART. Animal models have suggested that the manipulations involved in ART including the use of exogenous hormones to stimulate the ovaries, use of intracytoplasmic sperm injection (ICSI), *in vitro* culture of embryos and cryopreservation of embryos may have an effect on gene imprinting.[88] However, subfertility alone, rather than the techniques of ART themselves, may explain the increased incidence of conceiving a child with an imprinting disorders after ART.[90,91] While further studies are needed to confirm these findings, the overall low absolute risk of imprinting disorder diseases can provide some reassurance for patients undergoing ART.

GENES AFFECTING THE DEVELOPMENT AND FUNCTION OF REPRODUCTIVE ORGANS

Central Compartment

During embryologic development, gonadotropin-releasing hormone (GnRH) neurons migrate along with olfactory neurons from the olfactory placode into the forebrain. The cells then dissociate from the olfactory neurons and migrate from the preoptic area to their final position in the mediobasal hypothalamus.[92] Crucial to this migration is the correct spatial and temporal expression of several key proteins (Table 2) including fibroblast growth factor, nasal embryonic luteinizing-hormone releasing factor, anosmin-1 (KAL1),[93] and prokineticin 2. (PROK2).[92]

The GnRH pulse generator is the central regulator of the hypothalamic-pituitary-gonadal axis and is an intrinsic property of these specialized cells. Gonadotropin-releasing hormone is suppressed from childhood until puberty by an imprecisely defined mechanism but at least two pathways are thought to be involved: leptin and kisspeptin/GPR54 signaling.[93]

Pubertal delay combined with low gonadotropins and sex steroids points to hypothalamic or pituitary dysfunction. After excluding pituitary tumors, functional etiologies (extreme weight loss, exercise, or eating disorders for example) and constitutional delay, the diagnosis of idiopathic hypogonadotropic hypogonadism (IHH) is made.[93] Kallman syndrome (KS) characterizes IHH associated with anosmia or hyposmia suggesting that normal migration of the GnRH and olfactory neurons has been disrupted. Normosmic IHH is rare and genetically heterogeneous, involving genes that regulate development and GnRH secretion or action.[94] A discussion of the genetic factors follows, categorized by hypothalamic or pituitary compartments, which is associated with both KS and normosmic IHH.

Hypothalamic Compartment

Kallman syndrome is five times more common in men than women, but while transmission may be X-linked recessive, this is not the exclusive mode of inheritance.[95] Five to ten percent of patients with KS have a KAL1 mutation.[94] *KAL1* encodes for an extracellular glycoprotein, anosmin1 and is located on the pseudoautosomal Xp region. Mutation in *KAL1* may be a gene deletion,[96,97] intragenic deletion[98] or point mutation.[99] In addition to hypogonadism and anosmia, other clinical features include synkinesia (up to 70%) and unilateral renal agenesis (30–50%).[95]

Ten to seventeen percent patients with the KS phenotype may have a deletion on chromosome 8 coding for the fibroblast growth factor receptor 1 (FGFR1, also known as KAL2).[92,100] At least 39 documented mutations in FGFR1 have been described.[101-103] Unlike *KAL1* mutations, loss of FGFR1 function may also be associated with normosmic IHH. Affected patients may have neurologic abnormalities and midline facial clefting defects.

PROK2 gene encodes prokineticin 2, a peptide that signals via a G-protein coupled receptor, PROKR2. Mutations in both PROK2 and PROKR2 have been identified in 9% of patients with KS but admittedly some mutations have been demonstrated in normal patients as well.[104]

Mutations in the G-protein coupled receptor 54 (GPR54) present in GnRH neurons have been identified as causative of autosomal recessive IHH.[105,106] Four mutations were identified in consanguineous families with multiple members affected by IHH. Kisspeptins (KISS1 being the first identified) are the endogenous ligand for GPR54.[107,108] Kisspeptins are present in the anteroventral periventricular and arcuate nuclei of the hypothalamus, which project into the preoptic area of the hypothalamus responsible for GnRH secretion. No mutations have been identified in kisspeptins but signaling is disrupted by mutations in the associated receptor GPR54.[109] Knockout mice for GPR54 maintain normal hypothalamic architecture but are hypogonadal.[106]

Leptin (LEP) is a protein secreted by white adipose tissue and important in regulating metabolism. Leptin binds a hypothalamic leptin receptor (LEPR) and may exert influence by acting on KISS1 neurons in the arcuate nucleus of the hypothalamus.[109,110] Leptin and LEPR mutations have been identified in studies of families where affected individuals presented with early onset obesity and IHH.[111-113] Hypogonadism from LEP

Table 2 Gene mutations associated with IHH

Gene	Gene Product	Phenotype of Mutation
KAL1	Anosmin1	Kallman syndrome
FGFR1 (KAL2)	Fibroblast growth factor receptor 1	Kallman syndrome or nIHH
PROK2/PROKR2	Prokineticin 2 and its receptor	Kallman syndrome or nIHH
GPR54	Kisspeptin receptor	nIHH
LEP/LEPR	Leptin and its receptor	Early onset obesity, nIHH
LHβ	Luteinizing hormone beta-subunit	Isolated LH inactivation, nIHH
FSHβ	Follicle stimulating hormone beta-subunit	Isolated FSH deficiency, nIHH
GNRHR	Gonadotropin releasing hormone receptor	nIHH
HESX1	Homeobox protein	Septo-optic dysplasia, nIHH
PROP1/LHX3/LHX4	Homeobox proteins	Combined pituitary hormone deficiency, short stature, nIHH
NROB1	DAX1	Congenital adrenal hypoplasia, nIHH

nIHH: normosmic IHH

gene defects can be overcome with exogenous GnRH, human chorionic gonadotropin (hCG)[112] or lEP[113] but no treatment exists for LEPR mutations.

Pituitary Compartment

Follicle-stimulating hormone, LH and thyroid stimulating hormone (TSH) are pituitary glycoprotein hormones which, along with hCG, are heterodimers with a common α subunit and a unique β subunit. The β subunit confers specificity of action. No mutations of the α subunit have been identified but β subunit mutations have been described in the gonadotropes.

While rare, several mutations in the LH beta-subunit (LHβ) gene have been identified resulting in impaired bioactivity of LH, although by different mechanisms. The *Q54R* mutation was present in a male with hypogonadism and elevated but biologically inactive LH due to impaired binding of the heterodimeric hormone to the receptor.[114] A *G36D* mutation on the other hand, resulted in IHH with low serum LH levels due to failure of alpha-beta heterodimerization.[115] There is one reported case of a woman with an inactivating LHβ mutation. This patient underwent normal pubertal development, followed by secondary amenorrhea and anovulation.[116]

Mutations in the FSH-β subunit mutations are also very rare. Males present with hypogonadism and azoospermia.[117] Females have partial or absent puberty and infertility.[117,118] While LH levels are concomitantly elevated, no hyperandrogenism or hirsutism is observed, as is the case in PCOS.

While no mutations have been identified in GnRH protein, mutation of the GnRH receptor (GNRHR) is a frequent cause of normosmic IHH with a prevalence of 3.5–10.6%.[119] Gonadotropin-releasing hormone receptor is a G-protein coupled receptor present on pituitary gonadotropes. Its stimulation by GnRH causes the release of FSH or LH via inositol triphosphate triggered intracytoplasmic calcium release.[93] At least 21 mutations have been described affecting all domains of the receptor (extracellular, transmembrane and intracellular).[93] The mode of transmission is autosomal recessive with heterozygotes being phenotypically normal. The two most common mutations are of Arg262Glu (15.2% alleles) and Glu206Arg (32.6% of alleles).[119]

During development, a complex process of activation and repression of genes encoding the homeobox class of transcription factors is essential for proper differentiation and proliferation of the specialized cell types of the anterior pituitary.[120] Mutations in a number of these genes (*HESX1*, *PROP1*, *LHX3* and *LHX4*) have been identified that result in a spectrum of phenotypes that can include hypogonadism. Inheritance of a homozygous *HESX1* mutation results in septo-optic dysplasia, a triad of agenesis of the corpus callosum, panhypopituitarism and optic nerve hypoplasia,[121] while heterozygotes have a milder phenotype of pituitary hypoplasia.[122] *PROP1*, *LHX3* and *LHX4* mutations result in combined pituitary hormone deficiency.[123-126] Short stature is a common feature due to deficient TSH and GH levels.[93]

Adrenal Compartment

The NROB 1 locus (discussed above Section II) codes for the protein DAX1. Males with *NROB1* mutation present with an X-linked congenital adrenal hypoplasia typically diagnosed in childhood[127] but occasionally later in life.[128] DAX1 regulates both hypothalamic and pituitary genes[129] and inhibits SF-1. Conditional knockout of NROB1 homolog in the mouse (Nrob1) results in spermatogenic disruption.[130]

Mutations in steroidogenic enzymes may affect gonadal function or development. Mutations in the P450 enzyme CYP17, with both 17-hydroxylase and 17,20-desmolase activity, results in deficiencies of androgens, progestins, and estrogen in both sexes. While glucocorticoids (cortisol) are also diminished, mineralocorticoid activity is exaggerated causing hypertension and hypokalemic alkalosis. Additionally, 46, XX CYP17 mutation homozygotes show absent breast development, primary amenorrhea, elevated gonadotropins and hypoplastic vagina, uterus and ovaries. Patients with a 46, XY CYP17 mutation have a similar phenotype, however, Müllerian derived structures are absent due to anti-Müllerian harmone (AMH) production by the testes and sexual ambiguity may be present if the deficiency is partial.[131]

Aromatase (CYP19) defects are autosomal recessive in inheritance. They are characterized by the inability to convert androgens to estrogen. The 46,XX female with such a deficiency has signs of virilization at birth (clitoromegaly) with intraabdominal ovaries. At puberty, multicystic ovaries develop in a clinical hypergonadotropic hypogonadal state. As such thelarche and menarche do not occur.[132] Interestingly, no disruption in spermatogenesis has been observed in men.[133] This is as opposed to defects in enzymes responsible for testosterone synthesis; 17 hydroxysteroid dehydrogenase 3 (HSD17B3)[134] and 5-α reductase 2 (SRD5A2).[135] These defects cause male feminization and infertility.

Congenital adrenal hyperplasia (CAH) is also a recognized cause of adrenal dysfunction and infertility. The classical 21-hydroxylase deficiency results in either a salt-wasting or simple virilizing phenotype. The milder, nonclassical phenotype manifests as infertility and hyperandrogenism, but without disruption of mineralocorticoids (aldosterone) or glucocorticoids (cortisol).[136] A more severe form of CAH is the result of a mutation of the steroidogenic acute regulatory protein. This mutation, while very rare, results in congenital lipoid hyperplasia with deficiency of all steroid hormones and an infantilized female phenotype. These patients are also prone to the development of ovarian cysts following puberty and primary ovarian insufficiency.[137]

Gonadal Compartment

Developmentally, expression of Wilms tumor 1 (WT1) is crucial to development of gonads. Mutations or deletions in the *WT1* gene (11p13) result in human genitourinary syndromes, such as Frasier syndrome,[138] Denys-Drash syndrome and WAGR syndrome.[139] Wilms tumor 1 is a key transcription factor with four zinc fingers with splice variants containing or missing a lysine-threonine-serine (KTS) between the third and fourth zinc fingers. Presence of KTS (WT+KTS) prevents binding of the fourth finger to DNA and decreases gene transcription.[140] WT(-KTS) mutations result in streak gonads due to increased apoptosis due to lack of regulation of steroidogenic factor 1 (SF-1)[141] and WT(+KTS) mutants showing male to female sex reversal due to reduced SRY and SOX9 expression. In XY gonads, WT1 acts downstream on sex-determining region of chromosome Y (SRY) to transiently increase protein expression. *SRY* activity upregulates expression of *SOX9* (SRY-box containing gene 9),[142,143] which encourages development of testes. Loss of function mutations of *SOX9* causes severe bone disease, campomelic dysplasia and male-to-female sexual reversal.[144,145]

The ovarian differentiation pathway downstream of SF-1 involves transcription of R-spondin homolog 1 (RSPO1). R-spondin homolog 1 induces WNT4, which in turn stimulates β-catenin[146] although RSPO1 can directly stimulate some β-catenin signaling.[147] WNT4 allows β-catenin to translocate to the nucleus where it causes transcription of genes, such as follistatin (FST).[148] β-catenin is a target of gonadal development as SOX9 binding causes their mutual degradation and SRY directly binds to and inhibits β-catenin transcription.[149,150] It therefore stands to reason that SOX9 over-expression causes XX female-to-male sex reversal[151] and loss of function RSPO1 mutations causes palmoplantar hyperkeratosis and phenotypic males, whether XX or XY.[152] β-catenin, therefore, acts as a major pro-ovary regulatory factor such that over-expression in mice results in XY male-to-female sex reversal[153] and conditional XX knockouts develop coelomic vessels in the gonads.[154]

Outflow Tract Compartment

The urogenital system arises early in embryogenesis and subsequently differentiates into male or female structures. In females, the müllerian ducts generate the fallopian tubes, uterus, cervix and upper vagina. Sex differentiation is dependent on the presence of the testis determining gene *SRY* (present either on the intact Y chromosome or translocated to an X chromosome). *SRY* presence promotes generation of the male gonadal cells (Sertoli and Leydig) via SOX9, as discussed above. *SOX9* binds to the AMH promoter on chromosome 19 to initiate transcription of its product AMH otherwise known as müllerian inhibiting substance (MIS). Müllerian inhibiting substance protein belongs to the TGFβ family and acts through two specific receptors to cause regression of müllerian structures. In testes, WT1 interacts with orphan nuclear receptor SF-1 (steroidogenic factor) to promote transcription of MIS. In the ovary DAX1 complexes with SF-1, thereby blocking the WT1/SF-1 and preventing induction of MIS.[155] Expression of MIS with an XX genotype results in absence of the müllerian structures, and Wolffian duct structures do not develop as they rely on the presence of testosterone.

Mayer-Rokitansky-Kuster-Hauser (MRKH) is a syndrome of müllerian agenesis in an otherwise phenotypically normal 46,XX female. Most cases of MRKH are sporadic but some families have shown clustering of related phenotypes. Multiple gene mutations have been proposed to result in this syndrome including CFTR mutation[156] and Wnt4a mutation as identified in one patient.[157] Murine experiments using mutants null for the *Wnt, Hox* and *Hox* cofactor genes have failed to generate a phenotype similar to MRKH. Mutational analysis of *WNT* genes in women with müllerian agenesis also failed to demonstrate a link[158] and so the elucidation of genetic causes of MRKH remains to be demonstrated.

Mutations in the *HOXA13* gene have been shown to cause the uterine abnormalities observed in hand-foot-genital syndrome.[159] This mutation is transmitted in an autosomal dominant manner, while not directly causative of infertility, may result in recurrent pregnancy loss (RPL) given abnormal uterine structure. The homeobox A genes *HOXA10* and *HOXA11* have also been demonstrated to be induced in the endometrium, upregulating factors conducive to implantation.[160] Such activity is believed to be orchestrated by steroid hormones acting via their receptors over the course of the menstrual cycle.

Studies have investigated the role of ovarian steroids on uterine receptivity and an emerging area of interest examines prostaglandins and lysophosphatidic acid (LPA). Lysophosphatidic acid has been shown to interact through five different receptors, of which the LPA3 receptor is crucial in implantation.[161] Lpa3 null (Lpa3 -/-) mice demonstrate reduced litter sizes and abnormal spacing of implantation sites with clustering close to the cervix.[161] This phenotype was accompanied by decreased levels of prostaglandin E2 (PGE2) and prostaglandin I2 (PGI2). The delayed implantation noted in Lpa3 null mice uteri can be overcome with exogenous prostaglandins but abnormal spacing is maintained. Lysophosphatidic acid is therefore postulated to influence normal uterine contractility and therefore is implicated in normal embryo spacing.[162] Human studies examining markers of uterine receptivity noted progesterone regulation of *LPA3, HOXA10*, glycodelin A and osteopondin.[163] In women with endometriosis, LPA3 expression decreased in the middle and late secretory phase.[163] Additionally, a role in placentation for LPA has been suggested through induction of IL-8[164] but more studies are needed.

Clinically, incomplete or inappropriate development of the vagina can be caused by loss of function mutations in steroid enzyme genes and disrupted gonadogenesis, as discussed in preceding sections. An important disruption that results in a blind ending vaginal pouch is that of the androgen receptor (AR) in genotypic males (46, XY).[165] Because the Y chromosome is intact, müllerian inhibiting substance/AMH is produced and müllerian regression ensues. At puberty, breasts develop but adrenarche is impaired even though testes (intra-abdominal or inguinal) may produce normal levels of testosterone. Various degrees of androgen insensitivity give a spectrum of phenotypes, generally caused by missense mutations of the androgen receptor.[166]

GENETICS IN THE EVALUATION OF THE INFERTILE COUPLE

Our understanding of the genes affecting fertility has dramatically improved following the sequencing of the human genome. Many genetic tests are now commercially available that can assist in exploring the causes of infertility and inform couples about risk for transmission of genetic abnormalities. There are heritable diseases that warrant screening in couples attempting conception (for example, Sickle Cell Anemia, Tay Sachs) based on family and personal history but these conditions will not be discussed here. Routine chromosomal screening in all couples presenting for an infertility evaluation is not, however, advocated so the question naturally arises: which patients should be selected for screening? A thorough medical and reproductive history and a physical exam are key components for directing diagnostic testing. A history of prior fertility and plausible cause for current infertility, such as chemotherapy or prolonged illness, make a genetic etiology less likely (Table 3).

Karyotype Analysis

The frequency of karyotype abnormalities in infertile men is about 7% and is inversely proportional to sperm count: 10–15% in azoospermic men, 5% in oligospermic men and less than 1% in normospermic men.[54] The diagnosis of nonobstructive azoospermia or severe oligospermia (less than 10 million/mL) warrants a peripheral blood karyotype, as well as testing for Y chromosome microdeletions (discussed above).[54] In women, karyotype analysis may be helpful or indicated in patients presenting with primary amenorrhea, premature ovarian failure and RPL.

Cystic Fibrosis Transmembrane Regulator Mutation

The findings of azoospermia combined with bilateral or unilateral absence of the vas deferens on physical exam strongly suggest a mutation in the cystic fibrosis transmembrane regulator (*CFTR*) gene and should prompt CF carrier screening for the female partner. Affecting approximately 1% of infertile males, this condition is characterized by dysplastic, atrophic or aplastic seminal vesicles leading to a low seminal pH (6.5) and low volume with absent sperm (azoospermia).[167] The *CFTR* gene coded on chromosome 7q regulates fluid secretions in the lung and pancreas. When two mutant alleles are inherited, males may develop clinical CF with systemic pulmonary and pancreatic disease or isolated CBAVD in an otherwise healthy appearing individual. A spectrum exists for *CFTR* mutation classified in severity from I to V and with as many as 1,000 abnormalities documented.[168] The most common mutation combination for *CFTR* is the ΔF508/5T[169] accounting for 66% of CF mutations but limiting testing to just this allele greatly decreases the sensitivity of testing. Many private mutations exist accounting for the remainder of *CFTR* mutations and these are differentially clustered based on the ethnicity of the population studied. For example, 25 different mutations account for more than 75% of CF in gateway nations like Spain, as opposed to the 10.2 mutations identified in mainland European countries where the population is more homogenous.[168] Expanded testing is therefore needed to identify compound heterozygotes for *CFTR* mutations who may have a mild phenotype but will transmit an affected allele to their offspring.[170] If CBAVD is identified in a man, expanded testing is indicated in his partner in order to appropriately counsel regarding the risks to future offspring. Due to the heterogeneity of mutations in the CFTR gene, screening must take into consideration: (1) the ethnic make-up of the individual being tested and, (2) the fact that two different (private) mutations may exist in carrier parents resulting in an affected offspring if both mutations are inherited. While sperm may be extracted from the testes (TESE) for ICSI, this intervention would directly transmit the gene to offspring.

Table 3 Considerations for genetic testing of infertile couples

Phenotype	Testing
Male	
Non-obstructive azoospermia or severe oligospermia (concentration < 10 million/mL)	Karyotype, Yq microdeletions
Azoospermia and congenital absence of the vas deferens (CAV)	Expanded CFTR carrier screening in female partner
Idiopathic hypogonadotropic hypogonadism	Consider mutations in KAL1, FGFR1, and GNRHR
Female	
Primary amenorrhea	Karyotype, FMR1 premutations
Premature ovarian failure	Karyotype, FMR1 premutations
Recurrent pregnancy loss	Karyotype
Idiopathic hypogonadotropic hypogonadism	Consider mutations in FGFR1 and GNRHR

Fragile X Mental Retardation 1 Screening

As noted above, premutation in the fragile X mental retardation (*FMR1*) gene is associated with diminished ovarian reserve and premature ovarian failure. The American Society for Reproductive Medicine Practice Committee opinion, as of 2008, does not support routine screening for *FMR1* mutation in women with infertility or diminished ovarian reserve under the age of 40. However, patients presenting with primary ovarian insufficiency (also known as premature ovarian failure) should be offered such testing, as the possibility exists that offspring or relatives may be at risk. The National Fragile X Foundation goes further to recommend that FMR1 screening be offered to all women with infertility (www.fragilex.org/testing.html). In females with diminished ovarian reserve, a detailed family history should be obtained to screen for fragile X associated tremor/ataxia syndrome, autism and mental retardation, all of which are associated with *FMR1* mutation. Genetic screening would be indicated to inform reproductive counseling for patients with a family history of *FMR1* gene mutation, undiagnosed mental retardation or a family history of primary ovarian insufficiency.[171] This gene mutation may worsen with subsequent generations.

Preimplantation Genetic Testing

Preimplantation genetic testing refers to the procedures for preconceptional genetic evaluation of embryos by evaluating polar bodies, blastomeres or trophectoderm[172] with the goal of transferring chromosomally normal embryos after *in vitro* fertilization (IVF). These procedures can be further categorized as preimplantation genetic diagnosis (PGD), for couples with a known genetic abnormality, or preimplantation genetic screening (PGS), for improving ART success in patients with underlying risk factors. Testing includes PCR for autosomal single gene mutations, X-linked single mutations or HLA matching. Flourescence *in situ* hybridization (FISH) is used to identify structural and numerical chromosomal abnormalities.

Preimplantation genetic diagnosis refers to testing of embryos prior to implantation for a known chromosomal abnormality due to a single gene mutation or structural chromosomal imbalances (translocations, inversions). Couples may or may not have the diagnosis of infertility. Biopsies are performed during embryo development. All patients opting for PGD screening should undergo genetic counseling, be informed of the risks associated with ART procedures and understand that a false negative rate exists. Further definitive testing, including chorionic villus sampling and amniocentesis, may be necessary prenatally. Even when known mutations exist, patients may opt to forgo PGD and proceed with use of their own undiagnosed gametes or avail themselves of donor gametes.[173]

Preimplantation Genetic Screening refers to preimplantation testing for aneuploidies in patients with underlying risk factors including advanced maternal age or a history of RPL with the intention of improving ART success. In most cases, selection of embryos for transfer relies on morphologic features alone. This unfortunately does not exclude the transfer of morphologically normal but chromosomally abnormal embryos. In PGS, chromosomal copy number can be evaluated by FISH but is usually limited to only testing of 9–11 chromosomes. Evaluation can be improved by use of CGH (see below) which has the capacity of evaluating all 23 chromosome pairs, but CGH requires 2–3 days for analysis.[174] Comparative genomic hybridization can detect aneuploidy in as many as 25% of embryos deemed normal by FISH.[175] The rate of aneuploidies among human embryos generated by IVF is estimated at 19.3–81%.[176] Aneuploidies may result from meiotic[177] or mitotic[178] events. As meiotic events precede fertilization, the embryo generated has an identical cell complement. Mitosis on the other hand, follows fertilization and may result in an unequal distribution of euploid and aneuploid cells in the resulting embryo or chromosomal mosaicism.[178-181] Evidence does not currently exist to support use of PGS to improve live birth rates in women with RPL,[182] advanced maternal age[183,184] nor repeated implantation failure,[185-187] but PGS may reduce the likelihood of miscarriage in selected couples.

When FISH was performed for homologues of human chromosomes 13, 16, 18 X and Y in rhesus monkey embryos, mosaicism was detected at a rate of 31.2%.[176] More importantly, the false negative rate was 23.1% with a single blastomere biopsy. These findings suggest that implantation failures or early pregnancy loss may be the result of embryonic mosaicism, which may escape conventional screening. Other limitations of FISH include technical difficulty of the slide fixation, potential hybridization failure and risk of overlapping or inadvertent split signals.[188]

Unexplained Miscarriage

While not a cause of infertility, unexplained miscarriage is common and involves a high frequency of genetic abnormalities. It is widely acknowledged that early pregnancy loss is most commonly associated with the presence of fetal aneuploidies. Among women with a history of RPL, euploid abort uses are more common.[189] Parental chromosomes are abnormal in approximately 5% of couples with RPL, with balanced translocations being the most common finding.[190] A discussion of this topic will be covered in detail in another chapter of this text.

THE FUTURE OF MOLECULAR AND GENETIC EVALUATION OF THE INFERTILE COUPLE

Polymerase Chain Reaction Based Strategies

Polymerase chain reaction is a method to exponentially amplify a particular DNA sequence by combining the sample DNA with target region complimentary DNA primers and DNA polymerase and then subjecting the sample to thermal cycling. Polymerase chain reaction-based whole genome amplification (WGA) is used to generate a representative amplification of the genomic DNA. Treff et al.[191] recently validated a protocol using PCR-based WGA combined with single nucleotide polymorphisms (SNP) genotyping arrays for single cell 24 chromosome aneuploidy screening for use with blastomeres, polar bodies or trophectoderm tissue. This analysis can be performed in a time frame that allows for fresh embryo transfer. The added advantage of this technique is that patients undergoing PGD for single gene disorders may screen the same embryo for chromosomal aneuploidy at the same time given that the testing is DNA-based.

Comparative Genomic Hybridization

Designed to screen the entire genome for variations in gene copy number, CGH first came to light in study of human tumors.[192] Stated simply, this methodology involves labeling of the test sample DNA and reference sample DNA with fluorescence tags. Repetitive sequences are silenced with cot-1 DNA, which is unlabeled human placental DNA enriched for repetitive sequences. Both genomic samples are then hybridized to a representation of the whole genome represented as all the chromosomes or to defined DNA probes. This allows for detection of binding of test and reference samples to several loci in the genome. If the reference sequence is identical to the genome, all signals are normalized to 1.0 (on a linear scale) or 0.0 (on a logarithmic scale) so that test sequence increase in copy number are greater than the reference point and deletions are less.[193] The accuracy of CGH increases with the amount of test DNA available which is a limitation in its use for PGD as the quantity of available DNA is typically very limited. This may be circumvented by use of PCR for DNA amplification. As the technology improves and smaller changes are detected, whole genomic screening may find variations which are yet to be classified as normal or resulting in phenotypic abnormality. Since the resolution of CGH is superior to standard karyotype analysis, it is logical to assume that in the future CGH will replace karyotype assessment for many fertility-related conditions, for instance RPL.

Single Nucleotide Polymorphism Microarrays

Single nucleotide polymorphism microarray technology has recently been used to establish the rates of aneuploidy when compared to traditionally used FISH.[194] Hundred percent sampling of embryos with blastomere randomized to FISH or SNP microarray, showed a 31% rate of mosaicism in contrast to 100% by FISH. Importantly, follow up studies examining a known balanced translocation and associated microdeletion supports the use of SNP microarray in identifying normal embryos.[195] This study also noted 100% consistency between FISH and microarray for assessing targeted regions, but FISH failed to identify a monosomy detected on comprehensive SNP microarray. In a more expanded role, SNP microarray-based haplotyping might also be used to detect chromosomal abnormalities in phenotypically normal carriers of translocations.[196] This method of screening has the potential to improve pregnancy rates and reduce miscarriage.

Epigenetics and Reproduction

Non-DNA sequence alterations in the genome are known to occur during folliculogenesis for female germ cells (oocytes)[197-199] and embryogenesis in male germ cells (spermatogonia).[200-202] As such alterations in both these processes as with ART, may result in epigenetic changes which may as yet undiscovered.[203] Though not thoroughly understood, toxicants, such as vinclozolin have been shown to have transgenerational effects in rats exposed *in utero* during critical stages in development.[204] Such effects persisted for up to four generations[204] and included adult onset diseases, such as infertility, tumors, prostate disease, kidney diseases and immune abnormalitites.[205] Such studies highlight the need for further examination of epigenetic changes that may not only impact on embryo survival but also the health of the generated offspring especially later in life. Because epigenetic changes may be the result of isolated events *in utero* or due to persistent exposure during growth and development, Geurrero-Bosagna and Skinner[206] proposed the terms intrinsic epigenetic transgenerational process for the former and extrinsic epigenetic transgenerational process to refer to the latter. The relevance of epigenetics to reproduction is evolving rapidly and warrants close observation.

Sequencing for Everyone?

The utility of each of the outlined techniques is reliant on the ability to link genotypic differences to a specific phenotype. In the future, rare phenotypes may be queried genotypically against the established background for putative target sequences causing such manifestations. While sequencing for infertile couples is not recommended at the moment, as technology improves, sequencing of the individual genome may play a greater role in the infertility evaluation.

CONCLUSION

Infertility can result from genetic abnormalities acquired during gametogenesis, embryogenesis or during development of relevant organ systems. Through a variety of methods, genetic causes of infertility have been identified. However, genome-wide strategies may need to be employed in order to identify genes causative of phenotypes with clinical implications, such as RPL. The standard strategy is to work from an established phenotype back to a causative gene, but the new high-throughput and next generation sequencing technologies may change this paradigm. Appreciation for the subtleties of genomic modification, or epigenetics, may increasingly be useful in identifying risk factors for infertility. New understanding and technology will likely expand the current genetic evaluation of couples with infertility resulting in improved diagnosis and treatment.

ACKNOWLEDGMENTS

Special thanks to Dr Alan DeCherney for critical support and guidance.

REFERENCES

1. Redon R, Ishikawa S, Fitch KR, et al. Global variation in copy number in the human genome. Nature. 2006;444(7118):444-54.
2. Flores M, Morales L, Gonzaga-Jauregui C, et al. Recurrent DNA inversion rearrangements in the human genome. Proc Natl Acad Sci USA. 2007;104(15):6099-106.
3. Korbel JO, Urban AE, Affourtit JP, et al. Paired-end mapping reveals extensive structural variation in the human genome. Science. 2007;318(5849):420-6.
4. Fruhmesser A, Kotzot D. Chromosomal variants in klinefelter syndrome. Sex Dev. 2011;5(3):109-23.
5. Layman LC, Reindollar RH. Diagnosis and treatment of pubertal disorders. Adolesc Med. 1994;5(1):37-56.
6. Simpson JL, Rajkovic A. Ovarian differentiation and gonadal failure. Am J Med Genet. 1999;89(4):186-200.
7. Vogt PH, Edelmann A, Kirsch S, et al. Human Y chromosome azoospermia factors (AZF) mapped to different subregions in Yq11. Hum Mol Genet. 1996;5(7):933-43.
8. Repping S, Skaletsky H, Lange J, et al. Recombination between palindromes P5 and P1 on the human Y chromosome causes massive deletions and spermatogenic failure. Am J Hum Genet. 2002;71(4):906-22.
9. Zanaria E, Muscatelli F, Bardoni B, et al. An unusual member of the nuclear hormone receptor superfamily responsible for X-linked adrenal hypoplasia congenita. Nature. 1994;372(6507):635-41.
10. Mantovani G, Mancini M, Gazzano G, et al. Somatic mutational analysis of DAX1 in testes from men with idiopathic azoospermia. Fertil Steril. 2005;84(5):1542-4.
11. Achermann JC, Gu WX, Kotlar TJ, et al. Mutational analysis of DAX1 in patients with hypogonadotropic hypogonadism or pubertal delay. J Clin Endocrinol Metab. 1999;84(12):4497-500.
12. Wittenberger MD, Hagerman RJ, Sherman SL, et al. The FMR1 premutation and reproduction. Fertil Steril. 2007;87(3):456-65.
13. Pieretti M, Zhang FP, Fu YH, et al. Absence of expression of the FMR-1 gene in fragile X syndrome. Cell. 1991;66(4):817-22.

14. Verkerk AJ, Pieretti M, Sutcliffe JS, et al. Identification of a gene (FMR-1) containing a CGG repeat coincident with a breakpoint cluster region exhibiting length variation in fragile X syndrome. Cell. 1991;65(5):905-14.
15. Zalfa F, Giorgi M, Primerano B, et al. The fragile X syndrome protein FMRP associates with BC1 RNA and regulates the translation of specific mRNAs at synapses. Cell. 2003;112(3):317-27.
16. Turner DJ, Miretti M, Rajan D, et al. Germline rates of de novo meiotic deletions and duplications causing several genomic disorders. Nat Genet. 2008;40(1):90-5.
17. Schnieders F, Dork T, Arnemann J, et al. Testis-specific protein, Y-encoded (TSPY) expression in testicular tissues. Hum Mol Genet. 1996;5(11):1801-7.
18. Giachini C, Nuti F, Turner DJ, et al. TSPY1 copy number variation influences spermatogenesis and shows differences among Y lineages. J Clin Endocrinol Metab. 2009;94(10):4016-22.
19. Mathias N, Bayes M, Tyler-Smith C. Highly informative compound haplotypes for the human Y chromosome. Hum Mol Genet. 1994;3(1):115-23.
20. Repping S, van Daalen SK, Brown LG, et al. High mutation rates have driven extensive structural polymorphism among human Y chromosomes. Nat Genet. 2006;38(4):463-7.
21. Vodicka R, Vrtel R, Dusek L, et al. TSPY gene copy number as a potential new risk factor for male infertility. Reprod Biomed Online. 2007;14(5):579-87.
22. Segars JH, DeCherney AH. Is there a genetic basis for polycystic ovary syndrome? J Clin Endocrinol Metab. 2010;95(5):2058-60.
23. Luense LJ, Carletti MZ, Christenson LK. Role of Dicer in female fertility. Trends Endocrinol Metab. 2009;20(6):265-72.
24. Bartel DP. MicroRNAs: genomics, biogenesis, mechanism, and function. Cell. 2004;116(2):281-97.
25. Bagga S, Bracht J, Hunter S, et al. Regulation by let-7 and lin-4 miRNAs results in target mRNA degradation. Cell. 2005;122(4):553-63.
26. Wu L, Fan J, Belasco JG. MicroRNAs direct rapid deadenylation of mRNA. Proc Natl Acad Sci USA. 2006;103(11):4034-9.
27. Place RF, Li LC, Pookot D, et al. MicroRNA-373 induces expression of genes with complementary promoter sequences. Proc Natl Acad Sci USA. 2008;105(5):1608-13.
28. Berger SL, Kouzarides T, Shiekhattar R, et al. An operational definition of epigenetics. Genes Dev. 2009;23(7):781-3.
29. Holliday R, Pugh JE. DNA modification mechanisms and gene activity during development. Science. 1975;187(4173):226-32.
30. Margueron R, Trojer P, Reinberg D. The key to development: interpreting the histone code? Curr Opin Genet Dev. Apr 2005;15(2):163-76.
31. Leonhardt H, Page AW, Weier HU, et al. A targeting sequence directs DNA methyltransferase to sites of DNA replication in mammalian nuclei. Cell. 1992;71(5):865-73.
32. Smith SS, Kaplan BE, Sowers LC, et al. Mechanism of human methyl-directed DNA methyltransferase and the fidelity of cytosine methylation. Proc Natl Acad Sci USA. 1992;89(10):4744-8.
33. Bestor T, Laudano A, Mattaliano R, et al. Cloning and sequencing of a cDNA encoding DNA methyltransferase of mouse cells. The carboxyl-terminal domain of the mammalian enzymes is related to bacterial restriction methyltransferases. J Mol Biol. 1988;203(4):971-83.
34. Kaneda M, Okano M, Hata K, et al. Essential role for de novo DNA methyltransferase Dnmt3a in paternal and maternal imprinting. Nature. 2004;429(6994):900-3.
35. Naveh-Many T, Cedar H. Active gene sequences are undermethylated. Proc Natl Acad Sci USA. 1981;78(7):4246-50.
36. Waechter DE, Baserga R. Effect of methylation on expression of microinjected genes. Proc Natl Acad Sci USA. 1982;79(4):1106-10.
37. Craig JM. Heterochromatin--many flavours, common themes. Bioessays. 2005;27(1):17-28.
38. Wallace JA, Orr-Weaver TL. Replication of heterochromatin: insights into mechanisms of epigenetic inheritance. Chromosoma. 2005;114(6):389-402.
39. Dong J, Albertini DF, Nishimori K, et al. Growth differentiation factor-9 is required during early ovarian folliculogenesis. Nature. 10 1996;383(6600):531-5.
40. Vitt UA, McGee EA, Hayashi M, et al. In vivo treatment with GDF-9 stimulates primordial and primary follicle progression and theca cell marker CYP17 in ovaries of immature rats. Endocrinology. 2000;141(10):3814-20.
41. Atkinson C, Stewart S, Upton PD, et al. Primary pulmonary hypertension is associated with reduced pulmonary vascular expression of type II bone morphogenetic protein receptor. Circulation. 2002;105(14):1672-8.
42. Aittomaki K, Lucena JL, Pakarinen P, et al. Mutation in the follicle-stimulating hormone receptor gene causes hereditary hypergonadotropic ovarian failure. Cell. 1995;82(6):959-68.
43. Beau I, Touraine P, Meduri G, et al. A novel phenotype related to partial loss of function mutations of the follicle stimulating hormone receptor. J Clin Invest. 1998;102(7):1352-9.
44. Toledo SP, Brunner HG, Kraaij R, et al. An inactivating mutation of the luteinizing hormone receptor causes amenorrhea in a 46,XX female. J Clin Endocrinol Metab. 1996;81(11):3850-4.
45. Wu SM, Leschek EW, Rennert OM, et al. Luteinizing hormone receptor mutations in disorders of sexual development and cancer. Front Biosci. Mar 1 2000;5:D343-352.
46. Beall S, Brenner C, Segars J. Oocyte maturation failure: a syndrome of bad eggs. Fertil Steril. 2010;94(7):2507-13.
47. Bar-Ami S, Zlotkin E, Brandes JM, et al. Failure of meiotic competence in human oocytes. Biol Reprod. 1994;50(5):1100-7.
48. Avrech OM, Goldman GA, Rufas O, et al. Treatment variables in relation to oocyte maturation: lessons from a clinical micromanipulation-assisted in vitro fertilization program. J Assist Reprod Genet. 1997;14(6):337-42.
49. Lincoln AJ, Wickramasinghe D, Stein P, et al. Cdc25b phosphatase is required for resumption of meiosis during oocyte maturation. Nat Genet. 2002;30(4):446-9.

50. Masciarelli S, Horner K, Liu C, et al. Cyclic nucleotide phosphodiesterase 3A-deficient mice as a model of female infertility. J Clin Invest. 2004;114(2):196-205.
51. Woods LM, Hodges CA, Baart E, et al. Chromosomal influence on meiotic spindle assembly: abnormal meiosis I in female Mlh1 mutant mice. J Cell Biol. 1999;145(7):1395-1406.
52. Revenkova E, Eijpe M, Heyting C, et al. Cohesin SMC1 beta is required for meiotic chromosome dynamics, sister chromatid cohesion and DNA recombination. Nat Cell Biol. 2004;6(6):555-62.
53. Lipkin SM, Moens PB, Wang V, et al. Meiotic arrest and aneuploidy in MLH3-deficient mice. Nat Genet. 2002;31(4):385-90.
54. Report on optimal evaluation of the infertile male. Fertil Steril. 2006;86(5 Suppl 1):S202-9.
55. Foresta C, Moro E, Ferlin A. Y chromosome microdeletions and alterations of spermatogenesis. Endocr Rev. 2001;22(2):226-39.
56. Pryor JL, Kent-First M, Muallem A, et al. Microdeletions in the Y chromosome of infertile men. N Engl J Med. 1997;336(8):534-9.
57. McLachlan RI, O'Bryan MK. Clinical Review#: State of the art for genetic testing of infertile men. J Clin Endocrinol Metab. 2010;95(3):1013-24.
58. Hopps CV, Mielnik A, Goldstein M, et al. Detection of sperm in men with Y chromosome microdeletions of the AZFa, AZFb and AZFc regions. Hum Reprod. 2003;18(8):1660-5.
59. Cram DS, Ma K, Bhasin S, et al. Y chromosome analysis of infertile men and their sons conceived through intracytoplasmic sperm injection: vertical transmission of deletions and rarity of de novo deletions. Fertil Steril. 2000;74(5):909-15.
60. Kamp C, Hirschmann P, Voss H, et al. Two long homologous retroviral sequence blocks in proximal Yq11 cause AZFa microdeletions as a result of intrachromosomal recombination events. Hum Mol Genet. 2000;9(17):2563-72.
61. Luddi A, Margollicci M, Gambera L, et al. Spermatogenesis in a man with complete deletion of USP9Y. N Engl J Med. 2009;360(9):881-5.
62. Kuroda-Kawaguchi T, Skaletsky H, Brown LG, et al. The AZFc region of the Y chromosome features massive palindromes and uniform recurrent deletions in infertile men. Nat Genet. 2001;29(3):279-86.
63. Vogt PH, Falcao CL, Hanstein R, et al. The AZF proteins. Int J Androl. 2008;31(4):383-94.
64. Yen PH. Putative biological functions of the DAZ family. Int J Androl. 2004;27(3):125-9.
65. Lahn BT, Tang ZL, Zhou J, et al. Previously uncharacterized histone acetyltransferases implicated in mammalian spermatogenesis. Proc Natl Acad Sci USA. 2002;99(13):8707-12.
66. Repping S, Skaletsky H, Brown L, et al. Polymorphism for a 1.6-Mb deletion of the human Y chromosome persists through balance between recurrent mutation and haploid selection. Nat Genet. 2003;35(3):247-51.
67. Visser L, Westerveld GH, Korver CM, et al. Y chromosome gr/gr deletions are a risk factor for low semen quality. Hum Reprod. 2009;24(10):2667-73.
68. Tapanainen JS, Aittomaki K, Min J, et al. Men homozygous for an inactivating mutation of the follicle-stimulating hormone (FSH) receptor gene present variable suppression of spermatogenesis and fertility. Nat Genet. 1997;15(2):205-6.
69. Gromoll J, Simoni M, Nieschlag E. An activating mutation of the follicle-stimulating hormone receptor autonomously sustains spermatogenesis in a hypophysectomized man. J Clin Endocrinol Metab. 1996;81(4):1367-70.
70. Kremer H, Kraaij R, Toledo SP, et al. Male pseudohermaphroditism due to a homozygous missense mutation of the luteinizing hormone receptor gene. Nat Genet. 1995;9(2):160-4.
71. Li X. Extending the maternal-zygotic effect with genomic imprinting. Mol Hum Reprod. 2010;16(9):695-703.
72. Tong ZB, Bondy CA, Zhou J, et al. A human homologue of mouse Mater, a maternal effect gene essential for early embryonic development. Hum Reprod. 2002;17(4):903-11.
73. Morisato D, Anderson KV. Signaling pathways that establish the dorsal-ventral pattern of the Drosophila embryo. Annu Rev Genet. 1995;29:371-99.
74. Newport J, Kirschner M. A major developmental transition in early Xenopus embryos: I. characterization and timing of cellular changes at the midblastula stage. Cell. 1982;30(3):675-86.
75. Tong ZB, Gold L, Pfeifer KE, et al. Mater, a maternal effect gene required for early embryonic development in mice. Nat Genet. 2000;26(3):267-8.
76. Wu X, Viveiros MM, Eppig JJ, et al. Zygote arrest 1 (Zar1) is a novel maternal-effect gene critical for the oocyte-to-embryo transition. Nat Genet. 2003;33(2):187-91.
77. Bortvin A, Goodheart M, Liao M, et al. Dppa3 / Pgc7 / stella is a maternal factor and is not required for germ cell specification in mice. BMC Dev Biol. 2004;4:2.
78. Burns KH, Viveiros MM, Ren Y, et al. Roles of NPM2 in chromatin and nucleolar organization in oocytes and embryos. Science. 2003;300(5619):633-6.
79. Christians E, Davis AA, Thomas SD, et al. Maternal effect of Hsf1 on reproductive success. Nature. 2000;407(6805):693-4.
80. Tashiro F, Kanai-Azuma M, Miyazaki S, et al. Maternal-effect gene Ces5/Ooep/Moep19/Floped is essential for oocyte cytoplasmic lattice formation and embryonic development at the maternal-zygotic stage transition. Genes Cells. 2010;15(8):813-28.
81. Li L, Baibakov B, Dean J. A subcortical maternal complex essential for preimplantation mouse embryogenesis. Dev Cell. 2008;15(3):416-25.
82. Yurttas P, Vitale AM, Fitzhenry RJ, et al. Role for PADI6 and the cytoplasmic lattices in ribosomal storage in oocytes and translational control in the early mouse embryo. Development. 2008;135(15):2627-36.
83. Torres-Padilla ME, Zernicka-Goetz M. Role of TIF1alpha as a modulator of embryonic transcription in the mouse zygote. J Cell Biol. 2006;174(3):329-38.

84. Maraldi T, Riccio M, Sena P, et al. MATER protein as substrate of PKCepsilon in human cumulus cells. Mol Hum Reprod. 2009;15(8):499-506.
85. Neumann B, Kubicka P, Barlow DP. Characteristics of imprinted genes. Nat Genet. 1995;9(1):12-3.
86. Li E, Beard C, Jaenisch R. Role for DNA methylation in genomic imprinting. Nature. 1993;366(6453):362-5.
87. Maher ER. Imprinting and assisted reproductive technology. Hum Mol Genet. 2005;14 Spec No 1:R133-8.
88. Manipalviratn S, DeCherney A, Segars J. Imprinting disorders and assisted reproductive technology. Fertil Steril. 2009;91(2):305-15.
89. Clayton-Smith J, Laan L. Angelman syndrome: a review of the clinical and genetic aspects. J Med Genet. 2003;40(2):87-95.
90. Ludwig M, Katalinic A, Gross S, et al. Increased prevalence of imprinting defects in patients with Angelman syndrome born to subfertile couples. J Med Genet. 2005;42(4):289-91.
91. Doornbos ME, Maas SM, McDonnell J, et al. Infertility, assisted reproduction technologies and imprinting disturbances: a Dutch study. Hum Reprod. 2007;22(9):2476-80.
92. Silveira LF, Trarbach EB, Latronico AC. Genetics basis for GnRH-dependent pubertal disorders in humans. Mol Cell Endocrinol. 2010;324(1-2):30-8.
93. Bhagavath B, Layman LC. The genetics of hypogonadotropic hypogonadism. Semin Reprod Med. 2007;25(4):272-86.
94. Bianco SD, Kaiser UB. The genetic and molecular basis of idiopathic hypogonadotropic hypogonadism. Nat Rev Endocrinol. 2009;5(10):569-76.
95. Topaloglu AK, Kotan LD. Molecular causes of hypogonadotropic hypogonadism. Curr Opin Obstet Gynecol. 2010;22(4):264-70.
96. Franco B, Guioli S, Pragliola A, et al. A gene deleted in Kallmann's syndrome shares homology with neural cell adhesion and axonal path-finding molecules. Nature. Oct. 1991;353(6344):529-36.
97. Legouis R, Hardelin JP, Levilliers J, et al. The candidate gene for the X-linked Kallmann syndrome encodes a protein related to adhesion molecules. Cell. 1991;67(2):423-35.
98. Bick D, Franco B, Sherins RJ, et al. Brief report: intragenic deletion of the KALIG-1 gene in Kallmann's syndrome. N Engl J Med. 1992;326(26):1752-5.
99. Hardelin JP, Levilliers J, Blanchard S, et al. Heterogeneity in the mutations responsible for X chromosome-linked Kallmann syndrome. Hum Mol Genet. 1993;2(4):373-7.
100. Dode C, Levilliers J, Dupont JM, et al. Loss-of-function mutations in FGFR1 cause autosomal dominant Kallmann syndrome. Nat Genet. 2003;33(4):463-5.
101. Albuisson J, Pecheux C, Carel JC, et al. Kallmann syndrome: 14 novel mutations in KAL1 and FGFR1 (KAL2). Hum Mutat. 2005;25(1):98-9.
102. Sato N, Katsumata N, Kagami M, et al. Clinical assessment and mutation analysis of Kallmann syndrome 1 (KAL1) and fibroblast growth factor receptor 1 (FGFR1, or KAL2) in 5 families and 18 sporadic patients. J Clin Endocrinol Metab. 2004;89(3):1079-88.
103. Pitteloud N, Meysing A, Quinton R, et al. Mutations in fibroblast growth factor receptor 1 cause Kallmann syndrome with a wide spectrum of reproductive phenotypes. Mol Cell Endocrinol. 2006;254-255:60-9.
104. Monnier C, Dode C, Fabre L, et al. PROKR2 missense mutations associated with Kallmann syndrome impair receptor signalling activity. Hum Mol Genet. 2009;18(1):75-81.
105. de Roux N, Genin E, Carel JC, et al. Hypogonadotropic hypogonadism due to loss of function of the KiSS1-derived peptide receptor GPR54. Proc Natl Acad Sci USA. 2003;100(19):10972-6.
106. Seminara SB, Messager S, Chatzidaki EE, et al. The GPR54 gene as a regulator of puberty. N Engl J Med. 2003;349(17):1614-27.
107. Ohtaki T, Shintani Y, Honda S, et al. Metastasis suppressor gene KiSS-1 encodes peptide ligand of a G-protein-coupled receptor. Nature. 2001;411 (6837):613-7.
108. Kotani M, Detheux M, Vandenbogaerde A, et al. The metastasis suppressor gene KiSS-1 encodes kisspeptins, the natural ligands of the orphan G protein-coupled receptor GPR54. J Biol Chem. 2001;276(37):34631-6.
109. Smith JT, Clifton DK, Steiner RA. Regulation of the neuroendocrine reproductive axis by kisspeptin-GPR54 signaling. Reproduction. 2006;131(4):623-30.
110. Smith JT, Acohido BV, Clifton DK, et al. KiSS-1 neurones are direct targets for leptin in the ob/ob mouse. J Neuroendocrinol. 2006;18(4):298-303.
111. Clement K, Vaisse C, Lahlou N, et al. A mutation in the human leptin receptor gene causes obesity and pituitary dysfunction. Nature. 1998;392(6674):398-401.
112. Strobel A, Issad T, Camoin L, et al. A leptin missense mutation associated with hypogonadism and morbid obesity. Nat Genet. 1998;18(3):213-5.
113. Licinio J, Caglayan S, Ozata M, et al. Phenotypic effects of leptin replacement on morbid obesity, diabetes mellitus, hypogonadism, and behavior in leptin-deficient adults. Proc Natl Acad Sci USA. 2004;101(13):4531-6.
114. Weiss J, Axelrod L, Whitcomb RW, et al. Hypogonadism caused by a single amino acid substitution in the beta subunit of luteinizing hormone. N Engl J Med. 1992;326(3):179-83.
115. Valdes-Socin H, Salvi R, Daly AF, et al. Hypogonadism in a patient with a mutation in the luteinizing hormone beta-subunit gene. N Engl J Med. 2004;351(25):2619-25.
116. Lofrano-Porto A, Barra GB, Giacomini LA, et al. Luteinizing hormone beta mutation and hypogonadism in men and women. N Engl J Med. 2007;357(9):897-904.
117. Layman LC, Porto AL, Xie J, et al. FSH beta gene mutations in a female with partial breast development and a male sibling with normal puberty and azoospermia. J Clin Endocrinol Metab. 2002;87(8):3702-7.
118. Matthews CH, Borgato S, Beck-Peccoz P, et al. Primary amenorrhoea and infertility due to a mutation in the beta-subunit of follicle-stimulating hormone. Nat Genet. 1993;5(1):83-6.
119. Bhagavath B, Ozata M, Ozdemir IC, et al. The prevalence of gonadotropin-releasing hormone receptor mutations in a large cohort of patients with hypogonadotropic hypogonadism. Fertil Steril. 2005;84(4):951-7.

120. Quirk J, Brown P. Hesx1 homeodomain protein represses transcription as a monomer and antagonises transactivation of specific sites as a homodimer. J Mol Endocrinol. 2002;28(3):193-205.
121. Dattani MT, Martinez-Barbera JP, Thomas PQ, et al. Mutations in the homeobox gene HESX1/Hesx1 associated with septo-optic dysplasia in human and mouse. Nat Genet. 1998;19(2):125-33.
122. Thomas PQ, Dattani MT, Brickman JM, et al. Heterozygous HESX1 mutations associated with isolated congenital pituitary hypoplasia and septo-optic dysplasia. Hum Mol Genet. 2001;10(1):39-45.
123. Kim SS, Kim Y, Shin YL, et al. Clinical characteristics and molecular analysis of PIT1, PROP1,LHX3, and HESX1 in combined pituitary hormone deficiency patients with abnormal pituitary MR imaging. Horm Res. 2003;60(6):277-83.
124. Netchine I, Sobrier ML, Krude H, et al. Mutations in LHX3 result in a new syndrome revealed by combined pituitary hormone deficiency. Nat Genet. 2000;25(2):182-6.
125. Sloop KW, Parker GE, Hanna KR, et al. LHX3 transcription factor mutations associated with combined pituitary hormone deficiency impair the activation of pituitary target genes. Gene. 2001;265(1-2):61-9.
126. Machinis K, Pantel J, Netchine I, et al. Syndromic short stature in patients with a germline mutation in the LIM homeobox LHX4. Am J Hum Genet. 2001;69(5):961-8.
127. Muscatelli F, Strom TM, Walker AP, et al. Mutations in the DAX-1 gene give rise to both X-linked adrenal hypoplasia congenita and hypogonadotropic hypogonadism. Nature. 1994;372(6507):672-6.
128. Mantovani G, Ozisik G, Achermann JC, et al. Hypogonadotropic hypogonadism as a presenting feature of late-onset X-linked adrenal hypoplasia congenita. J Clin Endocrinol Metab. 2002;87(1):44-8.
129. Achermann JC. The role of SF1/DAX1 in adrenal and reproductive function. Ann Endocrinol (Paris). 2005;66(3):233-9.
130. Yu RN, Ito M, Saunders TL, et al. Role of Ahch in gonadal development and gametogenesis. Nat Genet. 1998;20(4):353-7.
131. Yanase T, Simpson ER, Waterman MR. 17 alpha-hydroxylase/17,20-lyase deficiency: from clinical investigation to molecular definition. Endocr Rev. 1991;12(1):91-108.
132. Ito Y, Fisher CR, Conte FA, et al. Molecular basis of aromatase deficiency in an adult female with sexual infantilism and polycystic ovaries. Proc Natl Acad Sci USA. 1993;90(24):11673-7.
133. Bulun SE. Aromatase deficiency and estrogen resistance: from molecular genetics to clinic. Semin Reprod Med. 2000;18(1):31-9.
134. Geissler WM, Davis DL, Wu L, et al. Male pseudohermaphroditism caused by mutations of testicular 17 beta-hydroxysteroid dehydrogenase 3. Nat Genet. 1994;7(1):34-9.
135. Andersson S, Berman DM, Jenkins EP, et al. Deletion of steroid 5 alpha-reductase 2 gene in male pseudohermaphroditism. Nature. 1991;354(6349):159-61.
136. Jaaskelainen J, Tiitinen A, Voutilainen R. Sexual function and fertility in adult females and males with congenital adrenal hyperplasia. Horm Res. 2001;56(3-4):73-80.
137. Bhangoo A, Buyuk E, Oktay K, et al. Phenotypic features of 46, XX females with StAR protein mutations. Pediatr Endocrinol Rev. 2007;5(2):633-41.
138. Barbaux S, Niaudet P, Gubler MC, et al. Donor splice-site mutations in WT1 are responsible for Frasier syndrome. Nat Genet. 1997;17(4):467-70.
139. Le Caignec C, Delnatte C, Vermeesch JR, et al. Complete sex reversal in a WAGR syndrome patient. Am J Med Genet A. 2007;143A(22):2692-5.
140. Laity JH, Dyson HJ, Wright PE. Molecular basis for modulation of biological function by alternate splicing of the Wilms' tumor suppressor protein. Proc Natl Acad Sci USA. 2000;97(22):11932-5.
141. Wilhelm D, Englert C. The Wilms tumor suppressor WT1 regulates early gonad development by activation of Sf1. Genes Dev. 2002;16(14):1839-51.
142. Jakob S, Lovell-Badge R. Sex determination and the control of Sox9 expression in mammals. FEBS J. 2011;278(7):1002-9.
143. Sekido R, Bar I, Narvaez V, et al. SOX9 is up-regulated by the transient expression of SRY specifically in Sertoli cell precursors. Dev Biol. 2004;274(2):271-9.
144. Foster JW, Dominguez-Steglich MA, Guioli S, et al. Campomelic dysplasia and autosomal sex reversal caused by mutations in an SRY-related gene. Nature. 1994;372(6506):525-30.
145. Wagner T, Wirth J, Meyer J, et al. Autosomal sex reversal and campomelic dysplasia are caused by mutations in and around the SRY-related gene SOX9. Cell. 1994;79(6):1111-20.
146. Binnerts ME, Kim KA, Bright JM, et al. R-Spondin1 regulates Wnt signaling by inhibiting internalization of LRP6. Proc Natl Acad Sci USA. 2007;104(37):14700-5.
147. Wei Q, Yokota C, Semenov MV, et al. R-spondin1 is a high affinity ligand for LRP6 and induces LRP6 phosphorylation and beta-catenin signaling. J Biol Chem. 2007;282(21):15903-11.
148. Yao HH, Matzuk MM, Jorgez CJ, et al. Follistatin operates downstream of Wnt4 in mammalian ovary organogenesis. Dev Dyn. 2004;230(2):210-5.
149. Bernard P, Sim H, Knower K, et al. Human SRY inhibits beta-catenin-mediated transcription. Int J Biochem Cell Biol. 2008;40(12):2889-2900.
150. Bernard P, Fleming A, Lacombe A, et al. Wnt4 inhibits beta-catenin/TCF signalling by redirecting beta-catenin to the cell membrane. Biol Cell. 2008;100(3):167-77.
151. Huang B, Wang S, Ning Y, et al. Autosomal XX sex reversal caused by duplication of SOX9. Am J Med Genet. 1999;87(4):349-53.
152. Parma P, Radi O, Vidal V, et al. R-spondin1 is essential in sex determination, skin differentiation and malignancy. Nat Genet. 2006;38(11):1304-9.
153. Maatouk DM, DiNapoli L, Alvers A, et al. Stabilization of beta-catenin in XY gonads causes male-to-female sex-reversal. Hum Mol Genet. 2008;17(19):2949-55.

154. Liu CF, Bingham N, Parker K, et al. Sex-specific roles of beta-catenin in mouse gonadal development. Hum Mol Genet. 2009;18(3):405-17.
155. Christopoulos P, Gazouli M, Fotopoulou G, et al. The role of genes in the development of Mullerian anomalies: where are we today? Obstet Gynecol Surv. 2009;64(11):760-8.
156. Cheroki C, Krepischi-Santos AC, Szuhai K, et al. Genomic imbalances associated with mullerian aplasia. J Med Genet. 2008;45(4):228-32.
157. Biason-Lauber A, Konrad D, Navratil F, et al. A Wnt4 mutation associated with Mullerian-duct regression and virilization in a 46,XX woman. N Engl J Med. 2004;351(8):792-8.
158. Ravel C, Lorenco D, Dessolle L, et al. Mutational analysis of the WNT gene family in women with Mayer-Rokitansky-Kuster-Hauser syndrome. Fertil Steril. 2009;91(4 Suppl):1604-7.
159. Mortlock DP, Innis JW. Mutation of HOXA13 in hand-foot-genital syndrome. Nat Genet. 1997;15(2):179-80.
160. Eun Kwon H, Taylor HS. The role of HOX genes in human implantation. Ann N Y Acad Sci. 2004;1034:1-18.
161. Ye X, Hama K, Contos JJ, et al. LPA3-mediated lysophosphatidic acid signalling in embryo implantation and spacing. Nature. 2005;435(7038):104-8.
162. Hama K, Aoki J, Inoue A, et al. Embryo spacing and implantation timing are differentially regulated by LPA3-mediated lysophosphatidic acid signaling in mice. Biol Reprod. 2007;77(6):954-9.
163. Wei Q, St Clair JB, Fu T, et al. Reduced expression of biomarkers associated with the implantation window in women with endometriosis. Fertil Steril. 2009;91(5):1686-91.
164. Chen SU, Lee H, Chang DY, et al. Lysophosphatidic acid mediates interleukin-8 expression in human endometrial stromal cells through its receptor and nuclear factor-kappaB-dependent pathway: a possible role in angiogenesis of endometrium and placenta. Endocrinology. 2008;149(11):5888-96.
165. Brown TR, Lubahn DB, Wilson EM, et al. Deletion of the steroid-binding domain of the human androgen receptor gene in one family with complete androgen insensitivity syndrome: evidence for further genetic heterogeneity in this syndrome. Proc Natl Acad Sci USA. 1988;85(21):8151-5.
166. Patterson MN, Hughes IA, Gottlieb B, et al. The androgen receptor gene mutations database. Nucleic Acids Res. 1994;22(17):3560-2.
167. Walsh TJ, Pera RR, Turek PJ. The genetics of male infertility. Semin Reprod Med. 2009;27(2):124-36.
168. Bobadilla JL, Macek M, Fine JP, et al. Cystic fibrosis: a worldwide analysis of CFTR mutations—correlation with incidence data and application to screening. Hum Mutat. 2002;19(6):575-606.
169. Ratbi I, Legendre M, Niel F, et al. Detection of cystic fibrosis transmembrane conductance regulator (CFTR) gene rearrangements enriches the mutation spectrum in congenital bilateral absence of the vas deferens and impacts on genetic counselling. Hum Reprod. 2007;22(5):1285-91.
170. Stuppia L, Antonucci I, Binni F, et al. Screening of mutations in the CFTR gene in 1195 couples entering assisted reproduction technique programs. Eur J Hum Genet. 2005;13(8):959-64.
171. Position Statement: Indications for Fragile X Mental Retardation-1 (FMR-1) Genetic Testing. Birmingham, AL: American Society for Reproductive Medicine. 2008.
172. Handyside AH, Kontogianni EH, Hardy K, et al. Pregnancies from biopsied human preimplantation embryos sexed by Y-specific DNA amplification. Nature. 1990;344(6268):768-70.
173. Preimplantation genetic testing: a Practice Committee opinion. Fertil Steril. 2008;90(5 Suppl):S136-43.
174. Wilton L, Williamson R, McBain J, et al. Birth of a healthy infant after preimplantation confirmation of euploidy by comparative genomic hybridization. N Engl J Med. 2001;345(21):1537-41.
175. Wilton L, Voullaire L, Sargeant P, et al. Preimplantation aneuploidy screening using comparative genomic hybridization or fluorescence in situ hybridization of embryos from patients with recurrent implantation failure. Fertil Steril. 2003;80(4):860-8.
176. Dupont C, Segars J, DeCherney A, et al. Incidence of chromosomal mosaicism in morphologically normal nonhuman primate preimplantation embryos. Fertil Steril. 2010;93(8):2545-50.
177. Hassold T, Hunt P. To err (meiotically) is human: the genesis of human aneuploidy. Nat Rev Genet. 2001;2(4):280-91.
178. Bielanska M, Tan SL, Ao A. Chromosomal mosaicism throughout human preimplantation development in vitro: incidence, type, and relevance to embryo outcome. Hum Reprod. 2002;17(2):413-9.
179. Delhanty JD, Harper JC, Ao A, et al. Multicolour FISH detects frequent chromosomal mosaicism and chaotic division in normal preimplantation embryos from fertile patients. Hum Genet. 1997;99(6):755-60.
180. Wells D, Delhanty JD. Comprehensive chromosomal analysis of human preimplantation embryos using whole genome amplification and single cell comparative genomic hybridization. Mol Hum Reprod. 2000;6(11):1055-62.
181. Gonzalez-Merino E, Emiliani S, Vassart G, et al. Incidence of chromosomal mosaicism in human embryos at different developmental stages analyzed by fluorescence in situ hybridization. Genet Test. 2003 Summer;7(2):85-95.
182. Rubio C, Simon C, Vidal F, et al. Chromosomal abnormalities and embryo development in recurrent miscarriage couples. Hum Reprod. 2003;18(1):182-8.
183. Staessen C, Platteau P, Van Assche E, et al. Comparison of blastocyst transfer with or without preimplantation genetic diagnosis for aneuploidy screening in couples with advanced maternal age: a prospective randomized controlled trial. Hum Reprod. 2004;19(12):2849-58.
184. Mastenbroek S, Twisk M, van Echten-Arends J, et al. In vitro fertilization with preimplantation genetic screening. N Engl J Med. 2007;357(1):9-17.

185. Gianaroli L, Magli MC, Ferraretti AP, et al. Preimplantation diagnosis for aneuploidies in patients undergoing in vitro fertilization with a poor prognosis: identification of the categories for which it should be proposed. Fertil Steril. 1999;72(5):837-44.
186. Munne S, Sandalinas M, Escudero T, et al. Improved implantation after preimplantation genetic diagnosis of aneuploidy. Reprod Biomed Online. 2003;7(1):91-7.
187. Mastenbroek S, Twisk M, van der Veen F, et al. Preimplantation genetic screening: a systematic review and meta-analysis of RCTs. Hum Reprod Update. 2011;17(4):454-66.
188. Fiorentino F, Kokkali G, Biricik A, et al. Polymerase chain reaction-based detection of chromosomal imbalances on embryos: the evolution of preimplantation genetic diagnosis for chromosomal translocations. Fertil Steril. 2010;94(6):2001-11.
189. Stephenson MD, Awartani KA, Robinson WP. Cytogenetic analysis of miscarriages from couples with recurrent miscarriage: a case-control study. Hum Reprod. 2002;17(2):446-51.
190. Tulppala M, Palosuo T, Ramsay T, et al. A prospective study of 63 couples with a history of recurrent spontaneous abortion: contributing factors and outcome of subsequent pregnancies. Hum Reprod. 1993;8(5):764-70.
191. Treff NR, Northrop LE, Kasabwala K, et al. Single nucleotide polymorphism microarray-based concurrent screening of 24-chromosome aneuploidy and unbalanced translocations in preimplantation human embryos. Fertil Steril. 2011;95(5):1606-12.
192. Kallioniemi A, Kallioniemi OP, Sudar D, et al. Comparative genomic hybridization for molecular cytogenetic analysis of solid tumors. Science. 1992;258(5083):818-21.
193. Pinkel D, Albertson DG. Comparative genomic hybridization. Annu Rev Genomics Hum Genet. 2005;6:331-54.
194. Treff NR, Levy B, Su J, et al. SNP microarray-based 24 chromosome aneuploidy screening is significantly more consistent than FISH. Mol Hum Reprod. 2010;16(8):583-9.
195. Treff NR, Su J, Tao X, et al. Single-cell whole-genome amplification technique impacts the accuracy of SNP microarray-based genotyping and copy number analyses. Mol Hum Reprod. 2011;17(6):335-43.
196. Handyside AH, Harton GL, Mariani B, et al. Karyomapping: a universal method for genome wide analysis of genetic disease based on mapping crossovers between parental haplotypes. J Med Genet. 2010;47(10):651-8.
197. Obata Y, Kaneko-Ishino T, Koide T, et al. Disruption of primary imprinting during oocyte growth leads to the modified expression of imprinted genes during embryogenesis. Development. 1998;125(8):1553-60.
198. Lucifero D, Mann MR, Bartolomei MS, et al. Gene-specific timing and epigenetic memory in oocyte imprinting. Hum Mol Genet. 2004;13(8):839-49.
199. Hiura H, Obata Y, Komiyama J, et al. Oocyte growth-dependent progression of maternal imprinting in mice. Genes Cells. 2006;11(4):353-61.
200. Davis TL, Yang GJ, McCarrey JR, et al. The H19 methylation imprint is erased and re-established differentially on the parental alleles during male germ cell development. Hum Mol Genet. 2000;9(19):2885-94.
201. Ueda T, Abe K, Miura A, et al. The paternal methylation imprint of the mouse H19 locus is acquired in the gonocyte stage during foetal testis development. Genes Cells. 2000;5(8):649-59.
202. Li JY, Lees-Murdock DJ, Xu GL, et al. Timing of establishment of paternal methylation imprints in the mouse. Genomics. 2004;84(6):952-60.
203. Maher ER, Afnan M, Barratt CL. Epigenetic risks related to assisted reproductive technologies: epigenetics, imprinting, ART and icebergs? Hum Reprod. 2003;18(12):2508-11.
204. Anway MD, Cupp AS, Uzumcu M, et al. Epigenetic transgenerational actions of endocrine disruptors and male fertility. Science. 2005;308(5727):1466-9.
205. Anway MD, Leathers C, Skinner MK. Endocrine disruptor vinclozolin induced epigenetic transgenerational adult-onset disease. Endocrinology. 2006;147(12):5515-23.
206. Guerrero-Bosagna CM, Skinner MK. Epigenetic transgenerational effects of endocrine disruptors on male reproduction. Semin Reprod Med. 2009;27(5):403-8.

17

Female Reproductive Aging

Keri Kalmbach, Lin Liu, David Keefe

Chapter Contents

INTRODUCTION

Women experience an age-related decline in reproductive function before other organ systems begin to fail. Well before the onset of menopause, fecundity begins to decrease (Figure 1). The age of last conception typically occurs 10 years before menopause even as several thousand primary oocytes remain within the ovary and regular cycling ceases. By age forty, half of women are sterile. The other half exhibits markedly decreased fecundity compared. Assisted reproductive technology not only provides the most effective treatment of human infertility but also provides an opportunity to study the pathobiology of reproductive aging because of the *in vitro* access to oocytes.

Maternal age provides the best predictor of oocyte quality and developmental capacity *in vitro* and *in vivo*. As women age, their chance of conception decreases while the risk of miscarriage and aneuploidy in the conceptus increases (Figure 1). The detrimental effects of aging on reproduction in women are abolished when oocytes are obtained from young donors. The profoundly beneficial effects of egg donation on human reproduction not only provide a highly effective treatment for older women intending to get pregnant, but also place the egg at the locus of reproductive aging in women. The localization of human aging to a single cell provides a unique opportunity to test hypotheses derived from model organisms about the cellular origins of aging.

The timing of age-related reproductive failure in women is a highly heritable trait. The heritability of age related reproductive failure, estimated from twin, mother-daughter and pedigree studies, ranges from 31 to 87%.[1] How failure of women to reproduce could confer selective advantage, however, remains unclear. The high mortality of pregnancy and parturition in older women, and the disruptive effects of maternal loss on the survival and reproduction of surviving offspring, no doubt, would provide positive selective pressure on reproductive senescence in women. Intriguingly, though the age of natural menopause is highly heritable, no consistent loci have been identified as the genetic source of variability in reproductive aging, in twenty-eight genome wide association studies.[1] The lack of consistent findings from these genome studies of reproductive aging may derive from genetic complexity, e.g. the reproductive aging phenotype may have emerged repeatedly during evolution and therefore involve

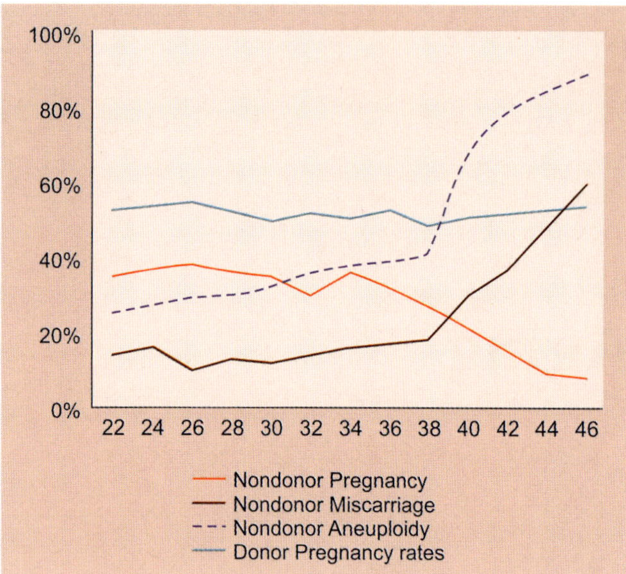

Figure 1 Risks of reproductive complications with advancing age in women

Source: Modified from Society for Assisted Reproductive Technology, 2000 and Centers for Disease Control and Prevention, 2000 data

small contributions from many genetic loci. It also may arise from the complex relationship between genes and environment.

The timing of reproductive aging also is linked to that of generalized aging. Mormon and French-Canadian women, who lived in societies where large families were prized and accessed to contraception limited, were far more likely to live past 100 years if they had children after the age of 40 years.[2] The event of having children late in life itself could confer survival advantage, however, a genetic link was suggested by the same study that found brothers (but not sisters-in-law) of these late-fertile women also enjoyed greater longevity than controls, who did not reproduce late in life.[2] Conversely, women that have early menopause are at greatly increased risk of early death.[3–5] Though the mechanisms underlying this genetic link are far from clear, the relationship between fertility in women and generalized aging highlights the urgency in understanding the mechanisms underlying reproductive aging.

THE OOCYTE THROUGHOUT DEVELOPMENT

Reproductive lifespan in women is influenced by two phases of germ cell development; a narrow window during gestation in which the female germ line proliferates and the subsequent 10–50 years of postmitotic-like arrest. A newborn female starts life with a finite population of primary follicles which sustain her entire reproductive lifespan. Each month, a cohort of these follicles is recruited. Only a small fraction reaches maturity, while most undergo atresia. This continual depletion of germ cells chips away at oocyte reserve until menopause ensues, when fewer than a thousand oocytes remain. The paucity of remaining primary follicles precludes normal recruitment and leads to cessation of the monthly cycle, ending the woman's natural reproductive lifespan.

While the female is still an embryo in the first trimester of development, a small group of primordial germ cells migrate from the epithelia of the yolk sac to the urogenital ridge. Upon arriving at the urogenital ridge, the germ cells differentiate to oogonia, the direct progenitors of oocytes. These progenitor germ cells undergo rapid mitotic expansion and eventually populate the ovary with six to seven million germ cells. Among those germ cells, a limited population of a few hundred thousand enters the initial stage of meiosis. Those that fail to enter meiosis undergo cell death by apoptosis. Thus, the greatest depletion of female reproductive tissue begins before birth. At birth, neonatal ovaries contain several hundred thousand germ cells. By puberty, only three hundred thousand cells remain.[6] Again, selection of a smaller population of cells from birth to puberty relies on apoptosis.[6]

Oocytes entering the early stage of meiosis tend to cluster in 'oocyte nests', which presumably arise from the same mitotically dividing precursor cell.[6] Not all oocytes survive. It is not known how the fate of germ cells is established in the ovary. Specifically, questions remain as to whether survival results from a vetting process that allows only the fittest cells to develop or whether this process is stochastic. Between birth and puberty, remaining oocytes enter a protracted phase of prophase arrest. Some cells remain in the state of meiotic prophase arrest for up to 50 years. During this time, oocytes recruit cells to become the supporting cumulus-corona and form primordial follicles.

Deoxyribo nucleic acid (DNA) labeling experiments conducted during the late 1960s and replicated by others followed the fate of mouse oocytes from the earliest developmental stages during gestation to ovulation. Those germ cells that first entered meiosis during fetal oogenesis were the first to ovulate in the adult.[7] The cellular basis of this production line of germ cell production in fetal development and subsequent aging in adult life remains poorly understood, though a number of other pathobiological processes have been implicated in age-related oocyte dysfunction, including mitochondrial dysfunction, free radical production, meiotic spindle dysfunction and genomic instability.

Interestingly, experimental telomere shortening recapitulates each of these reproductive aging phenotypes in mice, a species which normally do not exhibit appreciable age related oocyte dysfunction.

MITOCHONDRIA AND FREE RADICALS

Mitochondria contain their own chromosomes and are transmitted exclusively through the female germ line. Indeed, oocytes possess more mitochondria than any other cell in the body. Mitochondrial function has been linked to aging on the molecular level. The mitochondrial genome is highly susceptible to free radicals and genotoxic damage. Mitochondrial DNA (mtDNA) lacks nucleosomes, and the DNA damage repair pathways that protect against oxidative stress over the course of an organism's lifespan.[8] mtDNA is localized within the organelle compartment that primarily produces free radicals, which in turn may promote DNA mutations and exacerbate free radical production. Accumulation of damage during the prolonged prophase I arrest provides a compelling model for age-related changes in the oocyte. Indeed, mtDNA mutations in follicular cells increase with age.[9] Advancing age reduces the capacity mitochondria to produce ATP[10] and quality of preimplantation embryos is related to the ATP content.[11]

Mitochondrial dysfunction provides a compelling model for age-related pathologies observed in aged oocytes. The mtDNA from eggs of older women express the most common age-related deletion, a 5 kb deletion flanked by direct repeats.[13] In an attempt to model mitochondrial dysfunction in human embryos, chemically induced mitochondrial dysfunction[12] resulted in decreased ATP production, increased reactive oxygen and gross chromosome misalignment on the meiotic spindle, culminating in cell death. Other studies have described a relationship between oocyte function and mtDNA content. Oocytes with lower total mtDNA content demonstrate poor development,[13] and women with lower mtDNA copy number have lower ovarian reserve.[14] Depletion of mitochondrial organelle numbers through selective knockout of essential genes in mice, such as *Tfam,* fail to affect ovarian reserve, though they dramatically affect the ability to produce competent pregnancies.[15]

The bottleneck theory of mtDNA inheritance suggests that primordial follicles contain a limited number of copies of mtDNA that expand to populate a new organism. As the germ cell passes from oogonia to oocyte, mtDNA copy number increases from two hundreds to hundreds of thousands.[16] Theoretically, limiting inheritance initially to a few copies with later expansion would allow oogenesis to select for high quality mtDNA.[17] The consequence of selection for normal mitochondria would be deselection of abnormal mitochondria or infertility. While mtDNA pathology, as a cause of reproductive aging is attractive in theory, a recent study suggests that selection of mitochondria in primordial follicles is a random process,[18] allowing equal opportunity for mutated and normal mtDNA to pass on to subsequent generations.

SPINDLE ABNORMALITIES

Normally, only one oocyte attains maturation each month and is capable of responding to the preovulatory luteinizing hormone (LH) surge. The LH surge signals resumption of meiosis in the oocyte. A meiotic spindle forms and one kinetochore on each homologous chromosome captures microtubules to nucleate the spindle. Homologous chromosomes congress to the metaphase plate of the meiotic spindle, then segregate. Normally, one chromosome from each pair of homologues is extruded in the first polar body. Immediately, thereafter, another meiotic spindle forms and the remaining chromosomes, each consisting of two sister chromatids, align. At this point, however, the egg arrests at metaphase of meiosis II until fertilization signals the final separation of the sister chromatids. Spindle disruption can predispose to mis-segregation and aneuploidy at either stage of spindle formation. Errors in spindle assembly or chromosome alignment may result in cell cycle arrest, or produce aneuploidy and genetic instability. Some evidence suggests that mammalian oocytes have a more lax checkpoint preceding anaphase,[9] contributing to the increased incidence of aneuploidy of maternal origin.

Unlike in mitotic cells, the spindle apparatus in meiotic cells is responsible for separation of homologous chromosomes during meiosis I and separation of sister chromatids during meiosis II to produce normal haploid oocytes. Integrity of the meiotic spindle is inversely associated with maternal age.[20] In naturally, cycling women over the age of 40 years, nearly 80% of oocytes exhibit abnormal spindles or chromosome alignment, with one or more chromosomes displaced from the meiotic metaphase plate. In contrast, less than 20% of oocytes from women under 25 years exhibited these abnormalities. These age-related spindle and chromosome abnormalities could contribute to the higher prevalence of aneuploidy in older women. Spindle abnormalities in human oocytes also can be detected noninvasively using polarized light microscopy (the Polscope).[21] Absence, abnormal timing of appearance, shape, location and birefringence of the meiotic spindle imaged with the Polscope during *in vitro* fertilization

(IVF) have been associated with poor IVF outcome.[22]

discussed elsewhere in the chapter with respect to chromosome cohesin content, mitochondrial dysfunction and telomere length.

CHROMOSOME ABNORMALITIES; CHIASMATA, COHESIN

Chiasmata, the physical sites of recombination during meiosis, play a role in genetic recombination and in countering spindle pulling forces. Their number and/or location along the chromosome contribute to chromosome nondisjunction. Studies in experimental models as diverse as yeast, mice and humans demonstrate that chiasmata located too far from or too close to the center of the chromosome are more prone to nondisjunction.[23] Sites of crossover are established within the fetal ovary, which suggested a possible link with the first-in, first-out production line model of ovarian aging during fetal development.

Cohesins are the molecular pinions that hold the meiotic chromosomes together throughout a woman's reproductive lifespan. Cohesins are a class of protein that join sister chromatids during meiosis and mitosis. In meiosis, cohesins facilitate attachment and segregation of homologous chromosome pairs during meiosis I. Their normal function is essential for meiotic recombination and correct segregation at meiosis I. Cohesin complexes consist of four subunits, Scc1, Scc3, Smc1 and Smc3, which together form a ring-like structure that tethers the chromosomes together. The structural maintenance of chromosomes (SMC) proteins bind chromatids in an ATP-dependent fashion. The regulatory Scc1 and Scc3 subunits stabilize the ring structure that encloses the chromosome. Somatic and meiotic cells are differentially regulated from cell-type to cell-type and organism to organism and have accordingly, different cohesin subunits. The meiotic correspondent to Scc1 is Rec8, Smc1 is SMC1β and Scc3 is SA3/STAG3.[24] To facilitate proper segregation, cohesins at the kinetochore interact with microtubules derived from opposing poles. The force of tension emanating from the poles activates the anaphase-promoting complex to promote the cleavage of the cohesin complexes between the sister chromatid.

Some evidence implicates disruption of cohesion function with reproductive aging. Smc1β depleted mice show progressive loss of chromosomal integrity during the female's protracted prophase[25] in an age-dependent manner. Loss of bivalent integrity, or cohesion between sister chromatids, coincided with an increasing loss of chiasmata in metaphase I and with complete loss of meiotic sister chromatid cohesion by metaphase II.[25] Rec8-deficient female mice are born lacking oocytes, suggesting an early and essential role of the Rec8 subunit in the development of oocytes.[26] Premature separation of sister chromatids has been detected in cytogenetic studies of human oocytes and embryos coincident with the age-related reduction of cohesin proteins, including Rec8, SA3, and SMC1 β.[27] Sgo2, a regulatory protein that protects cohesin from removal, thereby maintaining the integrity of meiotic chromosomes, shows an age-related decline in a long-lived mouse strain.[28] Additionally, aging mice are increasingly ineffective at reloading cohesins on the chromosomes.[29] Why cohesins and their associated molecules might be especially susceptible to the effects of aging remains an enigma. They not only turnover in the long-lived, postmitotic oocyte but also not particularly exposed to common contributors to cellular aging, such as reactive oxygen, nor do they suffer the strain of repeated use.

A TELOMERE THEORY OF REPRODUCTIVE AGING

Telomeres are the repetitive sequences of DNA that cap and protect the ends of chromosomes. All linear chromosomes, including human, possess specialized structures that consist of repeat-enriched DNA and proteins that tether the chromosome ends into a protective loop. Telomere repeats are lost over the course of an organism's lifespan. In model systems, telomere shortening triggers senescence, apoptosis and genomic instability.[30] In humans, short telomeres have been associated with diabetes and obesity,[31] cardiovascular disease,[32] liver disorders,[33,34] cancer[35] and old age.[36] Telomere length is regulated by three mechanisms: genetic predisposition, mitotic cell division and oxidative stress. Telomere length is heritable both as a complex trait and markedly abnormal telomere length can be inherited in a Mendelian fashion. Mutations in genes encoding telomere associated proteins can lead to aplastic anemia, pulmonary fibrosis and dyskeratosis congenital, resulting from an insufficiency of progenitor cells in the specific tissues.[37]

Age-related changes in telomere length more commonly arise from a combination of replication-linked attrition and oxidative stress. During every round of cell division, the chromosome end loses a small amount of DNA as a result of the inability of the lagging strand to replicate the footprint of the RNA primer seeding replication. Thus, cells that underwent a high replication rate at least sometime during their lifespan and/or those with a finite supply are particularly sensitive to reduced telomere reserve. Free radicals can further deplete telomere length, even in nondividing cells because the guanine-rich sequence of telomeres is readily oxidized which promotes an excision repair of DNA damage response.

Telomerase is a reverse-transcriptase that extends telomeric DNA. Humans do not express appreciable levels of telomerase activity except in stem cells, male germ cells and cancer cells. Oocytes, eggs, zygotes and preimplantation embryos do not exhibit appreciable levels of telomerase until the blastocyst state of development.[38] In contrast, laboratory strains of mice express telomerase constitutively, leading to very long telomeres. Telomerase knockout (TelKO) mice lacking either the RNA or reverse-transcriptase component of the enzyme have been used to model aging in mice. After several generations, the telomere length of TelKO mice approaches that of humans. Oocytes in this mouse model faithfully recapitulate the age-related changes observed in female reproduction, including reduced chiasmata and synapsis,[39] mitochondrial dysfunction,[40] spindle abnormalities and misaligned chromosomes.[41] Spindle abnormalities as a phenotype of telomere attrition may result from the central role telomeres play in meiosis. In species as diverse as plants, yeast, mice and man, telomeres play an indispensable role in bouquet formation during early meiosis.[42]

The telomere theory of reproductive aging posits that there are two "hits" to telomeres in the germ line of women.[43] The first hit takes place during early development, when telomeres are sensitive to attrition during rapid mitotic oogonial divisions. The second hit arises during the prolonged interval between germ cell formation and ovulation, when reactive species, the inevitable byproducts of metabolism in living cells, further shorten telomeres. The Telomere theory provides a parsimonious way to explain many of the otherwise disparate observations of reproductive aging in women. For instance, the production line model posits that ovarian aging occurs prenatally, during the period of oogonial proliferation. The telomere theory predicts that late proliferating oogonia, which give rise to late ovulating oocytes, have depleted their telomere reserve during the many mitotic divisions that preceded their entry into meiosis. Expression of telomerase in these precursor cells might be expected to attenuate telomere attrition in oogonia, but even adult stem cells, which also express telomerase, are not spared the effects of senescence.[43] Telomere shortening progresses over the decades preceding ovulation, from the inevitable effects of reactive oxygen exacerbated by lifestyle factors, such as obesity[44] and smoking,[45] that have similarly detrimental effects on female fertility.[46,47]

In humans, a number of recent studies have implicated telomeres in reproductive success and provided evidence to support the Telomere Theory of Reproductive Aging. For instance, amongst a small sample of women undergoing IVF, those that became pregnant had greater relative telomere length than those that did not conceive.[48] Telomere length also predicted fragmentation in embryos after IVF.[49] Additionally, mothers of Down Syndrome newborns[50] and women that experience recurrent pregnancy loss[51] have shorter telomere length than unaffected controls. Further, implicating telomeres in the quality of oocytes and embryos, aneuploid oocytes have less telomeric DNA content than sister oocytes that were euploid from the same IVF patient and cycle.[52] Thus, in addition to studies in mice, a growing number of clinical studies implicate telomere length in oocyte quality.

OVARIAN RESERVE TESTING AND OVARIAN AGING

In a normally cycling woman, the anterior pituitary is stimulated by gonadotropin releasing hormone from the hypothalamus to secrete follicle stimulating hormone (FSH). In women of advanced reproductive age, who have depleted ovarian reserve, FSH levels progressively rise as a consequence of decreased negative feedback from inhibins and estradiol. Thus, early follicular FSH levels provide a useful clinical indicator of ovarian reserve. FSH is negatively associated with the probability of a woman conceiving, independent of age.[53] That is, both young and older women with high FSH have a reduced probability of conception. Some evidence exists that rising FSH levels also may contribute to accelerated female reproductive aging.[54] Anti-müllerian hormone (AMH), a peptide produced by early antral follicles, provides another biomarker of ovarian reserve. Paralleling the decline in antral follicle count with age, AMH levels decline with age.[53] AMH also is predictive of the age of menopause.[55]

Biomarkers of ovarian reserve such as AMH, FSH and antral follicle count provide valuable points of discussion in counseling the older woman attempting to conceive, though clinical management of the reproductive health of older woman also must consider lifestyle and genetic factors. Biomarkers of ovarian reserve also are valuable to patients who have been diagnosed with cancer. Radio and/or chemotherapies can have detrimental effects on the reproductive function of even young, fertile women,[56] including heightened risk of infertility and menopause at a younger age. Loss of oocyte number and quality may result from the effects of chemotherapy[57] on the ovary.

OTHER GENETIC MODELS

The genes encoding the BRCA family of proteins were identified by their link to heritable forms of breast and ovarian cancer. Intriguingly, both BRCA1 and BRCA2 proteins localize to telomeres and are involved in DNA damage repair.[58,59] Given their functional and structural link to telomeres and of telomeres to reproductive aging, we hypothesized that BRCA mutations might affect ovarian reserve. Our registry based study failed to demonstrate a relationship between BRCA mutations and reduced fertility, but the registry approach was limited by the tendency of women harboring known mutations in *BRCA* genes not to seek fertility late in life. We speculated that the effects of BRCA mutations on reproduction in women would be apparent only in later stages of reproductive life.[60] Another study examined the responses to ovarian stimulation of women undergoing fertility preservation before chemotherapy. Those with BRCA1 mutations had lower response to ovarian stimulation with fewer oocytes and lower peak estradiol compared to those with BRCA2 mutations or no known genetic mutation.[61] The mutant BRCA1 protein likely interacts with other factors to predispose women to subfertility or infertility.

Apoptosis is thought to be the primary mechanism of clearance of atretic follicles. In somatic cells, apoptosis can take place through a number of pathways, though the most common involves a balance between pro- and antiapoptotic proteins, such as Bax and Bcl-2 respectively. In mouse models that overexpress proapoptotic or are depleted of antiapoptotic factors, ovarian follicles are excessively lost and conversely, absence of proapoptotic factors or abundance of antiapoptotic signals exhibit delayed ovarian aging.[62–65] Interestingly, a genetic linkage study implicated a Bcl-2 locus in premature ovarian failure in women (reviewed in [1]).

The forkhead box (FOX) family of proteins consists of transcription factors important in embryonic development, cellular proliferation, mitosis and longevity. Specifically, the FOXO subfamily members have been implicated in genetic studies of female reproductive aging. In one genome wide association study, a locus including FOXO3 appeared high on the candidate list[66] (reviewed in [1]). FOXO3 suppresses follicular activation, suggesting that disruption in FOXO3 expression may lead to premature expenditure of primary follicles and early onset of menopause. FOXO3 along with FOXO1 mutations are also enriched in patients with premature ovarian failure.[67]

CLOSING REMARKS

Female reproductive capacity is limited foremost by age, so women have a limited period to make decisions about starting or expanding their family. Regular cycles begin in the early teenage years and fertility peaks through the late 20s. After 35 years, however, the risk of miscarriage and aneuploidy related complications increases exponentially. During this period, women will increasingly experience difficulty in conceiving until there is no further chance of natural conception at menopause. While oocyte preservation and egg donation afford more options to women, a deeper understanding of the mechanisms underlying reproductive aging will lead to better biomarkers and help inform those personal and clinical decisions about a woman's reproductive choices. Additionally, these same mechanisms may inspire the development of improved contraception options. Lastly, a further understanding of reproductive aging may elucidate the underlying biology of cellular aging.

REFERENCES

1. Voorhuis M, Onland-Moret NC, van der Schouw YT, et al. Human studies on genetics of the age at natural menopause: a systematic review. Hum Reprod Update. 2010;16(4):364-77.
2. Smith KR, Gagnon A, Cawthon RM, et al. Familial aggregation of survival and late female reproduction. J Gerontol A Biol Sci Med Sci. 2009;64(7):740-4.
3. Snowdon DA, Kane RL, Beeson WL, et al. Is early natural menopause a biologic marker of health and aging? Am J Public Health. 1989;79(6):709-14.
4. Cooper GS, Sandler DP. Age at natural menopause and mortality. Ann Epidemiol. 1998;8(4):229-35.
5. Mondul AM, Rodriguez C, Jacobs EJ, et al. Age at natural menopause and cause-specific mortality. Am J Epidemiol. 2005;162(11):1089-97.
6. Hartshorne GM, Lyrakou S, Hamoda H, et al. Oogenesis and cell death in human prenatal ovaries: what are the criteria for oocyte selection? Mol Hum Reprod. 2009;15(12):805-19.
7. Henderson SA, Edwards RG. Chiasma frequency and maternal age in mammals. Nature. 1968;218(5136):22-8.
8. Wilding M, Di Matteo L, Dale B. The maternal age effect: a hypothesis based on oxidative phosphorylation. Zygote. 2005;13(4):317-23.
9. Seifer DB, DeJesus V, Hubbard K. Mitochondrial deletions in luteinized granulosa cells as a function of age

in women undergoing in vitro fertilization. Fertil Steril. 2002;78(5):1046-8.

10. Shigenaga MK, Hagen TM, Ames BN. Oxidative damage and mitochondrial decay in aging. Proc Natl Acad Sci USA. 1994;91(23):10771-8.
11. Van Blerkom J, Davis PW, Lee J. ATP content of human oocytes and developmental potential and outcome after in vitro fertilization and embryo transfer. Hum Reprod. 1995;10(2):415-24.
12. Thouas GA, Trounson AO, Wolvetang EJ, et al. Mitochondrial dysfunction in mouse oocytes results in preimplantation embryo arrest in vitro. Biol Reprod. 2004;71(6):1936-42.
13. Reynier P, May-Panloup P, Chrétien MF, et al. Mitochondrial DNA content affects the fertilizability of human oocytes. Mol Hum Reprod. 2001;7(5):425-9.
14. May-Panloup P, Chrétien MF, Jacques C, et al. Low oocyte mitochondrial DNA content in ovarian insufficiency. Hum Reprod. 2005;20(3):593-7.
15. Wai T, Ao A, Zhang X, et al. The role of mitochondrial DNA copy number in mammalian fertility. Biol Reprod. 2010;83(1):52-62.
16. Wai T, Teoli D, Shoubridge EA. The mitochondrial DNA genetic bottleneck results from replication of a subpopulation of genomes. Nat Genet. 2008;40(12):1484-8.
17. Bentov Y, Yavorska T, Esfandiari N, et al. The contribution of mitochondrial function to reproductive aging. J Assist Reprod Genet. 2011; 28(9):773-83.
18. Inoue K. Generation of mice with mitochondrial dysfunction by introducing mouse mtDNA carrying a deletion into zygotes. Nat Genet. 2000;26(2):176-81.
19. Nagaoka SI, Hodges CA, Albertini DF, et al. Oocyte-specific differences in cell-cycle control create an innate susceptibility to meiotic errors. Curr Biol. 2011;21(8): 651-7.
20. Battaglia DE, Goodwin P, Klein NA, et al. Influence of maternal age on meiotic spindle assembly in oocytes from naturally cycling women. Hum Reprod. 1996;11(10):2217-22.
21. Keefe D, Liu L, Wang W, et al. Imaging meiotic spindles by polarization light microscopy: principles and applications to IVF. Reprod Biomed Online. 2003;7(1):24-9.
22. Kilani S, Cooke S, Tilia L, et al. Does meiotic spindle normality predict improved blastocyst development, implantation and live birth rates? Fertil Steril. 2011;96(2):389-93.
23. Hassold T, Hall H, Hunt P. The origin of human aneuploidy: where we have been, where we are going. Hum Mol Genet. 2007;16(Spec No. 2):R203-8.
24. Wood AJ, Severson AF, Meyer BJ. Condensin and cohesin complexity: the expanding repertoire of functions. Nat Rev Genet. 2010;11(6):391-404.
25. Hodges CA, Revenkova E, Jessberger R, et al. SMC1 beta-deficient female mice provide evidence that cohesins are a missing link in age-related nondisjunction. Nat Genet. 2005;37(12):1351-5.
26. Xu H, Beasley MD, Warren WD, et al. Absence of mouse REC8 cohesin promotes synapsis of sister chromatids in meiosis. Dev Cell. 2005;8(6):949-61.
27. Liu L, Keefe DL. Defective cohesin is associated with age-dependent misaligned chromosomes in oocytes. Reprod Biomed Online. 2008;16(1):103-12.
28. Lister LM, Kouznetsova A, Hyslop LA, et al. Age-related meiotic segregation errors in mammalian oocytes are preceded by depletion of cohesin and Sgo2. Curr Biol. 2010;20(17):1511-21.
29. Jessberger R. Deterioration without replenishment—the misery of oocyte cohesin. Genes Dev. 2010;24(23):2587-91.
30. de Lange T. How telomeres solve the end-protection problem. Science. 2009;326(5955):948-52.
31. Murillo-Ortiz B, Albarrán-Tamayo F, Arenas-Aranda D, et al. Telomere length and type 2 diabetes in males, a premature aging syndrome. Aging Male. 2011.
32. Fitzpatrick AL, Kronmal RA, Kimura M, et al. Leukocyte telomere length and mortality in the cardiovascular health study. J Gerontol A Biol Sci Med Sci. 2011;66(4):421-9.
33. Hartmann D, Srivastava U, Thaler M, et al. Telomerase gene mutations are associated with cirrhosis formation. Hepatology. 2011;53(5):1608-17.
34. Calado RT, Brudno J, Mehta P, et al. Constitutional telomerase mutations are genetic risk factors for cirrhosis. Hepatology. 2011;53(5):1600-7.
35. Martinez-Delgado B, Yanowsky K, Inglada-Perez L, et al. Genetic anticipation is associated with telomere shortening in hereditary breast cancer. PLoS Genet. 2011;7(7):e1002182.
36. Chen W, Kimura M, Kim S, et al. Longitudinal versus cross-sectional evaluations of leukocyte telomere length dynamics: age-dependent telomere shortening is the rule. J Gerontol A Biol Sci Med Sci. 2011;66(3):312-9.
37. Calado RT, Young NS. Telomere diseases. N Engl J Med. 2009;361(24):2353-65.
38. Wright WE, Piatyszek MA, Rainey WE, et al. Telomerase activity in human germline and embryonic tissues and cells. Dev Genet. 1996;18(2):173-9.
39. Liu L, Franco S, Spyropoulos B, et al. Irregular telomeres impair meiotic synapsis and recombination in mice. Proc Natl Acad Sci USA. 2004;101(17):6496-501.
40. Liu L, Trimarchi JR, Smith PJ, et al. Mitochondrial dysfunction leads to telomere attrition and genomic instability. Aging Cell. 2002;1(1):40-6.
41. Liu L, Blasco MA, Keefe DL. Requirement of functional telomeres for metaphase chromosome alignments and integrity of meiotic spindles. EMBO Rep. 2002;3(3):230-4.
42. Scherthan H. Telomere attachment and clustering during meiosis. Cell Mol Life Sci. 2007;64(2):117-24.
43. Keefe DL, Marquard K, Liu L. The telomere theory of reproductive senescence in women. Curr Opin Obstet Gynecol. 2006;18(3):280-5.
44. Zannolli R, Mohn A, Buoni S, et al. Telomere length and obesity. Acta Paediatr. 2008;97(7):952-4.
45. Strandberg TE, Saijonmaa O, Tilvis RS, et al. Association of telomere length in older men with mortality and midlife body mass index and smoking. J Gerontol A Biol Sci Med Sci. 2011;66(7):815-20.

46. Shah DK, Missmer SA, Berry KF, et al. Effect of obesity on oocyte and embryo quality in women undergoing in vitro fertilization. Obstet Gynecol. 2011;118(1):63-70.
47. Murin S, Rafii R, Bilello K. Smoking and smoking cessation in pregnancy. Clin Chest Med. 2011;32(1):75-91.
48. Keefe DL, Liu L, Marquard K. Telomeres and aging-related meiotic dysfunction in women. Cell Mol Life Sci. 2007;64(2):139-43.
49. Keefe DL, Franco S, Liu L, et al. Telomere length predicts embryo fragmentation after in vitro fertilization in women—toward a telomere theory of reproductive aging in women. Am J Obstet Gynecol. 2005;192(4):1256-60.
50. Ghosh S, Feingold E, Chakraborty S, et al. Telomere length is associated with types of chromosome 21 nondisjunction: a new insight into the maternal age effect on Down syndrome birth. Hum Genet. 2010;127(4):403-9.
51. Hanna CW, Bretherick KL, Gair JL, et al. Telomere length and reproductive aging. Hum Reprod. 2009;24(5):1206-11.
52. Treff NR, Su J, Taylor D, et al. Telomere DNA deficiency is associated with development of human embryonic aneuploidy. PLoS Genet. 2011;7(6):e1002161.
53. Buyuk E, Nejat E, Neal-Perry G. Determinants of female reproductive senescence: differential roles for the ovary and the neuroendocrine axis. Semin Reprod Med. 2010;28(5):370-9.
54. McTavish KJ, Jimenez M, Walters KA, et al. Rising follicle-stimulating hormone levels with age accelerate female reproductive failure. Endocrinology. 2007;148(9):4432-9.
55. Broer SL, Eijkemans MJ, Scheffer GJ, et al. Anti-mullerian hormone predicts menopause: a long-term follow-up study in normoovulatory women. J Clin Endocrinol Metab. 2011;96(8):2532-9.
56. Letourneau JM, Ebbel EE, Katz PP, et al. Acute ovarian failure underestimates age-specific reproductive impairment for young women undergoing chemotherapy for cancer. Cancer. 2011.
57. Buttiglieri S, Ruella M, Risso A, et al. The aging effect of chemotherapy on cultured human mesenchymal stem cells. Exp Hematol. 2011.
58. Ballal RD, Saha T, Fan S, et al. BRCA1 localization to the telomere and its loss from the telomere in response to DNA damage. J Biol Chem. 2009;284(52):36083-98.
59. Badie S, Escandell JM, Bouwman P, et al. BRCA2 acts as a RAD51 loader to facilitate telomere replication and capping. Nat Struct Mol Biol. 2010;17(12):1461-9.
60. Pal T, Keefe D, Sun P, et al. Fertility in women with BRCA mutations: a case-control study. Fertil Steril. 2010;93(6):1805-8.
61. Oktay K, Kim JY, Barad D, et al. Association of BRCA1 mutations with occult primary ovarian insufficiency: a possible explanation for the link between infertility and breast/ovarian cancer risks. J Clin Oncol. 2010;28(2):240-4.
62. Kim MR, Tilly JL. Current concepts in Bcl-2 family member regulation of female germ cell development and survival. Biochem Biophys Acta. 2004;1644(2-3):205-10.
63. Kugu K, Ratts VS, Piquette GN, et al. Analysis of apoptosis and expression of bcl-2 gene family members in the human and baboon ovary. Cell Death Differ. 1998;5(1):67-76.
64. Hsu SY, Lai RJ, Finegold M, et al. Targeted overexpression of Bcl-2 in ovaries of transgenic mice leads to decreased follicle apoptosis, enhanced folliculogenesis, and increased germ cell tumorigenesis. Endocrinology. 1996;137(11):4837-43.
65. Ratts VS, Flaws JA, Kolp R, et al. Ablation of bcl-2 gene expression decreases the numbers of oocytes and primordial follicles established in the post-natal female mouse gonad. Endocrinology. 1995;136(8):3665-8.
66. Cupples LA, Arruda HT, Benjamin EJ, et al. The Framingham Heart Study 100K SNP genome-wide association study resource: overview of 17 phenotype working group reports. BMC Med Genet. 2007;8 (Suppl 1):S1.
67. Watkins WJ, Umbers AJ, Woad KJ, et al. Mutational screening of FOXO3A and FOXO1A in women with premature ovarian failure. Fertil Steril. 2006;86(5):1518-21.

18

Ovarian Reserve Testing

Vasiliki A Moragianni, David B Seifer

CHAPTER CONTENTS

INTRODUCTION

A combination of environmental factors, social behaviors and unlimited access to contraception has led to the social phenomenon of delayed and 'timed' childbearing that has been becoming more prevalent in westernized societies over the last 20–30 years. As a result, couples and single women now, more often than even before in human history, postpone their decision to start a family until other societal and personal factors are aligned.[1] This societal shift necessitates access to information about appropriate timing and potential to successfully reproduce at any given time, and this is where markers of ovarian reserve act as surrogates for such information.

WHAT IS OVARIAN RESERVE?

By the time a female is born, she has already lost the majority of her reproductive potential. The peak of oocyte quantity is *in utero*; when at 20 weeks of gestation, a female fetus has 6–7,000,000 primary oocytes, while at birth this number is already reduced to 700,000–2,000,000. When a female reaches her early reproductive age, she has only 300,000–500,000 remaining oocytes that are available to be ovulated every month and ultimately lead to a pregnancy.

The number and quality of remaining oocytes are thus critical pieces of information for women trying to assess their reproductive capacity. Ovarian reserve should be perceived as a continuous spectrum that is influenced by multiple factors—primarily age, genetic predisposition and environmental exposures. It begins with normal ovarian function and gradually progresses to subfertility, sterility, irregular menses and ultimately menopause.[2]

Classic studies of natural populations, such as the Hutterites,[3] as well as recent data from the general population indicate that the peak of ovarian endowment, and thus fertility of a woman lies in her late teens and early twenties. At the age of 30 years, it begins to decline, the rate of decline increases after age 35 years, until it practically ceases at the age of 40 years. The mean age for the birth of the last child in natural fertile populations has been stable across time at the 40–41 years of age and pregnancies after the age of 45 years are extremely rare.

The rate or trajectory of any given patient's irreversible decline in reproductive capacity that begins *in utero* cannot be accurately predicted, but several surrogate markers exist and are used clinically. However, despite extensive research into the development and efficacy of these markers, they certainly remain imperfect and, in most instances, only give an estimate of the number of remaining oocytes, with quality being a much more elusive concept to fully characterize.

We review here all available tests of ovarian reserve by outlining their key strengths and weaknesses, and describing their value in special populations.

PROPERTIES OF SCREENING TESTS

Since tests of ovarian reserve are used to screen for diminished ovarian quality and/or quantity, they should be kept to the same basic standards as other screening tests in medicine, for example:

1. Reproducibility and validity: The results of a screening test should be able to be reproduced reliably and to measure what they are designed to measure. An ideal screening test for ovarian reserve should not be affected by the phase of menstrual cycle or hormonal status of the patient. We review this individually for each existing test of ovarian reserve.
2. High prevalence: The tested condition should have a reasonably high prevalence to justify screening in that population, namely the population of subfertile couples, who wish to conceive.
3. Cost-effective: Screening tests should be affordable and their cost should justify testing of all populations.
4. Minimally invasive: An ideal screening test should ideally be conducted in a noninvasive manner such as with ultrasounds and/or blood draws.
5. Early diagnosis: A screening test should lead to the diagnosis of the tested condition, in this case diminished ovarian reserve (DOR), at an early enough stage that intervention can still be warranted.
6. Treatment available: Once timely diagnosis of the tested condition is established there should be a treatment modality available. In the case of DOR, such treatments would primarily include ovulation induction and assisted reproductive technology (ART).

AVAILABLE TESTS OF OVARIAN RESERVE

Follicle Stimulating Hormone

One of the first tests that were used to monitor ART cycles and offer an outcome prediction was the basal or early follicular phase follicle-stimulating hormone (FSH) level.[4] FSH is measured during cycle day 2–3, while the ovarian hormone levels are not yet elevated and a normal value is typically cited as lesser than 10 mIU/ml. The first menstrual cycle day is defined as the first day of full flow. The FSH level offers a reasonable understanding of the hypothalamic-pituitary-gonadal axis, as it responds to feedback from estradiol and progesterone.

Advantages

- This test is relatively cheap ($150) and only involves a blood draw
- The results are usually available within 1–2 days
- It has a very high specificity, upwards of 95%
- At very high levels, FSH values are accurate predictors of poor response to ART treatment and failure of pregnancy,[2] as they correlate with lower oocyte yield, higher rates of cancellation and lower rates of implantation and pregnancy.[5]

Disadvantages

- False negatives: FSH values have to be interpreted in conjunction with an estradiol of lesser than 75–80 pg/ml, to exclude a false lowering of FSH in response to an elevated estradiol, such as in cases of oral contraceptive use or pregnancy[6]
- False positives: Although rare (~ 5%), cases of false positive FSH levels have been described.[7] In the reported cases, patients with normal ovarian reserve had markedly elevated FSH values, as a result of either autoimmune or heterophile anti-FSH antibodies. Hence, clinical judgment is paramount in the interpretation of this test
- Both the FSH and estradiol values are laboratory-specific and practice-specific and should be interpreted individually in the setting of each patient's clinical scenario
- FSH has a pulsatile and circadian pattern of secretion that introduces the potential for measurement variability.

Inhibin B

Inhibin B is one of the two subunits of inhibin, a 32 kDa dimeric glycoprotein member of the transforming growth factor-beta (TGF-β), superfamily that is produced by the granulosa cells of preantral follicles and early antral follicles. Whereas inhibin B is the dominant subunit present during the early- to mid-follicular phase of the menstrual cycle, inhibin A levels rise during the late-follicular and mid-luteal phases. Inhibin acts primarily by binding and inhibiting, as its name implies, activin and thus decreasing FSH production at the level of the anterior pituitary.[8] As a result of this interaction, inhibin B has been developed as a marker of ovarian reserve.

Advantages

- This test is relatively cheap (US$ 150–200) and only involves a blood draw
- The results are usually available within 1–2 days.

Disadvantages

- There is a lack of reliable assays. Only recently have second-generation assays been described, but they have not yet being incorporated into clinical practice[9]
- It has little value in predicting menopause,[10] ovarian response and ART treatment outcomes.[2]

Anti-Müllerian Hormone

Similar to inhibin B, anti-müllerian hormone (AMH) is another dimeric glycoprotein member of the TGF-β superfamily and is produced by the granulosa cells of follicles that are up to six mm in diameter. Once follicles mature AMH is no longer secreted and this is reflected in its levels across life: AMH is barely detectable at birth, reached a peak after puberty and progressively decreases after that until it returns to undetectable levels in menopause.[11] AMH promotes FSH-dependent ovarian follicular growth and inhibits primordial follicle pool depletion.[12-14] Serum levels greater than 0.7 ng/ml are considered normal, whereas values less than 0.3 ng/ml indicate DOR. Age-specific values are also available[11,15-17] for AMH.

Advantages

- This test is relatively cheap (US$ 75) and only involves a blood draw
- AMH is the earliest and most sensitive biomarker of ovarian reserve decline with changes noted well before changes in FSH or inhibin B: Nelson SM, Anderson RA, Broekmans FJ, Raine-Fenning N, Fleming R, La Marka A. Anti-Müllerin hormone: clairvoyance or crystal clear? Hum Reprod. 2012 Jan 11. [Epub ahead of print]
- Perhaps the most valuable quality of AMH as a test of ovarian reserve is its low intracycle and intercycle variability. Unlike most other markers of ovarian reserve, AMH can be measured at anytime during the menstrual cycle as its value does not fluctuate.[18] This allows for much higher scheduling flexibility and is not affected by cycle irregularities or difficulties with documentation.
- AMH levels are independent of the hormonal status of the patient, i.e. pregnancy, use of oral contraceptives or gonadotropin-releasing hormone agonist treatment.[19-21] It can thus be measured and reliably interpreted during any of these states, without unnecessarily delaying diagnosis and initiation of treatment.
- AMH age-specific values are potentially more informative than other markers where 'normal' ranges are based on a cross-section of women independent of age.[11,15-17]
- AMH is a useful measure of ovarian reserve even in the context of elevated baseline FSH values[22] and it allows for individualized ovulation induction protocols.[23-24]
- AMH is also a reliable predictor of ovarian response to treatment, ovarian hyperstimulation syndrome as a result of ART and the onset of menopause.[25-27]

Disadvantages

- AMH is run using ELISA assays, as opposed to an automated platform, therefore requiring outsourcing for labs that may not run it daily. This in turn limits the test's widespread use because of a longer than 1–2 day waiting time to obtain results.
- Its value may be limited in certain populations, namely patients with obesity and polycystic ovary syndrome, as they are both characterized by ovulatory dysfunction. Whereas polycystic ovary syndrome patients tend to have higher AMH values, obese patients have lower AMH levels than their nonobese counterparts.[28-29]
- Limited data exists on the predictive value of serum AMH in predicting pregnancy,[23,30,31] although this is rapidly changing.

Antral Follicle Count

- Antral follicle count (AFC) is an ultrasonographic marker of ovarian reserve, whereby an early follicular phase transvaginal ultrasound is used to determine the number of follicles measuring between 2 mm and 10 mm in diameter. Normal values are considered to be greater than or equal to 5–10 antral follicles.

Advantages

- AFC has been shown in several studies to correlate strongly with response to IVF and conception rates, as well as decrease significantly with age.[32-33] A more recent meta-analysis has confirmed that AFC is accurate in predicting poor response but at a low threshold levels[2]
- Along with AMH, AFC is one of the earliest markers of DOR

Disadvantages

- This is a more invasive and expensive test as it requires the use of transvaginal sonography
- This test is very operator-dependent as it relies highly on the experience of the sonographer as well as the body habitus and pathology of the patient. AFC is also characterized by moderate interobserver and intercycle variability.[33]

Clomiphene Citrate Challenge Test

Since clomiphene citrate challenge test (CCCT) was originally describes in the late 1980s,[27] this provocative test has been used to assess ovarian reserve. Typically, 100 mg of clomiphene citrate are administered on cycle days 5–9 and baseline (days 2–3) as well as post-treatment (days 9–11) levels of estradiol and FSH are measured. Patients with DOR have impaired inhibition of the clomiphene citrate-induced FSH secretion and thus persistently elevated post-treatment FSH values.

Advantages

- Similar to early follicular FSH, the CCCT is not operator-dependent. The results are usually available within 1–2 days following each blood draw.
- It offers the additional post-treatment FSH values, which correlate even better than cycle day 2–3 FSH with treatment response and outcomes, and thus improve sensitivity.

Disadvantages

- It is one of the most expensive modalities of assessing ovarian reserve, costing approximately US$ 550–600.
- It requires two blood draws on two separate days.
- Patients are required to take a medication that has potential, albeit rare, side effects for which they need to be monitored.
- It is cycle-day specific and has a rather high inter-cycle and intracycle variability.
- The CCCT has a low specificity which renders it no better of a marker than baseline FSH or AFC.[2]

Gonadotropin-Releasing Hormone Agonist Stimulation

This test is based on the physiologic principle that upon administration of a gonadotropin-releasing hormone agonist (such as leuprolide acetate on cycle day 2–3) there is an initial estradiol burst followed by a long-term suppression. One can thus assess both the pituitary and ovarian axes with this provocative test. Existing data on this test is limited but it demonstrates that it accurately predicts low response to treatment.[2]

SPECIAL CIRCUMSTANCES

Prediction of Age at Menopause

Accurate individualized prediction of the age at menopause would have great counseling value as it would afford patients the flexibility of planning their reproductive life with greater success, as well as facilitate health prevention. Thus far, the best proxy of cessation of reproductive potential has been the pool of primordial follicles each patient possesses at any given time, as reflected in AMH, AFC or baseline FSH values. A recent long-term follow-up study comparing these three modalities concluded that AMH in combination with age are the best predictors of age to menopause.[27]

Cancer Patients

The diagnosis of malignancy in a young patient of reproductive age is in itself devastating. Although in women the reproductive potential does not appear to be affected by the neoplastic process itself,[34] the chemotherapeutic agents administered to them markedly compromise their future potential. It is well-known that these life-saving treatments compromise their ovarian reserve, as demonstrated by a reflective reduction in AMH levels.[35-36] An accurate estimate of pretreatment ovarian reserve and post-treatment potential are thus paramount in the counseling of such patients. A recent study in patients with early breast cancer that compared several serum and sonographic markers (AMH, AFC, FSH, inhibin B and estradiol) demonstrated that pre-chemotherapy AMH levels accurately predict the long-term ovarian function at 4–5 years post-treatment.[37]

CONCLUSION

With the development of highly effective fertility treatments at a time that patients are more prone than ever before to postpone childbearing, the existence of accurate markers of ovarian reserve is absolutely warranted. Several tests exist currently and range from passive or provocative serum markers to sonographic surrogates for remaining fertility potential. Among them, AMH emerges as one of the most reliable tests as it correlates well with outcomes and is characterized by low variability and dependency on menstrual cycle timing. Further prospective follow-up studies will help shed more light in this area and provide invaluable tools for patient education and decision making.

REFERENCES

1. te Velde ER, Pearson PL. The variability of female reproductive ageing. Hum Reprod Update. 2002;8(2):141-54.
2. Broekmans FJ, Kwee J, Hendriks DJ, et al. A systematic review of tests predicting ovarian reserve and IVF outcome. Hum Reprod Update. 2006;12(6):685-718.
3. Teitze C. Reproductive span and rate of reproduction among Hutterite women. Fert Steril. 1957;8(1):89-97.
4. Muasher SJ, Oehninger S, Simonetti S, et al. The value of basal and/or stimulated serum gonadotropin levels in

prediction of stimulation response and in vitro fertilization outcome. Fertil Steril. 1988;50(2):298-307.
5. Roberts JE, Spandorfer S, Fasouliotis SJ, et al. Taking a basal follicle-stimulating hormone history is essential before initiating in vitro fertilization. Fertil Streil. 2005;83:37-41.
6. Licciardi FL, Liu HC, Rosenwaks Z. Day 3 estradiol serum concentrations as prognosticators of ovarian stimulation response and pregnancy outcome in patients undergoing in vitro fertilization. Fertil Steril. 1995;64:991-4.
7. Webster R, Fahie-Wilson M, Barker P, et al. Immunoglobulin interference in serum follicle-stimulating hormone assays: autoimmune and heterophilic antibody interference. Ann Clin Biochem. 2010;47(4):386-9.
8. Klein NA, Illingworth PJ, Groome NP, et al. Decreased inhibin B secretion is associated with the monotropic FSH rise in older, ovulatory women: a study of serum and follicular fluid levels of dimeric inhibin A and B in spontaneous menstrual cycles. J Clin Endocrinol Metab. 1996;81:2742-5.
9. Kalra B, Kumar A, Patel K, et al. Development of a second generation inhibin B ELISA. J Immunol Methods. 2010;362(1-2):22-31.
10. Sowers MR, Eyvazzadeh AD, McConnell D, et al. Anti-müllerian hormone and inhibin B in the definition of ovarian aging and the menopause transition. J Clin Endocrinol Metab. 2008;93(9):3478-83.
11. Seifer DB, Baker VL, Leader B. Age-specific serum anti-müllerian hormone values for 17,120 women presenting to fertility centers within the United States. Fertil Steril. 2011;95(2):747-50.
12. Weenen C, Laven JS, Von Bergh AR, et al. Anti-müllerian hormone expression pattern in the human ovary: potential implications for initial and cyclic follicle recruitment. Mol Hum Reprod. 2004;10(2):77-83.
13. Ledger WL. Clinical utility of measurement of anti-müllerian hormone in reproductive endocrinology. J Clin Endocrinol Metab. 2010;95(12):5144-54.
14. Seifer DB, Maclaughlin DT. Mullerian Inhibiting Substance is an ovarian growth factor of emerging clinical significance. Fertil Steril. 2007;88(3):539-46.
15. La Marca A, Sighinolfi G, Giulini S, et al. Normal serum concentrations of anti-müllerian hormone in women with regular menstrual cycles. Reprod Biomed Online. 2010;21(4):463-9.
16. Nelson SM, Messow MC, Wallace AM, et al. Nomogram for the decline in serum anti-müllerian hormone: a population study of 9,601 infertility patients. Fertil Steril. 2011;95(2):736-4.
17. Almog B, Shehata F, Suissa S, et al. Age-related normograms of serum anti-müllerian hormone levels in a population of infertile women: a multicenter study. Fertil Steril. 2011;95(7):2359-63.
18. Hehenkamp WJ, Looman CW, Themmen AT, et al. Anti-müllerian hormones levels in the spontaneous menstrual cycle do not show substantial fluctuation. J Clin Endocrinol Metab. 2006;91:4057-63.
19. La Marca A, Giulini S, Orvieto R, et al. Anti-müllerian hormone concentrations in maternal serum during pregnancy. Hum Reprod. 2005;20(6):1569-72.
20. Somunkiran A, Yavuz T, Yucei O, et al. Anti-müllerian hormone levels during hormonal contraception in women with polycystic ovary syndrome. Eur J Obstet Gynecol Reprod Biol. 2007;134(2):196-201.
21. van Rooij IA, Broekmans FJ, te Velde ER, et al. Serum anti-müllerian hormone levels: a novel measure of ovarian reserve. Hum Reprod. 2002;17(12):3065-71.
22. Buyuk E, Seifer DB, Younger J, et al. Random anti-müllerian hormone (AMH) is a predictor of ovarian response in women with elevated baseline early follicular follicle-stimulating hormone levels. Fertil Steril. 2011;95(7):2369-72.
23. Nelson SM, Yates RW, Fleming R. Serum anti-müllerian hormone and FSH: prediction of live birth and extremes of response in stimulated cycles–implications for individualization of therapy. Hum Reprod. 2007;22(9):2414-21.
24. Nelson SM, Yates RW, Lyall H, et al. Anti-müllerian hormone-based approach to controlled ovarian stimulation for assisted conception. Hum Reprod. 2009;24(4):867-75.
25. Broer SL, Dólleman M, Opmeer BC, et al. AMH and AFC as predictors of excessive response in controlled ovarian hyperstimulation: a meta-analysis. Hum Reprod Update. 2011;17(1):46-54.
26. Seifer DB, MacLaughlin DT, Christian BP, et al. Early follicular serum müllerian-inhibiting substance levels are associated with ovarian response during assisted reproductive technology cycles. Fertil Steril. 2002;77(3):468-71.
27. Broer SL, Eijkemans MJ, Scheffer GJ, et al. Anti-Müllerian Hormone Predicts Menopause: A Long-Term Follow-Up Study in Normo-ovulatory Women. J Clin Endocrinol Metab. 2011; 96(8):2532-9.
28. Pigny P, Merlen E, Robert Y, et al. Elevated serum level of anti-müllerian hormone in patients with polycystic ovary syndrome: relationship to the ovarian follicle excess and to the follicular arrest. J Clin Endocrinol Metab. 2003;88(12):5957-62.
29. Buyuk E, Seifer DB, Illions E, et al. Elevated body mass index is associated with lower serum anti-müllerian hormone levels in infertile women with diminished ovarian reserve but not with normal ovarian reserve. Fertil Steril. 2011;95(7):2364-8.
30. La Marca A, Nelson SM, Sighinolfi G, et al. Anti-Müllerian hormone-based prediction model for a live birth in assisted reproduction. Reprod Biomed Online. 2011;22(4):341-9.
31. Blazar AS, Lambert-Messerlian G, Hackett R, et al. Use of in-cycle anti-müllerian hormone levels to predict cycle outcome. Am J Obstet Gynecol. 2011.
32. Chang MY, Chiang CH, Hsieh TT, et al. Use of antral follicle cont to predict the outcome of assisted reproductive technologies. Fertil Steril. 1998;69:505-10.
33. Scheffer GJ, Broekmans FJ, Dorland M, et al. Antral follicle counts by transvaginal ultrasonography are related to age in women with proven natural fertility. Fertil Steril. 1999;72(5):845-51.

34. Das M, Shehata F, Moria A, et al. Ovarian reserve, response to gonadotropins, and oocyte maturity in women with malignancy. Fertil Steril. 2011;96(1):122-5.
35. Aslam MF, Merhi ZO, Ahmed S, et al. Changes in plasma müllerian-inhibiting substance and brain-derived neurotrophic factor after chemotherapy in premenopausal women. Fertil Steril. 2011;95(5):1790-3.
36. Yu B, Douglas N, Ferin MJ, et al. Changes in markers of ovarian reserve and endocrine function in young women with breast cancer undergoing adjuvant chemotherapy. Cancer. 2010;116(9):2099-105.
37. Anderson RA, Cameron DA. Pretreatment serum anti-müllerian hormone predicts long-term ovarian function and bone mass after chemotherapy for early breast cancer. J Clin Endocrinol Metab. 2011;96(5):1336-43.

4

In Vitro Fertilization

Section Contents

19

Controlled Ovarian Hyperstimulation for In Vitro Fertilization

David Frankfurter

Chapter Contents

INTRODUCTION

The history of human *in vitro* fertilization (IVF) spans over three decades. While the first three IVF deliveries resulted from eggs retrieved during spontaneous ovarian cycles, the overwhelming majority of IVF babies are the result of stimulated ovarian cycles, i.e. controlled ovarian hyperstimulation (COH) cycles.[1]

The objectives of this chapter are:

- To describe the major pharmaceutical agents used in modern IVF
- Illustrate several commonly used COH protocols for IVF
- Propose indications for using different protocols.

Little doubt remains regarding the ability to undertake IVF during a natural cycle. Benefits of this strategy include a reduced cost of drugs, it avoids agents that cause severe ovarian hyperstimulation syndrome, and it avoids daily injections. However, natural cycle IVF has a high rate of cancelation, requires frequent follicular monitoring and usually yields a single oocyte.[2,3] Observed pregnancy rates are a fraction of that seen with COH-IVF cycles and there is no opportunity to freeze supernumerary embryos for future use. The remainder of this chapter will address the use of COH in IVF cycles.

COH for IVF is predicated on two competing principles:

1. Minimizing the potential for a premature luteinizing hormone (LH) surge with subsequent ovulation;
2. Optimization of multifollicular recruitment.

The more effective is the ovulatory inhibition, the greater is the chance of blunting the ovarian response. COH protocols rely on a combination of suppressive and stimulating medications designed to enhance or diminish one of these aspects in accordance with the infertility diagnosis and ovarian reserve of the patient undergoing treatment. Agents are classified as to whether they inhibit the hypothalamic-pituitary-ovarian response or stimulate ovarian follicular recruitment. In addition, medications are administered to allow the oocytes to complete meiosis I.

Several adjuvant agents targeting the lining or aimed at fine tuning the follicular response have been employed in IVF-COH protocols.

STIMULATING AGENTS

The drugs used to enhance follicular recruitment must ultimately increase the granulosa cell follicle-stimulating hormone (FSH) response. An agent can do this indirectly by enhancing the pituitary discharge of FSH or directly by binding to the FSH receptor.

Indirectly Acting Agents

The prototypical indirectly acting ovarian stimulating agent is clomiphene citrate.[4] First utilized in 1962 for ovulation induction, clomiphene citrate is a synthetic estrogen agonist/antagonist. In the estrogenic individual, clomiphene citrate competitively binds to hypothalamic estrogen receptors leading to a decrease in estradiol effect. As such, hypothalamic negative feedback is reduced so that there is a change in gonadotropin-releasing hormone (GnRH) pulsatility facilitating an increase in FSH discharge by the pituitary gland. When administered in the follicular phase, the elevated FSH acts to enhance follicular recruitment and generation of multiple dominant follicles.[4] In a similar vein, tamoxifen will antagonize the hypothalamic estrogen receptor causing a similar rise of FSH as that seen with clomiphene.[5] There are some data to suggest that tamoxifen may actually outperform clomiphene with regards to ovulation induction.[6] Raloxifene hydrochloride acts centrally in a similar fashion to both clomiphene and tamoxifen. However, there is limited data on its efficacy in enhancing follicular dominance and because of its antagonistic effects on the endometrial lining with limited histological data it has not been well explored as a hyperstimulating drug.[7]

Aromatase inhibitors can drive pituitary FSH release by reducing granulosa cell estradiol production thereby undermining the hypothalamic, estrogen driven, negative feedback mechanism. With inhibition of estrogen synthesis and concomitant hypoestrogenemia, GnRH pulsatility within the arcuate nucleus leads to enhanced pituitary FSH release.[8] Letrozole, an aromatase inhibitor, has been widely studied for its ability to induce a multifollicular response. In head-to-head trials, it has shown superior efficacy when compared to clomiphene with regards to its ability to induce ovulation, facilitate a multifollicular response and yield a pregnancy.[8] While early data suggested an increased likelihood of birth defects following letrozole use when compared to clomiphene, subsequent trials have failed to demonstrate a relationship between letrozole and congenital anomaly risk.[9,10] Given letrozole's short half-life (30–60 hours) relative to clomiphene (5–7 days), its biologic plausibility as a teratogen when used outside of pregnancy remains in question.[10] Despite this, letrozole's manufacturer, Novartis, has indicated that letrozole should only be prescribed to postmenopausal women.[11]

GnRH agonists, i.e. leuprolide acetate, can be used to enhance multifollicular recruitment when administered during the follicular phase of ovulating women. This so called 'flare' response occurs when the agent first binds to the pituitary gonadotroph's GnRH receptor leading to the transduction of an agonist signal.[12,13] Given that the gonadotroph generally responds to pulsatile signaling, ultimately chronic activation of the GnRH receptor leads to internalization and down regulation of the GnRH receptor.[14] A 'flare' response can also be elicited when a GnRH agonist is given to a woman with a World Health Organization Class II ovulation defect unless appropriate measures are taken to blunt the GnRH response.

Directly Acting Agents

Controlled ovarian hyperstimulation can be achieved with the administration of exogenous FSH. With this strategy, the pituitary gland is bypassed. Because FSH is a heterodimeric glycoprotein, it cannot be taken orally. Parenteral administration will allow FSH to reach the granulosa cells where it binds and acts on its receptor. FSH injections result in the rescue of multiple recruitable follicles and multifollicular dominance.

Pharmaceutical companies use high performance chromatography to purify FSH containing supernatants.[15-17] Such supernatants derive from either postmenopausal urine or human FSH transfected Chinese hamster ovary cell line culture media. Whether urinary derived or recombinant FSH (recFSH), the end product acts very similarly. Advantages of recFSH include less batch-to-batch variability, absence of LH activity, lower total dose necessary and less frequent local reactions.[18] However, some have argued that the presence of LH and potentially trace human chorionic gonadotropin (hCG) found in urinary FSH may afford an advantage in some IVF stimulation regimens.[19]

SUPPRESSIVE AGENTS

Gonadotropin-Releasing Hormone Agonists

As already discussed, GnRH agonists lead to the down regulation of the gonadotroph GnRH receptor. In so doing, the gonadotroph becomes unresponsive to ovarian feedback and fails to mount an LH surge.[12-14]

Several synthetic GnRH agonists have been produced. Like GnRH, these synthetic analogues are decapeptides, but differ from the native peptide at positions 6, 9 and 10.[12-14] Alterations in the amino acid compositions at these positions change the half-life and binding affinity of the synthetic compound. If the daily administration of synthetic GnRH analogues is initiated following ovulation (during the luteal phase of the menstrual cycle), multifollicular recruitment can be avoided. As such, luteal GnRH analogue use results in GnRH receptor downregulation with concomitant ovarian suppression.[12-14]

Gonadotropin-Releasing Hormone Antagonists

Gonadotropin-releasing hormone antagonists act by competitive inhibition of the GnRH receptor leading to an uncoupling of the dimeric receptor protein.[20] These agents act immediately and do not lead to internalization and destruction of the GnRH receptor proteins. As a result, once the antagonist is metabolized, the receptors redimerize and become active.[20] The onset GnRH antagonism is rapid and the termination of GnRH action is relatively rapid. Extended dose formulations are available but many centers rely on daily dosing to take advantage of the more modest suppressive effects of GnRH antagonists relative to agonists. Recent studies suggest that pituitary GnRH antagonists may have agonistic properties in other tissues. Such findings support tissue specific actions, the consequences of which remain to be determined.[20]

Oral Contraceptive Pills

Combined oral contraceptive pills (OCPs) work to suppress the pituitary through negative feedback on the gonadotroph. In this fashion, both gonadotropin synthesis and secretion is reduced. Because of this, suppression is slow to achieve and relatively slow to abate. Low dose OCPs also allow for synchronizing menses with the start of ovarian stimulation and incur minimal risk of the break through bleeding seen with ultralow dose and phasic OCPs preparations.

Dehydroepiandrosterone

Weak androgens may enhance ovarian responsiveness by providing substrate for granulosa cell driven aromatization to estradiol. When used by individuals with poor ovarian reserve, dehydroepiandrosterone (DHEA) has been shown by some to enhance oocyte yield.[21] While excessive androgens are known to cause apoptosis within rodent follicles, androgen action in the primate granulosa cell appears to be more complex. Response appears to be dose and time related with studies suggesting that androgens may enhance granulosa cell FSH sensitivity.[22] Most commonly, patients self administer 75 mg of DHEA daily for 16 weeks prior to initiating COH for IVF.[23] In this manner, Barad et al. demonstrated more fertilized eggs, higher mean embryo scores and more embryos available for transfer.[23,24] However, these findings remain inconclusive.

Human Chorionic Gonadotropin

Human chorionic gonadotropin is used in IVF as a proxy for LH. LH and hCG share a common alpha subunit and differ with regards to their respective beta subunits only with regards to the increased length and glycosylation of then termini of hCG. This difference enhances the half-life of hCG and allows for its use to simulate the effect of the LH surge on releasing the oocyte from meiosis I arrest.

CONTROLLED OVARIAN HYPERSTIMULATION PROTOCOLS IN *IN VITRO* FERTILIZATION

Protocols for COH in IVF can be grouped into those for normal responders, those for hyper responders and those for poor responders. Regardless of the response prediction, all protocols couple ovarian stimulation with pituitary suppression. Depending on the prognostic group, the regimen leans more towards suppression or stimulation. Because of the exhaustive number of protocols currently employed, this chapter considers a limited number of examples (Figure 1).

Normal Responders

The long luteal agonist suppression is most commonly used for normal responders (Figure 1). Starting the agonist between 7 days and 10 days postovulation, avoids a flare response. After 10–12 days of an agonist like leuprolide acetate 1 mg sc q day (1 mg subcutaneous every day), ultrasound, hCG and estradiol levels are assessed for confirmation of ovarian suppression. With suppression, the agonist dose is reduced to 0.25 mg scq day and gonadotropin administration commences. The dose of gonadotropin is dependent upon the patient's age and prognosis. There is evidence that using mixed FSH/LH protocols improves IVF outcomes, however, the optimal ratio of FSH to LH remains to be elucidated.[25] Gonadotropin dose is adjusted based upon periodic monitoring and ultimately administering hCG to allow the oocyte to complete meiosis I.

It is not unusual to employ an antagonist protocol for normal responders (Figure 1). Using OCPs has been shown to make scheduling of the cycle and retrieval

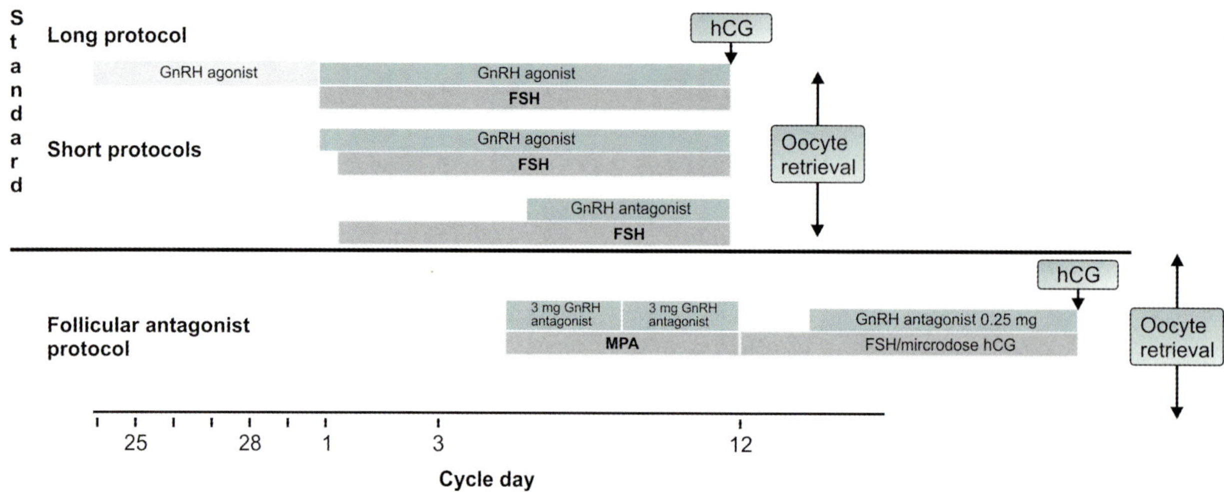

Figure 1 Schematic of long and short protocols

FSH: follicle-stimulating hormone; GnRH: gonadotropin-releasing hormone; hCG: human chorionic gonadotropin; MPA: medroxyprogesterone acetate

Source: Frankfurter D, Dyal M, Dubay A, Peak D, Gindoff P. Fertil Steril. 2007 Nov;88(5):1442-5

more user friendly, but the effect on outcome remains unclear though it does not appear to be detrimental.[26-28] Monophasic OCPs are started by cycle day 6 and continued for 14 days. At this time, ultrasound, hCG and estradiol levels are assessed for confirmation of ovarian suppression. With suppression, OCPs are stopped and stimulation with gonadotropin (generally a mixed FSH/LH preparation) starts day 4 post OCP stop. The dose of gonadotropin is dependent upon the patient's age and prognosis and the gonadotropin dose is adjusted based upon periodic monitoring. Either a fixed or flexible GnRH antagonist start can be prescribed. With the fixed start, GnRH antagonist is begun on stimulation day 6 while with a flexible start, GnRH antagonist administration commence when a lead follicle of 12–14 mm is observed. Either strategy yields acceptable outcomes, but the flexible start may reduce the dose of gonadotropin needed.[29] Gonadotropin dose is adjusted based upon periodic monitoring and ultimately administering hCG to allow the oocyte to complete meiosis I. With the use of a GnRH antagonist, completion of meiosis I can be accomplished using a GnRH agonist, i.e. leuprolide acetate.

High Responders

Because of concerns related to the potential of severe ovarian hyperstimulation, protocols can be altered for those at risk for hyper response. The dose of gonadotropin should be minimized and if a GnRH agonist is used, it can be maintained at a higher dose, i.e. 0.5 mg scq day after suppression is established. The flow of either the luteal suppression or GnRH antagonist protocols are the same, but consideration for withholding hCG, freezing all embryos or using a GnRH agonist for triggering completion of meiosis I must be considered. IVF practitioners must follow monitoring criteria, consistent with standard of care, to minimize the potential of severe ovarian hyperstimulation.

Poor Responders

Multiple strategies for stimulating resistant ovaries have been attempted. There is no single protocol that works for everyone and at times a trial and error approach is needed.

The flare is the most commonly used poor responder protocol. As described above, it employs the use of a GnRH agonist during the early follicular phase of the cycle. After ultrasound, hCG and estradiol levels are assessed to confirm lack of pregnancy and follicular recruitment, GnRH agonist (full dose or microdose) begins by day 3 of the cycle. Gonadotropin is added the day after agonist start. LH use can be avoided because the flare commonly leads to a discharge of LH from the pituitary gland. Gonadotropin dose is adjusted based upon periodic monitoring and ultimately administering hCG to allow the oocyte to complete meiosis I. One can also use the GnRH antagonist protocols for poor responders (see above).

A variation on the luteal suppression protocol for poor responders is the GnRH agonist stop protocol. This flows as a hybrid of the luteal suppression and the GnRH antagonist protocol. With this regimen, the agonist is started in the luteal phase as described above, however, after suppression is noted, the agonist is stopped and gonadotropins started. A GnRH antagonist can be used as the cycle progresses to minimize the potential for a spontaneous LH surge.

Attempts at minimizing the suppressive effects of OCPs and GnRH agonists have lead to the development of more novel protocols. Two such examples include the estrogen priming protocol (EPP) and the follicular antagonist protocol (FAP). In the EPP, luteal estrogen may provide modest negative feedback on pituitary gonadotrophs thereby delaying spontaneous follicular recruitment and assertion of follicular dominance.[30] Initially, patients monitor for an LH surge either by assessing serum LH levels or with a urinary LH kit at home. On day 10 post LH surge 0.1 mg transdermal estradiol patch is applied and changed every other day until menses. On second day of patches (day 11 post LH surge) the patient uses 0.25 mg of a GnRH antagonist for 3 days. On day 2 of menses, the patient has a baseline evaluation and stops changing the estradiol patch allowing the last patch to fall off on its own (or is removed with hCG trigger). On day 2 post menses, the patient begins at least 150 IU FSH and at least 150 IU mixed FSH/LH. The GnRH antagonist is restarted with either estradiol more than 300 pg/ml, lead follicle of 13 mm mean diameter or day 7 of stimulation. This protocol may improve follicular development and pregnancy rates in poor responders.[30]

The FAP also servers to delay spontaneous follicular recruitment and assertion of follicular dominance.[31] The protocol relies on pituitary suppression prior to selection of follicular dominance in the early follicular phase. With this protocol, a GnRH antagonist is initiated early in the follicular phase in combination with medroxyprogesterone acetate (MPA) (Figure 1). The GnRH antagonist serves to suppress pituitary gonadotropin release and prevent follicular recruitment. The purpose of the MPA is to suppress endometrial development and allow for endometrial proliferation in synch with the ovarian stimulation phase of this protocol. The GnRH antagonist is continued for 8–10 days after which baseline ultrasound, beta hCG and estradiol monitoring is performed. Once suppression is noted, the GnRH antagonist is held and MPA discontinued. Stimulation with mixed FSH/LH begins at this point. From this point forward the protocol is executed in a similar fashion to a standard GnRH protocol. When compared to either the flare or standard GnRH protocol, limited data reveal that the FAP may yield more oocytes and embryos for transfer.[31]

CONCLUSION

Medical practice continuously evolves. Moving from natural cycles to medicated stimulation, IVF proves this rule. A wide array of stimulatory, suppressive and adjuvant agents can be used to manipulate the ovarian cycle in hopes of optimizing oocyte yield. In a broad sense, protocols differ based on their relative suppressive or stimulatory potential. Each has its strengths and weaknesses, and no single protocol proves effective for all patients. Because of this, combinations of medications can be tailored to suit the individual need of a patient. Regardless of the regimen selected close monitoring is essential to ensure safety as well as optimize oocyte yield and maturity.

REFERENCES

1. Trounson A, Conti A. Research in human in-vitro fertilisation and embryo transfer. Br Med J (Clin Res Ed). 1982; 285(6337):244-8.
2. Pelinck MJ, Vogel NE, Arts EG, et al. Cumulative pregnancy rates after a maximum of nine cycles of modified natural cycle IVF and analysis of patient dropout: a cohort study. Hum Reprod. 2007;22(9):2463-70.
3. Pelinck MJ, Hoek A, Simons AH, et al. Efficacy of natural cycle IVF: a review of the literature. Hum Reprod Update. 2002;8(2):129-39.
4. Kousta E, White DM, Franks S. Modern use of clomiphene citrate in induction of ovulation. Hum Reprod Update. 1997;3(4):359-65.
5. Messinis IE, Nillius SJ. Comparison between tamoxifen and clomiphene for induction of ovulation. Acta Obstet Gynecol Scand. 1982;61(4):377-9.
6. Boostanfar R, Jain JK, Mishell DR, et al. A prospective randomized trial comparing clomiphene citrate with tamoxifen citrate for ovulation induction. Fertil Steril. 2001;75(5):1024-6.
7. Reproductive endocrine and endometrial effects of raloxifene hydrochloride, a selective estrogen receptor modulator, in women with regular menstrual cycles. J clin Endocrinol Metab. 1998;83(1):6-13.
8. Requena A, Herrero J, Landeras J, et al. Use of letrozole in assisted reproduction: a systematic review and meta-analysis. Hum Reprod Update. 2008;14(6):571-82.
9. Biljan MM, Hemming R, Brassard N. The outcome of 150 babies following the treatment with letrozole or letrozole and gonadotropins. Fertil Steril. 2005;84 (suppl 1):O-231.
10. Tulandi T, Martin J, Al-Fadhli R, et al. Congenital malformations among 911 newborns conceived after infertility treatment with letrozole or clomiphene citrate. Fertil Steril. 2006;85(6):1761-5.

11. Fontana PG, Leclerc JM. Contraindication of Femara® (letrozole) in premenopausal women. [online] Available from http://www.novartis.ca/products/en/pharmaceuticals-f.shtml
12. Belchetz PE, Plant TM, Nakai Y, et al. Hypophysial responses to continuous and intermittent delivery of hypothalamic gonadotropin-releasing hormone. Science. 1978;202(4368):631-3.
13. Cutler GB Jr, Hoffman AR, Swerdloff RS, et al. NIH Conference. Therapeutic applications of luteinizing hormone-releasing-hormone and its analogs. Ann Intern Med. 1985;102(57):643-57.
14. Mathias JR, Clench MH, Reeves-Darby VG, et al. Effect of leuprolide acetate in patients with moderate to severe functional bowel disease. Double-blind, placebo-controlled study. Dig Dis Sci. 1994;39(6):1155-62.
15. Recombinant follicle stimulating hormone: development of the first biotechnology product for the treatment of infertility. Hum Reprod Update. 1998;4:862-81.
16. le Cotonnec JY, Porchet HC, Beltrami V, et al. Clinical pharmacology of recombinant human follicle-stimulating hormone (FSH). I. Comparative Pharmacokinetics with urinary FSH. Fertil Steril. 1994;61(4):669-78.
17. Lunenfeld B. Historical perspectives in gonadotrophin therapy. Hum Reprod Update. 2004;10(6):453-67.
18. Vandervorst M, Devroey P. Recombinant FSH: results in assisted reproduction. In: Filicori M, Flamigni C (Eds). Ovulation Induction: Update '98: The Proceedings of the 2nd World Conference on Ovulation Induction. Carnforth: Parthenon Publishing Group; 1997. pp. 137-46.
19. Bassett R, Lispi M, Ceccarelli D, et al. Analytical identification of additional impurities in urinary-derived gonadotrophins. Reprod BioMed Online. 2009;19(3):300-13.
20. Tarlatzis BC, Fauser BC, Kolibianakis EM, et al. GnRH antagonists in ovarian stimulation for IVF. Hum Reprod Update. 2006;12(4):333-40.
21. Increased oocyte production after treatment with dehydroepiandrosterone. Barad DH, Gleicher N. Fertil Steril. 2005 Sep;84(3):756.
22. Nielsen ME, Rasmussen IA, Kristensen SG, et al. In human granulosa cells from small antral follicles, androgen receptor mRNA and androgen levels in follicular fluid correlate with FSH receptor mRNA. Mol Hum Reprod. 2011;17(1):63-70.
23. Barad D, Gleicher N. Effect of dehydroepiandrosterone on oocyte and embryo yields, embryo grade and cell number in IVF. Hum Reprod. 2006;21(11):2845-9.
24. Sönmezer M, Ozmen B, Cil AP, et al. Dehydroepiandrosterone supplementation improves ovarian response and cycle outcome in poor responders. Reprod BioMed Online. 2009;19(4):508-13.
25. Scobey MJ, Raike E, Marshall DC. Mixed protocols: multiple ratios of FSH and LH bioactivity using highly purified, human-derived FSH (BRAVELLE) and highly purified hMG (MENOPUR) are unaltered by mixing together in the same syringe. Reprod Biol Endocrinol. 2005;3:61.
26. A randomized prospective trial comparing gonadotropin-releasing hormone (GnRH) antagonist/recombinant follicle-stimulating hormone (rFSH) versus GnRH-agonist/rFSH in women pretreated with oral contraceptives before in vitro fertilization. Barmat LI, Chantilis SJ, Hurst BS, Dickey RP. Fertil Steril. 2005 Feb;83(2):321-30.
27. Kolibianakis EM, Papanikolaou EG, Camus M, et al. Effect of oral contraceptive pill pretreatment on ongoing pregnancy rates in patients stimulated with GnRH antagonists and recombinant FSH for IVF. A randomized controlled trial. Hum Reprod. 2006;21(2):352-7.
28. Huirne JA, van Loenen AC, Donnez J, et al. Effect of an oral contraceptive pill on follicular development in IVF/ICSI patients receiving a GnRH antagonist: a randomized study. Reprod BioMed Online. 2006;13(2):235-45.
29. Al-Inany H, Aboulghar MA, Mansour RT, et al. Optimizing GnRH antagonist administration: meta-analysis of fixed versus flexible protocol. Reprod BioMed Online. 2005;10(5):567-70.
30. Dragisic K, Davis O, Fasouliotis SJ, et al. Use of a luteal estradiol patch and a gonadotropin releasing hormone antagonist suppression protocol before gonadotropin stimulation for in vitro fertilization in poor responders. Fertil Steril. 2005;84(4):1023-26.
31. Frankfurter D, Dayal M, Dubey A, Peak D, Gindoff P. Fertil Steril. 2007 Nov;88(5):1442-5.

20

Procedures and Protocols in In Vitro Fertilization Laboratory

Douglas Peak, Reem Khaldi, Anil K Dubey

Chapter Contents

- In Vitro Fertilization Equipment
- Supplies (Media and Disposables)
- Quality Management Program
- Training and Protocols

INTRODUCTION

Since the advent of *in vitro* fertilization (IVF) and the birth of the first baby, the procedures and techniques which make IVF possible have become highly refined. Unique in the medical field, the treatment of a patient requires a symbiotic relationship between the clinic and lab. Clinicians cannot have a strong clinical practice without a solid IVF laboratory, and they cannot have a strong IVF lab without a solid clinical practice. Clinic and laboratory must work together to provide optimal results, a live birth, for a patient. A superior lab is made up of several key components: equipment, supplies (media and disposables), quality management, training and protocols.

IN VITRO FERTILIZATION EQUIPMENT

In vitro fertilization laboratory equipment comes in various shapes and sizes. Every laboratory staff member has particular equipment that he or she favors. Preferences are often individual. Sometimes that preference is based on science and sometimes that reason is purely because he or she feels something 'just works better'. Whatever reason a clinician use to choose a particular piece of equipment, keep in mind that no matter how good or how highly recommended a piece of equipment is, everything breaks and will need maintenance. Clinicians need to investigate the technical support in their area for that piece of equipment. Make certain you ask questions, such as: How long will it take to get a service technician to work on your machine? How much will it cost? Let us look closer at the primary equipment an IVF lab requires.

The Incubator

The incubator is the heart of the IVF laboratory. In essences, it will act as a pseudo female reproductive system providing a safe protective environment that will nurture the oocyte and sperm while it morphs into an embryo. The embryo is then cultured in an incubator until day 2 through day 6 depending on the day of transfer. There are three common varieties of incubators currently available based on the type of gases they use: carbon dioxide and air, carbon dioxide, air and nitrogen (also known as tri-gas) or tri-gas premixed. An incubator that uses a carbon dioxide tank will allow the lab to be able to alter the percent CO_2 in the incubator. This allows the lab the ability to control the pH of the culture medium as it might change from one lot to another. Clinicians will not have this ability if they use a premixed gas.

A tri-gas incubator includes the ability to connect a nitrogen tank to the incubator in addition to the CO_2 tank for the purpose of creating a low oxygen environment. The nitrogen is used to displace the oxygen in the air so that inside the incubator there would be a tri-gas mixture of, for example, 6% CO_2, 5% O_2 and 89% N_2. Is a tri-gas incubator necessary? This is one of those examples of personal preferences. There is research indicating that a tri-gas incubator will reduce fragmentation thus increasing the number of cells seen in a blastocyst. Other research indicates that a tri-gas incubator is only useful after day 2 of embryo culture. A tri-gas incubator is not needed for an IVF lab as evidenced by the hundreds and thousands of successful labs that do not use them. Additionally, these incubators use a lot of nitrogen which can be an added expense for a laboratory. To compensate for the added expense rather than purchase individual tanks of nitrogen, labs often use nitrogen generators or draw nitrogen directly from a liquid nitrogen tank.

The premixed tri-gas has become more popular with the introduction of a new smaller type of benchtop incubator. These incubators are specifically designed for IVF culture plates and are only large enough to hold a couple of dishes, in essence one or two patients per incubator. The smaller size allows for faster recovery of both temperature and gas environment in comparison to the larger standard incubators. Their design allows them to often save floor space in the IVF lab. However, since these use a premixed gas, the culture system's pH cannot be readily altered by adjusting the gas mixture. Additionally, the premixed gas must be purchased from a reliable gas company.

Microscopes

Microscopes (Figure 1) are the eyes of the laboratory. An IVF lab needs 3 types of microscopes: a phase contrast microscope, an inverted microscope with micromanipulator and a stereo dissecting microscope. The phase contrast microscope should have a 10x and 20x lenses for sperm counting and a 100x oil emersion lens for morphological analysis. The inverted scope should be equipped with 4x, 10x, 20x and 40x lenses, a heated work stage and a micromanipulator for intracytoplasmic sperm injection (ICSI) and assisted hatching (AH). Additionally, the inverted scope can be set up with a camera and monitor (with or without image capture), or be outfitted with a laser for AH which includes a video capture system. The stereo dissecting scope has a transmitted illumination base used for the visualization of the oocytes and embryos. Lower magnification (7x–15x) can be used to scan follicular fluid and aid in the movement of the embryo from culture dish to culture dish. Higher magnification (30x–70x) allows for oocyte classification and pronuclear identification. A stereoscope can be free standing with a heated working stage or mounted into a heated hood.

Hood/Work Surface

Tissue culture hoods or laminar flow hoods (Figure 2) are all different terms for biological safety cabinets. All should use high efficiency particulate air filters to treat exhaust air to protect the lab worker and environment from contamination. It is an enclosed benchtop often made of stainless steel that provides a work surface for

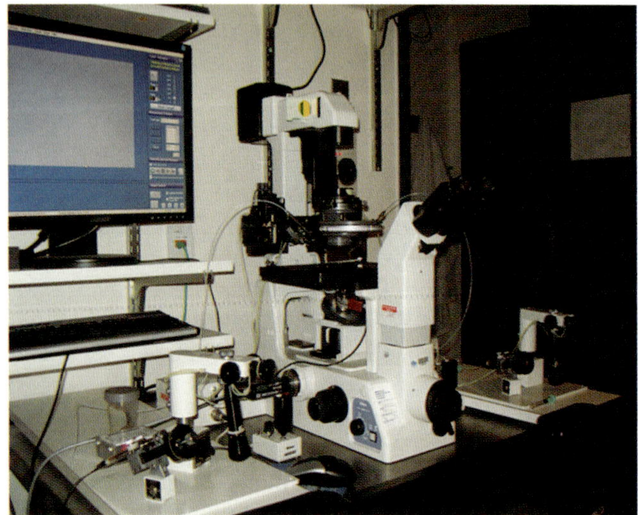

Figure 1 Microscope

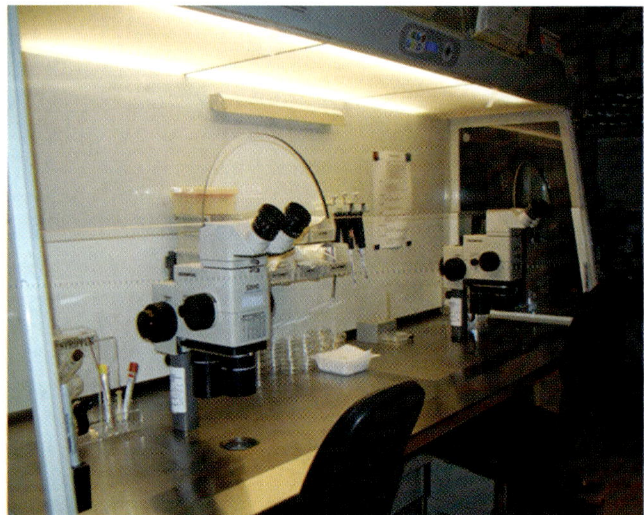

Figure 2 Laminar flow hood

the IVF lab. Ones manufactured specifically for an IVF lab can be heated or unheated. Maintaining a consistent temperature of 37°C is vital in the IVF lab because oocytes and embryos are sensitive to temperature shock. All surfaces that any oocyte or embryo can come in contact with must be at 37°C. A hood with a heated work surface is ideal. If not cost effective, an unheated hood may be used with slide warmers placed inside to preheat petri dishes and culture media.

SUPPLIES (MEDIA AND DISPOSABLES)

When laboratory teams first started culturing oocytes, sperm and embryos, they used plates and media designed for general tissue culture. Much has been learned through trial and error since the early days of IVF culture. Materials have become specialized in order to meet the specific needs of the IVF laboratory. Clinicians know now that care needs to be taken in selecting the supplies for the IVF process.

In vitro fertilization supplies can be categorized as disposables (plates, dishes, pipettes, tubes, etc.) and media. Choice of supplies becomes a very personalized issue in the IVF lab. Each lab has a slightly different method of culturing the gametes and embryos, which will affect the choices of culture plate and media used. Each embryologist has a distinct idea about what he or she thinks works best. Companies spend a lot of money sending their representative to the various labs in the hopes that the lab will switch products.

Culture Systems

Gametes and embryos have been successfully cultured in a variety of methods: test tubes, four well plates, petri dishes and organ culture dishes. Originally cultured in test tubes, hence the term test tube babies, today most labs use some type of dish. Culture systems can be separated into two distinct variants; opened and closed.

In an open system, the culture medium is directly exposed to the gases in the incubator. One of the advantages of this type of system is that it allows for the rapid equilibration of the medium, however, when out of the incubator the medium will also lose CO_2 just as rapidly. Care needs to be exercised to minimize the time the plates are out of the incubator when using this type of culture system.

A closed system uses medium often in micro drops of 10–20 µl overlayed with equilibrated mineral or paraffin oil. The oil acts as a buffer between the medium and the environment delaying gas diffusion, medium evaporation and filtering any air borne particles. A closed system will maintain pH, temperature and osmolarity better than an open system. All major IVF media suppliers now offer some type of oil to be used as an overlay, be careful in choosing your oil. Over the years, several companies have had manufacturing problems with their oil resulting in compromised results in the IVF lab.

Disposables

Depending on the manufacturing process, material the product is made from, sterilization process and storage conditions, some supplies are toxic to gametes and embryos. Today several companies manufacture supplies that are specifically intended for usage in IVF labs. These products come with certificates of analysis verifying that the lot of products has passed some form of mouse embryo testing. Whenever possible use supplies that are specifically designed for the IVF lab. If a certified product cannot be used, then the laboratory must test the product with a bioassay such as, mouse embryo testing or sperm survival testing prior to using the product in the laboratory. Each new lot of product received needs to be retested to ensure product quality.

Media

The early days of IVF offered very few choices for culture media. Today, many companies offer a variety of different media depending on how you would like to culture. This is again one of the areas of personal choice since all of the media seem to work well. In general, the different media can be grouped as sequential or nonsequential, single step. Additionally, each medium will either be bicarbonate or N-(2-hydroxyethyl)-piperazine-N′-2-ethanesulfonic acid (HEPES) buffered. Bicarbonate buffered media needs to be equilibrated in CO_2 to achieve the proper pH while HEPES buffered media can be used in room air. Care should be taken to avoid prolong exposure of the oocyte or embryo to the HEPES for a long period of time as it can be toxic over the long term. HEPES buffered media are most often used for oocyte and embryo manipulation, such as denuding, ICSI or AH.

Sequential medium is based on the concept that as an embryo develops from day of fertilization to blastocyst, it will have different nutritional needs. Sequential media are designed to work as a group. This is usually a combination of two or three different media that are designed to meet the nutritional needs of the embryo depending on its developmental stage: one medium for fertilization, one medium for day 1–3 and finally one medium for day 3–6.

Nonsequential medium or single step medium is specially designed to meet all nutritional needs for each stage of development. Proponents for the nonsequential medium claim that one medium will provide the optimum environment with no osmolality and pH shifts or shocks like those that can be experienced when changing medium in the sequential system. Opponents claim that one medium cannot meet the changing nutritional needs of the embryo (Table 1).

Which is the best system to use? Many posters and publications have been devoted to this topic. Each seems to work well depending on clinicians' lab setup and the type of incubators they choose to use. It is best to trial each system and the different types of media offered by the different companies to find out what works best in your laboratory.

No matter what media a clinician choose, always start with the manufacture recommendations and then optimize its usage for the lab. Prior to using any new medium, or for that matter new lot of a medium, that the clinicians are currently using, check the pH. Allow the medium to equilibrate in the incubator for at least 3–4 hours, but preferably overnight. After equilibration, test the pH. Optimal culture conditions are a pH of 7.2–7.4, with current thinking preferring the lower end of the range. There is an inverse relationship between the pH and the percent CO_2. The pH of the media can be decreased by raising the CO_2 and increased by decreasing the CO_2.

QUALITY MANAGEMENT PROGRAM

The objective of a quality management program is to provide an ongoing process for monitoring and evaluating quality and appropriateness of care in the IVF lab. By defining indicators and developing threshold values, important aspects of care may be studied in a planned and systematic method. The results of this regular analysis will be used to identify problems, highlight opportunities for improvement in quality and serve as a vehicle for communication between lab and clinical staff. The ultimate goal of the IVF lab is to provide the patient with the highest quality embryos possible in sufficient numbers that will contribute to the ultimate outcome of a successful pregnancy and live birth. Quality assurance in the IVF lab is the responsibility of the laboratory director of the IVF program.

The responsibilities of the IVF program director includes: delegating responsibility to the IVF lab supervisor and staff who collect and compile data for use in the monitoring and evaluation of the quality and appropriateness of care in the IVF lab; implementation of actions to improve the quality is also the responsibility of the director. The lab director ensures that all lab staff members are aware of the quality management responsibilities in the department. It is the responsibility of all lab personnel to know and follow the quality management process. The quality management process must be fully documented. Sources that will be used to provide the necessary information include:

- Patient oocyte/sperm sheet
- *In vitro* fertilization electronic medical records
- Quality control sheets—temperature records
- Instrument maintenance records
- Direct observation of patients or staff
- Documented written complaints
- Accident and incident reports

The IVF lab staff will collect and compile data on a monthly basis. After the data is organized and tabulated, the supervisor or director will use the information to prepare a report. Included in this report will be a monitor of the ongoing fertilization rate and pregnancy rate. These reports will be the basis of the monthly committee meetings which will be held in conjunction with the monthly lab meetings. At this time the reports will be submitted to the IVF laboratory director for review. The IVF team will meet once a week to review: positive and negative pregnancies, currently cycling patients and new patient cases. The meeting will include one member of the IVF Lab, all doctors and nurses in the IVF program and one clinical secretary. This meeting also presents the opportunity for the quality management report to be presented and discussed.

Laboratory Indicators and Thresholds

An indicator is a measurable parameter used to monitor an important aspect of care. A threshold is a pre-established level of performance related to a particular indicator. When the level of performance reaches the threshold, evaluation must be performed to determine if a problem exists or opportunity for improvement is present (Table 2). Developing indicators and revising

Table 1 Types of media offered by the different companies

Company	Product
Life Global	Global, HTF, Blastocyst
Irvine Scientific	P1, HTF, Multiblast, Single Step Medium, Early Cleavage Medium, Ham's F10
Sage	Quinn's Advantage: Fertilization, Cleavage, Blastocyst
COOK	Sydney IVF: Fertilization, Cleavage, Blastocyst
Vitrolife	G1, G2, G-IVF

Table 2 Laboratory indicators and thresholds

Lab indicators	Threshold	Patients
Percent GV, MI oocytes	> 50%	3
DG or fractured zona	> 5%	3
Percent fertilization	< 50% (0%)	4(2)
Percent 3 pronuclei (PN)	> 10%	3
Quality of embryos	> Type III	3
Development of blastocysts	< 30%	3
Pregnancy rate	< 10%	10
Multiple pregnancy rate	> 20%	10
% Viability post thaw	< 50%	10

thresholds represent a day to day, ongoing commitment to continual quality improvement.

Sentinel events will be evaluated immediately by the directors of the IVF program. Sentinel events are activities or outcomes that are so serious or unexpected that every case warrants evaluation. An example of a sentinel event would be failure of all of a patient's fertilized zygotes to divide. All information pertaining to the sentinel event will be included in a quality assurance review. Whenever a threshold is surpassed, an evaluation of an important aspect of care is triggered to determine if a problem exists or there is an opportunity for the improvement in quality.

TRAINING AND PROTOCOLS

Finding a well-trained embryologist is crucial to the overall program. Many IVF centers will not train an embryologist because of the inherent 'risk' with having a new person in the lab that might make a mistake. Throughout the training process, the trainee must observe all procedures before actually performing the task independently. Prior to being 'cleared' to perform a particular procedure, the trainee must be observed by a senior embryologist at all time. While every lab uses slightly different policies and protocols, there are some general procedures that should be followed by all labs:

- The assisted reproductive technology (ART) laboratory will be maintained as a separate unit. Only procedures directly related to oocyte, sperm and embryo culturing will be performed in the lab.
- Traffic in the lab will be kept to a minimum.
- No eating, drinking, smoking, manipulation of contact lenses, mouth pipetting or applying of make-up, fixing of hair will be allowed in the lab.
- Scrubs, hat and mask will be worn. Hands must be scrubbed before peforming any technical procedure.
- Protective powder free gloves will be worn prior to handling any sperm, oocytes or embryos.
- While working in the IVF lab, remember that a sterile environment is essential at all times. All procedures pertaining to culturing of oocytes, sperm and embryos are to be carried out using proper sterile technique and sterile materials.
- The temperature of the lab will be maintained from 20–25°C by and individually controlled thermostat. Incubators and thermoplate give off heat so the lab must have air conditioning with a thermostat located in the lab.
- The room is to be maintained under a positive air flow.
- The enviroment should be kept as dust free as possible. All housekeeping services will be performed by laboratory personnel.

All procedures involving human oocytes and embryos must be performed as rapidly as possible to ensure that they will be exposed to a less than ideal environment only when necessary.

Oocyte Retrieval

An oocyte retrieval is the process by which the physician aspirates ovarian follicles into test tubes. The aspiration is done using a transvaginal ultrasound transducer equipped with a needle guide. Through the needle guide, a single or double lumen needle is passed. There are different aspiration needles manufactured by various companies. Each needle has its advantages or disadvantages. The type of needle used and from which company it is purchased is an area of personal preference. In general, a single lumen has one bore while a double has two. The second outer channel in the double lumen allows for ease of flushing of the ovarian follicle. Naturally, this means that the double lumen will be smaller and more likely to clog or cause ruptured oocytes. When used in conjunction with a regulated vacuum suction system, the doctor will use the needle to aspirate follicular fluid into test tubes. It is then the responsibility of the embryologist to find the oocyte in the follicular fluid and to transfer the oocyte to the appropriate culture media for insemination.

The day before the retrieval, the embryologist needs to ensure that all the appropriate media is made and equilibrated. The lab should be stocked with all the needed culture dishes and disposables. The clinical staff must provide the lab with a written procedure request indicating the patient's and partner's names, dates of birth and unique identifying number, such as, a medical record number. Additionally, the form must indicate what procedures are being requested, such as ICSI, AH, blastocyst transfer and cryopreservation, preimplantation genetic diagnosis or preimplantation genetic screening. While not standard practice in some IVF centers, it is important to have the patient and partner prescreened for infectious diseases, such as HIV Types 1 and 2, HBV (HBsAg, anti-HBc – IgG + IgM), HCV, syphilis (RPR), chlamydia or gonorrhea. Patients testing reactive within the last 6 months must have their gametes and/or embryos cultured under isolation conditions. Ideally, this means in a separate incubator that can be decontaminated after the patient's case is completed.

The day of the retrieval, when the patient is brought into the IVF procedure room, the patient should identify herself to the laboratory staff. When the physician, procedure room nurse, anesthesiologist, medical technologist and embryologist(s) are all present in the room, there should be a 'time-out' pre-retrieval pause.

- The embryologist will read the patient's name, her date of birth, medical record number and procedure to be preformed. For example, "please confirm that this is Mrs Smith, date of birth 1/1/1965, MRN 9999999. She is here for retrieval with ICSI."
- The remaining staff will confirm this information.

Label the pre-equilibrated plates in the incubator with the name and a second identifier, such as, cycle number or medical record number as indicated during the timeout. Place a removable label with patient's name and second identifier on the outside of the glass door of the incubator identifying the patient's assigned location. The patient's chart should be placed in the IVF lab hood until the end of the retrieval. Tubes containing follicular aspirates will be passed through the window from the procedure room to the lab and placed in the block heater. The medical assistant placing the tube in the heater will again state the patient's name for the first tube. For example, 'first tube on Mrs Smith'. Pour out the contents of each tube into a petri dish. Scan the fluid for cumulus masses. Be sure not to overfill your dish as this makes finding an oocyte harder. If you find an oocyte, remove as much follicular fluid as possible from the petri dish. The cumulus/corona mass can now be scored.

Scoring Cumulus/Corona Masses

Additionally, gentle and quickly spread the cumulus out away from the inner oocyte and using the inverted microscope, try to assess the oocyte maturity (Figures 3 to 10).

After assessing the oocyte cumulus complex and/or the oocyte maturity, wash the oocyte cumulus complex twice in the appropriate medium, such as human tubal fluid (HTF) or modified HTF (mHTF) containing 10% human serum albumin (HSA), then transfer into a culture plate with appropriate medium, such as HTF+10% HSA. Make sure the plate is labeled with the patient's name and second identifier. Call out to the OR team the number of eggs the patient has, label the well with the oocyte number (01, 02, 03...) and record the information on the retrieval sheet. If a clinician does not find an oocyte after a minute or two, you should aspirate the fluid out of the dish and back into the tube with a 10 cc syringe. Clinician can look again after the case.

Preparation of Sperm for *In Vitro* Fertilization/ Intracytoplasmic Sperm Injection

Ejaculated semen is a viscous liquid made up of a combination of live sperm, dead sperm and cells, such as leukocytes and immature sperm cells suspended in various seminal secretions. The seminal secretions have been shown to inhibit capacitation and prevent fertilization. While the dead sperm and leukocytes are known to release reactive oxygen species which can

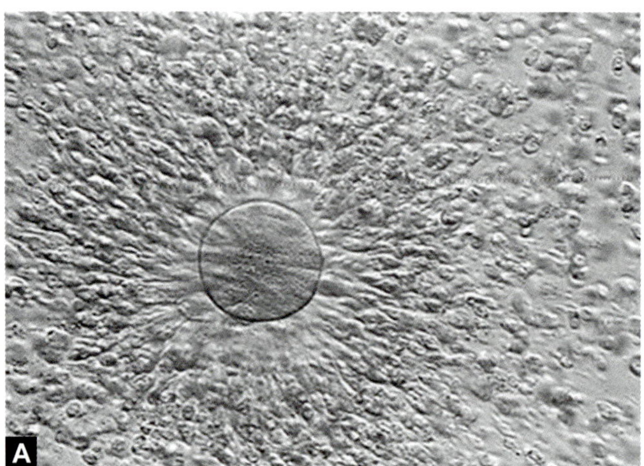

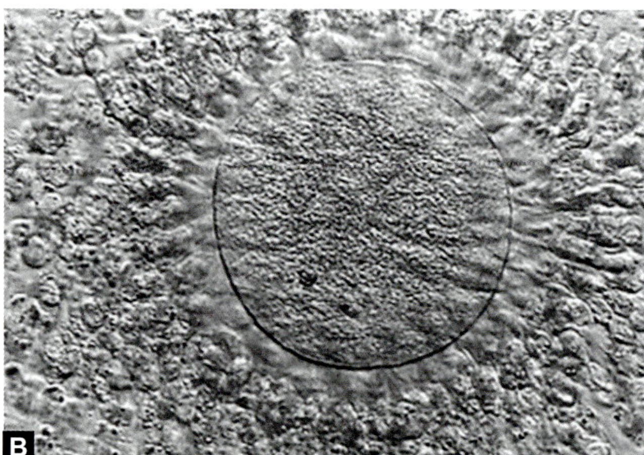

Figures 3A and B Type I oocytes: characterized by corona radiata, mature looking, expanded corona and cumulus

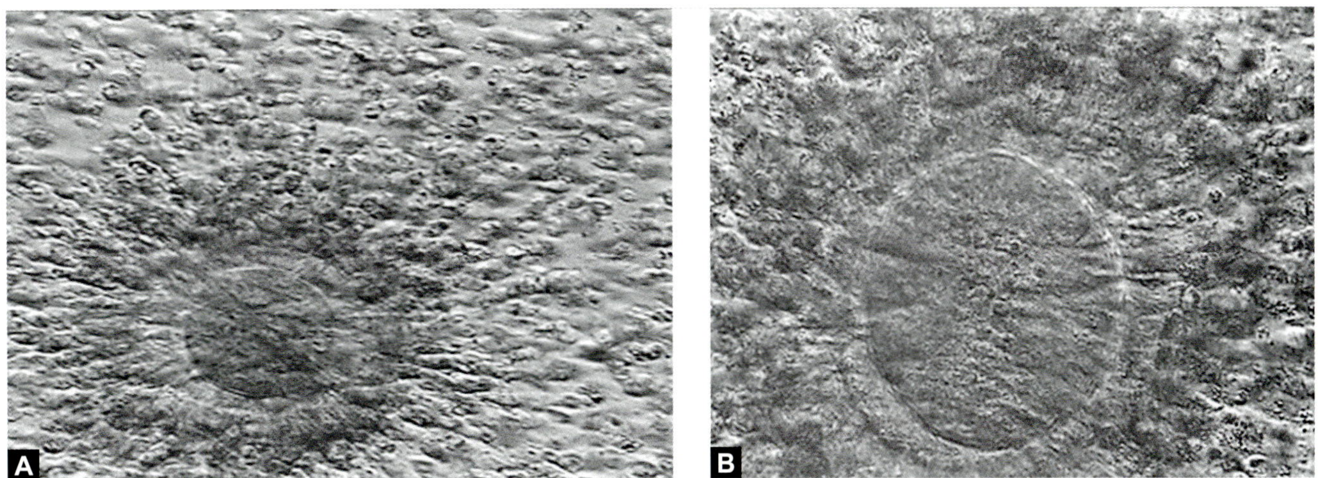

Figures 4A and B Type II oocytes: intermediate maturity, less expanded corona and cumulus

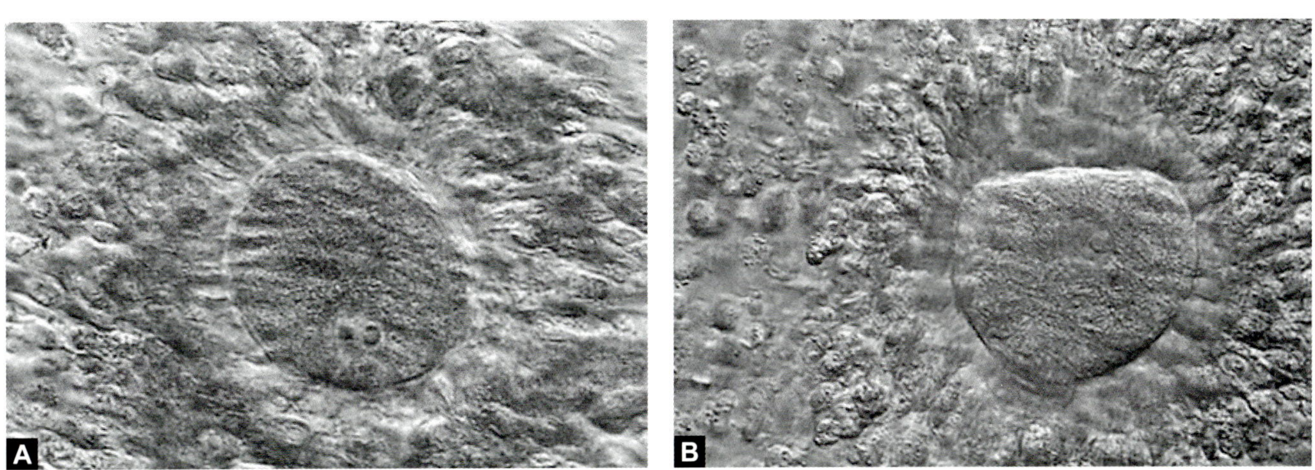

Figures 5A and B Immature oocytes (Prophase I-GV)

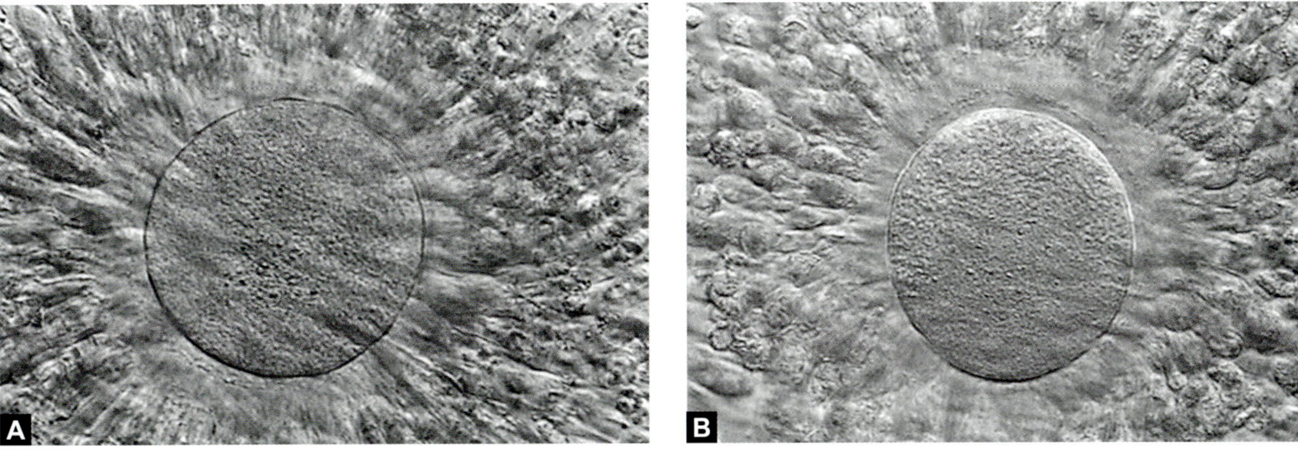

Figures 6A and B Immature oocytes (Metaphase I-MI)

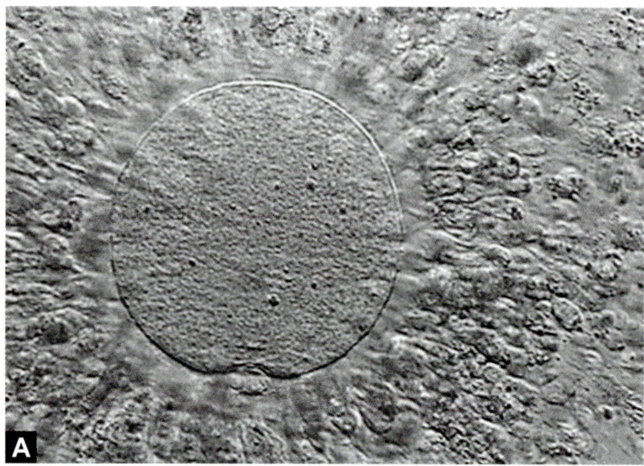

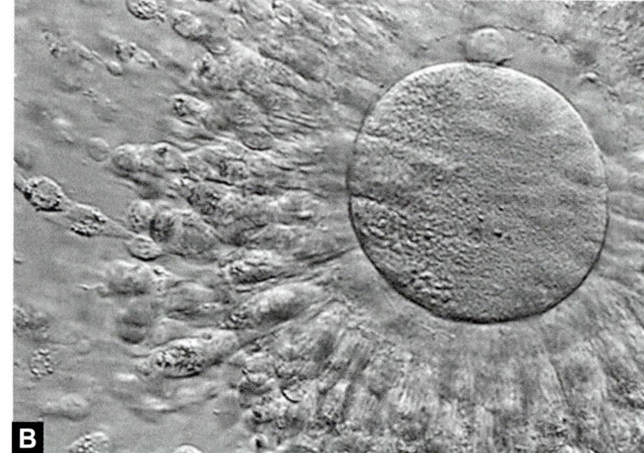

Figures 7A and B Mature oocyte (Metaphase II-MII)

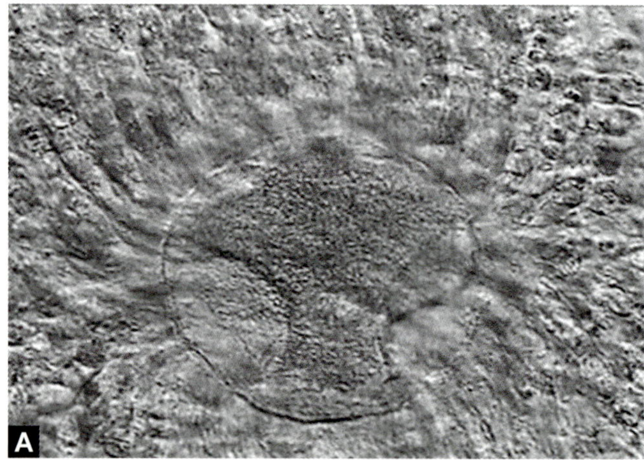

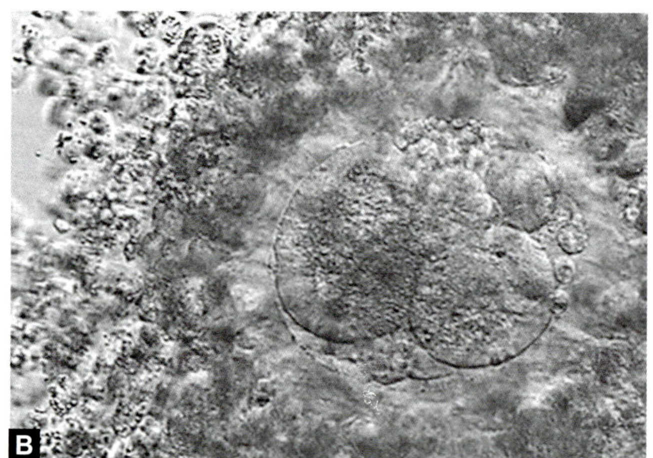

Figures 8A and B Degenerative oocyte

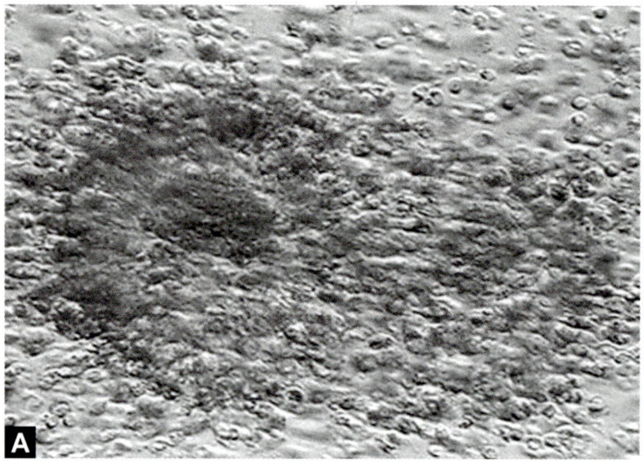

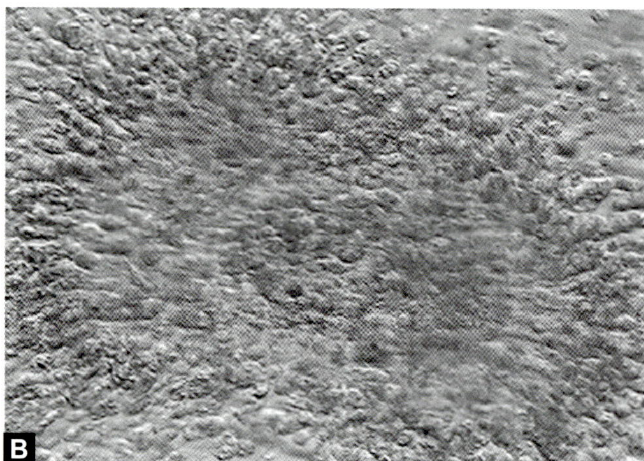

Figures 9A and B Ruptured oocyte

inhibit fertilization and cellular development. In order to inseminate an oocyte either through normal IVF or ICSI, the live motile sperm needs to be separated from the rest. This is accomplished through density gradient separation, a swim up technique or a combination of the two.

Many types of density gradients are available from commercial vendors. They can be a single 2 ml layer of 80% or 90%. Alternatively, many centers use two 1 ml layers of 40%/80% or 45%/90%. Care must be used not to mix the two layers during the making, storage and usage. The choice of a single or double layer gradient is

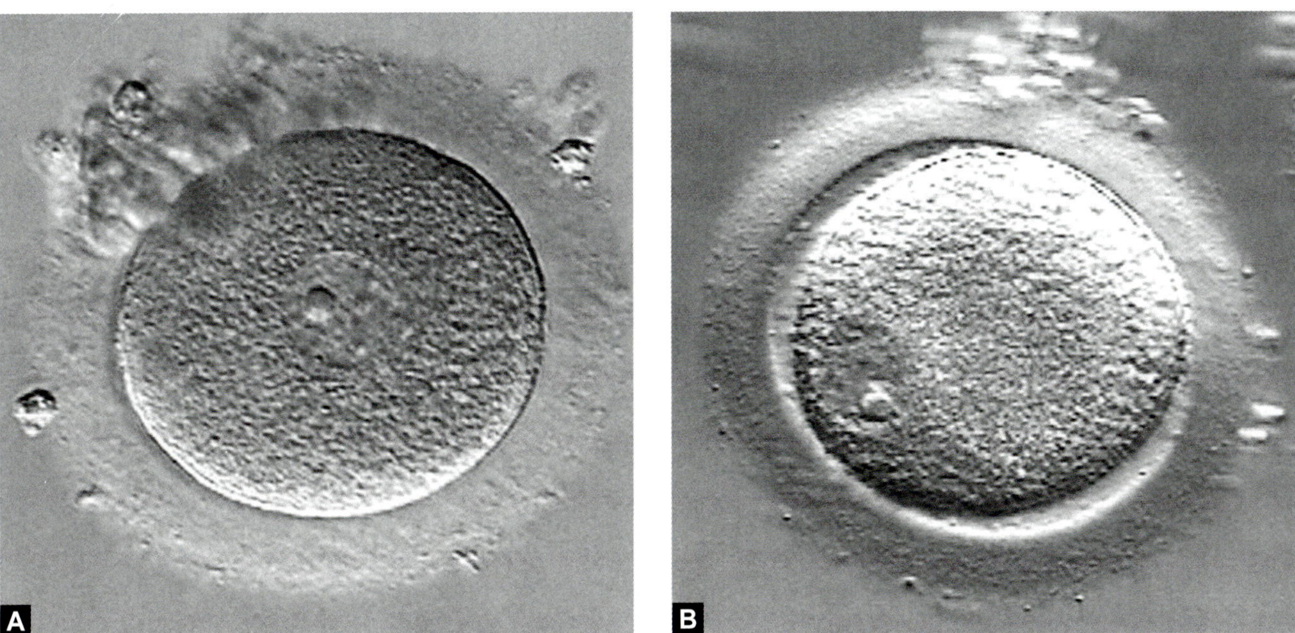

Prophase I Oocyte: Presence of a germinal vesicle (GV) indicates a completely immature oocyte. Takes more than 18 hours to mature.

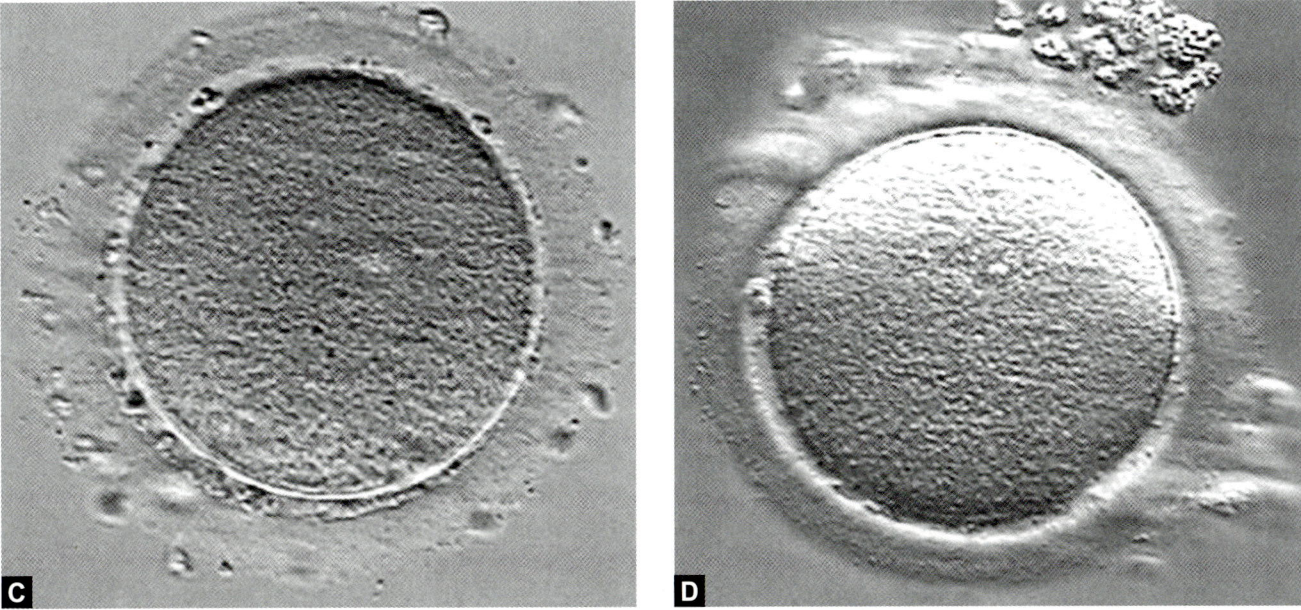

Metaphase I Oocyte: Lack of the GV and the lack of the first polar body indicates an immature MI oocyte
Takes about two hours to extrude the first polar body

Figures 10A to D

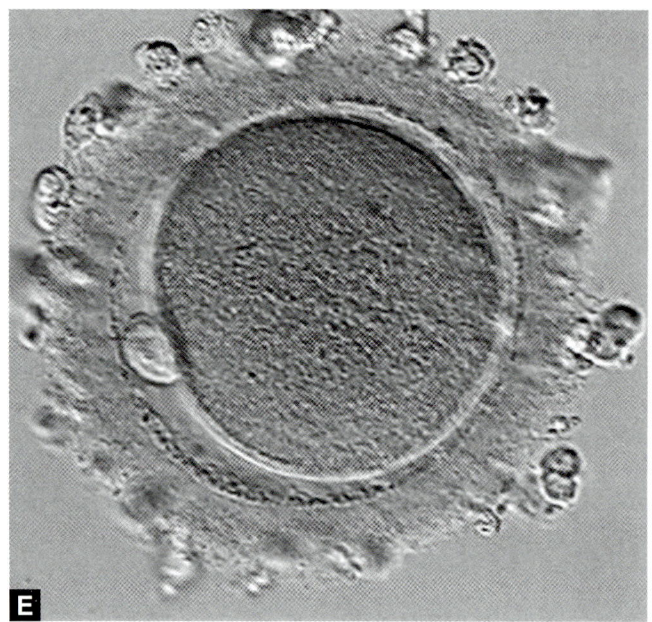

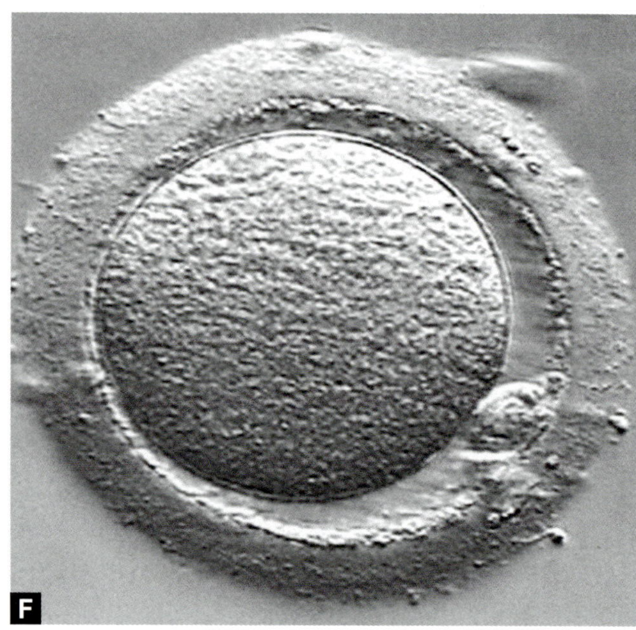

Metaphase II Oocyte: The presence of the first polar body indicates a mature MII oocyte that is ready for fertilization

Figures 10E and F

Figures 10A to F Maturity assessment

again one of personal preference and is often based on how the embryologist was trained.

Preparation of Fresh and Frozen Ejaculates

Tips, tricks and troubleshooting for semen sample is shown in the Table 3:

1. Place the patient's label on a tube rack.
2. Let the semen sample liquefy for at least 15–30 minutes or thaw in for at least 10 minutes at 37°C. Mix it well with a pipette. If it is too viscous, suck it up through an 18 gauge needle and a syringe to mix.
3. Take a drop of raw semen and check the concentration and motility. Record these numbers on the IVF sheet. If sperm concentration is very, very low (< 2 x 10^6 per ml), do 2x wash using appropriate medium such as HTF + 10% HSA or mHTF + 10% HSA. Do not use a gradient.
4. Layer the semen sample across 80–90% 2 ml gradient in a labeled 15 ml tube.
5. Centrifuge the suspension at 1,500 rpm for 10 minutes. Remove the pellet using a glass pipette.
6. Transfer to a 5 ml labeled tube containing 3–5 ml of appropriate medium. Resuspend the pellet and centrifuge again at 1,500 rpm for 5 minutes.
7. Discard the supernatant and add about 0.5 ml of appropriate medium. Transfer the solution to a labeled 5 ml falcon tube and spin down for 3 minutes. Place in the incubator for the swim-up. Transfer the rack label that is on the foam rack to the rack inside the incubator. Keep in the incubator for 0.5–3 hours.
8. Following the migration, remove the supernatant.
9. Follow the protocol for insemination.

Preparation of Testicular Tissue

1. Place the patient's label on a tube rack.
2. Obtain a sample of the testicular tissue in modified HTF + 10% HSA medium.
3. Cut the tissue into small pieces and use sterile glass tissue grinder to tease the tissue apart.
4. Place tissue and any fluid into a falcon tube. Add 3–5 ml of appropriate medium.
5. Centrifuge at 1,500 rpm for 5 minutes.
6. Remove the supernatant but leave 1 ml of medium. Resuspend the pellet.
7. Transfer the rack label to the rack inside the incubator.
8. Allow tube to sit in incubator for 1–2 hours.
9. Following incubation, add 3–5 ml of appropriate medium and centrifuge at 1500 rpm for 5 minutes.
10. Remove the supernatant but leave 1.0–0.1 ml of medium depending on the size of the pellet. Resuspend the pellet.
11. Follow the protocol for ICSI insemination.
12. Freeze all sample according to standard sperm freezing protocol.

Table 3 Tips, tricks and troubleshooting for semen samples

Problem	Probable Reasons	Response
Sperm counts very low % motility down as compared to previous sample	✓ Oligospermia ✓ Inappropriate abstinence time ✓ Cold, virus, infection ✓ On drugs	1. Obtain two ejaculates 2. Wash sperm by centrifugation and resuspension or tube migration 3. Isolate separation - multiple tube migration 4. Suggest ICSI 5. Microdrop insemination
Lower Migration	✓ Sperm antibody ✓ Lots of cellular debris ✓ Higher counts then normal	1. Ejaculate in EBSS 2. Multiple tube migration 3. Suggest ICSI
Ejaculate displays high viscosity with slow liquification	✓ Abnormal semen characteristics	1. Draw sample through a syringe several times with a 18 gauge needle 2. Use a Pasteur pipette to break up the sample 3. Use chymotrypsin protocol
Partner unable to provide a semen specimen	✓ Stress related factor(s)	1. Require that the semen sample be provided before the oocyte retrieval 2. Tell the partner to relax and assure him that you can wait for the specimen 3. Patient and partner can obtain the sample together at home
All sperm in the sample are dead	✓ Some factors involved in the method of semen collection ✓ Exposure of the sample in the extreme temperatures	1. Determine how he collected the sample and try to identify the problem 2. Change all plasticware which comes in contact with the semen sample 3. Request another sample later in the day for insemination

Preparation of Epididymal, Retrograde Ejaculation and Severe Oligospermia

1. Place the patient's label on a tube rack.
2. In a labeled 15 ml tube, mix the sample with appropriate medium, such as HTF or mHTF + 10% HSA volume to 10 ml.
3. Centrifuge the suspension at 1,500 rpm for 10 minutes. Discard the supernatant and add 3–5 ml of appropriate medium. Transfer to a 5 ml tube. Resuspend the pellet and centrifuge again at 1,500 rpm for 5 minutes.
4. Discard the supernatant and add about 0.5 ml of appropriate medium. Spin down for 3 minutes. Place in the incubator for the swim-up. Make sure the cap is loosened. Transfer the rack label to the rack inside the incubator. Keep in the incubator for 0.5–3 hours.
5. Following the migration, remove the supernatant.
6. Follow the protocol for ICSI.

Insemination for *in vitro* fertilization

Proper insemination of the oocytes is a critical step in the IVF procedure. Under insemination results in low fertilization rates while over insemination results in the formation of 3PNs. Techniques for insemination vary slightly from lab to lab, but generally fall under two categories: large volume culture insemination (> 500 µl) such as, in a 4 well plate and microdrop culture insemination (< 100 µl). Outlined below are some standard protocols for IVF insemination.

Large Volume Culture Insemination

1. Place the patient's chart whose oocytes you intend to inseminate in the IVF hood.

2. Remove that patient's sperm sample and label from the incubator. Verify that the name and secondary identifier on the tube match the information on the chart. Place the label on a rack under the hood containing the sample.
3. The goal is to inseminate one well of the 4-well NUNC plates (each well contains 1–5 oocytes) with 100,000–150,000 sperm.
4. After the sperm have swum (see semen preparation), take one drop and count the number of sperm per milliliter.
5. Calculate the number of sperm needed for insemination.
6. If you count 20 million motile sperm/ml and you wanted to inseminate with 150,000 sperm a clinician would need to use 7.5 µl

   150 / 20 = 7.5 µl
7. Pipette calculated volume from the sperm tube (aliquoted after migration) and mix it with the medium in a multiwell dish that contains no oocytes. Mix it well with pipette. Load a hemocytometer and check the number of motile sperm in 16 large squares. Take mean of four readings.

   (Concentration of motile sperm = 'mean of 4 readings' x 10,000)
8. If concentration is less than 150,000–200,000/ml, add more sperm to the test well. Repeat step 6 until count is correct. This is the volume you will use to inseminate all the oocytes.
9. Remove the 4-well plates that a clinician intend to inseminate. Make sure the name and secondary identifier on the 4-well plate match the information on the sperm prep tube and that both match the information on the chart in the IVF hood. This needs to be verified by 2 people.
10. Inseminate all wells containing oocytes regardless of assumed maturity. At the end of insemination check the sperm in wells by focusing at the bottom of the dish. Return the dish to the incubator.
11. Sperm survival should be checked between 3–4 hours following insemination.
12. Save the sample till the next day when fertilization can be confirmed. After fertilization is confirmed, discard the sample in the biohazardous trash.

Microdrop Culture Insemination

1. Place the patient's chart whose oocytes you intend to inseminate in the IVF hood.
2. Remove that patient's sperm sample and label from the incubator. Verify that the name on the tube and secondary identifier match the information on the chart. Place the label on a rack under the hood containing the sample.
3. The goal is to inseminate 50,000 sperm per 100 µl media drop with 1–2 oocytes per drop.
4. After the sperm has swum, (see semen preparation) take one drop and count the number of sperm per milliliter.
5. Calculate the number of sperm needed for insemination:

   If you counted 20 million motile sperm/ml and you wanted to inseminate with 50,000 sperm you would need to use 7.5 µl.

   50 / 20 = 2.5 µl
6. Set up a petri-dish containing 100 µl drops of equilibrated media and overlay with oil. Label it with the patient's name and secondary identifier as indicated on the chart.
7. Remove the 4-well plate that you intend to inseminate. Make sure the name and secondary identifier on the 4-well plates match the information on the sperm prep tube. And that both match the information on the chart in the IVF hood. This needs to be verified by two people.
8. Trim the cumulus of the oocytes to be placed in the drops.
9. Place 1–2 oocytes per drop.
10. Inseminate the drops with the proper number of sperm as calculated above.
11. Inseminate all drops containing oocytes regardless of assumed maturity. Return the dish to the incubator.
12. Sperm survival should be checked between 3–4 hours following insemination.
13. Save the sample till the next day when fertilization can be confirmed. After fertilization is confirmed, discard the sample in the biohazardous trash.

Decorinization

The oocyte is surrounded by cumulus mass of granulosa cells. In normal IVF (no ICSI), these cells need to be removed 18–20 hours post insemination in order to view fertilization (2PN formation) of the oocyte. Have several new dishes set up with appropriate medium, such as HTF + 10% HSA, at least 60 minutes prior to decorinization. The cumulus complex should mostly have been broken down by the sperm cells overnight, but the bottom of the plate often remains very sticky. Prepare a stripper pipette with a 130–140 µm tip. There are two common ways to prepare the tip. One is to prepare a glass pipette by heating up the tip over some form of flame, such as an alcohol lamp, and pulling it to the appropriate size of 130–140 µm. This is a learned skill and takes a lot of time to perfect. If not done properly, the pulled glass pipette can damage the oocyte. Fortunately, many commercial companies manufacture, sterilize and certify plastic or glass stripper tips of varying sizes to be used in common holders. Most commonly used to decorinize are the 130–140 µm tips. Fill pipette with the medium, locate oocyte and slowly flush out a stream of medium from the side and on top of the oocyte to dislodge it from bottom of the well. Transfer the oocyte to a fresh plate of appropriate medium once the oocyte is free from the bottom of the plate. Decorinization is carried out under the microscope by gently pipetting the oocyte in and out of the pipette tip. Once decorinized, follow the procedure for day 1 assessment—fertilization check.

For ICSI, the cumulus cells need to be removed in order for the embryologist to inject the oocyte. This is accomplished by placing the oocyte(s) in hyaluronidase. Again several commercial companies have hyaluronidase available. Have several new dishes set up with appropriate medium such as, HTF + 10% HSA, at least 60 minutes prior to decorinization. Also warm up some hyaluronidase and modified HTF + 10% HSA. Prepare a stripper pipette with a 130–140 µm tip. Using a 200 µl pipette tip make a 200–400 µl hyaluronidase drop. Transfer the oocyte(s) to the hyaluronidase solution. Decorinization is carried out under the microscope by gently pipetting the oocyte(s) in and out of the pipette tip. Watch for the cumulus to dissolve. Do not leave the oocyte(s) in the hyaluronidase for more than 30 seconds. Transfer the partially stripped oocyte(s) to modified HTF + 10% HSA media using the 130–140 µm stripper tip. Further decorinization can be carried out under the microscope by gently pipetting the oocyte(s) in and out of the pipette tip. After completing the decorinization, transfer the oocyte(s) to fresh HTF + 10% HSA culture media. Once decorinized, examine oocyte carefully and note the maturity of the oocyte [germinal vesicle (GV), metaphase I (MI), metaphase II (MII)]. Also note anything unusual about the oocyte (Figure 10A to F).

Intracytoplasmic Sperm Injection

Intracytoplasmic Sperm Injection involves the direct injection of a single 'normal' looking sperm into the cytoplasm of a mature (MII) oocyte. The procedure requires the use of a microscope with micromanipulator. Manipulators are generally oil filled or air filled. Each has its plusses and minuses, and the choice of the type of scope and manipulator is often based on what equipment you were trained on. The authors' preference is an oil filled system which they feel gives better control.

Setting-up the Micromanipulators (Figures 11A to D)

Two microinjectors control the suction on the holding and the injection pipettes. Both units consist of a syringe connected to the pipette holder by thin tubing. The whole system is filled with oil to give finer control. A pipette is attached to the end of the system and then a small amount of oil is injected into the pipette to remove any air from the system.

The two pipettes are put in their holders which are attached to the micromanipulator on either side of the stage. They are then moved into position using the coarse positioning controls while being viewed through the microscope at low magnification. Before using the pipettes, examine them at high power to make sure that they are not broken, damaged or blocked.

The two holders should be at an angle from the surface of the microscope stage. The angle used depends on the type of dish used, the angle of the pipette tips and the height of the stage warmer. This low angle requires that care be taken not to drag the edge of the pipette on the side of the petri dish on the stage. The Falcon #1006 dishes are very shallow and help eliminate this problem.

The injection pipette is lowered into the drop containing the sperm in media and, depending on the procedure and numbers of oocytes to be injected, a number of sperm are aspirated into the pipette. Sperm can be most easily picked up from the bottom of the dish, especially at the edges of the drop. Care must be taken not to damage the tip of the pipette during aspiration. The two pipettes are then raised vertically to get them out of the way. Tips, tricks and troubleshooting for micromanipulation are listed in Table 4.

Set-up of Intracytoplasmic Sperm Injection Plate (Figures 12A and B)

Use a shallow dish, such as the Falcon #1006 to prevent the holder and injector from hitting the sides of the plate. Even with a shallow dish, care must be taken to place your drops towards the center of the plate, else the sides of the dish will interfere with the microinjectors. One to two microliters of sperm are added to a 10 µl drop of 10% polyvinylpyrrolidone (PVP) media. Ready to use, 10% PVP solutions are now commercially available. The highly viscous PVP media helps to immobilize the sperm for easy pick up. Some people mix the sample with the PVP, some place the drops next to each other and make a bridge between the two drops and, some place the sperm in the middle of the PVP drop and allow the motile sperm to swim to the edges. Additionally, place several drops of a micromanipulation media, such as modified HTF + 10% HSA. Overlay with culture oil. Be careful not to allow the drops to dry out or evaporate. Any loss of water from the microdrop of media will quickly alter the osmolarity of the solution damaging the oocyte.

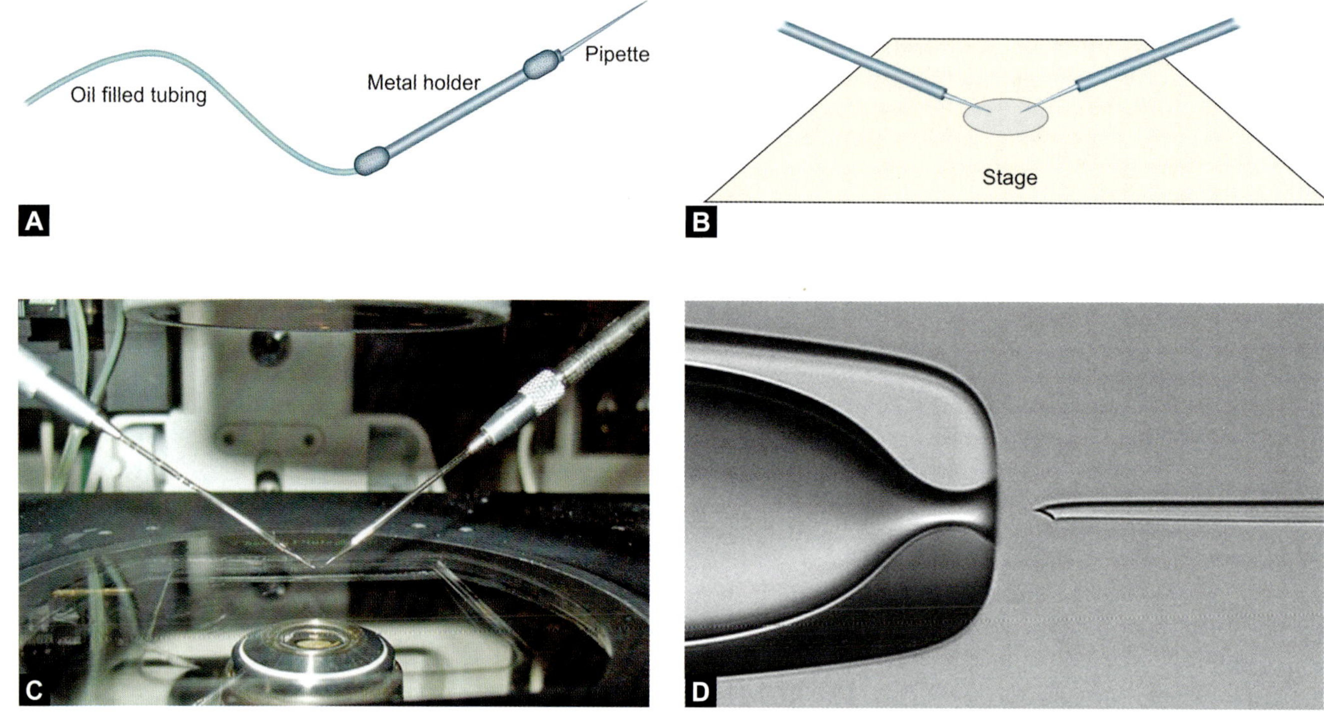

Figures 11A to D Setting-up the micromanipulators

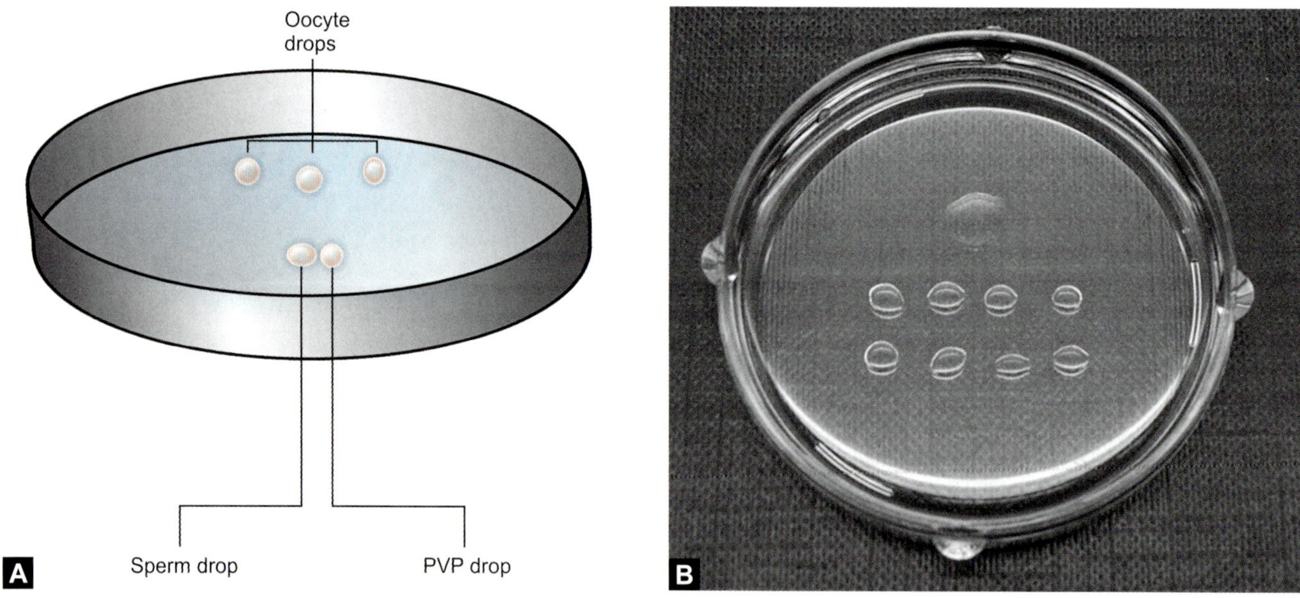

Figures 12A and B Set-up of intracytoplasmic sperm injection (ICSI)

Table 4 Tips, tricks and troubleshooting for micromanipulation

Problem	Probable Reasons	Response
Cannot push oil out from the micromanipulation syringe Pressure builds up in the line when the knob is turned	✓ An air bubble or piece of glass is blocking the passageway.	1. Take off the pipette and expel some oil. If you feel resistance, disassemble the pipette connection joint (plastic and metallic sleeve), clean and reassemble. Expel oil without resistance 2. Replace any parts that appear worn or scratched
Oil is leaking out of the lines	✓ Improper connection between the pipette and the holder/injector or between the holder/injector and the plastic tubing	1. Take apart connection which is leaking and fix
Cannot achieve fine control	✓ Micromanipulation syringe is too big ✓ Air bubble in the pipette between the oil and the culture media ✓ Line is leaking ✓ Plastic line is too big	1. Try a smaller syringe 2. Push the air bubble out of the pipette until the oil is flowing out. Then aspirate some culture media 3. Check all connections 4. Replace plastic line with a smaller gauge
The pipette tip is not in focus when at the bottom of the culture dish. It jerks when moved along the Y axis	✓ Pipette is not aligned and is hitting the bottom of the culture dish	1. Re-adjust the pipette to a sharper angle
Junk on the end of the ICSI needle	✓ Dirty pipette	1. Take the injection needle to the edge of the culture media droplet and drag it in and out of the media/oil till clean.
The pipettes do not move when the fine control knobs are moved	✓ The fine control knobs are below the zero line. All tension is lost	1. Start with the knobs at the midpoint between zero and five
Sperm like glue in PVP	✓ Inadequate washing after Isolate	1. Re-train
Increased degeneration after ICSI (> 15%)	✓ New service? New personnel? ✓ New PVP? New media batches? ✓ Temperature on microscope	1. Re-train 2. Decrease ICSI needle diameter 3. Change all medias
Decreased fertilization (< 50%)	✓ New service? New personnel? ✓ Polar body not at 12 or 6 O'clock ✓ Sperm treatment ✓ Oocyte treatment	1. Practice and re-training 2. Decrease hyaluronidase exposure 3. Check sperm immobilization 4. Check oocyte injection and cytoplasmic aspiration 5. Check PVP
Increased incidence of 1PN (> 10%)	✓ Oocyte activation	1. Sperm quality 2. Centromere problem 3. Temperature 4. pH / CO_2 5. Media
Increased multiple PN (> 5%)	✓ Poor technique: two sperm injected ✓ 60% failure to extrude PB	1. Re-train 2. Practice

Sperm Pickup (Figures 13A and B)

1. Focus on microscope on the border between the PVP and oil. This will help ensure that clinician's injector is not broken on the bottom of the dish.
2. Lower the injection pipette into the PVP drop containing the sperm.
3. Move the meniscus to near the end of the pipette but do not expel oil. Draw up some media.
4. Immobilize a sperm by touching, dragging the injection pipette over its midpiece. This crushing technique immobilizes the sperm and damages the cell membrane which is believed to be needed to induce sperm decondensation.
5. Pick up a single sperm, tail first by applying low suction at syringe, the sperm should be in the visual field all the time (turn counter clockwise).
6. Position the sperm in the pipette so that it is not too close to the tip. Adjust the suction until the sperm is no longer moving and then lift the pipette out of the droplet.
7. When injecting, bring sperm to the end of the pipette by increasing the pressure very slowly in tiny increments.

Intracytoplasmic Sperm Injection (Figures 14A to F)

1. The dish is placed on the microscope stage and the holding pipette is lowered down into the drop containing the oocyte. The oocyte is picked up by turning the microinjector control to create suction. The oocyte is held so that the polar body is at the 12 O'clock or 6 O'clock position. Once the oocyte is attached to the holding pipette, it is moved vertically upwards to lift the oocyte off the bottom of the dish.
2. The injection pipette is then moved into position near the holding pipette. Magnification is increased and the pipettes and oocyte are positioned so that they can be seen in the television monitor. The edge of the oocyte is then put in sharp focus. The tip of the injection pipette is brought into focus by adjusting its vertical position until it is at the same level as the oocyte. By gently poking the zona, the alignment of the injection pipette and the oocyte can be determined.
3. If all goes well there will be one or more sperm near the opening of the injection pipette. If not, then you can slowly expel media from the injection pipette

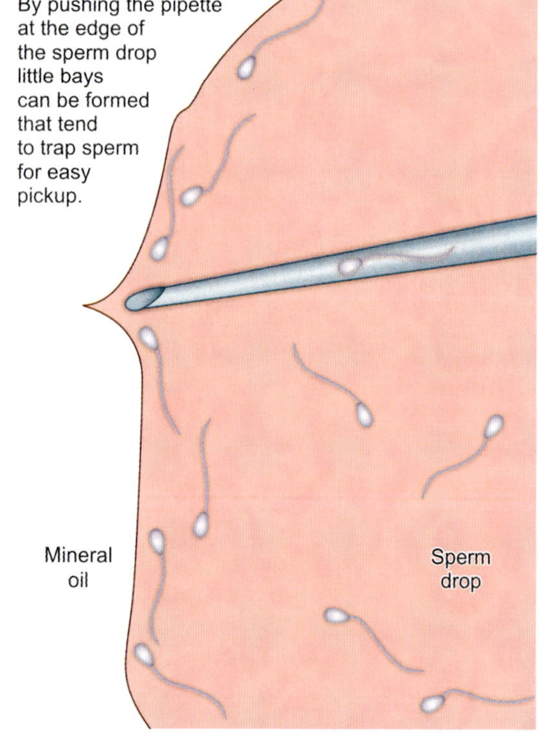

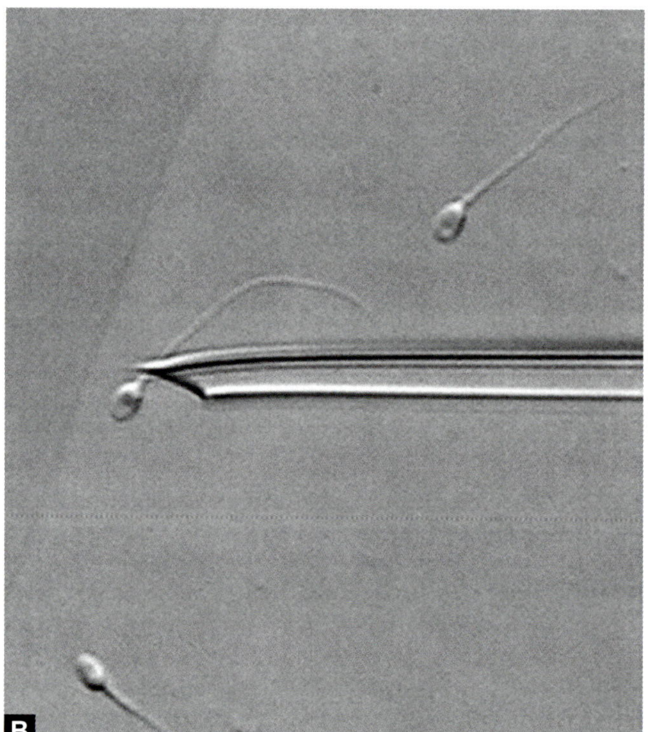

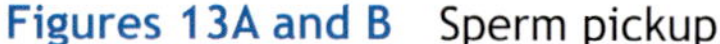
Figures 13A and B Sperm pickup

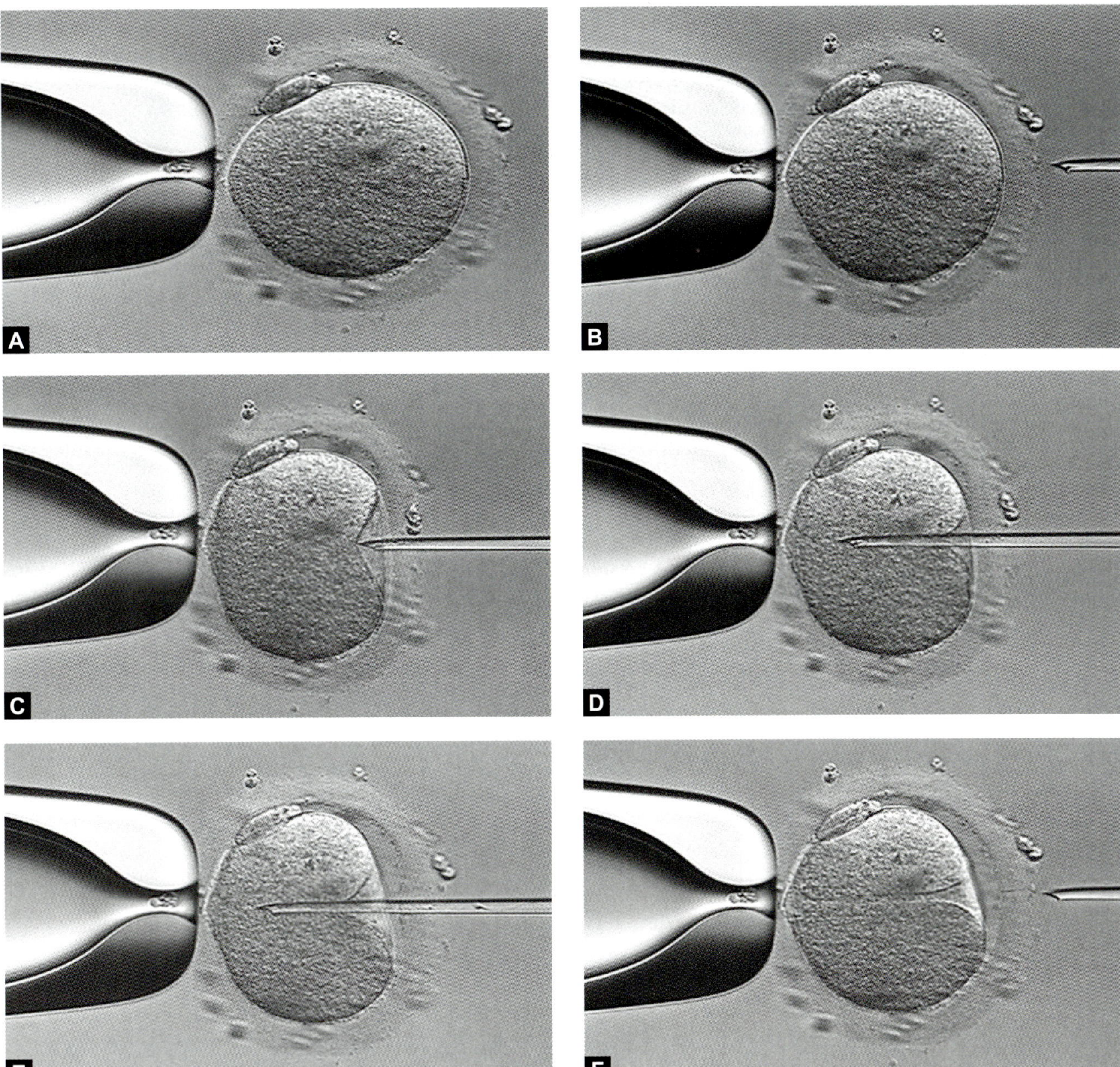

Figures 14A to F Intracytoplasmic sperm injection (ICSI)

until a sperm is seen. To see more of the injection pipette, it may be necessary to switch to a lower power magnification.

4. A single sperm is brought to the opening of the injection pipette which is positioned equatorially and then introduced into the oocyte. The pipette will need to be inserted almost all the way through the oocyte.
5. Prior to the injection of the sperm, draw in a small amount of ooplasm to ensure that the pipette has gone through the membrane. There is often a sudden pop as the membrane breaks.
6. Injection of the sperm is accomplished by turning the control on the injection pipette clockwise. Sperm is injected in a total volume of 1–2 picoliters. After successful injection of sperm, the injection pipette is withdrawn and the oocyte is removed from the holding pipette.
7. The oocyte is washed two or three times and placed in a fresh plate of media and put back into the incubator.

Day 1 Assessment—Fertilization Check

Proper embryo culturing and developmental scoring are extremely important for a successful IVF cycle. One of the most critical steps in embryo culturing is the medium and how it is prepared. While working with any medium remember to use sterile technique to avoid contamination. Every new shipment of medium must pass a bioassay test, such as, a sperm survival test, prior to usage to insure high quality. Additionally, the pH of the medium should be optimized prior to usage. Also remember to allow the medium to equilibrate in the incubator for a minimum of several hours prior to usage. None of these media should be used if kept at 37°C for longer than 48 hours because the proteins and nutrients in the media begin to breakdown. It is better to discard the old media and use fresh then risk a patient's embryos. Developmental scoring of an embryo is an indicator of implantation potential. An embryo that hits all of the developmental goals has a better chance of achieving pregnancy than one that misses some of the developmental goals. Tips, tricks and troubleshooting for oocyte fertilization are listed in Table 5.

Developmental Scoring—Day 1: 18–20 Hours Post Insemination (Fertilization Check) (Figures 15A to C)

- If needed strip the embryos according to protocol.
- Check each embryo for the presence of one or more PN.
- 2PN indicates proper fertilization. Anything more or less is considered to have fertilized abnormally and should be discarded (Figures 16A and B).
- Additionally each 2PN is assessed for symmetry.

Day 1: 24 Hours Post Insemination (Two-Cell Cleavage)

- Check each 0PN embryo for the presence of one or more PN. Discard polynucleated embryos.
- Check each 2PN embryo for the loss of the PN or the cleavage to the 2-cell stage.
- If the embryo has cleaved, grade it according to protocol.
- Additionally, note the nucleus in each blastomere of the embryo. If any blastomere exhibits polynucleation than note PN on the patients chart. If all the blastomeres exhibit mononucleation, then note MN on the patient's chart (Figures 17A and B).

Day 2 to 3 Assessment

Day 2: Cleavage Check

- Check each embryo for the presence of cleaving. An embryo not at the 2-cell stage should be discarded.
- If the embryo has cleaved, grade it according to protocol (Figure 18).
- Additionally, note the nucleus in each cell of the embryo and if a cell exhibit polynucleation.

Day 3: Cleavage Check

- Check each embryo for cleavage.
- Grade all cleaved embryos according to protocol .
- Additionally, note the nucleus in each cell of the embryo and if a cell exhibit polynucleation.

Tips, tricks and troubleshooting for early embryonic development are listed in Table 6.

Day 4 to 6 Assessment–Blastocyst Culture (Figures 19 and 20A to D)

In a normal IVF cycle, a patient's embryo(s) would be transferred back to the uterus on day 2 or day 3 post oocyte retrieval. However, in certain circumstances, such as a younger patient with more embryos in culture then are to be transferred, the physician may recommend to the patient to undergo a blastocyst transfer (day 5–7). This recommendation will be based on several factors which will include but not be limited to embryo quality, embryo quantity and patient's history. In general, you want at least 6 grade I embryos on day 3 prior to recommending blastocyst transfer. By culturing an embryo to blastocyst the lab is selectively omitting the embryos which might have looked good on day 3 but if transferred probably would have arrested *in vivo*. It should be noted that by choosing to culture the embryos to blastocyst the patient is at risk for not having any transfer, should the embryos fail to develop to the blastocyst stage.

Procedure

1. On day 3 following oocyte retrieval, the embryos are transferred to a blastocyst medium + 10% HSA or to a fresh single step medium, such as Global + 10% HSA, which has been pre-equilibrated in the incubator.
2. Label the culture plate with the patient's name, secondary identifying number and location of the embryos.
3. Remove one plate of patient's embryos from the incubator.
4. Record the stage of development and quality on the patient's egg sheet.
5. Carefully but quickly move the patient's embryos from the old medium to the new medium.
6. Return new plate to the incubator.
7. Check old plate to insure all of the embryos were transferred then discard in the biohazardous trash.
8. Do not remove more than one plate of embryos at a time to minimize the loss of CO_2 and temperature.
9. Transfer should occur when there is an expanded blastocyst usually on day 5. Any embryos not expanded can be cultured till day 6 and then frozen.

Table 5 Tips, tricks and troubleshooting for oocyte fertilization

Problem	Probable Reasons	Response
Failed fertilization— • No motile sperm • No cumulus dispersal • No PN • Motile sperm • Cumulus dispersal • Agglutinated sperm	✓ Male Factor ✓ Bad media batch ✓ Bad sperm or eggs ✓ Post or immature eggs ✓ Male factor ✓ Antisperm antibodies	1. Check equipment function 2. Check culture media 3. Reinseminate with fresh sample or remaining motile sperm using ICSI
Polyspermic fertilization	✓ Insemination with to high ✓ of a motile sperm concentration ✓ Immature or postmature oocytes	1. Suggest ICSI 2. Culture or freeze for QC purposes 3. Do NOT Transfer
Spontaneous cleaving of the oocyte—no fertilization seen	✓ Activation—spontaneous in aging oocytes	1. Culture but do NOT transfer 2. Suggest ICSI
Broken zona	✓ Excessive stress during aspiration ✓ Postmature oocytes ✓ Improper sized stripping pipette	1. Change vacuum pressure 2. Change retrieval needle 3. Make a larger stripping pipette 4. Do ICSI
Ruptured zona	✓ Same as above	1. Same as above 2. No insemination

Assisted Hatching

Embryos are surrounded by a zona pellucida. In order to achieve a pregnancy, the embryo must break out of the zona and implant into the uterine lining of the patient. Under certain circumstances, it is theorized that the zona 'hardens' preventing the embryo from breaking through and implanting. The lab can compensate for this by artificially creating a small hole (20 µm) in the zona. This gives the embryo a point of exit for implantation. The lab recommends AH for any patient over the age of 40, having failed a previous cycle with no implantation or all frozen embryo transfers. There are two methods for AH, are outlined below: acid tyrodes and laser.

Acid Tyrodes

Acid Tyrodes (pH 2.1–2.5) (Figures 21A to F) is used to create a small opening in the zona pellucida. Tyrode's solution is an acid. Use appropriate precautions.

Procedure

1. Attach the hatching pipette to the clear plastic tubing (old transfer catheter). Place the pipette in the empty holder.
2. Align the holder and hatcher under the microscope.
3. Attach a 10 cc syringe to the other end of the hatching tubing.
4. Place the hatching pipette in a drop of acid Tyrodes placed on a petri dish (not under oil).
5. Fill the hatcher by drawing back on the 10 cc syringe plunger until it locks in position. You should now see Tyrode's solution being drawn into the hatching pipette.
6. Set up a plate containing drops of modified HTF + 10% HSA overlayed with oil. Place the embryos in the drops.
7. Release the plunger on the 10 cc syringe. Draw back the plunger on a 250 µl gas tight syringe. Switch this with the 10 cc syringe.
8. The embryos are held by a holding pipette and the tyrode's pipette is brought to a position just short of touching the embryo. Position the embryo so that there is a space between the blastomeres and the zona at the position where the hatching will take place.
9. While observing the embryo, begin expelling the tyrodes solution by depressing on the plunger of the 250 µl syringe.
10. Advance the injection pipette slightly and watch for the zona to start dissolving.
11. Continue to advance the pipette until a small hole is made in the zona and the cell membrane.
12. As soon as the clinician breaks through the cell membrane draw the 250 µl syringe plunger back up to remove a Tyrode's solution which might have entered the embryo.
13. Withdraw the pipette and move the embryo through 3–4 washes of culture media to remove remaining acid Tyrode.

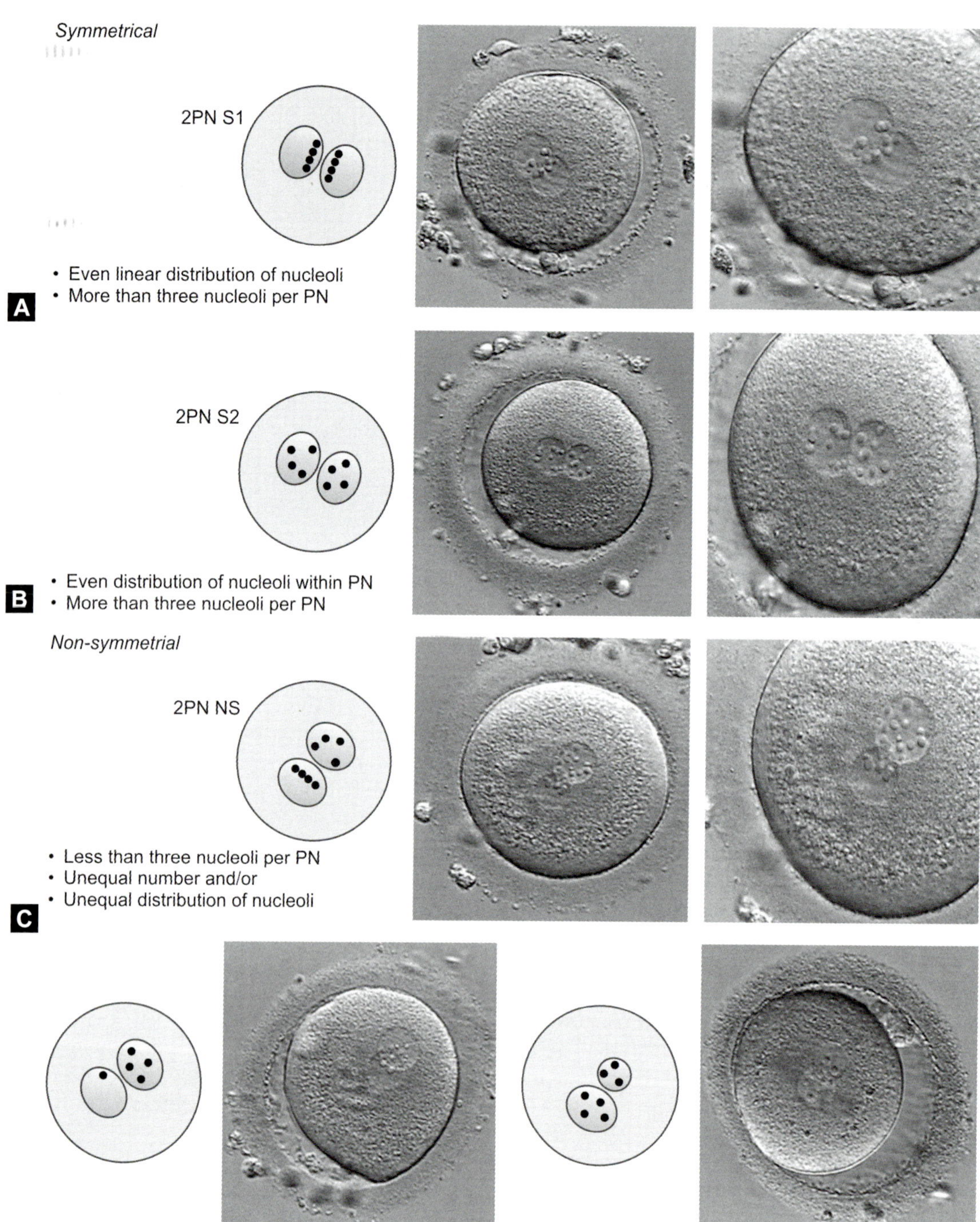

Figures 15A to C Fertilization check

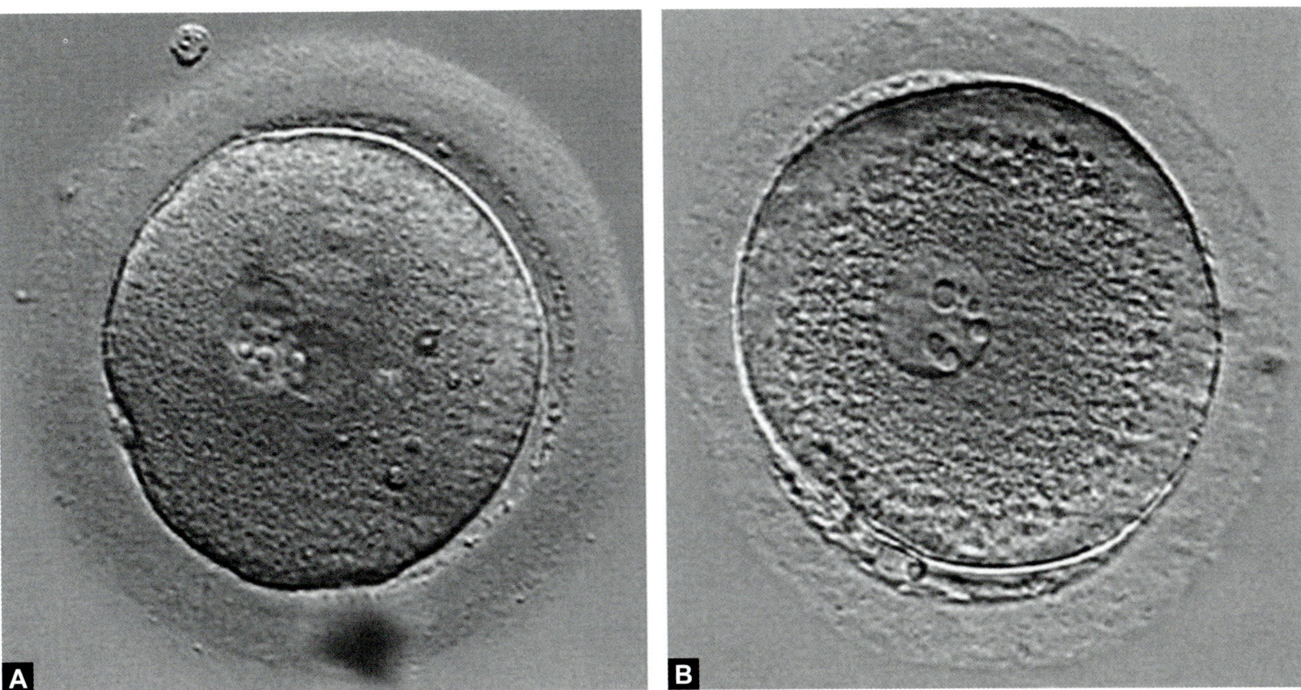

Figures 16A and B Abnormal fertilization

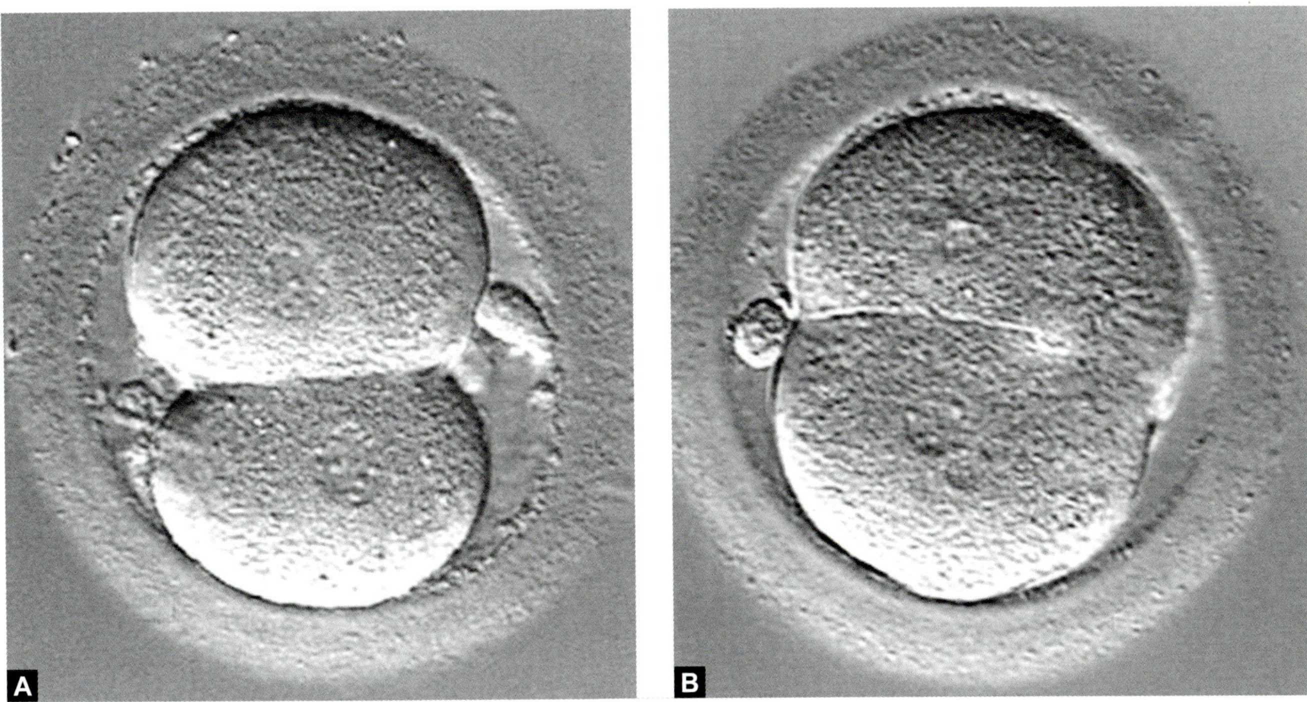

Figures 17A and B (A) 2-cell mononucleated blastomeres; (B) 2-cell polynucleated blastomeres

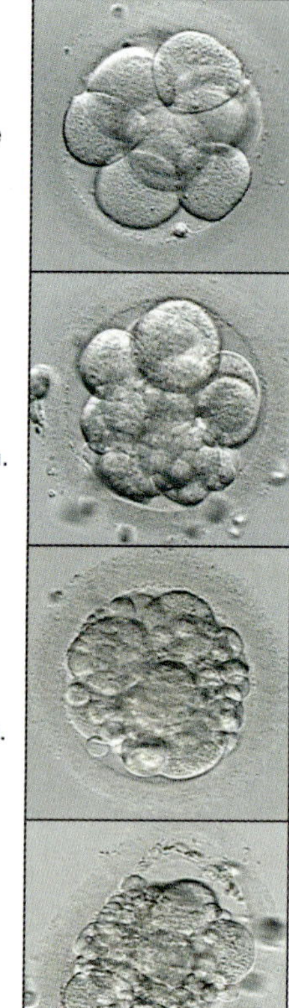

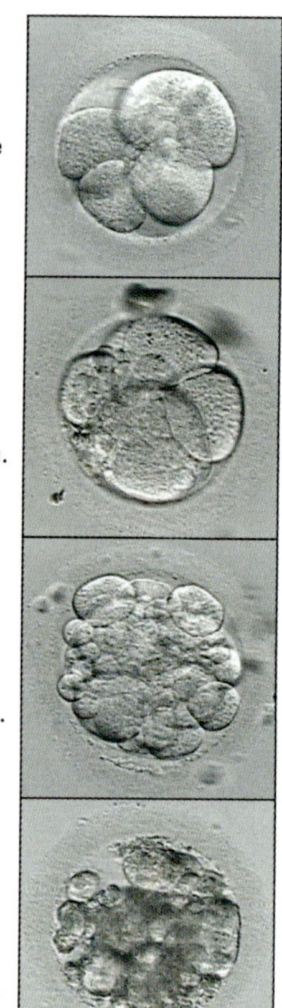

Figure 18 Grading cleavage stage of human embryos

Table 6 Tips, tricks and troubleshooting for early embryonic development

Problem	Probable Reasons	Response
Fail Cleavage - 2PN Cleavage arrest - multicellular	✓ Temperature shock ✓ pH/CO_2 shock ✓ Media problem ✓ Egg Factor ✓ Unknown causes	1. Change protocol next cycle 2. Suggest ICSI

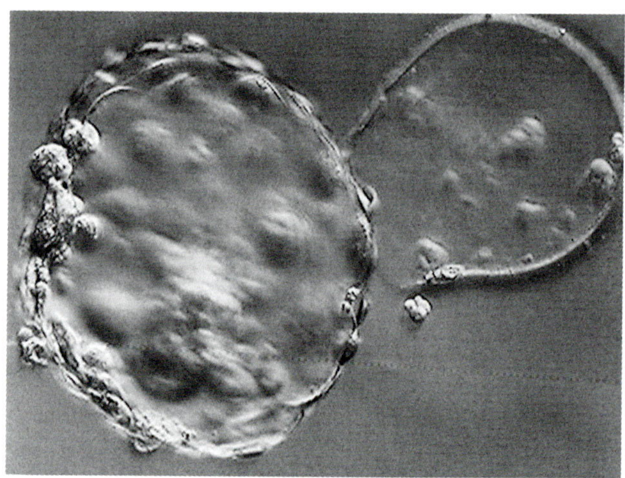

Figure 19 Blastocyst culture

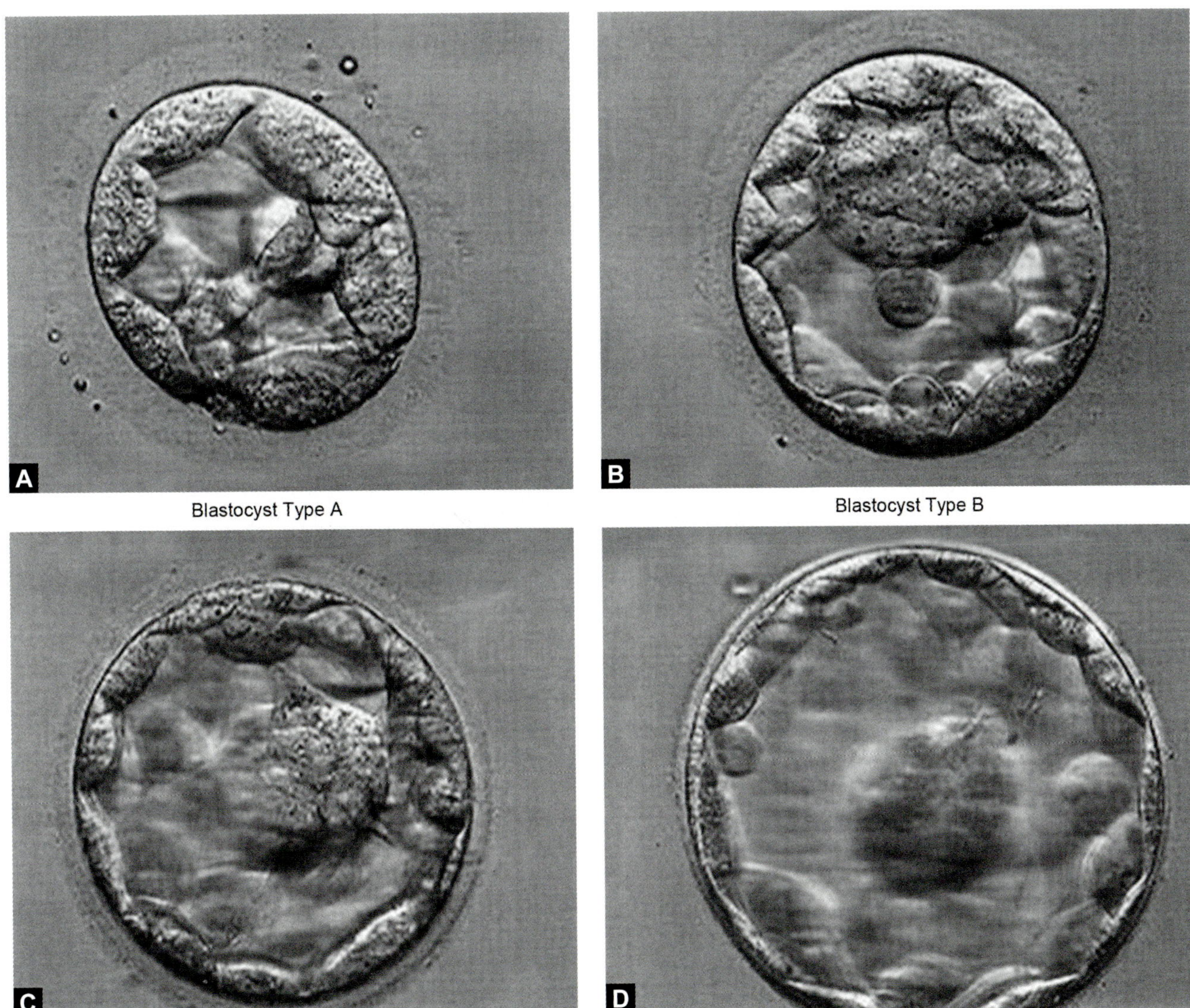

Figure 20A to D Stages of blastocyst development

Laser—Hamilton Thorne (Figures 22 and 23)

Procedure

1. Turn on computer and monitor.
2. Click 'ZILOS-tk' icon on desktop.
3. Place test plate with the marked cover slip onto the stage.
4. Focus on the edge of the marked square from low objective to the laser objective.
5. Move slightly towards center of marked square with the stage control.
6. Make sure the laser objective is in focus.
7. Click 'Target' and then click 'Align Target'.
8. Reduce pulse to 10 µs.
9. Click the foot pedal to blast a hole in the marker square.
10. If the target is not centered within the blasted hole, move the target with the mouse to the center of the blasted hole.
11. Once aligned to the center of the blasted hole, click 'Alignment OK'.
12. Move the stage to another spot and test the alignment.
13. Before beginning with laser hatching, make sure the pulse is set on 500 µs.
14. Set up a plate containing drops of modified HTF + 10% HSA overlayed with oil. Place the embryos in the drops.

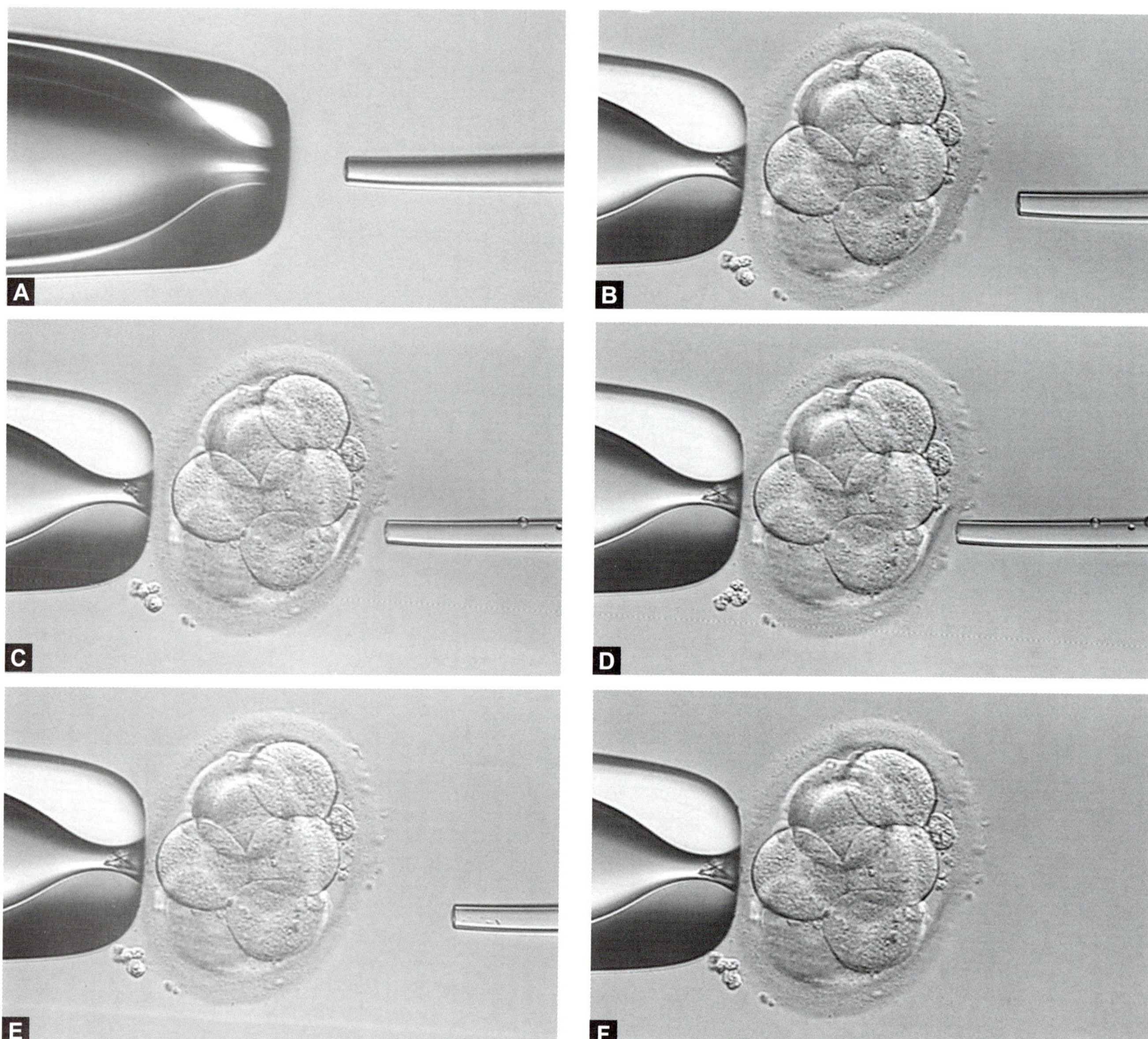

Figures 21A to F Acid tyrodes hatching

15. Position the embryo so there is a space between the blastomeres and the zona at the position where the hatching will take place.
16. Click the foot pedal to blast a hole in the marker square.
17. Move the embryo repeat as needed until a 20 µm hole is made in the zona. This is about the size of the green targeting circle.
18. Move the embryo through 3–4 washes of culture media.

Embryo Transfer

While a seemingly simple technique the embryo transfer is perhaps one of the most critical steps in the IVF process. Studies have shown that the pregnancy rates will vary depending on the doctor and embryologist doing the procedure. The embryo transfer can take place anytime between day 2 and day 6. Research varies regarding which day gives the best pregnancy rate. There are many variables that need to be taken into account such as embryo quality, embryo quantity, embryo developmental rate, patient age and previous cycles. Given all the variables, it is best to work out what day is best for the clinician's program.

Selection of embryos for transfer is most usually morphologically based. For example, most labs would agree that transferring a day three 8-cell I-S is better than an 8-cell III-NS. The issue becomes less clear when trying

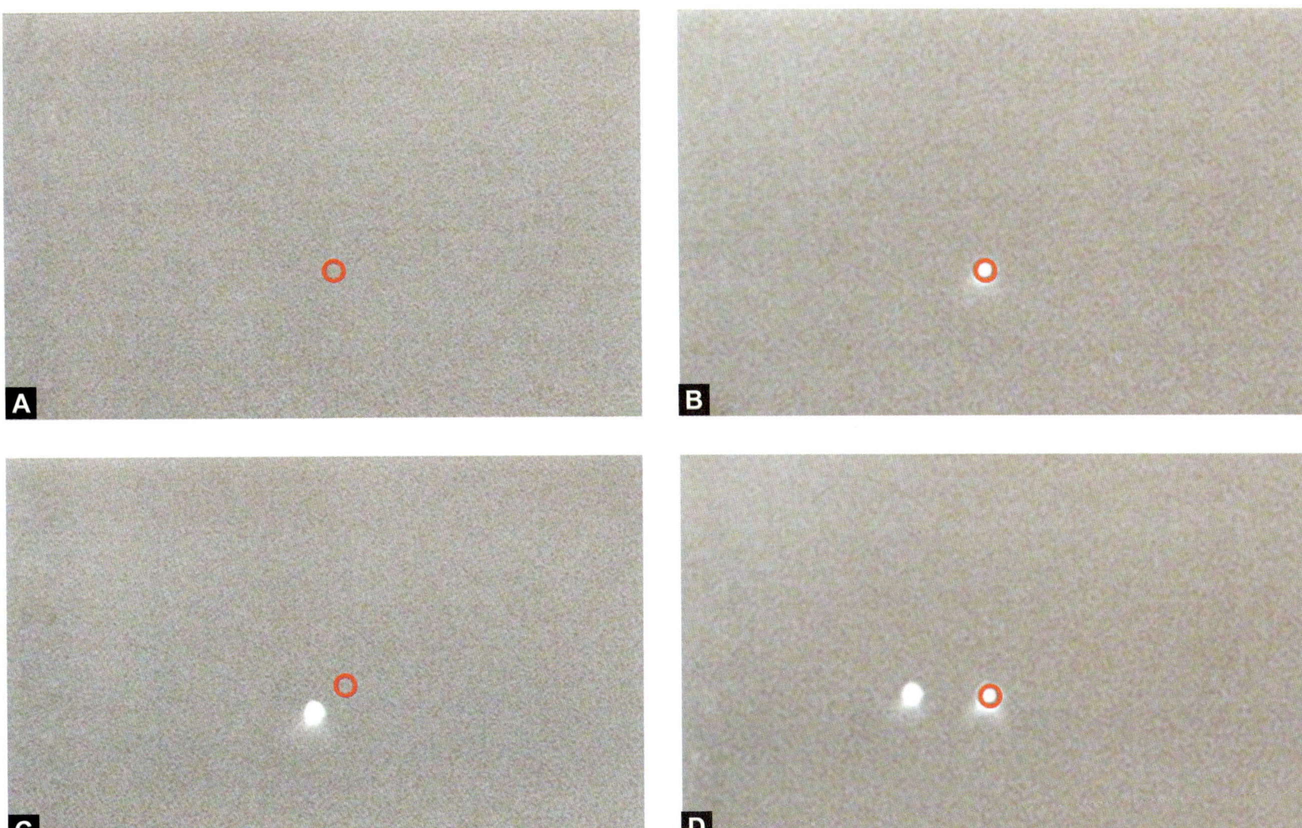

Figures 22A to D Laser Alignment—Hamilton Thorne

to decide between a day three 8-cell I-S and a 10-cell I-S or a day two 4-cell I-NS and a 6-cell I-NS. Under these circumstances, it is best to look at the developmental time line of the embryo taking into account patient age and the IVF labs 'normal' embryo development. In general, after exhibiting fertilization and 2PN development, the embryo will optimally be a 0PN or 2 cells at 24 hours post insemination, 4 cells at 48 hours and 8 cells at 72 hours. However, this will vary from lab to lab and it is best to know your labs 'normal' developmental time line.

How many embryos to transfer (Table 7)? This is again an IVF lab/clinic specific question. The goal of an embryo transfer should be a single live birth. Each lab should maintain statistics on its multiple pregnancy rates and attempt to limit multiple gestations. Many clinics are moving toward single embryo transfer without effecting live birth rates while many countries legislate the maximum number of embryos a clinic is allowed to transfer.

Procedure

1. Arrive at the ART lab early enough to have time to check the previous day's eggs for fertilization or cleavage. Before a clinician open the incubator, do the standard incubator quality control checks.
2. Place any media needed for washing the patient's cervix at 37°C so they will be warm at least 30 minutes prior to transfer.
3. Fill out an embryology report for the physician listing the number and quality of the embryos. It will be signed by the doctor and initialed by the patient. The report will be given to the embryologist as instructions for the number to be hatched, transferred and the disposition of the remaining embryo(s) (frozen, discard, research, etc.).
4. The embryologist should sign the embryology report prior to giving it to the physician for patient counseling. A picture of the embryo(s) should be taken to show to the patient and for the patient's record.
5. Prior to transfer, verify the name and date of birth of the patient who is in the procedure room. Note the verification on the embryo transfer form.
6. At this time, verify that the walking path into the ET room is clear and free of obstacles.
7. The physician will verify the name and date of birth of the patient in the room.
8. At this time, the physician will counsel the patients regarding the status of their embryo(s), if this has not already happened. Often the physician

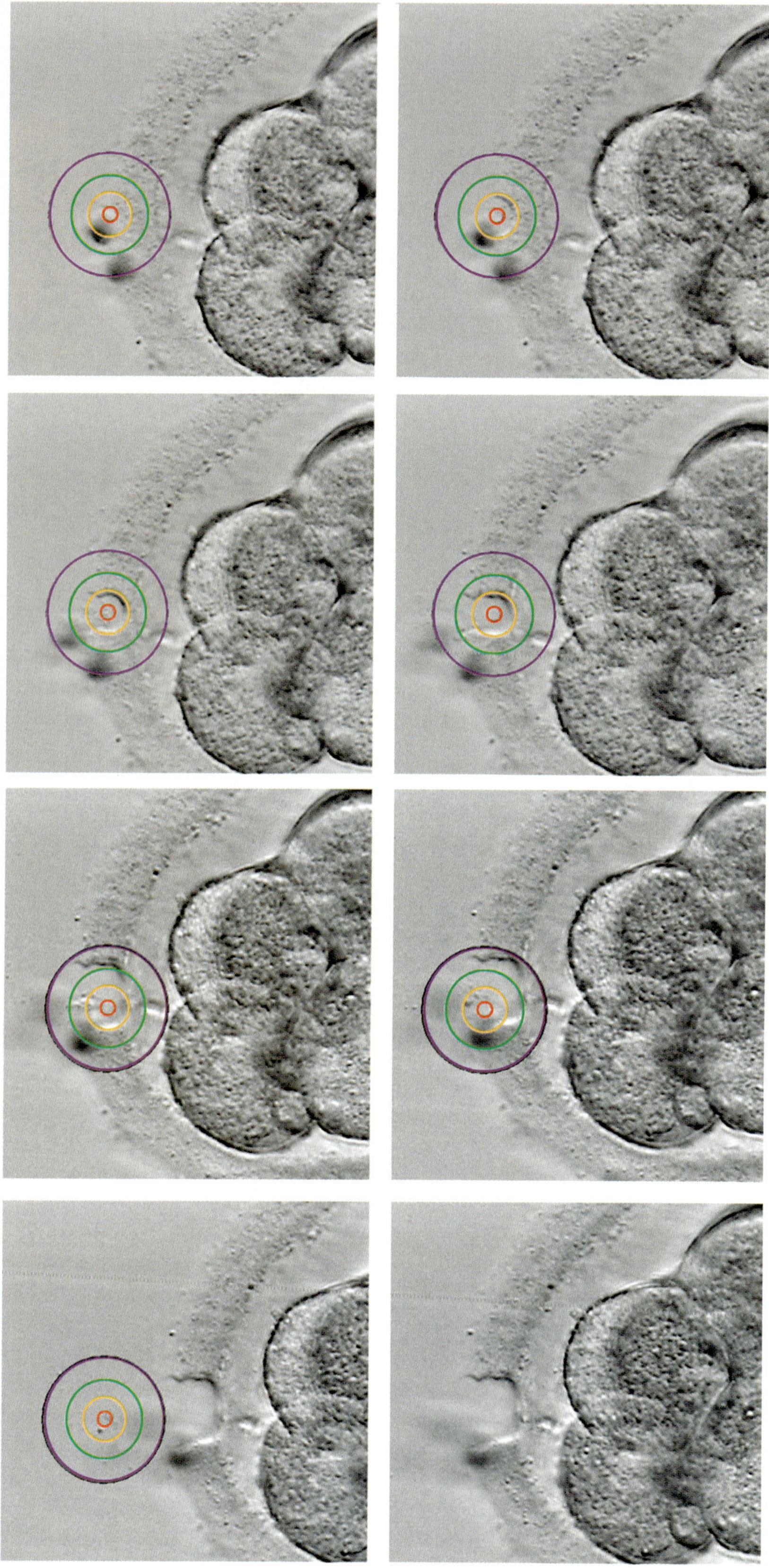

Figure 23 Laser assisted hatching

Table 7 Guidelines on number of embryos to be transferred

Day 2 or 3

	< 35	35-37	38-40	> 40
Favorable	1-2	1-2	≤ 3	≤ 5
Average	1-2	≤ 3	≤ 4	≤ 5

Blastocysts

	< 35	35-37	38-40	> 40
Favorable	1	1-2	1-2	≤ 3
Average	1-2	1-2	≤ 3	≤ 3

will counsel the patients prior to them entering the ET room at the bedside. Make sure both you and the physician still verify the name and date of birth of the patients while they are in the room prior to performing a 'time-out' procedure.

9. The physician is to write the name of the patient and the number of embryos being transferred on the dry erase board located by the door to the ET room including if there is any hatching.
10. The physician and the embryologist will have a 'time-out' meeting in which they will review:
    Patient's name
    Date of birth
    Embryology Report—including which embryos to be transferred, whether or not hatching is to be done and the disposition of the remaining embryos.
11. Hatching will be done now if indicated.
12. Move the embryo(s) to be transferred into one well containing the appropriate pre-equilibrated media before the transfer.
13. A prior mock transfer should have already been performed to determine the length and curvature of the patient's uterus. Depending on the patient's need or physician's preference or mock transfer, the doctor will choose a catheter. Several commercial vendors carry different types of catheters (Table 8). Each physician will have his/her preference. A prior mock transfer should have already been performed to determine the length and curvature of the patient's uterus.
14. Put on a pair of gloves and prepare the catheter for loading.
15. After the physician gives the permission to load, walk to the incubator and take out the dish with the embryo(s) and put it on the microscope stage under the hood.
16. While looking at the patient's plate, call out to the physician the name of the patient and the number of embryo(s) being loaded. For example, 'loading three embryos on Mrs Smith'.
17. A second embryologist if present needs to verify that the name on the transfer plate matches the name of the patient being transferred.
18. Loading the catheter:
    a. Load the catheter following the instructions below. It is important not to touch the distal end of the catheter at any time.

Table 8 Different types of catheter companies and their products

Company	Product
Sepal	Frydman
Irvine Scientific	Embryo view, Frydman
Sage	RG Edwards Embryo Transfer Catheter
COOK	Soft-Pass, Guardia
Rocket Medical	Genesis, EchoCath, Embryon

    b. Check the smoothness of the syringe and attach it firmly to the catheter.
    c. Fill the catheter with medium from the well that does not contain the embryo(s). While holding the catheter horizontally, remove the syringe from the media. Carefully, detach the syringe from the catheter and push the plunger down to the 0 ml setting so that there is no air in the syringe. Tightly fit the catheter back on to the syringe while continuing to hold the catheter horizontally.
    d. Draw in a little air to create a bubble between embryo(s) and medium in catheter.
    e. Hold the catheter tight with one hand and insert the catheter tip into the well until it touches the bottom of the well.
    f. Locate the tip of catheter while looking into the microscope and slowly advance it towards the cluster of embryo(s). Gently, aspirate the embryo(s) with a small volume of medium while maintaining precise control of the syringe. Make sure all of the embryo(s) are in the catheter.
    g. Withdraw the catheter slowly from the well until it is just above the medium surface and create another air bubble. Tilt the tip of catheter up and let the embryo(s) migrate down in the medium towards the air bubble.
19. Walk into the ET room and hand over the catheter with embryo(s) to the physician. While passing the catheter to him/her, again state the name of the patient and the number of embryo(s) in the catheter. For example, '3 embryos for Mrs Smith'.
20. After a few seconds (~60) the MD will give you the catheter. You should bring it back into the lab and check to see if all of the embryo(s) have been

successfully transferred. Rinse the catheter several times into a well. If there are no embryos present, state 'all clear'. If any embryo(s) remains, notify the physician how many came back and see if you should reload and repeat the transfer.

21. Note number of embryo(s) transferred, stage (cleavage), difficulty of transfer, presence of blood on catheter and time.

BIBLIOGRAPHY

1. Alukal JP, Lamb DJ. Intracytoplasmic sperm injection (ICSI)—what are the risks? Urol Clin North Am. 2008;35(2):277-88.
2. Ben-Yosef D, Shalgi R. Oocyte activation: lessons from human infertility. Trends Mol Med. 2001;7(4):163-9.
3. Bleil JD. In vitro fertilization. In: Wassarman PM, DePamphilis ML (Eds). Methods in Enzymology. New York: Academic Press; 1993. pp. 253-63.
4. Boone WR, Shapiro SS. Quality control in the in vitro fertilization laboratory. Theriogenology. 1990;33(1):23-50.
5. Booth PJ, Holm P, Callesen H. The effect of oxygen tension on porcine embryonic development is dependent on embryo type. Theriogenology. 2005;63(7):2040-52.
6. Cruz JR, Dubey AK, Patel J, et al. Is blastocyst transfer useful as an alternative treatment for patients with multiple in vitro fertilization failures? Fertil Steril. 1999;(2):218-20.
7. Dubey AK, Oates RD, Cardone VR, et al. A simplified method for processing sperm obtained during microsurgical epididymal sperm aspiration (MESA) for use in vitro fertilization. J Assist Reprod Genet. 1992;9(6):580-3.
8. Dubey AK, Wang HA, Duffy P, et al. The correlation between follicular measurements, oocyte morphology, and fertilization rates in an in vitro fertilization program. Fertil Steril. 1995;64(4):787-90.
9. Ebner T, Moser M, Sommergruber M, et al. Selection based on morphological assessment of oocytes and embryos at different stages of preimplantation development: a review. Hum Reprod. 2003;9(3):251-62.
10. Fasouliotis SJ, Schenker JG. Failures in assisted reproductive technology: an overview. Eur J Obstet Gynecol Reprod Biol. 2003;107(1):4-18.
11. Hornstein MD, Racowsky C. Assisted Reproduction. In: Strauss JF, Barbieri R. Yen and Jaffe's Reproductive Endocrinology, 6th edition. London: Saunders; 2009. pp. 725-57.
12. Johnson N, Blake D, Farquhar C. Blastocyst or cleavage-stage embryo transfer? Best Pract Res Clin Obstet Gynaecol. 2007;21(1):21-40.
13. Kea B, Gebhardt J, Watt J, et al. Effect of reduced oxygen concentrations on the outcome of in vitro fertilization. Fertil Steril. 2007;87(1):213-6.
14. Nanassy L, Peterson CA, Wilcox AL, et al. Comparison of 5% and ambient oxygen during days 3–5 of in vitro culture of human embryos. Fertil Steril. 2010;93(2):579-85.
15. Pacey AA. Male fertility and infertility. Obstet Gynecol Reprod Med. 2009;19(2):42-7.
16. Patrizio P, Sakkas D. From oocyte to baby: a clinical evaluation of the biological efficiency of in vitro fertilization. Fertil Steril. 2009;91(4):1061-6.
17. Pauli SA, Berga SL, Shang W, et al. Current status of the approach to assisted reproduction. Pediatr. Clin North Am. 2009;56(3):467-88.
18. Plachot M. Viability of preimplantation embryos. Baillierees Clin Obstet Gynaecol. 1992;6(2):327-38.
19. Schoolcraft WB, Surrey ES, Gardner DK. Embryo transfer: techniques and variables affecting success. Fertil Steril. 2001;76(5):863-70.
20. Setti PE, Cavagna M, Albani E, et al. Outcome of assisted reproductive technologies after different embryo transfer strategies. Reprod BioMed Online. 2005;11(1):64-70.
21. Zhao Y, Brezina P, Hsu CC, et al. In vitro fertilization: four decades of reflections and promises. Biochim Biophys Acta. 2011;1810 (9):843-52.

21

Cryopreservation of Human Embryos

Nina Desai, Faten Abdel Hafez

CHAPTER CONTENTS

INTRODUCTION

Embryo cryopreservation is now considered a vital part of a successful *in vitro* fertilization (IVF) program. The transfer of cryopreserved thawed embryos constitutes about 20% of all embryo transfers (ETs) worldwide[1]. Prior to the availability of cryopreservation technology, women producing excess oocytes had to choose between inseminating only a small portion of retrieved oocytes or having to discard excess untransferred embryos.[2] Embryo cryopreservation allows for storage of nontransferred embryos for a future treatment cycle. An effective cryopreservation program also encourages physicians and patients to transfer fewer embryos on the fresh transfer, thus helping to decrease multiple pregnancy rates and the associated obstetrical risk of complications. The development and improvements in embryo cryopreservation technology over the last two decades have helped to significantly increase overall clinical pregnancy rates from a single oocyte retrieval cycle along with decreasing overall costs.[3-7]

BACKGROUND

This discovery in 1948 by Polge et al. that fowl spermatozoa could survive freezing if glycerol was added to the medium, is a landmark in the history of cryopreservation.[8] The first live birth with cryopreserved mouse embryos was reported by Whittingham et al. in 1972[9]. Subsequent studies further elucidated the critical features for mammalian embryo cryopreservation.[10-14] Application of these principles to human embryos resulted in the first pregnancy with a frozen 8-cell embryo.[15] Although this pregnancy ended in a spontaneous loss, Zeilmaker and colleagues shortly thereafter reported the first term birth with a cryopreserved human embryo.[16] The first baby from frozen human oocytes was born 2 years later.[17]

Protocols for human embryo and oocyte freezing have continued to evolve as our understanding of the basic cryobiology of mammalian cells and the protective effects of different cryoprotectant agents (CPAs) has grown. Human embryos at all stages from pronuclear

(PN) through blastocyst have been successfully cryopreserved (Tables 1 to 4).

CRYOPRESERVATION TECHNIQUES

The two most commonly applied methods for embryo cryopreservation involve either slow cooling or else vitrification. The traditional slow rate cooling or equilibrium protocol involves the use of a programmable freezer to decrease the temperature in stepwise increments. This method has been successfully applied towards human embryo cryopreservation worldwide for over 20 years. The protocols have been well-standardized and used for domestic animal species, as well as human embryos. The key factors that affect results are the concentration of CPA, the rate of cooling (< 1°C/min to at least –60°C) and induction of ice crystal formation in the super cooled solution at a fixed temperature and away from the embryo.[9,13] Intracellular ice crystal formation during freezing can have extremely deleterious effects.[18,19] In general, with all slow cooling protocols, freezing of the sample takes 2–3 hours to complete as the typical rates of cooling used are 0.3–0.5°C/min.[9,20] The controlled rate of cooling allows exchange of solution between intracellular and extracellular fluids without osmotic shock, cell deformation and fracture or cytoskeletal alteration. It does, however, require the embryo to be exposed to non-physiological conditions for prolonged durations before final storage at –196°C in a biologically inactive state.

Table 1 Pronuclear and cleavage stage embryos—slow cooling

Author, year	Cell Stage	Transfers	Post thaw/ warm survival rate (%)	Clinical pregnancy rate (%)	Implantation rate (%)
Al-Hassani et al. 1996[134]	PN	204	77	17	–
Van den Abbeel et al. 1997[135]	PN	50	66	16	–
Senn et al. 2000[81]	PN CLV	329 192	80 73	20 11	11 6
Salumets et al. 2003[80]	PN	234	87	20	14
Tummon et al. 2006[136]	PN	653	95	44	22
Moragianni et al. 2010[82]	PN CLV	178 186	90 71	36 32	15 14
Mandelbaum et al. 1987 Mandelbaum, 1987 #921	CLV	185	61	19	15
Gabrielsen et al. 2004[112*]	CLV	136	–	18	11
Nagy et al. 2005 [137†]	CLV	44	64	54	26
Kuwayama et al. 2005[26]	CLV	536	91	32	NA
Balaban et al. 2006 [113*]	CLV	183	94	41	20
Salumets et al. 2006[138]	CLV	1242	79	14	18
Balaban et al. 2007[139]	CLV	101	95	43	19
Wilding et al. 2010[76]	CLV	48	87	35	14
Lin et al. 2010[89]	CLV	45	66	16	7

* Assisted hatching before transfer; † Lysed blastomeres removed before transfer

Table 2 Pronuclear and cleavage stage embryos—vitrification

Author, Year	Carrier	Transfers	Postwarming survival Rate (%)	Clinical pregnancy rate (%)	Implantation rate (%)
El-Danasouri et al. 2001[60]	Open pulled straw	36	49	31	10
Kuwayama et al. 2005[26]	Cryotop	504	98	27	NA
Rama Raju et al. 2005 [48]	Cryoloop	40	95	35	15
Desai et al. 2007 [54]	Cryoloop	77	85	44	20
Rezazadeh Valojerdi et al. 2009[140]	Cryotop	153	97	41	17
Hiraoka et al. 2009[91]*	Cryotop	60	96	47	32
Rama Raju et al. 2009[141]	Cryoloop	285	90	37	18
Desai et al. 2010[90]	Cryoloop	200	94	45	24
Sugiyama et al. 2010[67]	Plastic blade	1441	98	25	16
Aflatoonian et al. 2010[142]	Cryotop	187	96	42	25
Wilding et al. 2010[76]	HSV	51	93	35	14
Lin et al. 2010[89]	Cryotop	59	96	36	24

* Laser thinning of zona pellucida before transfer

Table 3 Blastocyst stage embryo—slow cooling

Author, year	Transfers	Post-thaw survival rate (%)	Clinical pregnancy rate (%)	Implantation rate (%)
Menezo et al. 1992[43]	101	75	21	9
Kaufman et al. 1995[95]	516	83	22	13
Pantos et al. 2001[143]	101	56	13	5
Virant-Klun et al. 2003[144]	288	81	30	18
Veeck et al. 2004[96]	211	79	59	39
Kuwayama et al. 2005[26]	98	84	51	31
Liebermann et al. 2006[29]	196	91	43	30
Richter et al. 2006[145]	268	NA	28	19
Shapiro et al. 2008[97]	73	99	59	38
Moragianni et al. 2010[82]	182	90	26	19

Table 4 Blastocyst stage embryos—vitrification

Author, year	Carrier	Transfers	Post-warming survival rate (%)	Clinical pregnancy rate (%)	Implantation rate (%)
Son et al. 2003[47]*	EM grids	25	90	48	29
Mukaida et al. 2003[52]	Cryoloop	207	80	37	20
Hiraoka et al. 2004[61]*	Cryotop	28	98	50	33
Kuwayama et al. 2005[26]	Cryotop	4745	90	53	NA
Takahashi et al. 2005[146]	Cryoloop	413	86	44	29
Zech et al. 2005[59]*	Hemi straw	20	82	45	26
Stehlik et al. 2005[62]	Cryotop	35	100	43	27
Mukaida et al. 2006[99]*	Cryoloop	266	97	60	47
Liebermann et al. 2006[29]	Cryotop	156	96	49	33
Lee et al. 2007[147]	EM grid	32	92	44	24
Raju et al. 2009[102]	Cryoloop	281	95	38	23
Vanderzwalmen et al. 2009[77]	VitriSafe plug	111	82	59	26
Hong et al. 2009[65]	EM grid	112	70	71	40
Keskintepe et al. 2009[100]*	Cryoloop	125	97	38	24
Liebermann et al. 2009[63]	HSV straw	277	97	45	31
Sugiyama et al. 2010[67]	Plastic blade	33	100	24	26

* Blastocysts were artificially collapsed before vitrification

Warming of the frozen cell and removal of the CPA are also critical in optimizing survival rates.

Vitrification, is an ultrarapid freezing technique first described by Rall and Fahy in 1985.[11] With vitrification, there is a conversion from the fluid to a solid-state without a phase change and in the complete absence of intra and extracellular ice crystallization. Viscosity of the solution increases as temperature is decreased and the sample is solidified in to a 'glass-like' state. This is usually accomplished through the use of relatively high concentrations of CPAs and/or very high cooling rates (15,000–20,000°C/min).[21-23] The optimal cooling rate allows the embryo to pass through the critical temperature zone from 15°C to –5°C extremely quickly to avoid cryoinjury. Water must be drawn out of the cell to 'vitrify' or freeze extracellularly. A practical limitation in the successful implementation of vitrification technology has been achievement of high cooling rates. The development of cryocontainers or carriers to sequester the embryo in miniscule fluid volumes of less than 1 µl, have been instrumental in facilitating high cooling rates[24-26] as the cells are immersed in liquid nitrogen (LN2) (–196°C). The LN2 vapor coat generated around the cell due to transient warming of the LN2 during immersion of the sample can reduce the actual cooling rate. This effect can be minimized by reducing fluid volumes. A device called the Vit Master uses slush nitrogen (–205 to –208°C) to further increase the cooling rate.[27] This cooling method for vitrification has not, however, gained much popularity.

Vitrification is rapidly becoming the technique of choice in IVF clinics around the world to cryopreserve embryos, as well as oocytes.[28] Current data suggests that it may be superior to conventional slow cooling methods.[29-33] This technique does not require expensive instrumentation. It is also far more efficient time-wise, requiring only a few minutes as opposed to the 2–3 hours needed with controlled rate freezing. Vitrification does, however, require expertise from laboratory personnel to obtain consistent successful outcomes.

CRYOPROTECTANT AGENTS

Cryoprotectant agents are divided into permeable and nonpermeable CPAs. Permeable CPAs are of low molecular weight, have a high solubility in water and permeate cells very quickly. They function by three basic mechanisms of action; dehydrating the cell, decreasing the freezing point and binding to intracellular water resulting in its slow release from the cell. Examples of permeable CPAs most commonly used for embryo and oocyte cryopreservation are ethylene glycol (EG), dimethylsulphoxide (DMSO), propanediol (PROH) and glycerol.

The nonpermeable CPAs include sugars and polymers. Sugar saccharides (e.g. sucrose, trehalose, raffinose, glucose, sorbitol and saccharose) can modify the properties of cryoprotectant solutions.[34] These agents do not enter the cell but instead draw water out through osmosis and thus aid in dehydration of the embryo. Cell injury from cryopreservation is generally a result of osmotic shock on warming. Water enters the cell at a faster rate than the intracellular solute, such as EG or glycerol can exit. During embryo warming, the added sugars act as osmotic buffers as the CPA is slowly diluted out.[1] They prevent too fast rehydration of the embryo by limiting transit of water back in to the cell.

Macromolecules, such as polyethylene glycol (MW = 8000), polyvinylpyrolidone (MW 360,000) and Ficoll (MW = 70,000), are also often added to cryoprotectant solutions. These macromolecules exert their cryoprotective effect by increasing the viscosity of the solution, therein decreasing the required concentration of permeable CPAs needed to successfully cryopreserve the embryo. Studies have shown the favorable effects of adding polymers during slow cryopreservations,[35] as well as the vitrification.[36-38]

The relative efficiency of different CPAs for cryopreservation is very much dependent on cell stage, specific membrane permeability characteristics, as well as toxicity threshold for the cell itself. For controlled rate freezing, PROH (1.5 M) combined with sucrose (0.2 M) has been favored for PN, as well as early cleavage stage embryos [39,40] and DMSO (1.5 M) for 8-cell embryos.[41] Glycerol (9%) with 0.2 M sucrose has been used for slow cooling of blastocysts.[2,43] Cryoprotectants at the 1–2 molar range used in slow freezing generally showed limited embryo toxicity.

Vitrification in contrast requires relatively high concentrations of solutes, typically 5–8 M (Fahy, 1984 #443; Ali, 1993 #431). A consensus as regards the best CPA and protocol for human embryo vitrification is yet to be reached. The CPAs used for vitrification can impact the outcome and further development of the transferred embryo. Rall et al. in his initial embryo vitrification work, observed that exposure to high concentrations of cryoprotectants was toxic to mouse embryos, inhibiting normal fetal development and birth of live young.[44].

With human embryos, EG at a concentration of as high as 40% has been successfully used for vitrification[45-48] but there have been concerns about potential cytotoxicity. Combining two permeable CPAs has been one approach that allows the use of lower concentrations of each CPA, without affecting their overall efficiency.[34,38,49-51] Vitrification protocols that combine EG with DMSO permit reduction of the final concentrations of the individual CPAs to 15% and have been shown to be quite effective for vitrification of human blastocyst[52,53] and cleavage stage embryos.[54] DMSO may have a protective effect on cell membrane integrity in vitrified mouse and human embryos.[55] Applying very high cooling and warming rates can further decrease the concentration of CPA necessary.[1]

CRYOSTORAGE VESSELS OR CARRIERS

During embryo cryopreservation, it is necessary to store the embryo in a vessel that allows temperature modulation during cooling and easy recovery on warming. For conventional slow cooled embryos, cryovials (1.5 ml) or 0.25 cc straws have been quite effective. The sample was usually frozen in relatively large fluid volumes of 25–300 µl. These conventional cryopreservation vessels have relatively thick walls that limit cooling and warming rates (around 2500°C/min). [51]

The successful application of vitrification techniques to human embryo/oocyte cryopreservation has been closely linked to the design and development of new vessels or carriers that permit extremely high cooling rates.[56,57] (Figure 1) This can be accomplished by reducing fluid volumes and preventing vessel walls from insulating the sample. Vitrification carriers sequester the cell in miniscule fluid volumes, typically 0.1–2 µl to maximize the rate of temperature decrease on immersion in LN2. Numerous carriers have been utilized for human embryo vitrification and have been classified as 'open' or 'closed' systems for vitrification.

Open vitrification carriers allow direct contact between the cell and LN2, thus allowing achievement of maximum cooling rates of over -20,000°C/min. Examples of 'open' systems used for human embryo vitrification are the hemi-straw,[58,59] the open pulled straw,[60] the cryotop-a thin plastic film,[26 61-63] the EM grid,[45,47,64,65] nylon mesh,[66] the plastic blade[67] and the cryoloop [24,48,52,54]. The cryoloop as a carrier is unique in that it allows vitrification without placing the embryo on any type of surface. Instead the embryo is deposited on a film of CPA before immersion in LN2.

Despite the successful use of 'open' carriers for human embryo vitrification, it can be argued that open systems have some inherent risks. There is the theoretical possibility of cross contamination among stored samples.[68] However, it should be noted that to date, there has never been a reported incidence of infection of reproductive tissues, as a result of cross-contamination in the LN2 storage tank. The other risk is related to direct contamination of the LN2 itself at the production facility or in the IVF lab through exposure to a contaminated

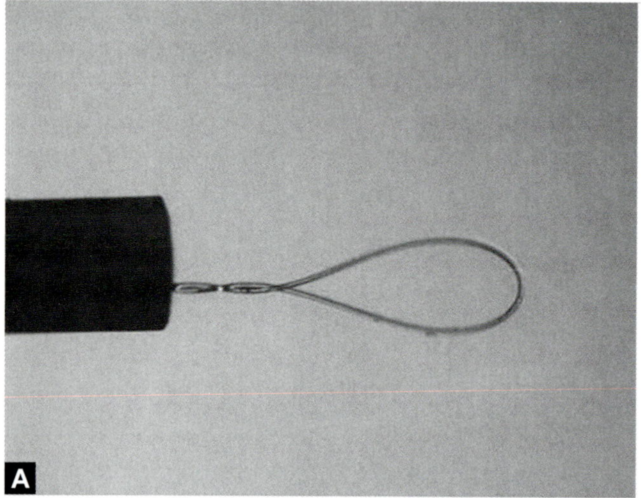

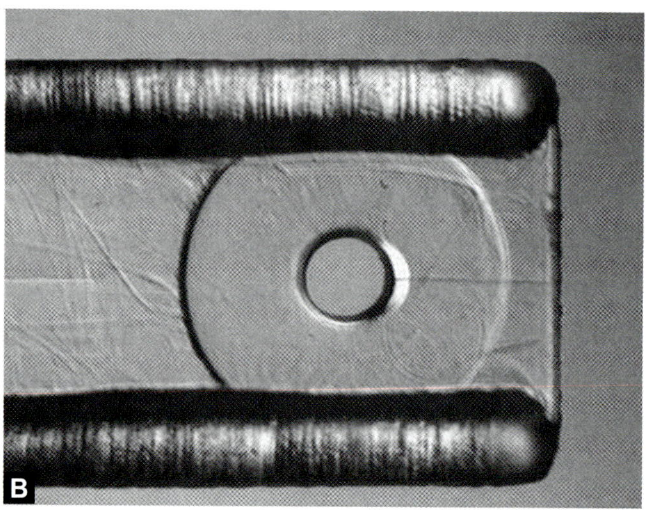

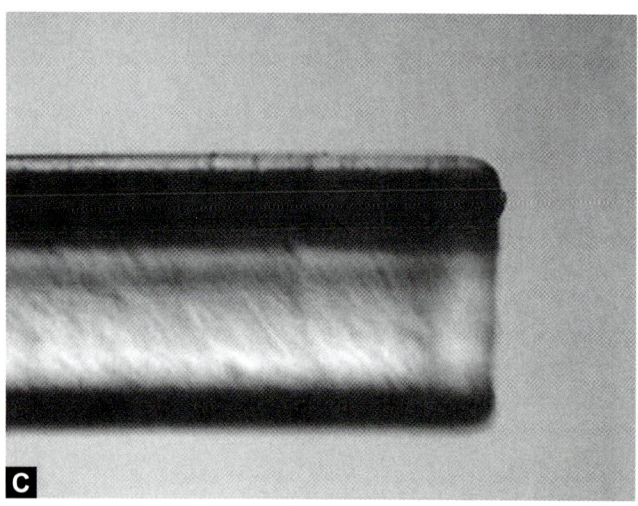

Figures 1A to C Examples of three vitrification systems: (A) Cryoloop, an open vitrification carrier. Embryo placed on a film of fluid covering a nylon loop and then immersed directly into a vial containing LN2; (B) Rapid I, closed carrier system. Embryo with miniscule fluid volume suspended in tiny eyelet hole formed at the end of a plastic wand. Rapid I carrier then dropped into a straw immersed in LN2 and heat sealed; (C) High Security Straw (HSV), closed carrier. Embryo with tiny fluid volume deposited on a capillary tube with a pre-cut gutter. The capillary tube is then placed into a straw and sealed before immersion in LN2

sample. Vapor phase storage of samples has been suggested as an option to get around this.[69] Yet it is possible that fungal contamination of samples stored in the vapor phase can still occur if the LN2 itself is contaminated.[70,71] One solution could be sterilization of LN2 by filtration or ultraviolet irradiation, followed by placement of the vitrification carrier with sample into a second sealable container before long term storage in LN2.[1,72,73] Routine screening of patients for infectious diseases before their treatment cycles and periodic disinfections of cryostorage tanks are good precautionary measures to reduce the possibility of LN2 contamination.

Elimination of direct contact between the biological sample and LN2 by using 'closed' vitrification carriers circumvents this potential risk. The concern has been that in sealed systems the cooling rates are somewhat lower. Numerous publications have however documented excellent outcomes with the new commercially available 'closed' carriers. Examples of these closed carrier systems include; cryotips (Irvine Scientific, CA, USA),[26,74] high security vitrification system (HSV) (Cryo Bio System, Paris, France),[63,75,76] VitriSafe (VitriMed, Austria),[77] Cryopette (Origio, Denemark)[78] and the Rapid-i ™ (Vitrolife Sweden AB).[79].

The European Union Tissue and Cells Directive, as well as US Federal Drug Administration regulations have mandated that reproductive tissue be isolated and handled so as to prevent cross-contamination. This is expected to greatly impact many of the techniques that are routinely used in IVF laboratories, including cryovessels acceptable for cryopreservation and most especially vitrification. The use of closed sealed systems is of course preferred if outcome data continue to suggest that the higher cooling rates attainable through direct contact with LN2 are not absolutely necessary for successful outcomes.

DEVELOPMENTAL CELL STAGE AND EMBRYO CRYOPRESERVATION OUTCOMES

Tables 1 to 4 present a sampling of published studies and clinical outcomes achieved with the transfer of cryopreserved embryos frozen either by slow cooling or more recently by vitrification. Studies are classified according to the cell stage at freeze. The question of what cell stage is best for embryo cryopreservation is yet to be answered. The size of the embryo, overall cell number, membrane permeability and response to different CPAs, all contribute to the embryos ability to withstand the cryopreservation process and maintain implantation potential. This is further complicated by the selected method of freezing; vitrification versus conventional slow cooling.

Pronuclear and Early Cleavage Stage Embryos

Pronuclear and early cleavage stage cryopreservation were initially more favored, as few labs were culturing embryos to day 5 (Table 1). The PN stage embryo tolerates conventional cryopreservation well and there are several studies suggesting better outcomes with this cell stage as opposed to early cleavage.[2,80,81] Higher post-thaw survival rates with PN stage as compared to both cleavage and blastocyst have also been reported.[82] The disadvantage of zygote stage freezing is that the embryo's developmental competence is unknown. With cleavage stage embryos, blastomere loss was shown to negatively impact successful outcomes.[83] Removal of necrotic blastomeres after thawing increased the subsequent developmental potential of partially damaged embryos and their ability to implant.[84] Resumption of mitosis within 24 hours of thawing is a key indicator of an embryo's potential and is a helpful tool for selecting embryos for transfer.[85]

Vitrification is also quiet effective for cryopreservation of early stage embryos from the zygote to the 8-cell stage (Table 2). High survival and a cardiopulmonary resuscitation (CPR) of 28% was reported for vitrified PN stage embryos.[86] Kuwayama reported higher survival rates with vitrification of 4-cell and PN stage embryos (98% and 100%, respectively) as compared to slow cooling (89% and 91%, respectively). Embryo vitrification on day 3 of culture at the 6–8 cell stage has also been successful with clinical pregnancy rates of 16–47%.[26,48,54,87-91] Vitrification at this cell stage permits further culture and monitoring of the warmed embryo for genomic activation before transfer. Progression to blastocsyt after 48 hours in culture is an excellent prognostic indicator of implantation potential.[54] Clinical pregnancy rate of 58% was noted if at least one of the transferred embryos reached this point by the time of transfer. The high compaction rate (78%) within 24 hours of warming was also indicative of the effectiveness of vitrification at this cell stage.

Blastocyst Stage Embryos

The first frozen blastocsyt pregnancy was established by Cohen and colleagues using slow cooling and a glycerol protocol.[42] One of the early limitations as regards freezing at the blastocyst stage, was the lack of suitable *in vitro* culture systems to produce high quality blastocysts. Co-culture of human embryos on monolayers of oviductal cells or Vero monkey kidney epithelial cells was one method initally used to cultivate blastocsyts.[92-94] Successful cryopreservation of human blastocsyts derived from co-culture systems was reported by several investigators.[43,95] More recently, the commercial availability of media formulations specifically designed for human blastocyst culture and the move towards blastocyst stage transfer, have spurred much interest in cryopreservation at this cell stage. Modifications of conventional slow freezing protocols have significantly improved outcomes with slow cooling of frozen blastocysts, leading to implantation rates as high as 30% per embryo in a few studies (Table 3).[29,96,97]

The current trend towards day 5 transfers and single ETs has focused much work on blastocyst stage vitrification. Success rates with vitrified-warmed blastocysts have ranged from 23% to as high as 71% (Table 4). Early stage blastocysts appear to withstand the vitrification procedure better than the more advanced blastocyst.[46,47,61,98,99] Higher birth rates per transfer were noted with vitrified morula (28%) and early blastocysts (27%) as compared to expanded blastocysts (14%).[46] Blastocoelic fluid in expanding blastocysts may be associated with poorer survival due to potential ice crystal formation. Artificial shrinkage of the fluid volume in the blastocyst cavity before vitrification is one avenue currently being applied in clinical labs to enhance outcomes with human blastocyst cryopreservation.[45-47,61,100]

Artificial shrinkage or collapse of blastocysts can be induced by mechanical means, such as repeated pipetting through different diameter micropipettes[61] or by use of needles.[46,47,99,101] A directed laser pulse can also be used for collapsing the blastocyst before vitrification.[99,101] (Figure 2) In 270 vitrification-warming cycles with either mechanical or laser collapse, Mukaida and colleagues (2006) achieved an impressive implantation rate of 47% per blastocyst transferred. Data suggest that artificial collapse before vitrification can reduce DNA damage and enhance postwarming re-expansion and cell proliferation in expanding blastocysts.[101]. The value of this intervention is still however controversial. Raju et al. reported that artificial collapse prior to vitrification did not enhance outcomes with expanded blastocsyts.[102]

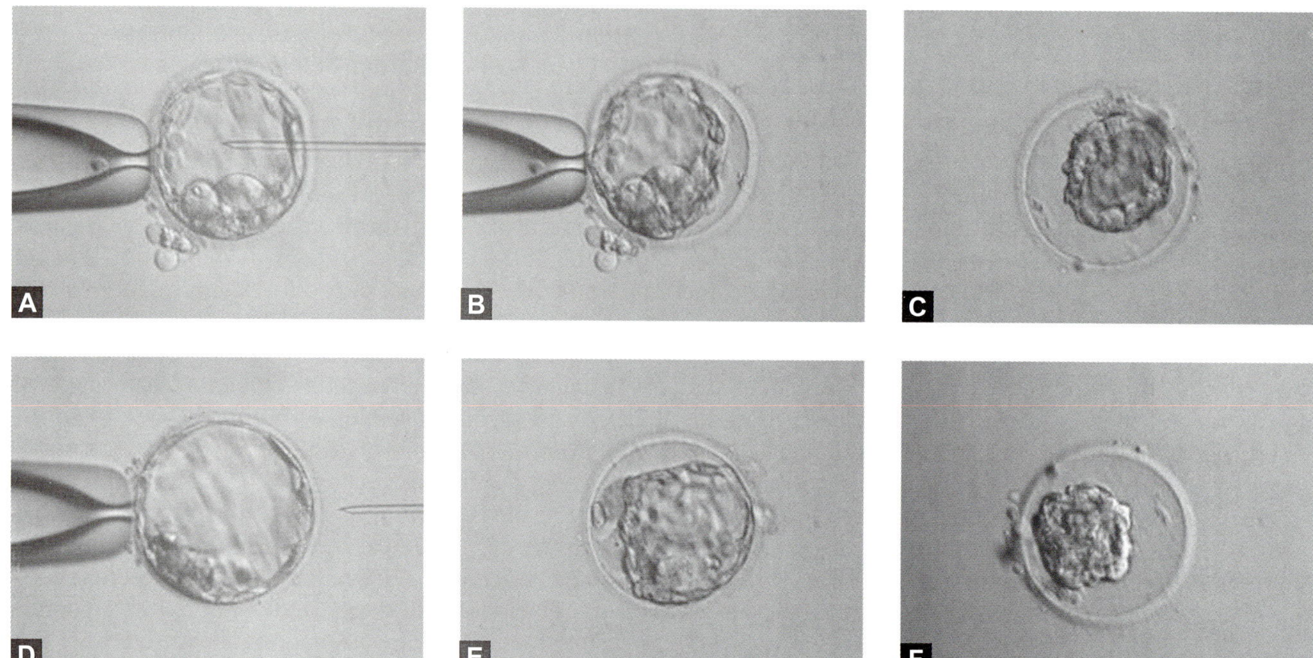

Figures 2A to F Mechanical collapse of expanded human blastocysts before vitrification using an ICSI needle. (A and D) Initial blastocyst morphology; (B and E) Penetration of blastocyst with ICSI needle to initiate collapse; (C and F) Blastocsyt morphology 5 minutes after mechanical collapse to reduce blastocelic fluid

Morula stage vitrification may be one way to circumvent the issue of blastocelic fluid and yet retain the advantage of cryopreservation after genome activation.[103]

Vitrification as a cutting edge technology for embryo freezing is gaining momentum and acceptance in clinics worldwide. The general consensus is that significant improvements in embryonic survival have been made possible through this methodology. This could ultimately translate in to higher pregnancy outcomes. Embryos biopsied for preimplantation genetic screening exhibited better survival with vitrification as compared to conventional slow cooling methods.[100,104,105] Wilding et al. observed less blastomere lysis with vitrification[76] but noted no difference in clinical outcomes.

Recent systematic reviews of published literature comparing both cryopreservation methods indicate that vitrification has a positive impact on postwarming survival of both cleavage and blastocyst stage embryos,[32,106] as well as pregnancy and implantation rates.[33] Developmental progression to blastocyst is also higher in vitrified cleavage stage embryos.[30] Clearly, additional prospective randomized controlled trials are needed to properly evaluate both methods and their impact on clinical pregnancy, implantation and live birth rates. Specific vitrification protocols, choice of CPA, stage of embryo, type of carrier and technical expertise are all likely to influence final outcomes and need to be given consideration in any comparative analysis.

ZONA OPENING AND/OR THINNING

It has been suggested that cryopreservation and exposure to high molar concentrations of CPAs may result in hardening of the zona pellucida, trapping the embryo and thus impeding subsequent implantation of the thawed embryo.[107] Thinning or opening of the zona through mechanical or laser assisted hatching should circumvent zona hardening and entrapment of the embryo. Whether this increases subsequent embryo implantation is still a matter of controversy. Some investigators have reported no improvements after hatching in frozen embryo transfer cycles.[108-111] Yet others have obtained significantly higher implantation rates after hatching of cryopreserved embryos before transfer.[112-115] Laser thinning and laser assisted removal of the zona also result in high clinical pregnancy (42% and 67%, respectively) and implantation rates (32% and 55%, respectively).[91,116] In contrast, Valojerdi et al. found that clinical outcome parameters were negatively impacted by laser thinning.[117]

The use of different methods for assisted hatching (i.e. mechanical, chemical and laser) may account for the variations observed as regard to the advantage of hatching frozen embryos. Location at which hatching is performed may also be important. In humans the hatching process seems to have polarity. Opening the zona closer to the inner cell mass (ICM) results in higher rate of complete hatching as compared to performing assisted hatching on the opposite side of the ICM.[118]

Noninvasive polarized light microscopy is one tool that has been used to study the impact of environment on the thickness and birefringence of the zona pellucida of embryos.[119-122] Birefringence of the trilaminar zona pellucida reflects the density, local fine structure and molecular order within the zona.[123] This technology has recently applied to slow frozen-thawed embryos to determine if their zona pellucidae differs from that of fresh embryos.[124] No significant change in zona pellucida birefringence has found before and after cryopreservation.

ENDOMETRIAL PREPARATION IN FROZEN THAWED CYCLES

There are various approaches for endometrial preparation before the frozen embryo transfer. Embryos can be replaced in natural cycles or after endometrial preparation with hormones.[125] In natural cycles the timing of transfer is determined by monitoring for the luteinizing hormone surge or else by administration of hCG to induce ovulation. Administration of estrogen and progesterone with or without gonadotropin releasing hormone agonist is also used to prepare the endometrium. The latter method allows the laboratory to have more control over the thaw and transfer dates. Two Cochrane systematic reviews failed to find any superiority of one regimen over the others.[125,126]

The day of embryo replacement in frozen transfers is determined by the cell stage at freeze. Blastocysts are generally transferred 5–6 days after ovulation or start of progesterone therapy. Pronuclear and early cleavage (2–4 cell) stage embryos are usually replaced on the 3rd day of progesterone treatment. With day 3 embryos frozen at the 6–8 cell stage, investigators have found that extended culture and transfer at the blastocyst stage is beneficial.[30,54]

SAFETY OF EMBRYO CRYOPRESERVATION

A systematic review on children born after cryopreservation found reassuring results regarding slow freezing of early cleavage embryos.[127] Obstetric outcomes, measured as preterm birth and low birth weight, for children born after cryopreservation were better or at least as good as those for children born after fresh IVF. Moreover, malformation rates between frozen and fresh were comparable.[127,128]

Wang et al. examined perinatal outcomes after transfer of fresh and thawed embryos at the cleavage or blastocyst stage.[129] The live birth rate from fresh transfers was higher than that with frozen embryos. To maximize the birth of a healthy baby from frozen embryos, the optimal practice was to freeze at the cleavage stage and culture to blastocyst before transfer. A recent meta-analysis of frozen blastocyst stage transfers concluded that live birth rates were lower with slow growing embryos, cryopreserved on day 6 versus those frozen on day 5.[130]

A recent Swedish study reported no difference in neonatal outcomes with embryo transfer of vitrified blastocsyts as compared to transfer of fresh blastocysts or slow frozen cleavage stage embryos. All three groups were comparable as regards preterm births, low birth weight and birth defects.[131] According to one report, cleavage stage vitrification results in a higher spontaneous abortion rate than transfer of fresh embryos but neonatal outcomes are similar.[132]

The sum of the data to date is encouraging as regards the safety of embryo cryopreservation. However, it is also clear that when compared to children from spontaneous pregnancies, children conceived from cryopreserved embryos after IVF are still at a higher risk for preterm birth, low birth weight, low APGAR score and admission to NICU.[133]

CONCLUSION

Embryo cryopreservation prevents the wastage of supernumerary embryos. It encourages transfer of fewer embryos per cycle and thus can lower the multiple pregnancy rates. With the establishment of a good cryopreservation program, the overall chance of conception and the cumulative pregnancy rate in an IVF program can be enhanced. Advances in our understanding of cryobiology and new techniques, such as vitrification, may help increase the efficiency and success of embryo cryopreservation. Continued monitoring of obstetric outcomes as freezing technology evolves is imperative. Finally, long term follow-up studies are still needed on infants born from vitrified embryos.

REFERENCES

1. Liebermann J, Dietl J, Vanderzwalmen P, et al. Recent developments in human oocyte, embryo and blastocyst vitrification: where are we now? Reprod Biomed Online. 2003;7:623-33.
2. Veeck LL. Does the developmental stage at freeze impact on clinical results post-thaw? Reprod Biomed Online. 2003;6:367-74.

3. Veeck LL, Amundson CH, Brothman LJ, et al. Significantly enhanced pregnancy rates per cycle through cryopreservation and thaw of pronuclear stage oocytes. Fertil Steril. 1993;59:1202-7.
4. Kjellberg AT, Carlsson P, Bergh C. Randomized single versus double embryo transfer: obstetric and paediatric outcome and a cost-effectiveness analysis. Hum Reprod. 2006;21:210-6.
5. Tiitinen A, Halttunen M, Harkki P, et al. Elective single embryo transfer: the value of cryopreservation. Hum Reprod. 2001;16:1140-4.
6. Schroder AK. Counselling on cryopreservation of pronucleated oocytes. Reprod Biomed Online. 2003;6:69-74.
7. Tatpati LL, Hudson SB, Gera PS, et al. High cumulative live births in oocyte donation cycles with cryopreservation of all embryos. Gynecol Obstet Invest. 2010;70: 76-81.
8. Polge C, Smith AU, Parkes AS. Revival of spermatozoa after vitrification and dehydration at low temperature. Nature. 1949;164:666-76.
9. Whittingham DG, LeiboSP, Mazur P. Survival of mouse embryos frozen to -196 degrees and -269 degrees C. Science. 1972;178:411-4.
10. Rall WF, Reid DS, Polge C. Analysis of slow-warming injury of mouse embryos by cryomicroscopical and physiochemical methods. Cryobiology. 1984;21:106-21.
11. Rall WF, Fahy GM. Ice-free cryopreservation of mouse embryos at -196 degrees C by vitrification. Nature. 1985;313:573-5.
12. Leibo SP. Fundamental cryobiology of mouse ova and embryos. Ciba Found Symp. 1977;20:69-96.
13. Wilmut I. The effect of cooling rate, warming rate, cryoprotective agent and stage of development on survival of mouse embryos during freezing and thawing. Life Sci II. 1972;11:1071-9.
14. Wood MJ, Farrant J. Preservation of mouse embryos by two-step freezing. Cryobiology. 1980;17:178-80.
15. Trounson A, Mohr L. Human pregnancy following cryopreservation, thawing and transfer of an 8-cell embryo. Nature. 1983;305:707-9.
16. Zeilmaker GH, Alberda AT, van Gent I, et al. Two pregnancies following transfer of intact frozen-thawed embryos. Fertil Steril. 1984;42:293-6.
17. Chen C. Pregnancy after human oocyte cryopreservation. Lancet. 1986;1:884-6.
18. Mazur P. The role of intracellular freezing in the death of cells cooled at supraoptimal rates. Cryobiology. 1977;14:251-72.
19. Pegg DE. The role of vitrification techniques of cryopreservation in reproductive medicine. Hum Fertil (Camb). 2005;8:231-9.
20. Willadsen SM. Factors affecting the survival of sheep embryos during-freezing and thawing. Ciba Found Symp. 1977;8-20:175-201.
21. Lane M, Bavister BD, Lyons EA, et al. Containerless vitrification of mammalian oocytes and embryos. Nat Biotechnol. 1999;17:1234-6.
22. Liebermann J, Tucker MJ. Effect of carrier system on the yield of human oocytes and embryos as assessed by survival and developmental potential after vitrification. Reproduction. 2002;124:483-9.
23. Liebermann J, Tucker MJ, Sills ES. Cryoloop vitrification in assisted reproduction: analysis of survival rates in > 1000 human oocytes after ultra-rapid cooling with polymer augmented cryoprotectants. Clin Exp Obstet Gynecol. 2003;30:125-9.
24. Lane M, Schoolcraft WB, Gardner DK. Vitrification of mouse and human blastocysts using a novel cryoloop container-less technique. Fertil Steril. 1999;72:1073-8.
25. Vajta G, Holm P, Kuwayama M, et al. Open Pulled Straw (OPS) vitrification: a new way to reduce cryoinjuries of bovine ova and embryos. Mol Reprod Dev. 1998;51:53-8.
26. Kuwayama M, Vajta G, Ieda S, et al. Comparison of open and closed methods for vitrification of human embryos and the elimination of potential contamination. Reprod Biomed Online. 2005;11:608-14.
27. Arav A, Zeron Y, Ocheretny A. A new device and method for vitrification increases the cooling rate and allows successful cryopreservation of bovine oocytes. Theriogenology. 2000;53:248.
28. Liebermann J, Nawroth F, Isachenko V, et al. Potential importance of vitrification in reproductive medicine. Biol Reprod. 2002;67:1671-80.
29. Liebermann J, Tucker MJ. Comparison of vitrification and conventional cryopreservation of day 5 and day 6 blastocysts during clinical application. Fertil Steril. 2006;86:20-6.
30. Balaban B, Urman B, Ata B, et al. A randomized controlled study of human day 3 embryo cryopreservation by slow freezing or vitrification: vitrification is associated with higher survival, metabolism and blastocyst formation. Hum Reprod. 2008;23:1976-82.
31. Son WY, Tan, SL. Comparison between slow freezing and vitrification for human embryos. Expert Rev Med Devices. 2009;6:1-7.
32. Loutradi KE, Kolibianakis EM, Venetis CA, et al. Cryopreservation of human embryos by vitrification or slow freezing: a systematic review and meta-analysis. Fertil Steril. 2008;90:186-93.
33. AbdelHafez F, Desai N, Abou-Setta AM, et al. Comparison of slow programmed freezing, vitrification and ultra-rapid freezing for the cryopreservation of human embryos: a systematic review and meta-analysis. Reprod Biomed Online. 2010;20(2):209-22. .
34. Kuleshova LL, MacFarlane DR, Trounson AO, et al. Sugars exert a major influence on the vitrification properties of ethylene glycol-based solutions and have low toxicity to embryos and oocytes. Cryobiology. 1999;38:119-30.
35. Dumoulin JC, Bergers-Janssen JM, Pieters MH, et al. The protective effects of polymers in the cryopreservation of human and mouse zonae pellucidae and embryos. Fertil Steril. 1994;62:793-8.
36. O'Neil L, Paynter SJ, Fuller BJ, et al. Vitrification of mature mouse oocytes: improved results following

addition of polyethylene glycol to a dimethyl sulfoxide solution. Cryobiology. 1997;34:295-301.

37. Shaw JM, Kuleshova LL, MacFarlane DR, et al. Vitrification properties of solutions of ethylene glycol in saline containing PVP, Ficoll, or dextran. Cryobiology. 1997;35:219-29.
38. Kuleshova LL, Shaw JM, Trounson AO. Studies on replacing most of the penetrating cryoprotectant by polymers for embryo cryopreservation. Cryobiology. 2001;43:21-31.
39. Lassalle B, Testart J, Renard JP. Human embryo features that influence the success of cryopreservation with the use of 1,2 propanediol. Fertil Steril. 1985;44:645-51.
40. Testart J, Lassalle B, Belaisch-Allart J, et al. High pregnancy rate after early human embryo freezing. Fertil Steril. 1986;46:268-72.
41. Van der Elst J, Van den Abbeel E, Jacobs R, et al. Effect of 1,2-propanediol and dimethylsulphoxide on the meiotic spindle of the mouse oocyte. Hum Reprod. 1988;3:960-7.
42. Cohen J, Simons RF, Edwards RG, et al. Pregnancies following the frozen storage of expanding human blastocysts. J In Vitro Fert Embryo Transf. 1985;2:59-64.
43. Menezo Y, Nicollet B, Herbaut N, et al. Freezing cocultured human blastocysts. Fertil Steril. 1992;58:977-80.
44. Rall WF, Wood MJ, Kirby C, et al. Development of mouse embryos cryopreserved by vitrification. J Reprod Fertil. 1987;80:499-504.
45. Cho HJ, Son WY, Yoon SH, et al. An improved protocol for dilution of cryoprotectants from vitrified human blastocysts. Hum Reprod. 2002;17:2419-22.
46. Vanderzwalme P, Bertin G, Debauche Ch, et al. Births after vitrification at morula and blastocyst stages: effect of artificial reduction of the blastocoelic cavity before vitrification. Hum Reprod. 2002;17:744-51.
47. Son WY, Yoon SH, Yoon HJ, et al. Pregnancy outcome following transfer of human blastocysts vitrified on electron microscopy grids after induced collapse of the blastocoele. Hum Reprod. 2003;18:137-9.
48. Rama Raju GA, Haranath GB, Krishna KM, et al. Vitrification of human 8-cell embryos, a modified protocol for better pregnancy rates. Reprod Biomed Online. 2005;11:434-7.
49. Ali J, Shelton JN. Design of vitrification solutions for the cryopreservation of embryos. J Reprod Fertil. 1993;99:471-7.
50. Mukaida T, Wada S, Takahashi K, et al. Vitrification of human embryos based on the assessment of suitable conditions for 8-cell mouse embryos. Hum Reprod. 1998;13:2874-9.
51. Vajta G, Nagy ZP. Are programmable freezers still needed in the embryo laboratory? Review on vitrification. Reprod Biomed Online. 2006;12:779-96.
52. Mukaida T, Nakamura S, Tomiyama T, et al. Vitrification of human blastocysts using cryoloops: clinical outcome of 223 cycles. Hum Reprod. 2003;18:384-91.
53. Mukaida T, Nakamura S, Tomiyama T, et al. Successful birth after transfer of vitrified human blastocysts with use of a cryoloop containerless technique. Fertil Steril. 2001;76:618-20.
54. Desai N, Blackmon H, Szeptycki J, et al. Cryoloop vitrification of human day 3 cleavage-stage embryos: Post-vitrification development, pregnancy outcomes and live births. Reprod Biomed Online. 2007;14:208-13.
55. Kartberg AJ, Hambiliki F, Arvidsson T, et al. Vitrification with DMSO protects embryo membrane integrity better than solutions without DMSO. Reprod Biomed Online. 2008;17:378-84.
56. Shaw JM, Jones GM. Terminology associated with vitrification and other cryopreservation procedures for oocytes and embryos. Hum Reprod Update. 2003;9:583-605.
57. Vajta G, Kuwayama M. Improving cryopreservation systems. Theriogenology. 2006;65:236-44.
58. Vanderzwalmen P, Bertin G, Debauche Ch, et al. Vitrification of human blastocysts with the Hemi-Straw carrier: application of assisted hatching after thawing. Hum Reprod. 2003;18:1504-11..
59. Zech NH, Lejeune B, Zech H, et al. Vitrification of hatching and hatched human blastocysts: effect of an opening in the zona pellucida before vitrification. Reprod Biomed Online. 2005;11:355-61.
60. El-Danasouri I, Selman H. Successful pregnancies and deliveries after a simple vitrification protocol for day 3 human embryos. Fertil Steril. 2001;76:400-2.
61. Hiraoka K, Hiraoka K, Kinutani M, et al. Blastocoele collapse by micropipetting prior to vitrification gives excellent survival and pregnancy outcomes for human day 5 and day 6 expanded blastocysts. Hum Reprod. 2004;19:2884-8.
62. Stehlik E, Stehlik J, Katayama KP, et al. Vitrification demonstrates significant improvement versus slow freezing of human blastocysts. Reprod Biomed Online. 2005;11:53-7.
63. Liebermann J. Vitrification of human blastocysts: an update. Reprod Biomed Online. 2009;19(Suppl 4):4328.
64. Park SP, Kim EY, Oh JH, et al. Ultra-rapid freezing of human multipronuclear zygotes using electron microscope grids. Hum Reprod. 2000;15:1787-90.
65. Hong SW, Sepilian V, Chung HM, et al. Cryopreserved human blastocysts after vitrification result in excellent implantation and clinical pregnancy rates. Fertil Steril. 2009;92:2062-4.
66. Nakashima A, Ino N, Kusumi M, et al. Optimization of a novel nylon mesh container for human embryo ultrarapid vitrification. Fertil Steril. 2010;93:2405-10.
67. Sugiyama R, Nakagawa K, Shirai A, et al. Clinical outcomes resulting from the transfer of vitrified human embryos using a new device for cryopreservation (plastic blade). J Assist Reprod Genet. 2010;27:161-7.
68. Bielanski A, Vajta G. Risk of contamination of germplasm during cryopreservation and cryobanking in IVF units. Hum Reprod. 2009;24:2457-67.
69. Cobo A, Romero JL, Pérez S, et al. Storage of human oocytes in the vapor phase of nitrogen. Fertil Steril. 2010;94:1903-7.
70. Fountain D, Ralston M, Higgins N, et al. Liquid nitrogen freezers: a potential source of microbial contamination of hematopoietic stem cell components. Transfusion. 1997;37:585-91.

71. Grout B W, Morris GJ. Contaminated liquid nitrogen vapour as a risk factor in pathogen transfer. Theriogenology. 2009;71:1079-82.
72. Vajta G, Lewis I, Kuwayama M, et al. Sterile application of the open pulled straw (OPS) vitrification method. Cryo-letters. 1998;19:389-92.
73. Parmegiani L, Cognigni GE, Filicori M. et al. Sterilization of liquid nitrogen with ultraviolet irradiation for safe vitrification of human oocytes or embryos. Fertil Steril. 2009;24:2969.
74. Cobo A, Pérez S, De los, et al. Effect of different cryopreservation protocols on the metaphase II spindle in human oocytes. Reprod Biomed Online. 2008;17;350-9.
75. Camus A, Clairaz P, Ersham A, et al. [The comparison of the process of five different vitrification devices]. Gynecol Obstet Fertil. 2006;34:737-45.
76. Wilding MG, Capobianco C, Montanaro N, et al. H man cleavage-stage embryo vitrification is compar ble to slow-rate cryopreservation in cycles of assisted reproduction. J Assist Reprod Genet. 2010;27(9-10):549-54.
77. Vanderzwalmen P, Ectors F, Grobet L, et al. Aseptic vitrification of blastocysts from infertile patients, egg donors and after IVM. Reprod Biomed Online. 2009;19:700-7.
78. Portman M, Nagy ZP, Behr B. Evaluation of blastocyst survival following vitrification/warming using two different closed carrier systems. Hum Reprod. 2010;25 (Suppl 1):375.
79. Tarakanov Y, Johansson B, Lehmann H, et al. in Proceedingsof the COMSOL Conference (Milan, Italy, 2009).
80. Salumets A, Tuuri T, Mäkinen S, et al. Effect of developmental stage of embryo at freezing on pregnancy outcome of frozen-thawed embryo transfer. Hum Reprod. 2003;18:1890-5.
81. Senn A, Vozzi C, Chanson A, et al. Prospective randomized study of two cryopreservation policies avoiding embryo selection: the pronucleate stage leads to a higher cumulative delivery rate than the early cleavage stage. Fertil Steril. 2000;74:946-52.
82. Moragianni VA, Cohen JD, Smith SE, et al. Outcomes of day 1, day 3, and blastocyst cryopreserved embryo transfers. Fertil Steril. 2010;93:1353-5.
83. Zhang S, Lu C, Lin G, et al. The number of blastomeres in post-thawing embryos affects the rates of pregnancy and delivery in freeze-embryo-transfer cycles. J Assist Reprod Genet. 2009;26:569-73.
84. Rienzi L, Ubaldi F, Iacobelli M, et al. Developmental potential of fully intact and partially damaged cryopreserved embryos after laser-assisted removal of necrotic blastomeres and post-thaw culture selection. Fertil Steril. 2005;84:888-94.
85. Ziebe S, Bech B, Petersen K, et al. Resumption of mitosis during post-thaw culture: a key parameter in selecting the right embryos for transfer. Hum Reprod. 11998;3:178-81.
86. Al-Hasani S, Ozmen B, Koutlaki N, et al. Three years of routine vitrification of human zygotes: is it still fair to advocate slow-rate freezing? Reprod Biomed Online. 2007;14:288-93.
87. Saito H, Ishida GM, Kaneko T, et al. Application of vitrification to human embryo freezing. Gynecol Obstet Invest. 2000;49:145-9.
88. Zhu GJ, Jin L, Zhang HW, et al. [Vitrification of human cleaved embryos in vitro fertilization-embryo transfer]. Zhonghua Fu Chan Ke Za Zhi. 2005;40:682-4.
89. Lin TK, Su JT, Lee FK, et al. Cryotop vitrification as compared to conventional slow freezing for human embryos at the cleavage stage: survival and outcomes. Taiwan J Obstet Gynecol. 2010;49:272-8.
90. Desai N, Abdelhafez F, Bedaiwy MA, et al. Clinical pregnancy and live births after transfer of embryos vitrified on day 3. Reprod Biomed Online. 2010;20:808-13.
91. Hiraoka K, Horiuchi T, Kusuda T, et al. Impact of the size of zona pellucida thinning area on vitrified-warmed cleavage-stage embryo transfers: a prospective, randomized study. J Assist Reprod Genet. 2009;26:515-21.
92. Menezo YJ, Nicollet B, Dumont M, et al. Factors affecting human blastocyst formation in vitro and freezing at the blastocyst stage. Acta Eur Fertil. 1993;24:207-13.
93. Wiemer KE, Cohen J, Tucker MJ, et al. The application of co-culture in assisted reproduction: 10 years of experience with human embryos. Hum Reprod. 1998;13 (Suppl 4):26-38.
94. Bongso A, Ng SC, Fong CY, et al. Cocultures: a new lead in embryo quality improvement for assisted reproduction. Fertil Steril. 1991;56:179-91.
95. Kaufman RA, Menezo Y, Hazout A, et al. Cocultured blastocyst cryopreservation: experience of more than 500 transfer cycles. Fertil Steril. 1995;64:1125-9.
96. Veeck LL, Bodine R, Clarke RN, et al. High pregnancy rates can be achieved after freezing and thawing human blastocysts. Fertil Steril. 2004;82:1418-27.
97. Shapiro BS, Daneshmand ST, Garner FC, et al. Contrasting patterns in in-vitro fertilization pregnancy rates among fresh autologous, fresh oocyte donor, and cryopreserved cycles with the use of day 5 or day 6 blastocysts may reflect differences in embryo-endometrium synchrony. Fertil Steril. 2008;89:20-6.
98. Park SP, Kim EY, Kim DI, et al. Simple, efficient and successful vitrification of bovine blastocysts using electron microscope grids. Hum Reprod. 1999;14:2838-43.
99. Mukaida T, Oka C, Goto T, et al. Artificial shrinkage of blastocoeles using either a micro-needle or a laser pulse prior to the cooling steps of vitrification improves survival rate and pregnancy outcome of vitrified human blastocysts. Hum Reprod. 2006;21:3246-3252.
100. Keskintepe L, Sher G, Machnicka A, et al. Vitrification of human embryos subjected to blastomere biopsy for pre-implantation genetic screening produces higher survival and pregnancy rates than slow freezing. J Assist Reprod Genet. 2009;26:629-35.
101. Desai N, Szeptycki J, Scott M, et al. Artificial Collapse of Blastocysts Before Vitrification: Mechanical vs Laser Technique and Effect on Survival, Cell Number, and Cell Death in Early and Expanded Blastocysts. Biopreservation and Biobanking. 2008;6:181-190.

102. Raju GA, Prakash GJ, Krishna KM, et al. Vitrification of human early cavitating and deflated expanded blastocysts: clinical outcome of 474 cycles. J Assist Reprod Genet. 2009;26:523-9.
103. Zhang X, Trokoudes KM, Pavlides C. Vitrification of biopsied embryos at cleavage, morula and blastocyst stage. Reprod Biomed Online. 2009;19:526-31.
104. Zheng WT, Zhuang GL, Zhou CQ, et al. Comparison of the survival of human biopsied embryos after cryopreservation with four different methods using non-transferable embryos. Hum Reprod. 2005;20:1615-8.
105. Kahraman S, Candan ZN. Outcomes of vitrified-warmed day 4 embryos after day 3 cleavage-stage biopsy. Reprod Biomed Online. 2010;21:636-41.
106. Kolibianakis EM, Venetis CA, Tarlatzis BC. Cryopreservation of human embryos by vitrification or slow freezing: which one is better? Curr Opin Obstet Gynecol. 2009;21:270-4.
107. Carroll J, Depypere H, Matthews CD. Freeze-thaw-induced changes of the zona pellucida explains decreased rates of fertilization in frozen-thawed mouse oocytes. J Reprod Fertil. 1990;90:547-53.
108. Ng, EH, Naveed F, Lau EY, et al. A randomized double-blind controlled study of the efficacy of laser-assisted hatching on implantation and pregnancy rates of frozen-thawed embryo transfer at the cleavage stage. Hum Reprod. 2005;20:979-85.
109. Sifer C, Sellami A, Poncelet C, et al. A prospective randomized study to assess the benefit of partial zona pellucida digestion before frozen-thawed embryo transfers. Hum Reprod. 2006;21:2384-9.
110. Petersen CG, Mauri AL, Baruffi RL, et al. Laser-assisted hatching of cryopreserved-thawed embryos by thinning one quarter of the zona. Reprod Biomed Online. 2006;13:668-75.
111. Primi MP, Senn A, Montag M, et al. A European multicentre prospective randomized study to assess the use of assisted hatching with a diode laser and the benefit of an immunosuppressive/antibiotic treatment in different patient populations. Hum Reprod. 2004;19:2325-33.
112. Gabrielsen A, Agerholm I, Toft B, et al. Assisted hatching improves implantation rates on cryopreserved-thawed embryos. A randomized prospective study. Hum Reprod. 2004;19:2258-62.
113. Balaban B, Urman B, Yakin K, et al. Laser-assisted hatching increases pregnancy and implantation rates in cryopreserved embryos that were allowed to cleave in vitro after thawing: a prospective randomized study. Hum Reprod. 2006;21:2136-40.
114. Ge HS, Zhou W, Zhang W, et al. Impact of assisted hatching on fresh and frozen-thawed embryo transfer cycles: a prospective, randomized study. Reprod Biomed Online. 2008;16:589-96.
115. Valojerdi MR, Eftekhari-Yazdi P, Karimian L, et al. Effect of laser zona pellucida opening on clinical outcome of assisted reproduction technology in patients with advanced female age, recurrent implantation failure, or frozen-thawed embryos. Fertil Steril. 2008;90:84-91.
116. Hiraoka K, Fuchiwaki M, Hiraoka K, et al. Zona pellucida removal and vitrified blastocyst transfer outcome: a preliminary study. Reprod Biomed Online. 2007;15:68-75.
117. Valojerdi MR, Eftekhari-Yazdi P, Karimian L, et al. Effect of laser zona thinning on vitrified-warmed embryo transfer at the cleavage stage: a prospective, randomized study. Reprod Biomed Online. 2010;20:234-42.
118. Miyata H, Matsubayashi H, Fukutomi N, et al. Relevance of the site of assisted hatching in thawed human blastocysts: a preliminary report. Fertil Steril. 2010;94:2444-7.
119. Pelletier C, Keefe DL, Trimarchi JR. Noninvasive polarized light microscopy quantitatively distinguishes the multilaminar structure of the zona pellucida of living human eggs and embryos. Fertil Steril. 2004;81(Suppl 1): 850-6.
120. Kilani SS, Cooke S, Kan AK, et al. Do age and extended culture affect the architecture of the zona pellucida of human oocytes and embryos? Zygote. 2006;14:39-44.
121. Rama Raju GA, Prakash GJ, Krishna KM, et al. Meiotic spindle and zona pellucida characteristics as predictors of embryonic development: a preliminary study using PolScope imaging. Reprod Biomed Online. 2007;14:166-74.
122. Madaschi C, Aoki T, de Almeida Ferreira Braga DP, et al. Zona pellucida birefringence score and meiotic spindle visualization in relation to embryo development and ICSI outcomes. Reprod Biomed Online. 2009;18:681-6.
123. Oldenbourg R. A new view on polarization microscopy. Nature. 1996;381:811-2.
124. Gu YF, Lu CF, Lin G, et al. A comparative analysis of the zona pellucida birefringence of fresh and frozen-thawed human embryos. Reproduction. 2010;139:121-7.
125. Ghobara T, Vandekerckhove P. Cycle regimens for frozen-thawed embryo transfer. Cochrane Database Syst Rev. 2008;CD003414.
126. Glujovsky D, Pesce R, Fiszbajn G, et al. Endometrial preparation for women undergoing embryo transfer with frozen embryos or embryos derived from donor oocytes. Cochrane Database Syst Rev. 2010;CD006359.
127. Wennerholm UB, Söderström-Anttila V, Bergh C, et al. Children born after cryopreservation of embryos or oocytes: a systematic review of outcome data. Hum Reprod. 2009;24(9):2158-72.
128. Li HZ, Qiao J, Chi HB, et al. Comparison of the major malformation rate of children conceived from cryopreserved embryos and fresh embryos. Chin Med J (Engl). 2010;123:1893-7.
129. Wang YA, Chapman M, Costello M, et al. Better perinatal outcomes following transfer of fresh blastocysts and blastocysts cultured from thawed cleavage embryos: a population-based study. Hum Reprod. 2010;25:1536-42.
130. Sunkara SK, Siozos A, Bolton VN, et al. The influence of delayed blastocyst formation on the outcome of frozen-thawed blastocyst transfer: a systematic review and meta-analysis. Hum Reprod. 2010;25:1906-15.
131. Wikland M, Hardarson T, Hillensjö T, et al. Obstetric outcomes after transfer of vitrified blastocysts. Hum Reprod. 2010;25:1699-707.

132. Aflatoonian A, Mansoori Moghaddam F, Mashayekhy M, et al. Comparison of early pregnancy and neonatal outcomes after frozen and fresh embryo transfer in ART cycles. J Assist Reprod Genet. 2010;27:695-700.
133. Pelkonen S, Koivunen R, Gissler M, et al. Perinatal outcome of children born after frozen and fresh embryo transfer: the Finnish cohort study 1995-2006. Hum Reprod. 2010;25:914-23.
134. al-Hasani S, Ludwig M, Gagsteiger F, et al. Comparison of cryopreservation of supernumerary pronuclear human oocytes obtained after intracytoplasmic sperm injection (ICSI) and after conventional in vitro fertilization. Hum Reprod. 1996;11:604-7.
135. Van den Abbeel E, Camus M, Van Waesberghe L, et al. A randomized comparison of the cryopreservation of one-cell human embryos with a slow controlled-rate cooling procedure or a rapid cooling procedure by direct plunging into liquid nitrogen. Hum Reprod. 1997;12:1554-60.
136. Tummon IS, Wentworth MA, Thornhill AR. Frozen-thawed embryo transfer and live birth: Long-term follow-up after one oocyte retrieval. Fertil Steril. 2006;86:239-42.
137. Nagy ZP, Taylor T, Elliott T, et al. Removal of lysed blastomeres from frozen-thawed embryos improves implantation and pregnancy rates in frozen embryo transfer cycles. Fertil Steril. 2005;84:1606-12.
138. Salumets A, Suikkari AM, Mäkinen S, et al. Frozen embryo transfers: implications of clinical and embryological factors on the pregnancy outcome. Hum Reprod. 2006;21:2368-74.
139. Balaban B, Yakin K, Isiklar A, et al. Utilization of high-security straws for embryo freezing in an in vitro fertilization program: a prospective, randomized study. Fertil Steril. 2007;87:691-6.
140. Rezazadeh Valojerdi M, Eftekhari-Yazd, P, Karimian L, et al. Vitrification versus slow freezing gives excellent survival, post warming embryo morphology and pregnancy outcomes for human cleaved embryos. J Assist Reprod Genet. 2009;26:347-54.
141. Rama Raju GA, Jaya Prakash G, Murali Krishna K, et al. Neonatal outcome after vitrified day 3 embryo transfers: a preliminary study. Fertil Steril. 92:143-8.
142. Aflatoonian A, Oskouian H, Ahmadi S, et al. Can fresh embryo transfers be replaced by cryopreserved-thawed embryo transfers in assisted reproductive cycles? A randomized controlled trial. J Assist Reprod Genet. 2010;27:357-63.
143. Pantos, K, Stefanidis K, Pappas K, et al. Cryopreservation of embryos, blastocysts, and pregnancy rates of blastocysts derived from frozen-thawed embryos and frozen-thawed blastocysts. J Assist Reprod Genet. 2001;18:579-82.
144. Virant-Klun I, Tomazevic T, Bacer-Kermavner L, et al. Successful freezing and thawing of blastocysts cultured in sequential media using a modified method. Fertil Steril. 2003;79:1428-33.
145. Richter KS, Shipley SK, McVearry I, et al. Cryopreserved embryo transfers suggest that endometrial receptivity may contribute to reduced success rates of later developing embryos. Fertil Steril. 2006;86:862-6.
146. Takahashi K, Mukaida T, Goto T, et al. Perinatal outcome of blastocyst transfer with vitrification using cryoloop: a 4-year follow-up study. Fertil Steril. 2005;84:88-92.
147. Lee SY, Son WY, Yoon SH, et al. Clinical-pregnancy outcome after vitrification of blastocysts produced from in vitro maturation cycles. Fertil Steril. 2007;88:1449-51.

22

Oocyte Donation Program

Brian A Levine, Mark V Sauer

CHAPTER CONTENTS

- Indications for Egg Donation and the Precycle Testing of Recipients
- Donor Screening and Safeguards
- Synchronization Schemes for Donors and Recipients
- Clinical Results and Pregnancy Outcomes
- Controversies that Surround the Use of Donor Eggs
- Future Use and Anticipated Role of Egg Donation in Assisted Reproduction

INTRODUCTION

Egg and embryo donation were first introduced as treatments for human infertility in 1983; and they have been widely practiced for nearly three decades.[1] Such services are available throughout the United States, and remain popular throughout the world, although access is restricted in many locations due to legal prohibitions. Egg donation cycles represent roughly 10% of all assisted reproduction techniques initiated, with nearly 10,000 attempts performed annually in the United States; in 2008 donor eggs or embryos were used in approximately 12% of all assisted reproductive technology (ART) cycles.[2]

In women utilizing donated eggs, pregnancies occur in over 50% of embryo transfers and represent the highest rates of success in the field of assisted reproduction. For instance, reviewing cycles completed in 2009 in which fresh donor eggs were used, more than 50% of the transfers resulted in a live birth (Table 1).[3] This is most remarkable since recipients are often older and typically would not be capable of conceiving with their own eggs. When reviewing the Centers for Disease Control (CDC) data from 2008, it is noted that comparatively, few women younger than age 40 years used donor eggs. However, the percentage of cycles performed with donor eggs increased sharply in women older than 40 years. Specifically, in women older than 48 years, nearly 90% of all ART cycles used donor eggs.[2] Interestingly, uterine receptivity to embryo implantation appears to remain unaltered in menopausal women, if these patients are adequately prepared with exogenous hormones prior to their embryo transfer.[4-6] This fact accounts for the high rate of implantation, high rate of multiple gestations and high rate of delivery in these older recipients. With that said, since donor cycles typically use eggs from women in their 20s or early 30s, the percentage of live births from donated eggs tends to be consistently greater than 50% regardless of the age of the recipient (Figure 1).[2]

This chapter reviews the practice of egg donation and its role in assisted reproductive technologies. It also includes indications for its use and the precycle testing of recipients, protocols for donor screening and safeguards, synchronization schemes for donors and recipients, and the expected clinical outcomes and pregnancy results of recipients. The chapter mentions the controversies that surround the method, and finally some thoughts regarding the anticipated role egg donation will play in the future of reproductive medicine.

INDICATIONS FOR EGG DONATION AND THE PRECYCLE TESTING OF RECIPIENTS

At the time of its introduction, and for nearly 10 years thereafter, egg donation was largely used as a treatment for infertility in younger women with either ovarian failure or other poor prognostic profiles to have children.[7] This trend was later changed once egg donation was applied to assist older women whose problems were a natural result of reproductive aging.[8] Many older recipients were frankly menopausal and brought with them additional health concerns that accompany advancing age. In fact, maternal deaths have rather unfairly been associated with oocyte donation in older patients, as most fatalities have occurred in younger recipients.[9] In reviewing the most recent data from the Society for Advanced Reproductive Technology (SART), nearly 45% of those utilizing oocyte donation, were assigned a diagnosis of diminished ovarian reserve, while nearly 20% had multifactorial infertility (Table 2).[3]

Table 1 The society for advanced reproductive technology data on oocyte donation outcomes (2009)[3]

Donor oocytes (all ages)	Fresh Embryos	Thawed Embryos
Number of transfers	9,485	5,614
Percentage of transfers resulting in live births	55.1	33.8
Average number of embryos transferred	2.0	2.1

Performing specific tests that may relate to the underlying reason for a woman's need for egg donation are pertinent, such as investigating associated autoimmunity in women with premature ovarian failure, as well as genetic testing for fragile X syndrome.[10] Patients known to have XY gonadal dysgenesis should undergo gonadal extirpation prior to conceiving since they are at increased risk for gonadal cancers.[11] Patients with Turner's syndrome are known to have a variety of unique health problems, particularly related to cardiac abnormalities and aortic aneurysm. There have been multiple case reports detailing the rupture of these aneurysms in pregnancy; and therefore, echocardiograms and ultrasound or MRI evaluation of the aorta is an essential part of their antenatal screening. If discovered,

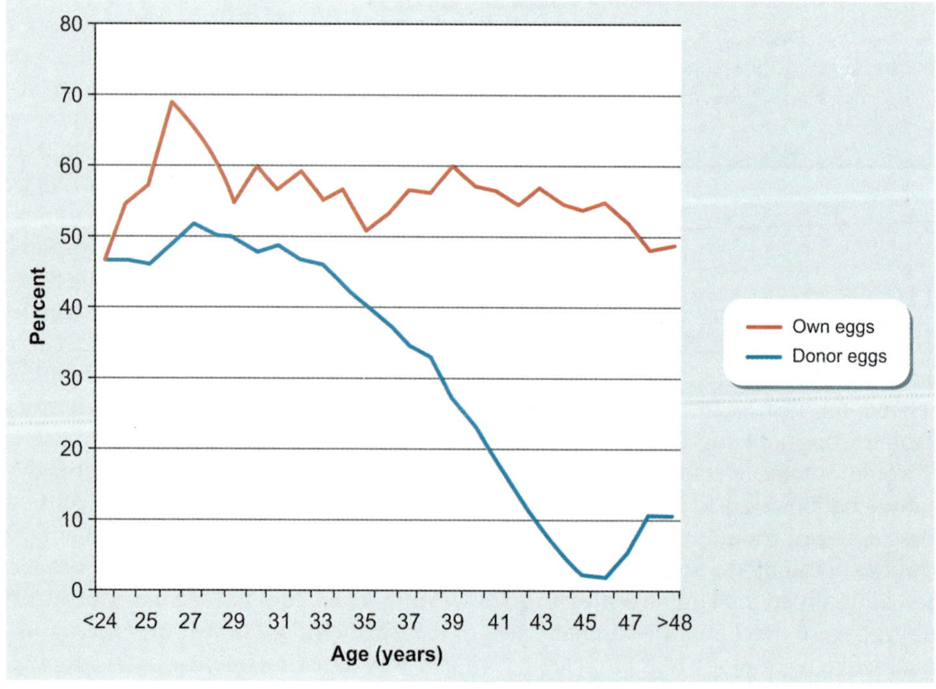

Figure 1 Percentages of transfers that resulted in live births for assisted reproductive technology cycles using fresh embryos from own eggs and assisted reproductive technology cycles using donor eggs, by age of woman (2008)[2]

Table 2 The society for advanced reproductive technology data regarding recipient diagnosis (2009)[3]

Diagnosis frequency	
Tubal factor	1%
Ovulatory dysfunction	2%
Diminished ovarian reserve	44%
Endometriosis	1%
Uterine factor	1%
Male factor	3%
Other factor	11%
Unknown factor	3%
Multiple factors	
Female factors only	17%
Female and male factors	17%

patients should be dissuaded from attempting pregnancy due to the propensity for rupture of the aneurysm and the catastrophic result to both mother and child.[12-14]

Cancer survivors often experience hypergonadotropic hypogonadism as a result of chemotherapy and/or radiation.[15] A full understanding of their previous disease, its stage and all components of its treatment needs to be disclosed to fully assess whether or not the patient should attempt pregnancy. For instance, the use of hormone therapy in survivors of advanced stage breast cancer and the effect of prolonged exposure to elevated pregnancy hormones may not be acceptable to many oncologists; and there is not a great deal of evidence based medicine to define the true safety of establishing pregnancy in these individuals.[16] In other cases, patients may have received enough pelvic radiation to destroy the regenerative capacity of the endometrium. Such individuals will not produce a normal decidual response to hormone replacement therapy and are unlikely to implant an embryo. Even women with an endometrial response may also be at risk for miscarriage, preterm labor, low birth weight infants and various placental abnormalities.[17] In such cases, gestational carrier surrogacy may represent a better and safer option for having a child.

As described with oocyte donors (see below), those seeking to become recipients have to go through a well-described screening process as recommended by the American Society for Reproductive Medicine (ASRM).[18] Older recipients are a unique population of patients and represent special challenges prior to attempting an embryo transfer. A thorough health evaluation should target organ systems that may be adversely, affected by age, with particular emphasis on the cardiovascular system.[19]

Leiomyomata are common in women over 40 years of age, and often recipients have undergone previous myomectomies, which may further render their uterus inhospitable to pregnancy. Implantation potential appears to be decreased when myomas are greater than 4 cm in diameter, regardless of their location; and therefore, such tumors may need to be removed to optimize outcomes. However, fibroid size, number and location also play a critical role in the decision to proceed with myomectomy. Therefore, a careful analysis of the overall clinical situation must be performed when creating a surgical plan.[20] It may be particularly difficult to recommend surgery to an asymptomatic middle aged woman, who despite her best efforts may subsequently, fail attempts at egg donation, and ultimately, question whether or not the pain and inconvenience of surgery were really in her best interest.[21]

DONOR SCREENING AND SAFEGUARDS

In the United States, egg donors have always been financially compensated for their participation. Screened much like their male counterparts serving as sperm donors, egg donors receive much higher rates of payment for their time and efforts. This is largely, due to the invasiveness and risks associated with the egg retrieval process combined with the high demand for eggs, which typically are used fresh and not cryopreserved. With the expansion of services to include older women, the demand for eggs has outpaced the supply of available donors. Consequently, the free market competition for services has progressively driven up the fees paid to these young women in hope of securing their services. In the 1980s, the typical egg donor was compensated approximately US$ 500 for each cycle of participation. Today, remuneration more commonly ranges from US$ 5,000 to US$ 8,000.[22]

The ASRM clearly states that compensation should be structured to acknowledge the time, inconvenience and discomfort associated with screening, ovarian stimulation and oocyte retrieval. However, the financial compensation should not vary according to the planned use of the oocytes, the number or quality of oocytes retrieved, the number or outcome of prior donation cycles, or the donor's ethnic or other personal characteristics.[22] With that said, there are many internet advertisements that claim to offer up to 10 times the reported national compensation rates.

Guidelines for the medical management of egg donors have been published by both ASRM and the European Society for Human Reproduction (ESHRE); and these recommendations have been revised several times over the years.[18,23] Landmark changes were implemented by the US government when implementing oversight control over donor gametes in 2005 followed by formal revised recommendations in 2008.[18] Additionally, several states have enacted legislation that either limit or provide tight controls over the clinical practice. For example, the New York State Department of Health requirements for practicing egg donation impose even more stringent regulations than those required by the US Food and Drug Administration (FDA).[24]

The screening of egg donors should address the woman's ability to participate in a variety of ways including her overall medical health, reproductive status, mental health, genetic background and social history. The 2008 ASRM guidelines for gamete donation clearly outlines the recommended screening.[18] Donors are required to respond to questions concerning high-risk behaviors related to infectious disease. Similarly, the FDA mandates that a comprehensive history be obtained and bloods be drawn to rule out individuals that might pass transmissible infections such as human immunodeficiency virus and hepatitis to a recipient.[25] Furthermore, since donors typically undergo oocyte retrieval under anesthesia, accurate reporting of current medications, alcohol use, cigarette smoking and illicit drug use is critically important for ensuring a good outcome. Most donors provide services anonymously and are often not told of the outcome of their efforts as it relates to whether or not a recipient conceived.

Complications are not only unsettling when occurring in a donor, but also present unique medical insurance coverage problems for payment of incurred expenses.[26] A recent report of 4,052 oocyte donor cycles demonstrated that egg donation is relatively safe, but that well-known complications do arise. Adverse events related to oocyte retrieval occurred in less than 0.5% of patients (intra-abdominal bleeding: n = 14, severe pain: n = 2, ovarian torsion: n = 1) with no cases of injury to pelvic structures or anesthesia complications reported. However, moderate to severe ovarian hyperstimulation syndrome (OHSS) was noted in approximately 20 patients, with half of them requiring hospital admission.[27] To avoid conflicts over the payment of medical bills, many programs including ours contract with an insurance carrier to underwrite the cost of incidental medical expenses that arise as a result of donor participation.

SYNCHRONIZATION SCHEMES FOR DONORS AND RECIPIENTS

Once donors are screened and found to be acceptable, they are placed on medications to hyperstimulate their ovaries as demonstrated in Figure 2. Usually, a combination of gonadotropins to effect multifollicular development (e.g. purified recombinant follicle-stimulating hormone or urinary gonadotropins) along with a gonadotropin-releasing hormone agonist (e.g. leuprolide acetate) or

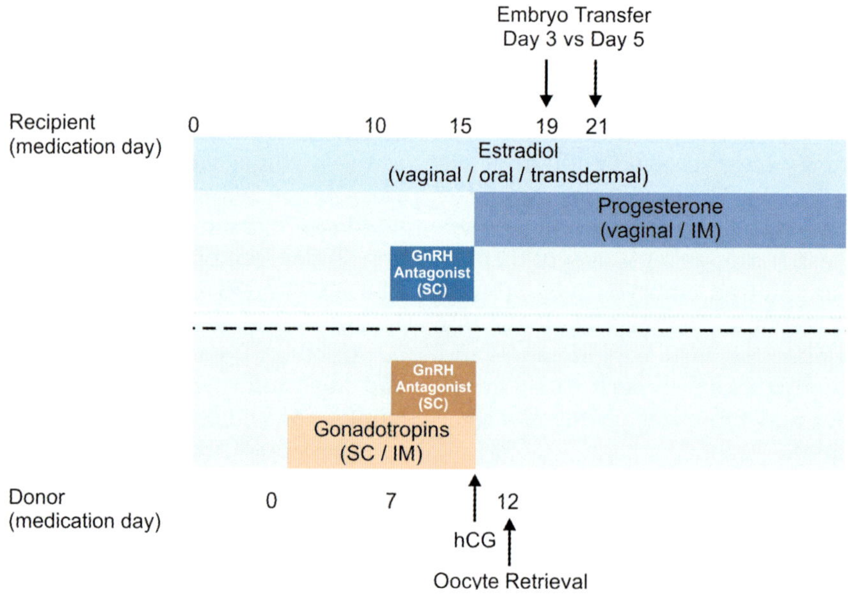

Figure 2 Hormonal synchronization between oocyte recipients and donors
GnRH: Gonadotropin-releasing hormone; IM: Intramuscular; SC: Subcutaneous

antagonist (e.g. ganirelix acetate) to prevent an inadvertent luteinizing hormone surge are prescribed. Drugs are administered daily and are parenterally delivered (subcutaneous or intramuscular) as they are fast acting and quickly metabolized. Most treatment cycles occur within a 2–3 week window of time and require frequent visits (8–10 times per cycle of participation) for monitoring of the response. Adequacy of response is gauged by daily transvaginal ultrasound examinations along with accompanying serum estradiol levels. Most donors will provide 10 to 20 eggs per retrieval. In our center, a response of less than seven dominant follicles is usually cancelled.

Egg retrieval is performed under conscious sedation with propofol and fentanyl, and usually takes less than 15 minutes. Bleeding is minimal and the procedure itself is largely painless. Although quite rare, complications may occur at the time of aspiration, which include excessive bleeding (particularly true in undiagnosed von Willebrand's disease), bladder atony, adverse anesthesia reactions, and pelvic hematoma.[27] As mentioned previously, more often (1% of cases) delayed problems arise as a result of OHSS. Fluid and metabolic instability in these cases may arise with the onset of nausea or difficulty in breathing 3–7 days later, and in severe cases, hospitalization is required to stabilize the patient.[27]

To synchronize the endometrial development in the oocyte recipients who are receiving the aspirated eggs, gonadotropin-releasing hormone agonists are used to downregulate and suppress endogenous ovarian activity in those with functioning ovaries (not necessary in women with premature ovarian failure or who are currently menopausal). The recipient is then treated with a schedule of exogenous estrogen and progesterone to allow for endometrial development, growth and maturation as demonstrated in Figure 2. In some centers, recipients undergo a mock treatment cycle to ensure the adequacy of the planned treatment regimen, although transvaginal ultrasonography is sensitive enough to monitor the real time endometrial thickness reflective of normal growth and development. If a woman does not respond appropriately, embryos can also be frozen after fertilization and used in a subsequent cycle once a normal appearing lining is demonstrated.[28-30]

CLINICAL RESULTS AND PREGNANCY OUTCOMES

The United States remains in the forefront of egg donation services. It can be assumed from reviewing the annual reported data of the CDC that approximately a quarter of a million cycles of egg/embryo donation have taken place in the United States since its introduction in 1984.[2,3] Currently, 10,000 to 12,000 attempts at donor *in vitro* fertilization (IVF) take place annually.[2,3] This is approximately 2–3 times the number reported per year in Europe or in Asia, where more restrictions on the practice are in place.[31]

The pregnancy rates of recipients of donated eggs and embryos remains as high, or higher than rates seen in younger women using autologous eggs and IVF.[2,3,31] This surprising fact was first documented in the late 1980s and remains true today.[8] This holds true even for patients 50 years of age and older, who would essentially have no success if attempting to conceive on their own. With the recent birth of babies to women in their seventies, it is fair to say that there is no biologic barrier to embryo implantation and pregnancy due to advancing age, even in a geriatric population.[32]

As important as pregnancy rates are in reflecting the success of the method, it is ultimately the obstetrical outcomes that matter most. When looking at Figure 3, one can appreciate that the percentage of transfers that resulted in live singleton births was lower than the percentage of transfers that resulted in live births.[2] This data demonstrates not only the prevalence of multiple gestations, but also serves as an important measure of IVF success since singleton births are associated with improved perinatal outcomes.

As might be expected, other than the increased rate of multiple births (also noted in women undertaking conventional IVF with autologous eggs), younger recipients of donated eggs and embryos appear to have no known unique risks to them or their offspring, although there have been reports of increased rates of pregnancy induced hypertension.[33] However, this is not the case for women of advanced reproductive age where considerable additional morbidity has been reported. Complications occur in this population roughly 20% of the time and include gestational hypertension, diabetes, small-for-dates infants, placental abnormalities and stillbirth.[9,19,34] The higher incidence and prevalence for problems has occurred despite the greater surveillance paid to them prenatally in their medical and obstetrical testing.

CONTROVERSIES THAT SURROUND THE USE OF DONOR EGGS

From the beginning, egg and embryo donation have been fraught with controversy. Payment for 'donation' has been criticized and has grown over the years as services have increased, and become more commercially competitive. Initial payments in 1984 of US$ 250 were

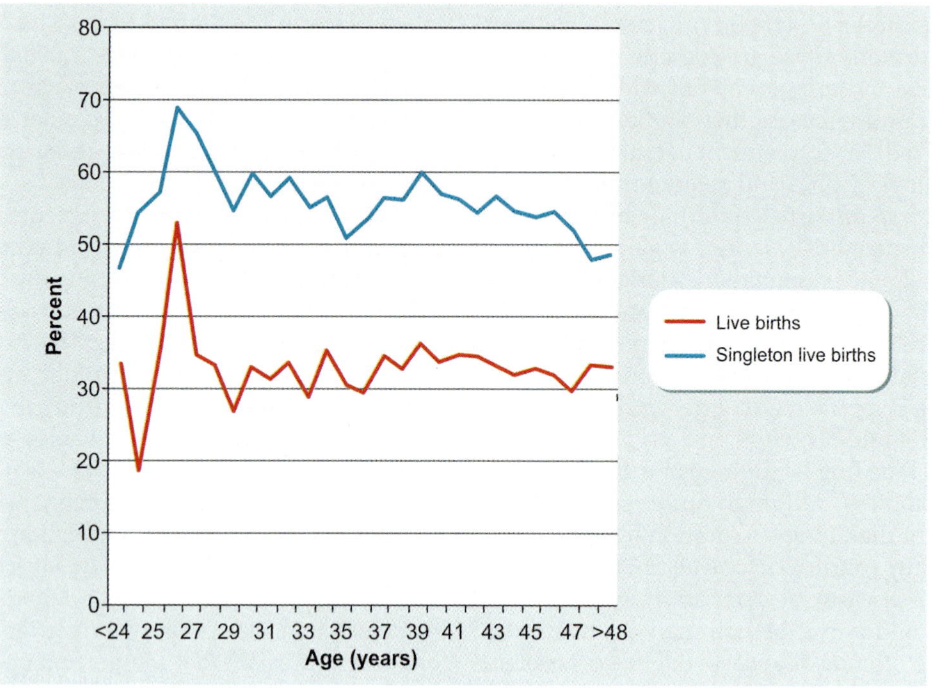

Figure 3 Percentages of transfers that resulted in live births and singleton live births for assisted reproductive technology cycles using fresh embryos from donor eggs, by age of woman (2008)[2]

actually considered excessive, yet pale in comparison to the US$ 8,000 per cycle paid to donors in Manhattan today. Concerns over coercion have fostered discussion on limiting payments by law, although no statutes have been passed in any state to control free market spending on donor services. The ASRM has proposed guidelines, which discourage payment over US$ 10,000 per cycle, but these are only recommendations and compliance is left up to the individual practitioners to enforce. As a result, clinicians may ignore them, if they choose, and not suffer penalty.[18] An impressive number of independent agencies have arisen to broker egg donor services, typically charging recipients large fees to secure the participation of donors; especially in cases where women with specific traits (e.g. race, religion) or pedigrees (e.g. advanced degrees, artistic talent) are sought. However, in many other countries such as Canada or Great Britain, payment of donors is restricted to reimbursement for daily expenses or is not permitted at all.[35]

Following the birth of a baby to a 'menopausal' 43-year-old woman, many ethicists argued that donor IVF was being used in 'unnatural' ways and should only be allowed in women of normal childbearing age. This argument gained momentum after 50-year-old and 60-year-old mothers delivered babies. Perhaps, the recent birth of twins to a 72-year-old woman in India seeking to provide a male heir for her family is the most poignant example of pushing the technology to its limit.[32] The main criticisms posed by older women having babies relate to the health risk of them carrying the fetus, and the uncertainty of their longevity after delivery to safely ensure that the child grows up in a nurturing home environment. Although the pregnancy and delivery outcome data is favorable, it remains to be seen if the children of these older parents reach adulthood without psychosocial or medical sequelae related to their unique circumstances.

Mandating the open disclosure of donors' identity has been suggested as a means to allow children an opportunity to know their biologic/genetic background. In the United Kingdom, when individuals born from gamete donations reach the age of 18 years or older, they have the right to ask the regulatory body (The Human Fertilization and Embryology Authority), if they were conceived using donated eggs or sperm; and if they were conceived after 2005, they can also request to know the identity of their donor.[36] Unfortunately, this practice has resulted in the stifling of volunteers for donation services. It is also unclear as to whether or not families actually desire such information. In cases of adoption or surrogacy, public records exist and formal adoption procedures and their public record are required; therefore, biologic parents and siblings may be discoverable. However, presently in the United States the record of the egg donor is protected by the Health

Insurance Portability and Accountability Act from disclosure and may be legally destroyed after a prescribed grace period defined under state law.

FUTURE USE AND ANTICIPATED ROLE OF EGG DONATION IN ASSISTED REPRODUCTION

More and more women are seeking donated oocytes as part of their infertility treatment plan and a shortage of available and willing egg donors remains. As such, various paradigms exist to maximize the resource in which women undergoing donor IVF can choose to share the donor's oocytes with other recipients. However, the shared donor also creates an interesting ethical conundrum for both the patient and the practitioner. For the patient, by sharing their cycle, they may save on the associated costs, but there may be fewer available embryos to use for implantation and/or cryopreservation. In a 2010 study that looked specifically at the risk to the recipient, it was noted that the probability of cryopreservation in a shared donor oocyte cycle is significantly reduced.[37] With fewer embryos available for cryopreservation, even successful patients may have to resort to using different egg donors for future cycles, which may be less than desirable when attempting to maintain genetic likeness amongst the children.

In some circumstances, an oocyte recipient has a directed oocyte donor (friend, family member, etc.) but may have no interest in fertility at this time. In such cases, oocyte cryopreservation may be useful in allowing women the opportunity to retain their designated donor and optimize the timing of their future IVF cycle to a time-frame of their choice. Oocyte cryopreservation has been shown to be a safe and effective modality for fertility preservation with no apparent increase in congenital abnormalities.[38] It was recently demonstrated that oocyte cryopreservation can approximate the success rates of fresh donor IVF when evaluated in a prospective randomized controlled clinical trial.[39] Banking of eggs would certainly simplify the synchronization of donors and recipients and allow programs to stockpile gametes for prospective recipients.

SUMMARY

Egg donation was introduced shortly after IVF with autologous eggs and has evolved alongside conventional fertility care. Evidence-based medical results have consistently demonstrated the method to be highly successful and on par with pregnancy rates witnessed in younger women undertaking autologous egg retrieval. Egg donation remains the treatment of choice for older women and younger patients with ovarian failure. Outcomes in the children born from this method have been uniformly good; however, obstetrical risk and complications in recipients are increased largely as a result of gestational hypertension and the exaggerated rate of multiple births. Guidelines for the safe and ethical use of donated eggs have been published by both ASRM and ESHRE and should be adhered to in order to optimize outcomes and minimize risk to participants.

REFERENCES

1. Blakeslee S. (1984). Infertile woman has baby through embryo transfer. [online]. Available from web address http://www.nytimes.com/1984/02/04/us/infertile-woman-has-baby-through-embryo-transfer.html [Accessed June 2011].
2. Centers for Disease Control and Prevention. (2008). Assisted reproductive technology report. [online]. Available from web address http://www.cdc.gov/art/ [Accessed June 2011].
3. Society for Assisted Reproductive Technology. (2009). Clinic summary report, 2009. [online]. Available from web address http://www.sart.org/frame/detail.aspx?id=3893 [Accessed June 2011].
4. Sauer MV. The impact of age on reproductive potential: lessons learned from oocyte donation. Maturitas. 1998;30(2):221-5.
5. Sauer MV, Paulson RJ, Lobo RA. Reversing the natural decline in human fertility. An extended clinical trial of oocyte donation to women of advanced reproductive age. JAMA. 1992;268(10):1275-9.
6. Davis OK, Rosenwaks Z. Preparation of the endometrium for oocyte donation. J Assist Reprod Genet. 1993;10(7):457-9.
7. Morris RS, Sauer MV. New advances in the treatment of infertility in women with ovarian failure. Curr Opin Obstet Gynecol. 1993;5(3):368-77.
8. Rosenwaks Z, Davis OK, Damario MA. The role of maternal age in assisted reproduction. Hum Reprod. 1995;10(Suppl 1):165-73.
9. Schutte JM, Schuitemaker NW, Steegers EA, et al. Maternal death after oocyte donation at high maternal age: case report. Reprod Health. 2008;5:12.
10. Reh A, Amarosa A, Licciardi F, et al. Evaluating the necessity for universal screening of prospective oocyte donors using enhanced genetic and psychological testing. Hum Reprod. 2010;25(9):2298-304.
11. Jorgensen PB, Kjartansdottir KR, Fedder J. Care of women with XY karyotype: a clinical practice guideline. Fertil Steril. 2010;94(1):105-13.
12. Chevalier N, Letur H, Lelannou D, et al. Materno-fetal cardiovascular complications in Turner syndrome after

oocyte donation: insufficient prepregnancy screening and pregnancy follow-up are associated with poor outcome. J Clin Endocrinol Metab. 2011;96(2):E260-7.
13. Hadnott TN, Gould HN, Gharib AM, et al. Outcomes of spontaneous and assisted pregnancies in Turner syndrome: the US National Institutes of Health experience. Fertil Steril. 2011;95(7):2251-6.
14. Boissonnas CC, Davy C, Bornes M, et al. Careful cardiovascular screening and follow-up of women with Turner syndrome before and during pregnancy is necessary to prevent maternal mortality. Fertil Steril. 2009;91(3): 929 e5-7.
15. Meirow D, Biederman H, Anderson RA, et al. Toxicity of chemotherapy and radiation on female reproduction. Clin Obstet Gynecol. 2010;53(4):727-39.
16. Kim SS, Klemp J, Fabian C. Breast cancer and fertility preservation. Fertil Steril. 2011;95(5):1535-43.
17. Wo JY, Viswanathan AN. Impact of radiotherapy on fertility, pregnancy, and neonatal outcomes in female cancer patients. Int J Radiat Oncol Biol Phys. 2009;73(5):1304-12.
18. Practice Committee of American Society for Reproductive Medicine, Practice Committee of Society for Assisted Reproductive Technology. 2008 Guidelines for gamete and embryo donation: a practice committee report. Fertil Steril. 2008;90(5 Suppl):S30-44.
19. Paulson RJ, Boostanfar R, Saadat P, et al. Pregnancy in the sixth decade of life: obstetric outcomes in women of advanced reproductive age. JAMA. 2002;288(18):2320-3.
20. Rackow BW, Arici A. Fibroids and in-vitro fertilization: which comes first? Cur Opin Obstet Gynecol. 2005;17(3):225-31.
21. Somigliana E, Vercellini P, Daguati R, et al. Fibroids and female reproduction: a critical analysis of the evidence. Hum Reprod Update. 2007;13(5):465-76.
22. Ethics Committee of the American Society for Reproductive Medicine. Financial compensation of oocyte donors. Fertil Steril. 2007;88(2):305-9.
23. ESHRE Task Force on Ethics and Law. III. Gamete and embryo donation. Hum Reprod. 2002;17(5):1407-8.
24. New York State Department of Health. (2011). Task force on life and the law. [online]. Available from web address http://www.health.ny.gov/regulations/task_force/reports_publications/#infertility_trt [Accessed June 2011].
25. US Food and Drug Administration. (2007). Guidance for industry: eligibility determination for donors of human cells, tissues, and cellular and tissue based products. [online]. Available from web address http://www.fda.gov/biologicsbloodvaccines/guidancecomplianceregulatoryinformation/guidances/tissue/ucm073964.htm [Accessed June 2011].
26. Maxwell KN, Cholst IN, Rosenwaks Z. The incidence of both serious and minor complications in young women undergoing oocyte donation. Fertil Steril. 2008;90(6):2165-71.
27. Bodri D, Guillén JJ, Polo A, et al. Complications related to ovarian stimulation and oocyte retrieval in 4052 oocyte donor cycles. Reprod Biomed Online. 2008;17(2):237-43.
28. Leon Speroff MAF. Clinical Gynecologic Endocrinology and Infertility, 7th edition. Philadelphia: Lippincott Williams & Wilkins; 2004.
29. Noyes N, Hampton BS, Berkeley A, et al. Factors useful in predicting the success of oocyte donation: a 3-year retrospective analysis. Fertil steril. 2001;76(1):92-7.
30. Glujovsky D, Pesce R, Fiszbajn G, et al. Endometrial preparation for women undergoing embryo transfer with frozen embryos or embryos derived from donor oocytes. Cochrane Database Syst Rev. 2010;(1):CD006359.
31. de Mouzon J, Goossens V, Bhattacharya S, et al. Assisted reproductive technology in Europe, 2006: results generated from European registers by ESHRE. Hum Reprod. 2010;25(8):1851-62.
32. BBC News. (2008). Woman in India 'has twins at 70'. [online]. Available from web address http://news.bbc.co.uk/2/hi/7491782.stm [Accessed June 2011].
33. Keegan DA, Krey LC, Chang HC, et al. Increased risk of pregnancy-induced hypertension in young recipients of donated oocytes. Fertil Steril. 2007;87(4):776-81.
34. Nelson SM, Lawlor DA. Predicting live birth, preterm delivery, and low birth weight in infants born from in vitro fertilisation: a prospective study of 144,018 treatment cycles. PLoS Med. 2011;8(1):e1000386.
35. Flower D. Assisted reproduction: should egg and sperm donors be paid? J Fam Health Care. 2010;20(2):69-71.
36. National Gamete Donation Trust. (2011). Donation and the law. [online]. Available from web address http://www.ngdt.co.uk/donation-and-the-law. [Accessed June 2011].
37. Mullin CM, Fino ME, Talebian S, et al. Comparison of pregnancy outcomes in anonymous shared versus exclusive donor oocyte in vitro fertilization cycles. Fertil Steril. 2010;93(2):574-8.
38. Noyes N, Porcu E, Borini A. Over 900 oocyte cryopreservation babies born with no apparent increase in congenital anomalies. Reprod Biomed Online. 2009;18(6):769-76.
39. Cobo A, Meseguer M, Remohí J, et al. Use of cryo-banked oocytes in an ovum donation programme: a prospective, randomized, controlled, clinical trial. Hum Reprod. 2010;25(9):2239-46.

23

Luteal Phase Supplementation in In Vitro Fertilization

Mindy S Christianson, Suheil J Muasher

Chapter Contents

INTRODUCTION

Luteal phase support is considered an integral part of contemporary *in vitro* fertilization (IVF) cycles. Almost all practitioners, utilize hormonal supplementation in the luteal phase, usually with progesterone (P_4), as it is considered essential for optimal success and possible support of pregnancy in the first trimester. Despite its widespread use, however, luteal phase support in IVF remains poorly studied. This has led to worldwide variability in regimens used with respect to type and modality of hormones used, dosage and duration of luteal phase supplementation. As a result, most practitioners today rely on clinical experience and poorly designed studies to choose the protocol for luteal phase support in IVF.

This chapter explores the rationale for luteal phase supplementation in IVF and reviews the various modalities and timing of P_4 supplementation during the luteal phase.

RATIONALE FOR LUTEAL PHASE SUPPLEMENTATION

It was originally postulated that hormonal supplementation with P_4 in IVF cycles was necessary due to aspiration of granulosa cells surrounding the oocytes at egg retrieval. The original luteal phase supplementation protocol described by Dr Howard W Jones in 1982, at the infancy of IVF, involved P_4 in oil, 12.5 mg intramuscular (IM) daily, starting on the day of embryo transfer (day 2). If the patient became pregnant, she was continued on 17-hydroxyprogesterone caproate, 250 mg IM once weekly, until 18 weeks gestation.[1]

Of interest, Dr Georgeanna Seegar Jones and the Norfolk IVF team did not necessarily advocate P_4 supplementation in IVF, as summarized in 1982, "Although it can be shown statistically that aspiration of follicles may be associated with a decreased luteal function in both estrogen and progesterone steroidogenesis, we do not believe that this is of clinical significance in most patients." They went on to conclude the following: "Once more, it should be emphasized that the average patient following IVF will not, in our experience, need supplementation of the luteal phase.[2]" This statement must be taken under consideration, since early IVF stimulation protocols gave rise to much lower peak estradiol (E_2) levels, fewer follicles and the widespread use of human chorionic gonadotropin (hCG) to trigger oocyte maturation.

Historically, it became common practice to supplement the luteal phase with P_4 before the contemporary use of gonadotropin-releasing hormone (GnRH) agonists. This was not supported by research with a 1988 meta-analysis, failing to support its use and previous studies failing to support the benefit of P_4 supplementation in IVF cycles stimulated with clomiphene citrate and human menopausal gonadotropin.[3-6]

With the development of current stimulation protocols, supraphysiologic levels of E_2, and suppression of luteinizing hormone (LH) with the use of GnRH agonist and GnRH antagonist protocols further supported the need for luteal phase supplementation. Since pituitary gonadotropins stay suppressed for 2–3 weeks after stopping the GnRH agonist, it made sense to supplement the luteal phase. Indeed, several studies have supported the need for luteal phase supplementation for IVF cycles stimulated with gonadotropins and suppressed with GnRH agonists.[7-9] Evidence also suggests a need for supplementation in GnRH antagonist cycles.[10-13] It is currently considered standard practice to supplement the luteal phase in GnRH agonist and GnRH antagonist cycles. While it is widely accepted to supplement the luteal phase in contemporary IVF cycles, controversy exists in route of administration, regimens and duration of treatment.

ROUTES OF PROGESTERONE ADMINISTRATION

The natural preparations of P_4 include progesterone, dydrogesterone and medrogestone. Primary modalities of administration include oral, vaginal and IM. P_4 is generally well tolerated with side effects often dependent on the route of administration. Vaginal and IM P_4 are the predominant modalities used today. A survey performed by IVF-Worldwide.com, which included 3,065 IVF programs, found that the majority of programs, 62%, used vaginal routes of P_4 administration (34% cream/gel and 28% capsule). Nineteen percent used both vaginal and IM P_4, 10% used IM P_4 exclusively and 2% used other modes such as oral P_4.[14]

Oral Preparations

When P_4 is taken orally, bioavailability is diminished by liver first-pass metabolism with 10% bioavailability and serum levels returning to baseline six hours after administration. Micronized P_4 formulations include Prometrium (Abbott Laboratories, North Chicago, IL) and Utrogest (Dr Kade/Besins Pharma GmbH, Berlin, Germany). Since oral P_4 forms sedative metabolites, patients may experience fatigue and drowsiness. Other side effects include headache and urinary frequency. While Prometrium is not approved in the United States for vaginal use, it is typically used vaginally due to side effects and diminished bioavailability from oral use.

Vaginal Preparations

Vaginal P_4 offers many benefits that make it widely used today. The vagina provides a local and systemic route for delivering hormones for uterine targeting. Due to the "uterine first-pass effect," P_4 concentrates in the uterus with low systemic exposure.[15] Serum P_4 levels remain elevated up to 48 hours. The three primary vaginal formulations of P_4 available in the United States are Crinone 8% gel (Watson Pharmaceuticals, Inc, Morristown, NJ), Endometrin (Ferring Pharmaceuticals, Inc, Suffern, NY) and Prometrium. Endometrin is a micronized, naturally derived vaginal P_4 tablet insert. While generally very well-tolerated, side effects of vaginal P_4 may include vaginal irritation, discharge and dyspareunia.[16] One randomized trial found that micronized P_4 forms and Crinone had similar rates of perineal irritation at 20%.[17] One study found Crinone 8% was better tolerated,easier to apply with less vaginal discharge than micronized P_4.[18]

Intramuscular Preparations

Intramuscular P_4 in oil results in a higher plasma concentration than vaginal or oral preparations and is maintained for a longer duration.[16] One main advantage of the IM route is that it can be administered once daily. The main preparation is P_4 in oil derived from sesame oil (Watson Laboratories, Inc, Phoenix, AZ). In cases of known sesame allergies, there is also a peanut oil preparation.[19] Drawbacks of IM administration include a rare risk for a severe allergic reaction, adult respiratory distress syndrome and eosinophilic pneumonitis. From case reports, pneumonitis typically starts 3 weeks following the first injection. Benzyl alcohol preservative may be responsible for allergic reactions.[20,21]

COMPARING ORAL PROGESTERONE WITH OTHER MODALITIES

Oral P_4 formulations are not commonly used secondary to systemic side effects, as supported by a prospective randomized study in which patients used with Crinone

8%, 90 mg vaginally or 300 mg micronized P_4 orally. The oral route was associated with a significantly increased incidence of drowsiness, although clinical pregnancy, delivery and miscarriage rates were comparable in both groups.[22] In comparison, another randomized trial found oral dydrogesterone and vaginal micronized P_4 to have similar pregnancy rates with the oral form better tolerated, and 10.5% of women receiving vaginal P_4, complaining of vaginal discharge and irritation.[23] Another study, comparing vaginal or oral micronized P_4, found significantly higher implantation rates with vaginal P_4, although there is not a statistically significant difference in clinical and ongoing pregnancy rates.[24] One prospective randomized study that compared oral micronized P_4 with 50 mg IM daily P_4 found significantly higher implantation rates per embryo transfer with IM P_4 (40.9% IM versus 18.1% oral), although clinical and ongoing pregnancy rates were not significantly different.[25]

Comparing Intramuscular and Vaginal Progesterone

A small number of studies compare IM and vaginal P_4 routes of administration, with conflicting results, leading to difficulty in determining which route is superior. One study compared the effects of both routes on the uterus, with both modalities showing similar histologic maturation and endometrial thickness on ultrasonography.[26] A randomized control trial, comparing Crinone 8% and IM P_4, found the IM P_4 group to have higher ongoing pregnancy and live birth rates per embryo transfer.[27] This finding was supported by a comparative study that also found a significantly higher clinical pregnancy rate in women used IM P_4 versus micronized vaginal P_4, although the dose was only 200 mg/day.[28] A 2002 meta-analysis also concluded that IM P_4 resulted in higher clinical and ongoing pregnancy rates.[29] Of note, a prospective randomized study, comparing Crinone 8% with 50 mg IM P_4, initially found higher implantation, clinical pregnancy and live birth rates with IM P_4. However, it was noted that the Crinone group had a higher proportion of women with 40 years of age or older so an interim analysis was performed, finding no significant improvement with IM P_4.[30]

Despite the studies that showed an advantage to IM P_4, a number of studies show no difference. A randomized study, comparing hCG, IM P_4 and vaginal P_4 for luteal supplementation, found no difference in clinical pregnancy rates among the three groups, although the vaginal P_4 was tolerated the best.[31] Five additional randomized trials showed similar pregnancy outcomes between vaginal and IM P_4.[32-36] A recent meta-analysis of randomized trials also showed that vaginal P_4 and IM P_4 were comparable in terms of pregnancy outcomes.[37]

Comparing Vaginal Preparations

Studies comparing vaginal preparations have not shown major differences regarding pregnancy outcomes, but some differences have been noted in patient tolerability. Two randomized controlled trials and one comparative study have found similar pregnancy rates with Crinone and micronized P_4 with two of the studies noting that Crinone gel was better tolerated by patients.[18,38-39] Similar findings were found in other studies comparing different vaginal preparations.[17,38] Other studies have compared Endometrin with other modalities. A large multicenter randomized trial, comparing Endometrin with Crinone, found similar clinical and ongoing pregnancy rates between the two.[39] A case-matched comparison study also found similar clinical outcomes between Endometrin, Crinone and IM P_4.[40] A meta-analysis investigating P_4 gel with other vaginal P_4 forms found no significant difference in pregnancy rates between gel and other forms when used for luteal phase support.[41]

OPTIMAL DOSE OF PROGESTERONE

The data are very limited regarding optimal dosing of P_4 for luteal phase supplementation. One study found no difference in IM P_4 doses when comparing 25 mg and 125 mg daily doses, and clinical and ongoing pregnancy rates.[42] Studies comparing 400 mg versus 600 mg micronized vaginal P_4 also found no difference in clinical pregnancy rates.[43] Clearly, more randomized control trials are needed to determine optimal doses of P_4 for luteal phase support (Table 1).

ADDITION OF HUMAN CHORIONIC GONADOTROPIN TO PROGESTERONE

Adding hCG to P_4 for luteal phase supplementation has been suggested, as it may rescue corpora lutea function in IVF cycles, leading to increased production of E_2 and P_4 by corpora lutea.[44] Currently, it is unclear whether P_4 alone, hCG alone or a combination of hCG and P_4 provides optimal luteal support. A number of studies have not shown a difference between either vaginal or IM P_4 and hCG in terms of pregnancy rates.[31,45-47] A meta-analysis, which included a total of 1,756 patients, found clinical pregnancy rates were similar when either hCG or P_4 was used for luteal phase support.[29] Another recent meta-analysis, which included

Table 1 Progesterone formulations available in the United States

Progesterone	Brand name	Manufacturer	Recommended dose
Intramuscular P_4	Progesterone in sesame oil	Watson Pharmaceuticals	25-100 mg intramuscular once daily
Vaginal P_4 gel	Crinone 8%	Watson Pharmaceuticals	90 mg vaginally once daily
Vaginal P_4 insert	Endometrin	Ferring Pharmaceuticals	100 mg vaginally twice or 3 times daily
Oral micronized P_4	Prometrium	Abbott Laboratories	200 mg vaginally 3 times daily*
Compounded P_4 suppositories	None	None	50 mg vaginally 3 times daily

P_4: Progesterone

* Not approved by US Food and Drug Administration for vaginal use

18 randomized trials, found that luteal support with either hCG or P_4 was associated with a significantly higher pregnancy rate than when no luteal support was used. A subanalysis of 5 trials found hCG superior to P_4. It should be noted, however, that this subanalysis included a trial, comparing hCG to oral P_4, with hCG resulting in significantly higher pregnancy rates than oral P_4.[48,49]

A limited number of trials have compared the combination of hCG/P_4 to P_4 alone. One study examined IM P_4 either alone or combined with hCG and found the hCG/P_4 combination was superior to P_4 alone. In this study, the pregnancy rate for the hCG/P_4 group was 32% compared to 14% for the P_4 only group.[50] Other trials comparing vaginal P_4 combined with hCG to P4 alone found no difference in pregnancy rates (Table 2).[51-53]

One potential downside to using hCG for luteal support is the increased risk of developing ovarian hyperstimulation syndrome (OHSS). The risk of developing OHSS with hCG has been estimated twice as high as P_4.[52] For this reason, supplementation with hCG should be limited to patients with low peak E_2 levels, who are not at risk for developing OHSS.

ADDITION OF ESTRADIOL TO PROGESTERONE FOR LUTEAL SUPPLEMENTATION

Since it is well known that implantation relies on an estrogen-dependent and P_4-dependent endometrial lining, some clinicians believe that adding E_2 to P_4 in luteal phase supplementation could maximize pregnancy outcomes. This is further substantiated by the hypothesis that hCG's benefit is due to stimulation of the corpus luteum to produce more E_2. While it's accepted that the endometrium is dependent primarily on estrogen during the follicular phase, the role of estrogen during the luteal phase is unclear. In IVF cycles, E_2 and P_4 levels drop in the mid-luteal to late-luteal phase.[54] Muasher et al., reported that a lower E_2 level after luteal day 11 was associated with lower pregnancy rates.[55] Another study showed that the higher the ratio of peak E_2 to midluteal E_2, the lower the implantation rate.[56]

Research currently shows mixed results regarding the benefit of adding E_2 to P_4 for luteal phase supplementation. One prospective randomized trial added 2 mg of E_2 orally twice daily to either IM P_4 injections or vaginal P_4. The E_2 was added on day 7 after embryo transfer. In the group of women receiving E_2 on long GnRH agonist protocols, pregnancy rates were higher for those receiving E_2 with P_4 than P_4 alone (39.6% vs 25.6%, $P<0.05$).[57] Another prospective randomized study compared varying doses of oral E_2 starting on the day of oocyte retrieval in addition to vaginal P_4 to P_4 alone. Patients were randomized to receive no E_2, 2 mg or 6 mg E_2 daily. Pregnancy rates were 51.3% in the 6 mg E_2 group, 32.8% in the 2 mg E_2 group and 23.1% in the no E_2 group.[58] Another prospective randomized study, comparing P_4 and 2 mg, 4 mg or 6 mg E_2, found no difference in pregnancy rates but a higher miscarriage rate when 2 mg E_2 was used.[59] Conversely, three prospective studies showed no difference in pregnancy outcome in comparing E_2 added to either vaginal or IM P_4.[60-63] Most recently, a meta-analysis of nine randomized controlled trials found that the addition of E_2 to P_4 for luteal phase support did not improve pregnancy outcomes in GnRH agonist and GnRH antagonist cycles.[64]

Table 2 Convenience and side effects of intramuscular progesterone versus vaginal progesterone

	Intramuscular	Vaginal
Route of Administration	One intramuscular injection daily	1-3 daily insertions per vagina
Minor Side Effects	Local reaction Discomfort	Messy Vaginal discharge Irritation Dysparunia
Serious Side Effects	Severe allergic reaction Acute respiratory distress syndrome Eosinophilic pneumonitis (rare)	None

DURATION OF LUTEAL PHASE SUPPLEMENTATION

The optimal times to begin and end luteal phase supplementation are currently not supported by research but rather by experience and comfort level of practitioners. Most IVF clinicians begin P_4 supplementation after oocyte retrieval. If the patient becomes pregnant, it is generally continued until 8–10 weeks gestation.[54] A survey conducted by IVF-Worldwide.com of 3,065 IVF programs found that 67% of practices continue P4 until 10–12 weeks gestation, 20% until a heart rate is detected and 13% until a positive pregnancy test.[14] A practice committee report by the American Society of Reproductive Medicine advocates that there is no evidence to indicate that maternal exposure to P_4 during pregnancy increases the risk of birth defects.[65]

Although the majority of clinicians continue P_4 support until 10–12 weeks gestation, the optimal time to begin luteal phase supplementation is unresolved by research. A randomized prospective trial found a significantly lower pregnancy rate when IM P_4 was started the day before oocyte retrieval versus on the day of retrieval.[66] A second randomized trial found a lower pregnancy rate when vaginal P_4 was started on day 6 versus day 3 of the luteal phase[67] while another study found no difference when P_4 was started on day of oocyte retrieval versus day of embryo transfer.[68] Finally, a 3-arm randomized prospective study found no significant differences in pregnancy rates when vaginal P_4 was started on day after hCG trigger, day of oocyte retrieval or day of embryo transfer.[69]

Once a patient has a positive pregnancy test, the optimal time to discontinue luteal phase support is unresolved with little research suggesting an ideal time to stop. Evidence is lacking to continue luteal support once there is a positive pregnancy test. One prospective study discontinued IM P_4 at 4 weeks gestational age if the serum P_4 was more than or equal to 60 ng/ml. There was no difference in delivery rates when patients discontinued the support at 4 weeks versus those who waited until 7 weeks to discontinue.[70] Another randomized prospective study showed similar findings,[71] as did a retrospective study of 400 patients.[72]

ROLE FOR GONADOTROPIN-RELEASING HORMONE AGONISTS IN LUTEAL PHASE SUPPLEMENTATION

Gonadotropin-releasing hormone agonists have been used as a substitute for hCG in patients at risk for OHSS and stimulated with a GnRH antagonist protocol. Two randomized prospective studies looking at this approach found a significantly lower pregnancy rate when patients were triggered with a GnRH agonist versus hCG.[73,74] Both studies hypothesized that the lower pregnancy rate could be due to an iatrogenic luteal phase defect. This theory was substantiated by a recent study that found no difference in pregnancy rates in donor oocyte recipients when donors were triggered with either a GnRH agonist or hCG.[75] These findings reflect the need for a different approach to luteal phase supplementation in IVF cycles with a GnRH antagonist protocol when a GnRH agonist is used to trigger ovulation.

One study examined the addition of a single dose of a GnRH agonist on luteal day 6 compared with placebo in donor oocyte recipients. The rationale for examining donor oocyte recipients was to examine a direct effect of the GnRH agonist on the endometrium and/or embryo to improve implantation as recipient cycles are suppressed and lack a corpus luteum. The group found a significantly higher pregnancy and delivery rate in the group that received the GnRH agonist.[76] The same group conducted a prospective randomized study in IVF patients stimulated with either GnRH agonist and GnRH antagonist protocols. A single GnRH agonist cycle given on luteal day 6 improved the pregnancy and delivery rates compared with placebo in both GnRH agonist and GnRH antagonist cycles, with a more pronounced effect in GnRH antagonist cycles.[77]

It is yet to be determined which patients will benefit most from GnRH administration in the luteal phase. The optimal dose and frequency will certainly be a future area of research.

CONCLUSION

Luteal phase supplementation in IVF cycles is a well-established practice. Ongoing pregnancy rates seem similar with IM and vaginal administration, patients seeming to prefer the vaginal route due to convenience and fewer adverse side effects. The different forms of vaginal administration demonstrate similar pregnancy rates. Most major randomized studies do not show a major difference in pregnancy rates when hCG is used alone or in addition to P_1 supplementation. It should be noted, however, that the use of hCG in the luteal phase increases the risk of OHSS in those at risk. Regarding timing of luteal phase supplementation, it is typically started after oocyte retrieval and before embryo transfer. There is no evidence to support continuing supplementation beyond the first positive hCG result. Using a GnRH agonist in the luteal phase, especially with patients on GnRH antagonist protocols, yields favorable pregnancy results when a GnRH agonist is used for ovulation trigger and is a promising area of future research.

REFERENCES

1. Jones HW Jr, Jones GS, Andrews MC, et al. The program for in vitro fertilization at Norfolk. Fertil Steril. 1982;38(1):14-21.
2. Edwards RG, Purdy JM. Human conception in vitro: proceedings of the first Bourn Hall meeting. London: Academic Press; 1982.
3. Daya S. Efficacy of progesterone support in the luteal phase following in-vitro fertilization and embryo transfer: meta-analysis of clinical trials. Hum Reprod. 1988;3(6):731-4.
4. Yovich JL, McColm SC, Yovich JM, et al. Early luteal serum progesterone concentrations are higher in pregnancy cycles. Fertil Steril. 1985;44(2):185-9.
5. Belaisch-Allart J, Testart J, Fries N, et al. The effect of dydrogesterone supplementation in an IVF programme. Hum Reprod. 1987;2(3):183-5.
6. Van Steirteghem AC, Smitz J, Camus M, et al. The luteal phase after in vitro fertilization and related procedures. Hum Reprod. 1988;3(2):161-4.
7. Smitz J, Devroey P, Camus M, et al. The luteal phase and early pregnancy after combined GnRH-agonist/HMG treatment for superovulation in IVF or GIFT. Hum Reprod. 1988;3(5):585-90.
8. Smith EM, Anthony FW, Gadd SC, et al. Trial of support treatment with human chorionic gonadotrophin in the luteal phase after treatment with buserelin and human menopausal gonadotrophin in women taking part in an in vitro fertilisation programme. BMJ. 1989;298(6686):1483-6.
9. Belaisch-Allart J, De Mouzon J, Lapousterle C, et al. The effect of HCG supplementation after combined GnRH agonist/HMG treatment in an IVF programme. Hum Reprod. 1990;5(2):163-6.
10. Albano C, Grimbizis G, Smitz J, et al. The luteal phase of nonsupplemented cycles after ovarian superovulation with human menopausal gonadotropin and the gonadotropin-releasing hormone antagonist Cetrorelix. Fertil Steril. 1998;70(2):357-9.
11. de Jong D, Macklon NS, Fauser BC. A pilot study involving minimal ovarian stimulation for in vitro fertilization: extending the 'follicle-stimulating hormone window' combined with the gonadotropin-releasing hormone antagonist cetrorelix. Fertil Steril. 2000;73(5):1051-4.
12. Kolibianakis EM, Bourgain C, Platteau P, et al. Abnormal endometrial development occurs during the luteal phase of nonsupplemented donor cycles treated with recombinant follicle-stimulating hormone and gonadotropin-releasing hormone antagonists. Fertil Steril. 2003;80(2):464-6.
13. Beckers NG, Macklon NS, Eijkemans MJ, et al. Nonsupplemented luteal phase characteristics after the administration of recombinant human chorionic gonadotropin, recombinant luteinizing hormone, or gonadotropin-releasing hormone (GnRH) agonist to induce final oocyte maturation in in-vitro fertilization patients after ovarian stimulation with recombinant follicle-stimulating hormone and GnRH antagonist cotreatment. J Clin Endocrinol Metab. 2003;88(9):4186-92.
14. Zeev Shoham, Milton Leong. (2009). Progesterone support in IVF patients. [online]. Available from web address http://www.ivf-worldwide.com/survey/survey-progesterone-results.html [Accessed June 2011].
15. Bulletti C, de Ziegler D, Flamigni C, et al. Targeted drug delivery in gynaecology: the first uterine pass effect. Hum Reprod. 1997;12(5):1073-9.
16. Posaci C, Smitz J, Camus M, et al. Progesterone for the luteal support of assisted reproductive technologies: clinical options. Hum Reprod. 2000;15(Suppl 1): 129-48.
17. Ng EH, Miao B, Cheung W, et al. A randomised comparison of side effects and patient inconvenience of two vaginal progesterone formulations used for luteal support in in-vitro fertilisation cycles. Eur J Obstet Gynecol Reprod Biol. 2003;111(1):50-4.
18. Ludwig M, Schwartz P, Babahan B, et al. Luteal phase support using either Crinone 8% or Utrogest: results of

a prospective, randomized study. Eur J Obstet Gynecol Reprod Biol. 2002;103(1):48-52.
19. Phy JL, Weiss WT, Weiler CR, et al. Hypersensitivity to progesterone-in-oil after in vitro fertilization and embryo transfer. Fertil Steril. 2003;80(5):1272-5.
20. Bouckaert Y, Robert F, Englert Y, et al. Acute eosinophilic pneumonia associated with intramuscular administration of progesterone as luteal phase support after IVF: case report. Hum Reprod. 2004;19(8):1806-10.
21. Veysman B, Vlahos I, Oshva L. Pneumonitis and eosinophilia after in vitro fertilization treatment. Ann Emerg Med. 2006;47(5):472-5.
22. Pouly JL, Bassil S, Frydman R, et al. Luteal support after in vitro fertilization: Crinone 8%, a sustained release vaginal progesterone gel, versus Utrogestan, an oral micronized progesterone. Hum Reprod. 1996;11(10):2085-9.
23. Chakravarty BN, Shirazee HH, Dam P, et al. Oral dydrogesterone versus intravaginal micronised progesterone as luteal phase support in assisted reproductive technology (ART) cycles: results of a randomised study. J Steroid Biochem Mol Biol. 2005;97(5):416-20.
24. Friedler S, Raziel A, Schachter M, et al. Luteal support with micronized progesterone following in vitro fertilization using a down-regulation protocol with gonadotrophin-releasing hormone agonist: a comparative study between vaginal and oral administration. Hum Reprod. 1999;14(8):1944-8.
25. Licciardi FL, Kwiatkowski A, Noyes NL, et al. Oral versus intramuscular progesterone for in vitro fertilization: a prospective randomized study. Fertil Steril. 1999;71(4):614-8.
26. Ragni G, Piloni S, Rossi P, et al. Endometrial morphology and ultrasound vascular findings. A randomized trial after intramuscular and vaginal progesterone supplementation in IVF. Gynecol Obstet Invest. 1999;47(3):151-6.
27. Abate A, Perino M, Abate FG, et al. Intramuscular versus vaginal administration of progesterone for luteal phase support after in vitro fertilization and embryo transfer. A comparative randomized study. Clin Exp Obstet Gynecol. 1999;26(3-4):203-6.
28. Perino M, Brigandi FG, Abate FG, et al. Intramuscular versus vaginal progesterone in assisted reproduction: a comparative study. Clin Exp Obstet Gynecol. 1997;24(4):228-31.
29. Pritts EA, Atwood AK. Luteal phase support in infertility treatment: a meta-analysis of the randomized trials. Hum Reprod. 2002;17(9):2287-99.
30. Yanushpolsky E, Hurwitz S, Greenberg L, et al. Comparison of Crinone 8% intravaginal gel and intramuscular progesterone supplementation for in vitro fertilization/embryo transfer in women under age 40: interim analysis of a prospective randomized trial. Fertil Steril. 2008;89(2):485-7.
31. Artini PG, Volpe A, Angioni S, et al. A comparative, randomized study of three different progesterone support of the luteal phase following IVF/ET program. J Endocrinol Invest. 1995;18(1):51-6.
32. Smitz J, Devroey P, Faguer B, et al. A randomized prospective study comparing supplementation of the luteal phase and early pregnancy by natural progesterone administered by intramuscular or vaginal route. Rev Fr Gynecol Obstet. 1992;87(10):507-16.
33. Chantilis SJ, Zeitoun KM, Patel SI, et al. Use of Crinone vaginal progesterone gel for luteal support in in-vitro fertilization cycles. Fertil Steril. 1999;72(5):823-9.
34. Anserini P, Costa M, Remorgida V, et al. Luteal phase support in assisted reproductive cycles using either vaginal (Crinone 8) or intramuscular (Prontogest) progesterone: results of a prospective randomized study. Minerva Ginecol. 2001;53(4):297-301.
35. Kahraman S, Karagozoglu SH, Karlikaya G. The efficiency of progesterone vaginal gel versus intramuscular progesterone for luteal phase supplementation in gonadotropin-releasing hormone antagonist cycles: a prospective clinical trial. Fertil Steril. 2010;94(2):761-3.
36. Yanushpolsky E, Hurwitz S, Greenberg L, et al. Crinone vaginal gel is equally effective and better tolerated than intramuscular progesterone for luteal phase support in in-vitro fertilization-embryo transfer cycles: a prospective randomized study. Fertil Steril. 2010;94(7):2596-9.
37. Zarutskie PW, Phillips JA. A meta-analysis of the route of administration of luteal phase support in assisted reproductive technology: vaginal versus intramuscular progesterone. Fertil Steril. 2009;92(1):163-9.
38. Germond M, Capelli P, Bruno G, et al. Comparison of the efficacy and safety of two formulations of micronized progesterone (Ellios and Utrogestan) used as luteal phase support after in vitro fertilization. Fertil Steril. 2002;77(2):313-7.
39. Doody KJ, Schnell VL, Foulk RA, et al. Endometrin for luteal phase support in a randomized, controlled, open-label, prospective in vitro fertilization trial using a combination of Menopur and Bravelle for controlled ovarian hyperstimulation. Fertil Steril. 2009;91(4):1012-7.
40. Khan N, Richter KS, Newsome TL, et al. Matched-samples comparison of intramuscular versus vaginal progesterone for luteal phase support after in vitro fertilization and embryo transfer. Fertil Steril. 2009;91(6):2445-50.
41. Polyzos NP, Messini CI, Papanikolaou EG, et al. Vaginal progesterone gel for luteal phase support in IVF/ICSI cycles: a meta-analysis. Fertil Steril. 2010;94(6):2083-7.
42. Check JH, Nowroozi K, Chase J, et al. Comparison of luteal-phase support with high and low-dose progesterone therapy on pregnancy rates in an in vitro fertilization program. J In Vitro Fert Embryo Transf. 1991;8(3):173-5.
43. Chanson A, Germond M, Lagnaux Y, et al. Comparison of two progesterone dose regimens for luteal phase support after embryo transfer: a prospective randomized study. Hum Reprod. 1996;11:170.
44. Hutchinson-Williams KA, DeCherney AH, Lavy G, et al. Luteal rescue in in-vitro fertilization-embryo transfer. Fertil Steril. 1990;53(3):495-501.

45. Golan A, Herman A, Soffer Y, et al. Human chorionic gonadotrophin is a better luteal support than progesterone in ultrashort gonadotrophin-releasing hormone agonist/menotrophin in vitro fertilization cycles. Hum Reprod. 1993;8(9):1372-5.
46. Araujo E Jr, Bernardini L, Frederick JL, et al. Prospective randomized comparison of human chorionic gonadotropin versus intramuscular progesterone for luteal-phase support in assisted reproduction. J Assist Reprod Genet. 1994;11(2):74-8.
47. Martinez F, Coroleu B, Parera N, et al. Human chorionic gonadotropin and intravaginal natural progesterone are equally effective for luteal phase support in IVF. Gynecol Endocrinol. 2000;14(5):316-20.
48. Buvat J, Marcolin G, Guittard C, et al. Luteal support after luteinizing hormone-releasing hormone agonist for in vitro fertilization: superiority of human chorionic gonadotropin over oral progesterone. Fertil Steril. 1990;53(3):490-4.
49. Nosarka S, Kruger T, Siebert I, et al. Luteal phase support in in vitro fertilization: meta-analysis of randomized trials. Gynecol Obstet Invest. 2005;60(2):67-74.
50. Fujimoto A, Osuga Y, Fujiwara T, et al. Human chorionic gonadotropin combined with progesterone for luteal support improves pregnancy rate in patients with low late-midluteal estradiol levels in IVF cycles. J Assist Reprod Genet. 2002;19(12):550-4.
51. Ludwig M, Finas A, Katalinic A, et al. Prospective, randomized study to evaluate the success rates using hCG, vaginal progesterone or a combination of both for luteal phase support. Acta Obstet Gynecol Scand. 2001;80(6):574-82.
52. Daya S, Gunby J. Luteal phase support in assisted reproduction cycles. Cochrane Database Syst Rev. 2004;(3):CD004830.
53. Mochtar MH, Hogerzeil HV, Mol BW. Progesterone alone versus progesterone combined with HCG as luteal support in GnRHa/HMG induced IVF cycles: a randomized clinical trial. Hum Reprod. 1996;11(8):1602-5.
54. Hubayter ZR, Muasher SJ. Luteal supplementation in in-vitro fertilization: more questions than answers. Fertil Steril. 2008;89(4):749-58.
55. Muasher S, Acosta AA, Garcia JE, et al. Luteal phase serum estradiol and progesterone in in-vitro fertilization. Fertil Steril. 1984;41(6):838-43.
56. Sharara FI, McClamrock HD. Ratio of oestradiol concentration on the day of human chorionic gonadotrophin administration to mid-luteal oestradiol concentration is predictive of in vitro fertilization outcome. Hum Reprod. 1999;14(11):2777-82.
57. Farhi J, Weissman A, Steinfeld Z, et al. Estradiol supplementation during the luteal phase may improve the pregnancy rate in patients undergoing in vitro fertilization-embryo transfer cycles. Fertil Steril. 2000;73(4):761-6.
58. Lukaszuk K, Liss J, Lukaszuk M, et al. Optimization of estradiol supplementation during the luteal phase improves the pregnancy rate in women undergoing in-vitro fertilization-embryo transfer cycles. Fertil Steril. 2005;83(5):1372-6.
59. Tonguc E, Var T, Ozyer S, et al. Estradiol supplementation during the luteal phase of in vitro fertilization cycles: a prospective randomised study. Eur J Obstet Gynecol Reprod Biol. 2011;154(2):172-6.
60. Smitz J, Bourgain C, Van Waesberghe L, et al. A prospective randomized study on oestradiol valerate supplementation in addition to intravaginal micronized progesterone in buserelin and HMG induced superovulation. Hum Reprod. 1993;8(1):40-5.
61. Lewin A, Benshushan A, Mezker E, et al. The role of estrogen support during the luteal phase of in vitro fertilization-embryo transplant cycles: a comparative study between progesterone alone and estrogen and progesterone support. Fertil Steril. 1994;62(1):121-5.
62. Tay PY, Lenton EA. Inhibition of progesterone secretion by oestradiol administered in the luteal phase of assisted conception cycles. Med J Malaysia. 2003;58(2):187-95.
63. Fatemi HM, Camus M, Kolibianakis EM, et al. The luteal phase of recombinant follicle-stimulating hormone/gonadotropin-releasing hormone antagonist in vitro fertilization cycles during supplementation with progesterone or progesterone and estradiol. Fertil Steril. 2007;87(3):504-8.
64. Jee BC, Suh CS, Kim SH, et al. Effects of estradiol supplementation during the luteal phase of in vitro fertilization cycles: a meta-analysis. Fertil Steril. 2010;93(2):428-36.
65. Practice Committee of the American Society for Reproductive Medicine. Progesterone supplementation during the luteal phase and in early pregnancy in the treatment of infertility: an educational bulletin. Fertil Steril. 2008;89(4):789-92.
66. Sohn SH, Penzias AS, Emmi AM, et al. Administration of progesterone before oocyte retrieval negatively affects the implantation rate. Fertil Steril. 1999;71(1):11-4.
67. Williams SC, Oehninger S, Gibbons WE, et al. Delaying the initiation of progesterone supplementation results in decreased pregnancy rates after in vitro fertilization: a randomized, prospective study. Fertil Steril. 2001;76(6):1140-3.
68. Baruffi R, Mauri AL, Petersen CG, et al. Effects of vaginal progesterone administration starting on the day of oocyte retrieval on pregnancy rates. J Assist Reprod Genet. 2003;20(12):517-20.
69. Mochtar MH, Van Wely M, Van der Veen F. Timing luteal phase support in GnRH agonist down-regulated IVF/embryo transfer cycles. Hum Reprod. 2006;21(4):905-8.
70. Stovall DW, Van Voorhis BJ, Sparks AE, et al. Selective early elimination of luteal support in assisted reproduction cycles using a gonadotropin-releasing hormone agonist during ovarian stimulation. Fertil Steril. 1998;70(6):1056-62.
71. Nyboe Andersen A, Popovic-Todorovic B, Schmidt KT, et al. Progesterone supplementation during early

gestations after IVF or ICSI has no effect on the delivery rates: a randomized controlled trial. Hum Reprod. 2002;17(2):357-61.
72. Schmidt KL, Ziebe S, Popovic B, et al. Progesterone supplementation during early gestation after in vitro fertilization has no effect on the delivery rate. Fertil Steril. 2001;75(2):337-41.
73. Humaidan P, Bredkjaer HE, Bungum L, et al. GnRH agonist (buserelin) or hCG for ovulation induction in GnRH antagonist IVF/ICSI cycles: a prospective randomized study. Hum Reprod. 2005;20(5):1213-20.
74. Kolibianakis EM, Schultze-Mosgau A, Schroer A, et al. A lower ongoing pregnancy rate can be expected when GnRH agonist is used for triggering final oocyte maturation instead of HCG in patients undergoing IVF with GnRH antagonists. Hum Reprod. 2005;20(10):2887-92.
75. Acevedo B, Gomez-Palomares JL, Ricciarelli E, et al. Triggering ovulation with gonadotropin-releasing hormone agonists does not compromise embryo implantation rates. Fertil Steril. 2006;86(6):1682-7.
76. Tesarik J, Hazout A, Mendoza C. Enhancement of embryo developmental potential by a single administration of GnRH agonist at the time of implantation. Hum Reprod. 2004;19(5):1176-80.
77. Tesarik J, Hazout A, Mendoza-Tesarik R, et al. Beneficial effect of luteal-phase GnRH agonist administration on embryo implantation after ICSI in both GnRH agonist- and antagonist-treated ovarian stimulation cycles. Hum Reprod. 2006;21(10):2572-9.

24

Fertility Preservation for Women

Ioanna Athanasiadis, Molina B Dayal, David Frankfurter

Chapter Contents

INTRODUCTION

In the United States, it was estimated that over 700,000 women were diagnosed with cancer in 2010 and roughly 8.4% of these diagnoses occurred in reproductive aged women.[1] Women of reproductive age present with concerns regarding their future fertility. As cancer survival rates improve, more and more survivors will be faced with reproductive choices.

For women, a cancer diagnosis can lead to a reproductive decline in various ways. Obviously, oophorectomy will result in sterility. Cancer treatments may involve gonadotoxic chemotherapy or radiation therapy that can affect ovarian reserve or cause ovarian failure.

TREATMENT AND OVARIAN FUNCTION

Although chemotherapy is vital in cancer therapy, many women develop menstrual/ovulatory irregularities or premature ovarian failure after completion of treatment. The incidence of diminished ovarian reserve depends on the age of the patient, the class of the chemotherapeutic agent (particularly alkylating agents) and its cumulative dose.

The number of primordial follicles in the ovary determines the ovarian reserve.[2] Chemotoxic agents are known to reduce this resting pool of follicles. Younger women have a higher number of primordial follicles and, therefore, have a decreased risk of chemotherapy-induced menopause relative to their older counterparts. Goodwin et al. demonstrated that the risk of menopause after chemotherapy in women under the age of 35 years was lower (approximately 15%) when compared to women at the age of 40 years (> 40%).[3]

The risk of ovarian damage seems also to be related to the type of chemotherapeutic agent used. Because, alkylating agents, such as cyclophosphamide, are not cell-cycle specific, they damage cells at different stages of the cell cycle and can, therefore, damage resting primordial follicles. Patients treated for breast cancer with cyclophosphamide, methotrexate and 5-fluorouracil (CMF), with or without tamoxifen, are at risk of menopause. This regimen results in amenorrhea in 5–40% in women lesser than or equal to 40 years old, and up to 76% for those more than or equal to 40 years old.[3]

Radiation therapy also damages ovarian follicles. High doses of radiation, as used to treat pelvic and abdominal malignancies (cervical cancer, rectal cancer, Wilms' tumor, and pelvic lymph nodes for hematologic malignancies such as Hodgkin's lymphoma) can lead to excessive ovarian radiation exposure. The toxicity of radiation to the ovary varies with the cell cycle, and primordial follicles appear to be more resilient to the effects of radiation than mature follicles.[4] The degree of ovarian damage seems to be related to the patient's age, radiation field, dose and the concurrent use of chemotherapy.[5]

In a study by Wallace et al., the dose required to destroy 50% of the resting follicle pool was less than 2 Gy.[6] In an effort to predict the age at which ovarian failure is likely to occur after irradiation, Wallace et al. conducted a follow-up study to account for age at treatment and exposure dose. The dose of radiation that led to premature ovarian failure immediately after treatment in 97.5% of patients or effective sterilizing dose was inversely related to age at treatment (Table 1).[7] These estimates may be useful in counseling patients prior to initiating radiation therapy. It is also important that consideration be given to transposing the ovaries outside of the radiation field in women of reproductive age who are seeking fertility preservation.

Pelvic radiation therapy also has a negative effect on reproduction in female patients by causing changes in both the musculature and blood flow to the uterus. This can lead to endometrial damage and a subsequent higher rate of obstetrical complications such as increased risk of spontaneous abortion, midrimester loss, and preterm birth.[8] The risk for these potential complications appear to be highest when conception occurs less than 1 year after radiation to the pelvis or abdomen has been completed.[9]

FERTILITY PRESERVATION TECHNIQUES

For many women, a cancer diagnosis elicits a serious concern with regard to the effect of treatment on the possibility for motherhood. In a survey of 757 breast cancer patients, Partridge et al. reported that 57% had concerns about their future fertility, with 29% of these patients admitting that these concerns influenced their treatment decisions. However, only 50% of these women reported that their physicians addressed their concerns adequately.[10] It cannot be overstated that physicians discuss the potential of therapy affecting fertility and fertility preservation options currently available. This is a conversation that must take place prior to initiating chemotherapy or radiation therapy. In 2006, the American Society of Clinical Oncology recognized the importance of fertility preservation and published guidelines recommending that all reproductive-age patients be offered referral to a reproductive endocrinologist to discuss options.[11]

Multiple fertility preservation strategies exist. These include ovarian transposition, gonadotropin-releasing hormone (GnRH) agonist therapy, ovarian tissue cryopreservation, oocyte cryopreservation and embryo cryopreservation.

Table 1 The impact of radiation on ovarian function with increasing age

Age at treatment	Effective sterilizing dose
Birth	20.3 Gy
10 years old	18.4 Gy
20 years old	16.5 Gy
30 years old	14.3 Gy

Gy: gray (unit of absorbed radiation dose)

OVARIAN TRANSPOSITION

Pelvic or abdominal radiation therapy can avoid ovarian exposure if transposition is performed prior to the start of irradiation. Either laparoscopic or open ovarian transposition should be performed just prior to radiation initiation as ovarian migration has been reported. The laparoscopic approach is generally preferred in patients for whom abdominopelvic surgery is unnecessary as part of the treatment such as those with hematologic malignancies.

Ovarian transposition involves moving the ovaries above the pelvic brim, out of the irradiation field. In order to estimate the amount of radiation that transposed ovaries are exposed to, Covens et al. performed dose calculations in patients, who received intracavitary radiation for cervical cancer. They compared these values to those that would have been obtained if the patients received external pelvic (45 Gy) with or without para-aortic nodal irradiation (45 Gy). Following treatment, the mean dose of radiation to each ovary (mean distance of transposition 14.4 cm on the right, 14.3 cm on the left) was 1.26 Gy in the intracavitary group, 1.35–1.90 Gy for pelvic radiation and 2.3–3.1 Gy for para-aortic lymph node irradiation. They noted that one patient developed ovarian failure after her transposed ovaries slipped back into the pelvis.[12]

Several published reports have investigated the efficacy of ovarian transposition on preservation of ovarian function and future fertility. Huang et al.

performed laparoscopic bilateral ovarian transposition in 14 premenopausal women with gynecologic malignancies. After a mean follow-up time of 72 months, 50% of these patients developed ovarian failure of which 6 (85.7%) were over the age of 40 years.[13]

Morice et al. assessed the efficacy of ovarian transposition prior to radiation therapy in 95 patients with cervical cancer. After a median follow-up of 31 months, the overall rate of ovarian function preservation was 83%.[14] Successful preservation of ovarian function is dependent on the patient's age and dose of radiation and should be offered to premenopausal patients, especially those less than 40 years old.

Ovarian transposition is not without complications. Adverse events include vascular compromise, infarction of the fallopian tubes, chronic ovarian pain, migration of ovaries back to anatomical position and formation of ovarian cysts (approximately 20%).[14,15]

GONADOTROPIN-RELEASING HORMONE AGONISTS

Gonadotropin-releasing hormone agonists induce reversible suppression of the hypothalamic-pituitary-gonadal axis. The use of GnRH agonists has been proposed as a method for fertility preservation. By reducing ovarian recruitment and possibly blood flow, such suppression may reduce the cytotoxic effect of chemotherapy on resting follicles, and thus decrease the risk of ovarian failure. The best candidates for GnRH agonists are postmenarchal patients.

Chemotherapeutic agents can lead to an increased rate of follicular destruction and diminished granulosa cell secretion of estradiol and inhibin. The decline in these factors leads to a loss of negative feedback resulting in an increase in follicle-stimulating hormone (FSH) secretion. The increase in FSH leads to enhanced recruitment of follicles, thus exposing them to the cytotoxic effects of chemotherapy. By administering a GnRH agonist, it is postulated that this cycle can be interrupted by inhibiting the increase in FSH concentration and temporarily preventing recruitment of follicles.[16] In doing so, FSH downregulation can lead to reduced vascular flow within the ovaries reducing chemotherapy exposure.

A limited number of trials have aimed to evaluate the efficacy of GnRH agonists as a means of fertility preservation in patients undergoing chemotherapy. Recchia et al. administered a GnRH analogue (goserelin) to 64 premenopausal breast cancer patients (median age 42 years) treated with adjuvant chemotherapy. Eighty six percent of these women had resumption of normal menses after a median follow-up of 55 months. One patient became pregnant and delivered a healthy child.[17] These same investigators performed a follow-up study of 100 consecutive premenopausal women undergoing a similar protocol for ovarian suppression. After a median follow-up of 75 months, normal menses resumed in all patients under the age of 40 years and in 56% of patients older than 40 years. Furthermore, 3 pregnancies that resulted in two normal deliveries and one elective termination were reported.[18]

In a prospective study by Urruticoechea et al. of 51 premenopausal patients treated with goserelin and chemotherapy, amenorrhea occurred in all but one patient. However, 45 patients (90%) recovered normal menses during the first year of follow-up, with a mean time to resumption of five months. Additionally, seven of ten attempting patients yielded eight pregnancies.[19]

A meta-analysis of nine studies reported an association between GnRH agonist administration and ovarian function preservation in women undergoing chemotherapy. When compared to patients who received concurrent GnRH agonist treatment, 93% resumed normal menses versus 48% of those who did not receive a GnRH agonist. Pregnancy rates between the two groups also differed and were found to be 22% in the treated group and 14% in women without GnRH therapy (RR = 1.65, CI 1.03–2.6).[20]

The German Hodgkin Study Group, however, found no ovarian function preservation in women (age 18–40 years), undergoing chemotherapy for advanced stage Hodgkin's lymphoma who were randomly assigned to receive a GnRH agonist or oral contraceptives. In both treatment groups, the antimüllerian hormone level was reduced below normal range, the ovarian preservation rate was 0%, and there were no reported pregnancies in a mean follow-up of 12 months.[21]

Evidence is still lack regarding the efficacy of GnRH agonists in preventing ovarian failure in patients undergoing chemotherapy. The above mentioned studies do not allow for definitive conclusions regarding this fertility preservation technique given the lack of randomization, small sample sizes, and few successful pregnancies. Additionally, there are some concern regarding the safety of GnRH agonists in terms of their potential to decrease the efficacy of chemotherapy by halting cancer cell proliferation, and thus decreasing tumor cell sensitivity to treatment. Therefore, the American Society of Clinical Oncology currently recommends that patients interested in GnRH suppression undergo treatment in the context of an approved clinical trial.[11]

OVARIAN TISSUE CRYOPRESERVATION

Ovarian tissue cryopreservation with future autotransplantation has become a promising fertility preservation technique. This modality appeals to patients that cannot delay treatment or do not currently have a male partner. For premenarchal females, ovarian tissue cryopreservation is an experimental technique that may provide the only reasonable chance for future fertility.

Upon completion of chemotherapy and with remission established, the frozen-thawed cortical strips may then be reimplanted orthotopically, near the ovary or infundibulopelvic ligament, or heterotopically with subcutaneous placement under the forearm or suprapubic area. Heterotopic transplantation may be preferred for patients at high risk for pelvic surgery such as those who received pelvic irradiation or have extensive adhesions. For patients at risk for ovarian metastases, the transplanted tissue can be closely monitored for any evidence of disease recurrence and can subsequently be easily removed.

The reimplantation of cryopreserved ovarian tissue provides a means for patients to resume ovulation, and thus maintain fertility. Resumption of ovarian function has been reported after both orthotopic and heterotopic transplantation of ovarian cortical strips. Sanchez et al. reimplanted cryopreserved cortical strips onto the contralateral ovarian medulla after the completion of chemotherapy. Two of four (50%) women regained ovarian function with no live births to date.[22] Schmidt et al. transplanted ovarian tissue orthotopically and heterotopically in 3 patients with premature ovarian failure after chemotherapy. All three women regained ovarian function as determined by resumption of menses, appearance of ovarian follicles on sonogram, and normalized FSH and estradiol levels.[23] Six years after ovarian cryopreservation, Oktay et al. transplanted ovarian tissue subcutaneously under the abdomen of a breast cancer patient. Three months later, the patient experienced return of ovarian function and embryos were eventually generated from the heterotopic tissue with one embryo transfer.[24] To date, there have been three reports of live births using this technique.[25-27]

The primary concern with this method of fertility preservation is the potential for introducing tissue with active metastases. Although the majority of cancers that occur in reproductive age women infrequently metastasize to the ovary, patients with hematological malignancies, such as leukemia, may have an increased risk of micrometastases. Additionally, BRCA1 and BRCA2 germline mutation carriers have a lifetime ovarian cancer risk of 40–60% and 15% respectively.[28] A very thorough histological analysis of the removed ovarian tissue should be performed in these patients when there is a significant concern for the possibility of ovarian micrometastases.

OOCYTE CRYOPRESERVATION

Embryo and oocyte cryopreservation are the most successful and well-studied methods of fertility preservation. Both of these strategies require mature meiosis II oocytes. Exogenous gonadotropins are utilized to stimulate ovarian follicular development. Once the desired ovarian response of multifollicular development has been obtained, human chorionic gonadotropin (hCG) is administered to the patient to provide final maturation of the oocytes. Oocyte retrieval is generally performed 36 hours after hCG administration under transvaginal ultrasound-guided oocyte aspiration. These mature oocytes are then cryopreserved and stored for future use. Oocyte cryopreservation is typically the preferred method of fertility preservation in women that do not have a male partner, or are uninterested in the use of a donor sperm.

Cryopreservation requires the use of cryoprotectant agents (such as propylene glycol, ethylene glycol, sucrose and trehalose) to prevent intracellular ice crystal formation. Oocyte cryopreservation has been available since 1986,[29] but initial success was limited due to the difficulties encountered from the slow freeze technique. Problems included intracellular ice crystal formation, hardening of the zona pellucida, osmotic swelling effect on oocyte and artificial activation of the mitotic spindle.[29,30]

Several adjustments have been made to the slow-freeze method including an increase in the sucrose concentration and a longer exposure time to the cryoprotectant during cryopreservation.[31] These allow for improved oocyte survival and clinical pregnancy rates. A clinical trial, including 96 patients, described the efficiency of the slow-freeze method using 1,769 cryopreserved oocytes. Out of a total of 1,502 thawed oocytes, 796 oocytes (54%) survived. There was a fertilization rate of 57.7% and 91.2% of the fertilized oocytes developed into cleavage stage embryos. Sixteen pregnancies were achieved including seven singleton and two twin live births.[31]

In order to improve fertility rates, the ultra-fast freezing (vitrification) technique was developed. Vitrification avoids ice crystal formation by modifying the cryoprotectant solution to include a higher sucrose concentration with added proteins and antioxidants to stabilize the media. Vitrified oocytes have higher survival rates and yield better pregnancy rates.[32] A meta-analysis of the vitrification technique revealed a fertilization rate of 74.2%, and live birth rates per injected oocyte and embryo transfer of 3.6% and 36.6%, respectively.[33]

In an effort to compare success rates between the slow-freeze and vitrification protocols, Smith et al. performed a randomized controlled trial including 78 patients (30 in the slow-freeze group and 48 in the vitrification group). There was a statistically significant increase in oocyte survival rates (81% vs 67%), fertilization rates (77% vs 67%), and clinical pregnancy rates per thaw cycle (38% vs 13%) after vitrification compared to slow-freezing.[34] However, there still is limited data available to recommend one oocyte cryopreservation technique over the other.

The advantage of slow-freeze cryopreservation is that it is technically similar to embryo cryopreservation and involves the same equipment. Vitrification, on the other hand, is more expensive to perform and its results may be dependent on the embryologist's experience with the new method. More data is required to determine if one technique should be preferred.

While there is a theoretical concern that disruption of the meiotic spindle during cryopreservation may predispose to aneuploidy, this has not been observed. It is estimated that more than 900 infants have now been born from cryopreserved oocytes, either with the slow-freeze or the vitrification technique. In this series, no increase in congenital anomalies was observed.[35]

Despite various improvements in the slow-freeze method, *in vitro* fertilization (IVF) with fresh oocytes remains superior to the slow-freeze technique. Oktay et al. published a meta-analysis comparing IVF success rates after oocyte cryopreservation via the slow-freeze protocol to IVF with unfrozen oocytes. They reported live birth rates per injected oocyte and embryo transfer to be 3.4% and 21.6% respectively, for slow-frozen oocytes 6.6% and 60.4% for IVF using unfrozen oocytes.[33]

EMBRYO CRYOPRESERVATION

Embryo cryopreservation is the most effective form of fertility preservation currently available. As in oocyte cryopreservation, the use of gonadotropin is common. The aim is to stimulate the ovaries for multifollicular recruitment. Once oocytes are mature, they are aspirated under transvaginal ultrasound guidance and subsequently combined with sperm to create embryos that are then cryopreserved.

Human embryos have up to 95% freeze-thaw survival rates. This is much higher than unfertilized oocytes.[36] The live birth rate using frozen-thawed embryos appears to be dependent on the age of the patient at the time her eggs were retrieved. In the United States, the average live birth rate with embryo cryopreservation is 27.7% per embryo transfer cycle.[37,38] Wilson et al. have reported successful pregnancies in patients, who had embryos that had been cryopreserved for more than 10 years.[39] Furthermore, embryo cryopreservation does not seem to have a negative impact on cognitive, psychomotor or neurodevelopmental outcomes in children born as a result of this technique.[40]

There are several legal and ethical concerns that arise when considering cryopreservation as a means for fertility preservation. In patients with potentially fatal diseases, the disposition of cryopreserved material after death should be addressed prior to undergoing the procedure. The issue of legal ownership of the tissue, oocytes and embryos also arises, and conflict between family members may occur if the patient's desires were not clearly documented before cryopreservation. Couples may discard unused embryos or donate them to infertile couples or for research. However, many couples may be faced with a moral dilemma of discarding embryos. Such couples may be served better with oocyte cryopreservation to avoid these dilemmas. Physicians offering fertility preservation techniques must discuss the final disposition of preserved materials prior to initiating treatment.

OOCYTE DONATION

While numerous fertility preservation techniques exist, oocyte donation remains a treatment option for many patients. The medical literature has repeatedly shown that the success rates of oocyte donation are dependent on the age of the oocyte rather than the age of the recipient.[41-43] The uterus seems to maintain its ability to successfully host a pregnancy despite advancing maternal age. The Centers for Disease Control and Prevention reported pregnancy rates of 17% in women over the age of 40 years undergoing assisted reproductive technology when using their own fresh embryos. This pregnancy rate increased to 47% when fresh embryos were created using donor oocytes.[44] Egg donation provides a reasonably high chance for successful pregnancy, and should be considered as an option, for those patients who meet criteria as potential candidates.

SUMMARY

There exist several fertility preservation techniques aimed at minimizing the risk of sterility following cancer treatment. Patients concerned with fertility preservation

Table 2 Commonly used chemotherapeutic agents and associated side effects

Drug	Regimen	Class	Side effect
Cyclophosphamide	CMF, FAC, FEC, AC	Alkylating agent	Ovarian toxicity, N/V, BM suppression, alopecia, hemorrhagic cystitis
5-Fluorouracil	CMF, FAC, FEC	Antimetabolite	Myelosuppression, mucositis, dermatitis
Methotrexate	CMF	Antimetabolite	Anemia, neutropenia, alopecia, hepatotoxicity, pulmonary fibrosis
Adriamycin	FAC, AC	Anthracycline	N/V, alopecia, cardiotoxicity
Epirubicin	FEC	Anthracycline	Fewer side effects than doxorubicin

AC: adriamycin, cyclophosphamide; BM: bone marrow; CMF: cyclophosphamide, methotrexate and 5-fluorouracil; FAC: 5-fluorouracil, adriamycin and cyclophosphamide; FEC: 5-fluorouracil, epirubicin and cyclophosphamide; N/V: nausea, vomiting

Table 3 Summary of fertility preservation techniques

Technique	Pros	Cons	Patient
Ovarian tissue cryopreservation	No male, no ovarian stimulation, unlikely to delay treatment	Very few pregnancies, may reimplant micrometastases	Premenarchal
Ovarian suppression with GnRH agonist	No male, noninvasive, unlikely to delay treatment	Side effects unknown, efficacy not confirmed	Postmenarchal, no male partner
Oocyte cryopreservation	No male	Requires ovarian stimulation, may delay chemotherapy, may transmit cancer susceptibility gene to offspring	Postmenarchal, no male partner
Embryo cryopreservation	Very effective in achieving pregnancy, PGD	Requires male, requires ovarian stimulation, may delay chemotherapy	Postmenarchal, has male partner
Egg donation	No ovarian stimulation, unlikely to delay treatment	Requires male	Poor ovarian reserve, ovarian failure, dominant genetic defect

GnRH: gonadotropin-releasing hormone; PGD: preimplantation genetic diagnosis

prior to undergoing treatment for malignancy or autoimmune disorders should be referred to a reproductive endocrinologist to allow timely discussion of available options prior to initiating chemotherapy or radiation therapy. Several factors will determine the most appropriate treatment option for these women including the patient's age, type of adjuvant treatment, time available before initiating therapy and the length of delay to childbearing. GnRH agonist treatment, ovarian tissue cryopreservation and oocyte cryopreservation are still considered experimental but may be the only feasible options for a specific patient population. Embryo cryopreservation and egg donation remain as the modalities with the highest pregnancy yield. However, these may not be the most appropriate options for some patients. Future studies are required to improve outcomes in both cancer survivors and otherwise healthy women.

REFERENCES

1. Altekruse SF, Kosary CL, Krapcho M, Neyman N, Aminou R, Waldron W, Ruhl J, Howlader N, Tatalovich Z, Cho H, Mariotto A, Eisner MP, Lewis DR, Cronin K, Chen HS, Feuer EJ, Stinchcomb DG, Edwards BK (Eds). SEER Cancer Statistics Review, 1975-2007. [online] SEER website. Available from http://seer.cancer.gov/csr/1975_2007/ [Accessed November 2009].

2. Oktem O, Oktay K. The ovary: anatomy and function throughout human life. Ann N Y Acad Sci. 2008;1127:1-9.
3. Goodwin PJ, Ennis M, Pritchard KI, et al. Risk of menopause during the first year after breast cancer diagnosis. J Clin Oncol. 1999;17:2365-70.
4. Ogilvy-Stuart AL, Shalet SM. Effect of radiation on the human reproductive system. Environ Health Perspect. 1993;101(Suppl 2):109-16.
5. Meirow D, Nugent D. The effects of radiotherapy and chemotherapy on female reproduction. Hum Reprod Update. 2001;7:535-43.
6. Wallace WH, Thomson AB, Kelsey TW. The radiosensitivity of the human oocyte. Hum Reprod. 2003;18:117-21.
7. Wallace WH, Thomson AB, Saran F, et al. Predicting age of ovarian failure after radiation to a field that includes the ovaries. Int J Radiat Oncol Biol Phys. 2005;62:738-44.
8. Critchley HO, Wallace WH. Impact of cancer treatment on uterine function. J Natl Cancer Inst Monogr. 2005;34:64-8.
9. Fenig E, Mishaeli M, Kalish Y, et al. Pregnancy and radiation. Cancer Treat Rev. 2001;27:1-7.
10. Partridge AH, Gelber S, Peppercorn J, et al. Web-based survey of fertility issues in young women with breast cancer. J Clin Oncol. 2004;22:4174-83.
11. Lee SJ, Schover LR, Partridge AH, et al. American Society of Clinical Oncology recommendations on fertility preservation in cancer patients. J Clin Oncol. 2006;24:2917-31.
12. Covens AL, van der Putten HW, Fyles AW, et al. Laparoscopic ovarian transposition. Eur J Gynaecol Oncol. 1996;17:177-82.
13. Huang KG, Lee CL, Tsai CS, et al. A new approach for laparoscopic ovarian transposition before pelvic irradiation. Gynecol Oncol. 2007;105:234-7.
14. Morice P, Juncker L, Rey A, et al. Ovarian transposition for patients with cervical carcinoma treated by radiosurgical combination. Fertil Steril. 2000;74:743-8.
15. Gabriel DA, Bernard SA, Lambert J, et al. Oophoropexy and the management of Hodgkin's disease. A reevaluation of the risks and benefits. Arch Surg. 1986;121:1083-5.
16. Blumenfeld Z. How to preserve fertility in young women exposed to 17. Chemotherapy? The role of GnRH agonist cotreatment in addition to cryopreservation of embryos, oocytes, or ovaries. Oncologist. 2007;12:1044-54.
17. Recchia F, Sica G, De Filippis S, et al. Goserelin as ovarian protection in the adjuvant treatment of premenopausal breast cancer: a phase II pilot study. Anticancer Drugs. 2002;13:417-24.
18. Recchia F, Saggio G, Amiconi G, et al. Gonadotropin-releasing hormone analogues added to adjuvant chemotherapy protect ovarian function and improve clinical outcomes in young women with early breast carcinoma. Cancer. 2006;106:514-23.
19. Urruticoechea A, Arnedos M, Walsh G, et al. Ovarian protection with goserelin during adjuvant chemotherapy for premenopausal women with early breast cancer (EBC). Breast Cancer Res Treat. 2008;110:411-6.
20. Clowse ME, Behera MA, Anders CK, et al. Ovarian preservation by GnRH agonists during chemotherapy: a meta-analysis. J Womens Health (Larchmt). 2009; 18:311-9.
21. Behringer K, Wildt L, Mueller H, et al. No protection of the ovarian follicle pool with the use of GnRH-analogues or oral contraceptives in young women treated with escalated BEACOPP for advanced-stage Hodgkin lymphoma. Final results of a phase II trial from the German Hodgkin Group. Ann Oncol. 2010;21:2052-60.
22. Sanchez M, Novella-Maestre E, Teruel J, et al. The Valencia programme for fertility preservation. Clin Transl Oncol. 2008;10:433-8.
23. Schmidt KL, Andersen CY, Loft A, et al. Follow-up of ovarian function post-chemotherapy following ovarian cryopreservation and transplantation. Hum Reprod. 2005;20:3539-46.
24. Oktay K, Buyuk E, Veeck L, et al. Embryo development after heterotopic transplantation of cryopreserved ovarian tissue. Lancet. 2004;363:837-40.
25. Demeestere I, Simon P, Emiliani S, et al. Fertility preservation: successful transplantation of cryopreserved ovarian tissue in a young patient previously treated for Hodgkin's disease. Oncologist. 2007;12:1437-42.
26. Donnez J, Dolmans MM, Demylle D, et al. Livebirth after orthotopic transplantation of cryopreserved ovarian tissue. Lancet. 2004;364:1405-10.
27. Meirow D, Levron J, Eldar-Geva T, et al. Pregnancy after transplantation of cryopreserved ovarian tissue in a patient with ovarian failure after chemotherapy. N Engl J Med. 2005;353:318-21.
28. Hickey M, Peate M, Saunders CM, et al. Breast cancer in young women and its impact on reproductive function. Hum Reprod Update. 2009;15:323-39.
29. Chen C. Pregnancy after human oocyte cryopreservation. Lancet. 1986;1:884-6.
30. Jain JK, Paulson RJ. Oocyte cryopreservation. Fertil Steril. 2006;86:1037-46.
31. Fabbri R, Porcu E, Marsella T, et al. Human oocyte cryopreservation: new perspectives regarding oocyte survival. Hum Reprod. 2001;16:411-6.
32. Tao T, Del Valle A. Human oocyte and ovarian tissue cryopreservation and its application. J Assist Reprod Genet. 2008;25:287-96.
33. Oktay K, Cil AP, Bang H. Efficiency of oocyte cryopreservation: a meta-analysis. Fertil Steril. 2009;91:1061-6.
34. Smith GD, Serafini PC, Fioravanti J, et al. Prospective randomized comparison of human oocyte cryopreservation with slow-rate freezing or vitrification. Fertil Steril. 2010;94:2088-95.
35. Noyes N, Porcu E, Borini A. Over 900 oocyte cryopreservation babies born with no apparent increase in congenital anomalies. Reprod biomed Online. 2009;18:769-76.
36. Seli E, Tangir J. Fertility preservation options for female patients with malignancies. Curr Opin Obstet Gynecol. 2005;17:299-308.
37. Center for Disease Control and Prevention (CDC). (2008) Assisted Reproductive Technology (ART) Report.

[online] CDC website. Available from http://www.cdc.gov/art/ART2008/section3.htm.
38. Society for Assisted Reproductive Technology, American Society for Reproductive Medicine. (2009) Assisted Reproductive Technology Success Rates: National Summary and Fertility Clinic Reports. Available from https://www.sartcorsonline.com/rpt CSR PublicMultYear.ear.aspx?ClinicPKID=0
39. Wilson C, Check JH, Summers-Chase D, et al. Successful pregnancies from embryos cryopreserved more than ten years: two case reports. Clin Exp Obstet Gynecol. 2006;33:79.
40. Pauli SA, Berga SL, Shang W, et al. Current status of the approach to assisted reproduction. Pediatr Clin North Am. 2009;56:467-88.
41. Stolwijk AM, Zielhuis GA, Sauer MV, et al. The impact of the woman's age on success of standard and donor in vitro fertilization. Fertil Steril. 1997;67:702-10.
42. Sauer MV, Paulson RJ, Lobo RA. Reversing the natural decline in human fertility. An extended clinical trial of oocyte donation to women of advanced reproductive age. JAMA. 1992;268:1275-9.
43. Noyes N, Hampton BS, Berkeley A, et al. Factors useful in predicting the success of oocyte donation: a 3-year retrospective study. Fertil Steril. 2001;76:92-7.
44. Center for Disease Control and Prevention. 2001 Assisted Reproductive Technology Success Rates: National Summary and Fertility Clinic Reports. US Department of Health and Human Services Centers for Disease Control and Prevention, 2003.
Guidelines for gamete and embryo donation. The American Society for Reproductive Medicine. Fertil Steril. 1998;70(4 Suppl 3):1S-13S.

25

Advanced Reproductive Age and ART

Paul R Gindoff

CHAPTER CONTENTS

INTRODUCTION

Advanced female reproductive age is an important factor when evaluating couples for infertility.[1] Reasons for this phenomenon include the aging of the baby-boom generation, deferment of childbearing to later years of reproductive life (because of changes in lifestyles) and increased exposure of patients to infertility services. This voluntary delay in childbearing not only poses a problem in terms of the 30–50% reduced pregnancy potential of older women, but other risks also have to be taken into account: the effect of pregnancy on other maternal illnesses, an increased risk of pre-eclampsia, hypertension and diabetes and an increased risk of chromosomal abnormalities, abortions and stillbirth.[2] The decrease of female fecundity beginning in the 30s, becoming more pronounced after 40, is well documented.[3-6] There is an approximately 50% decrease in the fertility rate of women attempting pregnancy at the age of 40 years or older compared with younger women, and a two fold to three fold increase in the rate of spontaneous abortions.[2] Reports of artificial insemination[6] and chromosomal analysis of unfertilized human oocytes[7] and embryos[8] in *in vitro* fertilization (IVF) suggest that the quality of the oocyte and the resulting embryo are affected seriously by age.

Various factors influence the decline in fertility of older women: prolongation of infectious, occupational and environmental exposures[9] which increases the risks of pelvic disease and reproductive organ dysfunction; an increase in embryonic chromosomal abnormalities; increased rates of early pregnancy wastage of both normal and abnormal fetuses; hypothalamic aging and de-synchronization of neuroendocrine signals which may contribute to accelerated rate of follicular loss;[10] an increased incidence of luteal phase dysfunction and;[11] oocyte senescence which seems to be the primary factor responsible for decrease in fertility. A measurable decline in fecundity can be seen to begin many years before the menopause (near end of fourth decade),[12,13] even though women may still have regular menstrual cycles. Senescence affects both the ovary (oocyte and granulosa cells) and the uterus, and defective vasculature of the uterus may be one of the causes of increased abortion rate in older patients.[14] Although oocyte quality and lifespan are fixed, the endometrium can retain its ability to respond to exogenous steroids and thus, provide a receptive environment for implantation and subsequent pregnancy for many years to come.[15] The superior pregnancy rates of oocyte donation patients of all ages suggest that aging of the nonovarian components of the reproductive axis has little impact on reproductive potential.[16-18]

Perimenopause is defined as the transition between normal reproductive life and the menopause, which has been characterized by increase in basal plasma follicle-stimulating hormone (FSH) levels when compared with younger women.[19] Changes in the hypothalamic-pituitary-ovarian axis during this period include a declining reproductive potential, increasing variability of the intermenses interval, decreasing ovarian response to stimulation by the gonadotropins and changes in both the quantity and quality of basal gonadotropins [FSH and luteinizing hormone (LH)] secretion.[20] Follicle stimulating hormone elevation in perimenopause is most marked during the early follicular phase, while increased basal levels of immuno active LH are less consistently observed.[21] The author[21] showed that perimenopausal women (defined as women > 35 years old with irregular menses) could be distinguished from normal cycling women of comparable age (pre-perimenopausal) and from menopausal women based on basal FSH, and that gonadotropin-releasing hormone (GnRH) stimulation could add further discriminating power for older women with irregular menses but with basal FSH levels within normal range. The author[22] also showed that by using the clomiphene citrate challenge test (CCCT), perimenopausal women could be distinguished from pre-perimenopausal women. Stimulated (post GnRH or CC) FSH was significantly higher and did not return to baseline levels in the perimenopausal group when compared to the pre-perimenopausal group in both studies, suggesting poor ovarian reserve reflected in significantly lower estrogen production or inhibin production from the aging follicle. Thus hormonal changes have been shown to parallel the menstrual changes in the transition to menopause.

OVARIAN RESERVE TESTING

The use of chronological age alone as a prognostic index of reproduction potential may be misleading because of individual variation.[15] The reproductive potential declines with age, and there are extensive data to indicate that the changes responsible for the age-related decline in reproductive potential begin within the ovary.[23,24] This decline correlates with the process of follicular depletion and diminished oocyte quality, factors which in aggregate may be referred to as diminished ovarian reserve,[25-27] the onset of which is highly variable.[28-30] In order to obtain an accurate prognosis of the patient's fecundity potential, various tools (most of them endocrine assays) have been invoked in order to estimate ovarian reserve. Clinicians most validate the threshold values with the assay system used in their own laboratory before the application of these tests.[28]

Follicle stimulation hormone secretion is inversely related to estradiol levels which decrease as the ovarian reserve decreases. Elevated FSH can also result from a reduced secretion of inhibin by the germ cell-depleted ovaries.[29] The group of IVF patients with elevated FSH developed fewer follicles, fewer oocytes and had fewer embryos transferred, suggestive of diminished ovarian reserve, even though the average age of the patients was approximately the same.[30]

One of the concerns about using basal FSH as a prognostic indicator of ovarian reserve is, how to interpret its intercycle variability.[31] It was noticed that patients with normal basal FSH (< 15 mIU/ml) had less inter-cycle variation than those patients with elevated FSH. In the same study, 28 patients had inter-cycle variations that resulted in the patient having a basal FSH in the normal or intermediate range during one cycle and an elevated FSH in another. Although by accepted convention, the basal FSH is evaluated on day 3 of the cycle. The author has[32] shown that FSH does not vary on day 1, 2, 3 or 4 during the menstrual cycle.

Elevation of day 3 estradiol (> 80 pg/ml) is also a poor prognostic sign, and it is theorized that elevated levels of FSH in the late luteal phase of the preceding cycle (caused by lower inhibin secretion by granulosa cells) may cause this change. The author[33] showed that higher cancellation rates and lower pregnancy rates occur in patients with elevated estradiol, in spite of normal day 3 FSH levels. Further evidence was obtained in perimenopausal studies.[22]

Reduced bioactivity of the FSH molecule is another theoretical mechanism that could result in an increased FSH requirement to sustain follicle development.

Other dynamic tests have been developed to evaluate ovarian reserve. Navot et al.[34] described the CCCT in a prospective study to assess the future fertility potential of women of advanced reproductive age. Clomiphene citrate (100 mg) was given daily from days 5–9 of the menstrual cycle, and FSH, LH and estradiol were measured before (day 3) and after (days 9–11) CC administration. Patients with stimulated FSH levels less than 26 mIU/ml were considered to have adequate ovarian response. The premise of the test is that, with normal ovarian reserve, the overall metabolic activity of the developing follicles should be able to overcome the impact of the CC on the hypothalamic-pituitary axis and suppress FSH levels back into the normal range by cycle day 10.[35] The CCCT thus unmasks an early hormonal insufficiency within the follicle, and may play an important role in determining the prognosis of an infertile patient who is over 35 years old.

Inhibin is a heterodimer that selectively inhibits FSH secretion. Klein et al.[36] revealed that follicular phase inhibin-B secretion was lower in older patients, who also demonstrated a monotropic rise in FSH, while inhibin-A secretion did not change. In view of these findings, Seifer et al.[37] conducted a study to describe the association between inhibin-B and fecundity potential, and found that women undergoing IVF with day 3 serum inhibin-B levels lower than 45 pg/ml had 70% of the estradiol response, 66.6% of the number of oocytes retrieved per patient, 28% of the clinical pregnancy rate per initiated cycle and 3 times the cancellation rate per initiated cycle when compared to women with higher inhibin-B levels. Despite normal day 3 FSH levels, they could also demonstrate differences in response to ovulation induction and outcome based on day 3 inhibin-B alone. Thus inhibin-B levels, as well as day 3 estradiol can be useful as prognosticators in addition to day 3 FSH levels.

Transvaginal ultrasound has also been used as a tool to measure ovarian reserve. Lass et al.[38] found that small ovaries (< 3 cm^3) were associated with a poor response to human menopausal gonadotropins (hMG) treatment, a high cancellation rate and a lower follicle yield and oocyte retrieval when studying 140 patients undergoing IVF. This suggests an inverse association between ovarian volume and ovarian reserve. Tomas et al.[34] reported that the number of small follicles present before ovarian stimulation was a better predictor of outcome than ovarian volume or age alone, and that ovarian volume correlated better with the number of follicles before stimulation rather than with the number of oocytes.

So far, assessment of the number of antral follicles by ultrasonography, the antral follicle count (AFC), best predicts the quantitative aspect of ovarian reserve.[39] However, measurement of the AFC requires an additional transvaginal ultrasound examination during the early follicular phase. Therefore, a serum marker that reflects the number of follicles that have made the transition from the primordial pool into the growing follicle pool, and that is not controlled by gonadotropins, would benefit both patients and clinicians.

Anti-Müllerian hormone (AMH), also known as Müllerian inhibiting substance (MIS), has been mainly studied for its regulatory role in male sex differentiation. Anti-Müllerian hormone, produced by the Sertoli cells of the fetal testis, induces the regression of the Müllerian ducts, the anlagen of the female reproductive tract. However, after birth, this sex-dimorphic expression pattern is lost and AMH is also expressed in granulosa cells of growing follicles in the ovary.

This inhibitory effect of AMH on FSH, sensitivity of follicles could play a role in the process of selection.

In young normal ovulatory women, early follicular phase hormone measurements at 3-year intervals revealed that serum AMH levels decline significantly whereas serum levels of FSH and inhibin-B and the number of antral follicles do not change during this interval.[40] Stratification for age revealed that both serum AMH levels and numbers of antral follicles decline with age. Importantly, a strong correlation of serum AMH levels with AFC was observed. This positive correlation was later confirmed and showed a stronger correlation between serum AMH levels and follicle count than between AMH and serum levels of inhibin-B, FSH and E2 on cycle day 3.

The results also suggest that changes in serum AMH levels occur relatively early in the sequence of events associated with ovarian aging.

On the one hand, correct identification of poor responders by assessment of their ovarian reserve before entering an IVF program is important. On the other hand, assessment of the ovarian reserve may also benefit patients that would generally be excluded from IVF programs because of advanced age. Several studies have shown that AMH is an excellent marker to determine ovarian responsiveness also in an IVF program. In agreement with the studies described above, AMH serum levels were shown to be highly correlated with the number of antral follicles before treatment and number of oocytes retrieved upon ovarian stimulation.[41] Serum AMH level can also serve as a marker in ovarian pathophysiology, such as polycystic ovary syndrome (PCOS), in which the antral follicle pool is enlarged. PCOS is one of the most common endocrine disorders in women of reproductive age.[42]

TREATMENT

During stimulation with exogenous gonadotropins, patients with decreased ovarian reserve develop fewer oocytes and achieve lower peak estradiol levels.[43] Horboy[44] studied the effect of age on outcome of controlled ovarian hyperstimulation/intrauterine insemination (COH/IUI) treatment in a group of 190 patients, who underwent 472 cycles. Pregnancy rate per cycle for patients less than 36 years old was 15.7%, whereas the rate for patients more than 36 years old was 7.2%. There are also limitations on IVF for women of advanced reproductive age. A poor ovarian response causes an increased cancellation rate and a reduced number of oocytes being retrieved. There is also an increased incidence of zona pellucida fractures and a decrease in the number of embryos transferred and the pregnancy rate.[45] Implantation and pregnancy rates do decrease while miscarriage rate increases, probably because of an increase in oocyte chromosome degeneration,[46] abnormalities of the oocyte meiotic spindle[47] and/or oocyte aneuploidy. Expression of the embryonic genome occurs only after the 4–8-cell stage and could account for the later wastage by failure of implantation and clinical miscarriage despite of apparently normal fertilization.[48] A recent study using sperm retrieval and intracytoplasmic sperm injection for couples with male factor infertility caused by azoospermia described the effects of female age and ovarian reserve.[49] It was shown that increased maternal age and diminished ovarian reserve had no effect on fertilization or embryo cleavage but dramatically affected embryo implantation, pregnancy and delivery rate.

Since oocyte quality and as result embryo quality, appears to be the most important factor affecting pregnancy rate in older women, several techniques have been developed to manipulate the embryos in order to increase the implantation rate. Assisted hatching (AH), the micro-surgical creation of an opening in the zona pellucida before transfer, has been suggested to facilitate implantation, thus resulting in increased pregnancy rate in older patients and in those with diminished ovarian reserve,[50] although these results have not been reproduced in other studies. Binder et al.[51] showed that AH in patients aged more than 38-year-old did not increase the take-home baby rate after IVF treatment. The author's experience has also been confirmatory. Selection of patients undergoing AH where only embryos with thick zonae are manipulated may be the key factor, since embryos with thin zonae may be jeopardized by the procedure.[52]

Defective ooplasm may be another cause of infertility in older women,[53] and in animals, restoration of normal developmental potential to eggs with ooplasma deficiencies has been achieved by transfer of ooplasm from a normal donor egg.[54,55] Cohen et al.[56] reported a pregnancy and live birth of an infant after cytoplasm (obtained from donor eggs) transfer to the oocytes of a 39-year-old woman with poor ovarian reserve and four previous failed attempts of assisted conception and embryo transfer. Further studies have to be done in order to establish the usefulness of this technique as a treatment and other options, such as the transfer of nuclear contents to an anucleate oocyte may have even more potential.

The increased incidence of early pregnancy loss and chromosomal abnormalities of the oocyte in older women are offered as evidence supporting a decrease in the biological quality of the oocyte with age. The reversal of decreasing pregnancy rates and increasing miscarriage rates by using oocyte donation, strongly supports this evidence.[57] Oocyte donation involves the aspiration of oocytes from donors undergoing COH for the purpose of IVF with the sperm of the recipient's partner. Resulting embryos are then transferred to the recipient whose endometrium has been hormonal with that of the donor.

The success rate after oocyte donation is age independent as long as embryos generated from ova obtained from young fertile women are transferred.[58] Recipient women more than 40-year-old in oocyte-donation programs have similar implantation rates when compared to the rates previously reported for women who are less than 40-year-old.[59] At least in the range of 30–53 years of age, the human uterus does not undergo substantial changes in terms of embryo implantation and nidation.[57] A report by Meldrum[78] did find that age negatively influences pregnancy rate in recipient patients more than 40 years of age in comparison to younger patients, but by administering higher progesterone doses during the transfer cycle, he was able to achieve identical results in both groups of patients.

Implantation failure which increases with age has been shown to be reflected in higher rates of aneuploidy in embryos from older women.[60-63] Approximately, 20% of morphologically normal embryos implant and produce a viable offspring, while about 50% of embryos cultured *in vitro* arrest development between post-retrieval day 1 and day 2, where aneuploidy accounts for a large percentage of arrested development. Aneuploidy can be observed for almost every chromosome in human spontaneous abortions, however, in live-born infants, aneuploidy is usually seen only for chromosomes 13, 18 and 21 and the sex chromosome. Preimplantation genetic diagnosis offers the patient and the clinician, the opportunity to obtain chromosomal and genetic information from the embryo prior to transfer. By removing a single cell from an 8-cell embryo and using polymerase chain reaction, fluorescent *in situ* hybridization or comparative genomic hybridization, genetic diseases and chromosomal aneuploidies in these embryos can be detected. When properly done, embryo biopsy does not decrease embryo viability or affect the living individual that results. This technique holds much promise for the future of IVF in all patients, particularly for those prone to increased aneuploidy, such as recurrent pregnancy loss.

SUMMARY

Recommendations for enrollment of women of advanced reproductive age into an advanced reproductive technology program should include an endocrine profile within the range considered normal for younger women.[64] Patients with elevated day 3 FSH or estradiol, or abnormal CCCT or GAST, have a poor potential for successful pregnancy after treatment, and should be counseled about ovum donation as a preferred option for treatment. Oocyte donation obviates the problems of inadequate response to stimulation and embryonic aneuploidy. Even though, a normal endocrine profile does indicate better long-term chances for a patient's conceiving by using her own oocytes, an age-related decline in fecundity remains and patient age should still be considered when counseling patients, who have normal screening results. On the other hand, women older than 40 years of age, who respond well to ovarian stimulation, the author recommend consideration of an empirical attempt at IVF before recommending oocyte donation for women with normal hormonal screens.[65] The transfer of higher numbers of embryos, if available in women more than 40-year-old, can improve their chances of pregnancy without the associated increased risks of multiple pregnancy.

REFERENCES

1. Mosher W, Pratt W. The demography of infertility in the United States. In: Asch RH, Studd JW (Eds). Annual Progress in Reproductive Medicine. New York: Parthenon Publishing Group; 1993. pp. 37-43.
2. Toner JP, Flood JT. Fertility after the age of 40. Obstet Gynecol Clin North Am. 1993;20: 261-72.
3. Leridon H. Human fertility. The basic components. Chicago, IL: University of Chicago Press; 1977. pp. 107.
4. Tietze C. Reproductive span and rate of reproduction among Hutterite women. Fertil Steril. 1957;8:89-97.
5. James W. The causes of the decline in fecundabiity with age. Soc Biol. 1979;26:330-4.
6. Schwartz W, Mayaux M. Female fecundity as a function of age: results of artificial insemination in 2193 nulliparous women with azoospermic husbands. Federation CECOS. N Engl J Med. 1982;306:404-6.
7. Plachot M, Veiga A, Montagut J, et al. Are clinical and biological IVF parameters correlated with chromosomal disorders in early life: a multicentric study. Hum Reprod. 1988;3:627-35.
8. Munné S, Alikani M, Tomkin G, et al. Embryo morphology, developmental rates, and maternal age are correlated with chromosome abnormalities. Fertil Steril. 1995;64:382-91.
9. Aral SO, Cates W. The increased concern with infertility. Why now? JAMA. 1983;250:2327-31.
10. Wise PM, Kashon ML, Krajnak KM, et al. Aging of the female reproductive system: a window into brain aging. Recent Frog Horm Res. 1997;52:279-303.
11. DeCherney AH, Berkowitz GS. Female fecundity and age. N Engl J Med. 1982;306:424-6.
12. Menken J, Trussell J, Larsen U. Age and infertility. Science. 1986;233:1389-94.
13. Klein NA, Battaglia DE, Fujimoto VY, et al. Reproductive aging: accelerated ovarian follicular development associated with a monotropic follicle-stimulating hormone rise in normal older women. J Clin Endocrinol Metabol. 1996;81:1038-45.
14. Pellicer A, Simón C, Remohí J. Effects of aging on the female reproductive system. Hum Reprod. 1995;10 (Suppl 2):77-83.
15. Kipersztok S, Gindoff P. Assisted reproductive management for the older woman. Assist Reprod Rev. 1991;1:77-83.
16. Scott R, Rosenwaks A. Oocyte donation. In: Sciarra JJ (Ed.). Obstet Gynecol, Volume 5. Philadelphia: JB Lippincott Co; 1990. pp. 1-14.
17. Rosenwaks Z. Donor eggs: their application in modern reproductive technologies. Fertil Steril. 1987;47:895-909.
18. Rotsztejn D, Asch R. Effect of aging on assisted reproductive technologies (ART): experience from oocyte donation. Semin Reprod Endocrinol. 1991;9:272-9.
19. Burger HG, Dudley EC, Hopper JL, et al. The endocrinology of the menopausal transition: a cross-sectional study of a population-based sample. J Clin Endocrinol Metab. 1995;80:3537-45.
20. Gindoff PR, Jewelewicz R. Reproductive potential in the older woman. Fertil Steril. 1986;46:989-1001.
21. Schmidt PJ, Gindoff PR, Baron DA, et al. Basal and stimulated gonadotropin levels in the perimenopause. Am J Obstet Gynecol. 1996;175:643-50.
22. Gindoff PR, Schmidt PJ, Rubinow DR. Response to clomiphene citrate challenge test in normal women through perimenopause. Gynecol Obstet Invest. 1997;43:186-91.
23. Henry L. Some data on natural fertility. Eugen Q. 1961;8:81-91.
24. Navot D, Drews MR, Bergh PA, et al. Age-related decline in female fertility is not due to diminished capacity of the uterus to sustain embryo implantation. Fertil Steril. 1994;61:97-101.
    Scott RT, Hofmann GE. Prognostic assessment of ovarian reserve. Fertil Steril. 1995;63:1-11.
25. Sherman BM, West JH, Korenmann SG. The menopausal transition: analysis of LH, FSH, estradiol, and progesterone concentrations during menstrual cycles of older women. J Clin Endocrinol Metab. 1976;42:629-36.
26. Rozenwaks Z, Damario M. Contemporary treatment strategies. Egg donation reproductive endocrinology, surgery, and technology. Philadelphia: Lippincott-New York: Raven Publishers; 1996. pp. 1432.
27. Scott RT, Toner JP, Muasher SJ, et al. Follicle-stimulating hormone levels on cycle day 3 are predictive of in vitro fertilization outcome. Fertil Steril. 1989;51:651-4.
28. Mosher WD, Pratt WF. Fecundity and infertility in the United States: incidence and trends. Fertil Steril. 1991;56:192-3.

29. Mosher W, Pratt W. Fecundity and infertility in the United States, 1965-1988 Advance Data from Vital and Health Statistics, No 192, Dec 4, 1990. Hyattsville, MD: National Center for Health Statistics. 33 US Congress, Office of Technology Assessment. Infertility. Medical and Social Choices. Washington, DC: US Government Printing Office; 1988, OTA-BA-358.
30. Maroulis G. Effect of aging on fertility and pregnancy. Semin Reprod Endocrinol. 1991;9:165-75
31. Scott RT, Hofmann GE, Oehninger S, et al. Intercycle variability of day 3 follicle-stimulating hormone levels and its effect on stimulation quality in in-vitro fertilization. Fertil Steril. 1990;54:297-302.
32. Gindoff P, Schmidt P, Kurl R, et al. Response to clomiphene citrate challenge test (CCCT) in the perimenopause. Abstract presented at the Annual Meeting of the Society of Gynecological Investigation, San Antonio, TX. Society of Gynecol Invest. 1992.
33. Smotrich DB, Widra EA, Gindoff PR, et al. Prognostic value of day 3 estradiol on in vitro fertilization outcome. Fertil Steril. 1995;64:1136-40.
34. Tomas C, Nuojua-Huttumen S, Martikainen H. Pretreatment transvaginal ultrasound examination predicts ovarian responsiveness to gonadotropins in in-vitro fertilization. Hum Reprod. 1997;12:220-3.
35. Scott RT, Hofmann GE. Prognostic assessment of ovarian reserve. Fertil Steril. 1995;63:1-11.
36. Klein N, Illingworth P, Groome N, et al. Decreased inhibin B secretion is associated with the monotropic FSH rise in older, ovulatory women: a study of serum and follicular fluid levels of dimeric inhibin A and B in spontaneous menstrual cycles. J Clin Endocrinol Metab. 1996;81:2742-5.
37. Seifer DB, Lambert-Messerlian G, Hogan JW, et al. Day 3 serum inhibin-B is predictive of assisted reproductive technologies outcome. Fertil Steril. 1997;67:110-4.
38. Lass A, Skull J, McVeigh E et al. Measurement of ovarian volume by transvaginal sonography before ovulation induction with human menopausal gonadotropin for in-vitro fertilization can predict poor response. Hum Reprod. 1997;12:294-7.
39. Scheffer GJ, Broekmans FJ, Looman CW, et al. The number of antral follicles in normal women with proven fertility is the best reflection of reproductive age. Hum Reprod. 2003;18:700-6.
40. de Vet A, Laven JS, de Jong FH, et al. Anti-müllerian hormone serum levels: a putative marker for ovarian aging. Fertil Steril. 2002;77:357-62.
41. van Rooij IA, Broekmans FJ, te Velde ER, et al. Serum anti-Müllerian hormone levels: a novel measure of ovarian reserve. Hum Reprod. 2002;17:3065-71.
42. Franks S. Polycystic ovary syndrome. N Engl J Med. 1995;333:853-61.
43. Romeu A, Muasher SJ, Acosta AA, et al. Results of in vitro fertilization attempts in women 40 years of age and older: the Norfolk experience. Fertil Steril. 1987;47:130-6.
44. Horbay G. Hyperstimulation and intrauterine insemination outcomes compared by age and diagnosis [Abstract 145]. Presented at the 46th Annual Meeting of the American Fertility Society, Washington, DC, 1990.
45. Hughes EG, Robertson DM, Handelsman DJ, et al. Inhibin and estradiol responses to ovarian hyperstimulation: effects of age and predictive value for in vitro fertilization outcome. J Clin Endocrinol Metab. 1990;70:358-64.
46. Lim AS, Tsakok MF. Age related decline in fertility: a link to degenerative oocytes? Fertil Steril. 1997;68:265-71.
47. Battaglia DE, Goodwin P, Klein NA, et al. Influence of maternal age on meiotic spindle assembly in oocytes from naturally cycling women. Hum Reprod. 1996;11:2217-22.
48. Hull MG, Fleming CF, Hughes AO, et al. The age-related decline in female fecundity: a quantitative controlled study of implanting capacity and survival of individual embryos after in vitro fertilization. Fertil Steril. 1996;65:783-90.
49. Silber SJ, Nagy Z, Devroey P, et al. The effect of female age and ovarian reserve of pregnancy rate in male infertility: treatment of azoospermia with sperm retrieval and intracytoplasmatic sperm injection. Hum Reprod. 1997;12:2693-700.
50. Cohen J, Elsner C, Malter H, et al. Impairment of the hatching process following IVF in the human and improvement of implantation by assisted hatching using micromanipulation. Hum Reprod. 1990;5:7-13.
51. Bider D, Livshits A, Yonish M, et al. Assisted hatching by zona drilling of human embryos in women of advanced age. Hum Reprod. 1997;12:317-20.
52. Cohen J, Munne S, Palermo G. Microsurgery in preimplantation embryology reproductive endocrinology, surgery, and technology. Philadelphia: Lippincott-New York: Raven Publishers; 1996. pp. 2376.
53. Van Blerkon J, Davis PW, Lee J. ATP content of human oocytes and developmental potential and outcome after in-vitro fertilization and embryo transfer. Hum Reprod. 1995;10:415-24.
54. Flood JT, Chillic CF, van Uem JF, et al. Ooplasmic transfusion: prophase germinal vesicle oocytes made developmentally competent by microinjection of metaphase II egg cytoplasm. Fertil Steril. 1990;53:1049-54.
55. Levron J, Willadsen S, Bertoli M, et al. The development of mouse zygotes after fusion with synchronous and asynchronous cytoplasm. Hum Reprod. 1996;11:1287-92.
56. Cohen J, Scott R, Schimmel T, et al. Birth of infant after transfer of anucleate donor oocyte cytoplasm into recipient eggs. Lancet. 1997;350:186-7.
57. Balmaceda JP, Bernardini L, Ciuffardi I, et al. Oocyte donation in humans: a model to study the effect of age on embryo implantation rate. Hum Reprod. 1994;9:2160-3.

58. Sauer MV, Paulson RJ, Lobo RA. A preliminary report on oocyte donation extending reproductive potential to women over 40. N Engl J Med. 1990;323:1157-60.
59. Paulson RJ, Sauer MV, Lobo RA. Embryo implantation following human in vitro fertilization: importance of endometrial receptivity. Fertil Steril. 1990;53:870-4.
60. Munné S, Sultan KM, Weier HU, et al. Assessment of numerical abnormalities of X, Y, 18 and 16 chromosomes in preimplantation of human embryos before transfer. Am J Obstet Gynecol. 1995;172:1119-9.
61. Munné S, Dailey T, Sultan KM, et al. The use of the first polar bodies for preimplantation diagnosis of aneuploidy. Hum Reprod. 1995;10:1014-20.
62. Munné S, Alikani M, Cohen J, et al. Embryo morphology, developmental rates, and maternal age are correlated with chromosome abnormalities. Fertil Steril. 1995;64:382-91.
63. Munné S, Alonso ML, Grifo J. Unusually high rates of aneuploid embryos in a 28-year-old woman with incontinentia pigmenti. Cytogenet Cell Genet. 1996;72:43-5.
64. Scott RT, Toner JP, Muasher SJ, et al. Follicle-stimulating hormone levels on cycle day 3 are predictive of in vitro fertilization outcome. Fertil Steril. 1989;51:651-4.
65. Widra EA, Gindoff PR, Smotrich DB, et al. Achieving multiple-order embryo transfer identifies women over 40 years of age with improved in vitro fertilization outcome. Fertil Steril. 1996;65:103-8.

26

Preimplantation Genetic Screening/Diagnosis

Anil K Dubey, Gary L Harton, Santiago Munne

CHAPTER CONTENTS

INTRODUCTION

Since the birth of the first *in vitro* fertilization (IVF) baby in 1978, the field of assisted reproductive technology (ART) has expanded overwhelmingly. Over the past 30 years, live birth rates following IVF have been improved with the use of drugs for controlled ovarian hyperstimulation of multiple follicles during the IVF cycle, improved culture media in the laboratory and cryopreservation of embryos for use in future cycles. The microsurgical manipulation of oocytes, sperm and embryos has opened up a new era in the field of ART. Micromanipulation technology has also provided the means whereby a single blastomere or polar body can be successfully removed and used in analysis.[1]

Twenty years ago, preimplantation genetic diagnosis (PGD) became a reality when 2 women with X-linked recessive traits gave birth to a female child after undergoing embryo biopsy for identification of the Y chromosome.[2] Experts in the nascent field predicted that PGD would be used primarily as a method of prenatal testing to prevent inherited genetic diseases in offspring, thus averting the use of selective abortion after invasive genetic testing of the fetus. They did acknowledge the possible use of PGD in the older female population as a method of aneuploidy screening, also known as preimplantation genetic screening (PGS) with the overall hope of improving live birth rates. However, they did not foresee a widespread use of PGD for aneuploidy screening. "Pre-implantation genetic screening would not be widely applied to all IVF patients, but only in order to detect the specific disease or diseases for which a particular couple is at high risk."[3] Nevertheless, PGS is widely used in IVF centers as a method to improve IVF outcomes by removing aneuploid embryos from the cohort before embryo transfer with an eye toward increasing implantation success and therefore pregnancy rates. Although, its use in preventing transmission of known genetic disorders from parents to offspring is well established, its use in the diagnosis of aneuploidy in chromosomally normal genetic parents is controversial. This group includes habitual aborters, patients with advanced maternal age, unexplained infertility and severe male factor.[4]

In the early years of clinical PGS testing, the technique showed great promise,[5,6] however, these studies had limitations, such as inclusion of patients with altered karyotypes[5] and nonrandomization.[6] By the early 2000s, studies were beginning to question the use of PGS for improved success in IVF.[7] Staessen et al.[8] published a randomized controlled trial of 400 patients who were 37 years of age or older where no statistical difference was seen in the implantation rate between PGS and control group using fluorescence *in situ* hybridization (FISH) for chromosomes X, Y, 13, 16, 18, 21 and 22.[8] In 2007, a paper published by Mastenbroek et al.[9] ignited even more controversy. This randomized controlled trial not only showed no statistical difference between the PGS versus a control group, but also demonstrated a significantly lower rate of ongoing pregnancy of the PGS group compared to the control group.[9] The authors concluded that PGS may actually be harmful for IVF outcomes. Since the Mastenbroek study,[11] randomized controlled trials have shown no improvement in IVF outcomes with PGS in poor prognosis patients.[9] Does this mean that doctors should abandon the use of PGS since it did not improve IVF outcomes? This topic remains highly divisive.

The discipline of molecular genetics has expanded remarkably over the past several decades. Before the advent of recombinant DNA technology, the diagnosis of a genetic disorder was based largely on the observation of the phenotype, the construction of pedigrees, and the empiric determination of recurrence risk. Chromosomal analysis, first with metaphase banding and more recently with prometaphase (extended) banding, provided a major advance in the characterization of genetic diseases. Although, these techniques remain an integral part of the diagnosis of genetic disorders, molecular biology has permitted finer resolution of the genetic defect. Through the use of techniques, such as Southern blotting, polymerase chain reaction (PCR), allele-specific oligonucleotide (ASO) probes and DNA sequencing, gene mutations may be effectively screened and characterized. Until recently, genetic diagnosis has been limited to the post implantation period by chorionic villus sampling (CVS) or amniocentesis. However, minute amounts of DNA now may be studied through the use of highly specific PCR tests allowing for preimplantation diagnosis of specific genetic diseases from a single embryonic cell.

The incidence of severe congenital anomalies and genetic disorders that can cause early death or lifelong chronic disease range from 15–45 per 1,000 live births.[10] Currently, prenatal diagnosis of inherited disorders involves the recovery of cells from fetal origin by amniocentesis between 15 and 20 weeks or CVS at 9–12 weeks of gestation. These cells are then subjected to cytogenetic, biochemical and molecular analysis. If the fetus is abnormal, selective reduction may be an option for some couples. Other couples may prefer delivery under planned, controlled circumstances, if fetal survival is desired. Preimplantation genetic diagnosis is particularly beneficial for couples who are at high risk of producing affected offspring, such as autosomal recessive or autosomal dominant disorders. Because PGD is performed before implantation, this technique might be more acceptable to patients, who would not consider abortion.[11,12]

While the use of amplification-based methods to detect and diagnose monogenic diseases is well-accepted throughout the world, the use of PGS to select euploid embryos remains controversial. The safety, diagnostic accuracy and pregnancy rate following PGS in various patient populations must be critically evaluated. This chapter will review the various methods used for PGS and summarizes the current state of PGS of human embryos in ART and the future directions.

HUMAN OOCYTES AND EMBRYO BIOPSY

Several methods for obtaining preimplantation material have been reported in the literature; however, the degree of viability of the embryo following biopsy varies. Although, these have been reviewed in detail elsewhere,[1,11,12] the basic principles of the biopsy of polar bodies (PBs), blastomeres, and trophectoderm cells will be briefly discussed. All of these procedures are carried out in the IVF laboratory with the aid of a micromanipulation setup on an inverted microscope. The basic principle of biopsy remains unchanged for cell types; however, the size of the holding and biopsy pipette differ in diameter for each procedure. The polar body removal (PBR) procedure needs to be carried out on the day of oocyte retrieval, whereas blastomere and blastocyst biopsies are carried out on day 3 and on day 5 or day 6, respectively, following oocyte insemination.

Polar Body Removal

To perform PBR from an oocyte, a holding pipette with an inner diameter of 15–30 µm is filled with light paraffin oil and connected to the suction syringe using the micropipette holder. The beveled pipette with an inner diameter of 15–18 µm is attached to the injector or aspirator syringe. Before micromanipulation, it is necessary to align the tools on the microscope. The oocyte is placed in a droplet of media in the concave portion of a depression slide and covered with paraffin oil. The microtools are then lowered into the medium under direct vision. The oocyte is located and picked up by the holding pipette and secured in the biopsy position by gentle adjustment of the vacuum. The ideal biopsy position for the polar body is at the 12 O'clock position. The beveled micropipette should be placed and inserted as shown in Figure 1A. The zona of the oocyte should be free from other cells. Gentle suction is applied to aspirate the polar body into the micropipette, and the micropipette is removed carefully to avoid any damage to the oocyte. The polar body is then carefully injected into a microcentrifuge tube, which is then transferred to the laboratory performing the genetic analysis. Extreme care must be taken to avoid any contamination of the sample with exogenous sources of DNA. The biopsied oocytes are then inseminated with sperm and cultured. The absence of any significant detrimental effect of PBR on fertilization and pre-embryonic development suggests that the first PB does not play a role in embryo development.[1,13,14]

Blastomere Biopsy

The blastomere biopsy from the cleavage stage embryo can be performed as soon as the embryo reaches the 6–8-cell stage on day 3 post insemination. This procedure is usually performed using aspiration or extrusion techniques (Figure 1B). In the aspiration technique, the blastomere is removed by gentle suction/aspiration of the micropipette. The sampling micropipette passes through the zona either by gentle force, through a hole in the zona made with the help of acid Tyrode's solution, or by a sharpened pipette. In the extrusion method, a beveled pipette is used to create two small holes at two different locations on the zone. The blastomere(s) are disconnected/displaced gently by pushing medium near the cell-to-cell connections. This will enable one or two blastomeres to protrude out of the zona through the second hole and into the medium.

Biopsy of Trophectoderm Cells

Similar to the blastomere biopsy at cleavage stage, a trophectoderm cell biopsy can be performed on the blastocyst by stitch and pull methods (Figure 1C). Briefly, the zona is dissected above the trophectoderm cells opposite to the inner cell mass using the micromanipulation setup. The blastocyst is placed in culture until hatching begins, i.e. when there is a herniation of the trophectoderm cell mass through the cell membrane. The herniated piece of tissue is cut with the help of a sharp needle or blade.[2,14] The cells are then aspirated into the micropipette and transferred to a microcentrifuge tube.

Development of Biopsied Embryos

Numerous animal studies in mammals have not demonstrated any adverse effects of biopsies of embryos on the rate of cleavage and development into blastocyst, implantation or successful pregnancy. Similarly, in the human, biopsy of 1, 2, or 3 blastomeres from 4-, 6-, and 8-cell embryos, respectively, does not seem to affect development to the blastocyst stage when the biopsy is carried out on day 3 after insemination.[15] However, biopsy of 1 of 4 or 2 of 8 blastomeres on day 2 post-insemination at the 4- to 8-cell stages resulted in a retarded cleavage rate and a reduction of the ratio of the inner cell mass to trophectoderm cells at the blastocyst stage.[16,17] Unfortunately, very little is known about the potential of the biopsied embryo for implantation and development with a reduced number of cells. However, reports on cryopreserved embryos suggest that a 50% survival rate of the blastomeres in transferred embryos will result in live deliveries.[17] The only systematic study conducted demonstrated that the developmental capacity of a biopsied embryo in patients carrying an X-linked recessive disorder is not compromised by the biopsy of a day 3 embryo at the 8-cell stage.[18,19] Likewise, no detrimental effects on implantation were demonstrated.

Gardner and Edwards[20] were the first to biopsy rabbit blastocysts for genetic evaluation and confirmed the prediction of gender sexing of newborns. Since then, blastocyst biopsy has been successfully used in rodent,

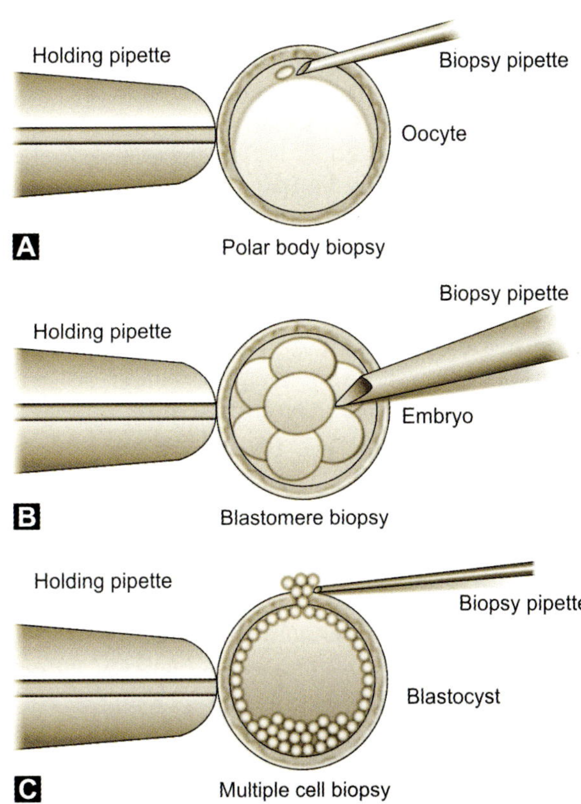

Figures 1A to C Diagrammatic illustrations of the method for (A) Polar body; (B) Blastomere; (C) Multiple cell biopsy of human oocyte and embryo

cattle, and nonhuman primates species for preimplantation genetic diagnosis and subsequent birth of normal offspring. The efficacy of trophectoderm biopsy and the development of human blastocysts were carried out by Dokras et al.[14] The pregnancy rate after blastocyst transfer are similar as compared to 4- to 8-cell stage embryo transfers. At the present time, trophectoderm cell biopsy for PGD from human blastocysts, is very promising but requires cryopreserving the blastocyst.

DNA TECHNIQUES USED IN PGD

Polymerase Chain Reaction

The use of PCR has revolutionized molecular biology, allowing for great leaps forward in the diagnosis and study of genes and gene products. PCR allows very small amounts of DNA to be faithfully reproduced in a very short amount of time. DNA analysis from a single cell was not possible until the advent of PCR. Prior to the advent of PCR, microgram amounts (typically 5–10 µg) were needed to study gene structure by Southern blot analysis. One hundred ng of DNA is sufficient for reproducible amplification by PCR in nearly all cases. Single cell PCR is more problematic, but has generally been successful (see below). PCR results in the amplification of a specific sequence of DNA among the 3 billion base pairs (bp) per haploid genome, so that hundreds of thousands to millions of copies of the desired sequence are produced. The sample is then subjected to electrophoresis on a polyacralymide gel, which would then be stained with ethidium bromide.

To perform PCR, the sequence of at least the boundaries of the region of DNA to be amplified must be known. With knowledge of the outer boundries, small runs of DNA are designed and synthesized as the starting point for DNA amplification. These small runs of DNA are termed primers and typically consist of 20–30 bp of DNA complimentary to the outer limits of DNA of interest. The primers are a necessary starting point for the DNA synthesis. Two other chemical components necessary for PCR are DNA polymerase and deoxyribonucleotides. DNA polymerase is a thermostable enzyme that copies single stranded DNA making double stranded copies. Deoxyribonucleotides are free neucleotides that are the building blocks of DNA. Following the mixture of a cocktail of the above reagents, template DNA is added to the mixture and the sample is heated and cooled through three distinct phases that make up PCR. The first step is denaturation of double-stranded DNA, which is accomplished by heating the sample to 94°C to render the DNA single stranded. The temperature is then lowered (in the 50–55°C range), which permits primer to anneal to the DNA template (Figure 2). The temperature is then increased to approximately 72°C allowing the DNA polymerase to read the single stranded DNA at the very end of the primer, find the free nucleotide that is next in the chain and attach this nucleotide to the chain. The polymerase then moves down to the next base in the chain, and attaches the next nucleotide. DNA polymerase can attach hundreds of bases in just a few seconds time. Each cycle of PCR allows for multiple copies of DNA.

After one cycle of denaturation, annealing and primer extension, the DNA content is doubled; two double-stranded pieces of DNA arise from one piece of double-stranded DNA. After 2 cycles there are four copies, whereas after 3 cycles there are eight. The amount of DNA being amplified increases exponentially with each cycle so that the amount of amplified DNA will be 2^n, when the process is completed. After 30 cycles, which is the typical number of cycles used, the gene of interest may be amplified well over 1 million fold (2^{30}). The amplified product is present in such enormous quantity that it may now be visualized as a band on an agarose gel without the need for a DNA probe. Fragments of several kilobase (kb) can be reproducibly amplified, but larger sequences may be successfully amplified. One important consideration with the use of PCR is the absolute necessity of controls. Both positive and negative controls are invaluable in the interpretation of PCR analysis. The negative control usually consists of all of the necessary reagents for PCR, excluding the DNA. If contaminant DNA is introduced anywhere in the process, the negative control will be positive. If this is the case, the data from the patient DNA is very suspicious and should be further studied. In addition, gloves should be worn at all times, handling of cells and reagents should be done under a tissue culture hood, positive displacement pipettes should be used, reagents should be pipetted in small amounts, and a separate area in the lab should be reserved for PCR only. A devoted pipettor set is another wise precaution to avoid contamination.

Polymerase chain reaction is largely responsible for the successful studies of genes in single cell analysis. Typically, the cell is boiled for 10–15 minutes to produce destruction of cellular proteins, while permitting the DNA to remain intact. When such small quantities of starting DNA template are used for PCR, either a larger number of cycles (between 60 and 75 cycles) may be necessary, or more often, two separate reactions are required to increase the copy number. In the first PCR, 25–35 cycles will not be sufficient to produce a product that can be visualized on a gel. Usually, a small aliquot (1 µl) from this reaction is then subjected to a second PCR to produce the necessary amount of DNA. Primer sets may differ in the two reactions. The primers from the second PCR may be complementary to sequences within the product in the first reaction, so that the product from the second PCR is smaller in size than that of the first reaction. These primers are termed as 'nested primers,' because they are located within the segment of DNA amplified in the first PCR. Quality control assumes particular importance in single cell PCR because any introduction of foreign DNA could cause serious misdiagnosis.

By employing PCR technology, several laboratories accurately predicted the sex of embryos from couples at risk for transmitting X-linked disorders. The first report was from Handyside et al.[18] who used PCR to amplify 149 bp of a 3.4-kb repeat sequence of the Y chromosome to determine the sex of seven embryos. From a single blastomere, the DNA was subjected to 60 cycles of PCR. The amplified samples (aliquot of 10 µl) were then resolved by 12% polyacrylamide gel electrophoresis (PAGE), stained with ethidium bromide, and visualized under ultraviolet light. This procedure was completed in only 5 hours from start to visualization of the PCR product. However, in this series of preimplantation diagnoses, one erroneous diagnosis occurred because of failed amplification of the Y-specific DNA sequence. Similarly, other studies of single cells from male and female embryos have shown that Y-specific sequences have the potential for failed amplification in 15% of the cases.[18]

GENETIC DIAGNOSIS BY PCR

Oocyte and Polar Bodies Diagnosis

Gamete analysis has been performed in humans. There seems to be differences in the frequency of chromosomal abnormalities between spermatozoa and oocytes.[39] Approximately, 5–13% of sperm possess chromosomal abnormalities, although structural abnormalities seem to be more common than numerical abnormalities (aneuploidies). Data concerning oocyte abnormalities are considerably more variable, but in general, aneuploidy is more frequently observed than structural abnormalities. Oocytes and sperm may be used for genetic diagnosis by PCR, but the procedure destroys the cell, which makes these cells impractical for diagnosis. The rates of structural anomalies and aneuploidy seem to be similar for fertile and infertile women, which suggest that zygote selection may be operative in human fertilization.

Of the potential modalities to diagnose genetic disorders before implantation, polar bodies and blastomeres are currently the most commonly studied cells. Unlike meiosis in the male, this result in four haploid spermatozoa, meiosis in the female yields only one mature oocyte with the remainder being PBs. Through the analysis of PBs, the genotype can be predicted for the oocyte, so the oocyte does not need to be studied. Only oocytes predicted to be euploid or containing normal alleles in the case of monogenic disease PGD will be used for fertilization, whereas those harboring mutant alleles or those that are anueploid would not be inseminated.

The basic premise of PB diagnosis relies upon the events taking place during normal meiosis. Normally, in meiosis I, 46 chromosomes are present, which then replicate and produce a 4n complement of genetic material. For an oocyte containing a normal allele and a mutant allele, the first meiotic division will result in one allele segregating to the oocyte and the other allele going to the PB. In the second meiotic division, the resulting cells will have a haploid number of chromosomes. If DNA analysis from the oocyte lacks the known mutation, then PB analysis by PCR should be abnormal. Similarly, if the oocyte possesses the mutation, the PB analysis should be normal. Performance of PCR on the first PB provides genetic diagnosis and spares the oocyte, which now may be used for insemination. It must be stressed, however, that PB diagnosis can only correctly identify mutant versus wild type alleles, if no crossing over occurs during meiosis. If crossing over occurs, both the oocyte and the PB will be heterozygous, so the genotype of the embryo cannot be accurately predicted. Crossing over is a much more common phenomenon at the telomeric regions of chromosomes than at the centromeres, so the gene location on the chromosome plays an important role.

The technique of PB diagnosis has been successfully used in humans for cystic fibrosis, hemophilia A, alpha-l-antitrypsin deficiency, Duchenne muscular dystrophy and Tay-Sachs disease.[13] Before PB diagnosis can be considered a standard of care, its success and risks must be evaluated. Verlinsky et al.[21 45] studied over 100 cases by PB diagnosis and did not find any change in monospermic fertilization rate (59% with PB removal; 64% without), dispermic fertilization rate (8% with PB diagnosis; 5% without), and the percentage of embryos cleaved (100% with PB analysis; 97% without). Failed PCR occurred in 15–20% of PBs with these disorders as a whole. As stressed before, extreme care must be taken when doing PCR on single cells, inasmuch as more cycles must be performed than for PCR using DNA from a number of cells. It is difficult to determine whether the PB diagnosis is correct, because most of the fertilized oocytes will not implant. False-positive results obtained by contamination during PCR amplification do occur and underscore the need for extreme care when PCR is performed from single cells. Much further study is necessary to increase the success of PCR of single cells, because 20% failure of amplification is too high to be of practical value to patients. Because PB diagnosis must be confirmed by blastomere diagnosis, perhaps blastomere biopsy may be preferable to PB diagnosis.

Genetic Diagnosis of Blastomeres

Polymerase chain reaction has been used for specific diagnosis associated with X-linked disorders and single gene defects. The first studies were reported by Handyside et a1.[18] using PCR technology to predict the sex of embryos from eight couples who were at risk for transmitting X-linked disorders. Approximately, 90% of the blastomeres could be sexed by amplifying a 149-bp fragment of a 3.4-kb repeat sequence on the Y chromosome. Sex distribution was approximately 50% male to female. Five embryos from each couple underwent biopsy and at least two female embryos were transferred. Five of the eight women became pregnant with two twin and three singleton implantations. The sex of each of the seven fetuses was female (later confirmed by CVS), except one, resulting in 85% efficiency.

To minimize misdiagnosis because of failure of amplification, duplex PCR has been used to coamplify X and Y chromosome-specific DNA sequence. Grifo et a1.[22] reported a case of a hemophilia carrier who underwent two IVF cycles and gave birth to a noncarrier female child. In this report, a total of 22 embryos were subjected to sexing, and Grifo et al.[33]could identify sex in 77.2% of embryos, but 22.7% of the embryos could not be sexed due to cell loss during the procedure or a weak signal on the gel.

The most important role of PCR methodology has been the detection of single gene defects in preimplantation diagnosis. Earlier studies were carried out on mice, [8,12] but more recently, human oocytes and embryos have been studied to detect single gene defects in disorders, such as Duchenne muscular dystrophy, cystic fibrosis, and sickle cell anemia.[31,36,47,48] Handyside et al.[34] used nested primer PCR to amplify a region of the cystic fibrosis transmembrane conductance regulator gene containing the 3-bp delta F508 deletion from a single blastomere. This initial series consisted of 3 patients, a total of 16 blastomeres obtained from 13 embryos. Amplification was successful in 75% (12/16) of the blastomeres analyzed. Unaffected embryos were transferred (2 each) to 2 different patients, resulting in the birth of an unaffected female child. Disappointingly, the rate of fertilization in this study was surprisingly low (38%).[23]

The use of PCR methodology and problems of diagnostic errors for PGD have been addressed by Navidi and Anaheim[24] using a mathematical model system. They analyzed the frequency of making mistakes in the diagnosis assuming a realistic range of PCR efficiency, cell transfer and contamination errors. Navidi and Arnheim concluded that, in general, analyzing a single blastomere is subject to less misdiagnosis than a PB analysis, except in the case of dominant diseases that are caused by genes located close to the centromere. Further, they stressed that the degree of unacceptable errors can be significantly lowered by analyzing more than one blastomere from a single embryo or by combining PB analysis with blastomere analysis. Moreover, they recommended that, after a successful implantation of the genetically normal embryo(s), the diagnosis should be reconfirmed by CVS or amniocentesis.

FLUORESCENCE IN SITU HYBRIDIZATION

Interphase FISH uses chromosome DNA probes that can signal the presence or absence of a chromosome in a mononucleated cell. These probes comprise of small pieces of DNA that match a sequence of DNA on the chromosome being analyzed and each probe fluoresces a different color. Fluorescent microscopy allows for five different colors to be identified at once. This limits the number of chromosomes that can be tested in a single assay and requires multiple assay rounds, thereby increasing errors. Chromosomes most involved in aneuploidy are 22, 16, 21 and 15.[25,26]

Testing of the critical chromosomes X, Y, 13, 15, 16, 18, 21, 22 demonstrates improved implantation.[13,14,17-20] A decrease in spontaneous abortion has been seen with five probes,[27] but the five chromosome test detects only about 30% of chromosome abnormalities (X, Y, 13, 18, 21). The nine probe test (X, Y, 13, 15, 16, 17, 18, 21, 22) has a 70% detection rate. A twelve probe test (prior eight chromosomes and 8, 14, 17, 20) (Figures 2 and 3) detects 80% of aneuploidies. This data is obtained from spontaneous abortions.[28-30] Comparative genome hybridization (CGH) technology improves the technology of FISH in PGS.[31] Array technology opens the opportunity for what experts in the field have been striving for, a method to test all 24 chromosomes and to identify the nearly normal embryo.

Some studies utilizing FISH-based strategies reported an improvement in implantation rates, reduction in spontaneous abortions and/or an increase in take home baby rate.[15,21,23-32] However, these studies were not randomized. Other studies, some performed in a randomized fashion, did not produce significant improvements or showed a detrimental effect of PGD for aneuploidy[33-36.] Several reasons for these conflicting results have been advanced.

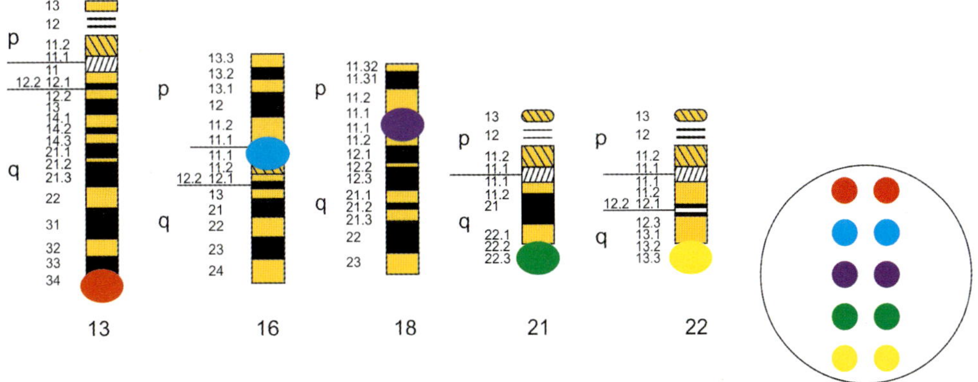

Figure 2 Schematic drawing of FISH probe localization for both 5-probe panel. Chromosomes 13, 16, 18, 21, and 22 are located using fluorescent probes specific to centromeric (16, 18) or subtelomeric (13, 12, 22) sections of each chromosome as seen above. Five colors are used in the 5-probe mix, spectrum red (13), spectrum aqua (16), spectrum blue (18), spectrum green (21) and spectrum gold (22)

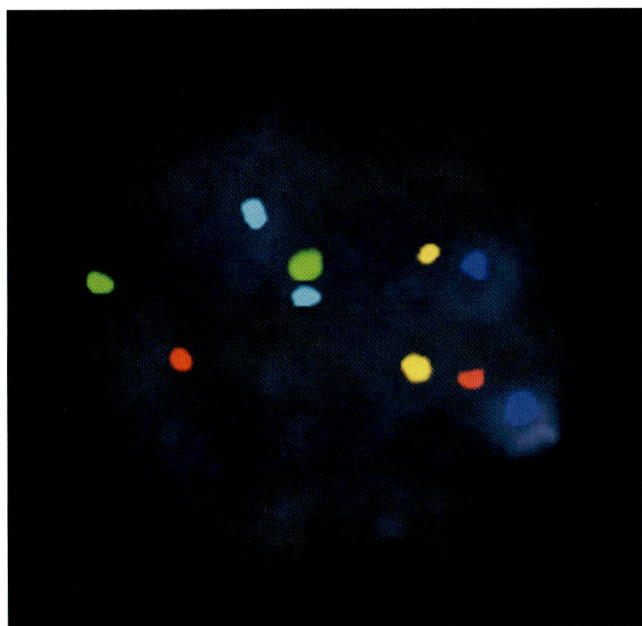

Figure 3 Composite image of 5-probe FISH on a single nucleus from a blastomere removed from a day 3 embryo. Two distinct spots can be seen for each of the colors used in this hybridization. As described above, spectrum red (13), spectrum aqua (16), spectrum blue (18), spectrum green (21), and spectrum gold (22)

The biological argument, which does not explain differences in reports, but attempts to understand why some studies observed a negative effect on outcome, argues that cleavage-stage embryos have such high rates of chromosomal mosaicism that any analysis based upon a single cell is unreliable. Although it is true that mosaicism is common in cleavage-stage embryos (about 30% according to FISH analyses),[1-4] the majority of these embryos display chromosome abnormalities in every cell. In such cases, the biopsied cell may not be chromosomally identical to the remaining cells of the embryo, they may contain errors affecting different chromosomes, but the clinical diagnosis of 'abnormal' is still valid. Large follow-up studies of preimplantation embryos diagnosed using FISH estimate only a 5–7% error caused by mosaicism,[15,37] and thus mosaicism is unlikely to be the primary cause of poor outcomes following PGD.

The most probable cause of intercenter differences in PGD results are variations in the embryological and genetic technologies employed. These encompass all aspects of the process and have been previously reviewed.[32] Here the authors will discuss briefly only a few of the key factors. Probably the most important variable in PGD is the embryo biopsy itself. One of the studies showing no difference in IVF outcome following PGD involved biopsy of two cells from each cleavage-stage embryo.[32] However, the same group later reported that 2-cell biopsy, in contrast to single-cell biopsy, is detrimental to embryo development.[32]

Even biopsying one cell in suboptimal conditions could be extremely damaging to embryo potential. A study conducted by Mastenbroek et al.[9] reported an astonishingly high rate of diagnostic failure (20%), resulting in many embryos being transferred without a diagnosis. The implantation rate of these undiagnosed embryos was 59% lower than the control. In this case, the only difference between the control and test groups appears to have been the biopsy, suggesting that embryo viability was drastically reduced by the biopsy procedures used in the clinics involved.

The second most important factor in obtaining good results can be summarized in the 'error rate'. The steps after biopsy involve fixation, FISH with a variety of potentially different protocols and probes, and cell scoring. However, the overall accuracy of these steps can be summarized in a single number, which is the error rate of a PGD laboratory. This error rate can be obtained by reanalyzing all the cells of nonreplaced embryos (abnormal embryos and arrested normal embryos) and determining if the original diagnosis was correct. Unfortunately, error rates vary widely, ranging from 4–5% to 40–50% depending on the PGD laboratory. As shown in a recent review, error rates around 50% will in fact decrease implantation rates.[30]

When performed using appropriate, well-validated methods, FISH can detect 90% of the chromosome abnormalities detected by CGH,[50] and some PGD laboratories do appear to obtain consistently good results with FISH and cleavage-stage embryo biopsy. Regardless, the field of PGD is evolving away from biopsying at this stage of embryo development and is increasingly focusing on biopsy of polar bodies from oocytes or zygotes or removal of trophectoderm cells from blastocysts. These embryonic stages may be more resilient to technical manipulation. Additionally, the limited chromosomal screening conveyed by FISH is increasingly being replaced by comprehensive methods of DNA analysis, which detect close to 100% of chromosomal abnormalities. The new wave of aneuploidy testing technologies are extremely redundant (each chromosome tested multiple times at different sites), readily automated, less subjective, and theoretically less prone to errors.

COMPREHENSIVE DNA ANALYSIS TECHNIQUES

Comparative genome hybridization was first applied to day 3 embryo biopsies.[33-36] However, CGH is time consuming and is incompatible with day 3 biopsy and transfer by day 5, necessitating cryopreservation of embryos while testing is carried out. At the time that it was first applied, embryo freezing was a relatively inefficient technique and the low survival rate of thawed embryos likely neutralized any beneficial effects of CGH. For these reasons, CGH was temporarily abandoned and not applied again until the development of vitrification.[31] In conjunction with vitrification, CGH has been clinically applied to polar bodies[37,39] and blastocyst biopsies.[31] The combination of CGH, blastocyst biopsy and vitrification significantly improved implantation rates in a recent study, from 46.5% in controls to 72.2% in cycles with screening, with nearly 100% of blastocysts surviving biopsy.[31] However, many clinics are not yet proficient at blastocyst culture and vitrification. Furthermore, freezing adds extra cost to the cycle and a majority of patients prefer to have a fresh cycle. Thus, for some laboratories this means day 3 biopsy combined with comprehensive chromosome analysis and fresh transfer on day 5 of embryo development. However, recent developments of regionalized laboratories with extra staffing has allowed for some laboratories to move to day 5 (trophectoderm) biopsy with fresh embryo transfer on the morning of day-6.

Three other techniques, microarray CGH (array-CGH or aCGH),[41-46] single nucleotide polymorphism (SNP) microarrays[47-49] and quantitative fluorescent PCR (QF-PCR), can be used for comprehensive chromosome analysis of single cells from day 3 biopsy, as well as trophectoderm samples from day 5 biopsy and yield results in 24 hours. The rapid turnaround time for these methods eliminates the need to cryopreserve embryos while testing is carried out.

Array-CGH (aCGH) is already widely used for the cytogenetic analysis of prenatal and postnatal samples[50-55] since it is rapid, cost effective and allows chromosomal regions to be screened at high resolution. Several types of aCGH platform are available for the purposes of aneuploidy screening (Figure 4). The variety most commonly used for the purpose of PGD utilizes bacterial artificial chromosome (BAC) probes, about 150,000 bp in length, covering all chromosome bands and giving a 4MB or lower resolution. Even higher resolutions are achievable, but not generally recommended since at that level the difference between clinically significant duplications/deletions and normally occurring copy number variations is less clear. A microarray recently validated for PGD had 4,000 probes and thus covered ~25% of the genome sequence.[52] Microarray-CGH has a similar accuracy rate to conventional CGH, and should therefore be capable of producing similar results to those obtained in the promising CGH study performed by Schoolcraft et al.[31]

CGH and aCGH provide a quantitative analysis based on comparing the relative amount of DNA from two different sources, one from the clinical sample (e.g. a cell from an embryo) and another from a chromosomally normal individual. DNA samples from the two sources are differentially labeled and hybridized to either metaphase chromosomes (CGH) or probes on a microarray (aCGH). In the case of aCGH, each probe reveals the relative amounts of these two DNAs at a single chromosomal site. Since multiple copies of each probe are placed on the microarray and each chromosome is tested at many distinct loci, the diagnosis is very accurate (Figures 5A to C).

Chromosome imbalances (aneuploidies, unbalanced translocations, deletions and duplications) are easily detected using CGH and aCGH, but a limitation of these approaches is that diploidy cannot be distinguished from changes involving loss or gain of an entire set of chromosomes (e.g. haploidy, triploidy, tetraploidy, etc). How important is this? In a recently submitted paper (Munne et al. personal communication) about 7.7% (n= 91,073) of the supposedly 2PN embryos tested were polyploid or haploid but the majority of them had additional abnormalities detectable by CGH or aCGH and only 1.8% of all embryos were homogeneously polyploid or haploid. Furthermore, of those, the majority arrested by day 4, leaving only 0.2% of developing embryos

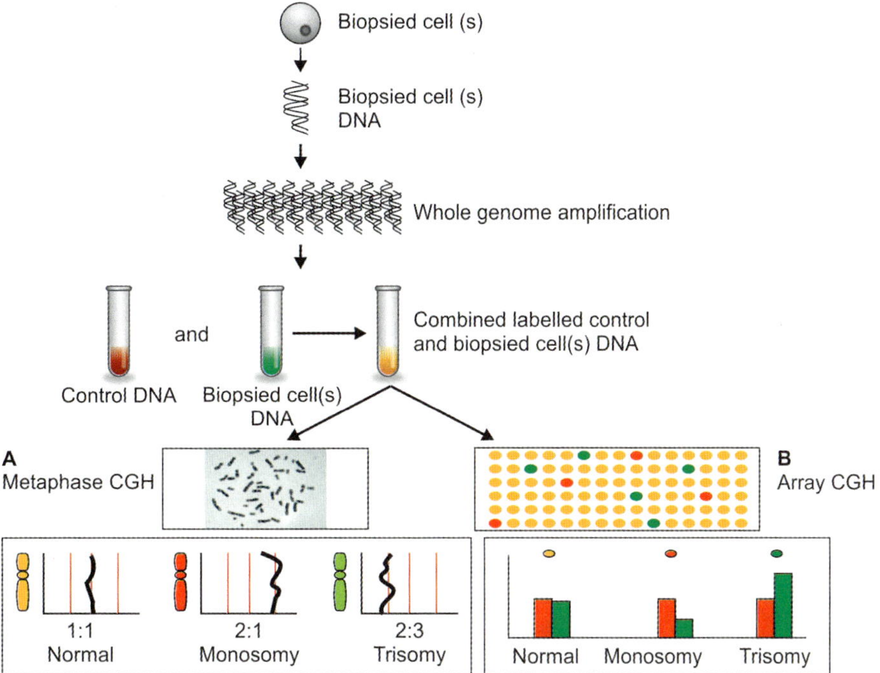

Figure 4 Comparative genomic hybridization; (A) Metaphase CGH and (B) Array CGH. First the biopsied material undergoes whole genome amplification and the embryonic DNA is labelled in green fluorescence. The samples are then cohybridized onto either (A) A metaphase spread or (B) An array platform. In both cases, a computer analyses the ratio of red to green fluorescence. Courtesy of Thalia Mamas and Leoni Xanthopoulou, UCL Centre for PG&D, UCL, Adapted from Harper and Harton, 2010

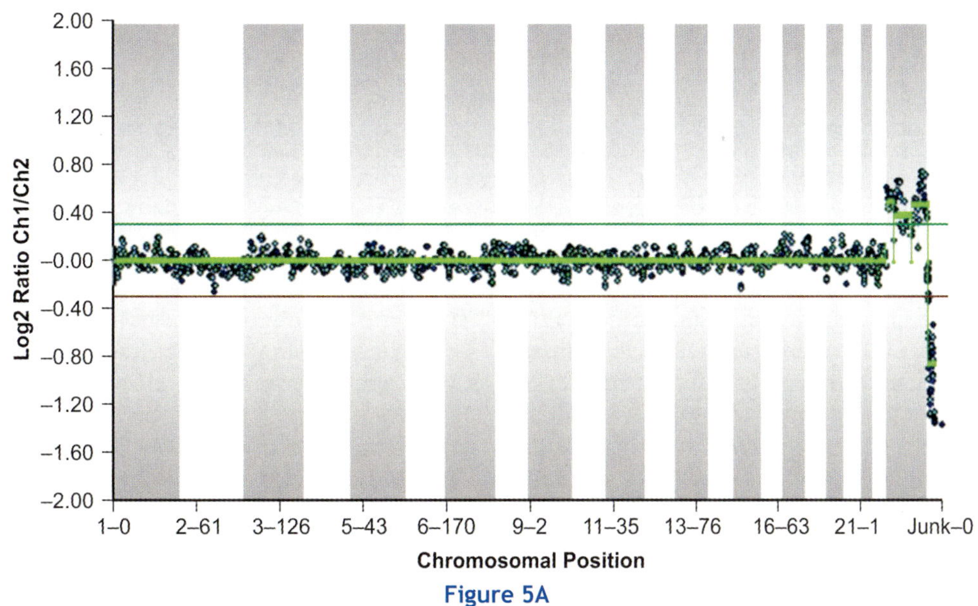

Figure 5A

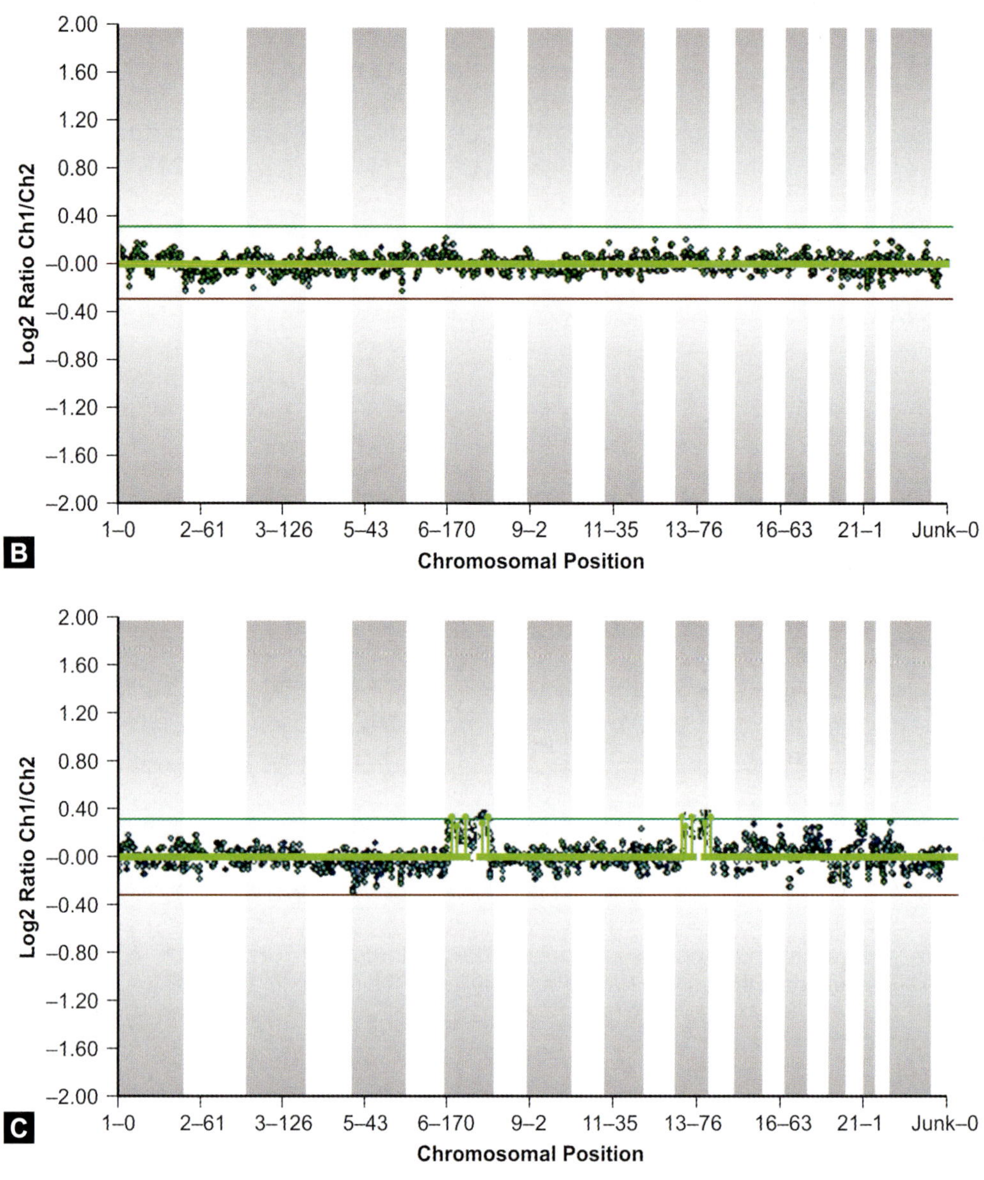

Figures 5B and C

Figures 5A to C Array CGH images following processing. Chromosome number can be found on the X axis (1-22, X, Y) and fluorescence intensity can be found on the Y axis. 1:1 ratio of green to red bright green line, 2:1 ratio of green to red above the dark green line (trisomy), 2:1 ratio of red to green below the red line (monosomy). Top is normal female, middle is normal male, bottom is abnormal, +7, +13.

uniformly polyploid or haploid. This suggests that failure to detect polyploid embryos may rarely lead to a misdiagnosis, but is unlikely to have a significant impact on the clinical efficacy of the screening using aCGH or CGH.

Single nucleotide polymorphisms are areas of the genome where a single nucleotide in the DNA sequence varies within the population. Most SNPs are biallelic, existing in one of two forms, and are found scattered throughout the genome. By determining the genotype of multiple SNPs along the length of each chromosome a haplotype (a contiguous series of polymorphisms on the same chromosome) can be assembled. This ultimately allows the inheritance of individual chromosomes or pieces of chromosomes to be tracked from parents to embryos. Current SNP microarrays simultaneously assay hundreds of thousands of SNPs, while utilizing powerful software to distinguish how many copies of each chromosome was inherited by an embryo.[53,55,57]

All of the new generation of chromosome screening methods (CGH, aCGH and SNP-microarrays) relies on whole genome amplification (WGA) to amplify DNA from cells. CGH can be performed in combination with a variety of WGA methods; however, SNP-microarrays are more sensitive to the type of amplification technique used and are not compatible with all methods. Currently, WGA methods like multiple displacement amplification (MDA), GenomePlex and PicoPlex are most commonly used for SNP-microarrays. These amplification methods allow for better overall coverage of the genome compared with earlier WGA methods (e.g. degenerate oligonucleotide primed PCR) and are less inclined to preferentially amplify some parts of the genome while leaving others unamplified or under amplified.

Currently, a few PGD groups around the world are validating SNP-microarrays and analysis software for clinical use in PGD for aneuploidy screening. It is expected that data from the clinical use of SNP-microarrays will closely match the data from CGH and aCGH testing. While the technologies differ greatly, both types of arrays (CGH-based and SNP-based) are trying to answer the same question; how many copies of each chromosome is present in a sample?

The small size of the SNP array probes can lead to poor hybridization efficiencies and low signal intensities for individual probes. This factor, coupled with the failure of WGA methods to amplify the entirety of the genome, can lead to many probes yielding no result (i.e. a low 'call rate'). Also, allele drop out (ADO) and/or preferential amplification (PA) of one SNP allele versus another can lead to a great deal of 'noise' in the system; which requires sophisticated computer-based interpretation. Several methods for the cleaning up of data from SNP-microarrays have been developed: Qualitative methods, looking only at the inheritance of specific SNPs and requiring comparison with parental DNA samples; quantitative approaches, assessing only the intensity of SNP calls; and techniques combining qualitative and quantitative methods, using both SNP intensity calls and inheritance patterns.

For qualitative approaches, it is necessary to assess parental DNA prior to clinical embryo testing. The key requirement is the deduction of the four parental haplotypes for each chromosome. Embryo testing is then focused on detecting the individual parental haplotypes, revealing how many chromosomes were inherited from each parent i.e. Karyomapping.[53] This approach has the disadvantage that mitotic abnormalities, in which only two haplotypes are present in a trisomy (i.e. caused by duplication of 1 of the 2 chromosomes in the embryo after fertilization), will not be detected. This can misdiagnose a substantial amount of embryos, since 30% of aneuploid embryos contain mitotic abnormalities (mosaics).[58] A quantitative approach compares the intensity of each SNP against the other SNPs. A purely quantitative approach for aneuploidy screening may not require parental testing ahead of the cycle, however, this approach would not be compatible with combination testing of single gene defects with aneuploidy screening (discussed below). This approach is currently the least developed. A qualitative/quantitative approach has also been applied clinically, and probably can obviate the issues mentioned above for purely qualitative or quantitative approaches.[57,58] All of the analysis approaches still share one limitation and that is the diagnosis of tetraploidies. In a tetraploid cell, only two haplotypes are present (i.e. a postmeiotic duplication of a euploid cell), therefore all SNPs will have the same intensity.

SNP-based microarrays offer some advantages over aCGH: (a) if qualitative analysis is employed, SNP-based microarrays can also detect the parental origin of any chromosome abnormalities. This may be valuable in rare instances of young couples producing many chromosome abnormalities, but of little relevance to cases of advanced maternal age where at least 90% of the aneuploidies will be maternal in origin; (b) SNP microarrays applied to PGD for chromosome rearrangements can differentiate between normal and balanced (carrier) embryos. However, because the rate of abnormalities in translocation cases is generally very high (> 80%),[59] the great majority of PGD cycles do not have a surplus of embryos with a balanced chromosome constitution. In most cases whatever balanced embryos are available are needed for transfer; (c) SNP arrays can directly produce a fingerprint of the embryo, allowing for assessment of which of the transferred embryos led to a pregnancy. However, if a laboratory is using aCGH, a similar test can be performed by utilizing a small aliquot of the DNA produced by WGA to perform conventional DNA fingerprinting; (d) Finally, qualitative SNP arrays can also detect uniparental disomy (UDP), although this is a very rare event (e.g. uniparental disomy 15 occurs in 0.001% of newborns (OMIM)).

A major disadvantage of a qualitative or combination approach to SNP array analysis is the need to assess parental DNA ahead of the PGD cycle. This complicates patient management, adds substantially to the cost of the test, and precludes ad hoc decisions on biopsy for PGD. Approximately, 20% of IVF cycles with planned PGD are cancelled on day 3 due to low embryo numbers. Thus, these patients would have spent money on pre-cycle parental testing that was ultimately unnecessary. In addition, a recent commentary by Bisignano et al.[60] questions the use of qualitative SNP arrays for aneuploidy screening in regards to data cleaning, and potential errors in assigning the parent of origin in errors, and UPD.

Also, at last year's American Society of Reproductive Medicine (ASRM) meeting, a quantitative polymerase chain reaction (qPCR) method was described and also showed similar advantages to aCGH and SNP array and very promising pregnancy results.[61] As the qPCR technique has not been published to date, comparing and contrasting this platform to aCGH and SNPa is impossible at this moment.

VALIDATION OF CGH AND SNP ARRAYS

Due to the intrinsic and often unforeseen problems with every new technology, a novel method should always be validated against other, more established methods.[62] Assessing a new approach against itself may preclude the detection of technique related flaws. Thus, validation by inadequate methods, such as the analysis of cell lines with defined chromosome abnormalities which cannot mimic mosaicism and other peculiarities of the cell being tested; analysis of eggs or embryos by one technique with analysis of polar bodies or the remainder of the embryo by the same technique which will preclude identifying abnormalities not detectable by that technique; blindly replacing undiagnosed embryos (either by single embryo transfer or fingerprinting the embryo) and following pregnancies and clinical losses to determine the fate of each tested embryo which does not account for the status of nonimplanted embryos; or using the SNP calls in one chromosome as internal controls for other SNPs in that same chromosome[62] may lead to false assumptions. In addition, the use of analysis tools that are qualitative in nature will miss the presence of two chromosomes of the same grandparental origin, and the errors caused by mosaicism will not be taken into account in this validation mode, resulting in bogus 99.9% confidence results.

In the authors opinion, the optimal method for validating a new technique is to reanalyze those embryos that were not transferred to the patient, either because they underwent arrest or because they were diagnosed chromosomally abnormal. The reanalysis of these embryos should be done with another well-established technique, the 'gold standard'. This would discern shortcomings of the new method under evaluation and account for issues related to embryo biology, such as mosaicism. The only problem with this approach is that euploid arresting embryos may become abnormal (karyokinesis without cytokinesis) from day 3 to day 5 before reanalysis[68,69] and there is a scarcity of non-replaced normal embryos.

To simplify comparison between studies, an error should be classified as diagnosing an embryo as euploid when reanalysis shows that it was abnormal or vice versa. Due to the extent of mosaicism, an error rate per chromosome has questionable relevance and no clinical importance compared to an error rate per embryo.

SNP-microarrays have undergone a variety of validation experiments, such as comparison of PGD results and analysis of babies born,[58] SNP-microarray reanalysis of embryos previously analyzed by SNP arrays,[54] and using data from one set of SNPs as internal controls for another set of SNPs.[55] To date, no studies have confirmed the original diagnosis by reanalyzing the remaining embryonic cells with a different technique.

Microarray-CGH for PGD has been validated by analysis of single cells from known cell lines (Dagan Wells, personal communication) and by analyzing eggs with aCGH and comparing them to the results obtained using aCGH of the corresponding PBs.[63] In a recent study, day 3 embryos analyzed by PGD with aCGH that were not replaced because of chromosome or morphological abnormalities were reanalyzed in most of their remaining cells by FISH using 12 probes for the most common chromosome abnormalities plus probes for any chromosomes found abnormal according to aCGH. Only 1.9% (1/54) of embryos were found to be incorrectly diagnosed.[64]

CLINICAL RESULTS

Of the techniques discussed, CGH is the one for which the greatest quantity of clinical data is available[31-40] with one study reporting a 74% ongoing pregnancy rate per transfer and 63% per retrieval in women with an average age of 37.5 years. For patients of a similar age, receiving blastocyst transfer, Schoolcraft et al.[31] detected a significant increase in implantation rates, from 46.5% to 72.2% ($p < 0.001$) following embryo selection using CGH. Interestingly, both studies showed high implantation rates and both avoided cleavage stage embryo biopsy and transferred embryos that had previously been cryopreserved in a later cycle. In addition to the potential benefits of transferring euploid embryos, there may be additional advantages associated with transfer in a nonstimulated cycle[34,36,37] Loss of blastocyst stage embryos after devitrification in the study by Schoolcraft et al. was minimal (0.7%).[31]

Less clinical data is available from SNP-/CGH-microarrays and QF-PCR. In presentations at ASRM, Schlenker et al.[74] reported that CGH- and SNP-microarrays provided the same high implantation rates after blastocyst biopsy and vitrification.

Regarding day 3 biopsy followed by aCGH and day 5 replacement, the authors' most recent data[61] showed that only 118/151 PGD cycles had normal embryos for transfer in a population of 38 years of age. The pregnancy rate was 59% per transfer compared with 38% in controls with a transfer ($p < 0.001$). The ongoing pregnancy rate for the PGD group was 54% per transfer, compared with 31.1% in controls with a transfer ($p < 0.001$). These results are encouraging, but not as impressive as the day-5 (blastocyst) biopsy results. It is probable that the difference between clinical results obtained using CGH and aCGH is related to the stage at which biopsy was carried out rather than to differences in the method of chromosome screening. It is very likely that aCGH will replicate the results obtained by CGH when applied in conjunction with blastocyst biopsy. In summary, although data on the clinical application of comprehensive chromosome analysis techniques is preliminary, all studies suggest a significant improvement in ART results.[65-68]

Neither CGH-microarrays, nor the SNP-microarrays in current use can directly detect gene defect mutations. However, SNP-microarrays can be used to indirectly infer the presence or absence of a chromosome segment containing a mutant gene (i.e. identification of the same SNP haplotype as the parental chromosome carrying the mutation). A diagnosis can be performed based upon this sort of information, indeed, this approach has recently been applied clinically for the simultaneous detection of gene defects and chromosome abnormalities.[69]

In the case of aCGH, although gene defects cannot be detected directly, enough DNA is produced during the WGA step of the procedure that an aliquot can be used for aCGH analysis of chromosome abnormalities and another taken for PCR-based analysis of gene defects.

The high levels of ADO recorded after WGA mean that direct detection of a mutation using a microarray is likely to be less reliable than existing forms of PGD. Microarray-based diagnosis will be safer using approaches, such as Karyomapping, where conclusions are based upon the results from multiple linked SNPs, rather than a single mutation site. While the sort of microarrays used for preconception screening are not currently suitable for PGD, it is anticipated that their use will significantly increase the identification of high risk couples and therefore lead to an increase in the usage of genetic testing modalities, such as prenatal testing and PGD.

SUMMARY

Preimplantation genetic diagnosis for aneuploidy or PGS has become a fairly routine part of ART worldwide. Although, the theory of aneuploidy screening makes scientific sense, there are no RCT that have shown a benefit of screening embryos for common chromosome anomalies. Here the authors discuss both the positive and negative aspects of current technology and review the literature to this point. Topics, such as mosaicism of early embryos, the limitations of older technology like FISH, as well as poor technique in the laboratories carrying out the embryology and genetic diagnostics, are discussed. New testing methodologies that allow analysis of the entire chromosome complement, including array-based testing platforms, as well as quantitative fluorescent PCR, have shown promise in a few recent publications and abstracts at scientific meetings. The two principal array-based platforms are explained, then compared and contrasted, followed by a discussion of validation strategies for new technologies. Finally, the current state of the clinical use of array-based testing is reviewed. A few reports have shown a benefit of aneuploidy screening using, array-based testing platforms, rekindling interest and hope in PGS.

CONCLUSION

Because it is still in the evolving phase of development, PGS/PGD is offered at only a few reference and clinical labs in the world at the present time. Initial experience suggests that PGD could be provided only in a few specialized centers where there is collaboration among many different specialties of medicine, such as reproductive endocrinology, embryology, cytogenetic, and clinical and molecular genetics. Such a team approach would be instrumental in establishing a PGD/PGS labs in major metropolitan cities around the world in association with IVF and specialized genetics programs.

The application of PGS/ PGD will also depend on the cost, which is currently too high to be affordable. However, with progress both in IVF and genetic analysis, the cost can probably be expected to decline. Moreover, it is too early to fully consider the cost effectiveness of this new option when considering the benefited which are vital for the couples at high genetic risk.

REFERENCES

1. Dubey AK, Layman LC. Preimplantation genetic diagnosis. Assist Reprod Rev. 1993;3:224-31.
2. Handyside AH, Kontogianni EH, Hardy K, et al. Pregnancies from biopsied human preimplantation embryos sexed by Y-specific DNA amplification. Nature. 1990;344(6268):768-70.
3. Whittingham DG, Penketh R. Prenatal diagnosis in the human pre-implantation period. Meeting held at the

Ciba Foundation on the 13th November 1986. Hum Reprod. 1987;2(3):267-70.
4. Harper J, Coonen E, De Rycke M, et al. What next for preimplantation genetic screening (PGS)? A position statement from the ESHRE PGD Consortium steering committee. Hum Reprod. 2010;25(4):821-3.
5. Gianaroli L, Magli MC, Ferraretti AP, et al. Preimplantation diagnosis for aneuploidies in patients undergoing in vitro fertilization with a poor prognosis: identification of the categories for which it should be proposed. Fertil Steril. 1999;72(5):837-44.
6. Munné S, Magli C, Cohen J, et al. Positive outcome after preimplantation diagnosis of aneuploidy in human embryos. Hum Reprod. 1999;14(9):2191-9.
7. Shahine LK, Cedars MI. Preimplantation genetic diagnosis does not increase pregnancy rates in patients at risk for aneuploidy. Fertil Steril. 2006;85(1):51-6.
8. Staessen C, Platteau P, Van Assche E, et al. Comparison of blastocyst transfer with or without preimplantation genetic diagnosis for aneuploidy screening in couples with advanced maternal age: a prospective randomized controlled trial. Hum Reprod. 2004;19(12):2849-58.
9. Mastenbroek S, Twisk M, van Echten-Arends J, et al. In vitro fertilization with preimplantation genetic screening. N Engl J Med. 2007;357(1):9-17.
10. Verlinsky Y, Kuliev AM. Preimplantation diagnosis of genetic diseases: A new technique in assisted reproduction. In: Verlinsky, Kuliev AM (Eds). New York: Wiley-Liss; 1992.
11. Train JJ, Handyside AH. Embryo biopsy strategies for preimplantation diagnosis. Fertil Steril. 1993;59:943-52.
12. Grifo JA, Boyle A, Lavy G, et al. Pre-embryo biopsy and analysis of blastomere by in situ hybridization. Am J Obstet Gynol. 1990;63:2013-9.
13. Verlisky Y, Cieslak J. Preimplantation diagnosis genetic diseases: A new technique in assisted reproduction. In: Verlinskr Y, Kuliev AM. (Eds). Embryological and technical aspects of preimplantation genetic diagnosis. New York: Wiley. Liss; 1992. pp. 49-67.
14. Dokras A, Sarocnt IL, Ross C, et al. Trophectoderm biopsy in human blastocysts. Hum Reprod. 1990;5:821-5.
15. Hardy K, Martin KL, Leese IU, et al. Human preimplantation development in vitro is not adversely affected by biopsy at 8-cell stage. Hum Reprod. 1990;5:708-14.
16. Hardy K, Handyside AH. Biopsy of cleavage stage human embryos and diagnosis of single gene defects by DNA amplification. Arch Pathol Lab Med. 1992; 116(4):388-92.
17. Simpson JL, Carson. SA. Preimplantation genetic diagnosis. N Eng J Med. 1992;327:951-3.
18. Handysicle AN, Kantogianni H, Hardy R, et al. Pregnancies from biopsied human preimplementation embryo sexed by Y-specific DNA amplification. Nature. 1991;344:768-70.
19. Handyside AH. Human embryo biopsy of the 2nd day after insemination for preimplantation diagnosis: Removal of a quarter of embryo retards. Fertil Steril. 1992;58:970-6.
20. Gardner R, Edwards PG Control of sex ratio at full term in rate rabbis by transferring seized blastocysts. 1968;215:346-8.
21. Verlinsky Y, Cieslak J, Evsikov S, et al. Reliability of preconception and preimplantation genetic diagnosis. Proceedings of the eight international congress of human genetics. Am J Hum Genet. 1991;49:22.
22. Grifo JA, Tang YX, Cohen J, et al. Pregnancy after embryo biopsy and coamplification of DNA from X and Y chromosomes. JAMA. 1992;268:727-9.
23. Handyside AH, Lesko LG, Train JJ, et al. Birth of normal girl after in vitro fertilization and preimplantation diagnostic testing for cystic fibrosis. New Eng J Med. 1992;327:902-9.
24. Navidi W, Amheim N. Using PCR in preimplantation genetic disease diagnosis. Hunt Reprod. 1991;6:836-49.
25. Harper JC, Coonen E, et al. Mosaicism of autosomes and sex chromosomes in morphologically normal, monospermic preimplantation human embryos. Prenat Diagn. 1995;15(1):41-9.
26. Munné S, Sultan KM, Weier HU, et al. Assessment of numeric abnormalities of X, Y, 18 and 16 chromosomes in preimplantation human embryos before transfer. Am J Obstet Gynecol. 1995;172 (4 Pt 1):1191-9.
27. Gianaroli L, Magli MC, Ferraretti AP, et al. Preimplantation diagnosis for aneuploidies in patients undergoing in vitro fertilization with a poor prognosis: identification of the categories for which it should be proposed. Fertil Steril. 1999;72(5):837-44.
28. Munné S, Bahçe M, Sandalinas M, et al. Differences in chromosome susceptibility to aneuploidy and survival to first trimester. Reprod Biomed Online. 2004;8(1):81-90.
29. Munné S, Sandalinas M, Escudero T, et al. Improved implantation after preimplantation genetic diagnosis of aneuploidy. Reprod Biomed Online. 2003;7(1):91-7.
30. Munné S, Fischer J, Warner A, et al. Referring Centers PGD Group. Preimplantation genetic diagnosis significantly reduces pregnancy loss in infertile couples: a multi-center study. Fertil Steril. 2006;85(2):326-32.
31. Schoolcraft WB, Fragouli E, Stevens J, et al. Clinical application of comprehensive chromosomal screening at the blastocyst stage. Fertil Steril. 2010;94(5):1700-6.
32. Munné S, Wells D, Cohen C. Technology requirements for preimplantation genetic diagnosis to improve assisted reproduction outcomes. Fertil Steril. 2010;94(2):408-30.
33. Wells D, Sherlock JK, Handyside AH, et al. Detailed chromosomal and molecular genetic analysis of single cells by whole genome amplification and comparative genome hybridization. Nucleic Acid Res. 1999;27:1214-21.
34. Voullaire L, Wilton L, Slater H, et al. Detection of aneuploidy in single cells using comparative genome hybridization. Prenat diagn. 1999;19:846-51.
35. Wells D, Delhanty JDA. Comprehensive chromosomal analysis of human preimplantation embryos using whole genome amplification and single cell comparative genomic hybridization. Mol Human Reprod. 2000;6: 1055-62.

36. Wilton L, Williamson R, McBain J, et al. Birth of a healthy infant after preimplantation confirmation of euploidy by comparative genomic hybridization. N Engl J Med. 2001;345:1537-41.
37. Wells D, Escudero T, Levy B, et al. First clinical application of comparative genome hybridization (CGH) and polar body testing for Preimplantation genetic diagnosis (PGD) of aneuploidy. Fertil Steril. 2002;78:543-5.
38. Hellani A, Abu-Amero K, Azouri J, et al. Successful pregnancies after application of array-comparative genomic hybri Treff N, Su J, Tao X, Miller K,, Levy B., Scott RT (2010) A novel single-cell DNA fingerprinting method successfully distinguishes sibling human embryos. Fertil Steril. 2010;93(7):2453-5.
39. Johnson DS, Gemelos G, Baner J, et al. Preclinical validation of a microarray method for full molecular karyotyping of blastomeres in a 24-h protocol. Hum Reprod. 2010;25(4):1066-75.
40. Sismani C, Kitsiou-Tzeli S, Ioannides M, et al. Cryptic genomic imbalances in patients with de novo or famililal apparently balanced translocations and abnormal phenotype. Mol Cytogenet. 2008;1(1):15.
41. Goobie S, Knijnenburg J, FitzPatrick D, et al. Molecular and clinical characterization of de novo and familial cases with microduplication 3q29: guidelines for copy number variation case reporting. Cytogenet Genome Res. 2008;123(1-4):65-78.
42. Dimova I, Vazharova R, Nikolova D, et al. Whole genome analysis by array-based comparative genomic hybridization in patients with congenital malformations. Balkan J of Medical genetics. 2008;11(1):33-40.
43. Beaudet AL, Belmont JW. Array-based DNA diagnostics: let the revolution begin. Annu Rev Med. 2008;59:113-29.
44. Heinrich U, Imma Rost, Anthony Brown, et al. Array comparative genomic hybridisation in clinical diagnostics: principles and applications. J Lab Med. 2009;33(5):255-66.
45. Stejskalová E, Malis J, Snajdauf J, et al. Cytogenetic and array comparative genomic hybridization analysis of a series of hepatoblastomas. Cancer Genet Cytogenet. 2009;194(2):82-7.
46. Hu DG, Webb G, Hussey N. Aneuploidy detection in single cells using DNA array-based comparative genomic hybridization. Mol Hum Reprod. 2004;10:283-9.
47. Le Caignec C, Spits C, Sermon K, et al. Single-cell chromosomal imbalances detection by array CGH. Nucleic Acids Res. 2006;34:e68.
48. Hellani A, Abu-Amero K, Azouri J, et al. Successful pregnancies after application of array-comparative genomic hybridization in PGS-aneuploidy screening. Reprod Biomed Online. 2008;17:841-7.
49. Fishel S, Gordon A, Lynch C, et al. Live birth after polar body array comparative genomic hybridization prediction of embryo ploidy-the future of IVF? Fertil Steril. 2010;93(3):1006.e7-10.
50. Gutiérrez-Mateo C, Colls P, Sánchez-García J, et al. Validation of microarray comparative genomic hybridization for comprehensive chromosome analysis of embryos. Fertil Steril. 2011;95(3):953-8.
51. Handyside AH, Harton GL, Mariani B, et al. Karyomapping: a universal method for genome wide analysis of genetic disease based on mapping crossovers between parental haplotypes. J Med Genet. 2009;47(10):651-8.
52. Treff N, Su J, Tao X, et al. A novel single-cell DNA fingerprinting method successfully distinguishes sibling human embryos. Fertil Steril. 2010;93(7):2453-5.
53. Johnson DS, Gemelos G, Baner J, et al. Preclinical validation of a microarray method for full molecular karyotyping of blastomeres in a 24-h protocol. Hum Reprod. 2010;25(4):1066-75.
54. Sismani C, Kitsiou-Tzeli S, Ioannides M, et al. Cryptic genomic imbalances in patients with de novo or familial apparently balanced translocations and abnormal phenotype. Mol Cytogenet. 2008;1(1):15.
55. Goobie S, Knijnenburg J, FitzPatrick D, et al. Molecular and clinical characterization of de novo and familial cases with microduplication 3q29: guidelines for copy number variation case reporting. Cytogenet Genome Res. 2008;123(1-4):65-78.
56. Dimova I, Vazharova R, Nikolova D, et al. Whole genome analysis by array-based comparative genomic hybridization in patients with congenital malformations. Balkan J of Medical genetics. 2008;11(1):33-40.
57. Beaudet AL, Belmont JW. Array-based DNA diagnostics: let the revolution begin. Annu Rev Med. 2008;59:113-29.
58. Colls P, Escudero T, Zheng X, et al. Increased efficiency of preimplantation genetic diagnosis for infertility through reanalysis of dubious signals. Fertil Steril. 2007; 88:53-61.
59. Munné S, Sandalinas M, Escudero T, et al. Outcome of preimplantation genetic diagnosis of translocations. Fertil Steril. 2000;73:1209-18.
60. Bisignano A, Wells D, Harton G, et al. PGD and aneuploidy screening for 24 chromosomes: advantages and disadvantages of competing platforms. Reprod Biomed Online. 2011;23(6):677-85.
61. Scott RT, Tao X, Taylor D, et al. A prospective randomized controlled trial demonstraing significantly increased clinical preznancy rates following 24 chromosome aneuploidy screening: biopsy and analysis on day 5 with fresh transfer. Fertil Steril. 2010;94:S2(O-65).
62. Gutiérrez-Mateo C, Colls P, Sánchez-García J, et al. Validation of microarray comparative genomic hybridization for comprehensive chromosome analysis of embryos. Fertil Steril. 2011;95(3):953-8.
63. Munné S, Alikani M, Grifo J, et al. Monospermic polyploidy and atypical embryo morphology. Human Reprod. 1994;9:506-10.
64. Geraedts J, Montag M, Magli MC, et al. Polar body array CGH for prediction of the status of the corresponding oocyte. Part I: clinical results. Hum Reprod. 2011;26(11):3173-80.

65. Scott TR. Choosing the best embryo for transfer. 2010 syllabus, Pacific Coast Reproductive Society, 2010. pp. 51-63.
66. Shapiro BS, Daneshmand ST, Garner FC, et al. High ongoing pregnancy rates after deferred transfer through bipronuclear oocyte cryopreservation and post-thaw extended culture. Fertil Steril. 2009;92:1594-9.
67. Munné S, Danzer H, Grifo J, et al. Preimplantation Genetic Diagnosis using array CGH significantly increases ongoing pregnancy rates per transfer. Fertil Steril. 2010;94: S81.
68. Schlenker T, Stevens J, Rawlins M, et al. Clinical success with vitrification following trophectoderm biopsy for comprehensive chromosomal screening. Fertil Steril. 2009;92:S71.
69. Handyside A, Grifo J, Gabriel A, et al. First clinical application of karyomapping for PGD of Gaucher Disease Combined with 24 Chromosome Screening. Reprod Biomed Online. 2010;20:S16.

27

Third Party Reproduction: Current Status and Future

Gautam N Allahbadia, Rubina Merchant, Gandhi Goral

CHAPTER CONTENTS

INTRODUCTION

Third party reproduction (TPR) involves the use of donor gametes (sperm and oocytes), embryos or surrogates by couples who may not be able to conceive with self gametes or gestate a fetus, respectively. The rapid evolution and progress in the various assisted reproduction techniques (ART) during the last 25 years, namely, genetic material donation (oocyte, sperm, embryo and pre-embryo donation), human embryo cryo-preservation and surrogacy have extended the possibilities of assisted reproduction to benefit childless couples,[1,2] in both traditional and non-traditional relationships. However, the extension of ART to non-medical causes (single individuals, unmarried and gay couples desirous of a child, postmenopausal women and postmortem artificial insemination) has not only resulted in ambiguous genetic and biological relationships between parents and children and generated complex ethical, medico-legal, social, religious and psychological complications, but also in an increasing demand for donor gametes, embryos and surrogates, the inevitable commodification of genetic material and the threat of exploitation. Intrafamilial (intragenerational and intergenerational) donation of genetic material to preserve the genetic inheritance of the family has led to problems of uncest, undue coercion and exploitation.[3] Large differences in ethical, legal and religious frameworks world over have presented unique challenges. Genetic material donation, age limitation, selective embryo reduction, preimplantation genetic diagnosis (PGD), surrogacy and cloning are interpreted differently in the various countries, as their definition and application are influenced by social factors, religion and law.[4] This, in addition to the resultant stratification in the extent of quality of ART services offered, and the desperate pursuit for a child irrespective of marital bonds, has resulted in cross border reproductive tourism to overcome local restrictions in the acceptance and practice of TPR, and hence, in globalization of the technology. Amidst a heated debate on ethical and legal issues that surrounds TPR, the practice continues to soar owing to the lack of a uniform legal regulatory framework within and across geographical borders. Nevertheless, though successful both medically and technically, these techniques have fragmented reproduction, exposed the human egg to intervention yet unknown[5] and opened a Pandora's box of ethical, legal, religious and social issues, often without clear answers that must be urgently addressed.[3] In this chapter, the authors have attempted to detail the domains of TPR, the complex problems they have presented, consequences of differences in global perspectives of TPR and the significant role of counseling prior to undertaking TPR.

THIRD PARTY REPRODUCTION

Categories

Third party reproduction may be distinguished into:

1. Sperm donation: The third party is a sperm donor, who provides sperm that can be used for insemination of the future mother or to fertilize an oocyte during *in vitro* fertilization (IVF) with the transfer of the resulting embryo into the mother or a surrogate mother.
2. Oocyte donation: The third party is an oocyte donor, who donates oocytes for IVF with the transfer of the resulting embryo into the mother or a surrogate mother.
3. Embryo donation: The third party is an embryo donor, donating surplus embryos for use by a couple in need or a commissioned surrogate after the woman for whom they were originally created has successfully carried one or more pregnancies to term, or embryos specifically created for donation using donor eggs and donor sperm.
4. Surrogacy: The third party is surrogate woman, used to carry a baby through pregnancy to term for a woman/couple incapable of doing so.

Third party reproduction separates sex from reproduction, motherhood from pregnancy and third, it separates the unity of one couple into the involvement of a third person within the potential family relationship.[6]

Indications

Gamete Donation

Sperm donation: Sperm donation may be indicated in severe male factor infertility due to the lack of sperm in the ejaculate due to:

- Severely impaired spermatogenesis (non-obstructive azoospermia)
- Irreparable reproductive tract obstruction (obstructive azoospermia)
- The presence of acrosomeless or immotile spermatozoa
- High risk of fertilization failure
- Subnormal sperm samples—semen parameters below the threshold for standard IVF treatment, e.g. oligoasthenoteratozoospermia (OAT), severely oligozoospermic and teratozoospermic men (strict normal sperm morphology ≤ 5%) with a very high (> 70%) frequency of defective sperm-ZP interaction and hence, a high risk of low or zero fertilization rate in IVF
- Sperm autoimmunity (high titers of antisperm antibodies/sperm-bound antibodies-interference with gametes interaction)
- Two previous fertilization failures with conventional IVF
- When PGD is indicated in pregnancies that are at high risk of aneuploidy because of genetic factors associated with azoospermia, to avoid contamination by extraneous DNA in the case of PCR-based testing and to increase the number of embryos available for testing.[7]
- HIV serodiscordant couples, where the male is HIV positive.

Causes of non-obstructive azoospermia include germ cell aplasia, maturation arrest and tubular sclerosis/atrophy, all with focal spermatogenesis, Sertoli-cell only syndrome, persistent azoospermia post chemotherapy, history of orchidopexy, spinal cord injury and seminiferous tubule dysgenesis (Klinefelter's syndrome 47, XXY). Obstructive azoospermia may be attributed to congenital absence of the vas deferens, acquired vas obstruction, irreparable epididymal obstruction, postinfectious epididymal obstruction, conservatively untreatable ejaculatory disturbances or failed microsurgical reversal for vasectomy.[7] Though microfertilization with intracytoplasmic sperm injection (ICSI), often combined with surgical procedures like microsurgically extracted epididymal or testicular sperm offers a readily available and successful option for bearing a biologically related child, ICSI often carries the risk of propagating the inherent disorder to the offspring, leaving sperm donation a safe alternative.

Oocyte donation: The indications for oocyte donation presently include:[8]

- Premature ovarian failure (POF)
- Carriers of genetic disorders, e.g. 46, XY pure gonadal dysgenesis, Turner's syndrome (45, XO)
- Severe endometriosis
- Poor responders to ovarian hyperstimulation
- Repeated IVF failure with autologous oocytes
- Surgical castration/conservative bilateral gonadectomy
- Advanced maternal age
- Postmenopausal women
- Contraindications for spontaneous or induced ovulation, such as those with von Willebrand's disease.
- Female survivors of childhood cancer and adolescents treated with bone marrow transplantation including total body irradiation (TBI), X-ray therapy or chemotherapy
- Surrogacy programs involving same-sex couples.

However, it must be mentioned that though oocyte donation is a successful option for achieving conception in these patients, the high risk of complications associated with pregnancies thus obtained, especially in women with genetic disorders and advanced maternal age, makes strict criteria for the selection of such patients and rigid protocols for the medical management of such pregnancies an absolute requirement.[8] For instance, though patients with Turner's syndrome may achieve high pregnancy rates comparable to that observed in patients with other indications requiring oocyte donation, high miscarriage rates, potentially severe cardiovascular complications during pregnancy, early implantation failure, possibly associated with a deficiency of X-linked genes regulating endometrial receptivity, and a high rate of Cesarean section are commonly observed.[8]

Change in societal trends, the increase in the average childbearing age in industrialized nations to late 30s to early 40s, the consequent decline in fertility with increasing female age and the decrease in success of various ART treatment options,[9] has resulted in an increased dependence on oocyte donation with hormone replacement therapy to achieve conception. However, the increase in maternal and fetal morbidity, mortality with advanced maternal age and the pregnancy-related complications (gestational diabetes, chronic and pregnancy-induced hypertension, antepartum hemorrhage, placenta previa, multiple gestation, prelabor rupture of membranes, preterm labor, complications of malpresentation, fetopelvic disproportion, abnormal labor, Cesarean section, instrumental delivery, sphincter rupture, and postpartum hemorrhage)[10,11] can hardly be ignored.

Embryo Donation

Embryo donation may be medically indicated in couples with double sterility, i.e. where both sperm and oocyte donation is mandatory to achieve conception, in unexplained genetic disease, ART failures (due to poor fertilization or poor embryo quality), in candidates eligible for oocyte donation when the delay is too long for the couples or now, as an option in single parents and homosexuals desirous of a child. The embryos may be sourced from couples consenting to donate their surplus embryos following self use or specifically created by using a chosen sperm and oocyte donor.

Surrogacy

Surrogacy is a reproductive technology involving one woman (surrogate mother) carrying a child for another person(s) (commissioning person/couple), based on a mutual agreement requiring the child to be legally relinquished to the intended parent(s) or the commissioning couple/person following birth. Surrogacy has given a new dimension to the concept of the 'traditional family' and not only has it separated genetic and gestational links between parents and children, but also created distinctions between social relationships and interpersonal ties within families.[12]

Surrogacy can be offered as a treatment option in women with non-functional reproductive organs, congenital (Mayer-Rokitansky-Küster-Hauser syndrome) or surgical absence of the uterus, postpartum hysterectomy, repeated IVF failure, high-order unexplained habitual abortions with a maternal cause, hysterectomy for menorrhagia, severe medical conditions, such as severe heart or renal disease, in which pregnancy is contraindicated or life-threatening, in gynecological cancers (uterine, ovarian, cervical, vaginal, and vulvar),[12] or following treatment modalities for numerous oncological and non-oncological conditions that result in gonadal insufficiency and infertility.[13] Pelvic-abdominal radiation may result in uterine damage resulting in poor reproductive outcomes, such as preterm birth, low birth weight and spontaneous abortion in adult survivors of childhood cancers,[13] leaving TPR with surrogacy as the only successful treatment option. Though ART using cryopreserved gametes or embryos offers a valid treatment option in patients with gynecologic cancers anxious to conceive after treatment, a reduction in the size of the uterus, possible uterine vasculature damage leading to decreased feto-placental blood flow or alteration or damage to the hypothalamic-gonadal hormonal axis, where the pelvis is not involved post-therapy, all of which may increase the risk for pregnancy-related complications, including spontaneous miscarriages, preterm labor and delivery, low birth weight infants, and placental abnormalities, may render these women unable to gestate, leaving surrogacy as the only option.[14] Even if such women can conceive after surgery (radical vaginal trachelectomy), the incidence of premature delivery is high.[15]

The indications for surrogacy today, have extended beyond genuine medical causes as they are increasingly being used by single, gay, divorced, remarried, unmarried partnered people to create reproductively assisted families with little resemblance to the traditional nuclear family.[12]

Rokitansky syndrome is a developmental defect. It is not commonly transmitted as a dominant genetic trait. Gestational surrogacy for patients with Rokitansky syndrome, characterized by agenesis of the uterus and vagina but normal gonads and secondary sexual characters, is reported to yield clinical pregnancy rates of 42.9% per embryo transfer and 54.5% per oocyte retrieval and live birth rates of 21.4% per embryo transfer, 27.3% per retrieval and 50% per patient. However, both commissioning and surrogate couples should be properly screened and counseled, their treatment approved by the clinic internal review committee (ethics committee) and supported to be able to have a family using their own genetic gametes.[14] Hysterectomized women demonstrate varying patterns of response to assisted conception treatment, however, gestational surrogacy generally appears to be a feasible option, especially in young patients with reported pregnancy rates of 37.5% per patient and embryo transfer and 27.3% per cycle of treatment commenced.[15] Patients with congenital absence of the uterus are shown to respond better to ovulation induction than patients who underwent a hysterectomy, perhaps due in part to ovarian compromise from previous surgical procedures.[16]

Types of surrogacy: Surrogacy may be of two types: (i) Traditional surrogacy, where the surrogate or birth mother is also the oocyte donor, and hence, the genetic mother and the intended father is the genetic father; pregnancy may be achieved by artificially inseminating the surrogate with the intended father's sperm and, (ii) IVF or gestational surrogacy, where the gametes from the intended parents or commissioning couple (the couple requesting surrogacy) are fertilized *in vitro* and the embryo transferred into the surrogate, who only rents the womb. In other words, the surrogate is not genetically linked to the child in any way. The child is legally adopted by the commissioning couple following delivery. The burgeoning of gestational surrogacy salvaged many of the significant disadvantages associated with traditional surrogacy that disabled the genetic link between the intended mother and the child. With gestational surrogacy, unless the intended couple requires gamete donation or embryo donation, they can retain the genetic link with the offspring, retaining the surrogate as only the birth or gestational mother.

In addition to differentiating surrogacy by parental roles, surrogacy can also be classified into two types based on financial compensation. Altruistic surrogacy does not financially compensate the surrogate for her role, though the intended parent or couple may cover any fees and costs associated with bringing an embryo to term. This type of surrogacy is most common among family members or close friends (e.g. a woman serving as a surrogate for her sister). The decision to be a surrogate stems from love, not from personal gain or even avarice. Commercial surrogacy financially compensates a surrogate beyond expenses associated with the pregnancy, i.e. the surrogate is paid for her gestational 'services'. Gestational surrogacy is typically arranged by surrogacy agencies, which collect a fee from intended parents and are responsible for the exchange of money between the intended parents and surrogate.[15]

Intrafamilial medically assisted reproduction: For different motives, couples in need of third party assisted reproduction sometimes prefer the help of a family member over an unrelated collaborator. Intrafamilial medically assisted reproduction (IMAR) may vary depending on whether: (i) the assistance would be intra- or intergenerational and familial closeness between the collaborator and the person whose reproductive contribution he or she replaces, (ii) the relationship between the collaborator and the fertile partner, which may or may not be consanguineous and, (iii) the material (sperm and oocytes) that is donated and the services (surrogacy) that are offered.[17]

ISSUES IN THIRD PARTY REPRODUCTION

The scientific breakthroughs resulting in the delivery of Louise Brown in 1978 have opened the floodgates for an ongoing bioethical discussion about medically assisted reproduction. While IVF has established itself as a successful and ethically justifiable procedure to alleviate infertility with the majority, the tremendous unwarranted and largely unregulated ramifications of the technology has left clinicians, psychologists, law-makers and society on the whole grappling with dire consequences for the so created children, the traditional family, and, indeed, for society as a whole.[18] Lack of informed consent, providing procedures not medically indicated for financial gain, practice by unqualified personnel, injury to patients and donors, failure to screen donated gametes and inadequate medical record keeping are some of the unfortunate consequences that the unfettered use of reproductive technologies can create.[19]

While sperm donation appears to generate little that is ethically new when coupled with IVF, involvement of third parties (gamete donation and gestational surrogacy) is more complex and raises new ethical questions that need close individual attention and continuing analysis.[20]

The encouragement of single parenthood by the use of TPR has been viewed by some as a negative impact on society that would go against the interests of the children born out of such an arrangement that, they would be deprived of the traditional family links important for the upbringing of any child. As this cannot be provided by gay or lesbian couples or individuals, children born to such couples or individuals may lack confidence and be adversely affected in the long run.[21]

Ethical Issues

Oocyte Donation

There is an increasing trend in the use of donor eggs by women unable to otherwise conceive. As the flexibility of the treatment options increase, the recruitment and management of donors, the maximal age for treatment, donor selection, the financial commitments involved and the lack of consensus on reimbursement issues make the practice of donor egg IVF ethically, medically and financially complex with exploitation as the inevitable outcome. Third party reproduction, specifically IVF with donor eggs, has particular ethical issues including possible conflict of interest between provider, donor and recipient, completeness of informed consent, legal representation of the donor and follow-up support.[22] In most countries, such as France for instance, despite the procedure being conducted within the legislative framework, the major difficulties encountered in the daily practice of oocyte donation concern the recruitment and management of donors and above all, the lack of optimal means to exercise this medical specialty, due to the lack of recognition of the organizational duties incurred, which are the cornerstone of the character-specific functioning of this type of ART.[23]

Intrafamilial Gamete Donation

Familial egg donation (intragenerational and intergenerational), practiced to preserve the family's genetic inheritance has resulted in confusing relationships and distorting family dynamics. Common risks inherent to the procedure include exploitation, undue coercion and incest (sexual intercourse, reproduction with gametes of first-degree relatives, symbolic incest). Impregnation of donor eggs fertilized with spermatozoa of the woman's brother with the intention of raising the child as social mother and father (intentional incest) has particularly been condemned.[24] The practice of intrafamilial (father to son) sperm donation to retain the genetic link and maintain kinship similarly threatens potential parental conflicts of interest, coercion of the prospective donor and unhealthy family dynamics[25] and suffers potential medical, ethical and emotional risks.[12]

Surplus Embryos

Reducing the number of eggs or embryos transferred to two when the egg or embryo quality is high are measures that have been taken to reduce the incidence of multiple pregnancies, especially triplets.[26] The generation of surplus embryos in the practice of TPR opens avenues for a number of potential uses, such as human embryo cryopreservation, embryo donation, and embryonic stem cell research, to prevent wastage of these embryos.

Embryo donation: Genetic material donation has become an integral part of the management of infertility, however, the practice of pre-embryo donation raises several unique issues, such as the status of the pre-embryo and its well-being.[2] Embryo donation presents a viable option to conceive and an ethically and legally acceptable way for infertile couples to form families,[27] however, the future of embryos created for assisted reproduction has confronted ethical, legal and moral issues with regard to wastage of surplus embryos not intentionally created for future use or donation.[12] Ethical issues may be related to financial compensation and mixing of gametes from different sources while legal issues may be related to whether embryo donation is viewed as gamete donation or adoption, the rearing rights and duties of donors and recipients towards the resulting offspring, liability, compensation issues and the legality of monetary compensation for donors.[28] In order to alleviate misunderstandings regarding the source of gametes despite the approval of the embryo donation law in Iran, a new term 'both-gamete donation' was defined to segregate it from 'embryo donation' The Iranian law now permits only embryo donation including surplus embryos from other infertile couples and not both-gamete donation. However, as gamete donation is practised in Iran upon decrees of clergy leaders, there is no law or legislation against both-gamete donation though there are many ethical, legal and religious questions about both-gamete donation to be answered compared to embryo donation. Alternatively, embryo sharing has been proposed as a good way for donation of fresh embryos.[29]

Cryopreservation: Cryopreservation of gametes (sperm and oocytes), embryos and reproductive tissues (ovarian and testicular tissues) is a significant area of reproductive medicine today that adds tremendous flexibility to the practice of ART. Successful cryopreservation of cells and tissues for future ART use offers an attractive option for preserving fertility in cancer patients undergoing chemo and radiotherapy. It provides an opportunity to limit the numbers of embryos transferred while enabling supernumerary embryos to be used in subsequent treatment cycles, thereby increasing the cumulative pregnancy rate, reduces the potential risk of hyperstimulation syndrome, enables patients to space the timing of sibling pregnancies and improve their potential of achieving a pregnancy at an advanced maternal age.[30] However, though embryo freezing has made a small but important contribution to overall pregnancy rates by enabling patients to use excess eggs and embryos, freezing human embryos breaks new ethical ground, particularly in the options it generates beyond a narrowly defined medical domain and it generates social and legal concerns that require new ethical and legal considerations.[20,26] The ultimate fate of these embryos can only be decided by the couple donating the gametes. If the couple is in a marital relationship, the decision becomes clear, however, if the gametes involve different sources, decision-making becomes complex and must be carefully buttressed both ethically and legally by the existing laws pertinent to the place. Due to the possibility of storing gametes and pre-embryos, conflicts over the use of pre-embryos and post-mortem insemination have found their way into the courts. Case law allows parties to conclude a binding agreement as to the destination of their pre-embryos in case of divorce or death.[31]According to an evaluation of the preferred fate of embryos cryopreserved for more than 2 years by Van Voorhis et al.[32] 44% couples elected to continue storage of their embryos for future use, 34% elected to discard their embryos while a minority elected to donate their embryos either to infertile couples (11%) or for research (10%).[32]

Embryonic stem cell research: While embryo cryopreservation serves as a potentially useful technology to preserve future fertility, embryonic stem cell research raises ethical, moral and religious issues, such as, the moral status of the embryo, commodification and rights of women as experimental subjects and donors and possibilities of exploitation, which hinders the universal acceptance of embryonic stem cell research.[33] However, arguments in favor of embryonic research suggest that as long as experimentally manipulated embryos are not returned to the womb, or artificially gestated to a stage at which they might become sentient research on human embryos produced *in vitro*, is not a wrong. Nevertheless, the large scale therapeutic or commercial use of human embryos might endanger women's rights.[34] According to Tangwa,[35] the ethical crux of reproductive technologies is linked to the issue of the moral status of the human embryo and a morally significant line of demarcation cannot be drawn between embryos and other categories of humans. Hence, if bound by thorough pre-procedure counseling and consent, embryonic research might be carried out without complications.[35]

Postmenopausal Motherhood

The increasing application and success of oocyte donation with hormone replacement therapy in women of advanced maternal age (≥ 40 years) and postmenopausal women has generated a medical, ethical and social debate. Despite the soaring success of oocyte donation to women over 50 years of age, a community survey to evaluate attitudes toward oocyte and embryo donation, suggests that only 54.6% of the participants felt that it was acceptable for a woman to have her own embryos transferred after menopause, while 37.9% were in favor of the donation of eggs or embryos to postmenopausal women. There were no significant differences in response amongst different religious groups or in relation to gender or income level.[36] It is opined that there are no compelling reasons for a systematic ban on the use of donated oocytes in postmenopausal women[28] and neither success rates, fault, parental competence, medical urgency or waiting time justify discrimination against postmenopausal women.[36] However, to streamline the practice and to optimize healthy live births and minimize multiple pregnancies in this sub-group of women, the Canadian Task Force on the periodic health has devised guidelines on the number of embryos that should be transferred in an IVF-ET cycle. They recommend that: (i) in women aged 35–39 years, no more than three embryos should be transferred in a fresh *in vitro* fertilization-embryo transfer (IVF-ET) cycle (III-B), (ii) in women over the age of 39 years, no more than four embryos should be transferred in a fresh IVF-ET cycle (III-B) and (iii) in older women with high-quality embryos in excess of the number to be transferred, consideration should be given to the transfer of three embryos in the first IVF-ET cycle (III-B). In women with obstetrical or medical contraindications to multifetal gestation, fewer embryos should be transferred to minimize the chance of multifetal gestation.[37]

Commodification of Third Party Reproduction

Commodification of reproductive bodies within this trade has reduced reproduction to exchange value with intensification and globalization in the stratification of reproduction. These inequalities are illustrated though discussion of the trade in poor women's bodies for surrogacy and ova donation.[38] Commercial gamete donation has triggered a fierce debate and resulted in a prolific growth of the practice fuelled both, by the demand for gametes, as well as the money. While sperm donation is not particularly problematic, except for when familial donation is involved, oocyte donation, because of the inherent medical risks involved, client emphasis on donor selection for superior traits and geographical and religious differences in the approach to donor egg IVF has resulted in extensive commodification of the technology. Race and ethnicity of the donor, educational qualifications, employment status and career and physical attributes and stature are significant in determining the value of compensation to donors. The shortage of egg donors from some ethnic groups, such as East Asians and Jews, has resulted in higher reimbursement rates for donors of such ethnicity.[39]

The commodification of gametes has incited an ethical and moral debate, with some authors opining this to be ethically unacceptable and incompatible with human dignity that nullifies the reproductive paradigm, irretrievably replacing it with a manufacturing paradigm,[40] while others maintaining that this is morally acceptable as long as it is regulated and not extended to zygotes, embryos or genomes.[41] This is particularly worrying because: (i) for-profit genetic enhancement and under conditions of economic necessity, it exploits poor by coercing them, in effect, to part with reproductive material they would otherwise prefer not to sell for money, and (ii) the market valuation and exchange of sperm, eggs, and embryos would distort the meaning and degrade the worth of those procreative goods.[42] Steinbock[43] maintains that some payment to donors is ethically acceptable and that donors should not be paid for their eggs, but rather they should be compensated for the burdens of egg retrieval. Making the distinction between compensation for burdens and payment for a product has the advantages of limiting payment, not distinguishing between donors on the basis of their traits and ensuring that donors are paid regardless of the number or quality of eggs retrieved.[43] Moreover, it is argued that monetary reward is the only way to recruit sufficient numbers of donors and meet the existing demand for donor gametes[44] and an 'all-inclusive' financial allowance analogous to volunteers in medical trials could be considered to prevent a complete collapse of the system, if nonfinancial rewards of donors do not suffice to motivate candidates.[45] However, a high compensation fees for egg donors may attract the 'wrong women' to donate[46] and place them at a special risk of exploitation.[47] Hence, financial incentives, including direct and indirect payment and inheritance, should not be so substantial that they become inducements that may lead the prospective donor to discount the emotional risk associated with the procedure.[25] It is simultaneously feared that the dangers of inordinate compensation may only increase this possible dearth by deterring altruistic donors and that large payments may be especially prejudicial to the interests and welfare of children born as a result of gamete donation.[48]

Differences exist in donor reimbursement policies in various countries, particularly in countries where the underlying principle of gamete donation is altruistic motivation and where reimbursement is given only for direct 'out-of-pocket' expenses, i.e. travelling costs, where there is a lack of clear and coherent internationally-binding legislation and regulatory guidelines overseeing the exchange of donor gametes across international borders.[49] Financial compensation to egg donors for their time and inconvenience in donating is established in the United States as ethically and legally acceptable.[50] The current situation of oocyte donation in the USA serves as a useful paradigm for a *laissez-faire* free-market model of egg donor reimbursement, based on supply and demand as is observed in any country that has a free market approach to surrogacy.

Though the Warnock Committee reporting to the British Government in 1984 expressed that it is inconsistent with human dignity that a woman should use her uterus for financial profit and treat it as an incubator for someone else's child, these objections remain unanswerable even today. The proposed Bill, however, legalizes not only surrogacy *per se* but even commercial surrogacy or surrogacy 'for monetary compensation' or 'on mutually agreed financial terms'. Whatever the intentions, its inevitable consequence would be the creation of a market specializing in the sale and purchase of babies or as the Court of Appeal in England put it in 1985, in "a kind of baby-farming operation of a wholly distasteful and lamentable kind." The only proper way to pursue the Bill would be to abandon it. In some states in Australia, arranging commercial surrogacy is a criminal offence and any surrogacy agreement giving custody to others is void. In Canada and New Zealand, commercial surrogacy has been illegal since 2004, although altruistic surrogacy is allowed.[21]

Financial compensation for embryonic stem cell research: The use of donated eggs for cloning-based stem cell research and financial compensation for the same is yet another area that has triggered a vigorous debate about the ethics of paying women for their eggs.[51,52] While commodification of reproductive labor or tissues is an inevitable reality that may interfere with the voluntariness among potential egg providers,[36] payment would undermine tendencies for domestic and international black and gray egg markets for stem cell research to develop.[52] Payment to British women undergoing IVF treatment for sharing their eggs with stem cell researchers has been hailed by the Human Fertilisation and Embryology Authority (HFEA) as a 'win-win' arrangement benefiting both infertile women and couples and British science.[19] The new stem cell guidelines of The International Society for Stem Cell Research also legitimize both reimbursement of direct expenses and financial compensation for many women who supply eggs for research.[53]

Preimplantation Genetic Diagnosis

Preimplantation genetic diagnosis is a technique used to detect genetic inadequacies in embryos prior to implantation to prevent the risk of transmission of inheritable diseases to the offspring. Hence, pre-procedure counseling is a very integral part of the practice. Preimplantation genetic screening (PGS)/PGD and surrogacy present as useful options in the management of women with recurrent miscarriage. While the former PGS/PGD assumes that the embryo is chromosomally abnormal and that the mother should receive a chromosomally normal embryo, surrogacy assumes that the embryo is normal and that the maternal environment needs to be substituted.[54] However, the ability of PGD to detect nondisease traits risks the threat of misuse and opens up new ethical questions related to the current and foreseeable uses of PGD and the adequacy of regulatory structures to review new uses.[55,56] Hence, it is very essential to discriminate the applications of these approaches depending on the likelihood of an embryonic chromosome aberration. While PGS or PGD may be indicated in women with repeated fetal aneuploidy or in the older patient, in women with recurrent miscarriages or autoimmune pregnancy loss, surrogacy is indicated, however, in balanced parental chromosome aberrations, it is uncertain which treatment mode is indicated. Both techniques have a place, but probably only in those patients with a poor prognosis in whom ART will be shown to improve the subsequent live birth rate above the spontaneous rate.[54]

According to the HFEA and the Human Genetics Commission, there should be serious indications to execute PGD and clear demarcations in the criteria for selection against disease as against those for selective abortion.[57] Since it cannot be reconciled with the provisions of the Embryo Protection Law, PGD is not being practiced in the Federal Republic of Germany. The existing German laws do not explicitly permit or prohibit PGD but forbid the wasting of totipotent embryonic cells, fertilizing oocytes without transferring them in the same cycle, the use of micromanipulations that later may harm embryonic development, limit the number of oocytes that may be fertilized in each IVF cycle to three and prohibit research on embryos. However, within the framework of medical and sociopsychological counseling, PGD can be used to the benefit of the health of both the pregnant mother and the expected children.[58] However, proponents of PGD suggest that the choice between evaluative, moral and (still to be specified) species-ethical arguments is still open to question[46] and hence, speculations about potential future uses of PGD should not prevent otherwise acceptable current uses of PGD.[59]

Surrogacy

With advancements in the preservation and transfer of gametes, surrogacy (along with other ART options) has further challenged how we define parents.[15] This has resulted in ambiguous genetic and biological relationships between parents and children and psychological and medico-legal complications, which clinicians, psychologists, law makers and society as a whole find hard to regulate.[12] Like adoption, surrogacy separates the role of rearing mother from what the law has called the natural mother, but gestational surrogacy breaks the latter down into the roles of genetic mother and birth mother, leaving two women with biological connections to the child.[60] Though, the practice of surrogacy has already become a big market in most countries, owing to the legal, social and psychological complications it brews in a largely unregulated set-up, most authors condemn surrogacy as an alternative way of procreation[60] that can render the child a helpless pawn in the parental, emotional and legal strife.[18] Some of the most significant problems that could be a result of an improper regulatory framework to streamline the practice of surrogacy are: (i) failure to relinquish the baby immediately after birth, (ii) separation of a commissioning couple prior to treatment initiation, (iii) withdrawal of a patient from treatment following initial counseling of the implications of the treatment, (iv) poor responders to follicular stimulation, particularly after Wertheim hysterectomy,[61] and (v) the possibility of the birth of a handicapped or genetically disordered child and fear of rejection.[62]

Surrogacy arrangements are legally complex and challenging[63] that have created different perceptions of parenthood. While some believe that being causally implicated in the creation of a child is the key basis for being its parent, others claim that genetic relatedness is sufficient grounds for parenthood based on a causal connection between genetic parents and their offspring and prospects of familial intergeneration surrogacy further stir controversy.[64] An insight into the psychosocial aspects of surrogate motherhood suggests that surrogate and intended mothers appear to reconcile their unusual choice through a process of cognitive restructuring and the success or failure of this cognitive appraisal affects people's willingness to be open and honest about their choices.[65]

Legal Issues

Most surrogacy arrangements are bound by a surrogacy agreement or contract that involves three parental roles: the role of the intended or social parents, who intend to raise the child; the role of biological parents who are genetically related to the child; and the role of birth or gestational mother, that is, the woman who carries the fetus and ultimately gives birth to the child. There are numerous possible permutations for fulfilling these roles. The commissioning couple may be the genetic parents too if no donor gametes are involved.[15] Though the purpose of a surrogacy contract, like any other type of contract, is to bring the involved parties under a legal obligation to ensure that they are aware of and will adhere to the rules and their responsibilities, the legality and enforceability of such an agreement varies not only from country to country, but also from state to state within countries like the United States and Australia.[15]

Moreover, different interpretations of surrogacy in the various countries, based on their definition, application, social, religious and legal influences has complicated matters further and extending the practice across political borders and beyond judicial limits.[12] Surrogacy laws vary within and across borders and suffer loopholes, such as failure to address commodification of children, exploitation of women of low socioeconomic status, failure to impose responsibility of ownership of an impaired child on 'intended parents,' ignorance of possibility of divorce or death of the 'intended parents' before the child's birth and splitting motherhood.[66]

While the practice is ethically and legally regulated by the The Human Fertilisation and Embryology Act (1990) in UK,[67] Singapore,[68] Australia,[69] Canada[70] and Israel[66] permit surrogacy arrangements that are not adequately regulated. The only countries in Europe which allow surrogacy are the UK, Belgium, Holland and Finland.[71-73] In France, Germany and Italy, surrogacy is unlawful. The Ethics Committee of the Asia-Oceania Federation of Obstetrics and Gynaecology (AOFOG)[74] follows strict ethical guidelines and legislation for permitting gestational surrogacy and recommends that ART must be performed by a board certified gynecologist in a certification laboratory, restricts the practice of surrogacy for medical reasons only and prohibits commercialization.[74] However, the attitude and status of country member societies vary in a wide range and do not have formal legal codes in majority regulating the ethical aspects of ART, the use of ART and surrogacy being affected by local traditions, popularity in the use of such techniques and cultural/religious concerns.[74] Differences in the acceptance and practice of surrogacy and the legal situation in the various countries across the globe are discussed. International approaches to surrogacy can be categorized as free market, regulated and prohibited as in India, Israel and France, respectively.[15]

India

India epitomizes the free market approach to surrogacy that permits surrogacy with limited or no government regulation and individuals, brokers and clinics, rather than the government, determine what appropriate measures need to be taken in order to protect all involved parties.[75] Since commercial surrogacy was legalized in 2002, the only regulatory measure in India is the "National Guidelines for Accreditation, Supervision and Regulation of ART Clinics in India, 2005" formulated by the Indian Council for Medical Research, Ministry of Health and Family Welfare, Government of India, which have no legal binding.[76] This has resulted in there being few restrictions on who can partake in surrogacy (e.g. homosexuals, individuals, etc.) and has led to more flexibility in legally defining parents. For instance, a surrogate can relinquish her motherhood rights before giving birth and not have her name be on the original birth certificate. Additionally, it enables each clinic to be self-regulated and implement independent policies to assure a smooth transaction.[77] Though the guidelines do not have legal binding, they are regulatory measures that safeguard the rights of the intended parents, surrogates, as well as the hospitals.[76]

India's surrogacy boom began in January 2004 with a grandmother delivering her daughter's twins. The success spawned a virtual cottage industry in Gujarat. The ART (Regulation) Draft Bill, 2010 legalizes commercial surrogacy for single persons, married or unmarried couples. A legally enforceable surrogacy agreement, yet to come under the law, would necessitate foreigners or NRIs coming to India to rent a womb to submit documentation confirming the legal recognition of surrogacy in their country of residence and that it will give citizenship to the child born through the surrogacy agreement from an Indian mother. This comes after several legal battles that rendered the children thus born stateless due to mutual non-recognition of laws. However, the Draft Bill lacks the creation of a specialist legal authority for adjudication and determination of legal rights of parties by a judicial verdict and falls in conflict with the existing laws, pitfalls that need to be examined closely before enacting the legislation. In the absence of any law to govern surrogacy, the Indian Council of Medical Research guidelines (2005) for accreditation, supervision and regulation of ART clinics in India are often violated. Exploitation, extortion and ethical abuses in surrogacy trafficking are rampant and surrogate mothers are misused with impunity.[21]

Today, India boasts of being the first to legalize commercial surrogacy, soon to legitimise both intra-and inter-country surrogacy. Renting wombs has become an easy and cheap option in India as the relatively low cost of medical services, easy availability of surrogate wombs, abundant choices of donors with similar racial attributes and the lack of any law to regulate these practices is attracting both foreigners and NRIs to sperm banks and surrogate mothers. The would-be parents from the Indian diaspora in the US, the UK and Canada and foreigners from Malaysia, the UAE, Afghanistan, Indonesia, Uzbekistan, Pakistan besides Nepal are descending on sperm banks and IVF centers in India looking for South Asian genetic traits of perfect sperm donors. Surrogacy in the UK, the US and Australia costs more than US$ 50,000 whereas advertisements on websites in India give varying costs in the range of US$ 10,000 and offer egg donors and surrogate mothers. It is a free trading market, flourishing and thriving in the business of babies.[21] Surreptitiously, India has become a booming center of a fertility market with its 'reproductive tourism, industry reportedly estimated at Rs 25,000 crore today. Assisted reproduction has been in vogue in India since 1978 and today an estimated 200,000 clinics across the country offer artificial insemination, IVF and surrogacy.[21]

Israel

Israel has a regulated approach to surrogacy, which was achieved with the passage of the Surrogate Motherhood Agreements Law in 1996. All surrogacy agreements are pre-approved by a Committee for Approving Surrogate Motherhood Agreements, set up as part of this law, and that ensures their adherence to regulations in order to protect all parties involved in surrogacy. In addition to written legislative surrogacy regulations, there are precedents set by the committee that serve as unofficial regulations for surrogacy contracts.[78] Israel has several regulations regarding surrogacy to protect society and social values, future children, surrogates and intended parents. In order to the protect the interests of future offspring, only heterosexual couples who are married or living together to be the intended parents can partake in surrogacy agreements, the father must be younger than 59 years and the mother younger than 48 years.[78]

In order to protect the surrogates, it is required that surrogates be older than 22 years but younger than 40 years, must have given birth to at least one child to establish the experience of pregnancy and make the decision to relinquish the baby easy, but no more than five times, and must have undergone a maximum of two cesarean sections. The surrogate must undergo a mandatory physical and psychological examination and is entitled to 6 months of counseling paid for by the intended parents following birth of the child. The surrogate's legal rights are supported by a mandatory legal council from a lawyer independent of the intended parents.[78]

Intrafamilial surrogacy is prohibited in Israel and commercial surrogacy is encouraged.[66] The rights of the intended parents are protected by oversight from the Committee and they are expected to provide compensation above the costs of all the medical procedures to the surrogate for the time and burdens imposed. The Committee must pre-approve compensation to protect the intended parents from extra demands by the surrogate before, during and after the pregnancy. The parents are further protected by the requirement that the surrogate must appeal to the committee if she changes her mind and wants to keep the child at any point during the process. It is believed that the Committee will rule in the best interests of the child if such a dispute ever arises.[78]

France

France legally bans all types of surrogacy, outlawing surrogacy with the 1994 Act on bioethics, the status of which has been reaffirmed through additional court cases and legislation. The impetus for banning surrogacy in France was a 1991 court case involving an altruistic traditional surrogacy that permitted the intended father to assume custody of the child through his genetic relationship but failed the intended mother's adoption attempts as she was not genetically related to the child. Though a lower appeals court found the surrogacy contract legal and granted the adoption, the higher court overturned the decision, ruling that surrogacy violates the principle of inalienability of the human body and the principle of inalienability of individual status.[79] A 2002 court case upheld France's ban on surrogacy allowing fatherhood to be claimed through genetic tests but outweighing the bond created through pregnancy over genetic contribution for motherhood. A French court could grant an intended parent partial adoption, which restricts a parent's legal rights to the child. Not having full legal or custodial rights can be problematic for a mother if the couple gets a divorce or the father passes away, as the child may not be awarded to her.[79]

Italy

After a heated debate, the Italian parliament passed the law on assisted reproduction that forbids the creation of no more than three embryos at any one time and necessitates the transfer of all the embryos created together even if the couple does not need all the embryos. Embryo cryopreservation, the screening of embryos for genetic defects and TPR, research using human embryos, gamete donation, surrogacy and the provision of any ARTs for single women or same-sex couples is forbidden.[80,81] The new Italian law, regulating the use of assisted reproduction technologies, limits the use of ART to 'clinically infertile, stable heterosexual couples who live together and are of childbearing age', prohibits treatment widely practiced in Europe.[81]

United Kingdom

In the UK, the HFEA is required to license and monitor clinics undertaking the storage and use of gametes and embryos, and to provide them with guidelines on practical clinical matters and also the HFEA's policy on a number of social and ethical issues in a Code of Practice.

The regulatory system that works by consultation and cooperation between the HFEA and the scientists and clinicians, was set up to reassure the public, to protect the interests of potential children, patients and donors and to promote good practice in fertility research and treatment, has established itself as an effective regulator and adviser and has provided a basis for the development of policy in the field of fertility treatment.[82] The HFEA Act (1990)[67] has outlined the categories acceptable for treatment with surrogacy, motives considered unacceptable and general considerations which apply to all cases and clinics undertaking surrogacy in a HFEA Code of Practice. Social reasons and prospective genetic parents with severe health problems are considered unacceptable as motives for surrogacy under Section 30 of the HFEA Act (1990).[67] Surrogacy is allowed in the UK, provided it is consensual and involves the payment of no more than reasonable expenses. But in an increasingly globalized world, patients are crossing borders for treatment, often to places where such restrictions on the commerciality or enforceability of surrogacy arrangements do not apply. The resulting conflicts of law can be a minefield and this makes the maintenance of the UK's careful legal balance increasingly untenable.[83] In the UK, no contract or surrogacy agreement is legally binding.[21] Moreover, the removal of donor anonymity has resulted in a donor oocyte shortage, propagating cross border reproductive tourism.

Australia

The professional and legal regulation of ART in Australia is a vast maze of intersecting laws and guidelines, which place restrictions on the provision of services, such as infertility treatment, surrogacy, sex selection for social reasons, donor insemination, preimplantation diagnosis and human embryo research. However, differences exist in regulation of the technologies across states. For instance, New South Wales is a relatively unregulated State with a wider range of ART services while Victoria is a relatively highly regulated State with uniform restrictions on ART to single and lesbian women and social sex selection procedures. Reproductive tourism is prevalent and restrictions are circumnavigated by patients with assistance from clinics.[84]

United States

In most states in the US, compensated surrogacy arrangements are either illegal or unenforceable.[21] Differing surrogacy opinions among the different states in the US are reflected in the state laws. There is no federal legislation, leaving each state to determine how they want to regulate surrogacy.[21] New York has statutes that ban surrogacy contracts and make it a criminal offense to broker contracts or engage in commercial surrogacy. In contrast, California has no state legislation regarding surrogacy, thereby leaving the courts to solve individual conflicts.[75] Surrogacy laws in Florida require the intended couple to be over 18-year old and married, the intended mother must be incapable of gestating a pregnancy without physical risk to herself or the fetus and at least one of the intended parents must be biologically related to any resulting child. These requirements have to be fulfilled in order for any surrogacy contract to be legal and enforceable.[75] Finally, some states do not have any laws dealing with surrogacy. Recognizing the complexity of surrogacy, especially the numerous possibilities for surrogacy contracts, some states have concluded that legislation is not the best way to address this issue. Consequently, courts have been left with the burden of resolving conflicts and dictating informal policies within these states.[15]

Singapore

In Singapore, gestational surrogacy is restricted to parous married women with stable family relationships. Foreign women¸ except close relatives of the recipient couple, are excluded from acting as gestational surrogates, medical professionals are excluded from surrogate recruitment and reimbursement and/or compensation of gestational surrogates is based on a direct expenses model. The prospective recipient couple is legally bound by the surrogacy contract to accept even a congenitally deformed child and stringent guidelines are in place for combining surrogacy with egg donation from a third woman, who is neither the social nor gestational mother.[68]

Religious Issues

Developments in science and technology in reproduction raise new religious questions that do not always have clear answers. Despite the widespread use of assisted reproductive technology as a common means of achieving conception in couples afflicted with infertility, religious differences exist in attitudes to therapeutic procedures, such as IVF-embryo transfer, donation of genetic material (sperm, oocyte, embryo), cryopreservation of genetic material, surrogacy, posthumous reproduction, gender preselection, and reproductive and therapeutic cloning. Different religious arguments of the world's religions impose limitations on the therapeutic approach to infertility.[85]

Judaism allows the practice of all techniques of assisted reproduction when the oocyte and spermatozoon originate from the wife and husband respectively. Jewish religious authorities prohibit artificial insemination from a donor for reasons of incest, lack of genealogy and the problem of inheritance. With regard to egg donation, according to the Jewish law, the child is related to the woman who finished its formation, the one who gave birth. Full surrogacy is permitted but from the religious point of view, the child will belong to the father who gave the sperm and to the woman who gave birth.[85] There are objections to treating unmarried couples, single or lesbian women and to posthumous conception, because such households are not traditional families.[86] However, though the use of donor gametes is largely unacceptable to orthodox rabbis, progressive and conservative rabbis place more emphasis on the social attributes of parents and frequently approve of gamete donation and the Jewish status of children resulting from surrogacy or adoption can be settled by religious conversion.[86]

Though traditional Christian views forbid most assisted reproductive technologies on the basis of the view that the embryo has moral status as a human being, differences exist in attitudes toward reproductive practice among Christian groups. While the Catholic Church is strongly against all forms of assisted conception, particularly those associated with gamete donation and surrogacy, the Anglican Church is less rigid in its views and does not condemn the practice of surrogacy.[87]

Islam shares many foundational values with Judaism and Christianity[88] and presents a complete moral, ethical and medical framework that forms the basis of the ethical, moral and even juridical attitudes and laws towards any problem or situation.[89] In keeping with the beliefs of Islam, IVF-ET is acceptable if performed only for husband and wife,[90] the use of donor sperm is strictly forbidden, oocyte donation and surrogacy is disallowed except, perhaps, when it is performed between wives with the same husband. Treatment outside a marital relationship, for example, fertilization of an ovum from cryopreserved sperm after divorce of the couple or death of the husband is strictly forbidden.[91] According to Serour,[92] Islam encourages family formation and assisted reproduction, when indicated, within the frame of marriage. Organ differentiation and ensoulment are believed to occur at 42 days after fertilization at the earliest. As individuation of the embryo does not occur before 14 days from fertilization, research on surplus embryos during this period is allowed. Similarly, PGD, gene therapy and non-reproductive cloning for the benefit of humanity are ethically acceptable in Islam.[92] However, the debate continues and there are differences in the degree to which Muslims will adhere to the faith.[91] For instance, in Egypt, as in the rest of the Sunni Islamic world, assisted reproduction treatments are permitted but third parties in assisted reproduction are banned.[93] Despite authoritative *fatwas* enforcing the non-permissibility of third party donation (of sperm, eggs, embryos or uteruses) in the 1980s, since the late 1990s, however, divergences in opinion over third party gamete donation between Sunni and Shiite Muslims have resulted in the permissibility of gamete donation under certain conditions.[94] In multisectarian Lebanon, the Sunni/Catholic ban on third party reproductive assistance has been lifted because of Shia rulings emanating from Iran and today, third party reproductive assistance is provided in Lebanon to both Muslims and Christians, unlike in neighboring Egypt and Italy.[93] It must be emphasized that Muslims will vary in their degree of adherence to the faith and the practitioner should present all the options to the couple before conscientious objection to offering various modalities of assisted reproduction to their infertile patients[92] and without assuming which treatments they will or will not accept.[91]

Cross Border Reproductive Tourism

Cross border reproductive travel involves the movement of patients to undertake assisted reproductive treatment, such as IVF and associated procedures, otherwise denied to them due to cost, access or regulatory restrictions. The desire to find the ideal ethnic attributes in sperm and egg donors, avail lower costs of treatment, overcome donor shortages and the long waiting time to treatment are additional reasons for seeking cross border reproduction.[95] Hence, even reproductive body parts, oocytes, sperm and embryos are stratified-marketed according to place of origin, the characteristics of their donors and gender.[38] Frozen eggs can now be bought online, ordered from US storage banks by phone and shipped to clinics.[96] The shortage of donor oocytes due to inadequate monetary compensation and the threat of removal of donor anonymity, as is the current situation in the United Kingdom,[95] a ban on commercial oocyte donation, as well as an explicit disallowance of egg-sharing in Singapore, and unreasonable demands placed upon their personal liberties by various governments, have resulted in increasing reproductive tourism for egg donation or surrogacy[97] to places like the United States, where donated oocytes are readily available because of generous financial remuneration to oocyte donors,[95,97,98]donor selection is possible, donor information is unrestricted and for the right price, donors can be screened to match particular criteria.[99] India cherishes a similar situation and is among the reproductive friendly nations that promote reproductive tourism with no rigid law to hamper its progress.

Medical tourism may be obligatory or elective. The former occurs when necessary treatments are unavailable or illegal in the place of origin, while the latter includes elective and medically indicated procedures that, although available at the place of origin, may be delivered more quickly or in a more cost-effective manner in another location. International outsourcing of medical and surgical care offers a cost-effective solution to the unprecedented increase in costs, fulfils the task of providing care to an estimated 46 million uninsured or underinsured patients and satisfies the efforts of these patients, along with both insurers and employers, seeking to reduce the costs of treatment.[100] Moreover, legal and policy limitations have created a global environment where, in a rising number of instances, individuals and couples must travel elsewhere to procure fertility procedures that are unavailable back home. This has only been facilitated by low cost airfares, a growing number of 'medical cartographers' guiding the task and, physicians, legal experts and policy makers shaping how government and health care agencies should formally guide or regulate reproductive tourism.[101] US residents are now turning to these French associations to help link them with more inexpensive foreign clinics, notably in Spain and Greece for a small annual fee.[102] Cheaper prices, high quality health care and the availability of donor eggs and surrogates are drawing an increasing number of couples to Thailand, Eastern Europe, Russia, China and India. In the English-speaking world, India has a big advantage because of the availability of English-speaking doctors with the main advantage of relaxed laws.[95]

The diversity in regulations in different countries has led to the globalization of the technology as infertile patients cross legislative borders to seek treatment. Substantial differences in European legislations exist from the open-up *'laissez faire'* to the most restrictive ones.[97] Owing to the restrictions imposed on egg donation and surrogacy in Japan, it has been estimated that over 1,000 Japanese couples travel every year to California alone to seek egg donation.[101] A consequence of the new Italian law, based primarily on Catholic views, is an increase in 'reproductive tourism' out of Italy, observed by a 20% increase in Italian patients in some clinics in Spain, Austria and Switzerland and relocation of practices of Italian fertility doctors outside the country's borders.[81] Reproductive tourism has now been considered as a 'safety valve' in Europe that can help to avoid moral conflict.[103] The growing number of women turning to egg donation has helped to break down social taboos surrounding assisted reproduction technology.[96] More permissive nations are taking a cottage industry approach to promote fertility services that are attracting a growing international clientele.[104] A retrospective analysis of the trend in the influx of patients coming from abroad to the authors' center for ART, over a period of 3 years, from January 2004 to December 2006 revealed a progressive increase in the number of cycles performed for patients from abroad from 7.5% in 2004 to 10.6% in 2005 and 15.0% in 2006. The percentage of foreigners seeking surrogacy doubled from 11.8% in 2005 to 23.3% in 2006.[96] Today, the concept of 'patient-friendly' medically assisted reproduction that includes a robust set of clinical practice principles (cost-effectiveness, equity of access, minimal risk for mother and child and minimal burden for patients), to improve the quality of sub-fertility care has deeper meaning than the sole focus on effectiveness and high pregnancy rates in ART.[105,106]

However, transnational or international oocyte donation, or the outsourcing of oocyte donation to poorer countries to meet the rising demand, has raised numerous ethical concerns such as: (i) exploitation of underprivileged women from poorer countries, (ii) abdication of responsibility for the welfare of donors by fertility physicians from richer counties, (iii) resulting issues of contention in cases of transmission of disease or congenital defects to the oocyte recipient and the resulting offspring born from such a donation.[5] Moreover, the extent of 'IVF tourism' is unknown, since women seeking infertility care or surrogates can carry an embryo back home undetected.[95]

Surrogacy tourism has emerged to fulfill the need of those wanting to use surrogacy, but living in a place where it is highly regulated or banned.[75] While domestic surrogacy provides an option for people living in a state that bans surrogacy to travel to a neighbouring state that permits it as in the US, international surrogacy is another option that extends to people in countries where surrogacy is highly regulated or banned. Even people in places with a limited, regulatory or a free market approach to surrogacy may sometimes opt for international surrogacy because it is much cheaper than domestic surrogacy.[75] India is an attractive destination for surrogacy tourism for precisely this reason; the average cost of a surrogacy arrangement in India is approximately $25,000, which is significantly cheaper than a conservative estimate of $70,000 in the United States. The price for Indian surrogacy covers all medical procedures, payment to the surrogate, as well as airfare and hotel accommodations for two trips (the first trip to implant the embryo and the second one to collect the baby). The lower cost in India makes surrogacy a more feasible option for individuals or couples of a lower socioeconomic class. In addition to the lower cost, India, as discussed, has very few regulations on surrogacy and allows surrogates to waive their parental rights before birth, thus giving intended parents a higher level of assurance that they will receive the baby.[107]

Although international surrogacy tourism offers an attractive option for couples seeking ART with surrogacy, differences in rights entitled to the intended parents in the country of origin and destination may result in legal complications, reducing the intended parents' rights. For instance, in 2008, divorce of a Japanese couple, the intended parents, seeking surrogacy with an Indian surrogate, when the latter was still pregnant left a baby girl parentless—a 'surrogacy orphan'. Following the divorce, neither did the intended mother nor the surrogate want any claim to the baby. Though the intended father was willing to take custody of his biological daughter, he could neither do this under the Indian law that does not allow single men to adopt girls, nor could he do so under the Japanese law since the baby was still considered an Indian citizen. Hence, he was denied custody rights.[108] Such problems could however, be avoided if guidelines are in place to establish how a couple can establish citizenship for a child born through an international surrogate. The Australian embassy in India, for example, has outlined specific steps Australian parents need to follow in order to establish citizenship for their child after he or she is born from a surrogate in India. On its website, the embassy has the necessary forms available for download and lists recommending DNA testing labs in Australia to verify the genetic ties between the intended parents and the child.[109] Despite potential legal complications, the demand for surrogacy tourism continues to increase. In India, commercial surrogacy is growing so rapidly that the Indian Council of Medical Research predicts that it will soon become a $6 billion per year industry.[77] Moreover, increased chances of survival among cancer patients of reproductive age following treatment has increased the popularity of surrogacy as a treatment option among such patients who cannot gestate with the opportunity to have biological children, as long as they are able to overcome the legal barriers found in various geographic locations.[15]

Solutions

Regulatory safeguards should be put in place to prevent fertility clinics and medical professionals from indulging in 'brokerage' of donated human material by 're-selling' imported donor gametes at a profit to the patient.[50] The more widespread this phenomenon of reproductive tourism, the louder the call for international measures to stop these movements. Reproductive tourism is moral pluralism, realized by moving across legal borders. As such, this pragmatic solution presupposes legal diversity.[103]

Appropriate regulation of surrogacy arrangements minimizes the potentially exploitative aspects of surrogacy and provides legal protection to both parties in the agreement,[69] while failure to do so may lead to clinics dealing with them in an unsatisfactory manner.[71] Hence, the provision of detailed counseling to all the parties involved in surrogacy arrangements is of paramount importance.[62] The British Medical Association, 1996[110] has detailed issues for discussion with the commissioning couple and the surrogate. However, according to Dodds and Jones,[84] the risks associated with surrogacy, such as the surrogate mother's loss of control over her body and daily activities during the pregnancy, the powerlessness of having to give up a child to whom one may have formed a deep attachment and the normal dangers of pregnancy, seriously undercut the ability to make a fully informed and free choice to become a surrogate mother.[84,111] There should be greater control of surrogacy and if performed only within licensed clinics with the appropriate health screening and counseling, fewer complications would occur.[63] An efficient regulatory framework to seal discrepancies in surrogacy arrangements is mandatory to affect amicable solutions in the best interests of the offspring to be.

OUTCOMES OF THIRD PARTY REPRODUCTION

Impact on the Offspring

Although existing knowledge about the impact of assisted reproduction on parenting and child development does not give undue cause for concern, there remain a number of unanswered questions in relation to children born in this way.[15] Despite concerns regarding the potentially negative consequences of gamete donation for parent-child relationships, it has been shown that the absence of genetic or gestational link between parents and their child does not have a negative impact on parent-child relationship.[112-114] and more positive parent-child relationships accompanied with greater emotional involvement with the child has been observed among gamete donation than the natural conception parents.[112,115] No evidence of cognitive impairment in singleton children born at full term as a result of IVF and embryo donation,[114] increased risk of psychological problems,[113] difference in socio-emotional or cognitive development between surrogacy children and the natural conception children,[113,116] have been observed, although the findings regarding the cognitive development of ICSI children are currently unclear.[114] A study on the perinatal outcomes and developmental follow-up of children born after IVF surrogacy, generated by the Society of Assisted Reproductive Technology (SART) Registry between 1991 and 1995, reported that congenital abnormalities following IVF and IVF surrogacy was within the expected range for spontaneous conceptions. Birth weights for singleton pregnancies following IVF surrogacy and IVF were the same but birth weights of twins and triplets born from the IVF surrogates were significantly heavier than those delivered from conventional IVF patients. Speech delays were predominant in the multiple births but neither speech nor motor delays persisted at 2 years of age in children born after IVF surrogacy. The incidence of low birth weight was significantly lower in children born after IVF surrogacy than in those born after IVF, for all births recorded. These findings would imply that a gestational carrier would provide potential environmental benefits for the infant.[117]

Disclosure of Donor Identities

The issue of genetic inheritance and particularly, the contradictory rights of donors, recipients and donor offspring as to the disclosure of donor identities, is ethically complicated.[118] Serious inconsistencies exist between the claim that donor offspring have a right to know the identity of their gamete donor and the way such a right is currently met in practice.[119] According to Frydman et al.[118] guaranteeing anonymous oocyte donation has practical importance because, for many volunteer donors, it plays a crucial role in their decision to donate. Intense arguments about philosophical, ethical and economic issues related to ART and research on donor egg IVF (i.e. 'nongenetic') motherhood suggests that while socially and technologically acquired parenthood add a highly desired dimension to their social identities, a sense of loss appeared to persist in most of the women's personal identities.[118] Where non-anonymous donation is practised, the donor offspring retains the proclaimed right to his/her genetic identity to know the circumstances of their conception and the right to information identifying the gamete donor.[119] Donor programs increasingly offer an open-identity between donors and offspring, including children conceived through embryo donation surrogacy, and the psychological needs of gamete donors and their attitudes toward disclosure are increasingly given consideration.[112] In contrast to the findings of earlier investigations, the donor insemination and egg donation parents appeared to be more open toward disclosing the donor conception to the child[120] and the psychological well being of donor conceived children does not seem to be impacted by the disclosure decisions of their parents.[112]

FUTURE RECOMMENDATIONS AND SOLUTIONS

The Role of Counseling

The exponential increase in the use of TPR as a means of conception that is now widely available to a diverse category of people, ethnic, legal, religious and social differences in the practice of TPR and the commercialization of the technology, make it mandatory to safeguard all the parties involved and especially, the offspring to be by appropriate and detailed procedure, medico-legal, implications, emotional and financial counseling prior to undertaking the program. The emotional, medical and potential risks to the donor, impact on family relationships, the future role of the donor in the offspring's life, disclosure of the donor's identity and unfortunate circumstances, such as divorce or death of requesting individuals, should be addressed[25] and medical, ethical, legal and psychological issues related to surrogacy carefully examined.[121]

Overall, loss of fertility can be an emotionally challenging experience for women regardless of its cause. Cancer survivors have been found to have lower scores of physical quality of life and sexual function than non-cancer infertile women and unmet informational needs about reproductive options appeared to be associated with negative mood and increased distress. Hence, targeted interventions to increase knowledge about reproductive options could be of great assistance to women pursuing parenthood in cancer survivorship.[122] Alongside the options of fertility preservation, the need and relevance of surrogacy in the event of the loss of ability to gestate following treatment, including potential legal barriers in utilizing it across borders must be fully explained to cancer survivors before they make fertility preservation decisions prior to cancer treatment.[15] Ethical issues of embryo freezing and gestational surrogacy and practical issues of ovarian preservation and transposition should be considered when counseling a woman with early-stage cervical cancer about future fertility.[123] Informed consent protocols must address the desires of young cancer survivors who may have difficulty assessing whether parenthood will be important to them in the future.[124]

Human Immunodeficiency Virus (HIV) serodiscordant couples (in which only the male partner is HIV positive) suffer: (i) the potential risk of HIV infection to the mother and the fetus during the process of fertility treatment, (ii) possibility of premature death of the male partner due to HIV/AIDS. Hence, arrangements for third party parenting in the event of the male partner's death are an important aspect of decision making.[1] Irrespective of whether the payment is personal or funded via a third party, IVF is expensive. Clinical and drug costs are known and, if necessary, can be budgeted for. But, indirect expenses involved in participation also need to be considered. The study demonstrates that over and above medical and drug costs, significant extra expense in terms of time and money can be spent in an IVF cycle. Patients must be adequately counseled about the financial costs involved prior to commencing the program and all other issues being equal, geographical location should be part of the decision as to which clinic to attend.[125]

A written informed consent that carefully outlines the procedure, the obligations toward each party, the risks involved and the implications must be obtained from all third party participants (donors, recipients, surrogates and commissioning couples).[48] Nurses may have an important role in helping couples and third party participants obtain fully informed consent[48] and play a significant role in positively affecting the egg donor's experience by making sure that donor understands the risks, as well as the benefits of egg donation.[22] Consents built upon effective lines of communication between clinical staff and legal counsel, assuring that parentage, relinquishment and re-contact information in donor-recipient agreements are consistent with clinic consent documents and desires of both parties are mandatory in all gamete donation programs. All decisions must be adequately documented and honored and long-term counseling needs should be addressed.[126]

Counseling plays a significant role in TPR in providing treatment and care of patients, not simply when they are undergoing fertility treatment but also with their long-term emotional well-being and that of their children and the reproductive helpers who may assist them in achieving biologic or reproductive parenthood, and may be given by a psychiatrist or another health care professional. It plays an essential role in educating patients about the side effects of infertility treatment medications, the impact of hormone shifts on psychologic well-being and differential diagnoses among grief, depression, and stress; in assessing psychologic preparedness and in determining the acceptability and suitability of gamete donation, a gestational carrier or surrogacy as a family-building alternative for individuals, couples and reproductive collaborators.[51]

The British Medical Association, 1996[110] recommends the following issues for discussion with the commissioning couple:

- A review of all alternative treatment options and the implications of not having children in the future
- The possibility of adoption instead of surrogacy
- The usefulness and need for in-depth counseling
- The need to find their own host and where they might find one
- The potential practical difficulties of treatment by gestational surrogacy
- The full costs of treatment
- The potential medical and psychological risks of surrogacy
- The potential psychological risks, short and long-term, to a child born by surrogacy
- The implications of having a multiple pregnancy
- The degree of involvement that the host may wish to have with the child following the birth
- The possibility that the child may be born with a handicap
- The risks to the baby if the host smokes and drinks during pregnancy
- The possibility that the host may wish to retain the child after birth
- The fact that surrogacy contracts in the UK are not enforceable
- The importance of obtaining legal advice
- The genetic couple is advised to take out insurance cover for the surrogate.

The British Medical Association, 1996[110] recommends the following issues for discussion with the surrogate:

- The full implications of undergoing treatment by IVF surrogacy
- The possibility of multiple pregnancies
- The possibility of her family and friends being against her having treatment
- The medical risks associated with pregnancy and the possibility of delivery by Cesarean section
- The implications of feelings of guilt on both sides if the host should spontaneously abort a pregnancy
- The potential effect on her own children of acting as a surrogate
- The possibility that the host may feel a sense of bereavement when she gives the baby to the commissioning couple
- The possibility that the child may be born with a handicap
- The fact that hosts in the UK may only claim `reasonable expenses'.

Third party reproduction through oocyte donation is a long and labor intensive process with a significant amount of emotional, financial and physical involvement from all parties, and is quite often, a gratifying experience for everyone involved, which include oocyte donors, recipients, social workers, nurses and physicians.[9] In order to ensure safety and success of the procedure, all the participants must be extensively screened medically and psychologically and a detailed understanding of the process by all parties involved should be achieved. In spite of the reassuring studies that have been carried out on the effects of surrogacy on the host and on the commissioning couples, further large follow-up studies are required, especially on the long-term effects on the children born as a result of surrogacy arrangements.[127] More research is needed on whether participating in fertility preservation reduces long-term distress about cancer-related fertility. Better evidence-based programs to educate families and reduce decisional conflict are needed.[124]

Egg Sharing

Egg sharing is a mutually beneficial scheme that provides lower cost or free IVF treatment to women in exchange for oocyte donation to anonymous recipients. Compensated egg sharing, originally conceived as a patient self-help co-operative scheme to avoid overt 'commodification' of donor oocytes and prevent doctors and medical institutions from acting as 'brokers' of donated human material, is an ethically justifiable and much preferred alternative to commercialized oocyte donation.[128] While egg sharing enables two infertile couples to benefit from a single surgical procedure, it is a very constructive way of solving the problem of the shortage of eggs for donation and has the advantages of including a group of women who would otherwise be denied treatment.[129]

Pennings[130] has proposed a mirror exchange system that can alleviate the shortage of both sperm and egg donation in an ethically acceptable way. The partner of the person who has no usable gametes donates and receives the mirror gametes in return in an indirect exchange system so that the couple receives bonus points for their donation and their waiting time for the gametes is reduced or even fully cancelled. However, this system of strict reciprocity is rejected as unfair because it excludes categories of people from access to donor gametes. Moreover, candidate recipients, who for medical or psychological reasons do not qualify as donors, should have access to donor gametes on the basis of points collected on other criteria and not only contribution, and the wish to have a child should be taken into account when allocating donor gametes.[130]

Intrafamilial Gamete Donation

Intrafamilial sperm donation, especially involving minors under the age of 18 years, should be avoided because of potential parental conflicts of interest, coercion of the prospective donor and unhealthy family dynamics, and alternative methods to conceive, such as anonymous sperm donation, should be advised. Sperm donation should not be used to prevent genetic diseases. Marshall[25] suggests that if intrafamilial sperm donation must, after careful consideration be pursued, then all precautions should be taken to prevent medical, psychological and legal harm to the requesting couple or individual, the potential donor and the prospective child and the standards governing anonymous sperm donation should be followed without exception in evaluating the proposed sperm donor for infectious and genetic diseases.[25]

Legislative Solutions

Assisted reproductive technologies have changed life for the past 25 years and many ethical and social issues have emerged following this new method of conception.[97] The practice of TPR faces diverse restrictions and regulations world over making an understanding the complex interactions between law, religion, local moralities and reproductive practices for global bioethics a necessity.[93] A given method of surrogacy may well result in different procedures and outcomes regarding parental rights in different jurisdictions, suggesting the need for a uniform method to resolve parental rights where ART is involved.[131]

The demand for women's egg cells for therapy and research is increasing and is leading to reproductive tourism and transnational oocyte trafficking. In the wake of the burgeoning ART industry and the growing oocyte market, regulations for the human oocyte market, designed to protect and promote important social values, such as health, safety, liberty and respect for human life, have been proposed as the most prudent course of action.[132] Schneider[133] emphasizes the need for supranational regulation to protect both donor interests and the public good.[133] Medical problems, which need to be considered, include the selection of donors, evaluation of the recipients and quality control of the genetic material.[2] New government and professional guidelines, broader representation on ethics committees and expanded counseling about risks and benefits can help reduce the potential for litigation and enhance patient autonomy.[48]

Regulatory safeguards are needed to ensure against undue coercion, deception or manipulation of women into becoming oocyte or embryo donors, considering their ability to make autonomous decisions about donating oocytes or embryos for biomedical research following adequate information and appropriate procedural protections.[34] The relationship between the biological and social parents and safeguarding the interests of the offspring may be resolved by specific legislations pertaining to each country.[2] Potential pre-embryo banks should be subjected to licensing, should not be run by a commercial system and the medical profession and society should consider not only the interests of the infertile couple, but also the interests of the offspring in pre-embryo donation.[2] The currently proposed National Institutes of Health guidelines for stem cell research are too narrowly drawn and do not adequately protect the freedom of choice and health of women who donate embryos. They need to be expanded to cover not only the point of embryo donation, but also that of embryo creation.[134] In order to protect individuals against scientific and ethical abuses without inhibiting scientific progress, a specific legal framework is necessary.[97] While the need for a legal framework to regulate the use of reproductive technologies is becoming apparent, a conscientious effort in this direction would help resolve the many unsettling issues that they raise. Taking into account the patients, their future child and the interests of third party collaborators, such as gamete donors and surrogates, ESHRE has formulated a good practice guide for cross border reproductive care for centers and practitioners. It aims to ensure high quality and safe assisted reproduction treatment by including considerations of equity, safety, efficiency, effectiveness (including evidence-based care), timeliness and patient centeredness.[135]

The limited availability of resources mandates their judicious use throughout medicine. In a field like infertility, by many perceived as 'elective', the judicious use of resources seems even more necessary since it would permit the treatment of larger patient populations than have currently access to care without further expense to third party payments.[136]

According to Merlet,[97] in order to avoid ethical abuses, homogenization with regard to respect for human life and ban on commercial practices of human body parts, eugenic practices and any kind of cloning is necessary. It must be reasserted that human body parts should not be a source of financial gain.[97] The *Agence de la biomédecine* is a government agency that represents the French competent authority for medical and scientific aspects of ART and is one of the main tools of the French regulations created in 2004 to focus on improving the quality and the safety of ART management.[97]

While legalizing the practice of TPR with accountability at every step would help overcome the many problems and settle the controversies it has sparked, it is feared that with things becoming easier and legal, people might become overenthusiastic and have a baby for which they are not emotionally prepared on a long-term basis. Neglect and abuse of these children is an issue of concern and a mechanism should be put in place for monitoring their progress by social agencies.[21]

RECENT ADVANCES

Ooplasmic transfer (OT) and nuclear transfer (NT) are recent technologies proposed to prevent the transmission of mitochondrial DNA (mtDNA) mutations to overcome the limitations in prenatal diagnosis and preimplantation genetic diagnoses. OT involves the transfer of normal mitochondria to a carrier's oocyte containing mutant mtDNA, while NT involves enucleation of a donor oocyte and replacement with the nuclear DNA from a woman carrying an mtDNA mutation. Both OT and NT are radical in the sense that they do not entail genetic selection but genetic intervention to correct the genetic cause of the disease. NT can be performed both before and after IVF, respectively, with the nucleus of an unfertilized oocyte, with the pronuclei of the zygote or with the nucleus of a blastomere of an embryo. However, these techniques have raised serious conceptual and ethical issues, such as: (i) whether they amount to germline modification and human cloning, (ii) the significance of intervening in the mtDNA, (iii) the implications of having 'three genetic parents', (iv) the ethics of oocyte donation and, (iv) the health and safety risks for children conceived as a result of these techniques. Further interdisciplinary debate and research is needed to determine whether a clinical application of OT and NT can be morally justified, and if so, under which conditions.[137]

Vitrification or ultrarapid freezing is an efficient cryopreservation technique for freezing oocytes and all stages of embryos with increased survival and success rates and several advantages compared to the conventional slow freeze-thaw techniques. Cryopreservation by vitrification can likely blur the ethical and moral boundaries between compensated egg sharing and commercialized oocyte donation.[128] Banking of cryopreserved oocytes would obviate the need for donors and recipients in egg sharing to have coordinated and synchronized treatment cycles and enable fertility doctors and medical institutions to offer subsidized fertility treatment upfront to any patient willing to donate a portion of her retrieved cohort of oocytes for banking and subsequent donation. However, Heng[67] fears that it would inevitably result in overt 'commodification' of donated human material by facilitating the opportunity for fertility physicians to broker the transaction of oocytes between the donor and recipient and profit from the banking and storage of cryopreserved oocytes.[128]

Natural cycle IVF, modified natural cycle IVF and mild approaches to ovarian stimulation combined with single embryo transfer (SET) are new alternatives to conventional IVF to overcome the disadvantages of stimulated cycles including the high risk of multiple pregnancy, risk of hyperstimulation and behavioural changes due to the effects of drugs,[49,138] high costs and discomfort. Immature oocyte retrieval and *in vitro* maturation of oocytes in high responders to ovarian stimulation is an additional option to decrease the incidence of ovarian hyperstimulation syndrome.

CONCLUSION

Third party reproduction (sperm, egg and embryo donation and surrogacy) has carried the science of ART to new dimensions with promising answers for everyone who desires a baby today without inhibitions of sex, marital status, religion or genuine medical indications. This has only been nurtured further by the vast differences in ethical, social, religious and legal perceptions of TPR, not only across continents but even among countries and states of the same country, leading to an explosive increase in cross border reproductive tourism. While arduous efforts to find valid solutions to the highly debated ethical, legal, clinical and moral issues that TPR brews continue, the pace at which the technology is growing seems beyond reach. While certain countries have been successful in imposing rigid legislations to keep the practice within legal, ethical, religious, social and moral limits, they have been unsuccessful in controlling cross border travel to seek ART, which is now, more than rampant. While instituting a single recognized global, legislative framework to regulate TPR might seem impossible, it rests with providers of the technology to execute the practice with a sense of human responsibility and safeguard the interests of all parties concerned, especially the offspring. The assigning authorities should make a conscientious effort to license the practice judiciously with mandatory guidelines devoid of loopholes. Commercial exploitation should be kept at bay so that the benefits of a technology that holds the key to the happiness of innumerable lives today can be meted out to the genuinely needy who have thus far, been deprived of it.

REFERENCES

1. Schenker JG. Ethical aspects of advanced reproductive technologies. Ann N Y Acad Sci. 2003;997:11-21.
2. Eisenberg VH, Schenker JG. Pre-embryo donation: ethical and legal aspects. Int J Gynaecol Obstet. 1998;60:51-7.
3. Merchant R, Allahbadia GN. Ethical and religious considerations in third party reproduction. In: Gautam N Allahbadia (Eds). Donor Egg IVF. Jaypee Medical Publishers: New Delhi; 2009. pp. 345-64.
4. Fasouliotis SJ, Schenker JG. Social aspects in assisted reproduction. Hum Reprod Update. 1999;5:26-39.
5. Heng BC. Ethical issues in transnational "mail order" oocyte donation. Int J Gynaecol Obstet. 2006;95:302-4.
6. van den Akker O. The importance of a genetic link in mothers commissioning a surrogate baby in the UK. Hum Reprod. 2000;15:1849-55.
7. Merchant R, Gandhi G, Allahbadia GN. In vitro fertilization/intracytoplasmic sperm injection for male infertility. Indian J Urol. 2011;27:121-32.
8. Merchant R, Allahbadia GN. Can we define the Indications for Oocyte Donation? In: Gautam N Allahbadia (Ed). Donor Egg IVF. Jaypee Medical Publishers: New Delhi; 2009. pp. 11-19.
9. Luk J, Greenfeld DA, Seli E. Third party reproduction and the aging couple. Maturitas. 2010;66:389-96.
10. Eisenberg VH, Schenker JG. Pregnancy in the older woman: scientific and ethical aspects. Int J Gynaecol Obstet. 1997;56:163-7.
11. Montan S. Increased risk in the elderly parturient. Curr Opin Obstet Gynecol. 2007;19:110-2.
12. Merchant R, Allahbadia GN. Surrogacy: Ethical, Psychological and Legal Implications. In: Gautam N Allahbadia (Ed.). Donor Egg IVF. Jaypee Medical Publishers: New Delhi; 2009. pp. 297-309.
13. Oktay K, Oktem O. Fertility preservation medicine: a new field in the care of young cancer survivors. Pediatr Blood Cancer. 2009;53:267-73.
14. Beski S, Gorgy A, Venkat G, et al. Gestational surrogacy: a feasible option for patients with Rokitansky syndrome. Hum Reprod. 2000;15:2326-8.
15. Meniru GI, Craft IL. Experience with gestational surrogacy as a treatment for sterility resulting from hysterectomy. Hum Reprod. 1997;12:51-4.
16. Goldfarb JM, Austin C, Peskin B, et al. Fifteen years experience with an in vitro fertilization surrogate gestational pregnancy programme. Hum Reprod. 2000;15:1075-8.
17. ESHRE Task Force on Ethics and Law, de Wert G, Dondorp W, et al. Intrafamilial medically assisted reproduction. Hum Reprod. 2011;26:504-9.
18. Herz EK. Infertility and bioethical issues of the new reproductive technologies. Psychiatr Clin North Am. 1989;12:117-31.
19. Cohen CB. Unmanaged care: the need to regulate new reproductive technologies in the United States. Bioethics. 1997;11:348-65.

20. Grobstein C, Flower M. Current ethical issues in IVF. Clin Obstet Gynaecol. 1985;12:877-91.
21. Law Resource India. Legalising surrogacy—Boon or bane. Available from www.indialawyers.wordpress.com/2010/07/14/legalising-surrogacy-%E2%80%94-boon-or-bane [Accessed 2011]
22. Black JJ. Egg donation: issues & concerns. MCN Am J Matern Child Nurs. 2010;35:132-7.
23. Letur H. Current practices of oocyte donation in France and Europe. (Article in French). J Gynecol Obstet Biol Reprod (Paris). 2007;36:727-37.
24. Pennings G. Incest, gamete donation by siblings and the importance of the genetic link. Reprod Biomed Online. 2002;4:13-5.
25. Marshall LA. Ethical and legal issues in the use of related donors for therapeutic insemination. Urol Clin North Am. 2002;29:855-61.
26. Trounson AO, Wood C. IVF and related technology. The present and the future. Med J Aust. 1993;158:853-7.
27. Robertson JA. Ethical and legal issues in human embryo donation. Fertil Steril. 1995;64:885.
28. Smajdor A. The ethics of egg donation in the over fifties. Menopause Int. 2008;14:173-7.
29. Samani RO, Moalem MR, Merghati ST, et al. Debate in embryo donation: embryo donation or both-gamete donation? Reprod Biomed Online. 2009;19 (Suppl 1): 29-33.
30. Youssry M, Orief Y, Palapelas V, et al. Embryo cryopreservation: is vitrification ready to replace slow freezing? Expert Review of Obstet & Gynecol. 2008;3:455.
31. Zwart-Hendrikx N. Chilling aspects of procreation. Med Law. 2002;21:567-86.
32. Van Voorhis BJ, Grinstead DM, Sparks AE, et al. Establishment of a successful donor embryo program: medical, ethical and policy issues. Fertil Steril. 1999; 71:604-8.
33. Valenzuela CY. Scientific ethics of the origin of humans. (Article in Spanish). Rev Med Chil. 1997;125:701-5.
34. Warren MA. Embryo manipulation and experimentation. Baillieres Clin Obstet Gynaecol. 1991;5:591-609.
35. Tangwa GB. Third party assisted conception: an African perspective. Theor Med Bioeth. 2008;29:297-306.
36. Bowman MC, Saunders DM. Community attitudes to maternal age and pregnancy after assisted reproductive technology: too old at 50 years? Hum Reprod. 1994; 9:167-71.
37. Min JK, Claman P, Hughes E, et al. Guidelines for the number of embryos to transfer following in vitro fertilization No. 182, September 2006. Int J Gynaecol Obstet. 2008;102:203-16.
38. Whittaker A, Speier A. "Cycling overseas": care, commodification, and stratification in cross-border reproductive travel. Med Anthropol. 2010;29:363-83.
39. Heng BC. Factors influencing the reimbursement rate of egg donation within a competitive free-market system. Reprod Biomed Online. 2007;15:16-8.
40. Cohen CB. Selling bits and pieces of humans to make babies: The gift of the magi revisited. J Med Philos. 1999;24:288-306.
41. Resnik DB. The commodification of human reproductive materials. J Med Ethics. 1998;24:388-93.
42. Fox D. Paying for particulars in people-to-be: commercialisation, commodification and commensurability in human reproduction. J Med Ethics. 2008;34:162-6.
43. Steinbock B. Payment for egg donation and surrogacy. Mt Sinai J Med. 2004;71:255-65.
44. Daniels KR. To give or sell human gametes—the interplay between pragmatics, policy and ethics. J Med Ethics. 2000;26:206-11.
45. Pennings G. Commentary on Craft and Thornhill: new ethical strategies to recruit gamete donors. Reprod Biomed Online. 2005;10:307-9.
46. McCormick RA. Surrogacy: a Catholic perspective. Creighton Law Rev. 1992;25:1617-25.
47. Reame N. Informed consent issues in assisted reproduction. J Obstet Gynecol Neonatal Nurs. 1999;28:331-8.
48. Shenfield F. Too late for change, too early to judge, but an oxymoron will not solve the problem. Reprod Biomed Online. 2005;10:433-5.
49. Heng BC. Legal and ethical issues in the international transaction of donor sperm and eggs. J Assist Reprod Genet. 2007;24:107-9.
50. Burns LH. Psychiatric aspects of infertility and infertility treatments. Psychiatr Clin North Am. 2007;30:689-716.
51. Robertson JA. Compensation and egg donation for research. Fertil Steril. 2006;86:1573-5.
52. Thompson C. Why we should, in fact, pay for egg donation. Regen Med. 2007;2:203-9.
53. Baylis F, McLeod C. The stem cell debate continues: the buying and selling of eggs for research. J Med Ethics. 2007;33:726-31.
54. Carp HJ, Dirnfeld M, Dor J, et al. ART in recurrent miscarriage: preimplantation genetic diagnosis/screening or surrogacy? Hum Reprod. 2004;19:1502-5.
55. Klipstein S. Preimplantation genetic diagnosis: technological promise and ethical perils. Fertil Steril. 2005; 83:1347-53.
56. Robertson JA. Extending preimplantation genetic diagnosis: the ethical debate. Ethical issues in new uses of preimplantation genetic diagnosis. Hum Reprod. 2003;18:465-71.
57. Scott R. Choosing between possible lives: legal and ethical issues in preimplantation genetic diagnosis. Oxf J Leg Stud. 2006;26:153-78.
58. Ludwig M, Pergament D, Schwinger E, et al. The situation of preimplantation genetic diagnosis in Germany: legal and ethical problems. Prenat Diagn. 2000;20:567-70.
59. Robertson JA. Extending preimplantation genetic diagnosis: medical and non-medical uses. J Med Ethics. 2003;29:213.
60. Chang CL. Surrogate motherhood. Formos J Med Humanit. 2004;5:48-62.
61. Balen AH, Hayden CA. British Fertility Society survey of all licensed clinics that perform surrogacy in the UK. Hum Fertil (Camb). 1998;1:6-9.
62. Boivin J, Appleton TC, Baetens P, et al. Guidelines for counseling in infertility: outline version. Hum Reprod. 2001;16:1301-4.

63. Goold I. Surrogacy: is there a case for legal prohibition? J Law Med. 2004;12:205-16.
64. When baby's mother is also grandma—and sister. Hastings Cent Rep. 1985;15:29-31.
65. van den Akker OB. Psychosocial aspects of surrogate motherhood. Hum Reprod Update. 2007;13:53-62.
66. Frenkel DA. Legal regulation of surrogate motherhood in Israel. Med Law. 2001;20:605-12.
67. Human Fertilisation and Embryology Act (1990). Her Majesty's Stationary Office, London.
68. Heng BC. Proposed ethical guidelines and legislative framework for permitting gestational surrogacy in Singapore. Reprod Biomed Online. 2007;15 (Suppl 1): 7-11.
69. Chen M. Wombs for rent: an examination of prohibitory and regulatory approaches to governing preconception arrangements. Health Law Can. 2003;23:33-50.
70. Reilly DR. Surrogate pregnancy: a guide for Canadian prenatal health care providers. CMAJ. 2007;176:483-5.
71. Willmott L. Surrogacy: ill-conceived rights. J Law Med. 2002;10:198-220.
72. Johnson I. Regulation of assisted reproductive technology: the Australian experience. In: Brinsden PR (Ed.). A Textbook of In Vitro Fertilization and Assisted Reproduction. Parthenon, Carnforth and New York; 1999. pp. 424-7.
73. Cohen J, Jones H. [Assisted reproduction. Rules and laws. International comparisons]
74. Chen KC, Ng HT. Legal and ethical considerations of assisted reproductive technology and surrogate motherhood in AOFOG countries. J Obstet Gynaecol Res. 2001;27:89-95.
75. Kindregan C, McBrien M. Assisted reproductive technology: a lawyer's guide to emerging law & science. Chicago: American Bar Association. 2006.
76. http://indiansurrogacylaw.com/?gclid=CJ-Gx MWM6 ZgCFQ0Zegodi3Zt1A.
77. Chang M. Womb for rent: India's commercial surrogacy. Harvard Int Rev. 2009;3111.
78. Schuz R. Surrogacy in Israel: an analysis of the law in practice. In: Cook R, Sclater S, Kaganas F (Eds). Surrogate motherhood: international perspectives. Portland: Oxford; 2003. pp. 35-54.
79. Hunter-Henin M. Surrogacy: is there room for a new liberty between the French prohibitive position and the english ambivalence. In: Freeman M (Ed). Law and bioethics. New York: Oxford; 2008. pp. 329–57.
80. Fineschi V, Neri M, Turillazzi E. The new Italian law on assisted reproduction technology (Law 40/2004). J Med Ethics. 2005;31:536-9.
81. Crosignani PG. Looking to Europe: something's changed in Italy. Hum Fertil (Camb). 2005;8:71-3.
82. Deech R. Legal and ethical responsibilities of gamete banks. Hum Reprod. 1998;13 (Suppl) 2:80-3.
83. Gamble N. Crossing the line: the legal and ethical problems of foreign surrogacy. Reprod Biomed Online. 2009; 19:151-2.
84. Petersen K, Baker HW, Pitts M, et al. Assisted reproductive technologies: professional and legal restrictions in Australian clinics. J Law Med. 2005;12:373-85.
85. Schenker JG. Infertility evaluation and treatment according to Jewish law. Eur J Obstet Gynecol Reprod Biol. 1997;71:113-21.
86. Hirsh AV. Infertility in Jewish couples, biblical and rabbinic law. Hum Fertil (Camb). 1998;1:14-19.
87. McCormick RA. Surrogacy: a Catholic perspective. Creighton Law Rev. 1992;25:1617-25.
88. Daar AS, al Khitamy AB. Bioethics for clinicians: 21. Islamic bioethics. CMAJ. 2001;164:60-3.
89. Al-Aqeel AI. Ethical guidelines in genetics and genomics. An Islamic perspective. Saudi Med J. 2005;26:1862.
90. Schenker JG. Assisted reproductive practice: religious perspectives. Reprod Biomed Online. 2005;10:310-9.
91. Husain FA. Reproductive issues from the Islamic perspective. Hum Fertil (Camb). 2000;3:124-8.
92. Serour GI. Islamic perspectives in human reproduction. Reprod Biomed Online. 2008;17(Suppl 3):34-8.
93. Inhorn MC, Patrizio P, Serour GI. Third party reproductive assistance around the Mediterranean: comparing Sunni Egypt, Catholic Italy and multisectarian Lebanon. Reprod Biomed Online. 2010;21:848-53.
94. Inhorn MC. Making Muslim babies: IVF and gamete donation in Sunni versus Shi'a Islam. Cult Med Psychiatry. 2006;30:427-50.
95. Allahbadia GN, Seidman DS. Cross border or reproductive tourism with special emphasis on donor oocytes. In: Gautam N Allahbadia (Eds). Donor Egg IVF. Jaypee Medical Publishers: New Delhi; 2009. pp. 427-36.
96. Allahbadia GN, Kadam KS, Gandhi GN, et al. Sun, sand and eggs (the reproductive tourism story). Reproductive BioMedicine Online. Abstracts for the 4th World Congress of the World Association of Reproductive Medicine 17. 2008; (Suppl 2):S-26.
97. Merlet F. Regulatory framework in assisted reproductive technologies, relevance and main issues. Folia Histochem Cytobiol. 2009;47:S9-S12.
98. Sauer MV. Indecent proposal: $5,000 is not "reasonable compensation" for oocyte donors. Fertil Steril. 1999;71: 7-10.
99. Ethics Committee of the American Society for Reproductive Medicine. Financial compensation of oocyte donors. Fertil Steril. 2007;88(2):305-.9
100. Forgione DA, Smith PC. Medical tourism and its impact on the US health care system. J Health Care Finance. 2007;34:27-35.
101. Chu H. 'It's win-win. It's a completely capitalistic enterprise'. Toronto Star. 2006;A03.
102. Jones HW, Cohen J. IFFS Surveillance 07. Fertil Steril. 2007;87(4 Suppl 1):S1-67.
103. Pennings G. Reproductive tourism as moral pluralism in motion. J Med Ethics. 2002;28:337-48.
104. Mukherjee, K. Rent-a-womb in India fuels surrogate motherhood debate. Reuters. 2007. www.reuters.com/article/latestCrisis/idUSDEL298735.
105. van Empel IW, Nelen WL, Hermens RP, et al. Coming soon to your clinic: high-quality ART. Hum Reprod. 2008;23:1242-5.
106. Pennings G, Ombelet W. Coming soon to your clinic: patient-friendly ART. Hum Reprod. 2007;22:2075-9.

107. Gentleman A. India nurtures business of surrogate motherhood. New York Times. 2008.
108. Surrogacy Orphan Trapped in Red Tape After Mothers Abandon Her. The Times. Available from www.timesonline.co.uk/tol/news/world/asia/article4474231.ece [Accessed 2010].
109. Children born through Surrogacy Arrangements applying for Australian Citizenship by Descent. Australian High Commission: India. Available from www.india.embassy.gov.au/ndli/vm_surrogacy.html [Accessed September 2009]
110. British Medical Association. Changing Conceptions of Motherhood. The Practice of Surrogacy in Britain. London: BMA Publications; 1996.
111. Dodds S, Jones K. Surrogacy and autonomy. Bioethics. 1989;3:1-17.
112. Greenfeld DA. The impact of disclosure on donor gamete participants: donors, intended parents and offspring. Curr Opin Obstet Gynecol. 2008;20:265-8.
113. Golombok S, Murray C, Jadva V, et al. Non-genetic and non-gestational parenthood: consequences for parent-child relationships and the psychological well-being of mothers, fathers and children at age 3. Hum Reprod. 2006;21:1918-24.
114. Golombok S, MacCallum F. Practitioner review: outcomes for parents and children following non-traditional conception: what do clinicians need to know? J Child Psychol Psychiatry. 2003;44:303-15.
115. MacCallum F, Golombok S, Brinsden P. Parenting and child development in families with a child conceived through embryo donation. J Fam Psychol. 2007;21:278-87.
116. Golombok S, MacCallum F, Murray C, et al. Surrogacy families: parental functioning, parent-child relationships and children's psychological development at age 2. J Child Psychol Psychiatry. 2006;47:213-22.
117. Serafini P. Outcome and follow-up of children born after IVF-surrogacy. Hum Reprod Update. 2001;7:23-7.
118. Frydman R, Letur-Könirsch H, de Ziegler D, et al. A protocol for satisfying the ethical issues raised by oocyte donation: the free, anonymous, and fertile donors. Fertil Steril. 1990;53:666-72.
119. Frith L. Beneath the rhetoric: the role of rights in the practice of non-anonymous gamete donation. Bioethics. 2001;15:473-84.
120. Golombok S, Lycett E, MacCallum F, et al. Parenting infants conceived by gamete donation. J Fam Psychol. 2004;18:443-52.
121. Committee on Ethics. ACOG committee opinion number 397, February 2008: surrogate motherhood. Obstet Gynecol. 2008;111(2 Pt 1):465-70.
122. Carter J, Raviv L, Applegarth L, et al. A cross-sectional study of the psychosexual impact of cancer-related infertility in women: third-party reproductive assistance. J Cancer Surviv. 2010;4:236-46.
123. Duska LR, Toth TL, Goodman A. Fertility options for patients with stages IA2 and IB cervical cancer: presentation of two cases and discussion of technical and ethical issues. Obstet Gynecol. 1998;92(4 Pt 2):656-8.
124. Schover LR. Patient attitudes toward fertility preservation. Pediatr Blood Cancer. 2004;53(2):281-4.
125. Kelly J, Hughes CM, Harrison RF. The hidden costs of IVF. Ir Med J. 2006;99:142-3.
126. Lindheim SR, Porat N, Jaeger AS. Survey report of gamete donors' and recipients' preferences regarding disclosure of third party reproduction outcomes and genetic risk information. J Obstet Gynaecol Res. 2011;37:292-9.
127. Brinsden PR. Gestational surrogacy. Hum Reprod Update. 2003;9:483-91.
128. Heng BC. Advances in oocyte cryopreservation technology will eventually blur the ethical and moral boundaries between compensated egg sharing and commercialized oocyte donation. Reprod Biomed Online. 2006;12:280-1.
129. Ahuja KK, Simons EG, Fiamanya W, et al. Egg-sharing in assisted conception: ethical and practical considerations. Hum Reprod. 1996;11:1126-31.
130. Pennings G. Mirror gametes donation. J Psychosom Obstet Gynaecol. 2007;28:187-91.
131. Ciccarelli JK, Ciccarelli JC. The legal aspects of parental rights in assisted reproductive technology. J Soc Issues. 2005;61:127-37.
132. Resnik DB. Regulating the market for human eggs. Bioethics. 2001;15:1-25.
133. Schneider I. Oocyte donation for reproduction and research cloning--the perils of commodification and the need for European and international regulation. Rev Derecho Genoma Hum. 2006;25:205-41.
134. Cohen CB. Use of 'excess' human embryos for stem cell research: protecting women's rights and health. Womens Health Issues. 2000;10:121-6.
135. Shenfield F, Pennings G, De Mouzon J, et al. ESHRE's good practice guide for cross-border reproductive care for centers and practitioners. Hum Reprod. 2011; 26:1625-7.
136. Gleicher N. Cost-effective infertility care. Hum Reprod Update.2000; 6:190-9.
137. Bredenoord AL, Pennings G, de Wert G. Ooplasmic and nuclear transfer to prevent mitochondrial DNA disorders: conceptual and normative issues. Hum Reprod Update. 2008;14:669-78.
138. Hammond N, Holm S. Resolving the 'egg supply problem' in human embryonic stem cell derivation through technical means—a legal and ethical analysis. Med Law. 2008;27:167-78.

28

Natural Cycle In Vitro Fertilization: The Current Practice

John David Gordon, Michael DiMattina

Chapter Contents

INTRODUCTION

The modern era of fertility treatment was ushered in by the birth of Louise Brown in July, 1978. Although this event captured the imagination of the general public worldwide, most observers would have been unlikely to predict the widespread adoption of assisted reproductive technologies (ART) that has led to nearly 5 million children conceived in this manner by 2011. As further refinements in ART have led to such unanticipated techniques such as intracytoplasmic sperm injection (ICSI) and preimplantation genetic diagnosis (PGD), there has been a countercurrent of renewed interest in simplified approaches to ART such as unstimulated (or natural cycle) *in vitro* fertilization (IVF). Proponents of these simplified approaches champion the potential benefits including improved patient access, lower costs, elimination of ovarian hyperstimulation syndrome and near universal single embryo transfer.[1-7] Those physicians opposed to natural cycle IVF focus upon the lower success rates and the need for multiple initiated treatment cycles to achieve the same pregnancy rates as a single cycle of traditional IVF.[8] This chapter reviews many aspects of natural cycle IVF ranging from historical perspective to patient selection, and the protocols and techniques utilized by those fertility clinics employing natural cycle IVF. The reported success rates of this milder approach to IVF, and patient and physician opinions will also be examined.

HISTORICAL PERSPECTIVE

The birth of Louise Brown in 1978 represented the culmination of decades of research into reproductive physiology. Robert Edwards' research in human reproduction produced many milestones along the path that led to the birth of Louise Brown, and his contribution to the field of medicine was recognized by Dr Edwards being awarded the Nobel Prize in Medicine in 2010.

The path to success began in 1965 when, Edwards determined that human oocytes could be matured *in vitro* but required 24 hours of incubation.[9] Edwards was able to demonstrate fertilization of these *in vitro* matured oocytes by utilizing the buffer conditions described by Barry Bavister, one of his graduate students.[10] By 1970,

Edwards had decided that the use of *in vivo* matured oocytes may be the key to induce human embryos to develop beyond the 2-cell stage.[11] He contacted Patrick Steptoe, a pioneer in the newly described surgical technique of laparoscopy, who was working at Oldham and District General Hospital. This set the stage for a friendship and collaboration that lasted until the death of Steptoe in 1988. Realizing that laparoscopic retrieval of a single oocyte from a single preovulatory follicle would be technically demanding, Edwards elected to prime his patients with gonadotropins prior to surgery. By 1971, the team had demonstrated the ability to culture human embryos to the blastocyst stage in development. Success was elusive as more than one hundred embryo transfers failed to result in an ongoing pregnancy. Only later did Edwards realize that his choice of Primolut for luteal support was in fact, to blame for the lack of success.[12,13] Finally, in 1976 the team reported its first ongoing pregnancy but this was an ectopic pregnancy.[14] Edwards was concerned that disruption of the endometrium by the clomiphene/gonadotropin stimulation protocol may have been responsible for the implantation of the embryo in the fallopian tube, and thus they changed course and abandoned stimulated cycle IVF in favor of unstimulated or natural cycle IVF. The second patient treated with natural cycle IVF was Lesley Brown and her first attempt at IVF was successful leading to the delivery of her daughter on July 25, 1978. Ultimately, a total of 35 cases of natural cycle IVF were initiated at Bourn Hall with 83% (29 out of 35 cases) of egg collections yielding an egg of which 86% (25 out of 29 cases) fertilized normally and 96% (24 out of 25 cases) of these fertilized eggs developed into embryos for transfer. The pregnancy rate per embryo transfer was 25% (6 out of 24 cases).[13] However, other clinics were unable to reproduce the success that Edwards had demonstrated (Table 1). Most clinics adopted the use of either clomiphene, clomiphene/gonadotropins or gonadotropins alone, and were able to achieve pregnancies and live births (Lopata, 1978; Johnston, 1981 and Jones, 1982).

Eventually, most clinics elected to pursue clomiphene/gonadotropin stimulated IVF in order to improve the odds of retrieving an egg laparoscopically. The introduction of ultrasound guided follicle aspirations (transabdominal, transvesicle and ultimately transvaginal) led most clinics to abandon laparoscopic egg collections. Meanwhile, ovarian stimulation protocols became increasingly more complex and varied as gonadotropin-releasing hormone (GnRH) agonists and newer gonadotropin preparations became available.[18,19] However, persistent concerns about the cost, side effects and long-term safety of ovarian stimulation has sustained interest in natural cycle IVF.[2,3,6]

Although some physicians (almost exclusively in the United States) have expressed skepticism and seem to be of the opinion that natural cycle IVF should not be offered to patients under any circumstances,[8] a very small number of clinics in the United States and a larger proportion of clinics throughout the world have continued to offer unstimulated IVF. Several notable proponents of natural cycle IVF have emerged over the last decade including Robert Edwards himself.[13] Groups that have reported extensively on their experiences with natural cycle IVF include Nargund et al. in London,[20,21] Lenton et al. in Sheffield (United Kingdom),[22-25] Pelinck et al. in the Netherlands,[4,26-29] Kadoch et al. in Canada,[5,30-33] Schimberni et al. in Italy,[34,35] Nygren et al. in Sweden,[3] Tomazevic et al. in Slovenia,[36] Vlaisavljevic et al. in Slovenia[37] and our group in the United States.[38-41]

TERMINOLOGY—WHAT IS NATURAL CYCLE *IN VITRO* FERTILIZATION?

The actual definition of unstimulated IVF is more problematic than one would expect. For some practitioners, unstimulated IVF refers to IVF performed in a completely natural cycle with the timing of egg collection based upon a patient's endogenous luteinizing hormone (LH) surge.[41] In fact, this was the method used initially by Steptoe and Edwards, but scheduling based upon the LH surge can lead to egg collections around the clock, which is problematic for most clinics. Consequently, nearly all reports of natural cycle IVF describe the use

Table 1 Early attempts at natural cycle *in vitro* fertilization with laparoscopic retrieval (modified from Lenton et al.[15])

	England[13]	Australia[16]	United States[17]
Laparoscopies	35	107	41
Cycles with eggs (%)	29/35 (83%)	62/107 (57.9%)	19/41 (46.3%)
Eggs fertilized (%)	24/25 (96%)	31/66 (47%)	9/15 (60%)
Pregnancy rate/embryo transfer (%)	6/24 (25%)	0	0

of human chorionic gonadotropin (hCG) to induce final follicle maturation prior to retrieval, although a few groups have reported their extensive experience with natural cycle IVF without the use of hCG to schedule egg collection.[15,22-25] In an extensive review of 1,800 cycles of natural cycle IVF wide variations in technique are readily apparent with a multitude of approaches to the use and timing of hCG, aspiration techniques and luteal support.[4] Table 2 expands upon this 2002 paper and includes additional reports of unstimulated IVF.

Since 2002, many clinics have used GnRH antagonists to eliminate an endogenous LH surge in patients undergoing natural cycle IVF.[26-29,42-45] In order to counteract the profound drop in pituitary gonadotropins, most patients are simultaneously treated with recombinant FSH (usually 150 IU daily) until hCG trigger. Proponents of this approach, described as 'modified natural cycle IVF', report reduced cycle cancelation rates, but essentially no recruitment of supernumerary follicles.[46] The International Society for Mild Approaches in Assisted Reproduction (ISMAAR) has recommended standardization of the definitions of natural cycle and modified natural cycle IVF.[47] In 2009, the International Committee for Monitoring Assisted Reproductive Technology and the World Health Organization revised ART glossary incorporated these suggestions.[48] Therefore, this ART glossary defines natural cycle IVF as "an IVF procedure in which one or more oocytes are collected from the ovaries during a spontaneous menstrual cycle without any drug use." Similarly, the ART glossary defines modified natural cycle IVF as "an IVF procedure in which one or more oocytes are collected from the ovaries during a spontaneous menstrual cycle. Drugs are administered with the sole purpose of blocking the spontaneous LH surge and/or inducing final oocyte maturation." These 2009 definitions would thus label any cycle in which hCG is used as a modified natural cycle. However, in the United States, the use of any gonadotropin preparation during an IVF cycle (even when these are used to replace pituitary gonadotropins suppressed by administration of a GnRH antagonist in an unstimulated cycle) would require the clinic to identify that cycle as a stimulated cycle when reporting to the Centers for Disease Control and Prevention (CDC) database—as required of all ART clinics in the United States since the 1992 passage of the Fertility Clinic Success Rate and Certification Act (the so-called Wyden law). A survey of fertility clinics in the United States supports the hypothesis that the current methodology of ART reporting used to generate 'league tables' has contributed to the failure of IVF centers in this country to embrace natural cycle IVF.[41,49]

PATIENT SELECTION

First and foremost, patients considering or being considered as candidates for natural cycle IVF must have regular ovulatory cycles. Although patients with anovulation (usually polycystic ovary syndrome) can be considered for *in vitro* maturation (IVM) following retrieval of immature eggs during an unstimulated cycle, the consideration of IVM is beyond the scope of this chapter. Initial reports of natural cycle IVF usually focused upon application of this approach to younger patients with tubal factor.[22,23,50-53] However, patients at the other end of the reproductive spectrum have been offered natural cycle IVF as an option because of their failure (or anticipated failure) to respond well to gonadotropin stimulation.[34,35,42,43,45,54-57] Only a few clinics appear to offer natural cycle IVF as a standard therapy for all infertile couples across a wide range of diagnoses. One such clinic has been Pelinck's group in the Netherlands,[28] and their approach has evolved to the point where patients at their clinic are only offered stimulated cycle IVF if they have failed to conceive following an extensive trial of modified natural cycle IVF (usually up to nine cycles).

Other indications for unstimulated IVF include those patients with a previous adverse experience with stimulated cycle IVF or those for whom stimulated cycle IVF with the creation of supernumerary embryos may be unacceptable for religious/moral reasons. Case reports have described the use of natural cycle IVF in cancer survivors or in patients at risk for cancer.[58,59] Couples with severe male factor may also find natural cycle IVF to be an attractive option and several reports have described the use of ICSI in natural cycle IVF.[30,60,61]

In our own clinic, all patients with regular cycles are considered candidates for natural cycle IVF. Patients with diminished ovarian reserve are accepted into the program. Although the success rates are clearly age dependent, we have had a team delivery of a normal baby in a 48-year-old, who previously had failed to generate even a biochemical pregnancy following four initiated cycles of stimulated IVF. If natural cycle IVF is integrated into a clinic's standard approach to the infertile couple (rather than relegating its use to those poor responders unwilling to use egg donation) then pregnancy rates will likely rise along with clinician and patient acceptance of this option.

TECHNICAL ASPECTS

Transvaginal oocyte retrieval in an unstimulated cycle generates a unique set of challenges usually eliminated in stimulated cycle IVF through the use of GnRH agonists or GnRH antagonists, which usually prevent a premature LH surge and/or cycle cancelation secondary to ovulation. These special concerns have been addressed in a variety of ways by those practitioners pursuing natural cycle IVF. The following sections review cycle monitoring, timing of retrieval, oocyte aspiration and fertilization/culture choices in natural cycle IVF.

Follicle Monitoring

Cycle monitoring in natural cycle IVF requires careful assessment in order to avoid cycle cancelation secondary to an LH surge or ovulation. Sonograms for natural cycle IVF monitoring can be performed much quicker than during stimulated cycle IVF owing to the assessment of a single follicle. Near daily measurement of the emerging dominant follicle following cycle day 7 is necessary to ensure correct timing of hCG. Ultimately, the risk of an LH surge causing cancelation of the cycle must be weighed against triggering too early and ending up with an immature oocyte. In the first months of launching our unstimulated IVF program, many cycles were canceled secondary to an LH surge while waiting for a mean follicular diameter of 18 mm. Once we elected to trigger at a mean follicular diameter of 16 mm, then the rate of cycle cancelation was markedly reduced. Measurement of estradiol and LH on each day of monitoring revealed the need to trigger at follicle sizes that were much smaller than during our typical stimulated IVF cycle in order to avoid an LH surge. If an LH rise of more than twofold to threefold increase over baseline or a rise to a level of more than 15 IU/L was noted, then most of the cycles where hCG was given were ultimately canceled secondary to ovulation prior to the scheduled retrieval time. Criteria utilized for hCG trigger in cycles without GnRH antagonist are noted in Table 2. The use of GnRH antagonists nearly eliminates the risk of an endogenous LH surge and can enable a delay in hCG trigger until follicle size is more than or equal to 18 mm. However, since most proponents of this approach recommend the simultaneous addition of gonadotropins with GnRH antagonist, the increased cost and complexity of this treatment may not be acceptable to some patients. In addition, the use of any gonadotropins would necessitate that the clinic identify this treatment cycle as stimulated IVF when reporting to the CDC database, as required by law in the United States. Although most clinics measure serum levels of estradiol and LH, this approach is not universal and depends upon the resources available. Timing of egg collection varied as well across different clinics, ranging from 31 hours to 37 hours following hCG (Table 2). Clinics performing egg collection based upon endogenous LH surge, scheduled the aspiration based upon the time of the initial LH rise and changes in LH over time, but this approach can lead to scheduling of aspirations throughout the day including late afternoon and early morning which may be problematic for some clinics from a logistical standpoint.[25]

Oocyte Retrieval

Our patients undergo sonogram the day after hCG to ensure the presence of the follicle and again on the morning of egg collection. Rarely, a patient will ovulate between her confirmation sonogram and the actual retrieval. Most reports of natural cycle IVF describe successful egg retrieval in 80–90% of procedures (Table 2). Although the technique for egg collection is similar to that of stimulated cycle IVF some adjustments are usually made to ensure success in retrieving an oocyte from a single dominant follicle. Many published reports of natural cycle IVF do not specify whether follicle flushing is utilized. However, according to an informal survey of those physicians attending the 2006 First World Congress of Mild Approaches to IVF in London, practitioners of natural cycle IVF almost universally flush the follicle until the egg is identified in the aspirate. Flushing requires either the use of a double lumen needle or modifying the use of an existing single lumen needle (the approach of choice of the authors). Using the standard Cook aspiration needle, we initially enter the follicle and aspirate at a pressure of 100 mm Hg. Once the follicle has fully collapsed, the tube with the aspirated fluid is handed off and a non Luer lock syringe filled with human tubal fluid (HTF) at 37°C is attached to the adapter that exits the bottom of the stopper assembly. The follicle is gently flushed to refill nearly to its previous size and then the syringe is detached, and the next tube attached to allow for aspiration of the flush that now fills the follicle. Care must be taken to avoid touching the adapter tip with any nonsterile item. Our experience has revealed that most oocytes are found within the first four flushes (in addition to the initial aspirate); however, we have found an oocyte on occasion as late as the tenth or higher flush. We do not use any type of vaginal antiseptic preparation prior to aspiration and all patients ingest an oral antibiotic on the morning of aspiration (cephalexin 500 mg) and are treated with doxycycline (100 mg bid) from day of hCG until embryo transfer.

Fertilization

All reports concerning natural cycle IVF prior to the introduction of ICSI in 1992 were obviously limited to routine IVF but, even after the introduction of ICSI, many reports of natural cycle IVF specifically excluded those couples with male factor requiring ICSI.[20,24,25,29,36,44,51-53,62-74] Following the widespread acceptance of ICSI, reports of its use in natural cycle IVF began to appear.[5,30,34,35,39,42,54,55,57,75,76] Interestingly, some groups have utilized ICSI on 100% of the patients electing to pursue natural cycle IVF whereas others have excluded patients with male factor (and hence needing ICSI) from pursuing modified natural cycle IVF (Table 2). Since 2007, we have utilized ICSI in all of our natural cycle IVF cases unless both partners have proven fertility. Many of our treatment cycles have been performed for male factor including patients using cryopreserved testicular or epididymal sperm.[39]

Embryo Culture

Nearly all previous reports of natural cycle IVF have described day 2 or day 3 embryo transfer.[4] However, a few recent papers have described the application of extended embryo culture to natural cycle IVF.[36,37,39,44] Advantages of extended embryo culture include possible improvement in implantation resulting from embryo-endometrium synchronization. However, this potential advantage must be weighed against the possibility that a viable embryo could arrest between day 3 and day 5 as a result of suboptimal embryo culture techniques in the IVF laboratory. Trokoudes demonstrated impressive success with the application of blastocyst transfer to modified natural cycle IVF. He reported a blastocyst formation rate of nearly 50% with an implantation rate and pregnancy rate per initiated cycle that was superior to nearly all previous reports.[44] Within 2 years of launching our own natural cycle IVF program, we moved to a policy of 100% extended embryo culture. In many cases, a high quality embryo failed to advance to blastocyst while conversely an occasional low to moderate-quality embryo generated an excellent blastocyst and an ongoing pregnancy. Our experience has been that patients are very accepting of extended embryo culture and, from an emotional perspective, they prefer to cancel a transfer for failure of an embryo to grow to blastocyst rather than to undergo a day 3 transfer with an embryo that is unlikely to generate a pregnancy.

Luteal Support

The need for luteal support in downregulated stimulated cycle IVF is well known and accepted by nearly all ART practitioners.[77] The vast majority of patients undergoing natural cycle IVF receive luteal support, and this issue of correct luteal support has been championed by none other than Robert Edwards himself. Edwards blamed his early failures in IVF on his decision to use Primolut (a luteolytic) for luteal support in natural cycle IVF. However, luteal support in published series of natural cycle IVF range from no luteal support to vaginal progesterone to sequential low dose hCG (Table 2). No randomized trials have been performed, and it has been suggested that the need for luteal support may also depend upon the utilization of follicle flushing at egg collection, which has been hypothesized to disrupt corpus luteum function.[37] In our own program, we have elected to use progesterone suppositories (100 mg bid) and oral Estrace 2 mg daily starting after egg collection.

Table 2 Published results of unstimulated or natural cycle IVF

	Foulot[62] (1989)	Hillensjo[66] (1990)	Levy[63] (1991)	Svalander[74] (1991)	Paulson[72] (1992)	Claman[64] (1993)
Cycles	80	48	22	51	101	75
Oocyte retrievals attempted (%/cycle)	83%	75%	72.70%	62.70%	77.20%	53%
Successful retrieval (%/attempt)	92.60%	83.30%	81.30%	97%	NA	60%
Fertilization ICSI or IVF	IVF	IVF	IVF	IVF	IVF	IVF
Fertilization rate (%/oocyte)	NA	66.70%	84.60%	64.50%	72%	60%
Day of embryo transfer	D2	NA	D2	NA	D2	NA
Embryo transfer (n)	53	20	11	20	63	18

Contd...

Contd...

Embryo transfer (%/cycle)	66.30%	41.70%	50%	39.20%	62.40%	24%
Embryo transfer (%/OR attempt)	77.90%	55.60%	68.80%	62.50%	81%	45%
Pregnancy rate/ET (%)	32%	20%	0	30%	17.40%	11%
Pregnancy rate/Retrieval attempt (%)	25%	5.50%	0	18.75%	14%	5%
Pregnancy rate/cycle (%)	23%	4.20%	0	11.80%	11%	2.70%
GnRH-antagonist	N	N	N	N	N	N
rFSH add-back	N	N	N	N	N	N
Follicle Size/E2 level	> 18 mm > 180 pg/ ml	17 mm	>16 mm >160 pg/ ml	>17 mm >500-650 pmol/l	20 mm and 200 pg/ml 18 mm and 250 pg/ml 15 mm and 300 pg/ml	>18 mm; >180 pg/ml
Timing (LH or hCG)	Both	hCG	hCG	hCG	hCG	hCG
Timing of retrieval (hr)	34-36 h	35 h	NA	34 h	34-36 h	34-36 h
Type of needle (SL, DL, NA)	NA	NA	NA	NA	NA	NA
Flushing of follicle	NA	NA	NA	NA	NA	yes
Luteal support/Type	hCG 1500 IU day of ET then q 3 d	NA	NA	NA	Prog supp 50 mg bid	hCG 1500 D1, D4, D7

	MacDougall[51] (1994)	Aboulgar[52] (1995)	Daya[65] (1995)	Seibel[73] (1995)	Fahy[53] (1995)	Kim[68] (1996)	Lindheim[69] (1997)
Cycles	14	229	240	64	79	80	35
Oocyte retrievals attempted (%/cycle)	28.60%	48.50%	65%	75%	82%	83.80%	85.70%
Successful retrieval (%/attempt)	100%	87.50%	83%	75%	83%	96%	100%
Fertilization ICSI or IVF	IVF	IVF	IVF	IVF	IVF	IVF	IVF
Fertilization rate (%/oocyte)	100%	88%	71%	69.40%	79.60%	98%	89.10%
Day of embryo transfer	D2	D3	D2	NA	NA	D2	NA
Embryo transfer (n)	4	86	92	25	43	61	28
Embryo transfer (%/cycle)	28.60%	37.50%	38.30%	39%	54.40%	76.30%	80%
Embryo transfer (%/OR attempt)	100%	76.70%	59%	52%	66.10%	91%	93%

Contd...

Contd...

Pregnancy rate/ ET (%)	0	12.80%	12%	28%	14%	16.40%	17.90%
Pregnancy rate/ Retrieval attempt (%)	0	9.80%	7%	14.60%	9.20%	14.90%	16.70%
Pregnancy rate/ cycle (%)	0	4.80%	4.60%	10.90%	7.60%	12.50%	14.20%
GnRH-antagonist	N	N	N	N	N	N	N
rFSH add-back	N	N	N	N	N	N	N
Follicle Size/E2 level	> 17 mm	17 mm	> 16 mm	≥ 18 mm; > 200 pg/ml	LH	> 18 mm > 200 pg/ml	NA
Timing (LH or hCG)	hCG	hCG	hCG	hCG	LH	hCG	hCG
Timing of retrieval (hr)	35h	36	34-36 h	36	LH	34-36 h	36
Type of needle (SL, DL, NA)	NA	NA	BOTH	NA	DL	NA	NA
Flushing of follicle	NA	NA	Yes	NA	Yes	NA	NA
Luteal support/type	NA	Oral P4 300 mg	Prog supp 50 mg bid	NA	None	50 mg PIO	NA

	Zayed[24] (1997)	Feldman[55] (1998)	Bassil[54] (1999)	Janssens[67] (2000)	Nargund[20] (2001)	Ingerslev[76] (2001)	Ng[70] (2001)
Cycles	162	44	16	75	181	114	32
Oocyte retrievals attempted (%/cycle)	89.50%	63.60%	81.25%	81.30%	96.10%	64.90%	37.50%
Successful retrieval (%/attempt)	93%	57%	84.60%	82%	81%	87.80%	83%
Fertilization ICSI or IVF	IVF	ICSI	BOTH	IVF	IVF	BOTH	IVF
Fertilization rate (%/oocyte)	73%	62.50%	54.50%	74%	70%	47%	80%
Day of embryo transfer	NA	NA	D2-3	D2	NA	D2	D2
Embryo transfer (n)	89	10	6	35	96	29	8
Embryo transfer (%/cycle)	54.90%	22.70%	37.50%	46.60%	53%	25.40%	25%
Embryo transfer (%/OR attempt)	61.40%	35.70%	46.10%	57.30%	55%	39.20%	66.70%
Pregnancy rate/ ET (%)	18%	20%	50%	20%	23.90%	13.80%	50%
Pregnancy rate/ Retrieval attempt (%)	11%	7.10%	23%	11.50%	13%	5.40%	33%
Pregnancy rate/ cycle (%)	9.90%	4.50%	18.75%	9.30%	12.70%	3.50%	12.50%

Contd...

Contd...

GnRH-antagonist	N	N	N	N	N	N	N
rFSH add-back	N	N	N	N	N	N	N
Follicle size/E2 level	LH	NA	> 18 mm E2>100 pg/mL	≥ 18 mm	16-18 mm	> 17 mm	> 16 mm; 600-700 pmol/l
Timing (LH or hCG)	LH	hCG	hCG	hCG	hCG	hCG	hCG
Timing of retrieval (hr)	34-36	NA	35 h	35 h	36 h	35-36 h	36
Type of needle (SL, DL, NA)	NA	NA	NA	SL	NA	SL	NA
Flushing of follicle	yes	NA	NA	No	NA	Yes	Yes
Luteal support/Type	NA	NA	Oral progestin	NA	NA	None	hCG 1500 at ET and ET+6

	Feldman[55] (2001)	Omland[71] (2001)	Kolibianakis[42] (2004)	Morgia[34] (2004)	Trokoudes[44] (2005)	Elizur[43] (2005)	Papaleo[57] (2006)
Cycles	44	223	78	NA	138	52	26
Oocyte retrievals attempted (%/cycle)	64%	64%	68%	114/?	91%	69%	96%
Successful retrieval (%/attempt)	57%	85.30%	83%	77%	81%	NA	72%
Fertilization ICSI or IVF	ICSI	IVF	Both	ICSI	IVF	NA	ICSI
Fertilization rate (%/oocyte)	66.70%	71%	60%	84%	95%	80%	94%
Day of embryo transfer	D2-3	D2-3	NA	NA	Blast	?D3	?D3
Embryo transfer (n)	10	82	19	47	45	35	15
Embryo transfer (%/cycle)	22.7	36.70%	24.30%	47/?	32.60%	67.30%	57.70%
Embryo transfer (%/OR attempt)	35.70%	57.30%	35.80%	41.20%	35.70%	97%	60%
Pregnancy rate/ ET (%)	20%	17%	0	14.90%	53%	14.30%	20%
Pregnancy rate/ Retrieval attempt (%)	7.10%	9.80%	0	6.10%	19%	13.90%	12%
Pregnancy rate/ cycle (%)	4.50%	6.30%	0	7/?	17.40%	9.60%	11.50%
GnRH-antagonist	N	N	Yes	N	Some	Yes	Yes
rFSH add-back	N	N	Yes	N	N	Yes	N
Follicle size/E2 level	≥ 17 mm; > 40 mmol/l	≥ 15l mm; > 0.5 nmol/l	≥ 16 mm	≥ 16 mm	≥ 16 mm; ≥ 400 pmol/L	> 18 mm	≥ 16-18 mm; > 200 pg/ml

Contd...

Contd...

Timing (LH or HCG)	hCG	hCG	hCG	hCG	hCG	hCG	hCG
Timing of retrieval (hr)	30-32	34-36	32	36	33-36	36	36
Type of needle (SL, DL, NA)	NA	NA	DL	NA	DL	NA	SL
Flushing of follicle	NA	NA	Probably	NA	flush x 2	NA	NA
Luteal support/ Type	NA	None	Prog 200 mg PV TID	50 mg PIO	hCG 2000 on OR + 1 and Prog tab 200 mg bid PV	NA	NA

	Lenton[25] (2007)	Tomazevic[36] (2007)	Phillips[5] (2007)	Pelinck[29] (2008)	Kadoch[32] (2008)	Schimberni[35] (2009)
Cycles	775	397	NA	1048	255	NA
Oocyte retrievals attempted (%/cycle)	92.60%	92.70%	242/?	81.70%	87%	500/?
Successful retrieval (%/attempt)	79.50%	82.30%	72.70%	73%	77.9%	78.10%
Fertilization ICSI or IVF	IVF	IVF	Both	IVF	Both	ICSI
Fertilization rate (%/oocyte)	NA	NA	73%	72.50%	NA	NA
Day of embryo transfer	NA	Blast	NA	D3	D2	NA
Embryo transfer (n)	368	122	127	382	119	285
Embryo transfer (%/cycle)	47.40%	30.70%	NA	36.50%	46.70%	NA
Embryo transfer (%/OR attempt)	51.20%	33.10%	52%	44.60%	53.60%	57%
Pregnancy rate/ET (%)	14.40%	39.30%	18.90%	27.20%	18.50%	17.10%
Pregnancy rate/Retrieval attempt (%)	7.40%	13%	9.90%	12.10%	9.90%	9.60%
Pregnancy rate/cycle (%)	6.80%	12%	NA	9.90%	8.60%	48/?
GnRH-antagonist	N	N	Yes	Yes	Yes	No
rFSH add-back	N	N	Yes	Yes	Yes	No
Follicle size/E2 level	LH	> 16 mm; > 0.39 nmol/l	17 mm	18 mm	17 mm	≥ 16 mm
Timing (LH or hCG)	LH	hCG	hCG	hCG	hCG	hCG
Timing of retrieval (hr)	Varied	31-32	34	34	34	36
Type of needle (SL, DL, NA)	NA	SL	DL	SL	DL	NA
Flushing of follicle	NA	N	Yes	No	Yes	NA
Luteal support/Type	NA	hCG 1500 D9	hCG 2500 OR+2 and OR+4 ; prog 200 mg PV tid	hCG 1500 OR+5, OR+8, OR+11	hCG, P4 supp	50 mg PIO

	Aanesen[75] (2010)	DiMattina[39] (2010)
Cycles	129	243
Oocyte retrievals attempted (%/cycle)	69%	86.80%
Successful retrieval (%/attempt)	85.40%	88%
Fertilization ICSI or IVF	Both	Both
Fertilization rate (%/oocyte)	NA	75%
Day of embryo transfer	D2	Day-3, and Blast
Embryo transfer (n)	60	119
Embryo transfer (%/cycle)	46.50%	49%
Embryo transfer (%/OR attempt)	67.40%	56%
Pregnancy rate/ET (%)	26.70%	35%
Pregnancy rate/ Retrieval attempt (%)	18%	20%
Pregnancy rate/cycle (%)	12.40%	17%
GnRH-antagonist	N	N
rFSH add-back	N	N
Follicle Size/E2 level	17-19 mm E2>500-750 pmol/l	≥ 15 mm
Timing (LH or hCG)	hCG	hCG
Timing of retrieval (hr)	37 h	34
Type of needle (SL, DL, NA)	NA	SL
Flushing of follicle	Some	Yes
Luteal support/Type	NONE	Prog supp 100 mg, estrace 2 mg

D2: day 2; D3: day 3; E2: estradiol; ET: embryo transfer; GnRH: gonadotropin-releasing hormone; hCG: human chorionic gonadotropin; ICSI: intracytoplasmic sperm injection; IVF: *in vitro* fertilization; LH: luteinizing hormone; NA: not available; OR: oocyte retrievals; rFSH: recombinant follicle stimulating hormone

OUTCOME DATA

In considering the multitude of reports describing natural cycle IVF, it is apparent that this fertility treatment can result in good to excellent implantation rates even in couples with poor prognosis or with previous failed stimulated IVF. But the difference between these two treatment approaches to IVF is the attrition that can occur from initiated cycle to embryo transfer. Unlike stimulated cycle IVF in which the vast majority of patients initiating a treatment cycle undergo egg collection and embryo transfer, those electing to pursue natural cycle IVF may not reach the point of attempted egg collection because of a premature LH surge or ovulation prior to retrieval. Although both of these barriers were not uncommon in the early days of stimulated cycle IVF (prior to the widespread adoption of protocols utilizing GnRH agonists), those clinicians more recently trained in IVF are often unprepared for the reality of cycle cancelation prior to retrieval except for the indication of a poor response to gonadotropins. Furthermore, in natural cycle IVF, the single egg may not fertilize, and that fertilized egg may not develop into an embryo of sufficient quality to transfer. Therefore, in pursuing natural cycle IVF one must be prepared to counsel patients appropriately, and consider the percentage of initiated cycles that progress to retrieval, the percentage of retrievals that result in a mature/viable oocyte, the fertilization rate per retrieval, the cleavage rate per fertilized ovum retrieved, the percentage of cycles and retrievals that result in embryo transfer, and finally, the pregnancy/delivery rate as calculated per cycle initiated, per retrieval and per embryo transfer (implantation rate). Pregnancy rates in natural cycle IVF have been reported to range from 0–50%, but many of these reports were from less than 100 initiated cycles. In examining those reports describing over 200–250 initiated cycles, the pregnancy rates range from 10–17% per initiated cycle and up to 35–40% per embryo transfer, which many patients would likely view favorably given the advantages of natural cycle IVF.

Several authors have suggested that natural cycle IVF needs to be considered as a series of treatments when evaluating the cost-effectiveness of this approach.[4,5,20,65,75,78] Using life table analysis, the cumulative success rate of three cycles of natural cycle IVF can approach 50%, a success rate which many patients may find acceptable when making decisions about their fertility treatments.

UTILIZATION IN THE UNITED STATES

Although interest in natural cycle IVF remains strong in countries as varied as Japan, England, Norway, Slovenia and Cyprus; according to data from the SART, in the United States less than 2% of IVF cycles are performed in unstimulated cycles, and only 15% of clinics even offer natural cycle IVF to patients.[41] At the vast majority of those clinics, the percentage of patients undergoing natural cycle IVF is a fraction of the total IVF volume (Table 3). Given the large percentage of unstimulated cycles attempted in patients greater than 40 years old, it seems likely that natural cycle IVF is utilized by many US clinics, primarily in poor prognosis older patients for whom stimulated cycle IVF is no longer an option given diminished ovarian reserve and poor egg quality. Lack of interest in natural cycle IVF has been suggested by Heng[49] to result from: (1) Diminished profits compared with stimulated cycle IVF, (2) Reduction in success rates as published in 'league tables' and, (3) Inability to create supernumerary embryos for future use or donation.

In a recent survey of ART clinics in the United States, physicians were asked to identify their reasons for deciding against offering natural cycle IVF.[41] The most often cited reasons were poor success rates, not cost-effective and lack of patient interest. Improvements in cycle management along with the use of extended embryo culture and ICSI for male factor may lead to pregnancy rates that are considered acceptable to physicians and their patients. One study found that some patients have such a strong preference for natural cycle IVF over stimulated cycle IVF that pregnancy rates per initiated cycle of 10–15% would be readily viewed as reasonable.[79] Our experience has confirmed this hypothesis as we have treated patients from hundreds of miles away from our clinic in Arlington, Virginia, because these patients were unable to convince any local IVF clinics to consider attempting a cycle of natural cycle IVF. However, there is no doubt that establishing a natural cycle IVF program will adversely impact a clinic's pregnancy statistics as reported by entities such as the CDC in the United States. Currently, the CDC combines stimulated IVF and unstimulated IVF cycle results when reporting a clinic's IVF success rates. Given the lower pregnancy rates per initiated cycle for natural cycle IVF, there is no way that a clinic can offer natural cycle IVF without adversely impacting its published IVF success rates. In fact, almost 40% of ART clinics responding to a survey concerning unstimulated IVF indicated that they would likely or definitely consider offering unstimulated IVF, if the reporting procedures were changed so that stimulated and unstimulated IVF results were segregated.[41]

THE FUTURE

Our own experience with natural cycle IVF has been extremely favorable. Patients find the process much less intimidating than traditional IVF, and even those who do not achieve success, seem very pleased with their decision to attempt natural cycle IVF. Some of these patients have ultimately moved on to stimulated cycle IVF satisfied that they had attempted a less intense option before advancing into traditional IVF. Other patients have achieved success in spite of failure to respond to gonadotropins for stimulated IVF, or following suboptimal IVF cycles with poor embryo quality. Success rates for these patients may be lower than those obtained in ideal candidates, but for those couples unwilling to pursue donor egg IVF or adoption, natural cycle IVF may be a very reasonable option. Whether or not natural cycle IVF in the United States achieves the level of acceptance seen, in Europe and throughout much of the rest of the world, depends upon changes in the reporting methodology for ART clinics. It seems clear that patient interest and acceptance of natural cycle IVF remains high, and increased utilization of natural cycle IVF may be occur in the future if physicians consider offering this fertility treatment option to a broader cohort of patients.

Table 3 Utilization of unstimulated IVF in the United States[40]

	2006	2007
Clinics performing natural cycle IVF	44 (12.8%)	57 (15.9%)
Total of unstimulated IVF cycles (% of total ART cycles)	288 (0.34%)	507 (0.58%)
Mean of unstimulated IVF cycles at clinics performing unstimulated IVF	6.55	8.89
Percentage of unstimulted IVF as a percent of total ART cycles at clinics performing unstimulated IVF	0.99%	1.36%

ART: assisted reproductive technology; IVF: *in vitro* fertilization

REFERENCES

1. Hojgaard A, Ingerslev HJ, Dinesen J. Friendly IVF: patient opinions. Hum Reprod. 2001;16(7):1391-6.
2. Nargund G. Natural-cycle/mild IVF: a science-based and patient-centered approach for the future. Womens Health (Lond Engl). 2008;4(4):327-8.
3. Nygren KG. Single embryo transfer: the role of natural cycle/minimal stimulation IVF in the future. Reprod Biomed Online. 2007;14(5):626-7.
4. Pelinck MJ, Hoek A, Simons AH, et al. Efficacy of natural cycle IVF: a review of the literature. Hum Reprod Update. 2002;8(2):129-39.
5. Phillips SJ, Kadoch IJ, Lapensee L, et al. Controlled natural cycle IVF: experience in a world of stimulation. Reprod Biomed Online. 2007;14(3):356-9.
6. Nargund G, Frydman R. Towards a more physiological approach to IVF. Reprod Biomed Online. 2007;14(5):550-2.
7. Olivennes F, Frydman R. Friendly IVF: the way of the future? Hum Reprod. 1998;13(5):1121-4.
8. Flisser E, Scott RT Jr, Copperman AB. Patient-friendly IVF: how should it be defined? Fertil Steril. 2007;88(3):547-9.
9. Edwards RG. Maturation in vitro of human ovarian oocytes. Lancet. 1965;2(7419):926-9.
10. Edwards RG, Bavister BD, Steptoe PC. Early stages of fertilization in vitro of human oocytes matured in vitro. Nature. 1969;221(5181):632-5.
11. Edwards RG, Steptoe PC, Purdy JM. Fertilization and cleavage in vitro of preovulator human oocytes. Nature. 1970;227(5265):1307-9.
12. Fauser BC, Edwards RG. The early days of IVF. Hum Reprod Update. 2005;11(5):437-8.
13. Edwards RG. IVF, IVM, natural cycle IVF, minimal stimulation IVF - time for a rethink. Reprod Biomed Online. 2007;15(1):106-19.
14. Steptoe PC, Edwards RG. Reimplantation of a human embryo with subsequent tubal pregnancy. Lancet. 1976;1(7965):880-2.
15. Lenton EA, Cooke ID, Hooper M, et al. In vitro fertilization in the natural cycle. Baillieres Clin Obstet Gynaecol. 1992;6(2):229-45.
16. Johnston I, Lopata A, Speirs A, et al. In vitro fertilization: the challenge of the eighties. Fertil Steril. 1981;36(6):699-706.
17. Jones HW Jr, Jones GS, Andrews MC, et al. The program for in vitro fertilization at Norfolk. Fertil Steril. 1982;38(1):14-21.
18. Engel JB, Riethmuller-Winzen H, Diedrich K. Extrapituitary effects of GnRH antagonists in assisted reproduction: a review. Reprod Biomed Online. 2005;10(2):230-4.
19. Paulson RJ, Sauer MV, Lobo RA. Addition of a gonadotropin releasing hormone (GnRH) antagonist and exogenous gonadotropins to unstimulated in vitro fertilization (IVF) cycles: physiologic observations and preliminary experience. J Assist Reprod Genet. 1994;11(1):28-32.
20. Nargund G, Waterstone J, Bland J, et al. Cumulative conception and live birth rates in natural (unstimulated) IVF cycles. Hum Reprod. 2001;16(2):259-62.
21. Fauser BC, Nargund G, Andersen AN, et al. Mild ovarian stimulation for IVF: 10 years later. Hum Reprod. 2010;25(11):2678-84.
22. Lenton EA, Woodward B. Natural-cycle versus stimulated-cycle IVF: is there a role for IVF in the natural cycle? J Assist Reprod Genet. 1993;10(6):406-8.
23. Monks NJ, Turner K, Hooper MA, et al. Development of embryos from natural cycle in vitro fertilization: impact of medium type and female infertility factors. Hum Reprod. 1993;8(2):266-71.
24. Zayed F, Lenton EA, Cooke ID. Natural cycle in-vitro fertilization in couples with unexplained infertility: impact of various factors on outcome. Hum Reprod. 1997;12(11):2402-7.
25. Lenton EA. Natural cycle IVF with and without terminal HCG: learning from failed cycles. Reprod Biomed Online. 2007;15(2):149-55.
26. Pelinck MJ, Vogel NE, Hoek A, et al. Minimal stimulation IVF with late follicular phase administration of the GnRH antagonist cetrorelix and concomitant substitution with recombinant FSH: a pilot study. Hum Reprod. 2005;20(3):642-8.
27. Pelinck MJ, Vogel NE, Hoek A, et al. Cumulative pregnancy rates after three cycles of minimal stimulation IVF and results according to subfertility diagnosis: a multicentre cohort study. Hum Reprod. 2006;21(9):2375-83.
28. Pelinck MJ, Vogel NE, Arts EG, et al. Cumulative pregnancy rates after a maximum of nine cycles of modified natural cycle IVF and analysis of patient drop-out: a cohort study. Hum Reprod. 2007;22(9):2463-70.
29. Pelinck MJ, Knol HM, Vogel NE, et al. Cumulative pregnancy rates after sequential treatment with modified natural cycle IVF followed by IVF with controlled ovarian stimulation. Hum Reprod. 2008;23(8):1808-14.
30. Kadoch IJ, Phillips SJ, Hemmings R, et al. Ongoing pregnancy after ICSI of frozen-thawed PESA-retrieved spermatozoa and IVF in a controlled natural cycle. Reprod Biomed Online. 2005;10(5):650-2.
31. Kadoch IJ, Fanchin R, Frydman N, et al. Controlled natural cycle IVF: a novel approach for a dominant follicle during an in vitro maturation cycle. Reprod Biomed Online. 2007;14(5):598-601.
32. Kadoch IJ, Al-Khaduri M, Phillips SJ, et al. Spontaneous ovulation rate before oocyte retrieval in modified natural cycle IVF with and without indomethacin. Reprod Biomed Online. 2008;16(2):245-9.
33. Kadoch IJ, Jamal W, Phillips SJ, et al. Successful pregnancy in an ovarian agenesis patient after modified natural cycle IVF oocyte donation. Reprod Biomed Online. 2009;19(2):221-3.
34. Morgia F, Sbracia M, Schimberni M, et al. A controlled trial of natural cycle versus microdose gonadotropin-releasing hormone analog flare cycles in poor responders undergoing in vitro fertilization. Fertil Steril. 2004;81(6):1542-7.

35. Schimberni M, Morgia F, Colabianchi J, et al. Natural-cycle in vitro fertilization in poor responder patients: a survey of 500 consecutive cycles. Fertil Steril. 2009;92(4):1297-301.
36. Tomazevic T, Korosec S, Virant Klun I, et al. Age, oestradiol and blastocysts can predict success in natural cycle IVF-embryo transfer. Reprod Biomed Online. 2007;15(2):220-6.
37. Vlaisavljevic V. Embryo transfer and luteal support in natural cycles. Reprod Biomed Online. 2007;14(6):686-92.
38. Celia GF, Botes A, Gordon JD, et al. Natural cycle IVF produces similar implantation rates compared with stimulated IVF. Fertil Steril. 2010;94:S162.
39. DiMattina M, Gordon JD, Botes A, et al. 3-year experience of natural cycle IVF (NCIVF) in a US fertility practice. Fertil Steril. 2010;94:S157.
40. Gordon JD, DiMattina M, Botes A, et al. Utilization and success rates of unstimulated in vitro fertilization (IVF) in the United States: an analysis of the Society for Assisted Reproductive Technology (SART) database. Fertil Steril. 2010;94:S157.
41. Gordon JD, DiMattina M, Botes A, et al. Opinions regarding unstimulated IVF: a survey of clinics reporting to SART. Fertil Steril. 2010;94:S158.
42. Kolibianakis E, Zikopoulos K, Camus M, et al. Modified natural cycle for IVF does not offer a realistic chance of parenthood in poor responders with high day 3-FSH levels, as a last resort prior to oocyte donation. Hum Reprod. 2004;19(11):2545-9.
43. Elizur SE, Aslan D, Shulman A, et al. Modified natural cycle using GnRH antagonist can be an optional treatment in poor responders undergoing IVF. J Assist Reprod Genet. 2005;22(2):75-9.
44. Trokoudes KM, Minbattiwalla MB, Kalogirou L, et al. Controlled natural cycle IVF with antagonist use and blastocyst transfer. Reprod Biomed Online. 2005;11(6):685-9.
45. Ata B, Yakin K, Balaban B, et al. Embryo implantation rates in natural and stimulated assisted reproduction treatment cycles in poor responders. Reprod Biomed Online. 2008;17(2):207-12.
46. Philips SJ, Kadoch IJ. Natural cycle IVF: a question of semantics? Reprod Biomed Online. 2007;15(3):255-6.
47. Nargund G, Fauser BC, Macklon NS, et al. The ISMAAR proposal on terminology for ovarian stimulation for IVF. Hum Reprod. 2007;22(11):2801-4.
48. Zegers-Hochschild F, Adamson GD, de Mouzon J, et al. International Committee for Monitoring Assisted Reproductive Technology (ICMART) and the World Health Organization (WHO) revised glossary of ART terminology, 2009. Fertil Steril. 2009;92(5):1520-4.
49. Heng BC. Reluctance of medical professionals in adopting natural-cycle and minimal ovarian stimulation protocols in human clinical assisted reproduction. Reprod Biomed Online. 2007;15(1):9-11.
50. Paulson RJ, Sauer MV, Francis MM, et al. In vitro fertilization in unstimulated cycles: a clinical trial using hCG for timing of follicle aspiration. Obstet Gynecol. 1990;76(5 Pt 1):788-91.
51. MacDougall MJ, Tan SL, Hall V, et al. Comparison of natural with clomiphene citrate-stimulated cycles in in vitro fertilization: a prospective, randomized trial. Fertil Steril. 1994;61(6):1052-7.
52. Aboulghar MA, Mansour RT, Serour GA, et al. In vitro fertilization in a spontaneous cycle: a successful simple protocol. J Obstet Gynaecol (Tokyo 1995). 1995;21(4):337-40.
53. Fahy UM, Cahill DJ, Wardle PG, et al. In vitro fertilization in completely natural cycles. Hum Reprod. 1995;10(3):572-5.
54. Bassil S, Godin PA, Donnez J. Outcome of in vitro fertilization through natural cycles in poor responders. Hum Reprod. 1999;14(5):1262-5.
55. Feldman B, Levron J, Binder D, Shulman S, Sine S, Dor J. Unstimulted cycles in IVF treatment of patients with low ovarian response. Fertil Steril. 1998;70(Suppl 1):S327.
56. Ubaldi F, Rienzi L, Ferrero S, et al. Natural in vitro fertilization cycles. Ann N Y Acad Sci. 2004;1034:245-51.
57. Papaleo E, De Santis L, Fusi F, et al. Natural cycle as first approach in aged patients with elevated follicle-stimulating hormone undergoing intracytoplasmic sperm injection: a pilot study. Gynecol Endocrinol. 2006;22(7):351-4.
58. Brown JR, Modell E, Obasaju M, et al. Natural cycle in-vitro fertilization with embryo cryopreservation prior to chemotherapy for carcinoma of the breast. Hum Reprod. 1996;11(1):197-9.
59. Hirt R, Davy C, Guibert J, et al. Pregnancy after in vitro fertilization-intracytoplasmic sperm injection obtained with a modified natural cycle in a BRCA1 mutation carrier. Fertil Steril. 2008;90(4):1199 e25-8.
60. Norman RJ, Payne D, Matthews CD. Pregnancy following intracytoplasmic sperm injection (ICSI) of a single oocyte in a natural cycle. Hum Reprod. 1995;10(7):1626-7.
61. Omland AK, Abyholm T, Fedorcsak P, et al. Pregnancy outcome after IVF and ICSI in unexplained, endometriosis-associated and tubal factor infertility. Hum Reprod. 2005;20(3):722-7.
62. Foulot H, Ranoux C, Dubuisson JB, et al. In vitro fertilization without ovarian stimulation: a simplified protocol applied in 80 cycles. Fertil Steril. 1989;52(4):617-21.
63. Levy MJ, Gindoff P, Hall J, et al. The efficacy of natural versus stimulated cycle IVF-ET. Fertil Steril. 1991;56(Suppl 1):S15-6.
64. Claman P, Domingo M, Garner P, et al. Natural cycle in vitro fertilization-embryo transfer at the University of Ottawa: an inefficient therapy for tubal infertility. Fertil Steril. 1993;60(2):298-302.
65. Daya S, Gunby J, Hughes EG, et al. Natural cycles for in-vitro fertilization: cost-effectiveness analsis and factors influencing outcome. Hum Reprod. 1995;10(7):1719-24.
66. Hillensjo T, Hammer M, Nilsson L, et al. Natural cycle IVF: preliminary results and characteristics of 48 cycles with minimal monitoring. Hum Reprod. 1990;5 (Suppl 1):36.
67. Janssens RM, Lambalk CB, Schats R, et al. In vitro fertilization in a spontaneous cycle: easy, cheap and realistic. Hum reprod. 2000;15(2):314-8

68. Kim SH, Kim CH, Suh CS, et al. Simultaneous program of natural-cycle in vitro fertilization and cryopreserved-thawed embryo transfer. J Assist Reprod Genet. 1996;13(9):716-21.
69. Lindheim SR, Vidali A, Ditkoff E, et al. Poor responders to ovarian hyperstimulation may benefit from an attempt at natural-cycle oocyte retrieval. J Assist Reprod Genet. 1997;14(3):174-6.
70. Ng EH, Chui DK, Tang OS, et al. In vitro fertilization and embryo transfer during natural cycles. J Reprod Med. 2001;46(2):95-9.
71. Omland AK, Fedorcsak P, Storeng R, et al. Natural cycle IVF in unexplained, endometriosis-associated and tubal factor infertility. Hum Reprod. 2001;16(12):2587-92.
72. Paulson RJ, Sauer MV, Francis MM, et al. In vitro fertilization in unstimulated cycles: the University of Southern California experience. Fertil Steril. 1992;57(2):290-3.
73. Seibel MM, Kearnan M, Kiessling A. Parameters that predict success for natural cycle in vitro fertilization-embryo transfer. Fertil Steril. 1995;63(6):1251-4.
74. Svalander P, Green B, Haglund K, et al. Natural versus stimulated cycles in IVF-ET treatment for tubal factor infertility. Hum Reprod. 1991;6(Suppl 1):101-2.
75. Aanesen A, Nygren KG, Nylund L. Modified natural cycle IVF and mild IVF: a 10-year Swedish experience. Reprod Biomed Online. 2010;20(1):156-62.
76. Ingerslev HJ, Hojgaard A, Hindkjaer J, et al. A randomized study comparing IVF in the unstimulated cycle with IVF following clomiphene citrate. Hum Reprod. 2001;16(4):696-702.
77. Papaleo E, Quaranta L, Molgora M. Intramuscular vs intravaginal natural progesterone in patients undergoing in vitro fertilization-embryo transfer cycles. A retrospective observational, case-control study. Eur Rev Med Pharmacol Sci. 2010;14(2):103-6.
78. Shahin AY. The problem of IVF cost in developing countries: has natural cycle IVF a place? Reprod Biomed Online. 2007;15(1):51-6.
79. Pistorius EN, Adang EM, Stalmeier PF, et al. Prospective patient and physician preferences for stimulation or no stimulation in IVF. Hum Fertil (Camb). 2006;9(4):209-16.

29

Sperm Banking: Indications and Regulations

Alaa Hamada, Monika Wasik, Sajal Gupta, Ashok Agarwal

Chapter Contents

INTRODUCTION

Sperm banking is the process of freezing sperm at very low temperatures and storing it for future use in assisted conception. The process was first used in the 1950s to freeze and store bull semen in an effort to improve dairy cow breeding.[1,2] In 1953, Schermann et al. were the first to apply the technology to human assisted conception.[3] In their breakthrough study, artificial insemination utilizing human sperm, frozen in dry ice with glycerol (10%), resulted in three successful pregnancies with viable embryo development. It was not until 1964, however, when the first live birth was reported using thawed ejaculated sperm, persevered in glycerol freezing media and embedded in liquid nitrogen.[4]

Currently, sperm banking is used to preserve fertility in a variety of men, including those with cancer. In fact, it has garnered a lot of attention in recent years largely because cancer cure rates have dramatically improved along with reproductive medicine technologies. As a result, a new field called 'oncofertility' has been created to focus on fertility preservation and quality of life issues for cancer survivors. Additionally, as male reproductive health has deteriorated during the past century, the indications for sperm banking have become more broadly implemented. It is now widely viewed as an effective method of fertility preservation for a variety of men.

CHAPTER OBJECTIVES

This chapter comprehensively describes the various aspects of sperm banking starting from patient counseling and ultimately describing the use of a thawed sample in assisted reproductive technology (ART) procedures. It aims to clarify common misconceptions and offers the most up-to-date information regarding semen freezing, otherwise known as cryopreservation. It is important to continuously update clinicians about fertility preservation options and innovations, so that they can apply this knowledge in their practice. When nonreproductive medicine specialists are familiar with these options, they can effectively counsel their patients to avoid the potentially devastating effects of fertility loss caused by toxic treatments or other confounding factors. Additionally, patients can learn about these topics and initiate the conversation regarding fertility preservation options with their healthcare provider. Sperm banking is generally considered to be a safe, cost-effective and useful means to preserve fertility and should be offered to all patients, who may benefit from it.

WHO CAN BENEFIT FROM SPERM BANKING AND WHY?

Cancer patients of reproductive age are most commonly referred to sperm banks in the United States—they comprise about 44% of all referrals.[5] However, other male patients may benefit from this service including adolescents, pre-pubertal cancer patients, men with azoospermia, severe oligozoospermia or other rheumatic, neurodegenerative or hematologic diseases, those with occupational risks or limitations and biological males undergoing sex change surgery (Table 1).

In general, users of sperm banking are divided into two categories: autoconservation group and donors group. Patients who belong to the autoconservation group often preserve their sperm or testicular tissue for the purposes of fertility preservation or fertility treatment whereas, donors are recruited to become surrogate fathers for couples suffering from refractory male infertility problems or planning to prevent transmission of certain genetic diseases or infectious diseases in the husband or for single or lesbian women planning to mother a baby. These donors donate their semen to be preserved in sperm banks for future use in assisted reproductive techniques.

Referral rates in other countries tend to be lower than those in the United States, e.g. in China, the reported figure for the referred cancer patients is only 1.9%.[6] These discrepancies reflect variations in the level of awareness, current emphasis on improving quality of life among cancer patients in western countries and probably limited financial resources allocated for sperm banking practice.

Sperm Donors Group

For sperm donor group see the Table 1.

Autoconservation Group

This group can be divided into two large subgroups based on the purpose of sperm cryopreservation: fertility preservation and fertility treatment.

Fertility Preservation Group Includes the Following

Adult oncology patients: Cancer and its effects on male fertility: In 2011, The American Cancer Society reported that the 5-year relative survival rate for all cancers was 68% (based on data gathered between 1999 and 2006). This is a significant improvement, up from 50% in the 1970s,[7] and is due to the wide use of reliable screening procedures for earlier detection and successful application of aggressive cancer therapy. As such, more cancer patients are younger when first diagnosed and are more often cured, culminating in a larger number of cancer survivors than ever before.[8] Thus, the landscape of patient priorities surrounding cancer management is changing as there is a greater concern for the treatment's effects on fertility. Therefore, it is imperative that oncologists become familiar with fertility preservation options.

The most common cancers that affect males of reproductive age include testicular cancer, Hodgkin's disease, acute leukemia, non-Hodgkin's lymphoma and soft tissue tumors, such as sarcomas.[7] Cancer affects the entire body in many negative ways, systemically and locally, and it particularly impairs spermatogenesis.[9,10] Meanwhile, cancer therapies are also quite toxic to reproductive health, hindering normal testicular function and decreasing semen quality.[8] As such, high incidence of poor semen quality is observed among referred men with asthenospermia being the most common finding (64.2–86.3%).[11,12] Other common semen abnormalities among cancer patients who are referred to sperm banking include oligozoospermia (49.8–53%),[13-15] severe oligozoospermia (< 1 million sperm/ml) (22.6%),[15] azoospermia (9.7–21%)[13,15,14] and abnormal sperm morphology (22.8%).[12] Alternatively, a recent study showed that teratozoospermia is the most common abnormality (93.2%) among pretreatment cancer patients.[11] Interestingly, most of these semen abnormalities often resolve after cancer therapy. Moreover, the chromosomal aneuploidy rate in germ cells (as detected by fluorescent *in situ* hybridization) is increased in men with testicular cancer and Hodgkin's disease before they start therapy.[16]

Just how cancer affects male fertility and semen quality is still incompletely understood. Testicular cancers have local and systemic influences on spermatogenesis, perhaps because they are associated with the production of local paracrine factors, such as β-human chorionic gonadotropin (enhances estrogen production and suppresses gonadotropin levels)[17] and cytokines,[18] and the cancer itself disrupts the blood-testis barrier, resulting in abnormal immune sensitization against sperm.[19] Meanwhile, male infertility and testicular cancer may coexist in males with undescended testes and males with a history of *in utero* exposure to xenoestrogens. Likewise, others suggest that testicular cancer and male infertility are the manifestation of fetal testicular insults culminating in testicular dysgenesis syndrome.[20] This last theory is supported by a high incidence of carcinoma *in situ* (CIS) in testicular biopsies among infertile men (4%). CIS can transform into invasive cancer in 50% of cases.[20,21]

Table 1 **Indications for sperm cryopreservation**

A. Fertility Preservation

Patient Condition	What Makes them Eligible for Sperm Banking?	Sperm Collection Method
Adult cancer	Cancer and related therapies damage the gonads and impair spermatogenesis	Frequent ejaculation
Adolescent cancer	Same as above	Frequent ejaculation (when they are sexually mature) Penile vibratory stimulation Electroejaculation
Cancer in prepubescent males	Cancer treatment negatively affects spermatogenesis; testicular tissue extraction is a promising experimental procedure	Testicular tissue freezing
Preoperative surgical procedure to treat or induce infertility	Bilateral varicocele ligation, prior to vasectomy	Frequent ejaculation
Nonmalignant disease	Systemic stress may impair spermatogenesis; gonadotoxic therapies affect semen quality	Frequent ejaculation
Occupational risk	Exposure to harmful chemicals may decrease fertility or cause chromosomal damage in the germ cells; facing hazardous situations that may result in an accident that causes infertility	Frequent ejaculation
Posthumous sperm cryopreservation	Performed at the time of brain death-based upon the patient's will or family request	Electroejaculation Surgical removal of testes and epididymides
Sex change/ gender reassignment	Hormone therapy damages spermatogenesis; and gender reassignment surgery sterilizes the male	Frequent ejaculation Removal of testicular tissue

B. Fertility Treatment

Patient Condition	What Makes them Eligible for Sperm Banking?	Sperm Collection Method
Severe oligozoospermia (<5 million sperm/ml)	Progressive decline in sperm production and high chances of azoospermia	Frequent ejaculation
Obstructive and nonobstructive azoospermic	Absence of sperm in ejaculate; benefit from using sperm extraction techniques for ART	Surgical retrieval techniques from testes or epididymis
Spinal cord injuries	Anejaculation and poor semen quality with difficulty in transportation	Assisted ejaculation and surgical sperm retrieval from testis and epididymis
Donor semen insemination	Donor sperm use as therapeutic measure in a couple with sterile men, men with genetic or infectious diseases such as HIV and for insemination of single or lesbian women	Frequent ejaculation
Absence of the male factor during conduction of ART cycles	Frequently traveling husband	Frequent ejaculation

Systemic effects of malignant disease include fever (Hodgkin's disease, non-Hodgkin's disease, leukemia), malignancy-related malnutrition, abnormal immune response (lymphoma), altered hormonal milieu (testicular cancer, central nervous system tumor) and a generalized stress and inflammatory response leading to the production of cytokines, such as interleukins and tumor necrosis factor, all of which can have devastating consequences on testicular and sperm function.[10,22] These substances damage sperm before treatment and may result in chromosomal aneuploidy in the germ cells.[16] The precise mechanism by which tumors affect spermatogenesis is not fully known, and the clinical cancer stage has no relation with the severity of male infertility. Therefore, it is imperative for physicians to address each cancer patient's fertility risk, no matter the clinical diagnosis nor disease stage.[23,24]

In addition to the cancer itself, modern oncologic treatments are also highly toxic to the body and the testes. Gonadotoxic therapies are particularly harmful to the early stages of spermatogenesis, specifically to proliferating and differentiating spermatogonia, and could cause permanent damage.[25] Oncologists should strive to maintain a balance between the toxic effects of cancer therapy and the benefits they procure, as cancer treatment acts as a double-edged sword having harmful effects on a man's fertility as a byproduct of its therapeutic activity.

In general, the effects of oncologic treatments on fertility are quite unpredictable. A common side effect of toxic treatment is temporary or permanent azoospermia and severe oligozoospermia.[26] Although spermatogenesis can resume after treatment, practitioners do not know how long that may take if and when it does happen. For instance, in men with testicular cancer, it takes at least 2 years after cessation of (etoposide + bleomycin) therapy for spermatogenesis to recover. Ultimately, recovery occurs in 80% of patients within 8 years of treatment.[27,28] While normal parameters may recover, the ability to fertilize an oocyte may still be affected as has been observed with the use of vincristine.[29] Due to the uncertain nature of cancer treatment, it is prudent to bank sperm before the start of treatment to insure against potentially permanent loss of fertility. It has been widely accepted that pretreatment sperm cryopreservation is the most effective method for preserving fertility in young cancer patients.

Chemotherapy, which is generally considered a highly toxic treatment, specifically affects spermatogenesis. Chemotherapy regimens consisting of either a single or multiple therapeutic medications have variable effects on testicular function-based upon the toxicity profile of each agent, cumulative dose, coexistent radiotherapy and treatment duration. Alkylating agents, such as nitrogen mustard, cyclophosphamide, ifosfamide, busulfan, procarbazine and chlorambucil are notorious for having the most harmful effects on the body organs including the testes. The more toxic regimen used in therapy for Hodgkin's disease, which consists of nitrogen mustard, vincristine (Oncovin), procarbazine and prednisone (MOPP) is less commonly used in the United States and is reserved mostly for treatment of advanced disease and in cases where there is a risk of cardiac toxicity that precludes the use of adriamycin, bleomycin, vinblastine, dacarbazine (ABVD). Six cycles or more of MOPP that contain two alkylating agents, mustard and procarbazine, results in a high incidence of prolonged azoospermia in 83–97% of patients post therapy.[30,31] Fortunately, the less toxic ABVD, which is the treatment more commonly used today, causes significantly less damage to the reproductive organs.[30] In testicular cancer, 53% and 44% of men receiving a regimen consisting of BEP and cisplatin—the most commonly used regimen, develop oligozoospermia and azoospermia, respectively, after 2–4 cycles.[32]

Radiotherapy is similarly harmful to spermatogenesis. While damage to the testicles depends on the dose and method of exposure, the risk is high when treatment is targeted directly at the testicles (e.g. testicular irradiation for CIS or total body irradiation prior to bone marrow transplantation) or when there is a scatter effect (e.g. radiotherapy for pelvic organs).[33] Radiotherapy occasionally causes persistent sperm DNA fragmentation and reduced semen volume and damages cells in all areas of the male reproductive organs. Moreover, radiotherapy can obstruct the ejaculatory ducts and access to mature sperm.

The amount by which spermatogenesis is affected depends on the dosage. Four Gy appears to be the threshold for permanent azoospermia, as anything less presumably only causes temporary variations in semen parameters.[33] Radiation-induced transient alterations in spermatogenesis may disappear within 2 years. For Leydig cells, the toxic dosage is 20 Gy or more for prepubertal boys and more than 30 Gy in adult males, which will render men testosterone deficient.[34] Predictably, the detrimental effects of chemotherapy and radiotherapy are increased when the two are used in combination.[35] During combined therapy, the body is exposed to a variety of toxins that affect the male gonads differently depending on whether the treatment is localized or general.

Pediatric and adolescent cancer patients: Sperm banking is also a viable option for many adolescent cancer patients whose fertile years are still ahead of them at time of diagnosis. Cure rates for pediatric cancers have dramatically improved over recent years and are currently approaching 80%. With the increasing number of cancer survivors living today, long-term quality of life concerns are becoming an important part of pretreatment discussion.[36] As a result, adolescent and pediatric cancer patients are increasingly being provided with opportunities for sperm cryopreservation. Adolescents, who have already achieved sexual maturity (at least Tanner stage 2, and a testicular volume of 5 ml) are interviewed regarding their ability to masturbate.[37] If masturbation is not feasible, other methods are offered, such as penile vibratory stimulation and electroejaculation under general anesthesia.[37] Semen quality is also influenced by cancer in the same way as in adults and probably through the same mechanisms.

When azoospermia is encountered, onco-testicular sperm extraction (TESE) is a reasonable choice. In prepubertal males, fertility preservation is a challenging situation as there are no haploid sperm or even spermatids in testicular tissue. In these cases, testicular tissue freezing opens the door for preserving fertility after iatrogenic sterilization, hopefully through stem cell isolation and transplantation or through *in vitro* maturation and induced spermatogenesis.

Regardless, fertility preservation options should be discussed before treatment is started. Indeed, the American Society of Reproductive Medicine and the American Society of Clinical Oncology (ASCO) support this practice for adolescent cancer patients.[38] Patients' parents are also quite receptive to sperm banking, even though some of the procedures such as, immature testicular tissue freezing are considered experimental in young boys. Ginsberg et al. showed that parents' attitude towards sperm cryopreservation procedures is noteworthy and deserve undertaking the opportunity, even though there are no guarantees.[36] It can therefore be concluded that fertility preservation options are indicated for young cancer patients.

Impaired fertility resulting from other disease-related factors: Patients with other diseases can also benefit from sperm banking before serious treatment or before the disease becomes so debilitating that it disrupts spermatogenesis. For example, men with lupus, rheumatoid arthritis, ulcerative colitis, multiple sclerosis or hematologic diseases that are treated with bone marrow transplants may also consider sperm banking early in the disease process.[39] Men with such conditions should be aware of the possible effects of their disease on spermatogenesis and future ability to father a child. Many experts suggest that health care providers offer sperm cryopreservation to patients with nonmalignant diseases and urological pathologies, such as bilateral varicocele, testis torsion or necrosis, particularly when they are about to undergo surgery.[40] A systemic disease that damages the entire body is likely to affect testicular function. Men who are awaiting surgery, such as a urogenital procedure or vasectomy should preserve their sperm as a precautionary measure as described below.

Occupational risks: Some healthy men may wish to consider using sperm banking for fertility preservation to counteract certain occupational risks. Gupta et al. recommended that men who work with toxic chemicals, ionization radiation or biological hazards "consider banking sperm as these exposures may jeopardize their reproductive potential".[41] Radiation, a known carcinogen, may damage the germ cells and cause birth defects in offspring. Working with glycol ethers also poses a threat to male fertility and is associated with a low motile sperm count.[42] To avoid such outcomes, men in high risk occupations should bank sperm before these negative effects accumulate.

Sperm banking is increasingly being promoted to men in the United States Armed Forces. These men often travel extensively and are away from home for extended periods of time when deployed. If a military man is having trouble conceiving with his partner, he may want to consider banking his sperm to have it available for use in ART procedures during the female's time of ovulation. Sperm banking would also act as insurance against severe combat-related injury or chemical exposure that may impair spermatogenesis or even death. While there are few studies published on this topic, the practice has garnered media attention, as there is a growing number of cryobanks offering services to armed forces personnel. Many cryobanks have noticed an influx of military personnel, who wish to bank semen before deployment.[43] One such place is the California Cryobank which discounts sperm storage costs for military men.[44] The Florida Fertility Institute allows military service members going overseas into combat to store their samples completely free of cost. In some places, the service is even being expanded to first responders or men who work in security and are often in dangerous situations. The California Cryobank also offers services for civilians, such as firefighters and emergency medical technicians.[44]

Sex change and gender reassignment: Biological males, who are undergoing gender reassignment through hormonal or surgical therapy may also benefit from sperm banking. Estrogen has been shown to have detrimental effects on spermatogenesis and overall semen parameters,[45] and sex change surgery includes orchiectomy and penectomy, which renders the male sterile, as they are no longer able to ejaculate. After male-to-female sex change surgery, two-thirds of patients identify as lesbian and some may want to have biological children with their partner—either via the biological female partner or a surrogate. For this reason, it would be beneficial to counsel such patients on fertility preservation before irreversible biological changes are made with surgery.

Prior to undergoing surgical procedures for treating or inducing infertility: Certain surgeries performed to cure infertility, such as bilateral varicocele ligation and surgical relief of seminal duct obstruction, may be complicated postoperatively by reduced testicular blood supply or inadvertent vasal transaction, particularly when the surgery is performed on both sides of the testes. Fertility preservation may also be an option for men planning to do surgical contraception via bilateral vasectomy as they may change their mind regarding having children in the future.

Fertility Treatment Group

This group includes the following indications:

Severe oligozoospermia: Severe, very severe and extreme oligozoospermia are defined by a very low sperm count of less than 5 million/ml, less than 1 million/ml and less than 100,000 million/ml, respectively. Technically, cryobanking is conducted in these patients to preserve existing spermatozoa to ensure an adequate sperm supply for multiple ART cycles and to eliminate the possibility of not finding fresh sperm in the ejaculate on the day, it is needed for ART. Moreover, recent reports have suggested that a significant proportion of men with severe oligospermia will ultimately become azoospermic and experience a loss of testicular germ cells, which further supports the use of sperm banking in this population.[46,47]

Azoospermia: Azoospermia is the condition of not having sperm in the ejaculate. There are two kinds of azoospermia: obstructive and nonobstructive. Obstructive azoospermia (OA) is usually caused by post-testicular congenital or acquired obstructive lesions. In such conditions, spermatogenesis is often normal. For this reason, viable sperm can still be obtained through various extraction methods from the testes or epididymides, and testicular sperm retrieval is successful in almost 100% of cases. Nonobstructive azoospermia (NOA), on the other hand, usually implies the presence of a sperm production defect, and its cause is often more difficult to identify and treat. For men with NOA, TESE and microsurgical TESE are the preferred methods for obtaining sperm.

Men with temporary azoospermia (perhaps due to a systemic disease or acute testicular insult) may wish to cryopreserve their semen as soon as possible to ensure against further loss of fertility.[48] If the transient azoospermia is due to disease, it is recommended that semen be banked before the start of any potentially gonadotoxic treatment. Furthermore, men who experience periodic azoospermia and are undergoing ART procedures with their partners may wish to bank sperm before the procedure, so that the sample is viable on the day it is needed, thereby minimizing the chances of any delays or fertilization failure.

Absence of male factor during assisted reproductive technology cycles: this indication applies for men, who are absent from home for long periods because of military service or frequent travels overseas.

Ejaculatory dysfunction and spinal cord injured men: more than 90% of men with spinal cord injury are infertile and have poor semen quality due to a combination of adverse factors, such as anejaculation, retrograde ejaculation, semen stagnation, frequent genital infections and increased levels of seminal oxidative stress.

COUNSELING AND ETHICAL CONSIDERATIONS

Counseling patients on fertility preservation can prove to be difficult, especially at the time of an initial oncologic diagnosis. When a patient first discovers that he has a disease or has been exposed to agents that have endangered his fertility, he may initially be reeling with the implications of this news. Who is the best candidate then, for counseling this patient during such a difficult time? Many studies on cryopreservation in cancer patients have observed that the first line of information on fertility preservation is often the oncologist or physician delivering the diagnosis.[49] The difficulty with counseling cancer patients stems from patient's excessive distraction and concern about his primary diagnosis. The important task of the oncologist at this time is to clearly explain, in a compassionate manner, the disease, possible lines of therapy and probable implications of the disease and its effects on male infertility. As fertility preservation issues garner more attention, it is important to identify the "role of healthcare practitioners have in patient decision-making with regard to fertility preservation."[38] To facilitate this added responsibility for the physician, the authors recommend early and open communication with patients and the implementation of a multidisciplinary oncofertility team.

Who Should Counsel?

Because cancer and cancer treatment both adversely affect spermatogenesis, it is part of an oncologist's duty to discuss the effects treatments can have on fertility and fertility preservation options, with an emphasis on cryopreservation. Whose responsibility is it to keep oncologists up to date on the advances in reproductive technologies? Van Casteren argues that it is in fact the reproductive medicine specialist's responsibility to ensure that other physicians are aware of 'the new possibilities in fertility treatment and relatively good pregnancy outcomes using the cryopreserved semen'.[49] It is imperative that physicians outside reproductive medicine are educated enough to know when to refer a patient to a fertility specialist and to discuss sperm banking and subsequent future fertility options.[49] Oncologists should also be aware of current ART procedures and use descriptions of promising advances in reproductive medicine to inspire optimism in their patients regarding future fertility options.

One organization, www.savemyfertility.org, whose mission is to increase awareness of fertility preservation options among both providers and patients, provides informative materials that facilitate and stimulate discussions on the importance of sperm cryobanking.[50] Specifically, the website provides handouts and tips on fertility preservation counseling, tailored information for patients on how to initiate this discussion with their care provider and take-home information to review after the shock of an initial potentially devastating diagnosis has tapered.[50] These outside organizations also encourage patients to take initiative and responsibility for their future fertility. Generally, the authors recommend that physicians initiate and guide sessions on fertility preservation with their patients. An informed nurse and other healthcare provider staff, however, may be helpful in providing continuing support throughout oncologic treatment. After the initial discussion, the patient should be referred to a skilled reproductive medicine specialist. The oncologist should follow-up with the patient to prevent failure to follow on the referral and discuss the patient's decision to remain informed (Figure 1).

Barriers to Counseling

Despite the effectiveness of cryobanking, barriers to counseling patients on fertility preservation, however, continue to exist. One study emphasizes that sperm cryopreservation remains underutilized for a variety of reasons,[9] including lack of time during a patient's visit, anxiety at the time of diagnosis, conflicting cultural or religious views, loss to follow-up during referral to a specialist, an inadequately communicated sense of seriousness regarding fertility loss and lastly, a physician, who is poorly informed about fertility preservation options.[9] Discussing potential fertility loss can cause patients to become very anxious. Specifically, discussing gamete cryobanking at the time of diagnosis may prove challenging, as the patient can feel overwhelmed, and his or her mind is primarily flooded with questions relating to survival rates, treatment strategies and an uncertain future. For example, in a retrospective 2008 study, Anderson observed that up to 58% of patients felt that their levels of anxiety had affected their ability to think about fertility. Consequently, it may be beneficial instead for physicians to discuss fertility preservation options initially at the time of diagnosis, and again perhaps a week later but still before the start of treatment. Cultural or religious views that oppose masturbation or artificial insemination, for example, may also prevent fertility discussions from occurring productively.[38] Fortunately, the interdisciplinary nature of the growing field of oncofertility aims to counter such problems and increase the understanding between the patient and physician on these issues.[38]

Some authors, on the other hand, believe that physicians who do not work in reproductive medicine may have a suboptimal knowledge of the effects of cancer and its treatment on fertility. As such, this factor is considered to be the main reason why many patients do not receive fertility counseling.[51] Currently, most oncologists do not automatically consider fertility preservation options as part of the standard workup of males with a newly diagnosed cancer.[36] Correcting this 'discrepancy' will also require an adjustment in thinking on the part of oncologists and other physicians. The ASCO included discussions on fertility preservation as part of standard care for malignancies in their 2006 guidelines. Although this recommendation was voiced approximately 5 years ago, it is still not implemented as often as it should be. Presumably, it will take time for physicians to become accustomed to initiating these difficult discussions with their patients and integrate new knowledge regarding fertility preservation into their practice.

Counseling adolescent patients poses an additional challenge to healthcare providers. Common barriers include patient age, experimental techniques, advanced disease progression and inadequate banking facilities. Most commonly, the physician will broach the topic of fertility preservation. Sometimes, the parents will ask about options; the patient does so least often.[51] Very young patients and/or those with a high level anxiety at diagnosis and at discussion have a more difficult time producing a semen sample. Doctors must work to alleviate patient anxiety by considering biological issues and acknowledging the psychological needs and

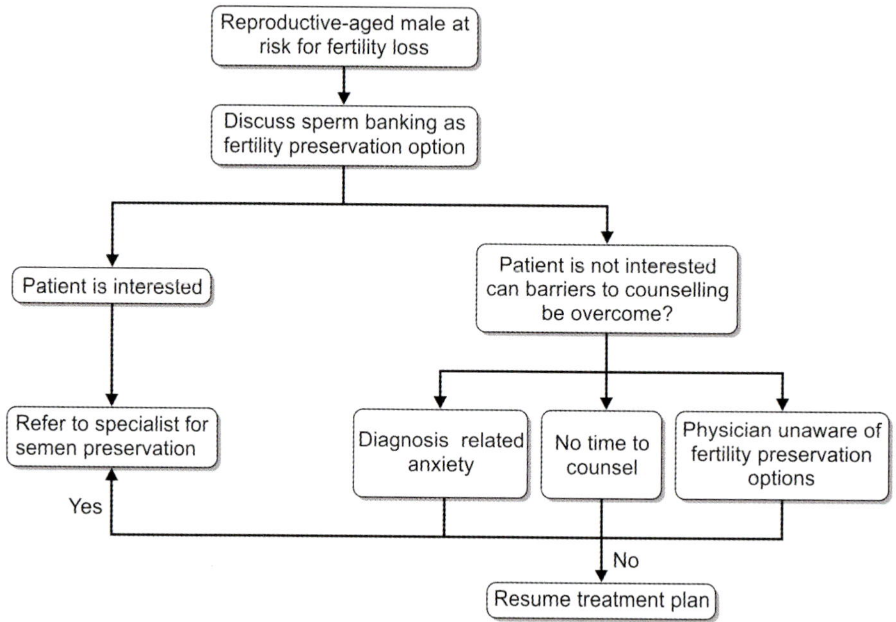

Figure 1 Counseling a reproductive-aged male at risk for fertility loss

individual situation when counseling each younger cancer patient, which can be quite a daunting task.[52] Uncertainty on how to navigate these legal and ethical issues may discourage them from appropriately counseling these patients.

Finally, if a patient has a very poor prognosis for survival, it is unlikely that fertility preservation will be considered important. It may be beneficial, however, for the care-provider to have a discussion regarding fertility preservation regardless of how seemingly hopeless the situation may be. By looking to the future, a patient may be able to foster an optimistic outlook to better focus on fighting the cancer. Anderson et al. noticed that many patients and their families make use of open and spontaneous discussion about fertility.[51] Such discussions can encourage patients to look to the future and reassure them that the aim of cancer therapy is to cure. It is possible, of course, that a patient may be so sick and have a prognosis so poor that he will be physically incapable of producing a sample—in this case, sperm cryobanking would not be worth the effort. Such possibilities again emphasize the need to discuss fertility preservation options on a case-by-case basis.

Ethical Issues Associated with Sperm Banking/ Difficulties Associated with Counseling

The topic of sperm cryobanking is often a very sensitive one for many patients. Future infertility, however, is not a problem of the individual, but of the couple and a product of a family. As a result, decisions regarding fertility preservation can impact others besides the patient. One particularly difficult case can occur when counseling an adolescent or pediatric cancer patient on fertility preservation. As minors, these patients have little autonomy to decide to bank sperm without their parents' approval.[36] Some families may not be comfortable discussing masturbation, sexuality or reproduction with their son. The boys themselves may feel particularly uncomfortable talking openly about these issues or providing a sample via masturbation or they may not fully understand the future implications of a more immediate loss of fertility, if they are too young to be thinking about having children. Asking them to produce a sample when accompanied by a parent may unduly embarrass them.

Another serious ethical issue surrounds is the postmortem period in cases where the patient did not use his semen sample. To whom does the sample belong? While the details of ensuring that the sample is properly handled is described in the section on 'disposing of the sample' below, it is important for physicians to be aware of this possibility and to address these conundrums. Because of the ethical dilemmas that may be encountered when discussing fertility preservation options, oncologists should carefully make sure to broach the topic with patients. Each patient and his family should be approached with specific consideration as to what the family will likely feel comfortable discussing, as well as the patient's given situation, as they have a right to be aware of fertility-threatening side effects and preventive options. Each clinical circumstance is unique and each individual patient's diagnosis, prognosis, current desires and future hopes, relationship status and (specifically in adolescents) maturity level must be taken into account when discussing fertility preservation options.

PROCESS OF CRYOPRESERVATION

Sperm cryopreservation is a tactful process that must be carefully performed. There are a variety of methods for obtaining the sample, and these range from masturbation to more invasive techniques. Freezing and thawing should be done in such a way as to minimize sperm damage. The field and associated methods of cryobiology are continuously changing, as evidenced by the variety of techniques currently in use. Finally, the cryobank facilities should be able to store the samples in a low-risk manner for long periods of time. There is little room for error in cryopreservation from beginning to end, as the samples being frozen are often a patient's only hope for being able to father a biological child.

Screening of Patients Prior to Banking

All sperm donors are required to complete a physical examination, including a genital exam, no more than 12 months prior to the first storage appointment. Most sperm banks also require every potential donor to schedule a physical semen analysis prior to sperm retrieval and storage. Donors are screened for infectious diseases with blood tests for HIV-1/2, HTLV-1/2, hepatitis B, hepatitis C, syphilis and sometimes CMV. Genetic testing of the sperm donor is required by certain states like New York. Some banks also request that donors complete an HIV risk assessment form, a personal and family health history form and undergo blood testing to identify blood type and Rh factor.

Obtaining the Sample

While there are a variety of methods to obtain sperm for cryopreservation, the most standard way is to collect the ejaculate via masturbation. This method is recommended for reproductive-aged patients, who are able to produce a viable sample for collection on their own. This method is quite convenient and safe although it is psychologically challenging. This is particularly a stressful issue for adolescents, whose parents often accompany them to the clinic. Some younger patients have described their experiences as being humiliating, stressful and emotionally draining.[53] To overcome the potential discomfort of having to produce a sample in a doctor's office at an already stressful time during initial diagnosis, some clinics, such as Cleveland Clinic, are pioneering home sperm banking kits. Using one of these kits, the patient can produce a sample at home and ship it immediately to a cryobank. This is a very convenient and attractive method that will undoubtedly make cryobanking an even more desirable option for fertility preservation.

The next set of methods is essentially assisted masturbation. These include penile vibratory stimulation and electro ejaculation and are most useful for men with spinal cord injury, anejaculation or young boys. For younger boys, whose testes are producing sperm but do not yet masturbate or for adolescent patients, who are anxious about producing a sample, penile vibratory stimulation or electroejaculation should be performed under general anesthesia to minimize psychological discomfort.[54]

If the patient is azoospermic, more invasive extraction and aspiration techniques should be contemplated. There are a variety of methods that can be used to extract sperm from the testes, including: fine needle aspiration, such as TESA (testicular sperm aspiration), TESE, micro-TESE. For men with OA, percutaneous epididymal sperm aspiration (PESA) or micro-epididymal sperm aspiration (MESA) can be performed.

For pre-pubertal boys, there is currently only one option for fertility preservation. A sample of testicular tissue, most often obtained during a testicular biopsy, can be cryopreserved for future use. Although the procedure is still considered experimental, the isolated stem cells from the tissue could be reimplanted again into the patient once thawed or they could be used to enhance *in vitro* maturation of spermatogenesis. Such procedures have been conducted in animal studies and will take some time to be translated into commonplace clinical practice.[36,55,56] A 2010 study, conducted at a children's hospital, showed that parents of pediatric cancer patients are willing to pursue this technique, despite any unknowns.[36]

Freezing the Sample and Cellular Damage During Freezing

Sperm cryopreservation is a controlled procedure. If not done properly, it can damage the sample, leaving it unusable for subsequent ART procedures post-thaw. Four kinds of clinical samples are cryopreserved for the purpose of sperm banking: ejaculated semen, aspirated epididymal fluid containing sperm, mature testicular tissue and immature testicular tissue.

Cryopreservation damage or cryoinjury to any cell is due to a combination of four factors: osmotic stress/dehydration, oxidative stress, intracellular ice formation and cryoprotectant toxicity (Figure 2). These factors are

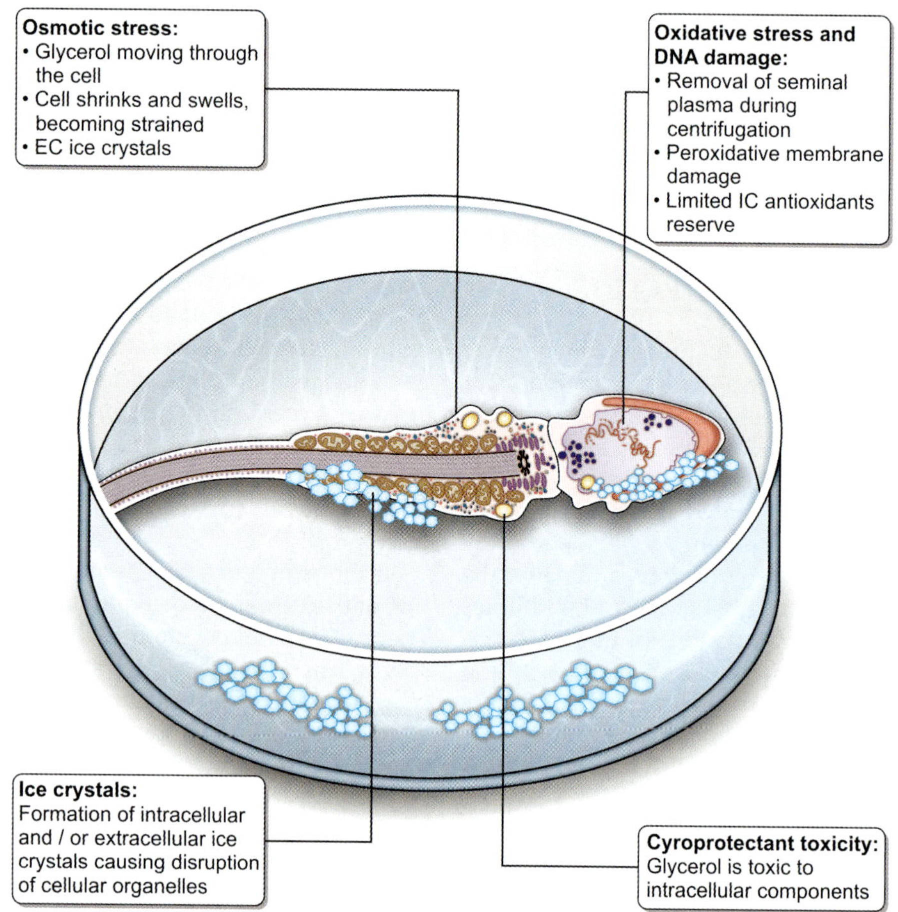

Figure 2 Potential factors responsible for sperm cryoinjury
Source: Reprinted with permission, Cleveland Clinic Center for Medical Art & Photography © 2011
EC: extracellular; IC: intracellular

responsible for a 25–75% loss of sperm motility, decrease in sperm cryosurvival and DNA fragmentation after thawing.[56,57] During cryopreservation and subsequent thawing, sperm are exposed to various challenging osmotic and oxidative situations that the sperm must overcome to survive. Sperm freezing and thawing results in osmotic stress, extracellular and intracellular ice crystals, production of reactive oxygen species (ROS), and resultant negative downstream effects on sperm motility, lipid phase change, membrane integrity, mitochondrial function, DNA integrity, cell signaling and metabolism. Apoptosis and necrotic cell death can also occur. Due to the relative stability of the frozen state, most of these negative effects mainly occur during thawing.

To minimize or avoid these effects, osmotically active cryoprotective agents (CPA) are added to the semen sample before it is frozen. The occurrence of excessive osmotic stress and intracellular ice formation depend on which cooling rate is selected. During rapid cooling rate, most intracellular water remains inside the cell and thereby forms intracellular ice whereas slow freezing dehydrates the cell resulting in shrinkage. Similarly, in response to the slow thawing process, after dilution of extracellular fluid, the cell swells in volume because of intracellular fluid hypertonicity, precipitating another form of osmotic stress (Figure 3).

A single spermatozoon has minimal and maximal cell volume limits between which the cell can withstand increased extracellular and intracellular fluid hypertonicity, respectively. These volume limits should be strictly considered when selecting the proper regimen of sperm freezing. Otherwise, the exerted osmotic stress can result in irreversible cellular damage (Figure 4).

Intracellular ice formation is usually lethal to the sperm as it culminates in cell rupture. Both osmotic and oxidative stresses have been shown to induce ROS in sperm and contribute to cellular damage that may be lethal or sublethal.[58-60]

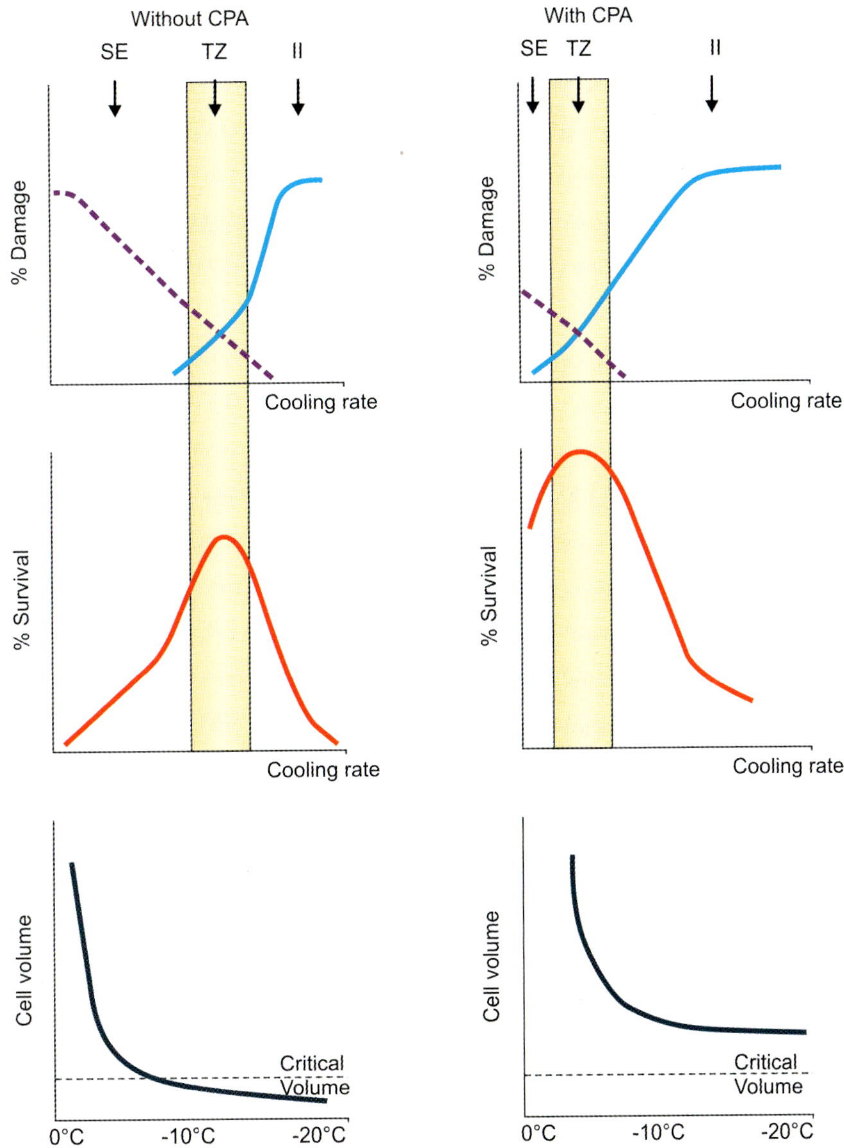

Figure 3 Cryodamage, survival, and cell volume changes during cryopreservation with and without CPA
Source: Brojandal L, Mortimer D, Barrat CLR, et al. Cambridge University Press, UK.[124]
SE: solution effect; TZ: transition zone; II: intracellular ice

Other sources of sperm damage during freezing can arise from exposure of sperm to cryoprotectants. Permeating cryoprotectants, such as glycerol, are foreign intracellular substances that can certainly poison the cell.[61] Such toxic effects might be masked or diminished by slow cell metabolism at very low freezing temperatures. Nonetheless, at relatively high temperature, such as 0°C, when very high concentration of these agents is used, substantial sperm toxicity effects might be evident.

Semen Sample

Semen samples destined for cryopreservation are usually obtained from two sources, either from the patient himself (autoconservation) or from the donor. Semen taken from a donor is used to inseminate single or lesbian women, treat couple with inability to find sperm in testicular biopsy or with frequent intracytoplasmic sperm injection (ICSI), failure due to sperm factors or prevent transmission of husband's known genetic or infectious diseases to the offspring. The whole

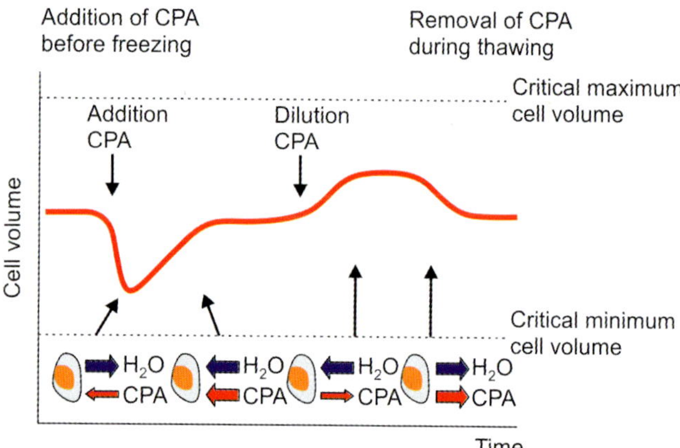

Figure 4 Effect of permeating CPA on cell volume
Source: Brojandal L, Mortimer D, Barrat CLR, et al. Cambridge University Press, UK.[124]
CPA: cryoprotective agent

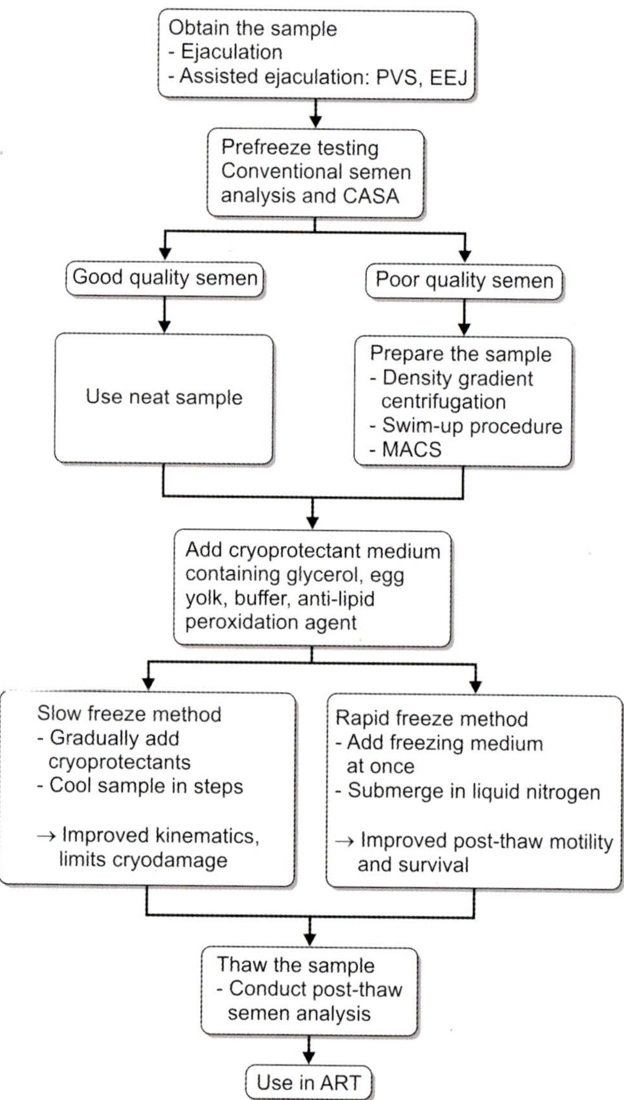

Figure 5 Lab work-up plan for preparing and freezing the sample PVS: penile vibratory stimulation; EEJ: electro-ejaculation; CASA: computer assisted sperm analysis; MACS; magnetic activated cell sorting; ART: assisted reproductive technique

laboratory work is shown in the flow diagram (Figure 5). At first, semen analysis is undertaken by experienced personnel after an adequate period of sexual abstinence (2–5 days) to check for adequate semen parameters, such as sperm count, motility and morphology. Although donors with a low sperm count or poor motility are primarily excluded from undergoing a cryopreservation protocol, this is not the case for those referred for autoconservation. Computerized assisted semen analyzer (CASA) can also be used for prefreezing and even post-thawing semen analysis (count and motility). CASA and computerized assisted sperm motion analysis can also provide additional information about the kinetic properties of prefreezing and post-thawing sperm, such as average path velocity (VAP), straight line velocity (VSL), curvilinear velocity (VCL), amplitude of lateral head displacement (ALH), straightness (STR) and linearity (LIN) (Figure 6). These kinetic measurements correlate well with frozen sperm fertilization outcomes using ART.[39]

Should sperm be washed before freezing? Given the high incidence of poor semen quality among cancer patients and infertile men, some authors prefer to subject semen samples to washing procedures before the samples are frozen. Sperm washing techniques aim to separate ejaculated spermatozoa from the seminal plasma and eliminate dead spermatozoa along with exfoliated epithelial cells, cellular debris, leukocytes and amorphous material.[62,63] Washing the sample not only improves post-thaw parameters, it also removes debris and some infectious diseases, such as HIV and improves acrosomal status.[64] It also allows for sample processing, which isolates the most viable and highly functioning sperm present in the sample, which is likely to improve ART success rates. Poor-quality samples are more likely to be damaged in the freeze-thaw process. As such, in patients with oligozoospermia and/or asthenospermia, semen washing is done to improve post-thaw motility and vitality.[57] For these reasons, the removal of seminal plasma is strongly recommended prior to freezing.

There is a number of semen washing protocols. In the swim-up technique, the centrifuged sperm pellet or uncentrifuged semen is layered below proper culture medium, Earle's balanced salt solution or sodium hyaluronate solution for 2 hours. This allows highly motile sperm to migrate inside the culture medium.

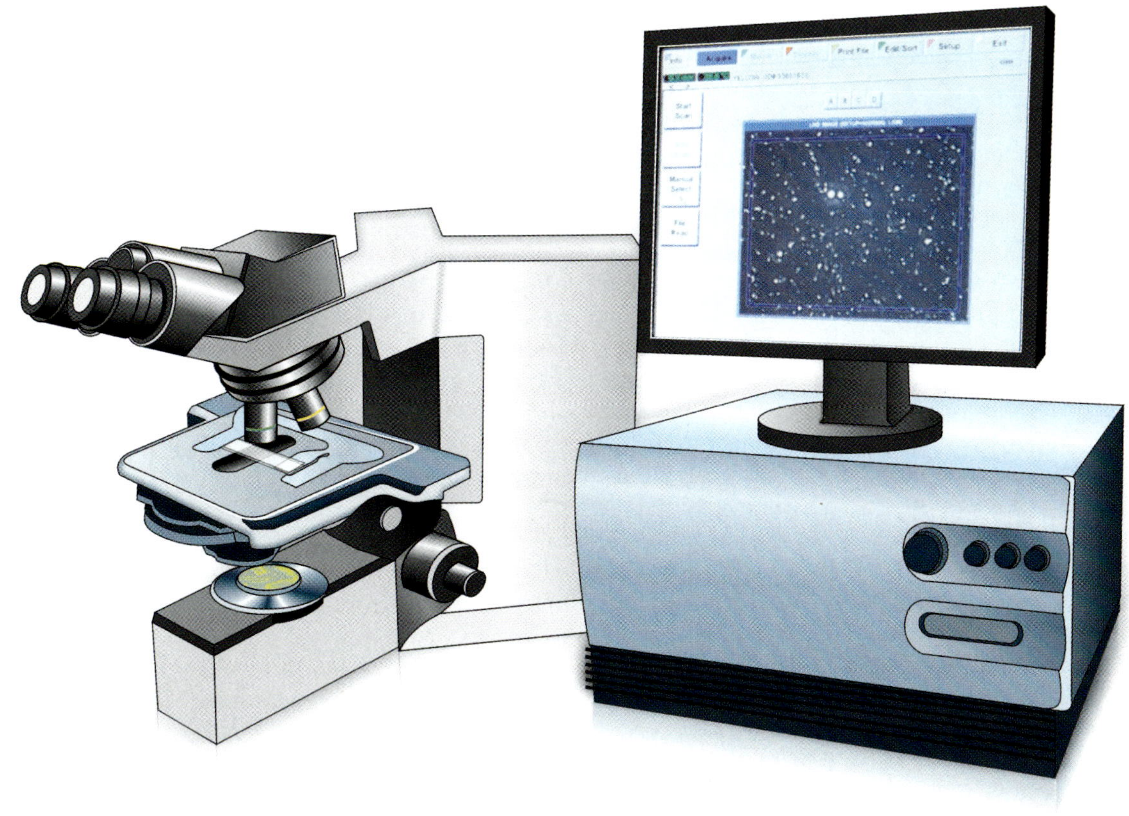

Figure 6 Computer-assisted semen analyzer for prefreeze analysis and post-thaw analysis of count and motility parameters (CASA and CAMA)

The supernatant containing the best sperm is aspirated, centrifuged and resuspended again to be stored.

In the density gradient method, two types of dense solutions—colloidal silica and a tri-iodinated derivative of benzoic acid—are commonly used to create the gradient either in a continuous fashion (a single layer of specific concentration of the dense solution) or in a discontinuous fashion (two layers of the same dense solution with different concentration). Semen is placed on the top of the dense solution and centrifuged for 30 minutes. Highly motile sperm penetrate the dense solutions and precipitate as pellets in the bottom of the tube while the seminal fluid and other cells remain on top. Sperm pellets are resuspended in a proper medium and prepared for the next step.

Magnetic activated cell sorting (MACS) is an alternative to semen washing that removes apoptotic cells and selects motile, viable, morphologically normal spermatozoa with high post-thaw survival rates and subsequent fertilization potential.[65,66] In this procedure, microbeads attached to annexin V—a phospholipid-binding protein, are used. Annexin V, in the presence of an adequate concentration of calcium, avidly binds with phosphatidylserine. This is an early marker of apoptosis and is expressed on the outer leaflet of the plasma membrane of apoptotic cells. The bound apoptotic sperm are then removed, leaving behind viable, intact sperm (neat sample). This method is still experimental and has not been used clinically. Nonetheless, most laboratories perform cryopreservation on neat semen even though the quality is not optimal. The advantage of using a neat sample is that the natural antioxidant enzymes (superoxide dismutase, catalase) and scavenging molecules (such as, ascorbate, urate, and albumin) are still present to protect against free radical damage during freezing.[57]

Addition of cryoprotective agents: The freeze-thaw cycle can induce cryodamage in sperm, resulting in poor vitality and motility post-thaw. To reduce such damage, CPAs are added to semen samples before freezing. Slow freezing initially induces extracellular ice crystal formation, which promotes cellular dehydration and shrinkage (osmotic stress). Rapid freezing, on the other hand, results in the propagation of intracellular crystal formation depending on the availability of intracellular water. Therefore, it is imperative to select the appropriate freezing rate and synchronize it with selecting a substance which can resist the damaging influences of freezing.

Cryoprotectants are substances that are added to prefrozen neat semen samples or the prep sperm to counteract extra- and intracellular ice formation during freezing. The mechanism of action is not entirely understood. However, these osmotically active agents lower the freezing point, reduce the size of ice crystals and prolong the time required for ice formation. CPAs are divided into one or two groups: penetrating or nonpenetrating. Penetrating CPAs are small, nonionic molecules that are lipophilic and highly miscible with water, giving them the ability to easily penetrate the plasma membrane. Examples include glycerol, dimethyl sulfoxide, propylene glycol, ethylene glycol and methylformamide.

Penetrating agents slowly permeate the cells and equilibrate within the cytoplasm, decreasing the volume of intracellular water without overtly dehydrating the cell. Furthermore, because CPAs are highly miscible with water, they act as solvents for other solutes in the remaining intracellular water, reducing their concentration and providing a buffer against freezing related salt-induced stress. These properties are attributed to the colligative nature of CPAs, which are responsible for reduction of the freezing point and osmotic pressure of solutes mixed in a solution.

Glycerol is the prototype of all penetrating CPAs and is most successfully used in the cryopreservation of human spermatozoa and that of other species including horse,[67] pig,[68] sheep,[69] dog,[70] and rabbit.[71] A final concentration of 5–10% has been shown to be an optimal concentration of glycerol for a freezing solution.

Examples of nonpenetrating CPAs include monosaccharide, disaccharide, polysaccharide and long-chain polymers (glucose, galactose, sucrose, trehalose, methylcellulose, raffinose, polyethylene glycol and hyaluronan)—these agents are unable to permeate the plasma membrane. Nonpenetrating CPAs can stabilize the lipid bilayer, form hydrogen bonds between hydrophilic sides, increase viscosity and lower the freezing point of the extracellular fluid even though they promote fast cellular dehydration. Egg yolk, which is composed of phospholipid, lipoproteins (low density lipoprotein), cholesterol and antioxidants, soy lecithin (phospholipid isolated from egg yolk and other sources), milk and albumin, are also considered nonpermeating CPAs that are included in every cryoprotective medium as they protect sperm membranes from cold injury. The mechanism of protection is unknown but it is thought that they maintain plasma membrane fluidity and constituents during freezing. Nonpenetrating CPAs have been used successfully as the sole cryoprotectant in the cryopreservation of red blood cells.[72,73] However, they are of limited value when used by themselves in the cryopreservation of nucleated cells, such as sperm. Alternatively, these high molecular weight CPAs are used synergistically with other penetrating CPAs to reduce the toxic concentration of penetrating CPAs.

Cryoprotective medium (CPM) is a solution used to dilute semen or prepared sperm—it is essentially composed of permeating CPAs and one or more of nonpermeating CPAs. Other components of CPM include plasma membrane protective agents, such as egg yolk, milk or soy lecithin, chelators, buffers and antilipid peroxidative agents (Table 2).

More than ten different CPMs are used in sperm banking. There are generally no specific advantages of one medium over another (Table 3). For a particular patient, different CPMs are used until the one that best suits his needs and the best post-thaw sperm parameters is identified. For donor cryopreservation, donors are selected based on their good post-thaw semen parameters in a particular single cryopreservative protocol and medium.

Nevertheless, the most common CPMs are Human Sperm Preservation Medium, Ackerman's Medium, Enhance Sperm Freeze and those containing strong pH buffer systems, such as zwitterions in Test yolk. TEST-

Table 2 Constituents of cryoprotective medium

- Permeating cryoprotective agent: glycerol, ethylene glycol, dimethyl sulfoxide, propylene glycol and methylformamide
- Nonpermeating cryoprotective agents: long chain polymers or sugars (methylcellulose, sucrose, raffinose, trehalose)
- Plasma membrane protecting agents: egg yolk, milk, soy lecithin and albumin.
- Chelating agents: EDTA and citrate chelate
- pH Buffers: Glycine, sodium citrate, TRIS or zwitterionic buffers, such as HEPES or TES
- Free radical scavenger (anti-lipid peroxidation agents): Butylated hydroxytoluene, glutathione and dithiothreitol have been reported to provide protection against peroxidation during cryopreservation, with improvements in post-thaw motility and acrosomal integrity
- Antibiotics: gentamicin

Table 3 Examples of common sperm cryopreservative media

Cryopreservative medium	Penetrating CPA	Nonpenetrating CPA	Plasma membrane protecting agents	Buffer	Free radical scavenger	Others
Test yolk buffer TBY (Irvin)	Glycerol 12%	Fructose	Egg yolk 20%	TES, TRIS	Monothioglycerol MTG	Gentamicin Sulfate or Penicillin-streptomycin
Enhance sperm freezing medium	Glycerol 15%	–	HSA	HEPES	–	–
Sperm freezing medium (Cooper Surgical, Trumbull, CT)	Glycerol	Sucrose Glucose	HSA	HEPES	–	Gentamicin
Ackerman medium (Cryobiosystem)	Glycerol 12%	Anhydrous Glucose	Egg yolk 20%	Citrate	–	–
Human sperm preservation medium Mahadevan and Tounson	Glycerol 15%	Sucrose	–	Glycine	–	–
Sydney sperm cryopreservation buffer (Cook Medical)	Glycerol	Glucose Sucrose	HSA	HEPES	–	Gentamicin
Tardigrade medium (Cryobiosystem)	Glycerol 24%	Glucose Sucrose	HSA	HEPES	–	–
Spermstore (Gynemed)	Glycerol 15%	–	HSA	HEPES	–	–
Sperm freezing medium (Life Global)	Glycerol 15%	Glucose Sucrose	HSA	HEPES	–	–
Cryosperm (Medicult)	Glycerol	Glucose, Raffinose	–	HEPES	–	Penicillin, streptomycin

yolk buffer is a combination of TES [*N*-Tris (hydroxymethyl) methyl-2-aminoethanesulfonic acid, pK 7.5] and Tris [(hydroxymethyl) aminomethane] and is combined with fresh egg yolk, dextrose and penicillin-streptomycin to form the cryobuffer known as TEST (TES and Tris)-yolk buffer (TYB).[74] TYB is the preferred cryoprotectant for men with good or poor semen quality as opposed to glycerol alone. TYB containing 12% glycerol is associated with higher post-thaw sperm motility and survival rates than glycerol alone.[47] TYB also promotes the recovery of a high percentage of motile sperm with normal shapes ($p = 0.04$), resulting in improved capacitation and sperm penetration. Furthermore, researchers at Cleveland Clinic compared TYB with other commercially available media, such as Sperm Freezing Medium (Cooper Surgical, Trumbull, CT) and Enhance Sperm Freeze (Conception Technologies, San Diego, CA), and found that the sperm cryopreserved in TYB had the greatest longevity.[75] Three possibilities may explain such findings: (a) sperm membranes may be stabilized by an altered phospholipid-cholesterol ratio imposed by the egg yolk content of TYB, (b) egg yolk has free radical scavenging properties resulting in less peroxidative damage to the sperm and, (c) TYB has a nearly optimal concentration of glycerol. Because sperm have critical volume limits, CPM should be added slowly and in a step-wise fashion with shaker assistance to reduce the risk of osmotic stress (Figure 7).

Options for packaging of the sample: semen samples are generally stored in cryovials and plastic straws. Syringes were traditionally used as they were easy to fill and could be prepared for insemination rather quickly. However, they are now obsolete due to their large size. Moreover, they are difficult to seal, which increases the risk of contamination. Cryovials are made of plastic material with either polypropylene or polyethylene screw caps which are manufactured as either an external or internal seal onto or into the vial. Cryovials are easily filled in an aseptic technique with 1 ml of semen plus cryoprotectant. However, there are two problems that arise with cryovial use. First, the heat exchange that occurs in the center of the vial is not equal to that in the periphery.[64] Secondly, the seals can leak resulting in liquid nitrogen ingress and a potential for explosion on vial removal and thawing.

Straws or paillettes, on the other hand, are small radius tubes that provide a uniform heat exchange system, efficient seal and less risk of contamination. At first, classic straws were made of polyvinyl chloride (PVC) or polyethylene terephthalate glycol (PETG). Polyvinyl chloride straws were withdrawn from the market in 1998, because the PVC disintegrated under radiation sterilization. Therefore, PETG straws replaced the old ones. Such straws can hold 0.25–0.5 ml of semen and are usually sealed from both ends by ultrasonic welding, solid plastic plugs or hematocrit tube sealant. These straws are easily filled with a sterile nozzle and are

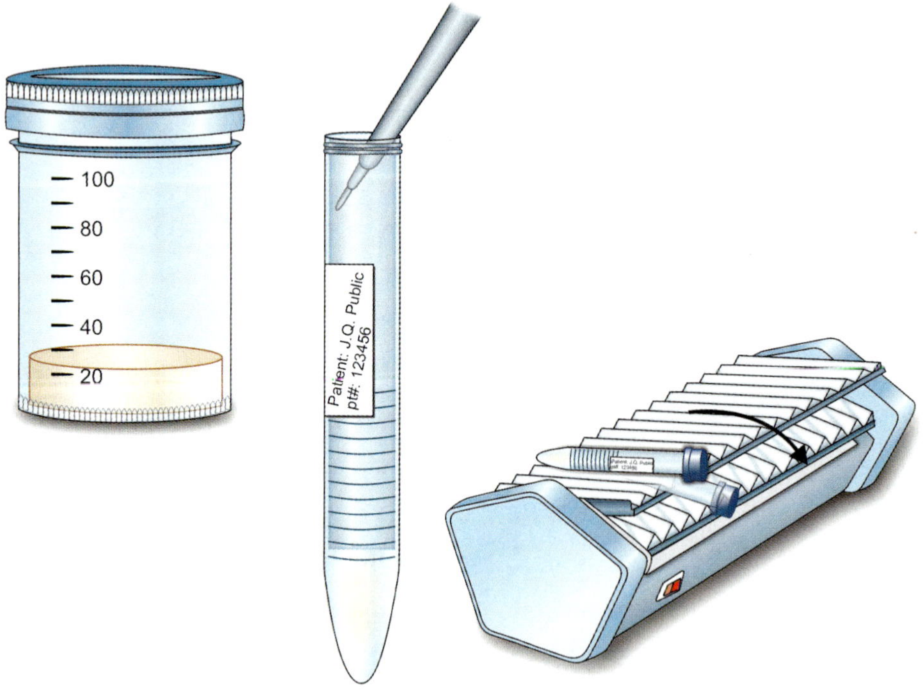

Figure 7 Cryopreservation protocol: shaker for the mixing of the cryoprotectants

free from contamination. Air space must be left to allow for expansion during cooling. Ionomeric resin straws made by Cryo Bio System (called high security straws) are characterized by enhanced tensile strength on cooling and secure sealing achieved via a thermal welding device (SYMS sealer) made by the same company.

Which freezing method is appropriate? There are a variety of methods used today to freeze semen samples, including slow freezing, rapid freezing and vitrification. Because there is debate over whether there is truly any considerable difference between the various freezing methods, each will be discussed here.

Slow freezing: Slow freezing allows the sperm cells to gradually adjust to new conditions and it places less osmotic strain on the cellular membrane. Cell membranes have a certain amount of flexibility when allowing fluids to cross in and out—this is referred to as the 'osmotic tolerance limit'.[76] The slow-freezing method used at Cleveland Clinic involves the gradual addition of cryoprotectants and step-wise freezing of the sample to increasingly colder temperatures before final storage in –196°C liquid nitrogen tanks. Some studies have shown that this method is superior to rapid freezing in regards to sperm kinematics.[41]

After the CPM has been slowly added to the samples (washed or raw semen), to achieve the final vol./vol. ratio of 1:1, they are loaded into straws or cryovials where they are exposed to a freezer temperature of –20°C for 8 minutes and to –96°C in liquid nitrogen vapor for another 2 hours. They are then placed in liquid nitrogen in –196°C for storage. This slow freezing rate can be achieved by manual freezing adjustment or by using the automatic freeze programmer.

Rapid freezing: Rapid freezing aims to minimize toxicity of the cryoprotectant and reduce osmotic membrane damage attributed to the formation of extracellular ice crystals. The most commonly recognized method is the Irvine Scientific Method during which the entire volume of freezing medium is added at one time—1:1 (vol./vol.) of freezing medium to ejaculate. The aliquots are placed in cryovials and then in nitrogen vapors at –96°C for 2 hours. The samples are finally immersed in liquid nitrogen at –196°C. Nallella et al. showed that compared with the slow freezing method, rapid freezing leads to better post-thaw motility and overall survival.[74] However, the same study also found that the slow freezing method was associated with better kinematics parameters, such as VCL; VSL; VAP; ALH in the slow freezing method.

Vitrification: Vitrification is a technique that rapidly cools sperm at a rate greater than 1,000°C per minute. This technique induces an extreme elevation in solution viscosity leading to glass-like solidification without ice crystal formation. Vitrification causes minimal cell damage, but the technique is quite difficult to execute for a number of reasons—it is difficult to cool the cell so rapidly, the cryoprotectants must be extremely concentrated and the procedure has not yet been standardized, leading to considerable variability depending on who is performing the technique.[52] Although this method is ideal for men with poor semen quality or for those in whom sperm retrieval yielded a very low number of sperm, a high concentration of cryoprotectant is harmful by itself to the cells.

Isachenko et al. introduced a new method of sucrose-based sperm vitrification utilizing 50 µl plastic capillaries containing 10 µl of prep specimen without any penetrating CPA.[77] This method was associated with better post-thaw sperm motility, plasma membrane integrity and acrosomal integrity than the conventional slow freeze method. Nevertheless, more studies are needed before this method can be widely implemented.

Epididymal Sperm

To obtain a large number of motile sperm in men with OA, MESA is generally used. It is preferable to PESA and carries a lower risk of blood contamination although it is more expensive. Epididymal aspirate is first checked for motile sperm with an inverted microscope, and when an adequate number of sperm number is found, the aspirate undergoes centrifugation at 1,800 gm for 5 minutes. The resultant pellets are resuspended in a nutrient-rich medium, such as human tubular fluid (HTF), and 4–6 samples of 0.5 cc are prepared for each patient. Each sample is mixed slowly with CPM such as Test-yolk buffer. At the authors' institution, the slow freezing method is applied. The samples should be placed in cryostorage within 1.5 hours of aspirate collection.

Peng et al. have conceptualized a method for preserving a few sperm cells at a time in a droplet of cryoprotectant for long-term storage.[78] In this study, the authors showed that a very small number of sperm are lost with high post-thaw sperm motility. It will be interesting to see that this method translated into clinical practice, as it seems particularly worthwhile for oligozoospermic men and patients, who are only able to bank a small number of cells.

Testicular Sperm

Testicular sperm are retrieved in men with OA and NOA. If surgeons are unable to aspirate sperm from the epididymis in patients with OA, then they should turn to the testes and perform TESA. Unfortunately, the aspirate usually yields a very low number of sperm and the sample might be contaminated by blood.

Sperm retrieved from the testes are frozen in the same manner as described for epididymal sperm. After mixing the aspirate with human tubal fluid (HTF), the mixture is centrifuged, and the pellets are resuspended with HTF. Cryovials are then filled with this suspension and an equal volume of CPM (e.g. Test-yolk buffer) is slowly added.

For sperm retrieval by TESE, the procedure is somewhat different from that used for testicular aspiration. In this case, tissue biopsies are taken and shredded into small pieces with a sterile 25-gauge needle or fine scissor, mincer or enzymatic digestion using type IV collagenase, trypsin and trypsin inhibitor. This allows the permeating cryoprotectant, such as glycerol, to fully penetrate testicular homogenate. Each tissue sample is assessed for the presence of motile spermatozoa with an inverted microscope. If there are no motile sperm in the testicular biopsy, further biopsies may be taken from the ipsilateral and contralateral testes until mature sperm are found.

The effluents and shredded biopsy tissue can be centrifuged. The pellet is resuspended in culture medium and prepared for freezing. CPM is added slowly in a drop-wise fashion to the testicular homogenate to allow proper mixing before the sample is frozen.

In many men with NOA, testicular biopsies often reveal a very low density of poorly motile sperm, and the cryopreservation method usually culminates in further deterioration of the harvested sperm. Alternatively, three other methods have been used in such cases that involve inserting testicular sperm inside: (1) Hamster egg's zona pellucida,[79,80] (2) Nylon microloops[81] or, (3) Vehicles made from the algae species Volvox globator[82] and then freezing . All three of these methods are experimental and future studies are required to refine these techniques.

Immature Testicular Tissue Preservation

As mentioned before, this procedure is used for children and prepubertal boys with cancer before receiving aggressive chemotherapy or radiotherapy. Gonadotoxic therapy can not only affect the rapidly proliferating differentiated spermatogonia but also the stem cell pool.[25] In some cases, testicular tissue is biopsied whereas in others, whole testes might be removed. Controlled slow-rate freezing with penetrating CPA such as 5% dimethyl sulfoxide proves to be the best approach to preserve human immature testicular biopsies.[83] Nevertheless, it is still an experimental procedure and there is currently no standard protocol. Extensive animal and human research is currently being performed in the field of fertility restoration including, stem cell transplantation, post-thaw testicular tissue transplantation and *in vitro* stimulation of sperm production.

Storing the Sample

Once the sample has been properly frozen, it must be safely stored for successful long-term (in practice, indefinite) preservation. Liquid nitrogen tanks are useful for short-term storage (Figure 8), while bulk refrigerators can be used for longer periods of time (Figure 9). Using liquid nitrogen tanks is reliable because the temperature remains constant. It is preferable to store sperm at temperatures lower than –96°C to prevent sperm damage. Long-term storage at –196°C is 'superior' to storage at any other temperature. It is of the utmost importance to ensure that samples are sealed well to prevent cross-contamination. To further decrease the risk of contamination, samples should be tested for infectious diseases prior to freezing.

Thawing the Sample

The thawing process must be performed carefully to minimize sperm damage. The objective of the thawing process is to obtain viable and motile sperm from the frozen specimen. Two important steps are followed. In the first step, the cryovial or straw is removed from the storage medium and allowed to rewarm. Although some authors prefer to adjust the rate of rewarming, so that it is in concordance with the freezing speed, others prefer rapid rewarming as it results in better recovery of motile sperm. This step is usually achieved by placing the cryovial or straw in room temperature for 5 minutes and then under water bath at 37°C for another 20 minutes. In the second step, the CPA is slowly removed from the cells along with the other constituents of the CPM, such as the buffer system. This step is performed using sperm washing medium, such as modified Biggers-Whitten-Whittingam (BWW) medium (HEPES-Biggers-Whitten-Whittingam, Irvine Scientific, Santa Ana, CA) (1:2, vol./vol.) enriched with 5% of human albumin or modified human tubal fluid. The sperm washing medium is added slowly over the rewarmed semen, followed by centrifugation at 350 g for 5–10 minutes. The pellets are resuspended and subjected to another round of centrifugation, resulting in sperm-concentrated pellets. Finally, the contents of these pellets are aspirated and resuspended in nutrient-rich media.

Semen analysis for the post-thawed frozen sample is conducted 24 hours after freezing to check the quality of frozen semen and measure the number of motile sperm which withstand the stress of freeze thaw cycle. Based on these results, patients will be asked to provide more samples to be banked.

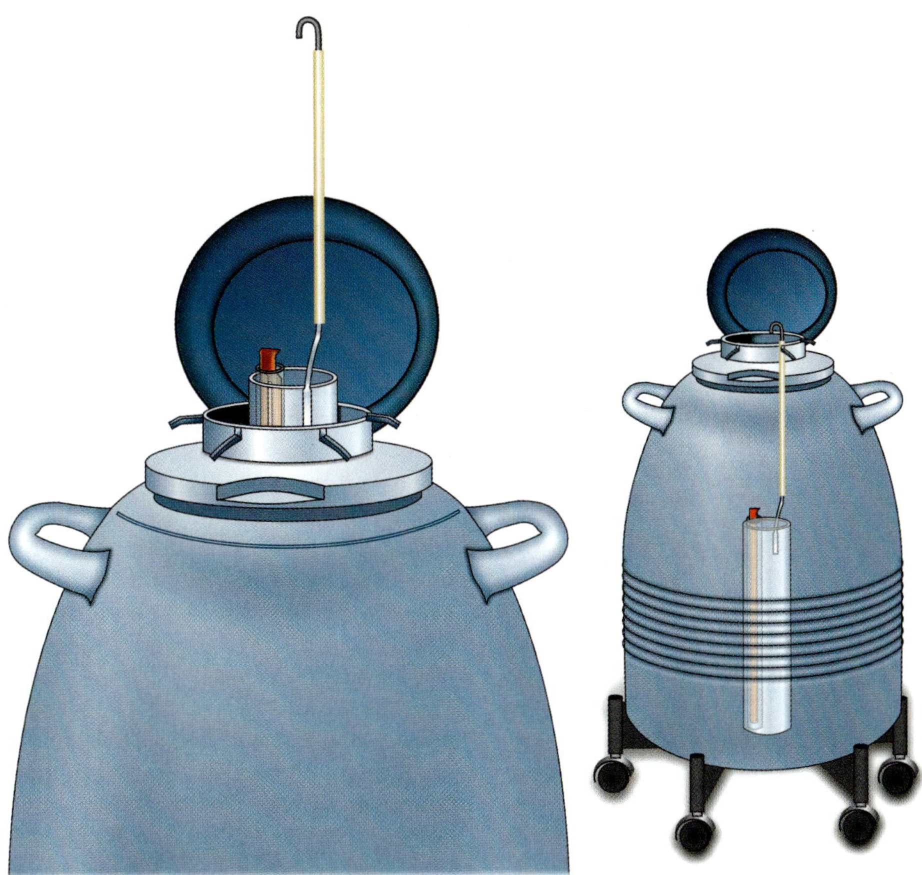

Figure 8 Short-term storage of semen sample in liquid nitrogen tanks

The thawing process can damage cell membranes and intracellular compartments, affecting metabolic activities and leading to decreased sperm motility. It also can cause DNA damage, possibly because the process increases production of ROS. To assess viability following thawing, hypo-osmotic swelling tests should be conducted, particularly in the presence of immotile sperm.[84] Poor sperm count and motility post-thawing may necessitate the addition of pentoxifylline and/or performing density gradient centrifugation to improve the quality of the thawed specimen in terms of sperm count and motility.

Utilization Rates

In discussing the usefulness and importance of sperm cryopreservation, it is important to examine utilization rates of banked samples. Overall, sperm cryopreservation remains underutilized for a variety of reasons. Studies report utilization rates ranging anywhere from 4.7–7.5%.[29,85,86] Despite these low rates, it is still recommended that all male cancer patients be counseled about this option, as sperm cryopreservation is a form of insurance for potentially irreversible health problems. The specific reasons why many men choose not to use their banked sperm or discard it, will be discussed at the end of this section. When looking at the rates of use of banked sperm, however, it is important to remember that without storage, none of these patients would have the opportunity to biologically father a child. Within this mindset, any rate of utilization can be considered a success.

Use of Cryopreserved Sperm in ART

Once the sample has been successfully thawed and the post-thaw semen parameters have been evaluated, the sperm is ready to be used in ART. Depending on each patient's situation and the quality of his sperm, different methods can be used to help him and his partner conceive. The success and type of the ART procedure will depend on a variety of factors; including the type of the sample (ejaculated semen, epididymal or testicular sperm) and the post-thaw sample quality. The highest-quality post-thaw ejaculated semen with adequate parameters can be used for intrauterine insemination

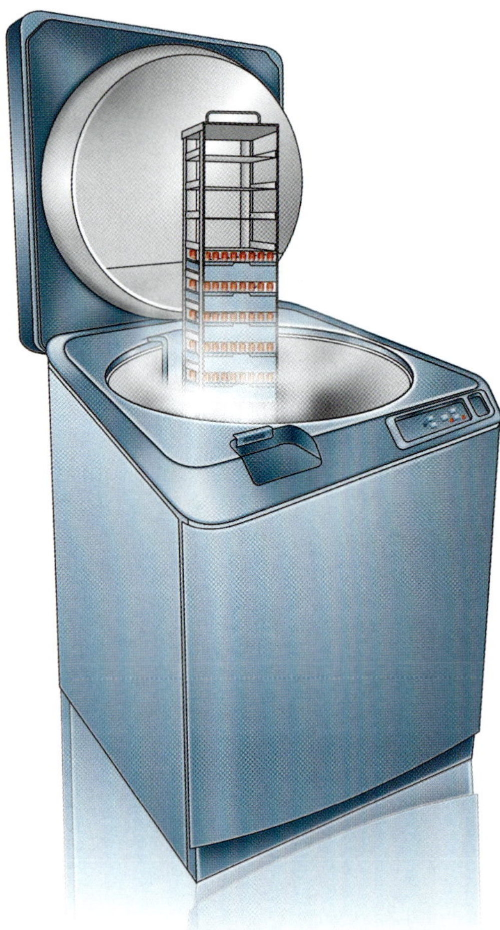

Figure 9 Long-term storage of semen sample in liquid nitrogen tank. The figure shows a metal canister containing boxes filled with cryovials

(IUI). This procedure is closest to natural conception, as sperm is injected into the woman's uterus. Poorer quality semen, as indicated by post-thaw parameters, epididymal sperm and testicular sperm should be used in assisted-fertilization procedures, such as *in vitro* fertilization (IVF) or Intracytoplasmic sperm injection (ICSI).

Fresh versus frozen ejaculated sperm and ART outcomes: despite the paucity of well-designed controlled trials on IUI outcomes using frozen ejaculated sperm, several studies have found that the fertilizing capability of frozen sperm is lower than that of freshly ejaculated sperm.[87,88] This finding can be interpreted on the basis of cryopreservation-related sperm dysfunction. However, one single study reported identical pregnancy rates between frozen and fresh ejaculated sperm used in artificial insemination when there was a sufficient number of progressively motile sperm in the post-thaw specimen and in absence of severe teratozoospermia and asthenospermia.[89] Several cases of allergic reactions to hen's egg yolk have been reported by women undergoing IUI.[64]

For conventional IVF, the data are also controversial. While Cohen et al. and Mahadevan et al. failed to show any difference in the fertility outcomes between cryopreserved ejaculated sperm and fresh sperm,[90,91] others have identified significant differences.[92-94] Nonetheless, good post-thaw semen quality has always correlated well with adequate outcomes.

Lastly, the advent and widespread use of ICSI has resulted in a tremendous modification in sperm banking practices as this procedure can overcome many limitations associated with sperm cryopreservation, such as poor post-thaw sperm quality and sperm dysfunction. Kuczyński et al. conducted well-designed controlled trials and found no difference in fertilization rates between cryopreserved and freshly ejaculated sperm.[95] Meanwhile, the authors reported higher ongoing pregnancy rates per cycle with fresh sperm (23.7%) versus frozen (35.2%).[95]

Fresh versus frozen epididymal sperm: the first pregnancy resulting from the use of fresh epididymal sperm (taken from a man with OA) occurred in 1995.[96] This breakthrough has since helped many infertile men, who were previously thought to be sterile to father biological children. Comparative studies between frozen and fresh epididymal sperm regarding ICSI outcomes have not detected major differences in regards to fertilization rates and ongoing pregnancy rates, particularly when motile sperm were used.[97]

Fresh versus frozen testicular sperm in ICSI outcomes: In general, there are no differences in ICSI outcomes in terms of fertilization rates, clinical pregnancy rates or ongoing pregnancy rates between fresh and frozen motile testicular sperm.[98,99,100] However, implantation rates are slightly better with the use of fresh motile testicular sperm.[100] Others have reported that such findings are more evident in men with OA than with NOA.[101] Motile testicular sperm are generally preferred for use in ICSI but when the testicular sperm are immotile, a common occurrence, it is important to verify their vitality. Viable sperm can be selected using the hypo-osmotic swelling test, via laser assisted immobilized sperm selection or by adding motility enhancing agents, such as pentoxifylline.[102]

Disposing of Samples

While ART procedures with cryopreserved sperm are often successful, not all men who bank sperm return to use their samples, as evidenced by the generally low utilization rates described above. Often, a cancer survivor who banked sperm will dispose of his sample following cessation of treatment—particularly, if he regains his fertility or his semen quality improves.[49] Others may wish to actively dispose of the banked samples for a variety of reasons, including patient death, financial restrictions or a lack of desire to father children.[103] Patients may also be concerned about whether they will be healthy enough in the future to be a good parent.[104]

Having a banked sample requires some amount of caution. While the patient is alive, he has full control over how the preserved sperm are used. If he dies unexpectedly or without ensuring the proper precautions to protect his sample, however, the situation could become fraught with legal and ethical problems. Who does the sample belong to when the patient passes away? It is therefore of the utmost importance that the patient signs a form stating the ownership and destination of the banked semen in case of his death.[49] Some important points to include in any such consent form include whether or not the sample should be disposed of after death and who else, if anyone is permitted to use it in ART procedures.

Additions of Antioxidants

Sperm are redox cells that can produce ROS. Meanwhile, sperm and seminal plasma possess enzymatic and nonenzymatic antioxidants that can scavenge ROS to prevent the precipitation of oxidative stress and cellular damage. Sperm are particularly susceptible to oxidative stress because their plasma membranes contain a large amount of polyunsaturated fatty acids and have a limited intrinsic reserve of cytoplasmic antioxidant enzyme systems. Therefore, sperm predominantly depend upon the antioxidant support of seminal plasma. As such, sperm preparation for cryopreservation, which often involves the removal of seminal plasma by centrifugation, increases the susceptibility of spermatozoa to oxidative stress. In addition, studies find that the antioxidant activity of the spermatozoa themselves may be decreased by cryopreservation.[105,106] Freeze-thawing of equine, human and bovine sperm was associated with an increase in ROS generation.[107-111] Recent studies on Rhesus Macaque cryopreserved sperm have shown that frozen-thawed sperm not only experience excessive ROS generation during the process but also severe DNA and chromosomal damage.[112] More recently, Gadea et al. identified decrease in the total seminal level of reduced glutathione (GSH) in human semen undergoing freezing-thawing cycles.[113]

Oxidative stress usually lowers sperm motility and viability and leads to ionophore-induced acrosome reaction and sperm-oocyte fusion. Hydrogen peroxide appears to be the primary ROS responsible for these adverse changes, and sperm plasma membrane lipid peroxidation is postulated to be an important mechanism of action.[114,115-118]

When plasma membrane lipid peroxidation occurs, the membrane loses the necessary fluidity and integrity required to participate in membrane fusion with an oocyte during fertilization. Moreover, lipid peroxidation can also damage DNA, resulting in chromatin cross-linking, base changes and DNA strand breaks.[114,119-121]

A recent study conducted by Kalthur et al. found that adding antioxidants to CPM in the form of Vitamin E during freezing significantly enhanced the total motility and progressive motility in post-thaw samples.[122] Such improvements in freezing procedures may ultimately lead to an increased conception rate in ART cycles.[121] Other authors have reported reduced oxidative stress markers with the use of antioxidants, including Gadea (who used reduced GSH) and Li et al. (who used ascorbate and catalase separately).[113] These significant findings should encourage the companies that produce CPM to add proper antioxidants supplementation, whether enzymatic or nonenzymatic, to their commercial preparations to enhance post-thaw sperm quality.

THE RISE OF ONCOFERTILITY AS A FIELD

The field of oncofertility has been growing rapidly since its official inception in 2006. It is a discipline that combines the fields of oncology and reproductive medicine which, until now, were kept separate. In fact, the field is a conglomeration of bioethics, social sciences, pediatrics and a multitude of other areas resulting in a highly interdisciplinary approach.[36,38,54] The union of these previously disjointed areas of study allows health-care providers to help resolve difficult ethical and legal issues that often arise in fertility preservation discussions. The field is developing in response to the discrepancy between the attention given to cure cancer and quality of life concerns and because infertility treatments have often been considered an enhancement rather than a necessary treatment that is covered by health-care insurance. This approach shifts reproduction from a privilege to a human right, acknowledging and addressing that, the desire to have a child is an overwhelming human emotion.[38] Oncofertility specialists also aim to raise awareness among patients about the detrimental effects of cancer on fertility and options for fertility preservation. The continual evolvement of this field will undoubtedly ease patient concerns regarding fertility during the already difficult time following a cancer diagnosis.

AVAILABLE RESOURCES ON FERTILITY PRESERVATION

Because of the growing awareness of fertility preservation both among providers and patients, there is an increasing body of knowledge on the topic as well as available informational resources. Oncologists treating reproductive-aged males would benefit from ready-to-use online provider handouts on counseling patients on fertility preservation. Likewise, patients can browse these websites to help ease diagnosis-associated anxiety and initiate a conversation with their provider on what fertility preservation option would be best for their specific case. Some organizations that provide these valuable resources include, the Oncofertility Consortium, Fertile Hope and the Livestrong Foundation.

CONCLUSIONS AND FUTURE RESEARCH

Although enormous strides have been made in the technologies of assisted reproduction, cryopreservation protocols, cancer research and in the new field of oncofertility, there are still many unknowns to be determined. Primarily, there is still much to be learned about what causes semen quality to decrease in patients with cancer and the mechanisms of how cancer affects spermatogenesis both locally and systemically. Ultimately, it is crucial to develop cancer therapies that are less harmful to fertility. This includes developing new therapies and ensuring that new chemotherapeutics are tested for gonadotoxicity prior to clinical prescription, as well as focusing on developing medications that have gonadoprotective properties.[38] The Oncofertility Consortium also strives to decrease the incidence of disease-related fertility loss by finding noninterventional or medical ways to eliminate a young person's risk of losing his fertility due to cancer treatment.[38] Experimental procedures, such as testicular tissue extraction and freezing for prepubescent cancer patients, require more formidable translation from animal research to real clinical human practice.[36] Finally, the field of oncofertility needs to continue gaining momentum, ensuring that all physicians are fully informed about fertility preservation options available to their patients. It is time for the awareness of the toxic effects of cancer treatments on future fertility to coincided with the rates of referral to sperm banks.

As the side effects of cancer therapy receive more attention and the field of oncofertility blossoms, the search continues for modern treatments that are less harmful to the body. Researchers in this area are generally looking at how to lower doses, use different treatment regimens and reduce 'drug-related toxicity without compromising cure rates.' For example, some specialists are looking at ways to make radiation therapies more localized to invasive cells, thereby minimizing damage to the rest of the body. One method of achieving this is to protect the gonads during treatment, to prevent radiation scatter and 'minimize the time required for spermatogenetic recovery following radiotherapy'.[26] In addition, researchers are looking at inhibiting spermatogenesis with hormone therapy prior to anticancer therapy to preserve fertility during treatment. Others are attempting to invent a molecular target therapy to combat cancer. For example, in lymphomas, researchers are looking at whether they can substitute epidermal growth factor or vascular endothelial growth factor for the toxic conventional chemotherapy to avoid their adverse effects. All of these projects are preliminary but promising nonetheless.[26]

Systemic diseases and chemotherapy disrupt fertility in general and spermatogenesis specifically. Kim et al. focused on hormonal disruptions by targeting the hypothalamic-pituitary-gonadal axis.[123] Specific endocrine therapy can be used to balance these changes and preserve fertility during treatment. A gonadotropin-releasing hormone analog can be administered either during or after treatment with procarbazine or radiotherapy.[123]

More research is still needed with larger groups using drugs that are used more commonly in humans. Overall, there is still much room for the improvement of cancer therapies. Ideally, these currently highly toxic treatments would become harsh enough to properly attack the cancerous, invasive cells while sparing the rest of the body, specifically, the gonads and fertility.

RECOMMENDATIONS

- Many men in various stages of life could benefit from utilizing sperm cryopreservation.
- It is advisable for any physician to engage in a discussion on cryobanking with any patient, who may be exposed to gonadotoxic factors at work, is severely oligo- or azoospermic, has cancer (regardless of age) or another disease that can directly or indirectly affect fertility or is undergoing hormonal therapy that may adversely impact semen quality.
- Such discussions can prevent patients' misconception about the sperm banking and regretting not taking the necessary precautions against potential fertility loss.

- It is preferable to offer the patient the option of fertility preservation rather than precluding his chance of fathering a biological child.
- Patients should have time to consider these issues rather than have their health care provider made decisions on their behalf.
- It is of the utmost importance to remember that specific fertility preservation recommendations must be made on a case-by-case basis.
- Sperm cryobanking has formally become part of the standard of care for reproductive-aged oncologic patients.
- Sperm cryopreservation is the most effective and the most strongly recommended option for fertility preservation prior to any treatment or occupational exposure that may pose a threat to a man's fertility.

REFERENCES

1. Bratton RW, Foote RH, Cruthers JC. Preliminary fertility results with frozen bovine spermatozoa. J Dairy Sci. 1955;38:40-6.
2. Polge C, Smith AU, Parkes AS. Revival of spermatozoa after vitrification and dehydration at low temperatures. Nature. 1949;164:666.
3. Bunge RG, Keettel WC, Sherman JK. Clinical use of frozen semen: report of four cases. Fertil Steril. 1954;5(6):520-9.
4. Sherman JK. Cryopreservation of human semen. In: CRC Handbook of the Laboratory Diagnosis and Treatment of Infertility. Keel BA, Webster BW (Eds). Boston: CRC Press; 1990. p. 229.
5. Tomlinson M. Therapeutic sperm cryopreservation. In: Björndahl L, Giwercman A, Tournaye L (Eds). Clinical Andrology EAU/ESAU Course Guidelines. London: Informa Health Care; 2010. pp. 124-133.
6. Ping P, Zhu WB, Zhang XZ, et al. Sperm banking for male reproductive preservation: a 6-year retrospective multi-centre study in China. Asian J Androl. 2010;12(3):356-62.
7. American Cancer Society. Cancer facts and figures, US, 2011. Available from www.cancer.org/acs/groups/content/@epidemiologysurveilance/documents/document/acspc-029771.pdf. [Accessed March 2011].
8. Steliarova-Foucher E, Stiller C, Kaatsch P, et al. Geographical patterns and time trends of cancer incidence and survival among children and adolescents in Europe since the 1970s (the ACCIS project): an epidemiological study. Lancet. 2004;364:2097-105.
9. Ragheb AM, Jones S, Sabanegh, et al. Implications of cancer on male fertility. Arch Med Sci. 2009;5, 1A:S63–9.
10. Agarwal A, Allamaneni SS. Disruption of spermatogenesis by the cancer disease process. J Nat Can Inst Monogr. 2005;34:9-12.
11. Amirjannati N, Sadeghi M, Hosseini Jadda SH, et al. Evaluation of semen quality in patients with malignancies referred for sperm banking before cancer treatment. Andrologia. 2011;43(5):317-20.
12. Crha I, Ventruba P, Petrenko M, et al. [Cryopreservation of sperm before neoplasm therapy—7 years' experience]. Ceska Gynekol. 2002;67(6):324-8.
13. Lass A, Akagbosu F, Abusheikha N, et al. A programme of semen cryopreservation for patients with malignant disease in a tertiary infertility centre: lessons from 8 years' experience. Hum Reprod. 1998;13:3256-61.
14. van Casteren NJ, Boellaard WP, Romijn JC, et al. Gonadal dysfunction in male cancer patients before cytotoxic treatment. Int J Androl. 2010;33(1):73-9.
15. Crha I, Ventruba P, Zakova J, et al. Survival and infertility treatment in male cancer patients after sperm banking. Fertil Steril. 2009;91(6):2344-8.
16. Tempest HG, Ko E, Chan P, et al. Sperm aneuploidy frequencies analysed before and after chemotherapy in testicular cancer and Hodgkin's lymphoma patients. Hum Reprod. 2008;23:251-8.
17. Morrish DW, Venner PM, Siy O, et al. Mechanisms of endocrine dysfunction in patients with testicular cancer. J Natl Cancer Inst. 1990;82:412-8.
18. Ho GT, Gardner H, DeWolf WC, et al. Influence of testicular carcinoma on ipsilateral spermatogenesis. J Urol. 1992;148:821-5.
19. Foster RS, Rubin LR, McNulty A, et al. Detection of antisperm-antibodies in patients with primary testicular cancer. Int J Androl. 1991;14:179-85.
20. Burns WR, Sabanegh E, Dada R, et al. Is male infertility a forerunner to cancer? Int Braz J Urol. 2010;36(5):527-36.
21. Rørth M, Rajpert-De Meyts E, Andersson L, et al. Carcinoma in situ in the testis. Scand J Urol Nephrol Suppl. 2000;205:166-86.
22. Perdichizzi A, Nicoletti F, La Vignera S, et al. Effects of tumour necrosis factor-alpha on human sperm motility and apoptosis. J Clin Immunol. 2007;27:152-162.
23. Viviani S, Ragni G, Santoro A, et al. Testicular dysfunction in Hodgkin's disease before and after treatment. Eur J Cancer. 1991;27:1389-92.
24. Fitoussi, Eghbali H, Tchen N, et al. Semen analysis and cryoconservation before treatment in Hodgkin's disease. Ann Oncol. 2000;11:679-84.
25. Bucci LR, Meistrich ML. Effects of busulfan on murine spermatogenesis: cytotoxicity, sterility, sperm abnormalities, and dominant lethal mutations. Mutat Res. 1987;176:259-68.
26. Ragheb AM, Sabanegh ES. Male fertility-implications of anticancer treatment and strategies to mitigate gonadotoxicity. Anti-Cancer Agents Med Chem. 2010;10:92-102.
27. Howell SJ, Shalet SM. Spermatogenesis after cancer treatment: damage and recovery. J Natl Cancer Inst Monogr. 2005;34:12-7.
28. Petersen PM, Skakkebaek NE, Giwercman A. Gonadal function in men with testicular cancer: biological and clinical aspects. APMIS. 1998;106(1):24-34.
29. Dobrzyńska MM, Czajka U, Slowikowska MG. Reproductive effects after exposure of male mice to vincristine and to a combination of X-rays and vincristine. Reprod Fertil Dev. 2005;17(8):759-67.

30. Viviani S, Santoro A, Ragni G, et al. Gonadal toxicity after combination chemotherapy for Hodgkin's disease. Comparative results of MOPP vs ABVD. Eur J Cancer Clin Oncol. 1985;21(5):601-5.
31. Ortin TT, Shostak CA, Donaldson SS. Gonadal status and reproductive function following treatment for Hodgkin's disease in childhood: the Stanford experience. Int J Radiat Oncol Biol Phys. 1990;19(4):873-80.
32. O'Flaherty C, Hales BF, Chan P, et al. Impact of chemotherapeutics and advanced testicular cancer or Hodgkin lymphoma on sperm deoxyribonucleic acid integrity. Fertil Steril. 2010;94(4):1374-9.
33. Wallace WH. Oncofertility and preservation of reproductive capacity in children and young adults. Cancer. 2011;117(10 Suppl):2301-10.
34. Shalet SM, Tsatsoulis A, Whitehead E, et al. Vulnerability of the human Leydig cell to radiation damage is dependent upon age. J Endocrinol. 1989;120:161-5.
35. Colpi GM, Contalbi GF, Nerva F, et al. Testicular function following chemo-radiotherapy. Eur. J. Obstet. Gynecol Reprod. Biol. 2004;113(Suppl 1):S2-6.
36. Ginsberg JP, Carlson CA, Lin K, et al. An experimental protocol for fertility preservation in prepubertal boys recently diagnosed with cancer: a report of acceptability and safety. Hum Reprod. 2010;25(1):37-41
37. Hagenäs I, Jørgensen N, Rechnitzer C, et al. Clinical and biochemical correlates of successful semen collection for cryopreservation from 12-18 year old patients: a single-center study of 86 adolescents. Hum Reprod. 2010;25(8):2031-8.
38. Woodruff TK. The Oncofertility Consortium—addressing fertility in young people with cancer. Nat Rev Clin Oncol. 2010;7:466-75.
39. Ranganathan P, Mahran AM, Hallak J, et al. Sperm cryopreservation for men with nonmalignant, systemic diseases: a descriptive study. J Androl. 2002;23:71-5.
40. Anger JT, Gilbert BR, Goldstein M. Cryopreservation of sperm: indications, methods and results. J Urol. 2003;170(4 Pt 1):1079-84.
41. Gupta S, Agarwal A, Sharma R, et al. Recovery, preparation, storage and utilization of spermatozoa for fertility preservation in cancer patients and subfertile men. J Reprod Stem Cell Biotech. 2011;1:150-68.
42. Cherry N, Moore H, McNamee R, et al. Occupation and male infertility: glycol ethers and other exposures. Occup Environ Med. 2008;65(10):708-14.
43. Families against cancer. Stop cancer before it starts. Available from www.familiesagainstcancer.org/?id=95 [Accessed July 2011].
44. War-Bound Soldiers Urged To Bank Sperm Before Deployment: California Cryobank Offers Discounted Semen Storage and Post-Mortem Retrieval Programs For All Military Men And First Responders. Available from www.cryobank.com/about-us/press-releases/template.cfm?id=1380 [Accessed July 2011].
45. Mishra DP, Shaha C. Estrogen-induced spermatogenic cell apoptosis occurs via the mitochondrial pathway: role of superoxide and nitric oxide. J Biol Chem. 2005;18:280(7):6181-96.
46. Bak CW, Song SH, Yoon TK, et al. Natural course of idiopathic oligozoospermia: comparison of mild, moderate and severe forms. Int J Urol. 2010;17(11):937-43.
47. Song SH, Bak CW, Lim JJ, et al. Natural course of severe oligozoospermia in infertile male: influence on future fertility potential. J Androl. 2010;31(6):536-9.
48. Walters EM, Benson JD, Woods EJ, et al. The history of sperm cryopreservation. In: Pacey AA, Tomlinson MJ (Eds). Sperm Banking: Theory and Practice. Cambridge: Cambridge University Press; 2009. pp. 1-10.
49. Van Casteren NJ, Santbrink EJP, van Izen W, et al. Use rate and assisted reproduction technologies outcome of cryopreserved semen from 629 cancer patients. Fertil Steril. 2008;90(6):2245-50.
50. Save My Fertility. Available from www.savemyfertility.org [Accessed July 2011].
51. Anderson RA, Weddell A, Spoudeas HA, et al. Do doctors discuss fertility issues before they treat young patients with cancer? Hum Reprod. 2008;23(10):2246-51.
52. Gosden RG. Fertility Preservation: definition, history, and prospect. Semin Reprod Med. 2009;27(6):433-7.
53. Edge B, Holmes D, Makin G. Sperm banking in adolescent cancer patients. Arch Dis Child. 2006;91:149-52.
54. Redig AJ, Brannigan R, Stryker SJ, et al. Incorporating fertility preservation into the care of young oncologic patients. Cancer. 2011;117:4-10.
55. Keros V, Rosenlund B, Hultenby K, et al. Optimizing cryopreservation of human testicular tissue: comparison of protocols with glycerol, propanediol and dimethylsulphoxide as cryoprotectants. Hum Reprod. 2005;20(6):1676-87.
56. Critser JK, Huse-Benda AR, Aaker DV, et al. Cryopreservation of human spermatozoa. III. The effect of cryoprotectants on motility. Fertil Steril. 1988;50:314-20.
57. Kalthur G, Adiga SK, Upadhya D, et al. Effect of cryopreservation on sperm DNA integrity in patients with teratospermia. Fertil Steril. 2008;89:1723-7.
58. Gandini L, Lombardo F, Lenzi A, et al. Cryopreservation and sperm DNA integrity. Cell Tissue Bank. 2006;7(2):91-8.
59. Bilodeau JF, Chatterjee S, Sirard MA, et al. Levels of antioxidant defenses are decreased in bovine spermatozoa after a cycle of freezing and thawing. Mol Reprod Dev. 2000;55(3):282-8.
60. McCarthy MJ, Baumber J, Kass PH, et al. Osmotic stress induces oxidative cell damage to rhesus macaque spermatozoa. Biol Reprod. 2010;82(3):644-51.
61. Fuller B, Paynter S. Fundamentals of cryobiology in reproductive medicine. Reprod Biomed Online. 2004;9:680-91.
62. Berger T, Marrs RP, Moyer DL. Comparison of techniques for selection of motile spermatozoa. Fertil Steril. 1985;43(2):268-73.
63. Esteves SC, Sharma RK, Thomas AJ, et al. Improvement in motion characteristics and acrosome status in cryopreserved human spermatozoa by swim-up processing before freezing. Hum Reprod. 2000;15(10):2173-9.
64. Mortimer D. Current and future concepts and practices in human sperm cryobanking. Reprod Biomed Online. 2004;9(2):134-51.

65. Said TM, Agarwal A, Zborowski M, et al. Utility of magnetic cell separation as a molecular sperm preparation technique. J Androl. 2008;29(2):134-42.
66. Grunewald S, Paasch U, Said TM, et al. Magnetic-activated cell sorting before cryopreservation preserves mitochondrial integrity in human spermatozoa. Cell Tissue Bank. 2006;7(2):99-104.
67. Nishikawa Y. Studies on the preservation of raw and frozen horse semen. J Reprod Fertil Suppl. 1975;(23):99-104.
68. Pursel VG, Johnson LA. Freezing of boar spermatozoa: fertilizing capacity with concentrated semen and a new thawing procedure. J Anim Sci. 1975;40(1):99-102.
69. Colas G. Effect of initial freezing temperature, addition of glycerol and dilution on the survival and fertilizing ability of deep-frozen ram semen. J Reprod Fertil. 1975;42(2):277-85.
70. Seager SW, Fletcher WS. Progress on the use of frozen semen in the dog. Vet Rec. 1973;92(1):6-10.
71. Fox RR. Preservation of rabbit spermatozoa: fertility results from frozen semen. Proc Soc Exp Biol Med. 1961;108:663-5.
72. Horn EP, Sputtek A, Standl T, et al. Transfusion of autologous, hydroxyethyl starch-cryopreserved red blood cells. Anesth Analg. 1997;85(4):739-45.
73. Connor W, Ashwood-Smith MJ. Cryoprotection of mammalian cells in tissue culture with polymers: possible mechanisms. Cryobiology. 1973;10:488-96.
74. Nallella KP, Sharma RK, Allamaneni SS, et al. Cryopreservation of human spermatozoa: comparison of two cryopreservation methods and three cryoprotectants. Fertil Steril. 2004;82(4):913-18.
75. Hallak J, Sharma RK, Wellstead C, et al. Cryopreservation of human spermatozoa: comparison of TEST-yolk buffer and glycerol. Int J Fertil Womens Med. 2000;45(1):38-42.
76. Walters EM, Men H, Agca Y, et al. Osmotic tolerance of mouse spermatozoa from various genetic backgrounds: acrosome integrity, membrane integrity, and maintenance of motility. Cryobiology. 2005;50(2):193-205.
77. Isachenko E, Isachenko V, Katkov LL, et al. Vitrification of mammalian spermatozoa in the absence of cryoprotectants: from past practical difficulties to present success. Reprod Biomed Online. 2003;6(2):191-200.
78. Peng QP, Cao SF, Lyu QF, et al. A novel method for cryopreservation of individual human spermatozoa. In Vitro Cell Dev Biol Anim. 2011;47:565-72.
79. Levi-Setti PE, Albani E, Negri L, et al. Cryopreservation of a small number of spermatozoa in yolk-filled human zonae pellucidae. Arch Ital di Urol Androl. 2003;75:195-8.
80. Cohen J, Garrisi GJ, Congedo-Ferrara TA, et al. Cryopreservation of single human spermatozoa. Hum Reprod. 1997;12:944-1001.
81. Desai NN, Blackmon H, Goldfarb J. Single sperm cryopreservation on cryoloops: an alternative to hamster zona for freezing individual spermatozoa. Reprod Biomed Online. 2004;9:47-53.
82. Just A, Gruber I, Wober M, et al. Novel method for the cryopreservation of testicular sperm and ejaculated spermatozoa from patients with severe oligospermia: a pilot study. Fertil Steril. 2004;82:445-7.
83. Keros V, Hultenby K, Borgstrom B, et al. Methods of cryopreservation of testicular tissue with viable spermatogonia in pre-pubertal boys undergoing gonadotoxic cancer treatment. Hum Reprod. 2007;22:1384-95.
84. Levron J, Madgar I, Shefi S, et al. IVF outcome with cryopreserved testicular sperm. Andrologia. 2011;43:48-51.
85. Tournaye H, Goossens E, Verheyen G, et al. Preserving the reproductive potential of men and boys with cancer: current concepts and future prospects. Hum Reprod Update. 2004;10(6):525-32.
86. Magelssen H, Haugen TB, von Düring V, et al. Twenty years experience with semen cryopreservation in testicular cancer patients: who needs it? Eur Urol. 2005;8:779-85.
87. Sherman JK. Synopsis of the use of frozen human semen since 1964: state of the art of human semen banking. Fertil Steril. 1973;24:397-412.
88. Richter MA, Haning RV, Shapiro SS. Artificial donor insemination: fresh versus frozen semen; the patient as her own control. Fertil Steril. 1984;41:277-80.
89. Keel BA, Webster BW. Semen analysis data from fresh and cryopreserved donor ejaculates: comparison of cryoprotectants and pregnancy rates. Fertil Steril. 1989;52(1):100-5.
90. Cohen J, Edwards RG, Fehilly CB, et al. In vitro fertilization using cryopreserved donor semen in cases where both partners are infertile. Fertil Steril. 1985;43(4):570-4.
91. Mahadevan MM, Trounson AO, Leeton JF. Successful use of human semen cryobanking for in vitro fertilization. Fertil Steril. 1983;40(3):340-3.
92. Englert Y, Delvigne A, Vekemans M, et al. Is fresh or frozen semen to be used in in vitro fertilization with donor sperm? Fertil Steril. 1989;51(4):661-4.
93. Yavetz H, Lessing JB, Niv Y, et al. The efficiency of cryopreserved semen versus fresh semen for in vitro fertilization/embryo transfer. J In Vitro Fert Embryo Transf. 1991;8(3):145-8.
94. Morroll DR, Matson PL, Troup SA, et al. The cryopreservation of donor semen by a simplified method: use in an IVF and GIFT programme. Int J Androl. 1990;13(5):352-60.
95. Kuczynski W, Dhont M, Grygoruk C, et al. The outcome of intracytoplasmic injection of fresh and cryopreserved ejaculated spermatozoa-- a prospective randomized study. Hum Reprod. 2001;16:2109-13.
96. Devroey P, Silber S, Nagy Z, et al. Ongoing pregnancies and birth after intracytoplasmic sperm injection with frozen-thawed epididymal spermatozoa. Hum Reprod. 1995;10(4):903-6.
97. van Steirteghem A, Nagy P, Joris H, et al. Results of intracytoplasmic sperm injection with ejaculated, fresh and frozen-thawed epididymal and testicular spermatozoa. Hum Reprod. 1998;13(Suppl 1):134-42.
98. Donoso P, Tournaye H, Devroey P. Which is the best sperm retrieval technique for non-obstructive azoospermia? A systematic review. Hum Reprod Update. 2007;13(6):539-49.
99. Van Peperstraten A, Proctor ML, Johnson NP, et al. Techniques for surgical retrieval of sperm prior to

ICSI for azoospermia. Cochrane Database Syst Rev. 2008;(2):CD002807.
100. Nicopoullos JD, Gilling-Smith C, Almeida PA, et al. Use of surgical sperm retrieval in azoospermic men: a meta-analysis. Fertil Steril. 2004;82(3):691-701.
101. Verheyen G, Vernaeve V, Van Landuyt L, et al. Should diagnostic testicular sperm retrieval followed by cryopreservation for later ICSI be the procedure of choice for all patients with non-obstructive azoospermia? Hum Reprod. 2004;19(12):2822-30.
102. Sereni E, Bonu MA, Fava L, et al. Freezing spermatozoa obtained by testicular fine needle aspiration: a new technique. Reprod Biomed Online. 2008;16(1):89-95.
103. Meseguer M, Molina N, Garcia-Velasco JA, et al. Sperm cryopreservation in oncological patients: a 14-year follow-up study. Fertil Steril. 2006;85(3):640-5.
104. Agarwal A, Ranganathan P, Kattal N, et al. Fertility after cancer: a prospective review of assisted reproductive outcome with banked semen specimens. Fertil Steril. 2004;81(2):342-8.
105. Bilodeau JF, Chatterjee S, Sirard MA, et al. Levels of antioxidant defenses are decreased in bovine spermatozoa after a cycle of freezing and thawing. Mol Reprod Dev. 2000;55(3):282-8.
106. Gadea J, Sellés E, Marco MA, et al. Decrease in glutathione content in boar sperm after cryopreservation. Effect of the addition of reduced glutathione to the freezing and thawing extenders. Theriogenology. 2004;62(3-4):690-701.
107. Chatterjee S, de Lamirande E, Gagnon C. Cryopreservation alters membrane sulfhydryl status of bull spermatozoa: protection by oxidized glutathione. Mol Reprod Dev. 2001;60(4):498-506.
108. Chatterjee S, Gagnon C. Production of reactive oxygen species by spermatozoa undergoing cooling, freezing, and thawing. Mol Reprod Dev. 2001;59(4):451-8.
109. Ball BA, Medina V, Gravance CG, et al. Effect of antioxidants on preservation of motility,viability and acrosomal integrity of equine spermatozoa during storage at 5 degrees C. Theriogenology. 2001;56(4):577-89.
110. Ball BA, Vo AT, Baumber J. Generation of reactive oxygen species by equine spermatozoa. Am J Vet Res. 2001;62(4):508-15.
111. Wang Y, Sharma RK, Agarwal A. Effect of cryopreservation and sperm concentration on lipid peroxidation in human semen. Urology. 1997;50(3):409-13.
112. Li MW, Meyers S, Tollner TL, et al. Damage to chromosomes and DNA of rhesus monkey sperm following cryopreservation. J Androl. 2007;28(4):493-501.
113. Gadea J, Molla M, Selles E, et al. Reduced glutathione content in human sperm is decreased after cryopreservation: Effect of the addition of reduced glutathione to the freezing and thawing extenders. Cryobiology. 2011;62(1):40-6.
114. Aitken RJ, Curry BJ. Redox regulation of human sperm function: from the physiological control of sperm capacitation to the etiology of infertility and DNA damage in the germ line. Antioxid Redox Signal. 1 2011;14(3):367-81.
115. Aitken RJ, De Iuliis GN, Finnie JM, et al. Analysis of the relationships between oxidative stress, DNA damage and sperm vitality in a patient population: development of diagnostic criteria. Hum Reprod. 2010;25(10):2415-26.
116. Alvarez JG, Storey BT. Role of Superoxide-Dismutase in Protecting Rabbit Spermatozoa from O-2 Toxicity Due to Lipid-Peroxidation. Biol Reprod. 1983;28(5):1129-36.
117. Barbas JP, Mascarenhas RD. Cryopreservation of domestic animal sperm cells. Cell Tissue Bank. 2009;10(1):49-62.
118. Tatone C, Di Emidio G, Vento M, et al. Cryopreservation and oxidative stress in reproductive cells. Gynecol Endocrinol. 2010;26(8):563-7.
119. Bailey JL, Bilodeau JF, Cormier N. Semen cryopreservation in domestic animals: a damaging and capacitating phenomenon. J Androl. 2000;21(1):1-7.
120. Baumber J, Ball BA, Linfor JJ, et al. Reactive oxygen species and cryopreservation promote DNA fragmentation in equine spermatozoa. J Androl. 2003;24(4):621-8.
121. Linfor JJ, Meyers SA. Detection of DNA damage in response to cooling injury in equine spermatozoa using single-cell gel electrophoresis. J Androl. 2002;23(1):107-13.
122. Kalthur G, Raj S, Thiyagarajan A, et al. Vitamin E supplementation in semen-freezing medium improves the motility and protects sperm from freeze-thaw- induced DNA damage. Fertil Steril. 2011;95(3):1149-51.
123. Kim HH, Schlegel PN. Endocrine Manipulation in Male Infertility. Urol Clin North Am. 2008;35:303-18.
124. Sperm cryobanking. In: Brojandal L, Mortimer D, Barrat CLR, et al (Eds). London: Cambridge University Press. 2010. pp. 189-217.

30

Ovarian Hyperstimulation Syndrome During Infertility Treatments

Jason Parker, NC Fayetteville

CHAPTER CONTENTS

INTRODUCTION

A degree of ovarian hyperstimulation is desired with all ovulation induction protocols using assisted reproductive technologies. This controlled ovarian hyperstimulation leads to an anticipated outcome forming an adequate number of mature oocytes for a pregnancy with usually minimal to mild complications. Ovarian hyperstimulation syndrome (OHSS) is usually an iatrogenic complication that results from enlarged ovaries in response to gonadotropins with a subsequent loss of fluid from the intravascular space. These physiologic changes may additionally be associated with multiple potential life-threatening disease sequelae resulting from ovulation induction.

The actual incidence of OHSS reported in the literature varies depending on data collection methods, population studied and the definitions, grading and classifications being used. Mild side effects of OHSS may include subjectively feeling uncomfortable, abdominal discomfort and pain associated with fluid shifts and ovarian enlargement. Nausea and vomiting along with hormonal changes that may include bloating, pelvic fullness, weight gain, headache, diarrhea, constipation and breast tenderness. Moderate OHSS will involve the same symptoms of mild OHSS along with ascities and other complications of enhanced vascular permeability[1,2] that may lead to dyspnea and pleural effusions. Severe forms of OHSS include the above in addition to alterations in blood volume, leading to hemoconcentration, coagulation abnormalities, electrolyte disturbances and reduced renal and hepatic function. Generally, mild and moderate OHSS is estimated to be around 6–12%, with the presentation of severe OHSS, is calculated to be about 0.1–3%.[3-7] Although, severe OHSS is relatively rare and self-limiting, severe OHSS may result in a potential life-threatening situation.[8]

Ovarian hyperstimulation syndrome is usually only associated with gonadotropin during ovulation induction, but can be seen with the use of clomiphene citrate,[9] and even in cases of spontaneous ovulation. Spontaneous forms of OHSS generally are reported to develop between 6 weeks and 12 weeks after ovulation and iatrogenic OHSS usually starts 1–3 weeks after ovulation. Other rare forms of OHSS presentation have been reported during multiple pregnancies[10] and in cases with hydatidiform moles,[11] secondary to elevated human chorionic gonadotropin (hCG) levels. Cases of OHSS have been associated with hypothyroidism and high levels of thyroid-stimulating hormone, being similar to hCG, perhaps.[12] Follicle stimulating hormone mutations also have been shown to cause OHSS.[13,14] Another rare disorder that can present with multicystic ovaries during pregnancy is hyper reactio luteinalis. This disorder can occur at any time during pregnancy and is usually also associated with elevated androgens.[15]

This chapter will review the pathophysiology of OHSS and the risk factors associated with OHSS. Those who are at risks of developing OHSS and the adverse complications that may occur from this iatrogenic condition will be discussed. Additionally, methods of avoiding OHSS and the treatment and management options that are available will be reviewed. Understanding the iatrogenic condition that lead to severe OHSS may allow healthcare providers, who provide fertility treatment for women with earlier recognition of the signs and symptoms of the disease process and earlier intervention to employ methods to avoid it.

PATHOPHYSIOLOGY

The increase in the size of the ovaries, which may mechanically facilitate capillary permeability, along with increased peripheral arteriolar dilatation[16] and other interactions between both endocrine and cytokines[17] have been proposed as causes of the hemodynamic alterations seen in OHSS. Reduction of colloid osmotic pressure resulting in vascular leaking and third spacing due to a combination of factors has been documented in leading to OHSS. These hemodynamic changes that occur appear to set into effect a cascade of subsequent disease processes. The leutinization of the multifollicular development during ovulation induction with gonadotropins in combination with triggering with hCG is the reason for the myriad of complications existing from vascular permeability as seen with OHSS.[7] The development of severe OHSS is a result of an alteration of an otherwise finely balanced physiological process.

Vascular endothelial growth factor (VEGF) is a peptide that is released from newly matured follicles as a result of ovulation induction. Angiogenesis, specifically in the ovaries and secondary to multifollicular recruitment, is a result of the characteristics of VEGF.[18-20] While VEGF promotes the growth of new capillaries, it also binds with the VEGF receptor 2 and induces the hyperpermeability of the capillaries.[21,22] Cellular actin fibers are also modified by VEGF resulting in compromising the tight cell junctions of the vessels leading to an additional increase of vessel permeability.[23]

Regard less of the relationship of the direct effects of VEGF leading to OHSS it appears that hCG plays a critical role in finalizing the last steps of OHSS in a susceptible woman.[24,25] The development of OHSS following ovarian stimulation with gonadotropins is mainly associated with the administration of hCG, as the syndrome rarely develops if it is withheld.[26-28] Pregnancy will increase the severity of OHSS.

Angiogenic cytokines growth factors (interleukins IL-2, IL-6, IL-8, IL-10, IL-18), basic fibroblast growth factor and tumor necrotic factor-α are produced by multiple corpora luteae[29,30] and are known to be implicated in the development of OHSS. These factors are associated with late follicular maturation and ovulation with subsequent corpus luteum formation and implantation.[31] Histamine, prolactin, prostaglandins and renin-angiotensin are also proposed in developing OHSS.[32]

Elevated estradiol levels have been implicated as a cause of developing OHSS,[33,34] although OHSS can develop in cases of low estradiol levels[35,36] demonstrating perhaps not a direct effect. Estradiol has been shown not to have direct vasoactive effects.[37] Women with low levels of estradiol can develop OHSS[38] implicating other factors. Elevated levels of estradiol will not lead to OHSS if hCG is not administered,[39,40] although high estradiol levels on the day of hCG injection are detrimental to uterine receptivity without affecting embryo quality[41] giving prudence to freezing embryos for a subsequent frozen embryo transfer, to avoid worsening symptoms of severe OHSS. Other factors resulting from high levels of estradiol may lead to OHSS. Cystic fibrosis transmembrane conductance regulator (CFTR) is upregulated by estradiol and may be the result of OHSS related to elevated estradiol levels. The function of CTFR has been shown to cause fluid shifts intrabdominally.[42] Elevated estradiol levels during ovulation induction are likely an expected finding with potential predictive value in determining that who will develop severe OHSS and potentially having a direct and/or indirect effect on causing OHSS, but more likely a result of OHSS.[43,44]

CLASSIFICATION

Ovarian hyperstimulation syndrome staging is based upon clinical symptoms and laboratory values to categorize the severity of disease. Classifications date back to as early as 1967,[7] and have gone through multiple modifications[8] that has led to categorizing and grading of OHSS. Ovarian hyperstimulation syndrome had been categorized as mild, moderate and severe and originally included six grades of severity. Later OHSS[9] classification was modified to include five grades.

Classifications and grading criteria are helpful in providing the ability to compare and document the incidence of OHSS. Classification and grading more importantly offer the clinician objective data points to determine the severity and prompt earlier treatment and may allow for standardized treatment plans to be initiated and to document recovery.

Ovarian hyperstimulation syndrome is classified by the degree of clinical and laboratory findings, as well as the severity of the symptoms. Mild OHSS is characterized by bilateral ovarian enlargement up to less than 6 cm and estradiol concentrations between 2000–4000 pg/ml along with abdominal discomfort and associated nausea and vomiting. Moderate OHSS will have worsening symptoms and have ovaries measuring 6–12 cm in size, worsening of ascites and estradiol levels of 4,000–6,000 pg/ml. Rapid weight gain also is an indicator and early sign of moderate OHSS. Severe OHSS is continued worsening of symptoms. The presence of large ovarian cysts and ovaries in excess of 12 cm, ascites and estradiol levels more than 6000 pg/ml. Other symptoms of severe OHSS may include electrolyte imbalance (hyponatremia, hyperkalemia), hypovolemia. This progresses to critical OHSS and includes hypovolemic shock, hemoconcentration, pleural and/or pericardial effusion.[2,29]

The progression of OHSS from mild through severe correlates with the underlying pathology of the disease and the different organs affected. Patients with abdominal and pelvic discomfort arise from abdominal distention and ascites increases as ovaries enlarge. Progression leads to nausea and vomiting and other gastrointestinal symptoms including paralytic ileus. Progressive ascites-lead to respiratory difficulty and pleural effusions. Continued ascites leads to decreased venous perfusion, decreased blood pressure and tachycardia. Decreased organ perfusion leads to hepatic and renal disorders that include hemoconcentration and alteration of proteins leading to coagulopathies and associated thrombotic disorders.

Recently, additional classification scheme have been introduced. Humaidan et al.[28] classification proposal allows for ease of categorizing based upon objective and subjective criteria with anticipated outcomes and guidance offered for the different classification schemes and recommendations for hospitalization and consultation. Individual clinical decisions are still required but the initial guidance is offered.

OHSS can develop at distinct times following ovulation. Two distinct types of OHSS are documented to develop, which additionally lead to further classification. Early OHSS occurs within a week of ovulation and late OHSS develops 2–3 weeks later.[45] Early OHSS occurs asa result of the exogenous hCG administration before oocyte retrieval and is usually related to an excessive ovarian response to gonadotropin stimulation.[46,47] Late OHSS is induced from endogenous hCG from the initiated pregnancy and in those with multiple gestations and may be more difficult to manage[45] identification of these distinctions of development of OHSS allows for recognition of the signs and symptoms and hopefully earlier intervention.

RISK FACTORS

Prior to initiating ovulation induction protocols, identifying features of patients that may be at a higher risk of developing OHSS allows for customized treatment regimens. The age of the patient is relevant and younger patients are at an increased risk of developing OHSS.[1,48] This factor of age may potentially be a result of the increased ovarian reserve and the increase in antral follicles that is generally exhibited by younger patients. Body mass index (BMI) has been evaluated with mixed results. One group demonstrated that lean patients were at greater risk of developing OHSS.[48] Others have found no correlation between BMI and OHSS.[49]

The etiology of infertility also plays a significant role in influencing OHSS. Women with the signs of polycystic ovary syndrome (PCOS), along with the presence of multiple (> 35) small and intermediate follicles, and excessively high levels of serum estradiol (> 4000 pg/ml) secondary to the multiple follicles on the day of hCG administration are at risk.[47] Women with PCOS also have an elevated serum anti-Müllerian hormone level[50] and OHSS also appeared to be associated significantly with ultrasonographic features of PCOS with the presence of multiple small follicles in the ovaries. Women with a prior history of developing OHSS are also at an increased risk of OHSS[51] and using ovulation induction protocols utilizing high doses of gonadotropins are implicated as leading to an increased development of OHSS.

PRESENTATION OF SYMPTOMS

Regardless of the classification system used, the signs and symptoms of OHSS and subsequent progression represent a spectrum of a disease process. Understanding the different symptoms, their etiology and consequences can allow for earlier intervention and treatment. Usually the enlarged ovaries will lead to the subjective feelings of abdominal fullness, pain, bloating, nausea and vomiting (Figures 1A and B). Constipation is often

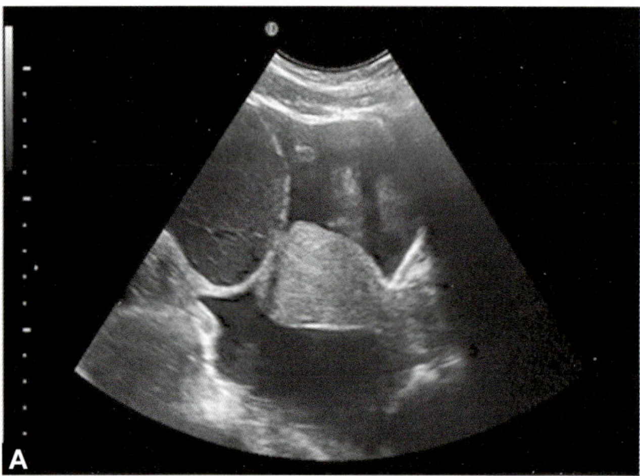

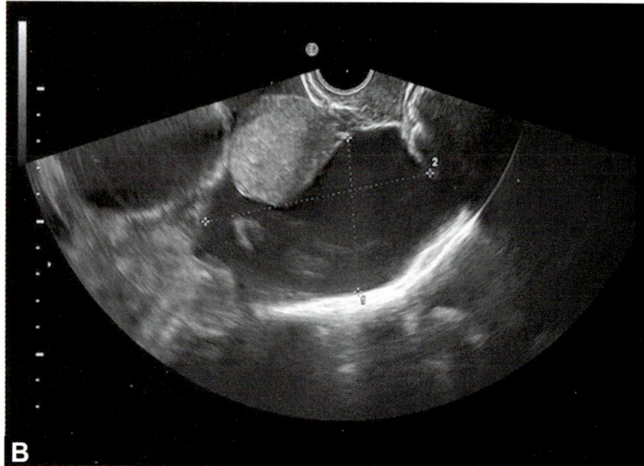

Figures 1A and B Ascites present in the pelvis and abdomen with uterus adjacent to enlarged ovary

common and may exacerbate the feelings of abdominal fullness and pressure. These symptoms will progressively worsen as the disease process continues and hCG levels increase. The hyperpermiability of ovarian vessels and dilation of the arteries leads to worsening ascites in OHSS[52] (Figures 2 and 3). The symptoms associated with the hypovolemia begin and may be manifested by tachycardia and hypotension. The continued hypovolemia leads to a hemoconcentration, electrolyte imbalance and decreased central venous pressure.

Decreased renal perfusion can occur as hypotension continues and ascites accumulate and leads to hemoconcentration. Oliguria and decreased glomerular filtration rate results from the hypotension. This also results in an increase of resorption of sodium and water leading to hyperkalemia and hyponatremia. Dyspnea occurs with increased ascites and abdominal pain secondary to an expanding girth and enlarging of the ovaries. The depth of inspiration may be limited and involuntary, secondary to avoiding pain which can lead to further atelectasis and pulmonary infiltrates. Dyspnea may also represent other symptoms of pulmonary effusion, pericardial effusion and/or a pulmonary embolism.

Pleural effusions represent significant complication related to OHSS. Pericardial effusions can develop with or without ascites being present. Acute respiratory distress syndrome is another complication that may result from severe OHSS. These respiratory findings may occur as a result of increased ascites and/or aggressive fluid hydration and the increased prostaglandins and cytokines associated with OHSS.

The enlarging ovaries, increased permeability of vessels and changed vascular pressure, all contribute to third spacing of fluid. Continued hypovolemia and loss of protein-rich exudates into the peritoneal cavity lead to hemoconcentration. The increase in hematocrit and leukocytosis is also considered to be associated with an inflammatory response. The hypovolemia and arterial dilation can lead to increased venous stasis. Hepatic perfusion is compromised[54] with hypotension resulting in decreased protein synthesis problems with hypercoagulability and precipitating thromboembolic events.

Ovarian torsion can also occur and a delay in diagnosis may be a result of having signs and symptoms similar to OHSS. The enlarged ovaries are hypervascularized and usually avoided by unnecessary manipulation, hence avoiding bimanual exams. Symptoms of ovarian torsion include a low grade temperature, elevated white blood cell count, abdominal pain and anemia.[53] Proper surveillance and monitoring and clinical suspicion need to be employed to avoid complication of a torsed ovary. Ovarian torsion usually occurs between the 6th week and 13th week of pregnancy[53] and if pain begins to increase when symptoms of OHSS should be decreasing, this may serve as an indication to intervene. Early intervention by untwisting the ovary should be the first line attempt prior to oophorectomy.[55]

PREVENTION

Early recognition of the signs and symptoms of OHSS allows for modifications in the ovulation regimen to prevent severe OHSS and gives the ability to offer recommendations and possible alternatives to cancelling a cycle. Providing these other alternatives builds upon the continued development of the patient-physician relationship.

Cycle cancellation by withholding hCG and subsequent treatment of symptoms allows for minimal physical side effects but is often met with emotional frustration and distress of the patient. Ovulation can still occur

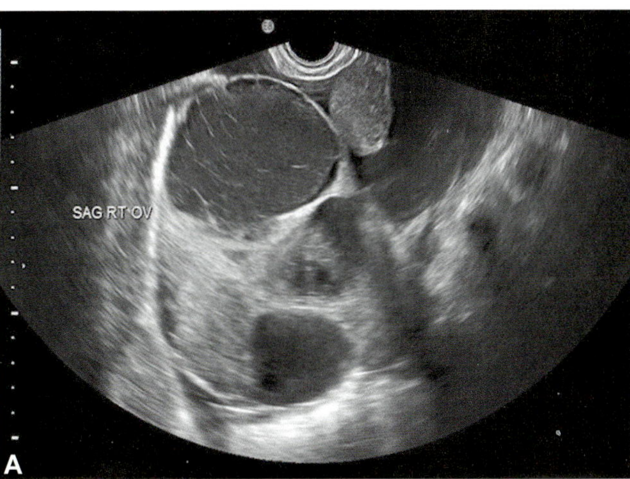

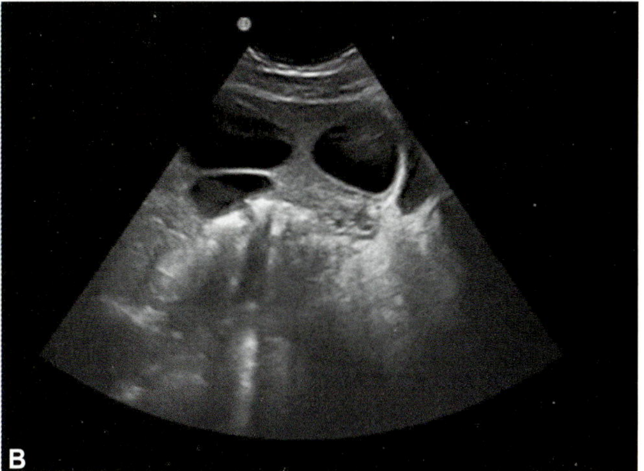

Figures 2A and B Ovarian enlargement during severe ovarian hyperstimulation syndrome with uterus adjacent to right ovary in the picture 'A'

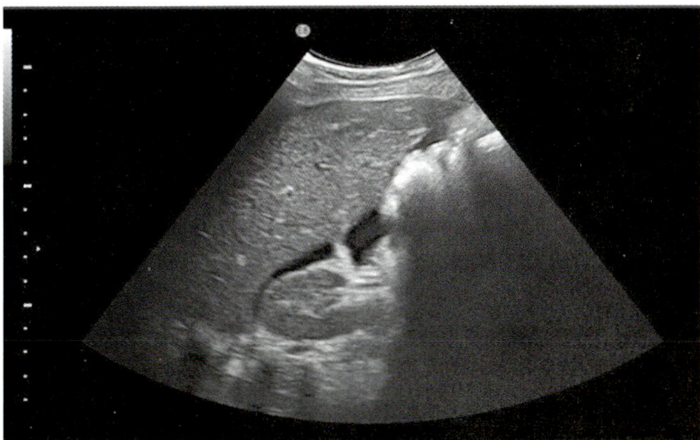

Figure 3 Ascites around liver

after withholding exogenous hCG and patients need to be counseled to refrain from unprotected intercourse to avoid multiple gestation. If concern for severe OHSS exists then refraining from intercourse should be recommended to avoid ovarian torsion or ovarian rupture. Taking a patient through retrieval and then freezing embryos allows for taking advantage of the oocytes being produced so that they may not be placed at the same risks in the future and then performing a frozen embryo transfer under better controlled situations may allow for similar pregnancy rates. Although, a Cochrane review has shown that there is insufficient evidence to support the use of cryopreservation to prevent OHSS.[56]

Short of cancelling the ovulation induction cycle is the option of coasting. Coasting delays the administration of hCG and allows for estradiol levels to fall into a range suitable for triggering ovulation. Coasting for 2–6 days resulted in a lower rate of OHSS while maintaining pregnancy rates.[57-61] Coasting is still controversial and some feel there is a limited benefit in effectively preventing OHSS[62] Coasting can be achieved through withholding gonadotropins or through administering gonadotropin-releasing hormone (GnRH) antagonist to decrease estradiol levels and allow for continued follicular growth[63] and maintaining the present growth of follicles.

Since exogenous hCG is the factor that begins the cascade of OHSS symptoms, using a decreased dose of hCG for ovulation induction, has been shown to be effective in decreasing OHSS risks.[64] GnRH agonists can also be used for ovulation induction with results as seen with hCG.[65] Using recombinant human luteinizing hormone can be used as the ovulatory trigger and has been demonstrated to not cause OHSS.[66]

Complete aspiration of follicles at the time of retrieval will decrease progesterone production but by itself does not prevent OHSS.[67] Unilateral ovarian aspiration at 12 hours post trigger and then at 36 hours of the other ovary did not decrease or prevent OHSS.[68]

Intravenous administration of 25% albumin given to women with elevated estradiol or a prior history of OHSS,[69,70] has been reviewed as a measure to decrease severe OHSS.[71] Treatment regimens when reviewe demonstrated that the majority of the time 20–50 g of albumin given at oocyte retrieval or immediately after demonstrates a decrease in developing OHSS.[72] These results demonstrate that 18 women would need to be treated to prevent one case of severe OHSS. The use of albumin is not without its own risks and side effects. Worsening of ascites, allergic reactions and viral transmission is among these side effects.[73,74]

The use of corticosteroid administration during ovarian stimulation in women at risks of developing

OHSS has been used but met with mixed results. One study demonstrated a decrease in developing OHSS from 44–10% in those treated with methylprednisolone from day 6 of stimulation cycle through 13 days post transfer.[75] The other study used glucocorticoids and found OHSS at 42% in both treated and untreated groups.[76] Another option is the use of dopamine agonist.

Dopamine agonist inactivates VEGFR-2 and prevents vascular permeability.[77] In a study of oocyte donors at high risk for OHSS [78] they were given daily cabergoline (0.5 mg) or placebo. Magnetic resonance imaging revealed that those receiving cabergoline had a decreased vascular permeability and reduced the rate of moderate OHSS. This may be helpful in donor cycles but further studies would need to be performed to determine pregnancy rates in fresh cycles in light of potential implantation effects with the decrease in vascular permeability that may occur at the level of the endometrium.

Using low dose aspirin initiated on the first day of ovarian stimulation was demonstrated in a randomized control trial to yield fewer cycles with OHSS.[79]

TREATMENT

Prevention of OHSS is the best treatment, but if that has failed then treatment should be centered on symptomatic relief and correction of medical complications. Close monitoring of the patient is required as progression of the disease from mild to severe OHSS can occur rapidly and early-onset OHSS can be treated only to have late-onset OHSS develop with an ongoing pregnancy. Generally, OHSS in its mild form can be treated on an outpatient basis. Proper education of the patient to enable them to determine early signs of OHSS is valuable.

Patients with mild forms of OHSS can be treated with symptomatic relief that may include pain medicine, counseling to avoid excessive exercise, antiemetics and proper fluid replacement will usually suffice. Home monitoring of weight and urinary output with close daily phone calls are also recommended. Beginning early on, the authors also recommend increasing fluid intake of electrolyte solutions and depending on their normal diet, increasing protein intake.

Treatment of moderate OHSS consists of continued close observation that should include a physical exam and ultrasound 2–3 times per week. At each visit a discussion should include informing the patient to continue the same monitoring of symptoms as with mild OHSS. Moderate OHSS will usually manifest itself with an increase in existing symptoms or the appearance of new symptoms. Serial monitoring of hematocrit, renal function, estradiol levels and hepatic function allow for recognition of hemoconcentration and electrolyte disturbances and these can be obtained at the time of examination. Discussion of decreasing activity to avoid risk of ovarian torsion or rupture, limiting or avoiding intercourse and reviewing an adequate fluid intake of electrolyte solutions continues to be recommended.

Severe OHSS usually will require prompt hospitalization secondary to the numerous systems involved and close active management of the sequelae of complications. Treatment of severe hyperstimulation will be directed at maintaining blood volume, resolving fluid and electrolyte balance and preventing thromboembolic events. Utilizing Table 2 as a guide for when to hospitalize patients is helpful, but other considerations may warrant hospitalization, as well as a combination of seemingly less impressive symptoms.

Upon hospitalization, determination of consulting other subspecialist can be made. Daily labs to monitor electrolytes, hemoconcentration, renal, hepatic function and estradiol levels, as well as serial vital signs, daily weights, fluid input and output monitoring and pulse oximeter should be performed. Radiographic test on admission would include an ultrasound to determine the size of the ovaries and amount of ascites present and a chest X-ray. An electrocardiogram is also indicated. An explanation of the diagnosis of severe OHSS to the patient and nursing staff also should be made upon hospital admission to avoiding any iatrogenic complications that may arise with inappropriate treatment. Discussion with the patient to make sure not to receive any bimanual examinations or aggressive abdominal exams to avoid damaging or rupturing ovaries by physicians or nursing staff that may be cross covering.

Once admitted to the hospital judicial fluid management should begin. The proper fluid administration is critical to improve the symptoms of hypotension and hypovolemia and to begin correcting electrolyte disturbances, although worsening of ascites may ensue from. Begin with strict monitoring of fluid intake and output. Administer normal saline with 5% dextrose to reverse hyponatremia. Hyperkalenia can be resolved with treatments involving insulin and glucose to move potassium into intracellular spaces. Emergently, use of calcium gluconate or kayexalate is warranted. Plasma expanders, albumin (200 ml of 25% albumin over 4 hours) and plasma (500–1000 ml over 24 hours), supplemented with appropriate electrolytes should be administered early and repeated as needed. Hematocrit should be monitored every 4–6 hours and repeated until the hematocrit is less than 38%. Once symptoms of OHSS are resolving then increasing oral intake of electrolyte solutions can resume. Diuretic agents are reserved for use after hypovolemia has resolved and if initiated too early will increase the risks of hemoconcentration.

Physical exam and ultrasound findings may reveal extensive ascites. This can be monitored by a serial increase in weight gain. Ascites will lead to an increased intra-abdominal pressure and subsequent pain. The intra-abdominal pressure may, as mentioned above, also have hemodynamic effects on maternal circulation and lead to a decreased pulmonary function. Improvement of renal function and correction of hemoconcentration, as well as weight loss in women with severe OHSS, treated with an abdominal paracentesis has been described.[80,81] Ultrasound guided vaginal paracentesis, similar to oocyte retrieval is the authors'method of choice. This allows for close observation of adjacent vascular structures and the ovaries and can remove the fluid in a slow and controlled manner to reduce the risks of ovarian torsion. Paracentesis resulted in a marked improvement of renal function, blood osmolarity and hemoconcentration, as well as relief of dyspnea and abdominal discomfort.[81] The symptomatic relief that comes from performing a paracentesis should be discussed with the patient as clinically indicated. Fluid will usually reaccumulate but at a much lower volume and requires a repeat paracentesis as indicated, and the patient may desire it for the symptomatic relief.[82] One study of 42 cases of severe OHSS treated by transvaginal sonographically guided aspiration of ascites and intravenous fluid infusion[83] was reviewed and this treatment relieved symptoms, reduced the hematocrit, improved renal clearance and urine output and shortened the duration of hospital stay.

A chest X-ray, electrocardiogram and pulse oximeter may reveal a hydrothorax pulmonary infection, thromboembolism or adult respiratory distress syndrome (ARDS) that may further complicate the clinical picture if not identified early. One study of patients with severe OHSS found 4% had lobar pneumonia, 2% had ARDS and 2% had pulmonary thromboembolism. Clinical manifestations included dyspnea, tachypnea, moderate hypoxemia, increased alveolar-arterial oxygen difference, hypocarbia, respiratory alkalosis, and metabolic compensation.[84] Pleural effusions should be drained to relieve dyspnea. Paracentesis may also be useful in alleviating breathing difficulties in patients with ascites and hydrothorax.[85] However, in cases of ascites, a paracentesis will usually resolve the hydrothorax and a thoracentis would be required for persistent pleural effusions.[85]

Thromboembolic events are the most serious, but the rarest complications of OHSS. Hemoconcentration, stasis, hypercoagulation and elevated estrogen concentrations are etiology of thromboembolic events. Thromboses in the arterial or venous circulations occur[86,87] and may lead to permanent neurologic injury or death.[88] Thromboembolic complications of OHSS have been reported in the internal jugular, subclavian, axillary and mesenteric vessels.[84,89] Incorporating anticoagulation with heparin or low molecular weight heparin in prophylactic dosing, in association with compression stockings should be used in the hospitalized patient.

CONCLUSION

Controlled ovarian hyperstimulation allows for couples to conceive in situations when different infertility etiologies may have otherwise kept them. Usually, the symptoms and side effects from ovulation induction are minimal and require only modest symptomatic relief. However, these mild symptoms can quickly progress into severe symptoms of OHSS with ramifications that necessitate prompt medical and/or surgical intervention to prevent death.

Despite an understanding of the etiology, risk factors and classification of OHSS, a patient may develop severe OHSS without warning. Monitoring the course of disease progression and being cognizant of the different presentations of OHSS may prevent serious surgical interventions. Looking for the symptoms of early and late onset OHSS is also critical.

Treatment of severe OHSS is aimed at providing symptomatic relief and correcting any other medical problems. Providing patients with the proper counseling and presenting treatment options provides information to patients that will benefit from the open and honest expectation of a cycle that result in severe OHSS. Early treatment and intervention is warranted and if caught early can usually be managed as an outpatient. The reversing of fluid imbalances that may lead to ascites complicated by respiratory and/or hypercoagulability-disturbances requires active management. Paracentesis and removing the ascites leads to quick resolution of symptoms and should be offered early in the treatment plan.

Patients with moderate or severe OHSS with symptoms resulting from ascites and hemodynamic changes should be managed with a transvaginal ultrasound guided paracentesis.

Anticoagulation therapy should be initiated to reduce the risk of thromboembolic events precipitated by OHSS.[36] Low molecular weight heparin at 40 mg twice a day at the time of diagnosing elevated hematocrit and/or leukocytosis should be initiated for 2–3 weeks and, as well if a paracentesis is performed. Most cases should be able to be successfully managed on an outpatient basis, which has been found to be the most cost-effective approach,[66] whereas patients who fail to tolerate oral fluids, are dehydrated or require supportive care, such as pain control, should be hospitalized.

REFERENCES

1. Golan A, Ron-El R, Herman A, et al. Ovarian hyperstimulation syndrome: an update review. Obstet Gynecol Surv. 1989;44:430-40.
2. Whelan JG III, Vlahos NF. The ovarian hyperstimulation syndrome. Fertil Steril. 2000;73:883-96.
3. Out HJ, Hannaerts BMJL, Driessen SGAJ, et al. A prospective, randomized, assessor-blind, multicentre study comparing recombinant and urinary follicle stimulating hormone (Puregon® versus Metrodin) in in-vitro fertilization). Hum Reprod. 1995;10:2534-40.
4. Enskog A, Henriksson M, Unander M, et al. Prospective study of the clinical and laboratory parameters of patients in whom ovarian hyperstimulation syndrome developed during controlled ovarian hyperstimulation for in vitro fertilization. Fertil Steril. 1999;71:808-14.
5. Devroey P, Boostanfar R, Koper NP, et al. A double-blind, non-inferiority RCT comparing corifollitropin alfa and recombinant FSH during the first 7 days of ovarian stimulation using a GnRH antagonist protocol. Hum Reprod. 2009;24(12):3063-72.
6. Delvigne A, Rozenberg S. Epidemiology and prevention of ovarian hyperstimulation syndrome (OHSS): a review. Hum Repro Update. 2002;8(6):559-77.
7. Vlahos NF, Gregoriou O. Prevention and management of ovarian hyperstimulation syndrome. Ann N Y Acad Sci. 2006;1092:247-64.
8. Mathur RS, Akande VA, Keay SD, et al. Distinction between early and late ovarian hyperstimulation syndrome. Fertil Steril. 2000;73:901-7.
9. Kristner RW. Further observations on the effects of clomiphene citrate in anovulatory females. Am J Obstet Gynecol. 1965;92:380-420.
10. Check JH, Choe JK, Nazari A. Hyperreactio luteinalis despite the absence of a corpus luteum and suppressed follicle stimulating concentrations in a triplet pregnancy. Hum Reprod. 2000;15:1043-5.
11. Ludwig M, Gembruch U, Bauer O, et al. Ovarian hyperstimulation syndrome (OHSS) in a spontaneous pregnancy with fetal and placental triploidy: information about the general pathophysiology of OHSS. Hum Reprod. 1998;13:2082-7.
12. Nappi RG, Di Nero E, D'Aries AP. Natural pregnancy in hypothyroid woman complicated by spontaneous ovarian hyperstimulation syndrome. Am j Obstet Gynecol 1998;178:610-11.
13. Vasseur C, Rodien P, Beau I, et al. A chorionic gonadotropin-sensitive mutation in the follicle-stimulating hormone receptor as a cause of familial gestational spontaneous ovarian hyperstimulation syndrome. N Engl J Med. 2003;349:753-9.
14. Smits G, Olatunbosun O, Delbaere A, et al. Ovarian hyperstimulation syndrome because of a mutation in the follicle-stimulating hormone receptor. N Engl J Med. 2003;349:760-6.
15. Foulk RK, Martin MC, Jenkins GL, et al. Hyperrectio lutenalis differentiated from severe ovarian hyperstimulation syndrome in a spontaneously conceived pregnancy. Am J Obstet Gynecol. 1997;176(6):1300-2.
16. Balasch J, Fabregues F, Arroyo V. Peripheral arterial vasodilation hypothesis: a new insight into the pathogenesis of ovarian hyperstimulation syndrome. Hum Reprod. 1998;13:2718-30.
17. Mathur R, Jenkins J. Ovarian hyperstimulation syndrome: an endocrinopathy? Curr Opin Obstet Gynecol. 2001;13:329-33.
18. Keck PJ, Hauser SD, Krivi G, et al. Vascular permeability factor, an endothelial cell mitogen related to PDGF. Science. 1989;246:1309-12.
19. Leung DW, Cachianes G, Kuang WJ, et al. Vascular endothelial growth factor is a secreted angiogenic mitogen. Science. 1989;246:1306-9.
20. Yamamoto S, Konishi I, Tsuruta Y, et al. Expression of vascular endothelial growth factor (VEGF) during folliculogenesis and corpus luteum formation in the human ovary. Gynecol Endocrinol. 1997;11:371-81.
21. Gille H, Kowalski J, Li B, et al. Analysis of biological effects and signaling properties of Flt-1 (VEGFR-1) and KDR (VEGFR-2). A reassessment using novel receptor-specific vascular endothelial growth factor mutants. J Biol Chem. 2001;276:3222-30.
22. Bates DO, Harper SJ. Regulation of vascular permeability by vascular endothelial growth factors. Vascul Pharmacol. 2002;39:225-37.
23. Gómez R, Simón C, Remohí J, et al. Administration of moderate and high doses of gonadotrophins to female rats increases ovarian vascular endothelial growth factor (VEGF) and VEGF receptor-2 expression that is associated to vascular hyperpermeability. Biol Reprod. 2003;68:2164-71.
24. McElhinney B, Ardill J, Caldwell C, et al. Ovarian hyperstimulation syndrome and assisted reproductive technologies: why some and not others? Hum Reprod. 2002;17:1548-53.
25. Al-Shawaf T, Grudzinskas JG. Prevention and treatment of ovarian hyperstimulation syndrome. Best Pract Res Clin Obst Gynecol Reprod. 2003;17:249-61.
26. Vardhana PA, Julius MA, Pollak SV, et al. A unique hCG-antagonist suppresses ovarian hyperstimulation syndrome (OHSS) in rats. Endocrinology. 2009;150:3807-14.
27. Nargund G, Hutchison L, Scaramuzzi R, et al. Low-dose HCG is useful in preventing OHSS in high-risk women without adversely affecting the outcome of IVF cycles. Reprod Biomed Online. 2007;14:682-5.
28. Humaidan P, Quartorolo J, Papanilolaou EG. Preventing hyperstimulation syndrome: Guide for clinician. Fertil Steril 2010,94:369-400.
29. Elchalal U, Schenker JG. The pathophysiology of ovarian hyperstimulation syndrome-views and ideas. Hum Reprod. 1997;12:1129-37.

30. Varnagy A, Bodis J, Manfai Z, et al. Low-dose aspirin therapy to prevent ovarian hyperstimulation syndrome. Fertil Steril. 2009;93(7):2281-4.
31. Rizk B. Ovarian Hyperstimulation Syndrome—Epidemiology, Pathophysiology, Prevention and Management, 1st edition. New York: Cambridge University Press; 2006. pp. 10-33.
32. Rizk B, Aboulghar M, Smitz J, et al. The role of vascular endothelial growth factor and interleukins in the pathogenesis of severe ovarian hyperstimulation syndrome. Hum Reprod Update. 1997;3:255-66.
33. Haning RV, Austin CW, Carlson IH, et al. Plasma estradiol is superior to ultrasound and urinary estriol glucorinide as a predictor of ovarian hyperstimulation during induction of ovulation with menotropins. Fertil Steril. 1983;40:31-6.
34. Asch RH, Balmaceda JP, Weckstein LN, et al. Severe ovarian hyperstimulation syndrome in assisted reproductive technology: definition of high risk groups. Hum Reprod. 1991;6:1395-9.
35. Villasante A, Pacheco A, Ruiz A, et al. Vascular endothelial cadherin regulates vascular permeability: Implications for ovarian hyperstimulation syndrome. J Clin Endocrinol Metab. 2007;92:314-21.
36. Pellicer A, Miró F, Sampaio M, et al. In vitro fertilization as a diagnostic and therapeutic tool in a patient with partial 17,20-desmolase deficiency. Fertil Steril. 1991;55:970-5.
37. Aboulghar MA, Mansour RT. Ovarian hyperstimulation syndrome: classifications and critical analysis of preventive measures. Hum Reprod Update. 2003;9:275-89.
38. Levy T, Orvieto R, Homburg R, et al. Severe ovarian hyperstimulation syndrome despite low plasma oestrogen concentrations in a hypogonadotrophic, hypogonadal patient. Hum Reprod. 1996;11:1177-9.
39. Meirow D, Schenker JG, Rosler A. Ovarian hyperstimulation syndrome with low oestradiol in non-classical 17 alpha-hydroxylase, 17,20-lyase deficiency: what is the role of oestrogens? Hum Reprod. 1996;11:2119-21.
40. Schenker JG. Prevention and treatment of ovarian hyperstimulation. Hum Reprod. 1993;8:653-9.
41. Simon C, Cano F, Valbuena D, et al. Clinical evidence for adetrimental effect on uterine receptivity of high serum oestradiol concentrations in high and normal responder patients. Hum Reprod.10, 2432-7.
42. Ajonuma LC, Tsang LL, Zhang GH, et al. Estrogen-induced abnormally high cystic fibrosis transmembrane conductance regulator expression results in ovarian hyperstimulation syndrome. Mol Endocrinol. 2005;19:3038-4
43. Aboulghar MA. Prediction of ovarian hyperstimulation syndrome. Estradiol level has an important role in the prediction of OHSS. Hum Reprod. 2003;18:1140-1.
44. Orvieto R. Prediction of ovarian hyperstimulation syndrome. Challenging the estradiol myths. Hum Reprod.2003;18:665-7.
45. Lyons D, Wheeler CA, Frishman GN, et al. Early and late presentation of the ovarian hyperstimulation syndrome: two distinct entities with different risk factors. Hum Reprod.1994;9:792-9.
46. Mathur R, Evbuomwan I, Jenkins J. Prevention and management of ovarian hyperstimulation syndrome. Curr Obstet Gynecol. 12:111-6.
47. Navot D, Bergh PA, Laufer N. Ovarian hyperstimulation syndrome in novel reproductive technologies: prevention and treatment. Fertil Steril. 1992;58:249-61.
48. Navot D, Relou A, Birkenfeld A, et al. Risk factors and prognostic variables in the ovarian hyperstimulation syndrome. Am J Obstet Gynecol. 1988;159(1):210-5.
49. Delvigne A, Dubois M, Battheu B, et al. The ovarian hyperstimulation syndrome in in-vitro fertilization: a Belgian multicentric study II. Multiple discriminate analysis for risk prediction. Hum Reprod. 1993;8:1361-71.
50. Cook CL, Siow Y, Brenner AG, et al. Relationship between serum mullerian-inhibiting substance and other reproductive hormones in untreated women with polycystic ovary syndrome and normal women. Fertil Steril. 2002;77:141-6.
51. Delvigne A, Dubois M, Battheu B, et al. The ovarian hyperstimulation syndrome in in-vitro fertilization: a Belgian multicentric study II. Multiple discriminate analysis for risk prediction. Hum Reprod.1993;8:1361-71.
52. Manau D, Balasch J, Arroyo V, et al. Circulatory dysfunction in asymptomatic in vitro fertilization patients. Relationship with hyperestrogenemia and activity of endogenous vasodilators. J Clin Endocrinol Metab. 1998;83:1489-93.
53. Mashiach S, Bider D, Moran O, et al. Adnexal torsion of hyperstimulated ovaries in pregnancies after gonadotropin therapy. Fertil Steril. 1990;53(1):76-80.
54. Fábregues F, Balasch J, Ginès P, et al. Ascites and liver test abnormalities during severe ovarian hyperstimulation syndrome. Am J Gastroenterol. 1999;94:994-9.
55. Chapron C, Capella-Allouc S, Dubuisson JB. Treatment of adnexal torsion using operative laparoscopy. Hum Reprod. 1996;11(5):998-1003.
56. D'Angelo A, Amso N. Embryo freezing for preventing ovarian hyperstimulation syndrome. Cochrane Database syst Rev. 2002;2:CD002806.
57. Grochowski D, Wołczyński S, Kuczyński W, et al. Correctly timed coasting reduces the risk of ovarian hyperstimulation syndrome and gives good cycle outcome in an in vitro fertilization program. Gynecol Endocrinol. 2001;15(3):234-8.
58. Waldenström U, Kahn J, Marsk L, et al. High pregnancy rates and successful prevention of severe ovarian hyperstimulation syndrome by 'prolonged coasting' of very hyperstimulated patients: a multicentre study. Hum Reprod. 1999;14(2):294-7.
59. Levinsohn-Tavor O, Friedler S, Schachter M, et al. Coasting-what is the best formula? Hum Reprod. 2003;18(5):937-40.
60. Mansour R, Aboulghar M, Serour G, et al. Criteria of a successful coasting protocol for the prevention of severe ovarian hyperstimulation syndrome. Hum Reprod. 2005;20(11):3167-72.
61. García-Velasco JA, Isaza V, Quea G, et al. Coasting for the prevention of ovarian hyperstimulation syndrome: much ado about nothing? Fertil Steril. 2006;85(3):547-54.

62. D'Angelo A, Amso N. 'Coasting' (with holding gonadotrophins) for preventing ovarian hyperstimulation syndrome. Cochrane Database Syst Rev. 2002;(3):CD002811.
63. Gustofson RL, Segars JH, Larsen FH. Ganirelix acetate causes a rapid reduction in estradiol levels without adversely affecting oocyte maturation in women pretreated with leuprolide acetate who are at risk of ovarian hyperstimulation syndrome. Hum Reprod. 2006;21(11):2830-7.
64. Whelan JG 3rd, Vlahos NF. The ovarian hyperstimulation syndrome. Fertil Steril. 2000;73:883-96.
65. Andersen CY, Humaidan P, Ejdrup HB, et al. Hormonal characteristics of follicular fluid from women receiving either GnRH agonist or hCG for ovulation induction. Hum Reprod. 2006;21(8):2126-30.
66. European Recombinant LH Study Group Human recombinant luteinizing hormone is as effective as, but safer than, urinary human chorionic gonadotropin in inducing final follicular maturation and ovulation in in-vitro fertilization procedures: results of a multicenter double-blind study. J Clin Endocrinol Metab. 2001;86(6):2607.
67. Friedman CI, Schmidt GE, Chang FE, et al. Severe ovarian hyperstimulation following follicular aspiration. Am J Obstet Gynecol. 1984;150:436-7.
68. Egbase P, Al-Awadi S, Al-Sharhan M, et al. Unilateral ovarian diathermy prior to successful in vitro fertilisation: a strategy to prevent recurrence of ovarian hyperstimulation syndrome? J Obstet Gynaecol. 1998;18(2):171-3.
69. Isik AZ, Gokmen O, Zeyneloglu HB, et al. Intravenous albumin prevents moderate-severe ovarian hyperstimulation in in-vitro fertilization patients: a prospective, randomized and controlled study. Eur J Obstet Gynecol Reprod Biol. 1996;70(2):179-83.
70. Shoham Z, Weissman A, Barash A, et al. Intravenous albumin for the prevention of severe ovarian hyperstimulation syndrome in an in vitro fertilization program: a prospective, randomized, placebo-controlled study. Fertil Steril. 1994;62(1):137-42.
71. Aboulghar M, Evers JH, Al-Inany H. Intravenous albumin for preventing severe ovarian hyperstimulation syndrome: a Cochrane review. Hum Reprod. 2002;17(12):3027-32.
72. Ben-Chetrit A, Eldar-Geva T, Gal M, et al. The questionable use of albumin for the prevention of ovarian hyperstimulation syndrome in an IVF programme: a randomized placebo-controlled trial.Hum Reprod. 2001;16(9):1880-4.
73. Ng E, Leader A, Claman P, et al. Intravenous albumen does not prevent the development of severe ovarian hyperstimulation syndrome in an in vitro fertilization programme. Hum reprod. 1995;10:807-10.
74. Ben-Chetrit A, Eldar-Geva T, Gal M, et al. The questionable use of albumin for the prevention of ovarian hyperstimulation syndrome in an IVF programme: a randomized placebo-controlled trial. Hum Reprod. 2001;16(9):1880-4.
75. Lainas T, Petsas G, Stavropoulou G, et al. Administration of methylprednisolone to prevent severe ovarian hyperstimulation syndrome in patients undergoing in vitro fertilization. Fertil Steril. 2002;78(3):529-33.
76. Tan SL, Balen A, el Hussein E, Campbell S, et al. The administration of glucocorticoids for the prevention of ovarian hyperstimulation syndrome in in-vitro fertilization: a prospective randomized study. Fertil Steril. 1992;58(2):378-83.
77. Gomez R, Gonzalez-Izquierdo M, Zimmermann RC, et al. Low-dose dopamine agonist administration blocks vascular endothelial growth factor (VEGF)-mediated vascular hyperpermeability without altering VEGF receptor 2-dependent luteal angiogenesis in a rat ovarian hyperstimulation model. Endocrinology. 2006;147(11):5400.
78. Alvarez C, Martí-Bonmatí L, Novella-Maestre E, et al. Dopamine agonist cabergoline reduces hemoconcentration and ascites in hyperstimulated women undergoing assisted reproduction. J Clin Endocrinol Metab. 2007;92(8):2931.
79. Varnagy A, Bodis J,Manfai Z, et al. low dose aspirin therapy to prevent ovarian hyperstimualtion syndrome. Fertil Steril. 2009.
80. Thaler I, Yoffe N, Kaftory JK, et al. Treatment of ovarian hyperstimulation syndrome: the physiologic basis for a modified approach. Fertil Steril. 1981;36(1):110-13.
81. Levin I, Almog B, Avni A, et al. Effect of paracentesis of ascitic fluids on urinary output and blood indices in patients with severe ovarian hyperstimulation syndrome. Fertil Steril. 2002;77(5):986.
82. Borenstein R, Elhalah U, Lunenfeld B, et al. Severe ovarian hyperstimulation syndrome: a reevaluated therapeutic approach. Fertil Steril. 1989;51(5):791-95.
83. Aboulghar MA, Mansour RT, Serour GI, et al. Management of severe ovarian hyperstimulation syndrome by ascitic fluid aspiration and intensive intravenous fluid therapy. Obstet Gynecol. 1993;81(1):108-11.
84. Abramov Y, Elchalal U, Schenker JG. Pulmonary manifestations of severe ovarian hyperstimulation syndrome: a multicenter study. Fertil Steril. 1999;71(4):645-51.
85. Rinaldi ML, Spirtos NJ. Chest tube drainageof pleural effusion correcting abdominal ascites in a patient with severe ovarian hyperstimulation syndrome: a case report. Fertil Steril. 1995;63:1114-7.
86. Stewart JA, Hamilton PJ, Murdoch AP. Thromboembolic disease associated with ovarian stimulation and assisted conception techniques. Hum Reprod. 1997;12(10):2167-73
87. Aboulghar MA, Mansour RT, Serour GI, et al. Moderate ovarian hyperstimulation syndrome complicated by deep cerebrovascular thrombosis. Hum Reprod. 1998; 13(8):2088-91.
88. Cluroe AD, Synek BJA fatal case of ovarian hyperstimulation syndrome with cerebral infarction. Pathology. 1995;27(4):344-6.
89. Tang OS, Ng EH, Wai Cheng P, et al. Cortical vein thrombosis misinterpreted as intracranial haemorrhage in severe ovarian hyperstimulation syndrome: case report. Hum Reprod. 2000;15(9):1913-16.

5

Practice Guideline for Infertility Treatments

Section Contents

31

Practice Guidelines for the Treatment of Patients with Infertility

Candice O'Hern Perfetto, Molina B Dayal, Anil K Dubey

Chapter Contents

INTRODUCTION

Worldwide, the protocols and techniques applied to assisted reproductive technology (ART) are incredibly diverse. In some countries, specific laws and regulations have been established by the government to direct management while, in others, unofficial guidelines play a larger role. In the United States, the government has not imposed laws on treatment of infertility with ART,[1] however, is the society of reproductive specialists that has evaluated the ethical, legal and medical issues within the field and has developed recommendations for treatment.

Given the impressive number of couples that suffer from infertility and the increasing number of states mandating *in vitro* fertilization (IVF) coverage, it is expected that more people will be seeking infertility treatment in the future. A general consensus amongst practitioners is that patients first should be offered the most minimally invasive technique appropriate for their diagnosis. Couples should initially be counseled on lifestyle modifications, including unprotected intercourse 2 to 3 times a week, eliminating smoking and drug abuse, consuming only one to two alcoholic drinks a week, maintaining a healthy weight and body mass index and obtaining the appropriate vitamin supplements.[2] Patients should also undergo an appropriate work-up to identify the cause of their infertility. Males must submit a semen sample for analysis. Women need an evaluation of their ovarian reserve, specifically day 3 follicle stimulating hormone (FSH), estradiol level, anti-Müllerian hormone (AMH) and antral follicle count.[3] The female patient also needs appropriate assessment of their pelvic anatomy, including hysterosalpingogram or laparoscopy/hysteroscopy and/or sonohysterogram as clinically indicated.[3] Once the cause of infertility has been identified, it is appropriate to consider a treatment intervention.

The objective of this chapter is to provide general clinical practice guidelines for the treatment of couples with infertility. Guidelines for undertaking ovulation induction (OI), controlled ovarian hyperstimulation, intrauterine insemination, IVF and associated ART are outlined. Specific details regarding each treatment intervention are discussed in detail in other chapters of this textbook.

Assisted reproductive technology encompasses all procedures that involve the manipulation of gametes outside of the human body in an effort to create a pregnancy. Multiple procedures exist that can be classified as ART, including: IVF, intracytoplasmic sperm injection (ICSI), assisted hatching (AH), preimplantation genetic testing, cyropreservation of embryos and gametes, gamete and embryo donation, gestational surrogacy and gamete and zygote intrafallopian tube transplantation[1] (GIFT/ZIFT). Although ART has the highest success rate for pregnancy and live birth rate, there are additional treatment options available for most causes of infertility. Intrauterine insemination (IUI), OI with oral medications or injectable gonadotropins and controlled ovarian hyperstimulation (COH) are not classified as ART. These are, however, less invasive and less expensive than all ART procedures.[4] If a couple wishes to proceed with treatment after a diagnosis of infertility, these non-ART treatments may be the most appropriate initial treatment option.

NON-ASSISTED REPRODUCTIVE TECHNOLOGY THERAPIES

General Guidelines for Ovulation Induction

Stimulation of ovulation can be accomplished with oral or injectable medications. Oral medications, specifically clomiphene citrate, are traditionally the first line treatment for those with anovulation, specifically polycystic ovarian syndrome. The goal of OI is the development of a single, dominant follicle, thus reducing the chance of a multiple pregnancy.

Clomiphene Citrate

A typical protocol begins with clomiphene citrate 50 mg daily on days 5 through 9 of a spontaneous or progestin induced flow. Patients then undergo ultrasound and hormonal assessments 3–4 days later. If the couple prefers timed intercourse without an ovulation trigger, a luteinizing hormone (LH) or ovulation kit can be used to better time intercourse once a follicle has achieved a mean diameter of 16–18. Once LH is detected in the urine, ovulation is expected in 18–36 hours later and sexual intercourse is recommended within 24–36 hours after the LH surge. If the couple opts for an ovulation trigger, the female patient will continue every other day or daily ultrasounds until a follicle is greater than 20 mm in diameter. Once the follicle is the appropriate size, ovulation can be triggered with human chorionic gonadotropin (hCG) with intercourse being timed accordingly.[5]

Injectable Gonadotropins

Ovulation induction with injectable medications is indicated in the same patient population as above, with the addition of women with hypogonadotropic anovulation (who seldom respond to clomiphene citrate) and those that fail to respond to clomiphene citrate.[4] The goal of OI with gonadotropins is to produce one mature follicle, which can be fertilized with either timed intercourse or IUI. For this purpose, patients receive a low dose of injectable gonadotropins [FSH/hMG (human menopausal gonadotropin) is started at 37.5–75 international units per day on cycle day 1].[6] An FSH formulation with some LH activity should be used in women with hypogonadotropic hypogonadism while a recombinant form can be used in those with polycystic ovary syndrome. The female patient returns for frequent sonographic and hormonal assessments to ensure that a single, dominant follicle is developing. If after 7 days of stimulation no follicle is greater than 10 mm in diameter, the daily dose of gonadotropins can be increased; rarely the dose will exceed 225 IU per day FSH/hMG.[6] The development of a mature follicle typically occurs within 10–12 days, however, many women require ovarian stimulation for more than 2 weeks. Once one or two mature follicles reach 16–18 mm, the patient should receive an ovulation trigger.[6] Specific ovulation triggers are discussed in greater detail in the IVF section. Ovulation will occur 36–40 hours after hCG administration. Patients should be instructed to engage in intercourse after the injection or to complete the IUI within 24–36 hours.[6] In addition, the likelihood of producing multiple (more than one) follicles is high and cycle cancellation should be considered if three or more mature follicles are noted to develop as this significantly increases the likelihood of multiple pregnancy.

The addition of injectable gonadotropins to the infertility treatment significantly increases the cost and risks to the female patient. The couple must be aware that there is a 5–10 fold increased risk of multiple gestations.[6] Given this risk, cycle cancellation or conversion to IVF, must be considered if more than three mature follicles (> 16–17 mm) are present, a large number of intermediate follicles (10–15 mm) are present or the serum estradiol level is greater than 1,000–1,500 pg/ml.[6] Due to these risks, many patients are counseled to consider IVF in lieu of OI with injectable gonadotropins as ovarian stimulation with IVF can be better controlled and a single embryo can be transferred, thus reducing the risk of a multiple pregnancy.

General Guidelines for Controlled Ovarian Hyperstimulation

The goal for COH is production of multiple (2–4) follicles, instead of a single dominant one, as these couples do not have ovulatory dysfunction. Production of multiple follicles can be achieved with the use of clomiphene citrate or injectable gonadotropins.

Clomiphene Citrate

A typical protocol with clomiphene citrate is 100 mg daily on days 3 through 7 of a spontaneous menstrual cycle. Initiating clomiphene citrate early in the menstrual cycle allows for recruitment of many follicles. Patients then undergo ultrasound and hormonal assessments 3–4 days later. Such monitoring provides a means to determine appropriate (2–4 follicles) or inappropriate (one follicle, suggesting no effect of medications or > 5, thus raising likelihood for a multiple pregnancy and/or ovarian hyperstimulation syndrome) response. Once 2–4 follicles are noted to be of appropriate size (approximately 20 mm in mean diameter), ovulation can be triggered with hCG with an IUI being timed accordingly.[5]

Injectable Gonadotropins

With injectable gonadotropins, the typical starting dose of FSH is 150 IU every night beginning on day-3 of the menstrual cycle. However, the dose can be adjusted based on the patient's age and ovarian reserve testing (specifically AMH level). Monitoring is performed in a similar fashion, beginning 3–4 days after initiation of injections followed by assessments every 1–3 days depending on the response of the patient. Once 2–4 follicles are noted to be of appropriate size (approximately 16–18 mm in mean diameter), ovulation can be triggered with hCG with an IUI being timed accordingly.[5]

Cancellation of treatment cycles should be strongly considered if the patients hyper-respond, indicated either with elevated estradiol levels (> 1500 pg/ml) or multiple follicles (five or more follicles measuring > 12 mm in mean diameter). In such situations, couples are also counseled to abstain from intercourse. Cancellation limits the likelihood of associated complications of multiple gestation and ovarian hyperstimulation syndrome. Another option for these over-responding patients is conversion to an IVF cycle; in these instances, a gonadotropin-releasing hormone (GnRH) antagonist is required to prevent an LH surge and gonadotropin stimulation is continued to further follicle growth. While the egg yield may not be as robust as a cycle initially planned for IVF, this intervention prevents cancellation of the COH/IUI cycle.

General Guidelines for Intrauterine Insemination

Couples suffering from unexplained infertility, specifically those with intact fallopian tubes and a normal semen analysis, have an increased cycle fecundity of 2.71 with IUI alone.[4] Although the studies on IUI are limited, a randomized controlled trial comparing timed intercourse to IUI found a significant, albeit minimal, improvement in conception with IUI (2.4% vs 4.1%).[4] According to the guidelines developed by the European Society of Human Reproduction and Embryology, most pregnancies occur within the first 6 cycles with only IUI and a patient should not exceed nine attempts.[7] This approach may be considered in women without a male partner or in couples where intercourse is difficult to consummate. For most couples, however, data suggests that IUI is more successful in combination with mild ovarian stimulation or COH.

Assisted Reproductive Technology Therapies

Guidelines for Considering In Vitro Fertilization

When couples fail multiple attempts with OI or COH/IUI, or if tubal disease, male factor or diminished ovarian reserve is present, patients must consider proceeding to ART. Assisted reproductive technology has become the gold standard for most infertility practitioners, as it has the highest likelihood of success. In 2009, the Society for Assisted Reproductive Technology (SART) noted the live birth rate per cycle to be 44% in women younger than 36-year old, a success rate that continues to steadily rise.[8] Although IVF is the most common procedure utilized in the category of ART, other techniques are often employed with IVF as well and they will be discussed in detail later in the chapter.

In vitro fertilization is effective for virtually all causes of infertility. It is indicated in couples who have failed less invasive treatment options, have unexplained fertility, as well as specific populations including men with moderate deficits in semen quality and women with documented tubal disease or advanced maternal age.[3] According to American Society for Reproductive Medicine (ASRM), it is appropriate to recommend IVF to a couple, if it is unlikely that a pregnancy will occur spontaneously, a less invasive form of treatment will most likely be ineffective and there will likely be a positive outcome from IVF.

In all couples considering IVF, practitioners must evaluate the various factors contributing to infertility, as well as how each will affect IVF outcome. Factors, such as maternal age, duration of infertility, pregnancy history and number of prior attempts and their associated cycle response must be considered and discussed with the couple when moving forward with an IVF cycle. Practitioners must use this information to determine which stimulation protocol, as well as which adjunct assisted reproductive procedures, should be employed to increase the likelihood of success.

Tubal disease is one diagnosis that may require additional treatment prior to proceeding with IVF. Multiple studies have confirmed that sonographically documented hydrosalpinges can adversely affect the IVF cycle, decreasing the live birth rate by 49%.[9] Given the poorer outcomes associated with hydrosalpinges, it is recommended that either a salpingectomy or proximal tubal occlusion be performed prior to initiating an IVF cycle. In addition, the presence of endometrial polyps and/or submucosal myomas may decrease IVF success. Resection of these endometrial filling defects should be strongly considered before proceeding with an IVF cycle. These clinical considerations are covered in further depth in the surgical techniques chapter.

Selecting an IVF Stimulation Protocol

Once the chance of success has been optimized and the couple understands the time commitment associated with IVF, the appropriate protocol is then chosen. Based on infertility diagnosis, patient characteristics (i.e. age, ovarian reserve testing, prior ovarian response), and infertility center preference, patients are placed into different protocols for ovarian stimulation.

Female patients with good ovarian reserve but male factor infertility, can consider a natural IVF cycle. Conversely, patients with poor ovarian reserve, documented with a single dominant follicle being recruited during a stimulated IVF cycle, are candidates for natural cycle IVF. Natural cycle IVF involves frequent monitoring of a spontaneous menstrual cycle with transvaginal ultrasounds and serum estradiol, LH and progesterone levels with the plan to retrieve a single oocyte prior to the LH surge. The retrieved oocyte is then fertilized with the partner's or donor's sperm using conventional IVF or ICSI. To decrease the chance of cycle cancellation secondary to a premature LH surge, the female patient can receive a GnRH antagonist. Timing for oocyte retrieval is optimized with administration of an hCG trigger. Although the success rate is low compared to other stimulated IVF cycles, 8% per cycle, it does decrease the cost of IVF by 75–80%.[3]

The vast majority of IVF protocols use ovarian stimulation with injectable gonadotropins. Dozens of protocols for IVF treatment exist. Selection of a specific protocol is dependent on the patient's age, ovarian reserve testing, etiology of infertility and prior response to ovarian stimulation. Prior to starting gonadotropin stimulation, many patients' hypothalamic-pituitary axis is downregulated. This provides a means for recruiting multiple follicles by preventing recruitment of a single dominant follicle and for preventing a premature LH surge. Downregulation can be achieved with oral contraceptive pills (OCP's), GnRH agonists or GnRH antagonists.[3] Other protocols without downregulation can be used.

Overview of a Typical IVF Cycle

In all protocols, close observation of follicle growth and hormone levels is required. Medication doses may be changed or decisions may be made about retrieval based on this monitoring. Typically, after 3–5 days of stimulation, transvaginal ultrasound and hormonal assessments are performed daily or every other day. Estradiol levels are correlated with ultrasound findings and suggest oocyte maturity. It is expected that each dominant follicle typically correlates with a serum estradiol level of 150–300 pg/ml.[6] Ultrasound is also necessary to evaluate the endometrial stripe; a trilaminar thickness of 8–9 mm is desired, with a thickness less than 6 mm and greater than 12 mm being associated with poor implantation.[3]

Multiple follicles 18–20 mm in diameter, multiple follicles measuring between 14–16 mm in diameter and an estradiol level greater than 2000 pg/ml signal the optimal time for ovulation trigger.[6] Depending on the initial protocol, multiple formulations exist for ovulation trigger. A single injection of 5,000–10,000 IU of hCG can be used in all protocols to initiate oocyte maturation. Women suppressed using GnRH antagonists have the option of using a GnRH agonist as a trigger instead; this is often useful in preventing ovarian hyperstimulation syndrome as no lingering effects of exogenous hCG are present. GnRH agonist triggers cannot be used in protocols where GnRH is being used to prevent the premature LH surge.

The patient then undergoes a transvaginal ultrasound guided oocyte retrieval 36 hours after the trigger injection. Some centers retrieve eggs 34 hours after the trigger; attempts at harvesting eggs before 34 hours may yield less mature oocytes.[3] The retrieval can occur under deep sedation, conscious sedation or general anesthesia, depending on the preference of the patient, practitioner and/or anesthesiologist. Patients typically begin progesterone supplements (either vaginal or intramuscular injection) the morning after the egg retrieval to provide luteal support to the endometrial lining. Progesterone supplementation continues until the pregnancy test is negative or if pregnant, until 10–12 weeks of gestational age.

The Egg Retrieval

The oocyte retrieval is completed under transvaginal ultrasound guidance with the patient in the dorsal lithotomy position. The patient is routinely given intravenous antibiotics 30–60 minutes prior to the procedure[3] or oral antibiotics beginning the day before egg retrieval. Povidone iodine is not used for prepping the perineum and vagina as it has been found to be toxic to oocytes, thus lowering the pregnancy rate; normal saline is used for vaginal irrigation and preparation.[3] Once the vagina is prepared, the transvaginal ultrasound identifies the ovarian follicles and a 16 or 17 gauge needle is introduced through the posterior vaginal fornix directly into the ovary. Ultrasound guidance decreases the likelihood of damaging the bowel, bladder, blood vessels or other pelvic structures. Using a vacuum suction of 100–120 mm Hg, each follicle is carefully punctured in an effort to obtain the greatest number of oocytes.[3] Although multiple techniques exist to optimize oocyte yield there are a few strategies that are most effective. Some practitioners advocate a gentle 'curettage' of the follicle by swiveling the needle in one place while others suggest flushing of the follicle with culture media. Regardless of the method used, it is important to minimize the number of punctures through the vagina to 1–2 per ovary. With each withdrawal, media should be flushed through the catheter to guarantee oocyte arrival in the test tube.[3] As the egg retrieval continues, the embryologists identify the oocytes within the aspirated fluid under a microscope and evaluate for maturity.

Fertilization

Mature oocytes are 'exposed' to sperm with conventional IVF or ICSI for fertilization.[3] The male partner is responsible for providing a semen sample on the day of oocyte retrieval. If a fresh sample is not available, a previously frozen sample can be thawed immediately before use. The semen undergoes density gradient centrifugation and preparation. After appropriate washing, the sperm are incubated for 0.5–4 hours in a specific protein media to facilitate capacitation.[3] For conventional IVF, the oocyte and 50,000 sperm are placed together in a 37° celsius incubator for 12–18 hours to facilitate fertilization.[3] For ICSI, cumulus cells are removed from the retrieved oocyte and a single sperm is injected into a mature, metaphase II oocyte. Fertilization is assessed approximately 14–16 hours later.

Intracytoplasmic Sperm Injection

Indications

Intracytoplasmic sperm injection has revolutionized assisted reproductive therapy. Prior to the advent of ICSI, couples with severe deficits in sperm quantity or quality had poor outcomes due to severely limited fertilization rates. In some cases, only sperm donation or adoption was option for family building.

The initial indication for ICSI was for couples where the male had low concentration (oligospermia), poor motility (asthenospermia) or low normal sperm morphology (teratospermia) on a semen analysis. Aspirated sperm from the epididymis or testes can be used for men with obstructive or nonobstructive azoospermia. For testicular sperm retrieval, sperm extraction is performed with a focus on identifying seminiferous tubules that appear wider in caliber and more opaque, which therefore may be more likely to harbor active spermatogenesis.[10] Otherwise, random sampling of the testis can be performed. Specimens from either procedure are immediately examined for the presence of sperm.

Since its advent, the indications for ICSI have become more varied. Intracytoplsmic sperm injection can be considered in couples with prior poor fertilization with conventional IVF or limited (< 5) egg yields. ICSI should be strongly considered in those couples that have had multiple unsuccessful COH/IUI cycles, as the underlying cause behind the failed treatments is presumed to be an occult fertilization problem. One of the newest indications for ICSI is for couples who desire prenatal genetic diagnosis or screening[10]. Because ICSI involves the injection of one sperm into one egg, any chance of polyspermy, resulting in false positive results, is eliminated.

Procedure

After preparation of the semen sample, a single sperm is injected directly into the oocyte. The sperm is immobilized, by compressing the tail with a pipette and then is drawn into the pipette, tail first. The oocyte, with the polar body stabilized at 6 or 12 O'clock, is then entered at the 3 O'clock position.[3] The pipette pierces the zona pellucida and the sperm is injected directly into the ooplasm. This manipulation triggers oocyte activation and fertilization occurs. After fertilization, the embryo is then handled and monitored similarly to a standard IVF cycle. The fertilization rate for ICSI/IVF is 45–75% per injected oocyte.[11]

In order to fully appreciate the success rate for this procedure, it must be understood that patients with severe male factor infertility rarely produce adequate motile sperm to allow any successful pregnancy with IUI or standard IVF. Since its development in 1992, very few complications have been attributed to this procedure. The only concerning evidence is what appears to be an increased incidence of congenital anomalies of the genitourinary system in male offspring.[11] Given the procedure has only been utilized in the last 2 decades; it is possible that more research and follow-up of the infants born through ICSI may lead to additional findings.

Assessment of the Embryo and the Embryo Transfer

After fertilization, embryos are monitored for development up to 5 days, depending on the couple and the infertility center's plan for embryo transfer. As the embryos mature *in vitro*, the culture media is sequentially changed. The developing embryos require slight changes in the culture media, as well as constant monitoring of carbon dioxide levels, pH and protein supplementation. Based on the number and appearance of the fertilized embryos, the female patients' age, prior IVF cycle outcomes, desire to reduce the likelihood of a multiple pregnancy, the decision is made about when, how many and which embryos to transfer. Cleavage stage embryos can be replaced on either day 2 or 3 with similar pregnancy rates.[12] Blastocysts are usually transferred on day- 5. Although evidence exists that blastocyst transfer has a significantly higher implantation rate than cleavage stage embryo transfer, only those women with presumed good prognosis have an elevated live birth rate with blastocysts.[13] Therefore, a detailed discussion between the provider and the couple determines which day will be the best for embryo transfer. Mock embryo transfer, either prior to the cycle or on the day of retrieval, has been shown to increase pregnancy rates. Other factors that have been attributed to higher pregnancy rate are 'easy' transfers, decreased mucus at the cervical os, no blood noted on the tip of the transfer catheter at completion of the transfer and use of soft catheters.[3] It is also advised to transfer the embryo under ultrasound guidance at the level of the mid-cavity. There is little, if any, evidence to support tubal transfer or bed rest after embryo transfer.[3]

Guidelines for Determining the Number of Embryos to Transfer

Specific guidelines, set by ASRM and SART, exist regarding how many embryos should be transferred. Although these guidelines are not laws set by the United States government, they are considered the standard of care for IVF centers. The recommendations set forth by these professional societies for the number of embryos to be transferred are based primarily on age of the patient, as well as their overall prognosis (Table 1)

- In women, who are younger than 35 years of age and have a favorable prognosis, a single embryo (either cleavage stage or blastocyst) should be transferred. A favorable prognosis includes the first IVF cycle, a good quality embryo, excess embryos available or a previously successful IVF outcome. For a less favorable prognosis, up to two cleavage stage or blastocyst stage embryos can be transferred.
- In women 35 to 37 years of age and a favorable prognosis, a maximum of two cleavage stage embryos should be transferred. The practitioner can transfer three cleavage stage embryos or two blastocysts in those with a less favorable prognosis.
- Women 38 to 40 years of age with a favorable prognosis can have 2–3 cleavage stage embryos or two blastocysts transferred. If the prognosis is unfavorable, four cleavage stage embryos and three blastocysts can be transferred.
- For women greater than 40 years of age, it is allowed to transfer up to five cleavage stage embryos and three blastocysts, regardless of prognosis.

The guidelines also comment that after two or more failed cycles, it is the practitioner's prerogative to consider the transfer of additional embryos. The guidelines set forth by ASRM and SART are designed to help minimize the most common complication of IVF multiple gestation.[14]

Other determining factors include the couple's openness to selective reduction (if clinically appropriate), current family size, maternal medical or surgical history, risk of ovarian hyperstimulation syndrome, ovarian response (or lack thereof) and embryo quality. For instance, the transfer of a single embryo in a woman with a history of cervical incompetence and subsequent preterm labor/delivery should be strongly considered.

Assisted Hatching

In vivo, the blastocyst undergoes a process of 'hatching' from the zona pellucida prior to implantation. There is a unique interaction between the embryo and uterus that leads to the dissolution of the zona pellucida. While the embryo develops *in vitro*, it does not experience the same interactions nor is it exposed to the same proteolytic enzymes. Assisted hatching, a more recent advancement for ART, attempts to mimic this process. It is an adjunct to traditional IVF that is performed immediately, prior

Table 1 American society for reproductive medicine—guidelines on number of embryos transferred

	Day 2 or 3				Blastocysts			
	<35	35–37	38–40	>40	<35	35–37	38–40	>40
Favorable	1 to 2	1 to 2	≤ 3	≤ 5	1	1 to 2	1 to 2	≤ 3
Average	1 to 2	≤ 3	≤ 4	≤ 5	1 to 2	1 to 2	≤ 3	≤ 3

to embryo transfer. Assisted hatching creates an artificial thinning or breach of the zona pellucida. A breach in the zona pellucida is performed using one of three techniques: (1) Drilling through the entire depth of the zona pellucida with acidified Tyrode's solution; (2) Partial dissection with either a glass microneedle, laser photoablation or a piezomicromanipulator and; (3) Thinning of the zona pellucida with proteolytic enzymes, acidified Tyrode's solution or LASER.

In clinical trials, the procedure was found to increase the implantation rate and clinical pregnancy rate in select patient populations. It is effective in those with one or more prior failed ART cycles,[14] poor embryo quality and female patients, who are older than 40 years of age.[15] While clinical pregnancy and implantation rates have been shown to improve, there is no evidence that it increases the live birth rate. Given the limited evidence on AH, current recommendations support its use in selected populations. This procedure is not without risks. One of the theoretical complications associated with AH include possible damage to the embryo which may reduce embryo viability. There is also a documented increase in monozygotic twinning.[16]

Preimplantation Genetic Diagnosis

Indications

Couples that are concerned about passing genetic mutations or chromosomal rearrangements onto their offspring can consider preimplantation genetic diagnosis (PGD). Preimplantation genetic diagnosis is indicated when one or both parents have a known gene sequence mutation or balanced chromosomal rearrangement. Although considered an ART, this technique can also be performed in patients that do not suffer from infertility. Couples that have been diagnosed with an autosomal dominant, autosomal recessive, X-linked mutation and chromosomal translocation, have the option to screen the oocyte or embryo for that specific gene defect prior to IVF transfer. Prior to PGD, couples would have prenatal testing via either chorionic villus sampling (CVS) or amniocentesis, and then have to make the difficult decision of whether to continue to carry the pregnancy. Preimplantation genetic diagnosis allows for detection of affected embryos prior to implantation; only embryos deemed 'normal' are transferred to the uterus. Such early evaluation of the oocyte or embryo reduces the chance of having an affected offspring; the reduction in risk is dependent upon the genetic disorder being tested.[17]

Procedure in Brief

The process requires the removal of one or more nuclei from the oocyte (polar bodies) or embryo (blastomeres or trophoectoderm cells). Similar to AH, the zona pellucida must be opened. A defect is created with a LASER, acidified Tyrode's solution or a sharpened glass needle as mentioned previously.[3] The polar body in an oocyte, 1–2 blastomeres in a day 3 cleavage stage embryo or mural trophoectoderm from a blastocyst are then extracted using a small suction pipette or gentle compression.[3] While the nuclei are being analyzed, the embryo can develop into a blastocyst in extended culture if biopsied on day 3 or undergo cryopreservation if biopsied as a blastocyst.

The genetic analysis for a specific gene mutation employs polymerase chain reaction (PCR) to amplify a gene segment. After amplification, restriction enzyme analysis, selective amplification of the abnormal sequences and direct comparison of normal and abnormal segments can be employed to detect the specific mutation.[17] Alternatively, fluorescent *in-situ* hybridization (FISH) is used to detect missing or excess chromosomal material. Although there have been many advances in PCR and FISH, there are still multiple challenges associated with PGD. In general, there is a very short interval available for analysis, as well as very little cellular data available. For PCR specifically, there is also the risk for misdiagnoses. Errors can occur, if specific DNA segments are not amplified appropriately, either from allele dropout or partial amplification. Either circumstance can lead to transfer of an affected embryo or the discard of a normal embryo.[3]

Prior to performing PGD, couples need to be counseled of the inherent limitations associated with the procedure. The couple will have to undergo IVF, even if they are not infertile. The embryo will also be exposed to extended culture and biopsy. Also, there is a small chance that an affected embryo may be transferred after it is falsely identified as normal, which has an incidence as high as 2% for recessive disorders and 11% for dominant disorders.[17] Knowing these inherent limitations, it is recommended that patients undergo chorionic villus sampling or amniocentesis once pregnant after a 'normal' embryo is transferred. In addition, according to one study, the pregnancy rate after PGD is also reduced compared to standard IVF. This reduced rate may be from the decreased number of embryos available for transfer after analysis either because abnormal embryos are discarded, normal embryos fail to progress to blastocysts or the normal embryos have decreased viability after the biopsy.[17]

Preimplantation Genetic Screening (PGS)

Indications

The most common cause of pregnancy failure or recurrent pregnancy loss is aneuploidy. Preimplantation genetic screening (PGS) involves the assessment of embryos for numerical abnormalities of the autosomes or sex chromosome, as opposed to assessment of a specific gene mutation (PGD). It is, therefore, frequently employed for those couples at the greatest risk of having an aneuploid embryo. Women with advanced maternal age, a history of recurrent pregnancy loss, multiple IVF failures and severe male factor infertility are relative indications for the procedure.[17] As with PGD couples must understand the risks associated with the procedure. These risks include risks specific to IVF, embryo culture, embryo biopsy and damage, a possible false positive or false-negative result and the limited evidence that exists on the procedure.

Procedure

The biopsy procedure for PGS is identical to that used in PGD. Preimplantation genetic screening employs FISH or comparative genomic hybridization for assessment of the biopsied cell. FISH for PGS/PGD can only evaluate 9–11 chromosomes in a single cell.[17] Comparative genomic hybridization, while can amplify the entire genome. The sample and reference chromosomes are amplified with red and green fluorochromes simultaneously. They are hybridized to normal male metaphase chromosomes for 2–3 days.[17] The quantity of red and green signaling is then analyzed for chromosome number and to identify any abnormalities. Both techniques provide results within 24–48 hours of biopsy. Advancement in these techniques is occurring rapidly; however, it is important to address the current limitations. Currently, FISH screens fewer than half of the chromosomes. It is important to note that up to 25% of aneuploid embryos may be falsely identified as normal by FISH and CGH.[17]

Embryo Cryopreservation

Cryopreservation of embryos is appropriate, if more embryos develop than can safely be transferred, if there is concern for ovarian hyperstimulation syndrome or if patients are awaiting results from genetic testing prior to transfer. Embryo cryopreservation can also be considered in women who would like to preserve their fertility before they undertake gonadotoxic treatment (i.e. chemotherapy, radiation therapy). The success associated with embryo cryopreservation has increased dramatically in the last decade. The introduction and advancement of vitrification protocols for rapid freezing is responsible for the marked improvement in frozen embryo survival rates. Vitrification employs a rapid freeze technique that minimizes intracellular water ice crystallization and therefore reduces intracellular damage. These embryos have higher survival rate, more than 75% and success approaches 50–67% that of a fresh embryo transfer.[3]

To proceed with frozen embryo transfer, the endometrium needs to be prepared and synchronized with the embryos for successful implantation. Patients can undertake a natural cycle cryothaw in a similar fashion to a natural IVF cycle; a spontaneous menstrual cycle is monitored with sonographic and hormonal assessments every 1–2 days. Once the LH surge is detected, embryos can be thawed and transferred in synchrony to the day of embryo freeze. In most situations, patients undertake a medicated cryothaw cycle which requires suppression of the hypothalamic-pituitary axis with a GnRH agonist followed by estrogen supplementation. Endometrial thickness is ascertained with a sonogram after 10–14 days of estrogen supplementation. Once the lining is trilaminar and a minimum of 6.5 mm in thickness, progesterone supplementation is initiated in synchrony to the day of embryo freeze. Embryos are subsequently, thawed and transferred accordingly.[3] Approximately, one-half to two-thirds of embryos survive the thaw at the cleavage stage while a greater percentage survives as blastocysts.

Oocyte Cryopreservation

Indications

Unlike cryopreservation of embryos, the cryopreservation of oocytes is considered experimental. Whereas embryo and sperm quality is mostly maintained during the freezing and thawing process, oocyte integrity and viability are at risk. The live birth rate per thawed oocyte is only 2% using the slow freeze method and 4% for vitrification.[18]

Current possible indications for egg freezing include elective fertility preservation, fertility preservation in those individuals with cancer prior to undertaking gonadotoxic therapies, fertility preservation in individuals with severe endometriosis prior to oophorectomy or the inability to obtain a sperm sample after an egg retrieval for IVF treatment.

Secondary to the low success rate associated with oocyte cryopreservation, female patients must receive extensive counseling if considering oocyte cryopreservation. As in a typical IVF cycle, the patient must undergo ovarian stimulation and oocyte retrieval prior to storage. In addition, once the decision is made to thaw the oocytes, they must be fertilized using ICSI. Patients need to be aware of the storage fees, expected survival and success rates for the facility, as well as have a plan for disposition of the oocytes, should they be not used or the facility were to close.[18] Given the extensive risks and limited success at this time, it is recommended that oocyte cryopreservation only be offered under guidance by the institutional review board.

Donation of Gametes

The most recent guidelines for gamete donation incorporate information from the United States Center for Disease Control and Prevention, the United States Food and Drug Administration and the American Association of Tissue Banks. The practice committee opinion published by ASRM and SART in 2008, established the protocols for screening and testing potential sperm and oocyte donors. In general, recommendations for sperm and oocyte donors are similar.

Donated Sperm

The use of donor sperm may be indicated in cases of severe deficits in semen quality, azoospermia, genetic or infectious diseases in the male, severe rhesus isoimmunization or female patients desiring fertility without a male partner.[19] As with all ART, prior to proceeding with insemination of donor sperm, the female partner needs to have a thorough infertility work-up. The female patient or couple also should undergo psychological counseling, routine preconception screening and communicable disease/sexually transmitted infection screening. Male donors should be in good health, less than 40 years of age and have an absence of any genetic abnormalities.[19] They also need to have a complete history and physical exam, psychological counseling and sexually transmitted infection screening. Screening is more extensive than routine bloodwork for hepatitis B and C, syphilis and HIV and examinations for gonorrhea and Chlamydia. Male donors must complete an extensive questionnaire about prior sexual experiences, travel, drug abuse and blood transfusions. Most sperm donors are screened for gene disorders based on their ethnic background (i.e. cystic fibrosis or an Ashkenazi Jewish panel). Even after completing the necessary examinations, anonymous donor specimens are quarantined for 1 year, at which time the donor is retested.[19] Of note, to limit the number of infants born from one genetic male, the current limitations are 25 births per 800,000 people in an area.[19]

Donated Eggs

Female patients with premature ovarian failure, advanced reproductive age, genetic or infectious diseases and prior IVF treatment failure may consider IVF using donor oocytes. Couples should receive psychological counseling and the female partner must complete a thorough infertility work-up to confirm that she can carry a pregnancy. Female patients with infertility secondary to reproductive aging, especially those greater than 45 years of age, should have a maternal fetal medicine consultation and obtain medical clearance before becoming pregnant. The ideal oocyte donor is between the ages of 21 years and 34 years old and although not required, it is preferred that she has proven fertility. Although the infectious disease screening is similar for female donors as for male donors, there are many more limitations and challenges associated with oocyte donation. First, the routine communicable disease screening must be completed within 1 year and within 30 days prior to the retrieval. Second, because cryopreservation of oocytes is not reliable, it is not possible to quarantine the donor gametes. Also, given the increased risks associated with COH for the donor, there are significantly larger risks associated with oocyte donation than for sperm donation.[19] It is imperative that the donor and the couple agree on appropriate compensation and discuss all possible outcomes and complications prior to beginning the cycle. It is inappropriate for the outcome to predicate the payment, which in average can be $2,500–$8,000 per cycle.[3]

Once the donor is medically and psychologically cleared, the egg donor will undergo ovarian stimulation with one of the IVF protocols previously mentioned. As previously mentioned, it is imperative that all communicable disease screens be completed within 1 year and within 30 days of retrieval. Eligibility forms delineating completion and review of these screens are necessary. Format of the donor form is given below.

Prior to initiation of the egg donor's stimulatory medications, the recipient's endometrium is prepared. For ovulatory recipients, a GnRH agonist is used to downregulate the hypothalamic-pituitary axis followed by estrogen supplementation to prepare the endometrial lining. For those with amenorrhea due to menopause, a GnRH agonist is not required and supplementation with estrogen can begin on any day. Typically, 10–14 days are required to prepare the uterine lining. On the day of the retrieval the recipient should be placed on vaginal or intramuscular progesterone to further prepare and synchronize the endometrial lining. It is expected that before initiation of supplemental progesterone, the recipients' endometrial thickness will be at

Donor Oocyte

Eligibility Determination: ☐ Determination Not Required
☐ Determination Required
Complete

Type: ☐ Anonymous ☐ Directed Donor ☐ Autologus

Donor Accession Number: ____________________

Recovery Method: ☐ Trans-vaginal aspiration

least 6.5 mm^3 and trilaminar in appearance. Because the recipient does not have a corpus luteum to support an ongoing pregnancy, she must remain on estrogen and progesterone until at least 10–12 weeks of pregnancy.[3]

Gestational Surrogacy

For those women without a uterus, with a uterus incapable of carrying a pregnancy or with a medical condition that puts her at increased risk of significant morbidity or mortality with childbearing, gestational surrogacy allows a woman to have a genetically related offspring. Gestational surrogacy can be performed by a relative, friend or a financially compensated female. It is not legal in all 50 states and is currently the cause of multiple legal battles in the United States. Given its serious legal, ethical and social complications, the parents and the surrogate must be encouraged to obtain legal counsel and decide on specific terms and conditions prior to proceeding. Once medical, psychological and legal clearances have been obtained, the surrogate undertakes endometrial preparation in a manner similar to a donor egg recipient.

Gamete Intrafallopian Transfer and Zygote Intrafallopian Transfer

Early in ART development, gamete and zygote transfer directly into the fallopian tubes had success rates similar to traditional IVF. Although extremely rare today, ZIFT uses laparoscopy to place a freshly fertilized zygote into the fallopian tube. Similarly, the GIFT process employed laparoscopy to transfer freshly retrieved oocyte and sperm, avoiding contact outside of the human body, 4 cm proximal to the fimbriae.[3] With the increased success of traditional IVF, GIFT and ZIFT have become less relevant. In 2007, only 0.1% of all ART procedures were ZIFT and less than 0.1% were GIFT.[3] While uncommon, indications for these procedures include religious objections for fertilization occurring outside the body (for GIFT), a history of cervical trachelectomy (for both GIFT and ZIFT), or in even more rare circumstances, an extremely difficult transcervical transfer (for both GIFT or ZIFT).

REFERENCES

1. Jones HW, Cohen J. IFFS Surveillance 07. Fertil Steril. 2007;87(1):S1-67.
2. Kamel RM. Management of the infertile couple: an evidence-based protocol. Reprod Biol Endocrinol. 2010;8:21.
3. Fritz MA, Speroff L. Assisted Reproductive Technologies. Clin Gynecol Endocrinol Infertility. 8th edition; 2010. pp. 1331-82.
4. Practice Committee of the American Society for Reproductive Medicine. Effectiveness and treatment for unexplained infertility. Fertil Sterility. 2006;86:S111-4.
5. American Society for Reproductive Medicine. ART medications. Available from www.asrm.org [Accessed April 2011].
6. Practice Committee of American Society for Reproductive Medicine. Use of exogenous gonadotropins in anovulatory women: a technical bulletin. Fertil Steril. 2008;90(5):S7-12.
7. Good Clinical Treatment in Assisted Reproduction—An ESHRE position paper. ESHRE. June 2008.
8. Society for Assisted Reproductive Technologies webpage. Available from www.sart.org [Accessed April 2011].
9. Salpingectomy for hydrosalpinx prior to in vitro fertilization. Fertil Steril. 2008;90(3):S66-8.
10. Intracytoplasmic sperm injection (ICSI). Fertil Steril. 2008;90(3):S187.
11. Practice Committee of American Society for Reproductive Medicine in collaboration with Society for Male Reproduction and Urology. The management of Infertility due to obstructive azoospermia. Fertil Steril. 2008;90(5):S121-4.
12. Dayal, M, Frankfurter,D, Athanasiadia , I. Peak, D Dubey, A, Gindoff, P. Day 2 embryo transfer (ET) and day 3 ET afford similar reproductive outcomes in the poor responder.Fertility and Sterility 95: 1130-1132, 2011.
13. Practice Committee of American Society for Reproductive Medicine, Practice Committee of Society for Assisted Reproductive Technology. Blastocyst culture and transfer in clinical-assisted reproduction. Fertil Steril. 2008;90(5):S174-7.
14. Practice Committee of Society for Assisted Reproductive Technology; Practice Committee of American Society for Reproductive Medicine. Guidelines on number of embryos transferred. Fertil Steril. 2008;90(5):S163-4.
15. Dayal MB, Dubey A, Frankfurter D, et al. Second cycle: To hatch or not to hatch? Fertil Sterility. 2007;88(3): 718-20.
16. Practice Committee of Society for Assisted Reproductive Technology, Practice Committee of American Society for Reproductive Medicine. The role of assisted hatching in in-vitro fertilization: a review of the literature. A Committee opinion. Fertil Steril. 2008;90(5):S196-8.
17. Practice Committee of Society for Assisted Reproductive Technology; Practice Committee of American Society for Reproductive Medicine. Preimplantation genetic testing: a Practice Committee opinion. Fertil Steril. 2008;90(5):S136-43.
18. Practice Committee of Society for Assisted Reproductive Technology, Practice Committee of American Society for Reproductive Medicine. Essential elements of informed consent for elective oocyte cryopreservation: a Practice Committee opinion. Fertil Steril. 2008;90(5):S134-5.
19. Practice Committee of American Society for Reproductive Medicine; Practice Committee of Society for Assisted Reproductive Technology. 2008 Guidelines for gamete and embryo donation: a Practice Committee report. Fertil Steril. 2008;90(5):S30-44.

32

Integrating Quality Management into a Fertility Practice

Michael M Alper

Chapter Contents

INTRODUCTION

Is your *in vitro* fertilization (IVF) program good? Do you consider it high quality? Are you patients satisfied? Most of us would answer 'yes', but how do you know?[1] After all, 83% of companies assume that their customers are happy with the service.[2] It is common for companies to make (erroneous) assumptions of what their customers really think of their service or product.

IVF centers are complex organizations. Although they often start as a simple doctor's office, they rapidly evolve into fairly complicated organizations involving the integration of many departments and skill sets. IVF centers are, in fact, like 'mini-hospitals'. A challenging aspect to providing the best care possible is to have the right systems in place that make all the pieces work together and towards the same goal. These systems take time and effort to establish and maintain.

An IVF Center can have a terrific group of doctors or an accomplished laboratory, but if the support elements are not well-established, then the professionals within the organization cannot function effectively. A top quality IVF center focuses on the entire entity, not just the doctors and not just the laboratory. Successful companies focus on quality; and IVF is not different.

WHAT IS QUALITY?

Many companies market their quality such as car manufacturers stating. "Quality is number one" or other similar phraseology. Although we intuitively know what we mean, when asked what is quality, it takes some thought to define it. But, quality is not some ill-defined or vague concept. Quality must be defined. For example, if you were to say that you wanted your IVF center to be the most 'accessible' IVF center, then you must decide what you mean by this. Do you mean good parking, or easy to contact via telephone? And when you are clear about what you mean, then you must be able to measure it. So, you would ask patients to rate your parking conditions or the people answering the phones. So, there must be a method to record and analyze whatever measurement of quality that is of interest.

DO HIGH PREGNANCY RATES MEAN HIGH QUALITY?

The IVF field is a competitive one. Most major cities have several IVF centers and, as one would expect, IVF programs are competing for the referral base. Pregnancy rates are numbers and it is intuitive for both referring physicians and patients alike to want to choose programs with the highest statistics. After all, is not a pregnancy rate of 45% better than 30%? And, is not a program with the highest pregnancy rate better quality? Well, may be not. Let me explain.

It is virtually impossible to compare IVF programs-based upon pregnancy statistics since there are many factors that affect statistics that are not available to the public. For example, the inclusion or exclusion criteria for IVF are a strong determinant of success. Some programs will not start an IVF cycle on patients with even modestly abnormal ovarian reserve testing. Others will not encourage patients to continue with treatment, if their expectation for pregnancy is below a certain percentage (that may differ from other programs). A most distressing consequence for IVF centers competing on pregnancy rates alone is the widespread use of transferring more embryos to have the highest pregnancy rate at the expense of multiple gestations. (Fortunately, this practice is becoming less common with the advent of national guidelines for the number of embryos to transfer).

Geographic and political boundaries alter practice patterns and statistics, making it impossible to use pregnancy rates as a measurement of quality. Some countries restrict the number of embryos to replace, or whether embryos can be frozen. In addition, certain local practices are influenced by insurance company requirements. For example, in Massachusetts some insurance companies require treatment with clomiphene or gonadotropin before approving IVF, thereby reducing IVF pregnancy rates (since many of the 'less infertile' patients are successful with simpler treatment).

As one can see, there are many factors affecting pregnancy rates so that a high pregnancy rates may actually mean that the IVF center is poor quality.[3] By restricting access to poor responders, replacing too many embryos and proceeding to IVF too quickly can all lead to a higher pregnancy rate but reflects poor practice.

QUALITY: BEYOND THE IN VITRO FERTILIZATION STATISTIC

There are numerous other important factors that patients should be aware of beyond pregnancy rates that affect their treatment. These include the consequences of ovarian hyperstimulation syndrome. This syndrome is potentially life threatening and is associated with some morbidity, but there is no way to ascertain whether overly aggressive stimulation protocols are present within a given IVF program.

Also, it is impossible for consumers to evaluate other factors such as whether the center is innovative and research oriented. Research is not simply measured by the number of abstracts or papers published, but research is part of a process of continuous improvement, which requires the analysis of data.

Another measure of quality is the compliance to protocols. Errors occur in all human endeavors; and the practice of infertility is no exception. It is of prime importance to have systems in place that result in a safe process. But, when an error occurs, is a system in place to catch it and prevent it from causing harm? Is there a process in place to deal with non-conformances? When a mistake is made, is there a system in place to recognize it, discuss it, and make improvement? Is there transparency, and are all mistakes brought to the group, or buried?

QUALITY IS WHAT THE CUSTOMER SAYS IT IS

In vitro fertilization, as with any business, must understand the needs of its customers (mainly patients). It sounds obvious, but no matter how impressed the doctors are with their IVF centers, if the patients are not content then they will not return. And, if there are no patients, then there is no IVF center. So, how does a medical practice know if their patients are satisfied? The answer is simple: Ask!

Patient surveys help to focus on the delivery of care in the various departments within the IVF center. I would recommend a comprehensive survey annually interspersed with briefer assessments throughout the year. Surveys can either be sent to the patients or distributed to be completed at the facility. Patients' experiences with particular services are rated and followed over time (Figure 1). It is common for patients to be satisfied with their doctor, yet be completely unhappy with services provided by others in the IVF process.

Sharing survey scores with the entire team is very important. If an area is substandard, then the root cause should be determined and corrected.

A WORD ABOUT THE RECEPTION DESK

First impressions are important. Patients, already nervous about visiting the doctor, are very sensitive and the

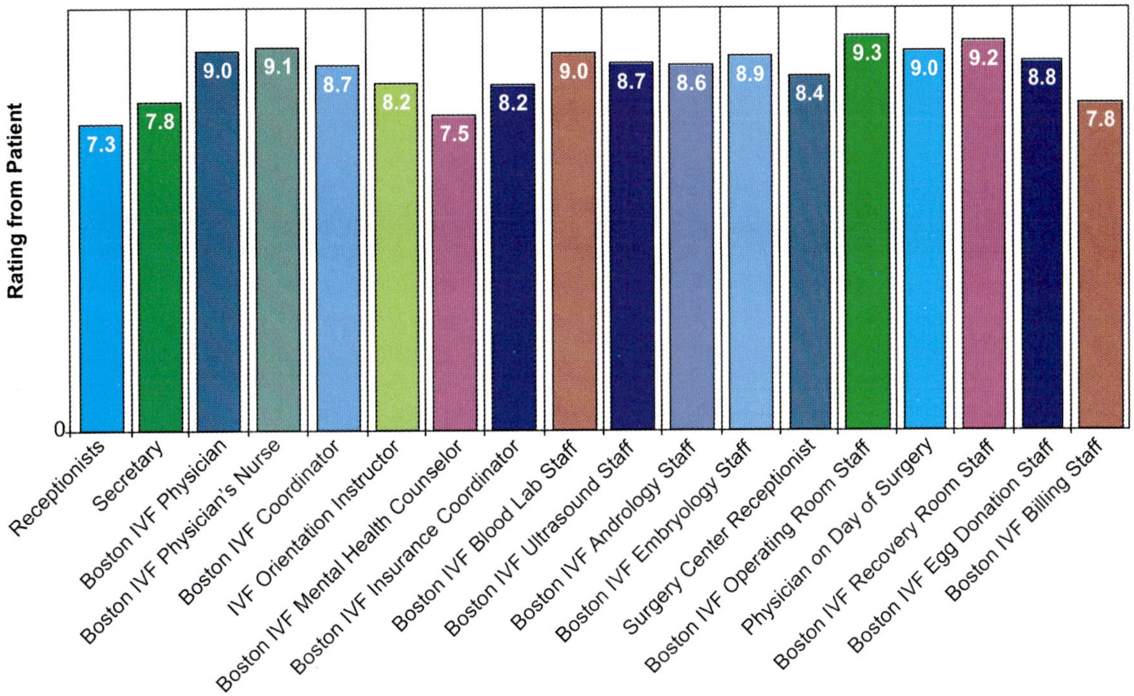

Figure 1 Patient survey scores assessing various aspects of service

first impression left by the receptionist is vital. Patients who are greeted with a smile and handled in a compassionate manner are left with a lasting impression of the IVF center. Unfortunately, the reception desk is often a neglected position. There are no educational requirements, little training, and it is often the least compensated entry positions within the organization. This is unfortunate since it is of vital importance. Several years ago, we achieved low scores for our reception desk. As a result, we hired a new receptionist who was upbeat, warm and customer focused. We set up standards for answering the phone, greeting patients and the like. We brought in customer service experts (such as done in the hotel industry) to train our receptionist and other staff. Books and CDs complemented the on-site training. It paid off for us—the complements followed, as did the survey scores. Of course, the medical and laboratory aspects of the IVF center are critical to success, but a grumpy receptionist can ruin an otherwise superb practice.

WHY A QUALITY MANAGEMENT SYSTEM?

A quality management system (QMS) is a set of principles that control quality within an organization. As opposed to accreditation or certification, which assures that an organization meets specific established criteria, a QMS sets a process in place that is somewhat generic for all entities and not specific for a particular industry. In simple terms, a quality system sets in motion goals for the company, a way of thinking about how the company functions, how it is managed, how problems and improvements take place.

What is ISO?

ISO is not an acronym, but is derived from the Greek word 'ISOs' meaning equal or standard. The official title is International Organization for Standardization. ISO is a nongovernmental organization of about 150 countries (including the USA), established in 1947 to promote the development of standardization to facilitate the international exchange of goods and services.

Between 1947 and the present-day, ISO has published more than 13,700 international standards, e.g. agriculture, construction, mechanical engineering, medical devices, information technology, telephone banking cards, etc. The need for these standards is obvious. ISO 9000 standards are the most popular since they are generic and can be applied to all businesses. The most recent revision was implemented in 2008; hence, the 'ISO 9000:2008' standard is the most current version.

In 2002, Boston IVF realized that it needed a better infrastructure to manage its quality. We spoke to colleagues in Europe, who had experience in implanting the ISO system into their IVF center and we were impressed with their experiences. In May 2003, Boston IVF became the first IVF practice in North America to be certified to the ISO 9000 system.

The ISO Process

Any QMS system, such as ISO, involves a process technique. The classic process approach modified for an IVF center is illustrated in Figure 2. Every organization starts with the needs of our customers (patients). Understanding their needs is important. We may think that the 'product' from our centers for infertile women is a baby; but it's much more than that. Sure, we want every patient to have a baby but many are unsuccessful despite everyone's best efforts. In fact, we do not only treat women, we treat mostly couples, so our customers are couples. And, since we cannot achieve 100% success, then the real product for any IVF center is the resolution of infertility (with a baby or not). We provide a service to our couples; and in order to satisfy them, we need to understand their needs. It is an interesting exercise to get to the bottom of this; but, only after understanding their needs can we put an effective system in place to address them.

Management is responsible to be certain that the organization has the physical plant, adequately trained staff, and equipment to perform its work. Only then can IVF treatment be performed. Management must determine if the treatment has been good from many different aspects (not just, whether a pregnancy ensued). Good treatment includes many different facets, e.g. nurse and doctor communication, ultrasound and blood testing, and laboratory functions (fertilization, embryo development and implantation).

Patient satisfaction and happiness with the service provided is the end result of what we do. As a reminder, babies are only part of the product. A patient, who is pregnant following IVF but is also angry with the staff because of many errors that occurred along the way, is not a happy patient necessarily. She may not refer patients to the IVF center despite having a 'positive' pregnancy test. Fertility specialists appreciate the patient who is grateful to the staff even in the absence of a positive pregnancy test.

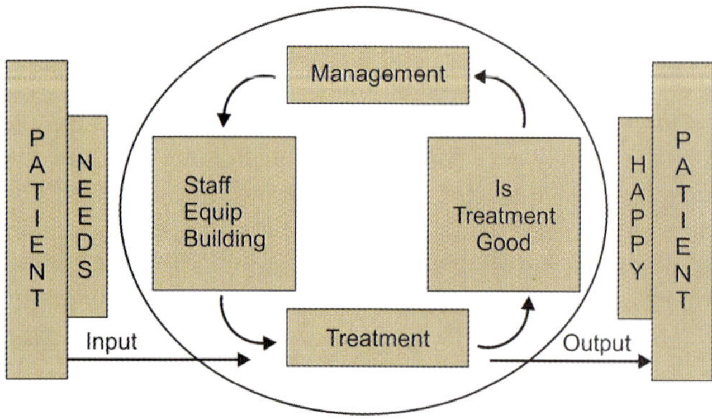

Figure 2 Implementation of a process approach

What are the Advantages of a Quality Management System in *in vitro* Fertilization?

There are numerous advantages of implementing a QMS. There is no better way to ensure high quality in an IVF center than to implement a QMS such as ISO. An important advantage is patient satisfaction. The focus of ISO is the customer and of course, the most important customers are our patients. Everyone in the organization is 'on the same page'; it is all about the patient and almost everything, we do, comes down to this. With a patient-focus approach paramount, patient satisfaction improves.

Another important customer of an IVF center is the referring physician. They must be understood in terms of their needs. Obviously, a report from a satisfied patient is the best feedback to the referring doctor; their needs go beyond this in terms of communication, involvement, integration, etc.

The essential goal of a QMS, such as ISO, is to ensure the reproducibility of all methods and competence in duties performed by the personnel. IVF centers are often large organizations, often with multiple offices. Consistency in how patients should be handled from office-to-office, nurse-to-nurse, doctor-to-doctor, or secretary-to-secretary. If there is consistency, then patients' expectations are anticipated and realized.

Since the emersion of IVF technology 30 years ago, IVF has become an established medical procedure, and most IVF programs are well-established and mature in nature. It is important to maintain excitement and passion in one's work environment to prevent complacency. There is not a better way to engage employees than to ask them to be part of the building of a QMS. Asking staff for their input motivates the team members in their work, knowledge and efficiency.

There are important business reasons to implement a QMS. ISO allows for efficiency by carefully working through workflow and other issues. Efficiency can lead to greater profitability and a competitive edge in gaining market share.

Implementing a QMS requires dedication and commitment. All employees must be familiar with the benefits and advantages of the system and 'buy in' to it. It also requires a financial commitment since it takes time. We highly recommend a consultant assist the organization to achieve the goal of certification, and the costs associated with this will vary based upon the size of the company and the existing systems in place. Although many books have been written about ISO, there are few that are specific to an IVF program.[4]

The ISO Requirements

The principles of ISO are, in fact, quite simple. ISO asks us to describe how you do things ('say what you do') and then be sure that you are doing things the way you said that you were going to do them ('do what you say').

Steps to ISO Certification

- Know the ISO standard
- Document a quality management system
- Implement the system
- Be surveyed (assessed) by an accredited registrar
- Be issued a certificate of conformity
- Be listed in the register of certified companines

Figure 3 The steps to ISO certification

The steps to ISO certification are listed in Figure 3. First, you must know the ISO system. Once familiar with the system, documentation of a quality system must follow. The master document for the QMS is the Quality Manual, a detailed analysis of the system parts. Once the documentation for all the processes in the organization is complete, they must be implemented. The next step is for a survey by an accredited ISO Registrar and the issuance of an ISO certificate. Regular future surveys are required for ongoing ISO accreditation.

1. Control of Documents
2. Control of Quality Records
3. Internal Audits
4. Control of Nonconformity
5. Corrective and Preventive Action

Figure 4 The procedural requirements for ISO

There are several ISO requirements as shown in Figure 4. Document control is an important element. It is an interesting exercise to collect all documents used in ones center. I was surprised to learn of the numerous piece of paper circulating; in fact, we had close to 3,000 documents, many of them old and superseded by newer versions of the same document. It was a mess, which needed to be cleaned up. A QMS system controls all documents by eliminating those that are not in use, organizing them, and placing one person in charge of that document and its revisions. Another QMS task is to control all the records associated with the organization. These include job descriptions, workflows, procedures and a master document, which describes the QMS.

It is important for any organization to be certain that a task is being performed according to the way it was designed. One way to ensure this is to audit the process. Typically, an internal audit involves someone in the organization (typically from another department) determining if the task is done according to its description. Nonconformities are errors or deviations from a plan; these must be collected and addressed. If errors occur, a corrective action and staff members must follow them. Also, staff must be able to raise methods to prevent errors or problems in the future ('preventative action').

SUMMARY

In vitro fertilization statistics alone cannot be used to reflect the quality of an IVF program. Good programs focus on patients as customers and strive to meet the needs of their customers. A quality management system establishes principles to ensure that processes and procedures are controlled and helps the organization meet the needs of their customers. A QMS, such as ISO, can be applied to any service business and, when applied to an IVF program, can improve the organization's ability to ensure that our patients are satisfied with the care that they receive.

REFERENCES

1. Alper MM, Brinsden PR, Fischer R, et al. Is your IVF programme good? Hum Reprod. 2002;17(1):8-10.
2. Furlong CB. Marketing for Keeps: Building Your Business by Retaining Your Customers. New York: John Wiley & Sons; 1993.
3. Alper MM. IVF outcomes: why doesn't anyone get it? Fertil Steril. 2004;81(3):514-6.
4. Bryce Carson, Michael Alper, Christoph Keck. Quality Management Systems for Assisted Reproductive Technology. London: Taylor & Francis Group; 2004.

6

Birth Defects and Assisted Reproductive Technology

Section Content

33

Assisted Reproductive Technology and Birth Defects

Erin Foran Wolff, Robert W Rebar, Alan H DeCherney

Chapter Contents

INTRODUCTION

Since the birth of Louise Browne in 1978, more than 3 million humans had been born by assisted reproductive technologies (ARTs) by 2006. The field of reproductive sciences is unique in that many of the clinical advances have occurred directly at the 'bedside' instead of at the 'bench'; in other fields, new techniques are introduced into clinical medicine only after rigorous testing under experimental protocols. The advent of *in vitro* fertilization (IVF) is also unique from a legal standpoint in that it became firmly established in clinical practice before the legalities were addressed, such as whether embryos are property or what name to put as 'mother' on the birth certificate of gestational carrier pregnancies. While some of these situations now have case law established to guide medical practice for reproductive therapies, science has not been afforded the opportunity to catch up. Rigorous hypothesis testing to examine possible effects of ART on women undergoing fertility therapy and their offspring has never occurred.

RESEARCH IN ASSISTED REPRODUCTIVE TECHNOLOGY IS DIFFICULT

The difficulty in performing IVF research using typical approaches is multifactorial. First, IVF research shares some commonalities with conducting research on pregnant women; the unsavory thought of randomly allocating half of the pregnant women in a study to a potentially inferior, or worse, harmful assignment exceeds the comfort zone of most institutional review boards and other regulators. An unanticipated side-effect of recent advances in our understanding of the fetal origins of disease has validated some of these concerns. Experimentation during IVF is a step away from pregnancy, where similar concerns often exist. Apprehension about experimenting on embryos has been confounded by a second factor hindering the highest levels of scientific rigor in our field: explicit federal legislation, such as the Dickey-Wicker Amendment, which prohibits research resulting in the intentional destruction of an embryo. This prevents basic research at the bench with federal funds, but has also been extended out of caution by institutions, such as the National Institutes of Health, to apply to any research that is applied to ART. Fear of loss of congressional funding prevents any IVF at the National Institutes of Health, who's funding is dependent on a continuing resolution vote every 2-year. Thirdly, in the United States, ART is expensive for patients, who often are paying out of pocket. Patients and providers are understandably reluctant to take the chance of gambling with this degree of financial investment.

CLINICAL EXPERIENCE WITH ASSISTED REPRODUCTIVE TECHNOLOGY

At first glance, it may seem preposterous that with such a common clinical practice worldwide, the answer to the question, "Is ART associated with congenital anomalies?" is not clear. ART has become standard of care despite the lack of a single rigorous, large scale, prospective, randomized trial to answer this question. We are left using weaker scientific evidence to answer this question indirectly, i.e. epidemiologic evidence (that is subject to inherent biases that occur through lack of randomization in a research setting). Much of the limited evidence that does exist was obtained after a decade or more of the use of ART. The good news is that in the first 30-year of anecdotal experience with ART, children born from this technology appear remarkably normal. In other words, if ART is associated with adverse outcomes like congenital anomaly rates, they are likely relatively small compared to real risks of multiple gestation and the accompanied sequelae.

THEORETICAL CONCERNS

Because assisted reproduction bypasses many of the naturally occurring steps in conception and reproduction, understandable concern exists about the potential impact of these interventions. First, there is concern that ART is subverting natural selection influences on reproduction.[1] Specifically, there is concern that couples, who are subfertile might harbor heritable factors that predispose to infertility/subfertility or other conditions that confer a negative survival advantage.[2,3] Second, there is concern that the ART treatments or the manipulation of the gametes in the *in vitro* environment will introduce damage or alterations to the resultant embryo.[4-10] For instance, the supraphysiologic hormonal levels achieved during ART may be detrimental to the pregnancy or developing child. We tend to think of the transient elevation in estradiol levels at the time of conception. However, there is also a supraphysiologic number of *corpus lutea* that remain hormonally active throughout pregnancy, with possibly unrecognized effects. Third, overcoming factors making it difficult to conceive may result in pregnancy in women not optimally fit for pregnancy. An unfavorable environment for pregnancy may lead to poor pregnancy outcomes in infertile women.

ANIMAL DATA

Many animal studies have demonstrated adverse effects of ART on offspring. Because culturing the embryo in media while *in vitro* is necessary for survival, gametes and embryos are obligated to come in direct contact with artificial environments. In animal data, it appears that there are effects at a variety of steps during ART: superovulation,[5,11,12] merely manipulating an *in vivo* conceived embryo and placing it back in a uterus without *in vitro* culture,[4] IVF,[13,14] ooplasm manipulation,[15] intracytoplasmic sperm injection (ICSI),[16] the media used,[17,18] culture of a developing embryo even if conceived *in vivo*,[19] and oxygen tension of the culture system used.[20] The effects of these factors have been described in placental development,[17] large offspring syndrome,[21-23] behavior,[24,25] altered gene methylation[26] and loss of imprinting.[4] However, vast differences in physiology between humans and rodents cannot be ignored; findings in animals do not always translate into similar effects in humans.[27] It is critical that the effects of ART are studied in humans to determine their true magnitude.

TWINS AND CONGENITAL MALFORMATIONS

With the advent of ART, it became clear early on that there were significant risks associated with multiple pregnancies resulting from ART.[28] This has lead to strict national legislation in some European countries, and greater awareness of the problem in the United States,[29] which has lead to decreasing multiple gestation rates.[30] Multiple gestations are associated with a host of adverse outcomes;[31-34] multiple gestation resulting from ART contribute greatly to the increased risk of spontaneous abortion,[35] preterm delivery,[36,37] preterm complications, low birth weight,[38] gestational diabetes, placenta previa, pre-eclampsia, vaginal bleeding, cesarean delivery,[39-41] neonatal intensive care unit admission, intraventricular hemorrhage,[42] and perinatal death.[43]

Twins and triplets have a higher rate of malformations than singletons,[44] and the increased rate of multiples accounts for much of the observed risk with ART.[45-49]

ADVERSE OUTCOMES IN SINGLETON ASSISTED REPRODUCTIVE TECHNOLOGY PREGNANCIES

Surprisingly, many of the adverse associations with ART were also present in singleton pregnancies.[34,45,50-52] However, many studies failed to control for underlying conditions that act as confounders of patients requiring ART[53] (e.g. advanced age, fibroids, uterine malformations, obesity, polycystic ovary syndrome, hormonal disorders and oligospermia). The largest of these effects are due to advancing maternal age at conception.[54-58]

There is extensive data which suggests that the effects of the underlying infertility or subfertility may also contribute to, or be the root cause of, adverse pregnancy outcomes associated with ART,[51,59-61] rather than the treatment effects. A notable exception to the evidence for this hypothesis was seen in a study of the entire population of Norway, where outcomes of ART pregnancies were compared to spontaneously conceived siblings.[62] No significant differences in birth weight, gestational age and preterm delivery were detected. Further evidence supporting an effect of the underlying infertility is a meta-analysis of surrogacy outcomes, which were associated with decreased rates of low birth weight deliveries and preterm deliveries in twin gestations.[63]

EARLY EVIDENCE OF BIRTH DEFECTS

Assisted reproductive technology has been implicated in many types of birth defects, but does appear to be stronger for some specific defects than others, such as chromosomal defects,[64,65] cardiovascular defects,[64,66-68] hypospadias,[69,70] genitourinary defects,[64,71] neural tube defects,[69,72] gastrointestinal defects,[68,69] cleft lip/cleft palate[68] and musculoskeletal defects.[64,66]

Many early studies on the association of ART and birth defects were conflicting, where some studies failed to detect an association.[73] However, many were limited methodologically due to sample size, comparison groups, or confounding factors.[53] In the New England Journal of Medicine, a publication by Hansen et al., in 2002,[64] a statistically significant difference in major birth defects (9% vs 4% for spontaneous conceptions) was detected in a Western Australian population after controlling for confounding factors including maternal age and parity. All birth defects were reported by a common national registry, and results were similar when controlling for pregnancy terminations for early detection of anomalies in IVF/ICSI pregnancies.

However, this and many other studies did not control for the effect of the underlying infertility on birth defects, which was found to be an important confounder of other adverse pregnancy outcomes observed with ART.

RECENT EVIDENCE: THE EFFECT OF UNDERLYING INFERTILITY

In subsequent studies, the effect of ART itself was begun to be teased apart from the confounding underlying fertility. In order to do this, a more appropriate control group would be infertile couples, who eventually spontaneously conceive. Ericson et al.[69] found similar increases in birth defects after ART as the Hansen study, but the association was lost after adjusting for infertility (i.e. involuntary childlessness). Similarly, in a study of the Danish national birth cohort, the effect of the underlying infertility on congenital malformation rate was again observed, but in this study, an independent effect of the infertility treatment itself was observed even when compared to infertile controls.[44] Of note, again an association specifically with genital organ abnormalities was detected (adjusted hazard ratio 2.32), even when using an infertile comparison group.

Remarkably, no differences in major malformations were detected in a study of surrogacy pregnancies, arguing against genetic influences of the underlying infertility.[63]

A genetic influence of the infertile male was seen in study comparing three groups: IUI with partners' sperm, donor IUI, and natural conceptions. Perinatal outcomes of low birth rate and preterm delivery were significantly more common in couples with IUI with the partners' sperm than natural conceptions. Interestingly, this difference was not seen in couples undergoing IUI with donor sperm.[74]

EPIGENETIC EFFECTS OF ASSISTED REPRODUCTIVE TECHNOLOGY

Angelman Syndrome

In humans, early clinical epigenetic concerns with ART arose around a specific subtype of epigenetic mechanisms: imprinting. This arose from early reports of ICSI offspring with a rare clinical syndrome, Angelman syndrome,[75,76] which occurs in only 1:15,000 births. Angelman syndrome is most frequently caused by non-epigenetic (i.e. genetic mutations) mechanisms, and only 5% are due to imprinting defects.[77] However, all of the early cases of Angelman syndrome in ART offspring were found to be caused by imprinting defects,[75,76,78] raising the question of whether ART induced epigenetic changes.

There was evidence that ART was not to blame. In 2005, Denmark National Registry published the outcomes of 25,000 children born after IVF and reported no cases of Angelman syndrome.[79] Again, the underlying infertility was implicated, where an identical increased risk of imprinting defects resulting in Angelman syndrome were reported in children born to subfertile couples, who did not have ART.[80] These findings were substantiated in a subsequent Dutch study; a similar rate of Angelman syndrome was detected in children born after ART (6.4%) as in infertile couples, who spontaneously conceived (6.8%) vs the general population (2.1%).[81] However, none of the ART cases were shown to be due to epigenetic mechanisms. Thus, the true nature of the association of ART with Angelman remains open to debate.

Beckwith-Wiedemann Syndrome

Beckwith-Wiedemann syndrome (BWS) is a rare growth disorder associated with abnormalities at chromosome 11p15, occurring in 1 of 13,700 births. This disorder was first linked to ART in 2003, where a BWS registry-based study identified a 4.6% rate of ART versus the 0.76% rate in the population,[82] which has been found in other registry-based survey studies.[81-85] The presence of a true association is strengthened by the fact that a consistent epigenetic abnormality was observed; most of the ART related BWS cases were found to be the result of altered methylation of multiple different genes in many studies,[21,82,84,86-89] though not all.[90-93] Once again, the underlying infertility was implicated as the true cause when more rigorous controls were used.[94]

OTHER EPIGENETIC EVIDENCE

Assisted reproductive technology has been linked to other imprinting disorders such as Prader-Willi syndrome, Silver-Russell syndrome, transient neonatal diabetes mellitus and maternal hypomethylation syndrome, but these conditions have weaker evidence.[95] Further, abnormal methylation patterns have been described in clinically normal children conceived by IVF,[96] raising the question, if abnormal methylation is a significant finding. This alternate hypothesis is supported by a study showing that methylation patterns vary greatly even in a given individual, and methylation status alters only 5% of imprinted gene expression.[10] Therefore, it is possible that ART is associated with epigenetic alterations, but these may not be clinically significant.

Male Factor Infertility

A well-described connection between infertility and heritable conditions is Y chromosome microdeletions associated with severe male factor infertility. Though this represents a small percentage of infertility patients, it validates concern that other heritable causes for infertility are being propagated by ART. Specifically, hypospadias in male offspring have been associated with ICSI[97] and IVF.[98] It is notable that the genital malformations, seen in the Danish national cohort, were associated exclusively with ART treatments associated with male factor infertility (IVF, ICSI, IUI) but not female hormonal treatment alone.[44] Similarly, no differences in outcomes were detected in women undergoing IUI with donor sperm, while adverse pregnancy outcomes were found in patients undergoing IUI with their partner's sperm.[74] Semen volume and sperm count have been inversely correlated with the male partner's parents' time to conception more than 1 year.[99] These findings provide scientific evidence that infertility treatment overcomes selective disadvantages that are propagated to the next generation where they have lower sperm concentrations, sperm count, smaller testis size, fewer motile sperm, fewer normal morphology sperm, lower testosterone levels and free androgen index.[100]

Progesterone Supplementation and Hypospadias

The association of hypospadias and ART also has historical literature that suggests an alternate pathway than genetic influences of ART on birth defects. Some studies,[101-105] but not all[105-115] detected an association with progesterone and hypospadias. Notably, the effect was always positive or even, but never reduced. This does have biologic plausibility, in that progesterone is a weak androgen and closure of the urethra is critically dependent on fetal androgens. Again, the optimal dose, duration and route for luteal supplementation in ART have not been determined with rigorous controlled studies. But the conflicting reports of the adverse effects of progesterone in pregnancy does highlight the fact that even treatments that are thought to be benign, could possibly have adverse effects—more is not always better.

A notable exception to the increased risks of congenital anomalies in multiples, which supports the progesterone effect on hypospadias, is a study that found that female IVF/ICSI twins actually experienced a lower risk of congenital abnormalities than spontaneously conceived female twins.[116] It is possible that the adverse effects of progesterone are most apparent in male fetuses. Further studies are needed to examine this association.

PATIENT COUNSELING

The complex interplay between infertility and infertility treatment may be hard to study, but it is even harder to explain to our infertility patients. Historically, the well-recognized multitude of adverse pregnancy outcomes associated with ART pregnancies have not played a large role in the informed consent and counseling before patients undergo treatment. At first, it was because there was not good evidence to provide patients. Then our understanding of the effects of underlying fertility became increasingly clear, which simultaneously exempted blame from our infertility treatments.

However, it is prudent to explain to infertile couples that, if they successfully become pregnant, they do have higher pregnancy risks and birth defect rates than a fertile population. This is important information for couples weighing risks and benefits of the viable alternatives to autologous fertility treatment: adoption, donor gametes, expectant management, or child free living.

CONCLUSION

In vitro fertilization has revolutionized the treatment of infertility and forever changed reproduction, allowing millions of people to have children. In general, children resulting from ART are remarkably normal. The adverse impact of multiple gestations resulting from assisted reproduction is real and far exceeds the risks to offspring resulting from ART to the best of our current understanding. The underlying condition of infertility in couples pursuing ART appears to account for much of the increased risk of birth defects. Patients should be counseled on the underlying risks and the alternatives to ART.

REFERENCES

1. Hawkins MM, Barratt CL, Sutcliffe AG, et al. Male infertility and increased risk of diseases in future generations. Lancet. 1999;354:1906-7.
2. Dowsing AT, Yong EL, Clark M, et al. Linkage between male infertility and trinucleotide repeat expansion in the androgen-receptor gene. Lancet. 1999;354:640-3.
3. Lopes FL, Fortier AL, Darricarrère N, et al. Reproductive and epigenetic outcomes associated with aging mouse oocytes. Hum Mol Genet. 2009;18:2032-44.
4. Rivera RM, Stein P, Weaver JR, et al. Manipulations of mouse embryos prior to implantation result in aberrant expression of imprinted genes on day 9.5 of development. Hum Mol Genet. 2008;17:1-14.
5. Fortier AL, Lopes FL, Darricarrère N, et al. Superovulation alters the expression of imprinted genes in the midgestation mouse placenta. Hum Mol Genet. 2008;17:1653-65.
6. Doherty AS, Mann MR, Tremblay KD, et al. Differential effects of culture on imprinted H19 expression in the preimplantation mouse embryo. Biol Reprod. 2000;62:1526-35.
7. Mann MR, Lee SS, Doherty AS, et al. Selective loss of imprinting in the placenta following preimplantation development in culture. Development. 2004;131:3727-35.
8. Khosla S, Dean W, Reik W, et al. Culture of preimplantation embryos and its long-term effects on gene expression and phenotype. Hum Reprod Update. 2001;7:419-27.
9. Khosla S, Dean W, Brown D, et al. Culture of preimplantation mouse embryos affects fetal development and the expression of imprinted genes. Biol Reprod. 2001;64:918-26.
10. Turan N, Katari S, Gerson LF, et al. Inter- and intra-individual variation in allele-specific DNA methylation and gene expression in children conceived using assisted reproductive technology. PLoS Genet. 2010;6:e1001033.
11. Sato A, Otsu E, Negishi H, et al. Aberrant DNA methylation of imprinted loci in superovulated oocytes. Hum Reprod. 2007;22:26-35.
12. Stouder C, Deutsch S, Paoloni-Giacobino A. Superovulation in mice alters the methylation pattern of imprinted genes in the sperm of the offspring. Reprod Toxicol. 2009;28:536-41.
13. Giritharan G, Talbi S, Donjacour A, et al. Effect of in vitro fertilization on gene expression and development of mouse preimplantation embryos. Reproduction. 2007;134:63-72.
14. Corcoran D, Fair T, Park S, et al. Suppressed expression of genes involved in transcription and translation in in-vitro compared with in vivo cultured bovine embryos. Reproduction. 2006;131:651-60.
15. Cheng Y, Wang K, Kellam LD, et al. Effects of ooplasm manipulation on DNA methylation and growth of progeny in mice. Biol Reprod. 2009;80:464-72.
16. Giritharan G, Li MW, De Sebastiano F, et al. Effect of ICSI on gene expression and development of mouse preimplantation embryos. Hum Reprod. 2010;25:3012-24.
17. Fauque P, Mondon F, Letourneur F, et al. In vitro fertilization and embryo culture strongly impact the placental transcriptome in the mouse model. PLoS One. 2010;5:e9218.
18. Rinaudo P, Schultz RM. Effects of embryo culture on global pattern of gene expression in preimplantation mouse embryos. Reproduction. 2004;128:301-11.
19. Corcoran D, Rizos D, Fair T, et al. Temporal expression of transcripts related to embryo quality in bovine embryos cultured from the 2-cell to blastocyst stage in vitro or in vivo. Mol Reprod Dev. 2007;74:972-7.

20. Rinaudo PF, Giritharan G, Talbi S, et al. Effects of oxygen tension on gene expression in preimplantation mouse embryos. Fertil Steril. 2006;86:1252-65, 65.e1-36.
21. Hori N, Nagai M, Hirayama M, et al. Aberrant CpG methylation of the imprinting control region KvDMR1 detected in assisted reproductive technology-produced calves and pathogenesis of large offspring syndrome. Anim Reprod Sci. 2010;122:303-12.
22. Young LE, Sinclair KD, Wilmut I. Large offspring syndrome in cattle and sheep. Rev Reprod. 1998;3:155-63.
23. Young LE, Fernandes K, McEvoy TG, et al. Epigenetic change in IGF2R is associated with fetal overgrowth after sheep embryo culture. Nat Genet. 2001;27:153-4.
24. Ecker DJ, Stein P, Xu Z, et al. Long-term effects of culture of preimplantation mouse embryos on behavior. Proc Natl Acad Sci USA. 2004;101:1595-600.
25. Fernández-Gonzalez R, Moreira P, Bilbao A, et al. Long-term effect of in vitro culture of mouse embryos with serum on mRNA expression of imprinting genes, development, and behavior. Proc Natl Acad Sci USA. 2004;101:5880-5.
26. Ceelen M, Vermeiden JP. Health of human and livestock conceived by assisted reproduction. Twin Res. 2001;4:412-6.
27. Mestas J, Hughes CC. Of mice and not men: differences between mouse and human immunology. J Immunol. 2004;172:2731-8.
28. Reynolds MA, Schieve LA, Martin JA, et al. Trends in multiple births conceived using assisted reproductive technology, United States, 1997-2000. Pediatrics. 2003;111:1159-62.
29. Stillman R, Richter K, Banks N, et al. Elective single embryo transfer: a 6-year progressive implementation of 784 single blastocyst transfers and the influence of payment method on patient choice. Fertil Steril. 2009;92:1895-906.
30. Pandian Z, Bhattacharya S, Ozturk O, et al. Number of embryos for transfer following in vitro fertilisation or intra-cytoplasmic sperm injection. Cochrane Database Syst Rev. 2004:CD003416.
31. Multiple gestation pregnancy. The ESHRE Capri Workshop Group. Hum Reprod. 2000;15:1856-64.
32. Choi SH, Park YS, Shim KS, et al. Recent trends in the incidence of multiple births and its consequences on perinatal problems in Korea. J Korean Med Sci. 2010;25:1191-6.
33. Fitzsimmons BP, Bebbington MW, Fluker MR. Perinatal and neonatal outcomes in multiple gestations: assisted reproduction versus spontaneous conception. Am J Obstet Gynecol. 1998;179:1162-7.
34. McDonald SD, Murphy K, Beyene J, et al. Perinatel outcomes of singleton pregnancies achieved by in vitro fertilization: a systematic review and meta-analysis. J Obstet Gynaecol Can. 2005;27:449-59.
35. Schieve LA, Tatham L, Peterson HB, et al. Spontaneous abortion among pregnancies conceived using assisted reproductive technology in the United States. Obstet Gynecol. 2003;101:959-67.
36. Pregnancies and births resulting from in vitro fertilization: French national registry, analysis of data 1986 to 1990. FIVNAT (French In Vitro National). Fertil Steril. 1995;64:746-56.
37. Westergaard HB, Johansen AM, Erb K, et al. Danish National IVF Registry 1994 and 1995. Treatment, pregnancy outcome and complications during pregnancy. Acta Obstet Gynecol Scand. 2000;79:384-9.
38. Schieve LA, Meikle SF, Ferre C, et al. Low and very low birth weight in infants conceived with use of assisted reproductive technology. N Engl J Med. 2002;346:731-7.
39. Tough SC, Greene CA, Svenson LW, et al. Effects of in vitro fertilization on low birth weight, preterm delivery, and multiple birth. J Pediatr. 2000;136:618-22.
40. McFaul PB, Patel N, Mills J. An audit of the obstetric outcome of 148 consecutive pregnancies from assisted conception: implications for neonatal services. Br J Obstet Gynaecol. 1993;100:820-5.
41. D'Souza SW, Rivlin E, Cadman J, et al. Children conceived by in vitro fertilisation after fresh embryo transfer. Arch Dis Child Fetal Neonatal Ed. 1997;76:F70-4.
42. Linder N, Haskin O, Levit O, et al. Risk factors for intraventricular hemorrhage in very low birth weight premature infants: a retrospective case-control study. Pediatrics. 2003;111:e590-5.
43. Venn A, Lumley J. Births after a period of infertility in Victorian women 1982-1990. Aust NZJ Obstet Gynaecol. 1993;33:379-84.
44. Zhu JL, Basso O, Obel C, et al. Infertility, infertility treatment, and congenital malformations: Danish national birth cohort. BMJ. 2006;333:679.
45. Helmerhorst FM, Perquin DA, Donker D, et al. Perinatal outcome of singletons and twins after assisted conception: a systematic review of controlled studies. BMJ. 2004;328:261.
46. Allen VM, Wilson RD, Cheung A, et al. Pregnancy outcomes after assisted reproductive technology. J Obstet Gynaecol Can. 2006;28:220-50.
47. Sutcliffe AG, Ludwig M. Outcome of assisted reproduction. Lancet. 2007;370:351-9.
48. Bergh T, Ericson A, Hillensjö T, et al. Deliveries and children born after in-vitro fertilisation in Sweden 1982-95: a retrospective cohort study. Lancet. 1999;354:1579-85.
49. Pinborg A. IVF/ICSI twin pregnancies: risks and prevention. Hum Reprod Update. 2005;11:575-93.
50. Jackson RA, Gibson KA, Wu YW, et al. Perinatal outcomes in singletons following in vitro fertilization: a meta-analysis. Obstet Gynecol. 2004;103:551-63.
51. Draper ES, Kurinczuk JJ, Abrams KR, et al. Assessment of separate contributions to perinatal mortality of infertility history and treatment: a case-control analysis. Lancet. 1999;353:1746-9.
52. Hansen M, Bower C, Milne E, et al. Assisted reproductive technologies and the risk of birth defects—a systematic review. Hum Reprod. 2005;20:328-38.
53. Schieve LA, Rasmussen SA, Buck GM, et al. Are children born after assisted reproductive technology at increased risk for adverse health outcomes? Obstet Gynecol. 2004;103:1154-63.

54. Chung K, Coutifaris C, Chalian R, et al. Factors influencing adverse perinatal outcomes in pregnancies achieved through use of in vitro fertilization. Fertil Steril. 2006;86:1634-41.
55. Cnattingius S, Forman MR, Berendes HW, et al. Delayed childbearing and risk of adverse perinatal outcome. A population-based study. JAMA. 1992;268:886-90.
56. Dulitzki M, Soriano D, Schiff E, et al. Effect of very advanced maternal age on pregnancy outcome and rate of cesarean delivery. Obstet Gynecol. 1998;92:935-9.
57. Hansen JP. Older maternal age and pregnancy outcome: a review of the literature. Obstet Gynecol Surv. 1986;41:726-42.
58. Milner M, Barry-Kinsella C, Unwin A, et al. The impact of maternal age on pregnancy and its outcome. Int J Gynaecol Obstet. 1992;38:281-6.
59. Gelbaya T. Short and long-term risks to women who conceive through in vitro fertilization. Hum Fertil (Camb). 2010;13:19-27.
60. Henriksen TB, Baird DD, et al. Time to pregnancy and preterm delivery. Obstet Gynecol. 1997;89:594-9.
61. Williams MA, Goldman MB, Mittendorf R, et al. Subfertility and the risk of low birth weight. Fertil Steril. 1991;56:668-71.
62. Romundstad LB, Romundstad PR, Sunde A, et al. Effects of technology or maternal factors on perinatal outcome after assisted fertilisation: a population-based cohort study. Lancet. 2008;372:737-43.
63. Serafini P. Outcome and follow-up of children born after IVF-surrogacy. Hum Reprod Update. 2001;7:23-7.
64. Hansen M, Kurinczuk JJ, Bower C, et al. The risk of major birth defects after intracytoplasmic sperm injection and in vitro fertilization. N Engl J Med. 2002;346:725-30.
65. Seifer I, Amat S, Delgado-Viscogliosi P, et al. Screening for microdeletions on the long arm of chromosome Y in 53 infertile men. Int J Androl. 1999;22:148-54.
66. Anthony S, Buitendijk SE, Dorrepaal CA, et al. Congenital malformations in 4224 children conceived after IVF. Hum Reprod. 2002;17:2089-95.
67. Koivurova S, Hartikainen AL, Gissler M, et al. Neonatal outcome and congenital malformations in children born after in vitro fertilization. Hum Reprod. 2002;17:1391-8.
68. Reefhuis J, Honein MA, Schieve LA, et al. Assisted reproductive technology and major structural birth defects in the United States. Hum Reprod. 2009;24:360-6.
69. Ericson A, Källén B. Congenital malformations in infants born after IVF: a population-based study. Hum Reprod. 2001;16:504-9.
70. Wennerholm UB, Bergh C, Hamberger L, et al. Incidence of congenital malformations in children born after ICSI. Hum Reprod. 2000;15:944-8.
71. Wood HM, Trock BJ, Gearhart JP. In vitro fertilization and the cloacal-bladder exstrophy-epispadias complex: is there an association? J Urol. 2003;169:1512-5.
72. Births in Great Britain resulting from assisted conception, 1978-87. MRC working party on children conceived by in vitro fertilisation. BMJ. 1990;300:1229-33.
73. Al-Fifi S, Al-Binali A, Al-Shahrani M, et al. Congenital anomalies and other perinatal outcomes in ICSI vs. naturally conceived pregnancies: a comparative study. J Assist Reprod Genet. 2009;26:377-81.
74. Gaudoin M, Dobbie R, Finlayson A, et al. Ovulation induction/intrauterine insemination in infertile couples is associated with low-birth-weight infants. Am J Obstet Gynecol. 2003;188:611-6.
75. Cox GF, Bürger J, Lip V, et al. Intracytoplasmic sperm injection may increase the risk of imprinting defects. Am J Hum Genet. 2002;71:162-4.
76. Ørstavik KH, Eiklid K, van der Hagen CB, et al. Another case of imprinting defect in a girl with Angelman syndrome who was conceived by intracytoplasmic semen injection. Am J Hum Genet. 2003;72:218-9.
77. Clayton-Smith J, Laan L. Angelman syndrome: a review of the clinical and genetic aspects. J Med Genet. 2003;40:87-95.
78. Sutcliffe AG, Peters CJ, Bowdin S, et al. Assisted reproductive therapies and imprinting disorders—a preliminary British survey. Hum Reprod. 2006;21:1009-11.
79. Lidegaard O, Pinborg A, Andersen AN. Imprinting diseases and IVF: Danish National IVF cohort study. Hum Reprod. 2005;20:950-4.
80. Ludwig M, Katalinic A, Gross S, et al. Increased prevalence of imprinting defects in patients with Angelman syndrome born to subfertile couples. J Med Genet. 2005;42:289-91.
81. Doornbos ME, Maas SM, McDonnell J, et al. Infertility, zassisted reproduction technologies and imprinting disturbances: a Dutch study. Hum Reprod. 2007;22:2476-80.
82. DeBaun MR, Niemitz EL, Feinberg AP. Association of in vitro fertilization with Beckwith-Wiedemann syndrome and epigenetic alterations of LIT1 and H19. Am J Hum Genet. 2003;72:156-60.
83. Maher ER, Brueton LA, Bowdin SC, et al. Beckwith-Wiedemann syndrome and assisted reproduction technology (ART). J Med Genet. 2003;40:62-4.
84. Gicquel C, Gaston V, Mandelbaum J, et al. In vitro fertilization may increase the risk of Beckwith-Wiedemann syndrome related to the abnormal imprinting of the KCN1OT gene. Am J Hum Genet. 2003;72:1338-41.
85. Bowdin S, Allen C, Kirby G, et al. A survey of assisted reproductive technology births and imprinting disorders. Hum Reprod. 2007;22:3237-40.
86. Rossignol S, Steunou V, Chalas C, et al. The epigenetic imprinting defect of patients with Beckwith-Wiedemann syndrome born after assisted reproductive technology is not restricted to the 11p15 region. J Med Genet. 2006;43:902-7.
87. Tierling S, Souren NY, Reither S, et al. DNA methylation studies on imprinted loci in a male monozygotic twin pair discordant for Beckwith-Wiedemann syndrome. Clin Genet. 2010;79(6):546-53.
88. Lim D, Bowdin SC, Tee L, et al. Clinical and molecular genetic features of Beckwith-Wiedemann syndrome associated with assisted reproductive technologies. Hum Reprod. 2009;24:741-7.
89. Katari S, Turan N, Bibikova M, et al. DNA methylation and gene expression differences in children conceived in vitro or in vivo. Hum Mol Genet. 2009;18:3769-78.

90. Tierling S, Souren NY, Gries J, et al. Assisted reproductive technologies do not enhance the variability of DNA methylation imprints in human. J Med Genet. 2010;47:371-6.
91. Manning M, Lissens W, Bonduelle M, et al. Study of DNA-methylation patterns at chromosome 15q11-q13 in children born after ICSI reveals no imprinting defects. Mol Hum Reprod. 2000;6:1049-53.
92. Neri QV, Takeuchi T, Palermo GD. An update of assisted reproductive technologies results in the United States. Ann N Y Acad Sci. 2008;1127:41-8.
93. Pinborg A, Loft A, Aaris Henningsen AK, et al. Infant outcome of 957 singletons born after frozen embryo replacement: the Danish National Cohort Study 1995-2006. Fertil Steril. 2010;94:1320-7.
94. Strawn EY, Bick D, Swanson A. Is it the patient or the IVF? Beckwith-Wiedemann syndrome in both spontaneous and assisted reproductive conceptions. Fertil Steril. 2010;94:754.e1-2.
95. Amor DJ, Halliday J. A review of known imprinting syndromes and their association with assisted reproduction technologies. Hum Reprod. 2008;23:2826-34.
96. Gomes MV, Huber J, Ferriani RA, et al. Abnormal methylation at the KvDMR1 imprinting control region in clinically normal children conceived by assisted reproductive technologies. Mol Hum Reprod. 2009;15:471-7.
97. Bonduelle M, Wennerholm UB, Loft A, et al. A multicentre cohort study of the physical health of 5-year-old children conceived after intracytoplasmic sperm injection, in vitro fertilization and natural conception. Hum Reprod. 2005;20:413-9.
98. Bertelsmann H, de Carvalho Gomes H, Mund M, et al. The risk of malformation following assisted reproduction. Dtsch Arztebl Int. 2008;105:11-7.
99. Ramlau-Hansen CH, Thulstrup AM, Olsen J, et al. Parental subfecundity and risk of decreased semen quality in the male offspring: a follow-up study. Am J Epidemiol. 2008;167:1458-64.
100. Jensen TK, Jørgensen N, Asklund C, et al. Fertility treatment and reproductive health of male offspring: a study of 1,925 young men from the general population. Am J Epidemiol. 2007;165:583-90.
101. Mau G. Progestins during pregnancy and hypospadias. Teratology. 1981;24:285-7.
102. Monteleone Neto R, Castilla EE, Paz JE. Hypospadias: an epidemiological study in Latin America. Am J Med Genet. 1981;10:5-19.
103. Calzolari E, Contiero MR, Roncarati E, et al. Aetiological factors in hypospadias. J Med Genet. 1986;23:333-7.
104. Aarskog D. Maternal progestins as a possible cause of hypospadias. N Engl J Med. 1979;300:75-8.
105. Harlap S, Prywes R, Davies AM. Letter: Birth defects and oestrogens and progesterones in pregnancy. Lancet. 1975;1:682-3.
106. Michaelis J, Michaelis H, Glück E, et al. Prospective study of suspected associations between certain drugs administered during early pregnancy and congenital malformations. Teratology. 1983;27:57-64.
107. Katz Z, Lancet M, Skornik J, et al. Teratogenicity of progestogens given during the first trimester of pregnancy. Obstet Gynecol. 1985;65:775-80.
108. Resseguie LJ, Hick JF, Bruen JA, et al. Congenital malformations among offspring exposed in utero to progestins, Olmsted County, Minnesota, 1936-1974. Fertil Steril. 1985;43:514-9.
109. Check JH, Rankin A, Teichman M. The risk of fetal anomalies as a result of progesterone therapy during pregnancy. Fertil Steril. 1986;45:575-7.
110. Yovich JL, Turner SR, Draper R. Medroxyprogesterone acetate therapy in early pregnancy has no apparent fetal effects. Teratology. 1988;38:135-44.
111. Sweet RA, Schrott HG, Kurland R, et al. Study of the incidence of hypospadias in Rochester, Minnesota, 1940-1970, and a case-control comparison of possible etiologic factors. Mayo Clin Proc. 1974;49:52-8.
112. Czeizel A, Tóth J, Erodi E. Aetiological studies of hypospadias in Hungary. Hum Hered. 1979;29:166-71.
113. Källén B, Winberg J. An epidemiological study of hypospadias in Sweden. Acta Paediatr Scand. 1982; 293(Suppl):1-21.
114. Polednak AP, Janerich DT. Maternal characteristics and hypospadias: a case-control study. Teratology. 1983;28: 67-73.
115. Martínez-Frías ML, Rodríguez-Pinilla E, Bermejo E, et al. Prenatal exposure to sex hormones: a case-control study. Teratology. 1998;57:8-12.
116. Klemetti R, Gissler M, Sevón T, et al. Children born after assisted fertilization have an increased rate of major congenital anomalies. Fertil Steril. 2005;84:1300-7.

7

Regulation of Assisted Reproductive Technology Laboratory

SECTION CONTENT

34

Regulation of Assisted Reproductive Technology Laboratory

Sangita Jindal

CHAPTER CONTENTS

INTRODUCTION

Assisted reproductive technology (ART) has become one of the most widely regulated medical specialties in the world and is of significant interest as a public health issue. Though difficult to calculate exactly, the number today worldwide of ART laboratories is in the hundreds of thousands. The term 'ART laboratory' refers generally to three types of specialties: embryology, andrology and chemistry, and the most widely used ART procedure is *in vitro* fertilization (IVF).

ART was first used to treat humans in the United Kingdom (UK) and not surprisingly, the UK has one of the most comprehensive regulatory mechanisms for this technology.[1] When regulation was first introduced, public sentiment regarding ART was mixed, as IVF was considered new and experimental. Thirty years after the advent of IVF, many countries now have decades-old regulations in place. Issues around reproduction continue to be increasingly complex and sensitive, suggesting a significant need for regulation, but the model, scale and scope of regulation are still open for debate.

As with all medical practices, safety in ART laboratories is assured through a combination of federal and state government regulation and peer oversight.[2] On the federal level in the United States, three agencies regulate ART. The Centers for Disease Control and Prevention (CDC) collects and publishes data on ART procedures.[3] The Food and Drug Administration (FDA) controls approval and use of drugs, biological products and medical devices, and has jurisdiction over screening and testing of reproductive tissues, such as donor eggs and sperm.[4] And finally, the Centers for Medicare and Medicaid Services (CMS) is responsible for implementation of the Clinical Laboratory Improvement Amendments (CLIA) to ensure the quality of laboratory testing.[5]

On the state level, individual departments of health may issue licenses to laboratory personnel and conduct inspections, and issue licenses for ART laboratories that do diagnostic testing. Additionally, the field of ART exercises significant self-regulation to help ensure the continuing competence of IVF laboratories. Continuing medical education and periodic re-examination are required to maintain certification. The American Society for Reproductive Medicine[6] (ASRM) and the College of American Pathologists[7] (CAP) administer a reproductive laboratory accreditation program for embryology laboratories to assure that they conform to high national standards of quality. An affiliate of ASRM, the Society for Assisted Reproductive Technology[8] (SART), strictly monitors member clinics for adherence to ASRM guidelines, accreditation of their embryology laboratories, qualification of their staff and submission of data to the CDC.[2]

The primary goal of regulation in the ART laboratory is ensuring patient safety and protection. Patients are being treated by their physician and have limited or no direct contact with the ART laboratory. Thus, it remains a 'black box' to most of them. However, the technical errors that occur in the IVF laboratory can be catastrophic for an infertile couple, and often become publicized in the media, leading to even more anxiety and discomfort for patients.

A second, but no less significant, goal of regulation is to provide protection for the laboratory personnel themselves. ART programs are extremely hierarchal, with a chain of command that moves from the medical director through the laboratory director and finally to the laboratory personnel. Embryologists and andrologists work with patient's gametes, a task which is technically complicated and requires a high degree of expertise. Without properly documented training, quality control, or protocols to follow, laboratory personnel would be vulnerable to miscommunication and misdirection.

MODELS OF ASSISTED REPRODUCTIVE TECHNOLOGY LABORATORY OVERSIGHT

There are three models of oversight for ART laboratories: (1) Regulation (binding and mandatory requirements), (2) Guidelines (nonbinding recommendations), and (3) Market driven forces (no regulations or guidelines). In an environment where laboratories are regulated, state and federal governments may impose mandatory requirements. Government officials qualified as inspectors may inspect laboratories and impose financial penalties or even close facilities, if deficiencies are found. In the United States, CLIA licenses are required for andrology and chemistry laboratories but not embryology laboratories. Different regulatory agencies accredit on behalf of CLIA, and they have specific requirements that must be followed by the laboratories.

Often, ART laboratories are under the oversight of a peer-run agency, such as ASRM or SART, which provide guidelines and recommendations that are not binding. Finally, but less commonly, some infertility programs are completely market-driven, operating within the law, but outside the existing boundaries of regulation or guidelines, in order to provide patients whatever, possible services they request.

At all times, laboratory personnel must be mindful of the public interest. Laboratorians are participating in a medical treatment for women and men that are loaded with emotional, ethical, legal, religious and cultural dilemmas. It is shortsighted to say that the ART laboratory serves only a technical purpose, or laboratorians provide only technical expertise with no responsibility to the patient. We know from many cases in the media and from documented legal cases of malpractice based on ART procedures that the role of the laboratory is central. The availability and high-cost of IVF worldwide continue to be controversial and much discussed, and only add to the emotional burden on the infertile couple. Legal issues, such as privacy, ownership, inheritance and malpractice, underlie the many functions that are carried out in the ART laboratory. In the laboratory, embryos are created, destroyed, frozen and used to generate pregnancy. Further enhancing public interest is the concept of third party reproduction involving donor eggs, donor sperms, donor embryos and surrogacy. In the future, the ART laboratory may be at the forefront of promising new technologies such as therapeutic cloning and stem cell research. These are the actions with direct ethical, religious, social and cultural implications that make the ART laboratory worthy of oversight and regulation.

Given the diversity of cultures, traditions and religions around the world, it is hard to imagine creating an international consensus of regulation and oversight for all ART laboratories.[9] However, in the absence of regulation, clinic-specific policies and protocols can seem haphazard and unduly influenced by patient demand. Private clinics that operate on a for-profit basis are motivated to treat as many patients as possible in order to maximize their revenues. On the other hand, these clinics attract patients with good success rates, so there may be a tendency to discriminate and select the best candidates from the patient pool. There may also be a tendency to overtreat the patient, offering more invasive and sophisticated procedures that are more expensive, but which come with higher success rates. As the economic climate rises and falls, the clinics' standards for patient care and specific treatment policies may also tend to change. An inconsistent or haphazard approach to patient management may be the result. Finally, as patients become more informed and experienced with IVF, they may request customized treatment that includes gender selection or procedures still deemed experimental. As a result, regulation and oversight of the ART laboratory is recommended at local and national levels, if not by worldwide consensus.

ASSISTED REPRODUCTIVE TECHNOLOGY LABORATORY OVERSIGHT WORLDWIDE

The process of ART regulation is not always separate from religious, historic or cultural issues. Further, in countries that strictly regulate ART laboratories, it is often assumed that the regulations are designed to reflect prevailing political pressure rather than scientific principles. An overview of ART regulation in various countries is presented here.

United Kingdom

In 1990, the Human Fertilization and Embryology Authority (HFEA) was created as a competent authority to oversee therapeutic use of human gametes.[1] This regulation was the result of a decade long discussion mostly around the moral status of an embryo. The main goals of HFEA are to protect patients and offspring, allay public concerns, safeguard scientific freedom and protect people working in the field of ART.[10] The HFEA imposes limits on the number of embryos transferred to the patient following IVF since the UK government financially supports both the cost of IVF cycles and the cost to the health care system of high-order multiple births. As a result of this strictly regulated environment, critics of HFEA say that it places undue limits on clinical discretion, mandates licensing procedures that are bureaucratic and time-consuming, and imposes a licensing fee. It is generally agreed that the HFEA has been an effective advocate for patient rights and protections, and a powerful regulatory model for all other countries engaged in the regulation of ART though difficulties and frustrations caused by mandated restrictions on clinical practice must be acknowledged.

Europe

The European Society for Human Reproduction and Embryology (ESHRE) operates in a similar way to the ASRM in the United States. ESHRE is the peer-regulated governing body for ART programs in Europe, and as part of its mission of education, it publishes guidelines for good practice in IVF laboratories.[11] These guidelines are designed to assist laboratorians in making good decisions for optimal clinical outcomes.

The Italian government passed the Medically Assisted Reproductive Law in 2004. It prohibits the destruction of embryos or freezing of embryos, which means that all embryos created from an IVF cycle must be transferred to the patient. A negative and inadvertent consequence of this strict regulation is a significant higher-order multiple birth rate from ART in Italy.

Spain-passed a law regulating ART in 1988, and the Royal Decree was passed in 1996 outlining specifically what ART laboratories were able to do.[12] IVF can occur only in authorized centers but is open to all women. Embryos are for procreation only, not research. Donor cycles are allowed but surrogacy is not; nor is sex selection. Embryo freezing is allowed, but destruction or donation of frozen embryos is prohibited.

The German Embryo Protection Act was passed in 1990, stipulating that only three eggs can be collected for fertilization. No embryo freezing or discard is allowed, so potentially all three embryos must be transferred to patient, including young women, who otherwise would be receiving only one or two embryos. Again, this has the negative and inadvertent consequence of higher-order multiples. Preimplantation genetic diagnosis is prohibited.

Canada

The Canadian government passed the Human Reproduction Act in 2004, providing for partial regulation of IVF including the prohibition of sex selection for family balancing, cloning, or the creation of embryos for research.[13] It is left up to the individual provinces to provide oversight, so that IVF clinics adhere to the national regulations. ART laboratories can also participate in a voluntary accreditation process called Accreditation Canada that offers a rigorous inspection process and a three-year accreditation.

Australia

The Fertility Society of Australia provides national accreditation of ART programs through the Reproductive Technology Accreditation Committee (RTAC) which administers a national code of practice. Using this code, RTAC sets professional and laboratory standards for ART clinical practice. RTAC-accredited ART programs must also have a state license to provide ART services.

India

The ART Regulation Bill was passed in 2008. Prior to this, ART in over 200,000 unlicensed clinics was subject only to ethical guidelines published by the government, with no enforcement.[14] There is much anecdotal evidence of exploitation of vulnerable patients. The Regulation Bill requires scrutiny and licensing of clinics, enforcement of quality standards and credentials for sperm banks, and surrogacy.

REGULATION AND ACCREDITATION OF ASSISTED REPRODUCTIVE TECHNOLOGY LABORATORIES AND PERSONNEL

United States Federal Laws and Regulations

Centers for Disease Control and Prevention

The CDC defines ART as all fertility treatments in which both eggs and sperm are handled, based on a 1992 federal act that endorses standard definitions, and requires annual reporting of ART cycle data.[3] This includes reporting from all programs academic or private, large or small, members or non-members of the ASRM and its affiliated society, SART. The data collected include the patients' infertility diagnoses, clinical information pertaining to the ART procedure and statistics on resulting pregnancies and births, all categorized by maternal age. Individual clinics and aggregate national data on infertility procedures and their success rates are generated, and consumer access to the report enables would-be parents to review details about ART clinics nationwide. The CDC and SART also serves the professional community by providing a way to monitor the operation of individual clinics and the number of multiple births, which are more dangerous for the infants and mothers and more costly for parents and society.[3]

Clinical Laboratories Improvement Amendments

In 1988, the United States federal government passed a law called the Clinical Laboratories Improvement Amendments, more commonly known as CLIA. The objective of the CLIA program is to ensure quality laboratory testing by establishing standards for accuracy, reliability and timeliness of patient test results. A laboratory is defined as any facility that tests specimens derived from humans for the assessment of health or the diagnosis, prevention and treatment of disease. CLIA regulations, published in 1992, are based on the complexity of the test method; thus, the more complicated the test, the more stringent the requirements.[5] Within the reproductive field, all US andrology laboratories that offer semen analysis, as well as chemistry laboratories that offer hormone testing on serum samples, must be licensed by CLIA. Embryology is not considered a testing laboratory; rather it serves a therapeutic service for patients. To comply with CLIA, laboratories must register and be surveyed to become certified. The survey process is outcome-oriented and utilizes a quality assurance focus to assess compliance. Once a laboratory is licensed by CLIA, it is able to operate, hire appropriate laboratory staff and bill patients for services. Laboratories must adhere to CLIA standards in order to be accredited for renewal, which is done on a regular basis. There are a number of regulatory agencies that may accredit reproductive laboratories on behalf of CLIA:

College of American Pathologists: This agency has specific checklists for reproductive laboratories, and conducts announced inspections every two years. Inspections are conducted by peers (i.e. laboratory directors of other reproductive laboratories) in a process that is intended to be collegial and educational, as well as a rigorous. The checklists are extremely comprehensive, making CAP the 'gold standard' accreditation that a reproductive laboratory can achieve.

The Joint Commission (TJC): The Joint Commission (TJC) commonly accredits large hospitals, but also inspects and accredits ART laboratories located in a hospital setting every three years. There are no specific checklists provided to reproductive laboratories by TJC; rather, the laboratory is expected to adhere to general quality control and patient control standards. All three types of reproductive laboratories are able to be accredited by TJC.

Commission on Office Laboratory Accreditation: The Commission on Office Laboratory Accreditation (COLA) was founded in 1988 as a private alternative to help laboratories stay in compliance with CLIA. Through its practical and educational accreditation methods, COLA gained authority to accredit laboratories by 1997 and is known for accrediting physician office laboratories as well as hospital and independent laboratories. COLA is able to accredit only chemistry laboratories within ART programs every two years.

Food and Drug Administration: The FDA is responsible for protecting the public health by assuring the safety, efficacy and security of drugs, biological products, and medical devices. Since 1995, the FDA has also had jurisdiction overscreening and testing of reproductive tissues, such as the eggs and sperm that will be implanted in human recipients.[15] The agency has strict requirements for egg and sperm donors, including thorough medical histories, identification controls and freedom from infectious diseases. In addition, the FDA conducts vigorous and unannounced inspections every two years of the facilities in which reproductive tissues are handled. Inspectors can order the recall or destruction of tissue that is infected with a communicable disease. The agency has established good tissue practices that are codified in an industry guidance document.[4]

United States State Laws and Regulations

In addition to federal regulations, a number of US states have imposed laws and restrictions on ART laboratories. In 1999, the CDC published requirements for certification of embryology laboratories. They include requirements for administration of a continuing certification program by the states, quality assurance and control standards, an inspection system, and conditions under which certification can be suspended or revoked. States may choose whether they wish to be part of this laboratory certification program.

New York State Department of Health

The New York state department of health has extensive policies that laboratories must follow in order to be accredited to operate within New York state. The New York state tissue bank regulates the screening, testing, labeling, distribution and storage of donor gametes, specifically donor eggs, sperm and embryos. New York state tissue bank makes unannounced inspections every 2 years and holds ART programs and their laboratories to strict standards. The recent federal involvement of the FDA in donor tissue use in ART was based on the model of the New York state tissue bank.

Each state in the United States has a department of health, each with varying degrees of oversight and regulation of ART laboratories. The state health departments of New York and California are particularly active in regulating ART laboratories and their personnel. In addition to setting individual state policies for insurance coverage for infertility patients, different states have different policies for CLIA laboratory inspections, use of donor tissue and licensure of ART laboratory personnel depending on whether the laboratory is part of a large medical institution or part of a small physician office.

United States Peer Oversight

American Association of Tissue Banks

To help ensure that tissue-banking activities are performed in a professional manner consistent with the American Association of Tissue Banks' standards, the association initiated an accreditation program for tissue banks in 1986. Tissue banks receive accreditation for retrieval, processing, storage and/or distribution of tissue following a comprehensive guidance document, similar to New York state department of health and FDA. The process is voluntary, with self-inspection followed by inspection from an outside expert.[16]

American Board of Bioanalysis

The American Board of Bioanalysis (ABB) certifies personnel working in high-complexity reproductive laboratories.[17] In order to be a member of SART, an ART laboratory must have a laboratory director, who is accredited by ABB as a high-complexity laboratory, director (HCLD), who can direct embryology, andrology and chemistry laboratories. Alternatively, an ART program may have an individual, accredited as an embryology laboratory director (ELD), responsible for directing the non-CLIA embryology laboratory only. In addition to the director level accreditation, the ABB also accredits laboratorians at the technical supervisor (TS) level (TS embryology and TS andrology) and at the general supervisor (GS) level (GS embryology and GS andrology). There is no specific supervisor accreditation for the moderate-complexity chemistry laboratory.

Laboratory Accreditation

The CAP and ASRM developed the Reproductive Laboratory Accreditation Program for embryology laboratories.[2] This program was established because the functions of ART laboratories are highly specialized. Recognized as an authorized accrediting agency, CAP uses multidisciplinary teams of practicing laboratory professionals as inspectors. The goal of the inspection teams is to ensure that reproductive laboratories conform to national standards for the education, certification, and expertise of laboratory personnel, as well as for their authority and responsibilities. The laboratory must have a performance improvement plan and a quality control program to anticipate and prevent errors. Its instruments must be properly maintained and calibrated, and it must have a proficiency testing system in place that assures test reliability through an interlaboratory comparison program. To maintain accreditation, laboratories are inspected regularly. They must also perform periodic self-evaluations and document any necessary corrective actions between site visits.

Society for Assisted Reproductive Technology

Society for Assisted Reproductive Technology (SART), an affiliate society of ASRM, includes more than 90% of American fertility clinics.[8] It has strict membership requirements. As a condition of membership, clinics must report their outcomes to the CDC as well as to SART, have accredited embryology laboratories, adhere to the Ethics and Practice Committee guidelines of ASRM, and have appropriately trained staff. Failure to adhere to these criteria can result in revocation of membership. Although this does not prevent the clinic from continuing to operate, the membership status of a clinic is included in the CDC's federally mandated annual report on ART success rates.

ASRM and SART membership is voluntary, and signifies a practitioner's commitment to adhering to the best practices in reproductive medicine. The societies may issue a warning or censure, or a suspension or revocation of membership for failure to maintain the requirements for membership, for ethical violations, or for any other cause, they deem sufficient. ASRM has published guidelines for ART laboratories that are strongly recommended but are not mandated by law.[18,19] The guidelines that pertain specifically to IVF laboratory and personnel are described in Table 1.

CONCLUSION

Ideally, standards set by our profession would provide a framework for self-regulation of ART. These standards would be based on broad principles that avoid including details that cannot keep pace with science. This evidence-based approach should be used to generate national practice guidelines similar to those already in place in the United States through ASRM and SART, in Australia through the Fertility Society of Australia and RTAC and in Europe through ESHRE. Admittedly, a self-regulated system would not be invulnerable to abuse. When professional guidelines are breached, as they were in the recent octuplet pregnancy and birth in California,[20] the public, spurred by sensationalized media coverage and largely unaware of the way medical practice is regulated in the United States, calls out for additional legal enforcements and punishments and restrictions.[2] The debate of autonomy versus regulation will undoubtedly continue.

In countries where the government provides financial support for ART, some regulation is acceptable, for example limiting the number of government-funded ART cycles one patient can have. A limit on the number of cycles is a benefit of regulation, ensuring that the tax dollars of all citizens are available to as many patients as possible seeking infertility treatment. An argument may be made that the government should also be able to regulate the number of embryos transferred to the patient, especially in a universal health care system where the costs of supporting newborns from high-order multiple births must be borne by the government. This additional level of regulation may become a burden, outweighing the benefit for a patient whose particular case (for example an older patient with reduced chances of success following IVF) does not fall within the strict limits established by a government agency. Further, the inadvertent negative consequences of regulating the number of embryos that may be transferred to the patient have been seen in countries such as Italy and Germany,

Table 1 Summary of ASRM minimal guidelines for ART laboratory (embryology), and laboratory personnel

ASRM Guideline	Description
Laboratory accreditation	• By CAP, TJC, or NYS Tissue Bank
Compliance	• With FDA, local, state, or federal licensing
Laboratory staffing	• Minimum of two qualified persons, who can perform all technical services
Embryo laboratory director	• Have PhD, MD, DO or be grandfathered in prior to 1999 • Be HCLD or ELD (ABB) since 2006 • Have 2 years experience in IVF • Have specialized training or expertise in IVF • Demonstrate technical competency • Have experience with problem solving, experimental design, statistics • Formulate laboratory policies and protocols • Communicate with medical director • Earn twelve hours continuing education units (CEU) per year
Embryo laboratory supervisor	• Day-to-day supervision of laboratory personnel performing ART procedures • BS or MS in chemical, physical, biological, medical technology, clinical or reproductive laboratory science from an accredited institution • Documented training, which includes performing, at a minimum, at least 60 ART procedures under supervision • Earn 12 CEU per year in ART or clinical laboratory practice • Perform at least 20 ART procedures per year
Embryology laboratory technologist	• BS or MS in chemical, physical, biological, medical technology, clinical or reproductive laboratory science from an accredited institution • Documented training, which includes performing, at a minimum, at least 30 ART procedures under supervision • Earn 12 CEU per year in ART or clinical laboratory practice • Perform at least 20 ART procedures per year

Contd...

Contd...

ASRM Guideline	Description
Personnel records	• Itemized list of all personnel • List of education, training and job qualifications of all laboratory personnel • Organizational chart documenting the chain of command • Training of personnel for each specific laboratory test offered; definitive training programs for all procedures should be established • Personnel participation in continuing education • Ongoing technical competency • Health status, physical examinations, or laboratory tests on personnel • Annual performance reviews for personnel
Laboratory space and design	• Adequate space to ensure safe and comfortable working conditions • Laboratory should be in low-traffic area proximal to procedure room • Adequate equipment to support patient volume • Separate media preparation area and separate office area recommended • Minimize or eliminate any toxic materials, aerosol use, etc.
Equipment and procedure manuals	• Require alarm systems, backup systems • Require measuring devices for daily monitoring of equipment • Use disposable materials when possible • Use nontoxic media within expiry • Detailed policies and procedures available to all staff, reviewed annually
Laboratory safety and infection control	• Policies and procedures available to all staff, reviewed annually • Use universal precautions • Should have exposure control plan • Material safety data sheets should be available
Quality control/Quality assurance	• Policies and procedures available to all staff, reviewed annually • Policies on sample preparation, labeling, handling, storage • QA program should look at the laboratory as a whole and identify problems or errors that exist in order to improve the entire process • Laboratory must participate in proficiency testing

ABB: American Board of Bioanalysis; ART: assisted reproductive technology; ASRM: American Society for Reproductive Medicine; BS: Bachelor of Surgery; CAP: College of American Pathologists; CEU: continuing education units; DO: Doctor of Osteopathic Medicine; ELD: embryology laboratory director; FDA: Food and Drug Administration; HCLD: high-complexity laboratory director; IVF, in vitro fertilization; MD: Doctor of Medicine; MS: Master of Surgery; NYS: New York State; PhD: Doctor of Philosophy; TJC: The Joint Commission

where cultural and religious influences impact the clinical management of the ART patient.

In the United States, government regulations take the form of the FDA's oversight of use of donor gametes. Because of the risk of infectious disease being transmitted from donor to recipient, regulation of this aspect of ART may help protect the donor, the recipient, the baby resulting from ART and the laboratory personnel. However, the risk to citizens from government regulation is that the response to changing clinical protocols and standards of care is slow, and regulations once designed to be beneficial can instead become a hindrance.

At all times, the ART laboratory and its personnel must be mindful of their responsibility to the patient. Laboratorians are called upon to provide scientific and technical services for patients; this should be accomplished without a paternalistic approach that fails to account for the autonomy of the patient, despite their vulnerability. Through peer review and self-regulation based on the highest standards of evidence-based medicine, laboratorians are encouraged to take a leadership role in determining guidelines and recommendations for the ART laboratory practice.

REFERENCES

1. English V. Autonomy versus protection--who benefits from the regulation of IVF? Hum Reprod. 2006;21(12):3044-9.
2. American Society for Reproductive Medicine. (2010). Oversight of assisted reproductive technology. [online]. Available from web address http://www.asrm.org/Oversight_of_ART/ [Accessed June 2011].
3. Centers for Disease Control and Prevention. (1992). Assisted reproductive technology (ART). [online]. Available from web address http://www.cdc.gov/art/ [Accessed June 2011].

4. Food and Drug Administration. (2007). Guidance for industry: eligibility determination for donors of human cells, tissues, and cellular and tissue-based products. [online]. Available from web address http://www.fda.gov/biologicsbloodvaccines/guidancecomplianceregulatoryinformation/guidances/tissue/ucm073964.htm [Accessed June 2011].
5. Centers for Medicare and Medicaid Services. (1992) Clinical laboratory improvement amendments (CLIA). [online]. Available from web address http://www.cms.gov/clia/ [Accessed June 2011].
6. American Society for Reproductive Medicine (ASRM). [online]. Available from web address www.asrm.org [Accessed June 2011].
7. College of American Pathologists (CAP). [online]. Available from web address www.cap.org [Accessed June 2011].
8. Society for Assisted Reproductive Technologies (SART). [online]. Available from web address http://www.sart.org/ [Accessed June 2011].
9. Schenker JG. Legal aspects of ART practice in Israel. J Assist Reprod Genet. 2003;20(7):250-9.
10. Human Fertilisation and Embryology Authority. (1992). First HFEA Annual Report 1992. [online]. Available from web address http://www.hfea.gov.uk/docs/Annual-Report-11th-2002.pdf [Accessed June 2011].
11. Gianaroli L, Plachot M, van Kooij R, et al. ESHRE guidelines for good practice in IVF laboratories. Committee of the special interest group on embryology of the European Society of Human Reproduction and Embryology. Hum Reprod. 2000;15(10):2241-6.
12. Boada M, Veiga A, Barri PN. Spanish regulations on assisted reproduction techniques. J Assist Reprod Genet. 2003;20(7):271-5.
13. Assisted Human Reproduction Act, Canada, 2004.
14. Allahbadia GN, Kaur K. Accreditation, supervision, and regulation of ART clinics in India—a distant dream. J Assist Reprod Genet. 2003;20(7):276-80.
15. Katayama AC. U.S. ART practitioners soon to begin their forced march into a regulated future. J Assist Reprod Genet. 2003;20(7):265-70.
16. American Association of Tissue Banks. AATB standards for tissue banking, 12th edition. Virginia: American Association of Tissue Banks; 2008.
17. American Association of Bioanalysts. (2011). American Board of Bioanalysis (ABB). [online]. Available from web address www.aab.org/aab [Accessed June 2011].
18. Practice Committee of Society for Assisted Reproductive Technology, Practice Committee of American Society for Reproductive Medicine. Revised minimum standards for practices offering assisted reproductive technologies. Fertil Steril. 2008;90(5 Suppl):S165-8.
19. Practice Committee of American Society for Reproductive Medicine, Practice Committee of Society for Assisted Reproductive Technology. Revised guidelines for human embryology and andrology laboratories. Fertil Steril. 2008;90(5 Suppl):S45-59.
20. James SD. (2010). Octomom lesson: more couples pressure doctors. [online]. Available from web address http://abcnews.go.com/Health/octomom-doctor-nadya-suleman-pressured-multiple-embryos/story?id=11962324 [Accessed June 2011].

8

Emotional and Social Aspects of Infertility Treatment

Section Content

35

Emotional and Social Aspects of Infertility Treatment

Kristin L Rooney, Alice D Domar

Chapter Contents

INTRODUCTION

The inability to conceive a child is experienced as a stressful and traumatic situation by individuals and couples across the globe. It is estimated that 72.4 million women are currently infertile worldwide.[1] Of these, 40.5 million are currently seeking infertility medical care.[1] Approximately, half of women undergoing fertility treatment rated infertility as the most stressful experience of their life.[2] The impact of infertility can have harmful social and psychological consequences on both the individual and couple. In the United States, specialists, who study infertility have noted that infertile couple are one of the "most neglected and silent minorities."[3]

With innovations in medicine and technology, health care professionals have been able to diagnose and successfully treat more cases of infertility. Research has made tremendous strides in the treatment of both female and male factor infertility, and the field of assisted reproductive technology is advancing every day. The success of infertility treatment has led health care providers to view infertility as an organic condition rather than a psychological one, although clinical research shows that psychological issues can have a significant impact on outcome, in terms of both pregnancy rates as well as the emotional stamina to continue with treatment. Individuals dealing with infertility may face both personal and social distress. The emotional burden of infertility can be profound.

In this chapter, the emotional and social aspects of infertility is reviewed including the emotional effect on the individuals experiencing infertility as well as the strain infertility treatment may have on relationships between partners, family and friends. The varying cultural views and how society shapes how individuals feel about infertility is presented. Finally, research on effective psychological interventions, including cognitive behavioral interventions, is discussed.

The goal of this chapter is to provide a better understanding of the emotional and social burden of infertility, and how to support patients so that they can cope more effectively with treatment stressors.

THE EMOTIONAL IMPACT OF INFERTILITY

Infertility affects all aspects of an individual's life including the couple's relationship, their sex life, their relationships with family and friends, their job, their financial stability and their spiritual or religious beliefs. The emotional aspects of not being able to conceive can be daunting and many infertility patients describe it as a major life crisis. Couples undergoing an infertility diagnostic workup and subsequent treatment may experience anxiety, guilt, inadequacy, poor self-esteem and depression. Although it is not a terminal illness, women experiencing infertility have comparable levels of anxiety and depression to women with heart disease, HIV positive status, or metastatic cancer.[4] Research has shown the prevalence of depressive symptoms with the infertile population is twice that of the general population.[5] An alarming 40.8% of infertile women suffer from depression, while in one study, 86.8% of the patients reported experiencing anxiety.[6]

One of the most difficult emotional consequences of infertility is the loss of control over one's life.[3] The loss of control can begin when one senses that they have no control over their own reproduction, as they experience difficulties trying to conceive. When conception does not occur, individuals may become confused, frustrated and angry. Infertile women may become so focused on conception that they place professional goals, life pursuits and social connections on hold, and solely focus on having a baby.[3]

For many women who assumed they would grow up to have children of their own, infertility can challenge her core female identity. A diminished sense of self-worth may develop, because not only her body has 'failed' her but also because her self-esteem has been damaged.[7] It is common for infertile women to feel guilty and view the infertility as a punishment for past sexual indiscretions, abortions and contraceptive use.[3]

Women are typically identified as the patient in fertility centers, regardless of which spouse carries the diagnosis. It is frequently the women, who undergo the majority of the invasive procedures, are responsible for daily monitoring and frequent office visits for the vigorous treatment regimens. As such, women carry the psychological burden of infertility, even when the infertility diagnosis lies with the husband.[8] Women, tending to be more outwardly emotional beings, often seek support through family, friends, or support groups. A meta-analysis, exploring gender differences in coping with infertility, found women used the strategies of seeking social support, escape-avoidance, planful problem solving and positive reappraisal to a greater degree than their partners.[9]

Although women carry much of the infertility burden on their shoulders, men experience the psychological repercussions as well. The majority of research focuses on the effects women experience with treatment and do not include men, which is why it may appear that women experience a greater amount of emotional angst.[9] Many husbands tend to suppress their emotions in an effort to support their wives.[10] Research on North American couples indicates that men tend to use fewer coping strategies overall. They tend to increase their involvement at work and other activities, are more optimistic and problem-solving oriented, and they are less apt to use social support.[9] In addition, men appear to negotiate the transition to a childless lifestyle more easily than their wives, who find it more difficult to resolve the dilemma of infertility.[3]

As infertility does affect both partners going through treatment, it may often lead to arguments and heartaches. Unfortunately, when partners are under stress, there is a tendency to take it out on the ones they love, specifically their partner. A study of 162 couples evaluated men and women seeking infertility treatment, looking at how accurately each was able to rate their partners' quality of life. The findings indicated each partner had a tendency to underrate the others' view of quality of life.[11] It is important for individuals and couples going through treatment to be considerate of their partner and understand that while both are feeling the frustrations of infertility, each individual may deal with their emotions differently.

For most couples, infertility is viewed as a temporary life crisis but psychological symptoms may linger long after treatment ends for many. Research found 15% of women and 6% of men reported severe depressive symptoms after 1 year of unsuccessful treatment.[12] Among men, low emotional support, lack of appreciation and extreme demands from the partner were highly correlated with the incidence of severe depressive symptoms. Among both women and men, severe depressive symptoms were affected by low appreciation and high excessive demands from family and friends.[12] Women tend to maintain high levels of distress from the onset of the initial evaluation throughout treatment procedures, which in turn has an effect on sexual and marital satisfaction; men's marital satisfaction is significantly influenced by the acute stress of treatment demands.[13,14] Another factor affecting marital satisfaction is the strict treatment schedules around infertility. The demands of timed intercourse can make sex become mechanic and result in a decreased desire for intimacy as well as more instances of sexual function. The long period of diagnostic testing and treatment procedures have been linked to a higher frequency of male sexual disturbances, specifically erectile dysfunction, ejaculatory disorders, loss of libido and a decrease in the frequency of intercourse.[15]

FINANCIAL AND DECISION-MAKING STRESSORS

Fertility treatment is not only emotionally draining, but also poses a significant financial challenge for many couples. The majority of states in the United States do not require the health insurance companies to cover the cost of fertility treatment. Paying for testing and treatment can strain a couple's financial resources and add pressure to an already distressed couple. Given that fertility treatment is not a guarantee of success, it can also become quite a conflict for patients when weighing out the cost of treatment and the money they will have to spend in their efforts to conceive a child.

The decision-making process contributes greatly to the distress of couples undergoing infertility. When the diagnosis of infertility is unexplained, this may lead to a sense of hopelessness on the part of a couple.[16] The lack of explanation alone may be stressful, and what may be even more frustrating is the persistent questioning of potential causes and decisions about when treatment should be discontinued.[14]

As a result of treatment, couples often find themselves making moral and ethical decisions; two of the most challenging are the use of a third party and embryo disposition. If using a third party (donor or surrogate) enters into the treatment plan, it can create significant psychological distress.[3] It is advisable for couples to consult a mental health counselor specializing in third-party reproduction when making such difficult decisions. The ethical decision of disposition of cryopreserved embryos, ooctyes, or sperm can be enormously difficult for *in vitro* fertilization (IVF) participants to comprehend. Studies found the majority of individuals, who had created embryos with their own oocytes either used their embryos (39%) or continued storage (35%).[17] Of those who did not use their remaining embryos 21% donated to other infertile couples, 11% donated to research, and 68% discarded.[17] Seeking advice from a mental health professional when making the choice regarding disposition of cryopreserved embryos may be advisable as it is a very difficult to judgment to make.

SOCIAL AND CULTURAL INFLUENCES OF INFERTILITY

Infertile couples often feel ostracized from family, friends and their community, in part due to societal views or lack of empathy around treatment from family and friends. One of the most difficult aspects that infertile women describe is dealing with social situations, such as dealing with feelings of jealousy and envy, when learning of another woman's pregnancy, or being in the presence of others who have children.[3] Many women opt to avoid these events altogether to avoid the distress and emotional angst. Sadly, many women choose to hide their distress because they are self-conscious of their feelings and do not want to be criticized for their thoughts. In fact, the majority of infertile individuals do not even tell family and friends that they have been unable to conceive.

Modern day society has brought about many changes in the area of reproduction. Postponing childbirth is becoming increasingly common in Western countries, especially among those who are highly educated. Establishing a career is now being prioritized ahead of starting a family, and developing financial stability is becoming more important. In a survey conducted among university students in Sweden, male and female students alike reported; that they planned to have children, but about half the women reported, they intended to have children after the age of 35 years. Of these women, most were not aware of the age-related decline in female fecundity.[18] It is important that the younger generation be educated on reproduction and infertility. Women and men may postpone childbearing with the potential false expectation that science will come up with new advancements in the field of reproductive technology to completely compensate the impact that aging has on egg and sperm quality.

Current society is highly dependent on the internet for much of the available information on health. The internet allows people the ability to seek out medical 'advice' effortlessly. Research shows, the majority of infertility patient turn to the internet for guidance. In fact, an internet search, using Google, found 13.8 million hits using the term 'infertility' and 'IVF' yielded 7.2 million.[19] Research indicates that 99% of respondents rely on the internet for infertility information and support; 91% rely on infertility specialists and only 32% mental health counselors.[19] It is crucial to have adequate accurate information available online for the patient regarding fertility treatment as well as emotional support.

Cultural factors play a large role in the experiences individuals or couples have in regard to infertility. While people across cultures may feel similar psychological distress, the reported sources of distress may differ depending on their cultural affiliation. Some cultures will ostracize women who cannot conceive; women may be criticized by both family and community for the inability to produce a child. An Iranian study found that 81% of women reported that the main stressor regarding their infertility were relatives' comments about their infertility.[20]

Certain cultures will allow a man to divorce his wife, if she is not able to conceive, while in societies where polygamy is acceptable, men may take a new wife in her place. Muslims and Christians in the Middle East believe that, since marriage is a contract between the wife and husband during the span of marriage, no third party is allowed to be used for reproduction (donor sperm, egg or surrogate).[21] For some infertile women, childlessness results in social stigmatization and places them at risk of serious social and emotional consequences. In a country like Rwanda, and other resource-poor countries, not being able to procreate has severe social and economic repercussions. Three hundred twelve infertility patients completed a survey study in Rwanda, and the results showed more infertility patients reported domestic violence, union dissolutions and sexual dysfunction than fertile couples.[22] Although women tend to experience the burden of suffering, the negative repercussions of infertility for men, especially at the level of the community, are considerable as well.[22]

STRESS AND TREATMENT OUTCOME

The relationship between stress and pregnancy rates has remained a subject of controversy for many years. A recent study on the impact of stress on fecundity indicated that distress significantly reduced the probability of conception in women just starting to attempt pregnancy.[23] The authors concluded that couples need to relax and minimize stress when attempting to conceive.

Many IVF patients report depressive symptoms prior to beginning their cycle. In fact, mild depressive symptoms were evident in 54% of patients prior to initiating an IVF cycle and 19% had symptoms in the moderate to severe range.[24] Most IVF patients state that IVF treatment is primarily a psychological stressor rather than a physical stressor.[25]

The impact of distress on treatment outcome is difficult to assess. A notable research study looked at various psychological factors of infertility treatment and their impact on the IVF outcome. The factors included not only how stressed the patients reported feeling, but also what factors about the treatment were the most stressful, as well as physical factors such as number and quality of oocytes retrieved, pregnancy outcomes and birth weight. The results show that baseline level of stress was significantly linked to outcome; stress levels were correlated to number of retrieved oocytes, percentage fertilized, pregnancy rates, live birth rates and birth weight. The subjects, who expressed the least baseline level of distress, were 93% more likely to have a live birth than the patients, who reported the most baseline level of distress.[26] In sum, this study supported the theory that the more distressed the patient is prior to starting IVF, the less likely she will conceive, the same conclusion reached by a number of other studies.

However, a recent meta-analysis[27] had the opposite conclusion. The meta-analysis included 14 studies, about half the number published. It showed no relationship between distress and pregnancy. However, distress was assessed at only one point in time (ranging from three months prior to cycle initiation to early in the cycle). There is preliminary research,[28] which shows that distress prior to cycle initiation may actually be beneficial, as long as distress falls while cycling. Thus, the relationship between psychological functioning and pregnancy rates in IVF remains unknown and it appears to be a complex one.

If treatment failure ensues, it is common for IVF patients to report symptoms of depression, anxiety and anger. Unfortunately, many of these symptoms may extend for a period of time. In one retrospective study of 86 couples who did not conceive with IVF, 66% of women and 40% of men reported symptoms of depression following their failed IVF cycle, and one-third reported depressive symptoms 18 months later.[29]

TREATMENT DISTRESS AND TERMINATION

Contrary to prior belief, distress is the leading reason insured patients discontinue IVF treatment. It had been previously assumed that patients discontinue treatment for two reasons: limited financial resources or physician censoring due to a poor prognosis. A cohort study investigating the reason patients discontinue treatment prior to conceiving found that the majority of couples discontinue treatment due to psychological burden (26%), followed by a poor prognosis (25%), spontaneous pregnancy (19%), physical burden (6%), serious disease (2%) and other unexplained reasons (7%).[30]

Two similar studies found the same results: psychological stress played the greatest role in patients' decisions to discontinue treatment. Both these studies used self-reported questionnaires and found that the most common reason for terminating treatment was stress, explicitly the toll it took on the couple's relationship and, as well as being too anxious and depressed to continue treatment.[31,32]

A study conducted in Massachusetts, an insurance mandated state with coverage for 6 IVF cycles for those 40 years and under, found that 38% of women under age 40 receiving IVF treatment did not initiate a third cycle and the top reason given was stress.[32] Stress is likely the reasons many patients never commence treatment at all. A study tracking patients daily during their IVF cycle indicated that the level of stress increased following the embryo transfer and peaked just before the pregnancy test. The stress experienced during this waiting period overwhelms many patients and may lead to the decision to discontinue treatment.[33]

COGNITIVE-BEHAVIORAL INTERVENTIONS

If one accepts the theory that stress can have a negative impact on IVF outcome, then interventions designed to decrease stress should have a positive effect on pregnancy rates. In fact, the limited research done to date does for the most part support this notion.

A cumulative review of psychosocial intervention studies analyzed the benefits of counseling during infertility treatment. The analyses concluded that group interventions, which emphasized education and skills training, were significantly more effective in comparison to interventions, which emphasized emotional support and discussion about thoughts and feelings related to infertility. Both men and women benefit equally from psychosocial intervention.[34] In fact, intervention participants were shown to communicate more often about infertility with their partner after the intervention.[35] Both men and women have been noted to receive psychological benefit from support groups; women reporting lessened anxiety and men greater optimism upon completion of the group.[36]

The first study to assess the effect of a mind/body program for infertility was conducted in 1990. The findings of this study recognized the need for stress reduction in the long-term treatment of infertility. In this study, the first 54 women to complete the program showed a significant reduction in anxiety, depression and fatigue and an increase in vigor.[37] Additionally, 34% of these women became pregnant within 6 months of completion of the program.[37]

The first randomized control trial to investigate the efficacy of a cognitive behavioral intervention on viable pregnancy rates was conducted in 2000; this study looked at women, who had been trying to conceive for less than 2 years. Participants were randomized to one of three groups: a 10 session cognitive-behavioral group, a standard support group, or a routine care control group.[38] Results of the study found significant differences between participants in the two intervention groups versus the control group leading the authors to conclude that group psychological intervention appears to lead to increased pregnancy rates in infertile women. The live birth rate was 55% for the cognitive group, 54% for the support group, and 20% for the control group.[38]

The cognitive behavioral approach for infertility has been utilized for over 20 years. The first mind/body program for infertility was developed in 1987 and, since then, programs have expanded internationally.[37] These programs are led by mental health professionals and meet for ten sessions. The content of these programs include relaxation techniques, stress management and coping skills, cognitive strategies, and group support. The goal of the program is to teach women basic skills to help reduce levels of distress. Participants report significant decreases in both psychological symptoms and physical symptoms, including depression, anxiety, hostility, fatigue, headaches, insomnia and abdominal pain.[37]

Multiple studies have been published which show a positive effect on pregnancy rates for those who participate in a mind/body program. The most recent study, published in 2011, showed that patients who were randomized to attend a 10-week mind/body program had significantly higher pregnancy rates than those who were not. The study found that 52% of women, who attended more than half of the 10-session program conceived in IVF cycle two, versus 20% of the control group.[39]

Internet-based stress reduction may be beneficial. In one study, the impact of an internet-based infertility patient education and stress management program was assessed. The research found that patients, who were exposed to 60–90 minutes of the online program, reduced their fertility problem distress and improved their self-efficacy in managing their treatment compared to patients who did not use this program.[40]

Advocacy organizations, such as Resolve, offer support groups, online support and information on reducing stress and gaining coping skills. These resources can be valuable for individuals and couples going through treatment. Not only the skills learned during these support groups useful tools, but also the bonds that participants make with fellow group members can offer much needed support and help individuals to feel less isolated as they undergo infertility treatment.[36]

Mental health professionals can be highly beneficial to infertile patients. The mental health professional is able to teach the patient, how to cope better with emotional aspects of infertility, work with couples to communicate more effectively, assist in evaluating treatment options and decisions, as well as explaining what to expect from the different treatment regimens. Unfortunately, some individuals are reluctant to seek mental health support out of fear of stigmatization and miss out on the benefits of professional support.[41] It seems that the most beneficial time for an individual with infertility to seek additional support from a mental health professional is prior to beginning IVF or in the earlier stages of treatment and throughout the duration.[42] Any coping strategies, learned to assist in dealing with the emotions and distress of infertility treatment, should be beneficial not only to individual's quality of life, but also may have a potential impact on success of the cycle.

SUMMARY

Infertility represents a significant emotional challenge to individuals and couples. The distress can be profound and can have a huge impact on quality of life. High levels of distress are associated with treatment termination even in insured patients. In addition, highly distressed patients may experience lower pregnancy rates. It is crucial to understand the emotional challenges facing infertility patients and to recommend psychological interventions, which are most likely to help them through this crisis.

REFERENCES

1. Boivin J, Bunting L, Collins J A, et al. International estimates of infertility prevalence and treatment-seeking: potential need and demand for infertility medical care. Hum Reprod. 2007;22(6):1506-12.
2. Freeman EW, Boxer AS, Rickels K, et al. Psychological evaluation and support in a program of in vitro fertilization and embryo transfer. Fertil Steril. 1985;43(1):48-53.
3. Domar AD, Siebel MM. Emotional aspects of infertility. In: Seibel MM (Ed). Infertility: A Comprehensive Text. Stamford: Appleton & Lange; 1997. pp. 29-44.
4. Domar AD, Zuttermesiter PC, Friedman R. The psychological impact of infertility: a comparison to women with other medical conditions. J Psychosom Obstet Gynaecol. 1993;14(suppl):45-52.
5. Domar AD, Broome A, Zuttermeister PC, et al. The prevalence and predictability of depression in infertile women. Italian (Italy) Fertil Steril. 1992;58(6):1158-63.
6. Ramezanzadeh F, Aghssa MM, Abedinia N, Zayeri F, et al. A survey of relationship between anxiety, depression and duration of infertility. BMC Womens Health. 2004;4(1):9.
7. Greil AL. Not Yet Pregnant: Infertile Couples in Contemporary America. London: Rutgers University Press; 1991.
8. Abbey A, Andrews FM, Halman LJ. Gender's role in responses to infertility. Psychol Women Q. 1991;15: 295-316.
9. Jordan C, Revenson TA. Gender difference in coping with infertility: a meta-analysis. J Behav Med. 1999;22(4): 341-58.
10. Berg BJ, Wilson JF. Psychological functioning across stages of treatment for infertility. Portuguese (Portugal) J Behav Med. 1991;14(1):11-26.
11. Chachamovich JR, Chachamovich E, Ezer H, et al. Agreement on perceptions of quality of life in couples dealing with infertility. J Obstet Gynecol Neonatal Nurs. 2010;39(5):557-65.
12. Lund R, Sejbaek CS, Christensen U, et al. The impact of social relations on the incidence of severe depressive symptoms among infertile women and men. Hum Reprod. 2009;24(11):2810-20.
13. Edelmann RJ, Humphrey M, Owens DJ. The meaning of parenthood and couples' reactions to male infertility. Br J Med Psychol. 1994;67(Pt 3):291-9.
14. Daniluk JC. Gender and infertility. In: Leiblum SR (Ed). Infertility, Psychological Issues and Counseling Strategies. New York: John Wiley & Sons; 1997;103-35.
15. Lenzi A, Lombardo F, Salacone P, et al. Stress, sexual dysfunctions, and male infertility. J Endocrinol Invest. 2003;26(3 Suppl):72-6.
16. Domar AD, Zuttermeister PC, Seibel M, et al. Psychological improvement in infertile women after behavioral treatment: a replication. Fertil Steril. 1992;58(1):144-7.
17. Hill GA, Freeman MR. Embryo disposition: choices made by patients and donor oocyte recipients. Fertil Steril. 2011;95(3):940-3.
18. Lampic C, Svanberg AS, Karlström P, et al. Fertility awareness, intentions concerning childbearing, and attitudes towards parenthood among female and male academics. Hum Reprod. 2006;21(2):558-64.
19. Kahlor L, Mackert M. Perceptions of infertility information and support sources among female patients, who access the Internet. Fertil Steril. 2009;91(1):83-90.
20. Noorbala AA, Ramazanzadeh F, Malekafzali H, et al. Effects of a psychological intervention on depression in infertile couples. Int J Gynaecol Obstet. 2008;101(3):248-52.
21. World Health Organization. Current Practices and Controversies in Assisted Production. Geneva: World Health Organization; 2001. pp. 45.
22. Dhont N, van de Wijgert J, Coene G, et al. 'Mama and papa nothing': living with infertility among an urban population in Kigali, Rwanda Portuguese (Portugal). Hum Reprod. 2011;26(3):623-9.
23. Buck Louis GM, Lum KJ, Sundaram R, et al. Stress reduces conception probabilities across the fertile window: evidence in support of relaxation. Fertil Steril. 2011;95(7):2184-9.
24. Demyttenaere K, Bonte L, Gheldof M, et al. Coping style and depression level influence outcome in in-vitro fertilization. Fertil Steril. 1998;69(6):1026-33.
25. Eugster A, Vingerhoets AJ. Psychological aspects of in vitro fertilization: a review. Soc Sci Med. 1999;48(5): 575-89.

26. Klonoff-Cohen H, Chu E, Natarajan L, et al. A prospective study of stress among women undergoing in vitro fertilization or gamete intrafallopian transfer. Fertil Steril. 2001;71:675-87.
27. Boivin J, Griffiths E, Venetis CA. Emotional distress in infertile women and failure of assisted reproductive technologies: meta-analysis of prospective psychosocial studies. BMJ. 2011;342:d223.
28. Domar AD, Backman K, Wiegand B, et al. The relationship between stress and IVF outcome. 2010;94(4):S66.
29. Baram D, Tourtelot E, Muechler E, et al. Psychological adjustment following unsuccessful in vitro fertilization. J Psychosom Obstet Gynaecol. 1998;8:181.
30. Olivius C, Friden B, Borg G, et al. Why do couples discontinue in vitro fertilization treatment? A cohort study. Fertil Steril. 2004;81(2):258-61.
31. Rajkhowa M, McConnell A, Thomas GE. Reasons for discontinuation of IVF treatment: a questionnaire study. Hum Reprod; 2006;21:358.
32. Domar AD, Smith K, Conboy L, et al. A prospective investigation into the reasons why insured United States patients drop out of in vitro fertilization treatment. Fertil Steril. 2010;94(4):1457-9.
33. Boivin J, Lancastle D. Medical waiting periods: imminence, emotions and coping. Womens Health (Lond Engl). 2010;6(1):59-69.
34. Boivin J. A review of psychosocial interventions in infertility. Soc Sci Med. 2003;57(12):2325-41.
35. Schmidt L, Tjornhoj-Thomsen T, Boivin J, et al. Evaluation of a communication and stress management training programme for infertile couples. Patient Educ Couns. 2005;59(3):252-62.
36. McNaughton-Cassill ME, Bostwick JM, Arthur NJ, et al. Efficacy of brief couples support groups developed to manage the stress of in vitro fertilization treatment. Mayo Clin Proc. 2002;77(10):1060-6.
37. Domar AD, Seibel MM, Benson H. The mind/body program for infertility: a new behavioral treatment approach for women with infertility. Fertil Steril. 1990;53(2):246-9.
38. Domar AD, Clapp D, Slawsby EA, et al. Impact of group psychological interventions on pregnancy rates in infertile women. Fertil Steril. 2000;73(4):805-11.
39. Domar AD, Rooney KL, Wiegand B, et al. Impact of a group mind/body intervention on pregnancy rates in IVF patients. Fertil Steril. 2011;95(7):2269-73.
40. Cousineau TM, Green TC, Corsini E, et al. Online psychoeducational support for infertile women: a randomized controlled trial. Hum Reprod. 2008;23(3):554-66.
41. Wasser SK, Sewall G, Soules MR. Psychosocial stress as a cause of infertility. Fertil Steril. 1993;59(3):685-9.
42. Terzioglu F. Investigation into effectiveness of counseling on assisted reproductive techniques in Turkey. J Psychosom Obstet Gynecol. 2001;22:133-141.

Index

Page numbers followed by *f* refer to figure and *t* refer to table

F

G

H

I

J

K

L

M

T